CAMBRIDGE LIBRARY COLLECTION

Books of enduring scholarly value

Classics

From the Renaissance to the nineteenth century, Latin and Greek were compulsory subjects in almost all European universities, and most early modern scholars published their research and conducted international correspondence in Latin. Latin had continued in use in Western Europe long after the fall of the Roman empire as the lingua franca of the educated classes and of law, diplomacy, religion and university teaching. The flight of Greek scholars to the West after the fall of Constantinople in 1453 gave impetus to the study of ancient Greek literature and the Greek New Testament. Eventually, just as nineteenth-century reforms of university curricula were beginning to erode this ascendancy, developments in textual criticism and linguistic analysis, and new ways of studying ancient societies, especially archaeology, led to renewed enthusiasm for the Classics. This collection offers works of criticism, interpretation and synthesis by the outstanding scholars of the nineteenth century.

Claudii Galeni Opera Omnia

Galen (Claudius Galenus, 129–c. 199 CE) is the most famous physician of the Greco-Roman world whose writings have survived. A Greek from a wealthy family, raised and educated in the Greek city of Pergamon, he acquired his medical education by travelling widely in the Roman world, visiting the famous medical centres and studying with leading doctors. His career took him to Rome, where he was appointed by the emperor Marcus Aurelius as his personal physician; he also served succeeding emperors in this role. A huge corpus of writings on medicine which bear Galen's name has survived. The task of editing and publishing such a corpus, and of identifying the authentic Galenic texts within it, is a hugely challenging one, and the 22-volume edition reissued here, edited by Karl Gottlob Kühn (1754–1840) and published in Leipzig between 1821 and 1833, has never yet been equalled.

Cambridge University Press has long been a pioneer in the reissuing of out-of-print titles from its own backlist, producing digital reprints of books that are still sought after by scholars and students but could not be reprinted economically using traditional technology. The Cambridge Library Collection extends this activity to a wider range of books which are still of importance to researchers and professionals, either for the source material they contain, or as landmarks in the history of their academic discipline.

Drawing from the world-renowned collections in the Cambridge University Library, and guided by the advice of experts in each subject area, Cambridge University Press is using state-of-the-art scanning machines in its own Printing House to capture the content of each book selected for inclusion. The files are processed to give a consistently clear, crisp image, and the books finished to the high quality standard for which the Press is recognised around the world. The latest print-on-demand technology ensures that the books will remain available indefinitely, and that orders for single or multiple copies can quickly be supplied.

The Cambridge Library Collection will bring back to life books of enduring scholarly value (including out-of-copyright works originally issued by other publishers) across a wide range of disciplines in the humanities and social sciences and in science and technology.

Claudii Galeni Opera Omnia

Volume 14

Edited by Karl Gottlob Kühn

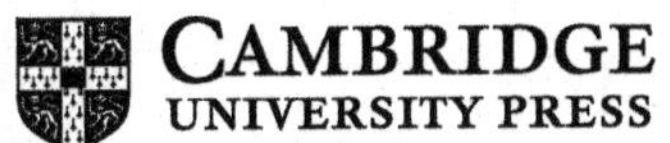
CAMBRIDGE
UNIVERSITY PRESS

CAMBRIDGE UNIVERSITY PRESS

Cambridge, New York, Melbourne, Madrid, Cape Town,
Singapore, São Paolo, Delhi, Tokyo, Mexico City

Published in the United States of America by Cambridge University Press, New York

www.cambridge.org
Information on this title: www.cambridge.org/9781108028400

This edition first published 1821-3
This digitally printed version 2011

ISBN 978-1-108-02840-0 Paperback

MEDICORVM GRAECORVM

O P E R A

Q V A E E X S T A N T.

EDITIONEM CVRAVIT

D. CAROLVS GOTTLOB KÜHN

PROFESSOR PHYSIOLOGIAE ET PATHOLOGIAE IN LITERARVM VNIVERSITATE LIPSIENSI PVBLICVS ORDINARIVS ETC.

V O L V M E N XIV.

CONTINENS

C L A V D I I G A L E N I T. XIV.

L I P S I A E

PROSTAT IN OFFICINA LIBRARIA CAR. CNOBLOCHII

1 8 2 7.

ΚΛΑΥΔΙΟΥ ΓΑΛΗΝΟΥ

ΑΠΑΝΤΑ.

CLAVDII GALENI

OPERA OMNIA.

EDITIONEM CVRAVIT

D. CAROLVS GOTTLOB KÜHN

PROFESSOR PHYSIOLOGIAE ET PATHOLOGIAE IN LITERARVM VNIVERSITATE LIPSIENSI PVBLICVS ORDINARIVS ETC.

TOMVS XIV.

LIPSIAE

PROSTAT IN OFFICINA LIBRARIA CAR. CNOBLOCHII

1827.

CONTENTA TOMI XIV.

ΓΑΛΗΝΟΥ ΠΕΡΙ ΑΝΤΙΔΟΤΩΝ ΒΙΒΛΙΑ ΔΥΟ. ΒΙΒΛΙΟΝ Α.

Ed. Chart. XIII. [865.] Ed. Baſ. II. (423.)

Κεφ. α΄. [Τί ἐστιν ἡ ἀντίδοτος καὶ πόθεν τὴν γένεσιν ἔχει ἡ θηριακή.] Τὰς ἰωμένας τὰ πάθη δυνάμεις οὐκ ἔξωθεν ἐπιτιθεμένας, ἀλλ' εἴσω τοῦ σώματος λαμβανομένας ἀντιδότους ὀνομάζουσιν οἱ ἰατροί. τρεῖς δ' αὐτῶν εἰσιν αἱ πᾶσαι διαφοραί. τινὲς μὲν γὰρ ἕνεκα τῶν θανασίμων προσφέρονται φαρμάκων, τινὲς δὲ τῶν ἰοβόλων ὀνομαζομένων θηρίων, τινὲς δὲ τοῖς ἐκ φαύλης διαίτης γιγνομένοις πάθεσιν ἀρήγουσιν. ἔνιαι δὲ τὰς τρεῖς ἐπαγγέλλονται χρείας, ὥσπερ καὶ ἡ θηριακὴ κα-

GALENI DE ANTIDOTIS LIBRI DUO. LIBER PRIMUS.

Cap. I. [*Quid ſit antidotus et unde theriaca originem habuerit.*] Quae remedia non extrinſecus corpori impoſita, ſed intro aſſumpta pravis affectibus medentur, antidota medici nominant. Tres autem in univerſum ipſorum ſunt differentiae. Quaedam etenim lethalium venenorum gratia offeruntur; quaedam ad virulentas quas appellitant feras *proficiunt;* quaedam affectibus ex pravo victu oborientibus auxiliantur; nonnulla hunc triplicem uſum pol-

λουμένη, συντεθεῖσα μὲν ὑπὸ Ἀνδρομάχου τοῦ ἰατροῦ, παρωσαμένη δὲ τὴν Μιθριδάτειον ὀνομαζομένην, καὶ αὐτὴν ἀπὸ τοῦ συνθέντος αὐτὴν οὕτω κληθεῖσαν. ὁ γάρ τοι Μιθριδάτης οὗτος, ὥσπερ καὶ ὁ καθ' ἡμᾶς Ἄτταλος, ἔσπευσεν ἐμπειρίαν ἔχειν ἁπάντων σχεδὸν τῶν ἁπλῶν φαρμάκων, ὅσα τοῖς ὀλεθρίοις ἀντιτέτακται, πειράζων αὐτῶν τὰς δυνάμεις ἐπὶ πονηρῶν ἀνθρώπων, ὧν θάνατος κατέγνωστο. τινὰ μὲν οὖν αὐτῶν ἀνεῦρεν ἐπὶ φαλαγγίων ἰδίως ἁρμόζοντα, τινὰ δὲ ἐπὶ σκορπίων, ὥσπερ ἐπὶ τῶν ἐχιδνῶν ἄλλα. καὶ ἐπὶ τῶν ἀναιρούντων φαρμάκων τὰ μὲν ἐπὶ ἀκονίτου, τὰ δὲ ἐπὶ λαγωοῦ τοῦ θαλαττίου, τὰ δ' ἐπ' ἄλλου τινὸς ἢ ἄλλου. πάντα δ' οὖν αὐτὰ μίξας ὁ Μιθριδάτης ἓν ἐποίησε φάρμακον, ἐλπίσας ἕξειν ἀρωγὸν ἐπὶ πᾶσι τοῖς ὀλεθρίοις. ὕστερον δὲ Ἀνδρόμαχος ὁ Νέρωνος ἀρχιατρὸς, ἔνια μὲν προσθεὶς, ἔνια δὲ ἀφελὼν, ἐποίησε τὴν θηριακὴν ὀνομαζομένην ἀντίδοτον, οὐκ ὀλίγην ἐχιδνῶν σάρκα μίξας τοῖς ἄλλοις, ἣν οὐκ εἶχεν ἡ Μιθριδάτειος. καὶ διὰ τοῦτο πρὸς

licentur, quemadmodum et quae theriace vocatur ab Andromacho medico composita, quaeque quod Mithridatium nominant, depulit, ipſum etiam, ab eo qui id compoſuit, ſic appellatum. Hic enim Mithridates, quemadmodum et apud nos Attalus, omnium prope ſimplicium medicamentorum experientiam habere studuit, quae perniciofis venenis adverſantur, facultates ipſorum in facinoroſis hominibus morte damnatis explorans. Quaedam igitur eorum comperit adverſus phalangia privatim convenire, quaedam in ſcorpiones, quemadmodum in viperas alia. Item adverſus perimentia venena quaedam in aconitum, nonnulla in leporem marinum, alia in aliud quippiam aut aliud *pugnant*. His itaque omnibus contemperatis Mithridates unum confecit medicamentum, ſperans ſe adverſus omnia lethalia habiturum praeſidium. Poſtea Andromachus Neronis primarius medicus quibusdam adjectis, nonnullis ademtis, theriacen dictum antidotum praeparavit, haud exigua viperarum carne, quam

μὲν τὰ τῶν ἐχιδνῶν δήγματα καλλίων ἐστὶν ἡ θηριακὴ τῆς Μιθριδάτειος ὀνομαζομένης· πρὸς τὰ ἄλλα δὲ οὐδὲν ἥττων ἡ Μιθριδάτειος, ἀλλ' ἔστιν ἐφ' ὧν καὶ βελτίων. οὐ τὴν αὐτὴν δὲ δύναμιν ἔχουσιν [866] ἐπιλαμβανόμεναι καὶ προλαμβανόμεναι (424) τῶν ἀναιρούντων φαρμάκων. ὃ γὰρ αὔταρκες αὐτῶν ἐστι μέγεθος εἰς τὸ μηδὲν παθεῖν προληφθέντων, τοῦτο αὐξηθὲν εἰς τετραπλάσιον ἢ πενταπλάσιον ἐπιδιδόμενον ὀνίνησι, καὶ οὐχ ἅπαξ γε τῆς ἡμέρας, ἀλλὰ δίς. εἰ δέ τις ἤτοι καθ' ἑκάστην τὴν ἡμέραν, ὡς ὁ καθ' ἡμᾶς γενόμενος αὐτοκράτωρ Αὐρήλιος Ἀντωνῖνος ἢ ὡς αὐτὸς ὁ Μιθριδάτης, λαμβάνοι τοῦ φαρμάκου, παντάπασιν ἀβλαβὴς ὑπὸ τῶν θανασίμων τε καὶ δηλητηρίων φαρμάκων ὀνομαζομένων ἔσται, ὥσπερ φασὶ καὶ τὸν Μιθριδάτην αὐτὸν, ἡνίκα προείλετο δι' ὀλεθρίου φαρμάκου μᾶλλον ἀποθανεῖν, ἢ ὑπὸ Ῥωμαίοις γενέσθαι, μηδὲν εὑρεῖν ἀνελεῖν αὐτὸν δυνάμενον. τὰ μὲν οὖν κατὰ Μιθριδάτην ἀκούομεν· αὐτοὶ δ' ἡμεῖς ἴσμεν κατὰ τὸν Ἀντωνῖνον, ὃς τὸ μὲν πρῶτον εἰς ἀσφάλειαν ἑαυτοῦ κατασκευάζων ἑκάστης

Mithridatium non habebat, aliis admixta. Atque ob id theriace ad viperarum morſus praeſtantior quam Mithridatium vocatum exiſtit. Ad alia vero Mithridatium nihilo minus valet, ſed eſt in quibus etiam praeſtantius inveniatur. At non easdem facultates habent et post deleteria medicamenta et ante aſſumpta. Quae enim magnitudo ipſorum, quum praeſumuntur, ſufficit ad nihil patiendum; ea quadruplo aut quintuplo aucta, quum postea datur, adjuvat; idque non ſemel quotidie, ſed bis. Verum si quis vel ſingulis diebus, quemadmodum noſtra tempeſtate factus imperator Aurelius Antoninus vel ut ipſe Mithridates, medicamentum capiat, omnino a lethalibus et deleteriis appellatis medicamentis erit ſecurus et immunis; ſicuti ajunt et Mithridatem ipſum, quum lethali medicamento interire potius, quam Romanorum ſubjici imperio maluit, nihil inveniſſe quod ipſum interimere potuerit. Quae jam Mithridati acciderunt audimus. Nos autem ipſi novimus Antonini tempore, qui primum theriacen in ſui

ἡμέρας, ὅσον Αἰγυπτίου κυάμου μέγεθος ἐλάμβανεν, ἢ καταπίνων ἄνευ μίξεως ὕδατος ἢ οἴνου ἢ τοιούτου μιγνύς. ἐπεὶ δὲ συνέβαινεν αὐτῷ νυστάζειν καρωδῶς ἐν ταῖς ὁσημέραι πράξεσιν, ἀφεῖλε τὸν ὀπὸν τῆς μήκωνος. πάλιν οὖν αὐτὸν συνέβη διὰ τὸ πρόσθεν ἔθος, ὡς ἂν αὐτῷ τε φύσει ξηροτέρας ὄντι κράσεως, καὶ ξηραῖνον φάρμακον ἐκ πολλοῦ προσφερόμενον, τό γε πλεῖστον μέρος τῆς νυκτὸς ἄγρυπνον διατελεῖν, καὶ διὰ τοῦτο ἠναγκάσθη προσφέρεσθαι, καὶ τοῦ τὸν ὀπὸν ἔχοντος ἤδη πως κεχρονικότος. εἴρηται γάρ μοι πολλάκις ἤδη τὰ τοιαῦτα φάρμακα χρονίζοντα πραότερον ἴσχειν αὐτόν. ἦν δὲ τηνικαῦτα διὰ τὸν Γερμανικὸν πόλεμον ἐν τοῖς περὶ τὸν Ἴστρον χωρίοις, ἐμοῦ παραιτησαμένου τὴν ἀποδημίαν ἐκείνην. ἐπεὶ δὲ τὴν ὑπὸ Δημητρίου τοῦ ἀρχιατροῦ σκευαζομένην ἀντίδοτον ἐπήνει, μετὰ θάνατον αὐτοῦ γράψας Εὐφράτει τῷ καθολικῷ, παρ᾽ οὗ τὰ πρὸς τὴν σύνθεσιν ἐλάμβανεν ἁπλᾶ φάρμακα, δηλῶσαι τίς αὐτῷ παρῆν τῶν λαμβανόντων σύνταξιν αὐτοκρατορικὴν, καὶ πυθόμενος ἐμὲ διὰ παντὸς αὐτῷ κατὰ πάσας τὰς συν-

tutelam praeparans, quotidie Aegyptiae fabae magnitudinem assumebat, vel citra aquae vinive aut ejusmodi misturam deglutiens. Quum autem ipsum in quotidianis actionibus comate corripi contingeret, papaveris succum ademit. Rursus quum accideret, ut propter consuetudinem pristinam, ceu qui siccioris temperamenti naturam haberet, et ob desiccans medicamentum a longo tempore oblatum, bonam noctis partem insomnem transigeret, coactus est propterea etiam, ex eo quod papaveris succum habet jam inveterato, adjicere. Dictum est autem a nobis saepe ejusmodi medicamenta inveterata mitiorem eum succum obtinere. Erat autem tunc imperator ob bellum Germanicum in Istri ripis, me profectionem illam aversato. At quum antidotum ab Demetrio archiatro compositum laudaret, post mortem ipsius literis ad Euphratem catholicum, a quo ad compositionem apta simplicia medicamenta accipiebat, missis ut indicaret quis ipsorum adesset, qui compositionem imperialem accepisset, rogavit

θέσεις παραγεγονέναι, σκευάζεσθαι μὲν ἐκέλευσεν ὑπὸ ἐμοῦ τὴν ἀντίδοτον. ἀρεσθεὶς δὲ αὐτῇ μόνῃ, παραγενόμενος εἰς Ῥώμην, ἐπυνθάνετο κατὰ τίνα συμμετρίαν τῶν ἁπλῶν φαρμάκων σκευάζοιμι, κἀγὼ τἀληθὲς αὐτῷ διῆλθον, ὡς οὐδὲν οὐδὲ τοὐλάχιστον, οὔτ' ἐνέλιπον, οὔτε προσέθηκα τῶν ἐμβαλλομένων ἐξ ἔθους παλαιοῦ τοῖς κατὰ τὴν αὐλὴν ἰατροῖς, ἐδήλωσά τε τὴν αἰτίαν, δι' ἣν ἀρέσκει μάλιστα αὐτῷ ἐμοὶ σκευασία, περὶ ἧς εἰπεῖν καὶ νῦν προθέμενος, ἐμνημόνευσα τῶν τότε πραχθέντων. ἅτε γὰρ ἑκάστης ἡμέρας λαμβάνων ὁ Ἀντωνῖνος ἅμα πολλῷ μέλιτι τοῦ φαρμάκου, ἀκριβέστατα διεγίνωσκε τήν τε κακίαν αὐτοῦ καὶ τὴν ἀρετήν.

Κεφ. β'. [Πῶς ἂν καλλίστη σκευάζηται ἡ θηριακή.] Γίνεται δὲ κάλλιστον τοῦτο, καὶ τὰ ἄλλα σχεδὸν ἅπαντα φάρμακα, διὰ τὴν τῶν ἐμβαλλομένων ἀρετήν τε καὶ ἀναλογίαν τῆς πρὸς ἄλληλα δυνάμεως. οἱ πολλοὶ δ' οὐδὲ τὴν ἀρχὴν ἴσασι δοκιμάζειν ἕκαστον αὐτῶν καταμόνας, εἰς ὅσον ἥκει κακίας ἢ ἀρετῆς, ὥστ' οὐδὲ τὴν ἀναλογίαν τῆς πρὸς ἄλληλα δυνάμεως ἐπίστανται. καὶ διὰ τοῦτο βάλλοντες

me ut femper ei in omnibus compofitionibus adeffem, praepararique antidotum a me juffit. Sed quia hoc folum ei placuerat, Romam profectus inquirebat, quanam fimplicium medicamentorum commoderatione conficerem, ac ego verum ei confeffus fum. Nam nihil etiam minimum vel reliqui vel adjeci iis, quae ex veteri confuetudine aulici medici immittunt, caufamque oftendi propter quam potiffimum mihi ipfi confectio placeat, de qua impraefentiarum dicere inftituens, eorum quae tunc gefta funt, commemini. Nam Antoninus, ut qui fingulis diebus medicamentum una cum melle copiofo affumeret, exactiffime et malitiam ejus et virtutem dignofcebat.

Cap. II. [*Quomodo optima theriaca componatur.*] Fit autem hoc praeftantiffimum, reliquaque prope univerfa medicamenta, tum propter eorum quae injiciuntur probitatem, tum ob virtutis inter fefe proportionem. Plerique neutiquam fingula ipfa privatim probare noverunt, quantum maligna probave exiftant. Quapropter neque virium

Ed. Chart. XIII. [866. 867.] Ed. Baſ. II. (424.)

ἐνίοτε τὰ πλεῖστα τῶν φαρμάκων ἀσθενῆ, ἢ διὰ χρόνον, ἢ διὰ γένος, ἔμιξαν αὐτοῖς τῶν ἰσχυροτάτων. ἐμβαλὼν γοῦν τίς ποτε ἐκ τῶν Θηβῶν τῶν Αἰγυπτίων ὀπὸν ἰσχυρότατον ὄντα, παραπλήσιον Φιλωνείῳ φαρμάκῳ καὶ τῇ γεύσει καὶ τῇ δυνάμει τὴν ἀντίδοτον εἰργάσατο. σμύρναν δὲ αὖθις ἐμβαλὼν, ἰσχυρότατον ἅμα τοῖς [867] πλείστοις ἀσθενέσιν, ἐπικρατηθῆναι τὴν ἀντίδοτον ὑπ᾽ ἐκείνης ἐποίησε, καί τις ἄλλος ὅμως ἐν κρόκῳ ταὐτὸν ἥμαρτεν, ὁ δὲ ἐν σαγαπηνῷ, καθάπερ γε πάλιν ἄλλος ἐν ἀσφάλτῳ καὶ χαλβάνῃ. τινὲς δὲ καὶ δύο καὶ τρία τῶν οὕτως ἰσχυρῶν ἀσθενέσι τοῖς ἄλλοις μίξαντες ὑπ᾽ ἐκείνων ἐπικρατουμένην τὴν ἀντίδοτον εἰργάσαντο. τὴν σκευασίαν μὲν οὖν αὐτὴν κἂν ἅπαξ τις ἤδη δριμὺς ἄνθρωπος εὐκόλως μαθήσεται· τῶν δ᾽ ἐμβαλλομένων φαρμάκων τὴν διάγνωσιν οὐχ ἅπαξ ἢ δὶς ἢ τρὶς, ἀλλὰ πάνυ πολλάκις ἑωρᾶσθαι δεῖται, κἂν ἀκριβῶς ὑπό τινος δεικνύντος τε ἅμα καὶ λόγου διδάσκοντος, ὁποῖόν ἐστι τὸ ἄριστον ἐκμάθοι, τῷ δὲ χωρὶς τοῦ δείξαντος ἐξ ἀναγνώσεως βιβλίου τινὸς, ὁποῖα τά θ᾽ Ἡρα-

inter ſe proportionem cognoſcunt. Unde factum eſt ut pluribus medicamentis imbecillibus aut temporis ſpatio, aut genere nonnunquam injectis, validiſſima ipſis admiſcuerint. Quidam enim aliquando liquorem qui ex Thebis Aegypti affertur valentiſſimo immittens antidoto, Philonio id medicamento et guſtu et viribus perſimile effecit. Rurſus myrrha indita maxime valenti, ſimul cum pluribus imbecillis, praestitit ut antidotum ab illa vinceretur, ac alius quidam ſimiliter in croco erravit, alius in ſagapeno, quemadmodum rurſus alius in bitumine et galbano, nonnulli et duo et tria tam valida aliis imbecillibus admiſcentes antidotum quod ab illis ſuperatur confecerunt. Quomodo igitur ipſum praeparetur vel uno verbo aliquis jam ſagax homo ex facili addiſcet. Porro medicamentorum dignotionem ac diſcrimina non ſemel aut bis ſerve, ſed admodum frequenter ſpectaſſe convenit, etſi accurate a quodam indicante ſimul, et rationem docente quale optimum ſit, poterit indipiſci. At ei qui ſine indice ex libro quodam

Ed. Chart. XIII. [867.] Ed. Baf. II. (424.)

κλείδου τοῦ Ταραντίνου Θηριακὰ καὶ Κρατεύα καὶ Διοσκορίδου καὶ Νίγρου καὶ Ἰόλλα καὶ Ῥούφου τοῦ Ἐφεσίου καὶ ἄλλων τινῶν ἐπὶ τὴν διάγνωσιν αὐτῶν ἥκοντι, πολὺ πλείονος αὐτοψίας δεῖ πρὸς τὸ διαγινώσκειν ἀκριβῶς ἑκάστου φαρμάκου τήν τε ἀρετὴν καὶ τὴν κακίαν. ἔνια μὲν γὰρ παραποιοῦσιν οἱ καπηλεύοντες οὕτω σαφῶς, ὡς καὶ τοὺς τριβακωτάτους ἐν αὐτοῖς λανθάνειν, ἐφ᾽ ὧν κάλλιστόν ἐστιν αὐτῶν ἐκ πολλοῦ παρεσκευάσθαι διὰ φίλον ἀνόθευτον ἐκ τοῦ χωρίου, καθ᾽ ὃ κάλλιστον γεννᾶται, πορίζεσθαι τὸ φάρμακον, ἢ ἅπαξ πορευθέντα παρασκευάσασθαι τὰ διαμεῖναι δυνάμενα πρὸς ὅλον τὸν βίον, ὁποία σχεδὸν ἅπαντά ἐστι τὰ μεταλλικὰ καλούμενα. Κύπρον γοῦν ἱστορῆσαι βουληθεὶς ἐγὼ διὰ ταῦτα, φίλον τε ἔχων τὸν ἐν αὐτῇ πολὺ δυνάμενον, ἑταῖρον ὄντα τοῦ προεστῶτος τῶν μετάλλων ἐπιτρόπου Καίσαρος, καδμείαν τε πολλὴν ἐκεῖθεν ἐκόμισα καὶ διφρυγὲς καὶ σπόδιον καὶ πομφόλυγα χαλκῖτίν τε καὶ μίσυ καὶ σῶρυ καὶ χάλκανθον, ὥσπερ γε πάλιν ἐκ τῆς Παλαιστίνης Συρίας ὀποβάλσαμον ἀκριβές.

perlecto, quales funt Heraclidis Tarentini Theriacae, Crateuae, Diofcoridis, Nigri, Iollae, Ruffi Ephefii et aliorum quorundam, dignotioni ipforum incumbit, multo magis fuifmet oculis infpicere opus eft, quo cujusque medicamenti virtutem et malitiam exacte internofcat. Nonnulla fiquidem inftitores tam callide adulterant, affimilantque veris, ut etiam exercitatiffimos in eis fallant, in quibus optimum eft, ex longo tempore ea praeparaffe atque per amicum fincerum ex regione qua praeftantiffimum nafcitur medicamentum exhiberi, aut femel eo profectum praeparare quae per totam vitam durare poffent, qualia fere omnia funt metallica nuncupata. Quum itaque Cyprum propterea invifere ftatuiffem, haberemque amicum in ea praepotentem, qui familiaris erat praefecti metallorum, commiffarii Caefaris, cadmiam copiofam illinc exportavi, item diphryges, fpodium, pompholygem, chalcitidem, mify, fori et chalcanthum, quemadmodum ex Palaeftina Syria opobalfamum exactum. Bitumen fane ne adulterari

ἄσφαλτος μὲν γὰρ οὐδὲ δολωθῆναι δύναται πανούργως, ὥσπερ οὐδὲ ὁ τοῦ ὀποβαλσάμου καρπὸς ἢ τὸ ξυλοβάλσαμον. ἔπλευσα δὲ καὶ εἰς Λῆμνον, ἴσασι δὲ οἱ θεοὶ, δι' οὐδὲν ἄλλο ἢ διὰ τὴν Λημνίαν, εἴτε γῆν ἐθέλει τις ὀνομάζειν, εἴτε σφραγῖδα, λέλεκται δὲ περὶ αὐτῆς αὐτάρκως ἐν τῷ περὶ τῆς τῶν ἁπλῶν φαρμάκων δυνάμεως ἐνάτῳ. ταύτην οὖν εἴτε Λημνίαν γῆν, εἴτε σφραγῖδα καλεῖν ἐθέλεις, παραποιοῦσιν, ὡς μηδένα δυνάσθαι διαγνῶναι τὴν ἀληθινὴν ἀπὸ τῆς παραπεποιημένης. καθάπερ γε τὸ καλούμενον Ἰνδικὸν Λύκιον, ἕτερά τε πολλὰ δυσκολωτάτην ἔχοντα διάγνωσιν ἀπὸ τῶν νενοθευμένων, ἃ χρὴ παρὰ τῶν εἰς τὰ χωρία πορευομένων, ἐπιτρόπων τε καὶ συγκλητικῶν ἀρξάντων τῆς χώρας ἀθροίζειν, ἢ καὶ τῶν κατοικούντων ἐν αὐτοῖς φίλων, ὥσπερ ἐμὲ ποιοῦντα τεθέασθε. κομίζεται γάρ μοι τὰ μὲν ἐκ τῆς μεγάλης Συρίας, τὰ δ' ἐκ τῆς Παλαιστίνης, τὰ δὲ ἐξ Αἰγύπτου, τὰ δὲ ἐκ Καππαδοκίας, ἐκ Πόντου δ' ἄλλα, καθάπερ γε καὶ Μακεδονίας τε καὶ τῶν πρὸς τὴν δύσιν χωρίων, ἔνθα Κελτοὶ καὶ Ἴβη-

quidem poteſt dolo, quemadmodum neque opobalſami fructus aut xylobalſamum. Navigavi autem in Lemnum quoque ob nullam (ita me dii ament) aliam rem quam Lemniam, ſive terram quis nominare velit, ſive ſphragida, quod eſt ſigillum. Porro diximus de ea abunde nono de ſimplicium medicamentorum facultate libro. Hanc igitur ſive Lemniam terram, ſive ſigillum malis appellare, adulterant, ut nemo veram a fucata falſaque poſſit dignoſcere. Quemadmodum et quod vocatur Indicum Lycium, aliaque multa dignoſci ab adulteratis difficillima: quae convenit ab iis qui in regiones proficiſcuntur tum commiſſariis tum ſenatoriis loci praeſidibus colligere, vel ab amicis qui ea loca inhabitant, quemadmodum me facere conſpexiſtis. Nam alia ex magna Syria, alia ex Palaeſtina, alia ex Aegypto, alia ex Cappadocia, ex Ponto mihi alia afferuntur. Quemadmodum etiam ex Macedonia et occidentalibus plagis, ubi Galli et Hiſpani habitant, a

ρες, οἵ τε κατὰ τὴν ἀντικειμένην χώραν οἰκοῦντες Μαυρούσιοι. τίνα μὲν οὖν ἐν ἑκάστῃ χώρᾳ γίνεται κάλλιστα φάρμακα, Διοσκουρίδης τε καὶ οἱ ἄλλοι γεγράφασιν ἀληθῶς. ἡμᾶς δ', ὡς ἔφην, χρὴ παρασκευάσασθαι καθ' ὃν εἴρηκα τρόπον αὐτὰ, καὶ μάλιστα ἐὰν ἐν Ῥώμῃ κατοικῶμεν, εἰς ἣν ἐξ ἁπάντων τῶν ἐθνῶν καθ' ἕκαστον ἐνιαυτὸν ἐξικνοῦνται πάμπολλα. τίνα δὲ καὶ κατ' αὐτὴν τὴν Ἰταλίαν τὰ μὲν αὐτοφυῶς γεννᾶται, τὰ δὲ κατασκευάζεται, καθάπερ ἐν Δικαιαρχίᾳ τῇ νῦν καλουμένῃ Ποτιόλοις, ἰὸς καὶ ψιμύθιον καὶ χαλκὸς καὶ λεπὶς χαλκοῦ καὶ ἄλλα τινὰ, κατὰ δὲ τὴν Ῥώμην αὐτὴν ἡ λιθάργυρος. ἔνια δὲ μόνον οὐχὶ καθ' ἑκάστην ἡμέραν κομίζεται, καθάπερ τά τ' ἐκ τῆς Σικελίας καὶ τῆς μεγάλης Λιβύης καθ' ἕκαστον ἐνιαυτὸν ὥρᾳ θέρους ἀπό τε Κρήτης πολλὰ, τῶν ἐκεῖ βοτανικῶν ἀνδρῶν ὑπὸ Καίσαρος τρεφομένων, οὐκ αὐτῷ Καίσαρι [868] μόνῳ, ἀλλὰ (425) καὶ πάσῃ τῇ Ῥωμαίων πόλει, πλήρη πεμπόντων ἀγγεῖα ταυτὶ τὰ πλεκτὰ καλούμενα, διὰ τὸ τῶν λυγῶν εἶναι πλέγματα. φέρεται δὲ ἀπὸ Κρήτης τὰ τοιαῦτα καὶ εἰς ἄλλα πολλὰ τῶν ἐθνῶν, ὡς μηδὲν τῶν ἀπ' αὐτῆς ἐνδεῖν,

Mauris, item qui oppofitam illis regionem incolunt. Quae vero in fingulis regionibus praeftantiffima medicamenta gignantur, Diofcorides aliique vere defcripferunt. Nos autem, ut dicebam, praeparare ea oportet quo docui modo, et praefertim fi Romae habitemus, quo ex omnibus gentibus fingulis annis permulta adveniunt. Nonnulla in ipfa quoque Italia partim fua fponte gignuntur, partim praeparantur, quemadmodum in Dicaearchia quae nunc vocatur Puteoli, aerugo, cerufa, aes, fquama aeris, ac alia nonnulla. In ipfa autem Roma argenti fpuma. Nonnulla tantum non quotidie afferuntur, ficuti quae ex Sicilia magnaque Libya et Creta fingulis annis aeftivo tempore multa apportantur, quum herbarii viri, qui illic a Caefare aluntur, non ipfi Caefari folum, fed toti quoque Romanorum urbi plena vafcula transmittant, quae πλεκτὰ dicuntur, quod viminum plexibus conftent. Feruntur ejusmodi a Creta etiam ad alias plerasque gentes, ut nihil ex iis quae

μήτε βοτανῶν, μήτε καρπῶν, μήτε σπερμάτων, μήτε ῥιζῶν, μήτε χυλῶν. τὰ μὲν οὖν ἄλλα πάντα εἰλικρινῆ· νοθεύονται δὲ ἔνιοι τῶν χυλῶν, ἀλλὰ καὶ τοῦτο σπανίως γίνεται. διὰ γὰρ τὸ πλῆθος τῶν γενομένων βοτανῶν ἐν τῇ νήσῳ οὐ πάνυ τι πανουργεῖν ἐπιχειροῦσιν οἱ κατ᾽ αὐτὴν βοτανικοὶ, οὐ μὴν οὐδ᾽ ἡ καινουργία μεγάλη, καθάπερ ἐπ᾽ ἄλλων, ἀλλ᾽ ἀντὶ τοῦ χυλὸν ἀψινθίου μόνου ποιήσασθαι πρασίου μιγνύουσιν, ἤ τι τοιοῦτον παραποιοῦσι μικρὸν, ὥστε τοὺς ἐν Ῥώμῃ μυροπώλας ὠνουμένους καθ᾽ ἕκαστον ἔτος τὰ πλήρη τῶν φαρμάκων ἀγγεῖα τὰ πλεκτὰ, πρῶτον μὲν ἕκαστον αὐτὸν διδάσκεσθαι γνωρίζειν, εἰ καὶ μὴ πρότερον ἑορακώς τις εἴη. πρὸς τούτῳ δὲ καὶ τὸ κάλλιστον ἐκ τῆς συνεχοῦς θέας, ὁποῖόν ἐστι διδάσκεσθαι. μεμνημένοι γὰρ ὧν ὠνήσαντο πέρυσι, ὅταν ἴδωσιν ἕτερον, ἄμεινον αὐτοῦ γνωρίζουσιν· ἐν μὲν ταῖς βοτάναις, ὅσαι μετὰ τοῦ καρποῦ προσκειμένου τοῖς ἀκρέμοσι κομίζονται, πολυκαρπότερον· εὐθαλέστερόν τε καὶ ἁδρότερον, ἐσφιγμένον τε κατὰ τὴν οἰκείαν οὐσίαν, ἔν τε τῷ χρόνῳ μὴ διαφθειρόμενον, ἐννοοῦντες

ab ea proveniunt defit, neque herbis, neque fructibus, neque feminibus, neque radicibus, neque fuccis. Alia igitur omnia fincera accipiuntur: nonnulli autem fucci adulterantur, fed et hoc raro accidit: nam propter copiam herbarum in infula nafcentium herbarii incolae non adeo fucum facere conantur, imo neque novitas magna quemadmodum in aliis exiftit, fed ut abfinthii fuccum duntaxat faciant, marrubium mifcent, aut ejusmodi quippiam exiguum immutant. Quare unguentorum inftitores Romani quum fingulis annis plena medicamentorum vafa plectilia coëmunt, primum unumquodque ipforum cognofcere docentur, etiamfi non prius aliquis viderit. Ad haec etiam quale pulcherrimum exiftat, ex continua infpectione apprehendunt. Memores autem eorum quae anno fuperiore emerunt, quum alterum eo praeftantius viderint, agnofcunt: inter herbas fane, quae cum fructu furculis adhaerente apportantur, foecundius, germinantius, magis amplum, fubftantia ipfius compactum et tempore non contabefcens,

εἶναι κρεῖττον τῶν ἀτροφωτέρων τε καὶ ἀκαρποτέρων, ἀραιῶν τε καὶ κούφων καὶ διαφθειρομένων ταχέως. ὄνος γὰρ ἂν εἴη σαφῶς ὁ μηδὲν τούτων ἐννοῆσαι δυνάμενος. ὥσπερ γε καὶ κατὰ τὴν γεῦσίν τε καὶ ὄσφρησιν οὐδὲν χαλεπὸν ἐννοῆσαι τὸ ἄριστον, ἑορακότας πολλάκις ταὐτόν. ἐν ᾧ γὰρ τῶν ἄλλων διαφέρει κατ᾽ ὀσμὴν ἢ γεῦσιν ἕκαστον τῶν φαρμάκων, ἐν ἐκείνῳ σφοδρυνόμενον πρωτεύει τῶν ὁμοειδῶν. οὕτω γοῦν καὶ τὸ μέλι λέγομεν ἄριστον εἶναι τὸ γλυκύτατόν τε καὶ δριμύτατον τῶν ἄλλων ἁπάντων, ἐπειδὴ τὸ γένος αὐτοῦ τὴν ἐν γλυκύτητι τοιαύτην ὑπεροχὴν ἔχειν φαίνεται. ὅταν οὖν ἐκ γλυκειῶν φύσει σταφυλῶν τὸ γλεῦκος εἰς ἥμισυ μέρος ἢ καὶ τρίτον ἑψηθείη, γλυκύτητι μὲν οὐδὲν ἀποδεῖ μέλιτος, ἀμβλὺ δ᾽ ἐστὶ καὶ ἄδηκτον, ὥσπερ τὸ ὕδωρ· ἀλλ᾽ οὐ τό γε μέλι τοιοῦτον· ἔχει γάρ τινα δριμύτητα μετὰ τῆς γλυκύτητος, ὥστε ἄριστόν ἐστι τὸ πρωτεῦον ἐν τούτοις, καὶ πρῶτά γε αὐτῶν τὰ γνωρίσματα τῆς οἰκείας ἀρετῆς ἐκ τούτων ἔσται. κατὰ συμβεβηκὸς δέ τι καὶ παρεπόμενον αὐτῇ κατὰ χροιὰν καὶ σύστασιν καὶ

intelligentes eſſe praeſtantius iis, quae macriora, minus fructuoſa, rara, levia et celeriter contabeſcentia viſuntur. Aſinus enim nimirum eſſet qui nihil horum poſſit intelligere, quemadmodum etiam guſtu odoratuque nihil negotii eſt optimum deprehendere, quum idem ſubinde viderimus. In quo enim ſingula medicamenta ab aliis odore aut guſtu differunt, in illo validum, principem inter ſimilia ſpecie, locum obtinet. Ita ſane et mel dicimus eſſe praeſtantiſſimum, quod dulciſſimum et acerrimum inter omnia alia habeatur, quoniam genus ipſius ejusmodi in dulcedine exceſſum obtinere apparet. Quum itaque ex dulcibus natura uvis muſtum ad dimidias aut etiam tertias fuerit incoctum, dulcedine quidem nihil a melle deficit, hebes autem eſt et morſus expers, quemadmodum aqua; verum mel non hujusmodi exiſtit, quippe acrimoniam quandam cum dulcedine refert. Quare laudatiſſimum eſt, quod in his praecellit ac primae ipſorum notae propriae virtutis, ex his ac ex accidenti ejusque conſequio petentur, juxta

ὀσμὴν καὶ τὴν οἷον ἀλληλουχίαν τῶν μορίων. ὠχρὸν μὲν οὖν ἐστι τῇ χροιᾷ, τῇ συστάσει δὲ οὔτε παχὺ καὶ θρομβῶδες οὔτε λίαν ὑγρὸν ἡνωμένον τε δι᾿ ὅλου καὶ γλίσχρον, ὡς ἐάν γε βαστάσας ἀπ᾿ αὐτοῦ τῷ δακτύλῳ ῥεῖν ἐπιτρέψῃς, κατατείνεσθαι συνεχὲς αὐτὸ, καθάπερ ἰξὸν, οὐ διασπώμενον, οὐδὲ ἀποῤῥηγνύμενον, ἀλλ᾿ οὐ διὰ ταῦτ᾿ ἔστιν ἄριστον, ἀλλ᾿ ὅτι τὸ κατὰ τὴν οἰκείαν φύσιν ἄριστον μέλι ταῦτ᾿ ἔχει συμβεβηκότα διὰ παντὸς ἑαυτῷ, καὶ διὰ τοῦτο γνωρίσματα γίνεται τοῦ βελτίστου. διὸ καὶ πολλάκις ἑωρᾶσθαί φημι δεῖν ἕκαστον τῶν ἁπλῶν φαρμάκων, ἵνα διὰ μνήμης ἔχωμεν εἰς ὅσον ἥκει δριμύτητος, ἢ γλυκύτητος, ἤ τινος τῶν ἄλλων αἰσθητῶν ποιοτήτων, ὧν τὸ ποσὸν ἀδύνατον λόγῳ δηλωθῆναι. προσέρχεται δέ τις καὶ ἄλλη κρίσις τῆς ἑκάστου φαρμάκου δυνάμεως ἐξ ἐμπειρίας πολυχρονίου, μηδὲν ὑπὸ τοῦ λόγου βοηθουμένη. τὸ γοῦν ἀπὸ Κνίδου κάλλιστον μέλι φαινόμενον οἷς εἶπον ἄρτι γνωρίσμασιν, ὡς ἐγγὺς εἶναι τῷ Θασίῳ τε καὶ Ὑμηττίῳ, κακίαν οὐ μικρὰν ἐνδείκνυται χρονίζον, εἰς οἰνώδη μεταβάλλον ποιότητα. παραπλήσιον

colorem, ſubſtantiam, odorem, et veluti particularum compagem. Colore igitur pallidum eſt, ſubſtantia neque craſſum et grumoſum, neque nimis liquidum, unitumque per tota et viſcoſum, ut ſi ex eo nonnihil digito geſtans fluere permiſeris, diſtendatur, ſibi contiguum, viſci modo, ne divellatur neque abrumpatur: verum non ideo eſt optimum, ſed quia ex peculiari natura mel optimum haec perpetuo ſibi accidentia vendicat, eaque de cauſa praeſtantiſſimae notae efficiuntur. Hinc igitur opus eſſe dico ſingula medicamenta ſimplicia ſubinde inſpexiſſe, ut in memoria habeamus, quantum acrimoniae ſortita ſint, aut dulcedinis, aut alterius cujusdam ſenſibilis qualitatis, quarum quantitas verbis nequit indicari. Jam et aliud quoddam cujusque medicamenti facultatis judicium ex longa experientia accedit, quod nihil ratione adjuvatur. Nam mel a Cnidio excellentiſſimum notis quas dixi nuper apparens, ceu prope accedat ad Thaſium et Hymettium, malitiam non mediocrem vetuſtate oſtendit, in vinoſam tranſiens

δέ τι πέπονθεν αὐτῷ καὶ τὸ Ῥόδιον. ὥστε τις ἐμβαλὼν τούτου τοῦ μέλιτος εἰς τὴν θηριακὴν [869] εἶτα μετὰ γʹ ἐνιαυτὸν εὑρὼν αὐτὴν οἰνίζουσαν, οὐ κατὰ τὴν γεῦσιν μόνον, ἀλλὰ καὶ κατὰ τὴν ὀσμὴν ἔδειξέ μοι, κἀγὼ θεασάμενος εἶπον τὸ γεγονὸς αὐτῷ παρὰ τοῦ βεβλημένου μέλιτος, ὥστε θαυμάσαι τὸν ἄνθρωπον. ἔτι δὲ προσεπυθόμην, εἴ γε ἐπὶ πλέον ἥψησέ τε καὶ ἀπήφρισεν αὐτό. προσωμολόγει δὲ καὶ ταῦτα, καὶ διὰ τοῦτο ἐθαύμαζε μὲν ὥς τι σοφὸν ἀκηκοὼς παρ᾽ ἐμοῦ, κατέγνω δὲ τῆς ἑαυτοῦ προπετείας, ἐπιχειρήσαντος σκευάζειν φάρμακον ἐκ μόνης τῆς γραφῆς. ἄλλως δ᾽ ὀξώδη γενομένην, ἣν ἐσκεύασε θηριακὴν ἔδειξέ μοι, πυνθανόμενος τὴν αἰτίαν. ἀκούσας οὖν παρ᾽ ἐμοῦ πλείονα τοῦ δέοντος ἐμβεβλῆσθαι οἶνον, καὶ τοῦτον οὐκ ἄριστον οὐδὲ παλαιὸν, ἴσως δὲ καὶ ἄρτου μὴ καλῶς κατεσκευασμένου, πλέον μεμίχθαι τῇ σαρκὶ τῶν ἐχιδνῶν, ὁμολογήσας οὕτως ἔχειν, ἑαυτοῦ κατέγνω τῆς προπετείας.

Κεφ. γʹ. [Ὁποῖον δεῖ τὸν οἶνον ἐμβαλεῖν ταῖς ἀντι-

qualitatem. Simile ipfi quippiam et Rhodio accidit. Quapropter quum aliquis mel hoc in theriacam mififfet, deinde poft triennium ipfam vinum refipientem deprehendiffet, non guftu modo, fed odore etiam mihi oftendit, ac ego contemplatus dixi, id ei ex melle indito accidiffe, ob quod homo me admirari coepit: praeterea interrogavi, an largius ipfum incoxiffet defpumaffetque. Confitebatur autem et haec, eoque admiratus eft ut qui fapiens nonnihil a me audiviffet. Caeterum fuam ipfe temeritatem ac praecipitantiam damnavit, quod ex fola fcriptura medicamentum praeparare effet aggreffus. Alius acidam quam praeparavit theriacen effectam mihi indicavit, caufam interrogans. Itaque quum a me audiviffet plus impendio vini effe injectum, ejusque non optimi neque veteris, forte etiam panis non probe confecti amplius quam convenit carni viperarum effe immixtum, confeffus ita fe rem habere, temeritatis fe damnavit.

Cap. III. [*Quod vinum in antidotis poni debeat.*]

δότοις.] Διὸ καὶ προνοητέον ἐστὶν οἶνον ἐμβαλεῖν τῷ γένει τοιοῦτον, ὁποῖος μὲν ἐκ τῆς ἐμπειρίας ἔγνωσται μονιμώτατος ὑπάρχειν, ἔπειτα δ' ἰσχυρὸν, ἔτεσι πλείοσιν ἤδη δεδωκότα βάσανον, ὡς οὐκ ἔτι μεταβληθήσοιτο. καὶ γάρ τοι καὶ ἀσθενέστατοί γε καὶ ὡς ἂν εἴποι τις ὑδατωδέστατοι τῶν οἴνων ἢ σφόδρα αὐστηροὶ, καὶ μάλιστα πάντων οἴνων ὀξυνόμενοι, φθάσαντες ἐν τοῖς πρώτοις ἔτεσιν ὀξυνθῆναι, διαμένουσι τοῦ λοιποῦ. χρόνος δὲ τῆς τοιαύτης κρίσεως ἄλλος ἄλλῳ οἴνων ἐστὶν, οὐ πολλῶν μὲν ἐτῶν τοῖς ὑδατώδεσιν· οὕτω δ' ὀνομάζουσι τοὺς λευκοὺς τῇ χρόᾳ καὶ λεπτοὺς τῇ συστάσει, καὶ μὴ πολλοῦ δεομένους ὕδατος ἐν τῷ κεράννυσθαι. πάντως δ' αὐτοῖς ὑπάρχει τοιούτοις οὖσιν, ὥσπερ οὐδ' ὅλως πλήττουσι τὴν κεφαλὴν, οὕτω μηδὲ θερμαίνειν σαφῶς τὸ σῶμα, μηδὲ πέψει τῇ κατὰ γαστέρα, καὶ φλέβας ἐναργῶς συντελεῖν τι, μηδὲ εὐτροφίᾳ συναίρεσθαι. τάχιστα πάντων οἴνων οὗτοι παλαιοῦνται. καλοῦσι δὲ οἱ περὶ ταῦτα δεινοὶ παλαιοῦσθαι τὸ μεταβάλλειν ἑτοίμως εἰς τὴν τοιαύτην ποιότητα τῶν παλαιουμένων. δρι-

Quare etiam profpiciendum venit, cujusmodi genere id immittas, quale fane experientia notum eft firmiffimum exiftere; deinde validum, quod pluribus jam annis probatum fuerit, quod non amplius immutetur. Etenim imbecillima et, ut fic dicam, aquatiffima vina aut vehementer auftera, et maxime omnium vinorum acefcentia, ubi primis annis exacuerint, reliquo tempore permanent. Verum hujusmodi judicii tempus aliud alii vino exiftit: non multis fane annis aquofis id accidit. Ita vero nominant alba colore tenuiaque fubftantia, et non multae inter temperandum aquae indiga. Omnino autem ea quae talia funt, uti nec caput omnino feriunt, ita neque corpus manifefto calefaciunt, neque concoctioni in ventriculo et venis evidenter quicqnam conferunt, neque alendo corpori fubminiftrant. Haec ex omnibus vinis celerrime inveterantur. Vocant autem harum rerum periti inveterari prompte in talem veterafcentium qualitatem immutari. Atque haec acrimonia eft cum calore manifefto.

μύτης δ' ἐστὶν αὕτη μετὰ τοῦ θερμαίνειν σαφῶς, ὕστερον δὲ καὶ πικρότης, εἰς ἣν μετέστη. ἐνίοτε δὲ καὶ τοὺς ὑδατώδεις οἴνους ἀφικνουμένους ἐστὶν ἰδεῖν, ὅταν γε μὴ φθάσωσιν ἐν τοῖς πρώτοις, ἢ τρισὶν, ἢ τέτρασιν ἔτεσιν ὀξυνθῆναι· τοῖς δ' ἰσχυροῖς τε ἅμα καὶ αὐστηροῖς καὶ λευκοῖς μετὰ πάχους οἴνοις καὶ μετὰ δεκαετίαν ἐνίοτε συνέπεσε μὴ καλῶς ἀποκειμένοις ὀξυνθῆναι. συνέβαινε δ' αὐτοῖς καὶ παλαιοῦσθαι χρόνῳ παμπόλλῳ· τοιοῦτοι κατὰ τὴν Ἰταλίαν εἰσὶν, ὅ τε Τιβουρτῖνος καὶ Σιγνῖνος καὶ Μάρσος καὶ Σουῤῥεντῖνος. ὁ μέντοι Τιβουρτῖνος καὶ Μάῤσος αὐστηροί τε, καὶ ῥᾳδίως ὀξυνόμενοι κατὰ τὴν ἀπρονόητον ἀπόθεσιν. ὁ δὲ Σιγνῖνος ἰσχυρότερός τε τούτων ὑπάρχει, καὶ ἧττον ὀξύνεται καὶ παλαιωθεὶς κάλλιστος γίνεται. περὶ δὲ τοῦ Σουῤῥεντίνου τί δεῖ καὶ λέγειν; ἅπαντες γὰρ τοῦτ' ἤδη γινώσκουσιν ὡς σχεδὸν πρὸ κ' ἐτῶν ἔτι ἐστὶν ἄπεπτος. ἀκμάζει δὲ τοσούτων ἐτῶν γιγνόμενος, ἐπὶ πολύ τε παραμένει πότιμος, οὐκ εὐκόλως ἐκπικρούμενος, συνάμιλλος κατ' ἀρετὴν ὑπάρχων τῷ Φαλερίνῳ. ἐναντία δὲ τούτοις τοῖς οἴνοις οἱ ὑδατώδεις πάσχουσιν, ὅ τε Σαβῖνος καὶ ὁ Ἀλβα-

Poſtea vero amaror, in quem tranſit. Nonnunquam et aquoſa vina perſeverantia eſt videre, quum non primis aut tribus aut quatuor annis ſubacuerint. At validis ſimul et auſteris albisque cum craſſitie vinis etiam poſt decennium interim, ſi non bene fuerint recondita, aceſcere accidit. Eadem quoque inveterari longo temporis ſpatio contingit. Ejusmodi in Italia ſunt Tiburtinum, Signinum, Marſum, Surrentinum. Et quidem Tiburtinum Marſumque auſtera ſunt, et ex facili ſi imprudentius condantur aceſcunt. Signinum vero et his valentius eſt et minus aceſcit, inveteratumque optimum redditur. De Surrentino quid opus eſt dicere? Omnibus enim hoc jam conſtat, id ante viginti prope annos adhuc eſſe crudum. Viget autem tot annis natum, diuque potulentum permanet, non ex proclivi amareſcens, Falerno viribus perſimile. Secus aquoſis accidit, Sabino, Albano,

νὸς καὶ ὁ Γαυριανὸς ἐν τῷ Ποτιόλων λόφῳ γενόμενος, ὅ τε ἐν Νεαπόλει κατὰ τοὺς ὑποκειμένους αὐτῇ λόφους, Ἀμιναῖος μὲν ὀνομαζόμενος, [870] ἀλλὰ λεπτὸς μὲν ὑπάρχων, οὐχ ὥσπερ οἱ κατὰ τὴν Σικελίαν τε καὶ Βιθυνίαν Ἀμιναῖοι, καίτοι κἀν τούτοις τοῖς ἔθνεσιν ὀλίγος μὲν ὁ ὑδατώδης καὶ λεπτὸς οἶνος γεννᾶται, οὐ μὴν ἀποδεῖ γε οὔτε τοῦ Σαβίνου κατὰ τὴν Ἰταλίαν οὔτε κατὰ τὴν Ἀσίαν Ἀρσινίου τε καὶ Τιτακαζηνοῦ καὶ τοῦ παρ᾽ ἡμῖν ὀνομαζομένου Τιβηνοῦ διὰ τὸ χωρίον ἐν ᾧ γεωργεῖται Τίβας ὀνομα-(426) ζόμενον. οὗτοι πάντες ῥᾳδίως μεταβάλλονται πρὸς τὰς ἐναντίας ποιότητας, ἤτοι τὴν ὀξεῖαν ἢ τὴν πικρὰν, ἐν μὲν ἀρχῇ τὴν ὀξεῖαν, ἐὰν δὲ διαμένωσι, τὴν πικράν. πολὺ δὲ εἰς ἑκάτερα τὴν ἀλλοίωσιν αὐτοῖς συμβάλλεται τὸ χωρίον ἐν ᾧ κεῖνται. καταρχὰς μὲν ἄριστόν ἐστι τὸ ψυχρὸν, ὕστερον δὲ τὸ θερμὸν, ἢ πάλιν ἱκανῶς θερμὸν ἐξ ἀρχῆς, ὡς τό γε χλιαρὸν ὀξύνει ῥᾳδίως αὐτούς. ἐὰν δὲ ἐν τῷ ψυχρῷ κείμενοι διαμένωσιν ἔτεσι β′ καὶ γ′, τοὐντεῦθεν ἱκανῶς θερμαίνεσθαι δέονται, τοῦ χλιαροῦ δὲ χωρίου καὶ

Gauriano quod in Puteolorum colle naſcitur. Item et quod in Neapoli in ſubjectis ei colliculis provenit, Aminaeum quidem appellatum, ſed tenue, non ſicuti in Sicilia et Bithynia Aminaea, etſi his gentibus paucum ſane, aquoſum, ac tenue vinum gignatur non tamen abeſt vel a Sabino in Italia, vel in Aſia, Arſinio, Titacazeno, et quod apud nos vocatur Tibenum propter regionem in qua colitur Tibas appellatam. Haec omnia facile in contrarias qualitates mutantur, vel acidam, vel amaram: inter principia quidem acidam; ſin autem permanſerint, amaram. At multum ad adulteram qualitatem regio, in qua ſita ſint, confert. Initio ſane optima eſt frigida, poſtea vero calida, aut e contrario, calida per initia. Nam tepida facile ipſa in acorem perducit Si autem in frigidiore ſita loco permanſerint annis duobus et tribus, illinc abunde calefieri deſiderant, tepidum autem locum et temperatura medium nunquam requirunt; nonnulla

Ed. Chart. XIII. [870.] Ed. Baſ. II. (426.)
τοῦ μέσου, κατὰ τὴν κρᾶσιν οὐδέποτε δέονται. τινές γε μὴν οὕτως ἀσθενεῖς εἰσι καὶ ὑδατώδεις, ὡς μηδ' ἐξ ἀρχῆς φέρειν τὸ ψυχρὸν, ἐφ' ὧν ὁ πατήρ μου πείρας ἕνεκεν εἰς θερμότατον οἶκον ἐμβαλὼν στοιβὴν πολλὴν καὶ θερμὴν ἐνέκρυψεν αὐτῇ πληρώσας κεράμια, καὶ τυχὼν τῆς ἐλπίδος οὐδέποτε ἔσχεν οἶνον ὀξυνόμενον, ἀλλὰ πάντας τάχιστα παλαιουμένους. ὅπως δ' ἄν τις οἴκημα παρασκευάσειε θερμὸν, ὡς ἐκεῖνος παρεσκεύασεν, καὶ δὴ φράσω. κατὰ τοὺς ἀγροὺς ἅπαντας παρ' ἡμῖν οἶκοι γίνονται μεγάλοι, τὴν μὲν ἑστίαν, ἐφ' ἧς καίουσι τὸ πῦρ, ἐν μέσοις ἑαυτῶν ἔχοντες, οὐ πολὺ δὲ αὐτῆς ἀπέχουσιν αἱ τῶν ὑποζυγίων στάσεις, ἤτοι κατ' ἀμφότερα τὰ μέρη, δεξιόν τε καὶ ἀριστερὸν, ἢ πάντως γε κατὰ θάτερον. εἰσὶ δὲ κρίβανοι συνεζευγμένοι ταῖς ἑστίαις κατὰ τὸ πρόσω μέρος ἑαυτῶν, ὃ πρὸς τὴν θύραν βλέπει τοῦ παντὸς οἴκου. τοιοῦτοι μὲν οὖν ἅπαντες οἱ κατὰ τοὺς ἀγροὺς οἶκοι κατασκευάζονται, κἂν εὐτελεῖς ὦσιν. οἱ δ' ἐπιμελέστερον αὐτῶν κατασκευαζόμενοι κατὰ τὸν ἔνδον τοῖχον ἔχουσι τὴν κατ' ἄντικρυ τῇ θύρᾳ τεταγμένην ἐξέδραν. ἑκατέρωθεν δ' αὐτῆς κοιτῶνα, καθ' ὃν ἄνω-

tamen adeo ſunt imbecillia aquoſaque, ut ne initio quidem frigus tolerent; in quibus pater meus cauſa experientiae ſtoebe copioſa calidaque in domum calidiſſimam injecta vaſa repleta occultavit, et aſſequutus id quod ſperabat, nunquam vinum habuit acidum, ſed omnia celerrime veteraſcentia. Quomodo autem domunculam calidam praepares, ut ille extruere ſolebat, etiam nunc indicabo: in agris omnibus apud nos domus fiunt praegrandes, focum in quo ignem excitant in medio ipſarum habentes, non multum autem ab eo diſtant jumentorum ſtabula, vel in utraque parte: dextra et ſiniſtra, aut certe in alterutra. Sunt et fornaces focis conjuncti juxta anteriorem ipſorum partem, quae totius domus oſtium reſpicit. In eum itaque modum omnes in agris domus conſtruuntur, etiamſi exiguae exiſtant; quae autem curioſius ex eis aedificantur interiore pariete exedram habent, oſtio ex adverſo oppoſitam; utraque autem ipſius parte lectum, in cujus ſu-

θέν ἐστιν ὑπερῷα οἰκήματα, καθάπερ καὶ κατὰ πολλὰ τῶν πανδοχείων ἐν κύκλῳ κατὰ τρεῖς τοίχους τοῦ οἴκου τοῦ μεγάλου, πολλάκις δὲ καὶ κατὰ τέτταρας. ἐκ τούτων οὖν τῶν οἰκημάτων τὸ μάλιστα σκεπόμενον ἑκατέρωθέν ἐστι, τὸ κατὰ τῆς ἐξέδρας ἐπικείμενον, ἐν ᾧ τὸν οἶνον ὁ πατήρ μου κατετίθετο, μετὰ τὸ κατὰ τοὺς πίθους ζέσαι. τὸ δὲ μονιμώτερον ἐπὶ τῶν κεραμίων ἀποτίθεται πρότερον, ὥσπερ καὶ τοὺς ἄλλους ἐστὶ παρ' ἡμῖν δι' ἔτους θερμαίνειν διόλου. ἀμείνων δὲ τῶν οἴκων ὁ πρὸς μεσημβρίαν μὲν ἐστραμμένος, ἀπεστραμμένος δὲ τὰς ἄρκτους. ἔστι δέ τις παρ' ἡμῖν γενομένη βοτάνη θαμνώδης, πάνυ θερμὴ καὶ δριμεῖα, καὶ ἀρωματίζον ἔχουσά τι, καλοῦσι δ' αὐτὴν οἱ ἐπιχώριοι κολυμβάδα, ἔνιοι δὲ στοιβὴν, ἐπιτηδειοτάτην οὖσαν εἰς φυλακὴν οἴνου. συντίθεται οὖν ἐν ταύτῃ τῇ βοτάνῃ τὰ κεράμια, καὶ τῶν οἴκων τῶν ὑπερῴων τοῦ μέρους τὸν ἕνα τοῖχον διετίτρα τρήμασιν ἀξιολόγοις, ἐστραμμένοις εἰς τὸν μέγαν οἶκον, ἐν ᾧ τόν τε κρίβανον ἔφην εἶναι καὶ τὴν ἑστίαν, προμηθούμενος, διὰ τῶν τρημάτων εἰσιέναι θερμασίαν εἰς τὸν οἶκον, ἐν ᾧ τὰ

periore parte domunculae sublimes ſunt, quemadmodum in multis omnigenarum rerum receptaculis orbiculatim juxta tres magnae domus parietes, saepe etiam juxta quatuor. Ex his igitur domunculis quae maxime spectatur utrobique, exedrae incumbit in qua vinum pater meus reponebat, poſtquam in doliis eſſerbuiſſet, at firmius in vaſis fictilibus prius reponitur, quemadmodum et alia licet apud nos per totum annum caleſacere. Praeſtantior autem domus eſt, quae meridiem ſpectat, a ſeptentrione remota. Porro herba quae apud nos naſcitur ſruticoſa admodum eſt, calida, acris et odoratum quippiam recipiens; vocant ipſam incolae Colymbadem, nonnulli Stoeben, ad vini conſervationem aptiſſimam. Condebat autem hac herba vaſcula, et domuncularum ſuperiorum partis unum parietem foraminibus notandis in majorem modum diductis, qua et fornacem et ſocum eſſe dixi, dividebat, conſiderans calorem per eadem foramina in domunculam pervenire, qua vini dolia reponebat. Itaque ex magnae domus calore et ſtoebe

κεράμια κατετίθετο. ἔκ τε οὖν τῆς κατὰ τὸν μέγαν οἶκον θερμασίας ἡ ἀποθήκη θερμαινομένη, κἀκ τῆς στοιβῆς θαλπομένη, διεφύλαττε πάντα τὸν οἶνον, ὡς μηδέποτε ὀξυνθῆναι. πρὸς δὲ τὸ μᾶλλον ἐπιτυγχάνειν, καὶ μηδέποτε ἁμαρτεῖν τοῦ σκοποῦ, τοῖς κεραμίοις ἐνέχει τὸν οἶνον οὐ καινοῖς, ἀλλ' ἐξ ὧν ἐκεκένωτό τις τῶν πεπαλαιωμένων. παραπλή[871]σιον δ' οἷς εἴρηκα καὶ κατὰ τὴν Ἰταλίαν εἶδον ἐν τοῖς περὶ Νεάπολιν, καὶ τὸν γειτνιῶντα λόφον αὐτῇ τῇ χώρᾳ γενόμενον, ὃν ὀνομάζουσι Τριφύλλινον. ἐπυθόμην δὲ καὶ κατ' ἄλλα πολλὰ χωρία τῆς Ἰταλίας οὕτω θερμαίνεσθαι τὸν οἶνον, ἀλλ' ὅ γε τοιοῦτος, ὥσπερ μόνιμος, οὕτω καὶ κεφαλαλγὴς γίνεται, διὰ τὴν ἐκ τοῦ καπνοῦ προσερχομένην αὐτῷ ποιότητα. φευκτέον οὖν σοι τοὺς τοιούτους ἅπαντας οἴνους ἐν τοῖς συντιθεμένοις φαρμάκοις, ἃ μέλλομεν εἴσω τοῦ σώματος λήψεσθαι. κατὰ δὲ τὰς ἐμπλάστρους καὶ τὰ ἄλλα τὰ ἔξωθεν ἐπιτιθέμενα φάρμακα, καὶ τοῖς τοιούτοις, οὐδὲν κωλύει χρῆσθαι, μὴ παρόντων ἀρίστων. αἱρετέον οὖν εἰς τὰς ἀντιδότους οἴνους φύσει μονίμους, ὧν πρῶτος οὐκ εἰς τοῦτο μόνον, ἀλλὰ καὶ τὴν ἄλλην ἅπασαν ἀρετὴν, ὁ Φαλε-

ſotu, theca vinaria incaleſcens vinum totum conſervabat, ut nunquam aceſceret. Quo autem magis id conſequeretur, et nunquam a propoſito aberraret, vaſis infundebat vinum non recentibus, ſed ex quibus aliquod inveteratum evacuarit. Perſimile iis quae dixi in Italia quoque vidi circa Neapolim ſieri, et collem eidem regioni vicinum, quem nominant Triphyllinum. Audivi etiam in multis Italiae locis vinum ita calefieri, ſed tale quemadmodum firmum et durabile, ita etiam doloris in capite efficax efficitur, propter qualitatem quae ipſi ex ſumo accedit. Itaque ejusmodi omnia vina in medicamentis componendis quae intra corpus aſſumpturi ſumus, evitabis. In emplaſtris autem, et aliis quae extrinſecus imponuntur medicamentis, etiam talibus uti optimorum penuria nihil prohibet. Deligi itaque vina debent in antidota natura firma, inter quae primum non ad hoc ſolum, ſed aliam quoque omnem virtutem ſalernum exiſtit: aſſumendum

ρινός ἐστιν. αἱρετέον δὲ καὶ τούτου τὸν μήπω πικρὸν ὑπὸ παλαιότητος, ὡς ἔνιοι καὶ κατὰ τοῦτο σφάλλονται τῶν τὴν θηριακὴν σκευαζόντων. ἀκηκοότες γὰρ ἀεὶ τὸν περιφερόμενον λόγον τοῦτον, ὡς τἄλλα πάντα γηρᾷ τῷ χρόνῳ πλὴν οἴνου, τὸν παλαιότατον ἐμβάλλουσιν, οὐδὲ τῆς ποσότητος ἔνιοι στοχαζόμενοι, διὰ τὸ μηδὲ γεγράφθαι τὴν συμμετρίαν αὐτοῦ κατὰ τὰς φαρμακίτιδας βίβλους. δυοῖν δ' ὄντοιν εἰδῶν αὐτοῦ, μηδὲν ἀλλήλων διαφερόντων ἀρετῇ, ἡδίονα τὴν ἀντίδοτον ὁ γλυκύτερος ἐργάζεται, καὶ καλοῦσιν αὐτὸν ἰδίως Φαυστιανόν. καθάπερ οὖν οἱ τὸν μεταβάλλοντα καὶ ὀξυνόμενον οἶνον ἐμβάλλοντες ἁμαρτάνουσιν, εἰ γὰρ καὶ μηδὲν ἔχον ἔγκλημα καθ' ἑαυτὸν ἀναμιχθείη τοῖς τῆς ἀντιδότου φαρμάκοις, ὀξύνεται πολλάκις, οὕτως ὁ παλαιότατος Φαλερῖνος, καὶ μάλισθ' ὅταν βραχὺ πλείων ληφθῇ, πικρὸν ἐργάζεται τὸ φάρμακον.

Κεφ. δ'. [Περὶ μέλιτος ταῖς ἀντιδότοις ἐμβληθῆναι δεομένου.] Εἷς δέ τις ἰατρὸς καὶ τὸ μέλι πάνυ παλαιὸν

vero et hujus generis eſt, quod nondum prae vetuſtate amareſcat, ſicut nonnulli qui theriacen praeparant in hoc quoque falluntur. Quum enim audiviſſent ſemper ſermonem hunc celebrari circumferrique, puta alia omnia praeter vinum tempore conſeneſcere, vetuſtiſſimum injiciunt, neque quantitatem aliqui conjectura aſſequentes, eo quod neque in libris medicamentariis menſura ipſius ſcripta inveniatur. Quum autem duplices ſint ipſius ſpecies, nihil viribus inter ſe differentes, ſuavius Antidotum, id quod dulcius eſt, efficit, ac vocant ipſum proprie Fauſtianum. In quibus igitur qui mutatum et aceſcens vinum miſcent, errant. Si enim vel nullo infectum vitio per ſe Antidoti medicamentis contemperetur, ſubinde aceſcit, ita ut vetuſtiſſimum falernum, et praeſertim quando paulo copioſius fuerit inditum, medicamentum reddit amarum.

Cap. IV. [*De melle componendis antidotis idoneo.*] Jam vero alius unus medicus etiam mel admodum vetus

ἐνέβαλεν ὁμοίως τῷ Φαλερίνῳ, κατὰ τοιόνδε τινὰ λογισμόν. οἰνῶδές ποτε μέλι τι γέγονε τὸ κεκραμένον, ἔμπροσθεν ἄριστον αὐτὸ φαινόμενον. ἀσφαλέστερον οὖν ἔδοξε, καθάπερ ἐπ' οἴνου τοῦ τῷ μήκει τοῦ χρόνου κεκριμένου ὡς ου φθείροιτο, μῖξαι τῷ φαρμάκῳ. τὸ δὲ ἦν ἄρα διὰ τὸν χρόνον ὑπόπικρον, εἶτα καὶ τὴν ἕψησιν προσλαβὸν ἐπὶ πλέον γενομένην, ἔτι μᾶλλον ἐδείχθη πικρὸν, ὅπερ ἅπαντι μέλιτι τῷ παλαιοτέρῳ συμβαίνει κατὰ τὴν ἕψησιν. καὶ θαυμαστὸν οὐδὲν, ὅπου γε καὶ χωρὶς τῆς ἑψήσεως ἐν τῷ χρόνῳ πικρότερον ἀντὶ τοῦ γλυκυτέρου γίνεται. καὶ παρά γε τῷ ἐμῷ πατρὶ μέλι τι πικρὸν οὕτως ἦν, οἷον ἐν τῷ Πόντῳ γίνεται κατά τινα τῶν χωρίων, ἐν οἷς αἱ μέλιτται συνάγουσιν ἀπὸ τῶν ἀψινθίων. αὐτὸ τοῦτο δ' ἔφασκε τὸ μέλι τὸ παρὰ Ἀθηναίοις ἄριστον χρόνῳ παμπόλλῳ παλαιωθὲν γεγονέναι πικρόν. ἐπεὶ δ' ἄχρηστον ἐφάνη μοι, καὶ μετὰ τὴν τελευτὴν τοῦ πατρὸς ἄχρι νῦν φυλάττω, πικρότερον μὲν ἔτι καὶ μᾶλλον, ἢ τότε ἦν γεγονὸς, ὥσπερ γε καὶ μελάντερον, οὐ μὴν παχύτερόν γε πολλῷ. καὶ τοῦτ' ἔοικεν ἐξαίρετον

falerno fimiliter injecit, tali quadam ratiocinatione ufus. Vinofum quandoque mel aliquod evafit temperatum, quod praeftantiffimum ante apparebat. Tutius itaque vifum quemadmodum in vino quod longitudine temporis indicatum eft non corrumpi, medicamento admifcere. Erat autem hoc utique propter tempus fubamarum, deinde ex coctura largiore magis adhuc amarum eft oftenfum, quod omni melli vetuftiori ex coctione accidit. At meri nihil eft, quum et citra cocturam tempore amarius pro dulciori evadat. Atque apud patrem meum mel quoddam amarum adeo erat, quale in Ponto nafcitur quibusdam locis, ubi apes ipfum ex abfinthio congregant; id ipfum dicebat, mel quod apud Athenienfes eft praeftantiffimum, multo tempore inveteratum amarum evafiffe. Quoniam vero inutile mihi vifum eft, etiam a patris obitu in hunc usque diem fervo, amarius quidem adhuc multo quam tunc erat redditum, ficuti et nigrius, non tamen multo craffius. Atque hoc optimo melli eximium adeffe videtur

ὑπάρχον τῷ καλλίστῳ μέλιτι. καὶ γάρ τοι καὶ τὸ ἐν Ἐλεοῦντι τῆς Χεῤῥονήσου κατὰ τὴν χώραν ἐκείνην ἔνθα τὸ ἡρῷόν ἐστι τοῦ Πρωτεσιλάου γενόμενον μέλι, πάντ᾽ ἔχον Ὑμηττίου μέλιτος, μέχρι πολλοῦ τὰ αὐτὰ, τῷ χρόνῳ προϊόντι, πρὸς τὸ παχύτερον γίνεσθαι, καὶ θρομβοῦται πολλάκις. μέλι μὲν οὖν πάντως ἐμβλητέον ἐστὶ τὸ κάλλιστον ταῖς ἀντιδότοις Ὑμήττιον ἢ Θάσιον ἢ πάντως γε Ἀττικόν· εἰ δὲ ἀποροῖμέν ποτε αὐτοῦ, τοῦ ἐν [872] ταῖς Κυκλάσι νήσοις γινομένου, ὅ τί περ ἂν ὁμοιότατον ᾖ τούτῳ. γίνεται δὲ κατὰ τὸν Ἰσθμὸν μέλι ἀγαθὸν, καὶ καλεῖταί γε τοῦτο Ἰσθμιακὸν ἰδίως ἀπὸ τοῦ χωρίου, καθάπερ καὶ Τούβρεον καὶ αὐτὸ τὴν ἐπωνυμίαν ἔχον. ἔνδοξα μὲν οὖν ταῦτα. γίνεται δὲ καὶ κατ᾽ ἄλλα χωρία κάλλιστον μέλι, διὰ βραχύτητα δ᾽ ἅπαν δαπανώμενον ὑπὸ τῶν ἐγχωρίων, ὡς μὴ περιττεύειν εἰς ἄλλην χώραν ἐξάγεσθαι, καὶ διὰ τοῦτ᾽ ἀγνοεῖσθαι. καὶ γὰρ οὖν ἐν τῇ παρ᾽ ἡμῖν χώρᾳ (427) τῇ μεταξὺ Περγάμου τε καὶ τῆς ἐπὶ θαλάττῃ πόλεως Ἐλαίας ἔστι τις λόφος θύμων μεστὸς, ἐν ᾧ κάλλιστον αἱ μέλιτται

Quinetiam in Eleonte Cherroneſi juxta illam regionem, ubi monumentum eſt Proteſilai, mel natum, quod omnia diu eadem quae Hymettion mel occupat, proceſſu temporis praeter quod craſſius efficitur, etiam ſubinde in grumum concreſcit. Itaque mel omnium optimum Antidotis injici debet Hymettion aut Thaſium aut omnino Atticum. Quod ſi penuria quandoque ſit ipſius, quod in Cycladibus inſulis naſcitur, quodque huic ſimillimum fuerit, admittendum eſt. Quin et in Iſthmo mel bonum gignitur, ac id a regione Iſthmiacum proprie nuncupatur, quemadmodum Tibenum et ipſum denominationem ſortitum Egregia nobiliaque haec ſunt. Caeterum et in aliis regionibus optimum mel provenit. Propter paucitatem autem ab incolis inſumptum, ut non poſſit ſuperfluum i aliam efferri regionem, ignoratur. Etenim in noſtro agro qui inter Pergamum et Elaeam urbem in mari ſitam habetur, collis quidam eſt thymis refertus, in quo apes laudatiſſimum mel componunt, quod inibi

συντιθέασι μέλι, δαπανώμενον αὐτόθι. κεῖται δὲ ὁ λόφος οὗτος ἀπὸ Περγάμου πορευομένῳ εἰς Ἐλαίαν ἐν τοῖς ἀριστεροῖς μέρεσιν, οὐ μὴν ἐγγὺς τῆς ὁδοῦ, καὶ κατὰ τὴν ὑπερκειμένην δὲ τῆς ἡμετέρας χώρας Μυσίαν, ἣν ὀνομάζουσι Βρῖττον, ἐθαύμασα θεασάμενος μέλι παραπλήσιον ἀκριβῶς Ἀττικῷ, καίτοι τοῦ ἄλλου μέλιτος ἀκριβῶς ἐν αὐτῷ φαυλοτάτου γενομένου. ἀλλὰ γὰρ κἀκεῖ λόφος τις ἦν οὐ μέγας, πετρώδης ὅλως, θύμων τε καὶ ὀριγάνων μεστός. ἄλλοθι δὲ κυτίσου μὲν ἦν τὸ χωρίον μεστόν. ἐγεώργει δ' ὁ δεσπότης αὐτοῦ μέλι γλυκύτατον, ὡς ὑπερβάλλειν ἐν τούτῳ τὸ Ἀττικὸν, οὐ μὴν δριμύ γε, καὶ διὰ τοῦτο ταχέως μὲν ἀποστρέφον τοὺς χρησαμένους αὐτῷ, ταχέως δὲ ναυτίαν κινοῦν, εἰ καὶ βραχὺ πλέον ληφθείη. καὶ γὰρ οὖν καὶ τοῖς γράψασι περὶ τῆς κυτίσου ταῦθ' ὁμολογεῖται πᾶσιν, ὡς πλεῖστον μέλιτος ἐκ τῶν ἀνθέων αὐτῆς αἱ μέλιτται δρέπονται. θαμνῶδες δ' ἐστὶ φυτὸν ἡ κύτισος, εἰς ὕψος ἀνῆκον ὅσον αἱ μυῤῥίναι. εἴρηται δέ μοι ταῦτα χρησιμώτατα τοῖς μὴ μόνον ἐν Ῥώμῃ κατοικοῦσιν ἰατροῖς, εἰς ἣν τὰ πάντα-

conſumitur. Jacet autem hic collis a Pergamo proficiſcenti ad Elaeam in ſiniſtra, non tamen propter viam. Ac in Myſia quae ſupra noſtrum agrum eſt, nominant Britton, demiratus ſum quum viderem mel omnino Attico perſimile, etſi illud mel longe praviſſimum in ea naſcatur. Sed enim et illic tumulus quidam erat non grandis, in totum petricoſus, thymis et origanis conſitus. Alibi locus erat Cytiſi plenus. Colebat autem dominus ejus mel dulciſſimum, ut excelleret hic Atticum, non tamen acre, atque ideo celeriter uſos eo avertit, ſubitoque nauſeam commovet, ſi etiam paulo copioſius fuerit aſſumptum. Etenim et iis qui de Cytiſo ſcripſerunt haec in confeſſo ſunt omnibus, quod bonam mellis partem ex floribus ipſius apes decerpunt. Fruticoſa autem planta eſt Cytiſus in altum excreſcens, myrtis ſimiliter. Haec ſane diximus utiliſſima iis, qui non ſolum Romam incolunt medicis, quo ex omni terra quotannis bona veniunt, ſed qui in qualibet orbis parte habitant, ut

χόθεν ἥκει καλὰ διὰ παντὸς ἔτους, ἀλλὰ καὶ τοῖς ἐν ἅπαντι μέρει τῆς οἰκουμένης, ὅπως εἰδότες τὰ γνωρίσματα τῶν ἀρίστων ἐκλέγοιντ' ἂν τῶν παρ' ἑαυτοῖς ἢ πάντως γε τῶν ἀστυγειτόνων ἢ ὁμοεθνῶν τὰ κάλλιστα. Φιλώνειον μὲν οὖν τις ἀντίδοτον ἤ τινα ἄλλην τῶν εὐτελῶν συντιθεὶς, οὐ πάνυ τι δεῖται τῶν εἰς ἄκρον ἀρίστων φαρμάκων. εἰ δὲ τὴν Μιθριδάτειον ἢ τὴν θηριακὴν ἤ τινα ἄλλην τῶν πολυμιγμάτων τε καὶ κιννάμωμον ἐχουσῶν συντιθείη, πάντων τῶν ἀρίστων δεῖται φαρμάκων. καὶ οὐκ ἂν εὐπορήσειεν ἐν ἄλλῳ χωρίῳ, καὶ διὰ τοῦτο ἐν Ῥώμῃ σκευάζουσι τὰς τοιαύτας ἀντιδότους οὐχ οἱ ἄριστοι μόνοι τῶν ἰατρῶν, ἀλλὰ καὶ οἱ μυροπῶλαι, πάντες μέντοι τῶν ἐν αὐταῖς ἁμαρτάνοντες ἔλαττον ἢ μεῖζον, ὅμως μὴ συντιθέντες ἄχρηστον φάρμακον. Ἀντωνίνου μὲν οὖν βασιλεύοντος τῶν πλουσίων ἡ θηριακὴ ἐσκευάζετο πολλοῖς, καὶ διὰ τοῦτο ἐνίοτε τῶν δυσπορίστων ἀπέλιπέ τινα· θαυμαστὸν γὰρ ὅπως οἱ πλούσιοι τὰ τῶν αὐτοκρατόρων ζηλοῦσιν, ἢ βούλονταί γε φαίνεσθαι ζηλοῦντες. ἐπεὶ δ' ἐκεῖνος ἐξ ἀνθρώπων ἀπῆλθεν,

cognitis optimorum notis, ex iis quae apud ſuos aut certe vicinos aut ejusdem gentis homines exiſtunt, optima deligant. Qui igitur Philonium Antidotum aut aliud quoddam exiguum componit, non adeo ſumme bonis medicamentis indiget. Si vero Mithridation aut Theriacen aut aliud quoddam multae miſturae et Cinnamomum recipiens conficiat, omnium praeſtantiſſimis opus medicamentis habet. Atque alio in loco eorum copia non datur, eoque Romae ejusmodi Antidota praeparant, non ſolum optimi medici, ſed etiam Myropolae, omnes utique in eis magis aut minus peccantes, non tamen inutile medicamentum componentes. Itaque Antonino imperante a divitibus plerisque Theriaca praeparabatur, atque ideo nonnunquam aliqua quae difficile poterant comparari, reliquerunt. Mirum enim quam divites principis ſtudia imitentur, aut cupiant ſaltem imitantes videri. Quum autem ille e vita exceſſit, pauciſſimi hoc Antidotum veluti

Ed. Chart. XIII. [872. 873.] Ed. Baf. II. (427.)

ὀλίγιστοι κατασκευάζουσι την ἀντίδοτον ταύτην, ὥσπερ γε καὶ τὴν Μιθριδάτειον. ὡς οὖν ἐν Ῥώμῃ τῶν ἀρίστων φαρμάκων ἁπάντων εὐπορῆσαι μᾶλλόν ἐστιν, ἢ κατ' ἄλλο χωρίον, οὕτως ἐν αὐτῇ τῇ Ῥώμῃ Καίσαρι σκευάζων τις, ἔτι μᾶλλον εὐπορεῖ πάντων τῶν εἰς ἄκρον ἀρετῆς ἡκόντων, οἴνου μὲν τοῦ Φαλερίνου καὶ μέλιτος Ὑμηττίου, ὀποβαλσάμου τε τοῦ Συριακοῦ καλουμένου. διὰ δὲ τὸν τόπον ἐν ᾧ γεννᾶται πλεῖστόν τε καὶ κάλλιστον, ἕτερον ὄνομα δεύτερον ἔχον, τὸ Ἐγγαδηνὸν γὰρ ὀνομάζεται, κρεῖττον ὂν τῶν ἐν ἄλλοις χωρίοις τῆς Παλαιστίνης γινομένων. ὅσῳ δ' ὁ οἶνος ὁ Φαλερῖνος ἀμείνων ἐστὶ τοῦ κατὰ τὰ καπηλεῖα, τοσούτῳ τοῦ κατ' Αἴγυπτον γενομένου. τῷ τοίνυν ἐπισταμένῳ γνωρίζειν ἀκριβῶς ἑκάστου τῶν φαρμάκων τὴν ἀρετὴν ἐὰν ὑπάρξῃ Καίσαρι [873] σκευάζειν ὡς ὑπῆρξεν ἐμοὶ, τὸ κάλλιστον σκευασθήσεται. κομιζομένων γὰρ τοῖς βασιλεῦσι τῶν ἀρίστων ἁπανταχόθεν, ἐξ αὐτῶν πάλιν τούτων τὸ κάλλιστον αἱρήσεται, ἔγωγέ τοι τῶν οἴνων τῶν Φαλερίνων ἑκάστου τὴν ἡλικίαν ἀναγινώσκων ἐπιγεγραμμένην τοῖς κεραμίοις,

et Mithridation praeparabant. Quemadmodum igitur Romae optimorum medicaminum omnium copia facilius quam alibi fuppeditatur, ita in ipfa Roma alicui Caefari Antidotum praeparanti multo magis adhuc omnia praeftantiffima fuppetunt, vinum fane Falernum, mel Hymettium, opobalfamum quod Syriacum appellatur; ex loco autem in quo generatur copiofiffimum optimumque aliud nomen fecundum obtinet, vocatur enim Engadenum praeftantius iis, quae in aliis Palaeftinae locis gignuntur. At quanto vinum Falernum excellentius eft eo quod in tabernis venditur, tanto etiam eo quod in Aegypto nafcitur. Quapropter fi exacte cognofcenti uniuscujusque medicamenti virtutem liceat Caefari praeparare, quemadmodum mihi licuit, optimum conficietur. Nam quum regibus praeftantiffima quaeque ex omni terra adferantur, ex his rurfus ipfis optimum eligetur. Ego vero vini Falerni uniuscujusque aetatem vafculis infcriptam relegens, guftu de-

εὐχόμην τῆς γεύσεως, ὅσοι πλειόνων ἐτῶν ἦσαν εἴκοσι, προερχόμενος ἀπ᾽ αὐτῶν ἄχρι τῶν οὐδὲν ὑπόπικρον ἐχόντων. ὁ γὰρ παλαιὸς τῶν οὐδέπω πικρότητα προσειληφότων ἄριστός ἐστιν, ὡς ἐφ᾽ ἡλικίᾳ. τοῦ δ᾽ Ὑμηττίου μέλιτος ἐν ταῖς αὐτοκρατορικαῖς ἀποθήκαις ὄντος πολλοῦ, τοῦ διετοῦς γευομένου, ἐκλέγων ἐξ αὐτοῦ πάλιν τὸ γλυκύτατον καὶ δριμύτατον. ἄμεινον γὰρ τοῦτο τοῦ προσφάτου καὶ παλαιοτέρου. ἐπεὶ δ᾽ οὐ μόνοις τοῖς βασιλικὴν ἀφθονίαν ἔχουσι τῆς τοιαύτης παρασκευῆς, ἀλλὰ καὶ τοῖς ἄλλοις ἅπασιν ἰατροῖς ὠφέλιμον εἶναι χρὴ τὴν γραφὴν, ὁ λόγος μοι γίνεται μακρότερος. αὐτίκα γέ τοι πολλὰ τῶν Ἀθήνησι πιπρασκομένων, ἔχει μόρια πολλὰ κατακεκρυμμένα μὲν ἐν τῷ βάθει, καὶ διὰ τοῦτο μὴ βλεπόμενα, δριμύτητα δὲ τῷ μέλιτι παρέχοντα, τῷ χρόνῳ δὲ ἐπιπολῆς γίνεται τὰ θύμα, καθάπερ καὶ τἄλλα ὅσα τῶν ἑτερογενῶν ἐμφέρεται τῷ μέλιτι, καὶ πολλὰ τῶν πιπρασκομένων ἐν Ῥώμῃ τοιαῦτα φαίνεται, πλὴν εἰ τρίβωνες ὄντες οἱ κομίζοντες αὐτὰ φθάσειαν ἀφελεῖν ὅσα τῶν θύμων ἐπεπόλασεν, ὡς τοὺς πολλοὺς ἐξαπατᾶσθαι γευο-

prehendi, quae plures quam viginti annos haberent, a quibus processi usque ad ea quae nihil subamari saperent. Nam vetus ex iis quae nondum amaritudinem assumpserunt, optimum est, quantum ad aetatem attinet. Hymettium autem mel quum in scriniis imperatoriis copiosum habeatur, bimulum gustans, delegi, ex eo quod esset dulcissimum et acerrimum, ut quod recenti et vetustiori sit praestantius. Quia vero non solum iis qui regiam hujus confecturae copiam habent, sed et aliis quoque omnibus medicis scripturam utilem esse convenit, sermo mihi sit prolixior. Statim namque multa quae Athenis emuntur particulas habent plerasque in imo reconditas, et propter hoc inspiciuntur, acrimoniam melli exhibentes. Tempore autem in superficie thymi erumpunt, quemadmodum etiam alia quae alterius generis melli respondent, ac multa quae Romae venduntur, talia apparent, praeterquam si exercitati qui adferunt ea exemerint, quae thymis supernatant, ut vulgares qui mel degustant, praepollenti thymorum

μένους τοῦ μέλιτος, ἐπικρατοῦσαν ἔχοντος τὴν τῶν θύμων ποιότητα. τοῦτο δ' οὐ γίνεται κατὰ τὸ μὴ δολωθέν. ἐάν ποτ' οὖν αἴσθῃ θύμου ὄζον τὸ μέλι, τὴν εἰρημένην ἄρτι πανουργίαν τεκμαίρου. τὸ γὰρ ἄριστον μέλι τὴν μὲν δριμύτητα τῶν θύμων ἐπισπᾶται, τὴν ὀσμὴν δ' οὐκ ἐκμάττεται, καθάπερ οὐδὲ τὸ τῆς γεύσεως σφοδρόν. περὶ μὲν οὖν τῆς μέλιτος ἀρετῆς αὐτάρκως εἴρηται. μέχρι γὰρ πόσου χρὴ ἕψειν αὐτὰ, ἐν τῷ τῆς σκευασίας εἰρήσεται λόγῳ. περὶ δὲ τῶν οἴνων λεκτέον ἐφεξῆς, ὅσα μικρῷ πρόσθεν ἀπελίπομεν.

Κεφ. ε'. [Ὅτι κατὰ πάσας τὰς χώρας ζητεῖν χρὴ τό τε μέλι καὶ τὸν οἶνον καὶ τὰς ἁπλᾶς δυνάμεις.] Ἐὰν γὰρ ἐν Ἀσίᾳ σκευάζων ἤ τινι τῶν ἐθνῶν τῶν ἄλλων δεηθῆς οἴνου χρησίμου τῷ φαρμάκῳ, τὴν μὲν χροιὰν ζητεῖν τὸν κιῤῥόν. οὐδεὶς γὰρ οὔτε τῶν μελάνων οὔτε τῶν λευκῶν, ἀλλ' οὐδὲ τῶν ἐρυθρῶν ἐπιτήδειος εἰς τὰς τοιαύτας ἀντιδότους ἐστὶ, τῇ συστάσει δὲ τὸν λεπτὸν, ὡς διαυγεῖσθαι, τῇ γεύσει δ', ὡς ἐπὶ τοῦ Φαλερίνου προείρηται, τὸν μηδέπω μὲν πικρὸν, οὐ μὴν ἄπεπτον ἔτι διὰ τὴν νεό-

qualitate praeditum, decipiantur. Hoc autem non accidit in eo quod dolum non fenfit. Si itaque aliquando thymum fenferis mel olfaciens, commemoratam modo fraudem conjicito. Nam optimum mel acrimoniam thymorum attrahit, odorem vero non exhaurit, ficuti nec guftus vehementiam. Etenim quatenus incoquere convenit, ubi de confectura agetur, exponemus. De mellis igitur virtute fatis eft difputatum. De vinis autem deinceps dicentur, quae paulo ante reliquimus.

Cap. V. [*Conquirenda effe quavis in regione mella, vina, fimplices medicinas.*] Nam fi in Afia aut apud alias quasdam gentes Antidotum praeparans vinum medicamento utile defideres, colore vermiculum quaerere oportet. Quippe nullum vel nigrum vel album vel rubrum ad hujusmodi Antidota eft accommodatum, verum fubftantia tenue, ut pelluceat, guftu, ficut in Falerno dictum, necdum amarefcens, non tamen crudum adhuc

τητα. γράψω δέ σοι καὶ παράδειγμα τῶν τοιούτων οἴνων ὀνομαστὶ, τῶν γε κατὰ τὴν ἡμετέραν Ἀσίαν γενομένων, καὶ πρὶν αὐξηθῆναι τὴν Ῥωμαίων δύναμιν, ἔνδοξον γεγενῆσθαι τὸν Φαλερῖνον, οἱ παλαιοὶ τῶν ἰατρῶν ἔγραψαν τὰς προσηγορίας. εἰσὶ δ' οὗτοι τρεῖς ἐν Ἀσίᾳ. γεννᾶται δὲ ὁ μὲν ἐπῃνημένος ὑπ' αὐτῶν Ἀριούσιος ἐν Χίῳ, τὴν προσηγορίαν ἀπὸ τοῦ χωρίου κτησάμενος ἐν ᾧ γίνεται. καθάπερ καὶ ὁ Λέσβιος ἀπὸ τοῦ τῆς νήσου πάσης ὀνόματος. ὁ δὲ Τμωλίτης ἀπὸ τοῦ λόφου καθ' ὃν γίνεται. Τμῶλος γὰρ αὐτῷ τοὔνομα. δῆλον δ' ὅτι τὸν ἄριστον αὐτῶν τούτων ἐκλέγεσθαί σε χρὴ κατὰ τὰ προειρημένα γνωρίσματα, καθάπερ ἐπὶ τοῦ μέλιτος εἶπον. ὄντος γὰρ ἅπαντος σχεδὸν τοῦ κατὰ τὴν Ἀττικὴν καλοῦ, τούτου πάλιν αὐτοῦ τὸ Ὑμήττιόν ἐστι κάλλιστον, εἶτ' ἐπ' αὐτῷ τὸ Θάσιον. οὕτως οὖν καὶ τῶν οἴνων πολλῶν ὄντων τῶν ἐν [874] Λέσβῳ γενομένων, ὁ κιῤῥὸς καὶ μὴ παχὺς, εὐώδης δὲ καὶ στύφων μὲν ἥκιστα, βραχυτάτην δὲ γλυκύτητα ἔχων, οὐ μὴν ἀσαφὲς τοῦτο, καλεῖται μὲν ἰδίως Λέσβιος. ἄριστος δέ ἐστιν ἐν Ἐρεσῷ

propter novitatem. Scribam autem ejusmodi vinorum nominatim tibi exemplum quae in Afia noftra proveniunt, et priusquam Romanorum potentia effet adaucta, ac Falernum inclaruiffet, veteres medici appellationes eorum literis prodiderunt. Sunt autem tria in Afia. Ariufium fane quod ab ipfis eft commendatum, nafcitur in Chio, nomenclaturam a loco ubi gignitur fortitum. Quemadmodum et Lesbium a totius infulae nomine vocatur. Tmolites a colle cui Tmolus nomen eft, ubi nafcitur. Porro conftat ex his ipfis optimum deligi fecundum praedictas notas oportere, veluti in melle dictum a me eft. Quum enim omne propemodum in Attica bonum exiftat, in hoc rurfus ipfo Hymettion eft laudatiffimum, mox Thafium, fic etiam inter multa vina quae in Lesbo nafcuntur, vermiculum, non craffum, odorum, minime aftringens, non exiguae admodum dulcedinis compos, quod nulli ignotum eft, vocatur proprie Lesbium. Excellentiffimum eft, quod tale in Erefo provenit; ab hoc deinde quod in Methymna;

γεννώμενος τοιοῦτος, εἶτα δεύτερος ὁ ἐν Μηθύμνῃ, καὶ τρίτος ὁ ἐν Μιτυλήνῃ. τὸν ἄριστον οὖν ἐν τούτοις ἐκλέξῃ, τοῖς εἰρημένοις γνωρίσμασι κρίνων. ὃς γὰρ ἂν ἐν τοῖς εὐωδεστέροις ᾖ τοῦ παραλαμβανομένου, καὶ γλυκύτερος, καὶ κατὰ τὴν σύστασιν λεπτότερος, οὗτός ἐστιν ἄριστος. τοῦ μὲν οὖν Λεσβίου τοιοῦτο τὸ εἶδός ἐστιν, ὥσπερ γε καὶ τοῦ Ἀριουσίου, βραχεῖαν διαφορὰν ἐν τῷ μᾶλλόν τε καὶ ἧττον ἐχόντων. οὐ μὴν τοῦτό γε Τμωλίτου, οὐδὲ (428) τοῦ Φαλερίνου. δύο γὰρ αὐτῶν εἴδη, γλυκὺς μὲν ὁ ἕτερος, ὁ δὲ ἕτερος ὥσπερ οὐ γλυκὺς, οὕτως οὐδ᾽ αὐστηρὸς, ἀλλ᾽ ἐν τῷ μέσῳ κατά γε ταῦτα τῶν τε αὐστηρῶν καὶ τῶν γλυκέων οἴνων. ἐμβάλοις οὖν τῇ θηριακῇ τὸν γλυκὺν, οὐχ ὡς εἰς τὴν ὅλην τοῦ φαρμάκου δύναμιν ὄντα βελτίονα προαιρούμενος, ἀλλ᾽ ἕνεκα τῆς ἐν τῷ γεύεσθαι χάριτος, ἧς χρὴ φροντίζειν ἐν τοῖς καταπινομένοις φαρμάκοις, ὅταν ἐν αὐτοῖς ἔχῃ πάμπολλα πικρὰ, καθάπερ ἡ Μιθριδάτειός τε καὶ ἡ θηριακή. καὶ τὰ ἄλλα δὲ πάντα φάρμακα διὰ πολλῆς πείρας κεκριμένα τοῖς ἰοβόλοις θηρίοις ἀντιτετάχθαι πικρὰ ταῖς ποιότησίν ἐστιν, ὡς κἀν τῷ περὶ αὐτῶν λόγῳ

tertium quod in Mitylena. Ex his optimum deliges, ſuperius enumeratis notis judicans. Quod namque inter odoratiora fuerit, eo quod aſſumitur et dulcius, et ſubſtantia tenuius, hoc eſt praeſtantiſſimum. Itaque Lesbii talis eſt ſpecies, quemadmodum et Ariuſii, quae exiguo diſcrimine ſecundum majoris minorisque rationem diſcrepant. Non tamen haec Tmolitis, neque Falerni exiſtit. Quippe duae ipſorum habentur ſpecies, alterum quidem dulce, alterum ut non dulce, ita neque auſterum, ſed in medio hic auſterorum dulciumque vinorum conſiſtit. Injicias itaque Theriacae dulce, non tanquam ad totam medicamenti virtutem melius deligens, ſed gratioris guſtus cauſa, cujus ſolicitudo in medicamentis quae deglutiuntur, eſt habenda, quum in ſe multa habeant amara, quemadmodum Mithridation et Theriace. Reliqua autem omnia medicamenta ex longo uſu virulentis beſtiis adverſari judicata qualitatibus amara ſunt, ut ſermone de ipſis

φανεῖται. Ὅμηρος δ', ὡς ἔοικεν, οἴεται καὶ τὰς ὀδύνας ἰώμενα τοιαῦτ' εἶναι πάντα. λέγει γοῦν οὕτως·

Ἐπὶ δὲ ῥίζαν βάλε πικρὴν
Χερσὶ, διατρίψας ὀδυνήφατον, ἥ οἱ ἁπάσας
Ἔσχ' ὀδύνας.

ἔμπειρον εἶναι συμβουλεύω τὸν ἰατρὸν, εἰ οἷόν τε πάντων φυτῶν. εἰ δὲ μὴ, ἀλλὰ τῶν πλείστων γε, καὶ ὧν ἡ χρεία πολλή. γένη δ' αὐτῶν, εἰ δὲ βούλει διαφορὰς ὀνομάζειν, αἵδε εἰσὶν, δένδρα καὶ θάμνοι καὶ πόαι καὶ ἄκανθαι καὶ φρύγανα. δυνάμενος γὰρ αὐτὰ γνωρίζειν ἀπ' ἀρχῆς εἰς τέλος, ἐν πολλοῖς τῆς γῆς εὑρήσεις τόποις, ὥσπερ κἀγὼ κατὰ τὴν Ἰταλίαν εὗρον ἐν πολλοῖς χωρίοις, ὅσα μήτε φυόμενα μήτε αὐξανόμενα γνωρίζουσιν οἳ τὰ ξηρανθέντα μόνα διαγινώσκουσιν. οὐδεὶς γοῦν ἐστι τῶν μυροπωλῶν, ὃς οὐκ οἶδεν τὰς ἐκ Κρήτης κομιζομένας βοτάνας, ὥσπερ καὶ τοὺς καρποὺς αὐτῶν, ἀλλ' ἐν τοῖς προαστείοις Ῥώμης ἐξ αὐτῶν οὐκ ὀλίγας φυομένας παντάπασιν ἀγνοοῦσι, καὶ διὰ τοῦτο κατὰ τὸν καιρὸν, ἐν ᾧ τοὺς καρποὺς αὐτῶν ἐκφέ-

apparebit. Homerus autem, ut videtur, omnia quae doloribus medentur talia esse autumat. Scribit itaque hunc in modum:

Radicem adjecit amaram
Contritam manibus, omnes quae auferre dolores
Apta.

Medicum igitur peritum esse consulo, si fieri potest, omnium stirpium; sin minus, at plurimarum et quarum usus multus est. Genera ipsarum, aut si malis, differentiae hae sunt, arbores, frutices, herbae, spinae, sarmenta. Nam quum ea ab initio ad finem poteris cognoscere, in multis terrae regionibus reperies, quemadmodum et ego in Italia offendi variis locis, quae neque nascentia, neque aucta noverunt, siccata tantum agnoscunt. Nullus itaque est unguentariorum, qui ignoret herbas quae ex Creta apportantur, sicuti et fructus ipsarum. Verum in suburbiis Romae earum non paucas nascentes omnino nesciunt, ac ideo quum fructus ipsarum efferunt, non inquirunt. Ego

ρουσιν, οὐκ ἐπιτηροῦσιν. ἐγὼ δ' εἶδον καὶ χαμαιπίτυν καὶ χαμαίδρυν καὶ θλάσπι καὶ κενταύριον, ὑπερικόν τε καὶ πόλιον, ἄλλα τε τοιαῦτα κατὰ τὸν καιρὸν ἐπιτηρῶν, ἀκμαῖα λαμβάνων, μήθ' ὑπερξηρανθέντα κατὰ τὸν θερινὸν ἥλιον, ἀλλὰ μηδὲ θᾶττον ἢ προσήκει ληφθέντα, τῶν καρπῶν ἀπέπτων ἔτι καὶ ἀτελῶν ὑπαρχόντων. ἡ γάρ τοι τῶν συνθέτων φαρμάκων ἀρετὴ ταῖς τῶν ἁπλῶν ἀρεταῖς ἕπεται, βραχείας τινὸς τῆς ἐν αὐτῇ τῇ σκευασίᾳ γιγνομένης διαφορᾶς, ἐφ' ἣν ἤδη μεταβήσομαι, προσγράψας τὴν συμμετρίαν τῶν μιγνυμένων ἀλλήλοις ἁπλῶν φαρμάκων. ἐπεὶ δ' ἔνιαι κακῶς εἰσι γεγραμμέναι, τινῶν μὲν ἐν τῷ τοῖς αἰτήσασι διδόναι τὰς γραφὰς ἑκοντὶ ψευδομένων, ἐνίων δὲ καὶ διαστρεφόντων ἃ παρά τινων ἔλαβον ἀντίγραφα. τὰ δὲ δὴ βιβλία τὰ κατὰ τὰς βιβλιοθήκας ἀποκείμενα, τὰ τῶν ἀριθμῶν ἔχοντα σημεῖα, ῥᾳδίως διαστρέφεται, τὸ μὲν πέντε ποιούντων ἐννέα, καθάπερ καὶ τὸ ο, τὸ δὲ ιγ, προσθέσει μιᾶς γραμμῆς, ὥσπερ γε καὶ ἀφαιρέσει μιᾶς ἑτέρας, διὰ τοῦτο ἐγὼ, καθάπερ ὁ Μενεκράτης ἔγραψε βιβλίον, ἐπι-

autem novi et chamaepityn et chamaedryn et thlafpi et centaurium hypericumque et polium, ad haec alia ejusmodi quum tempus eft inquirens, florentia capio neque reficcata aeftivo fole, fed neque citius quam convenit fumpta, dum fructus adhuc crudi imperfectique exiftunt. Nam compofitorum medicaminum virtus fimplicium vires comitatur, exigua quadam in ipfa confectione, differentia obveniente, ad quam modo digrediar, ubi fimplicium medicamentorum, quae invicem mifcentur, menfuram decentem adfcripfero. Quoniam vero nonnulla perperam funt fcripta, dum quidam ubi petentibus fcripturam exhibent, fponte mentiuntur, aliqui etiam pervertunt, quae a nonnullis acceperunt exemplaria, ifti libri qui in bibliothecis funt repofiti, numerorum notas habentes, ex facili pervertuntur, dum quinque mutantur in novem, ficut et *o*, quod eft octoginta, in *ιγ*, id eft tredecim, unius literae appofitu, quemadmodum et alterius ablatione. Quapropter ego, ficut Menecrates librum confcripfit, titulum

γράψας ὁλογράμματα αὐτοκράτορος, καθότι τὰ μὲν ζ, διὰ [875] δυοῖν γέγραπται συλλαβῶν, οὐ διὰ τοῦ ζ μόνον, τὰ δὲ κ διὰ τριῶν, οὐ διὰ τοῦ κ μόνον, τὰ δὲ τριάκοντα διὰ τεττάρων, οὐ διὰ τοῦ λ μόνον, καὶ τἄλλα ὁμοίως, οὕτω ποιήσω καὶ αὐτός. ἐπαινῶ δὲ καὶ τὸν Ἀνδρόμαχον ἐμμέτρως γράψαντα τὴν θηριακὴν αὐτὴν, ὥσπερ καὶ ἄλλοι τινές. ὁ δὲ Δαμοκράτης καὶ τἄλλα πάντα διὰ μέτρων ἔγραψεν ὀρθῶς ποιήσας. ἥκιστα γὰρ οἱ πανοῦργοι δύνανται διαστρέφειν αὐτά. καὶ πρῶτόν γέ σοι τὴν ἐκείνου γραφὴν ἔμμετρον ἐνταῦθα παραθησόμεθα.

Κεφ. στ'. [Ἀνδρομάχου πρεσβυτέρου θηριακὴ δι' ἐχιδνῶν, ἡ καλουμένη Γαλήνη.

Κλῦθι πολυθρονίου βριαρὸν σθένος ἀντιδότοιο,
Καῖσαρ, ἀδειμάντου δῶτορ ἐλευθερίης.
Κλῦθι Νέρων, ἱλαρήν μιν ἐπικλείουσι, Γαλήνην,
Εὔδιον, ἣ κυανῶν οὐκ ὄθεται λιμένων.

imponens, Hologrammatos Autocrator, quaſi dicas integris literis deſcriptis imperator, in quo ἑπτὰ, id eſt ſeptem, duabus ſyllabis ſcripta ſunt, non per ζ ſolum; viginti tribus ſyllabis, ut εἴκοσι, non per κ duntaxat exprimit; τριάκοντα, id eſt triginta quatuor ſyllabis effert, non per λ tantum, aliaque ſimiliter, ita faciam et ipſe. At laudo etiam Andromachum, qui carmine Theriacam ipſam, quemadmodum alii nonnulli, deſcripſit. Damocrates etiam alia omnia numeris incluſit, recte nimirum faciens. Minime ſiquidem fraudulenti illi poſſunt eos pervertere. Ac primum tibi illius ſcripturam verſibus comprehenſam hic apponemus.

Cap. VI. [*Andromachi ſenioris theriace ex viperis, Galena dicta.*]

Accipe quas habeat vires, clariſſime Caeſar,
Antidotus multis conſociata modis.
Accipe ſecurae Nero libertatis alumne
Magna ſalutiferae robora Theriaces.

Οὐδ' εἴ τις μήκωνος ἀπεχθέα δράγματα θλίψας,
  Χανδὸν ὑπὲρ στυγνῆς χεῖλος ἔχοι κύλικος.
Οὐδ' εἰ κωνείου πλήσοι γένυν, οὐκ ἀκονίτου,
  Μέμψατο δ' οὐ ψυχροῦ χυλὸν ὑοσκυάμου.
Οὐ θερμὴν θάψον τε καὶ ὠκύμορον πόμα Μήδης,
  Οὐδὲ μὲν αἱμηρῶν ἕλκεα κανθαρίδων.
Οὐ ζοφερῆς ἔχιός τε καὶ ἀλγεινοῖο κεράστου
  Τύμματα, καὶ ξηρῆς διψάδος οὐκ ἀλέγοι.
Σκορπίος οὐκ ἐπὶ τήνδε κορύσσεται, οὐδὲ μὲν αὐτὴ
  Ἀσπὶς, ἀδηρίτων ἰὸν ἔχουσα γόων.
Οὐ μὲν ἀπεχθόμενος καὶ δρύας ἀντιάσειε,
  Καὶ κατὰ φωλειὸν θερμὸς ἔνερθε μένοι.
Οὐκ ἀλέγοι δρύϊνα ἂν ἀναίμακτον δ' ἔχει ἰὸν
  Αἱμόῤῥους, τοιῷ δαμναμένη πόματι.
Οὐ μὲν ἀπεχθήεντα φαλάγγια σίνεται οὕτως
  Ἀνέρα, φρικαλέον δ' ἄχθος ἔθηκε πόνων,
Οὐχ ὕδρος, οὐκ ἐπὶ χέρσον, ὅθ' ὕδατα καρκίνος αἴθει
  Βοσκόμενος, θερμῆς ἤρξατο πρῶτον ἅλης,

Dicitur haec grajis Hilare, Eudios, atque Galene,
  Ad portus diros, haud medicina levis.
Nec, ſi Meconis perfrigida pocula ſucci
  Hauſeris, inſignem vim negat illa ſuam.
Nulla cicuta poteſt hanc vincere, nullum aconitum,
  Nullus frigidior ſuccus hyoſcyami.
Fervida non thapſus, letalia pharmaca Medae,
  Sanguineumque valent, ulcera cantharidum.
Vipera nigreſcens ictu, infeſtusque ceraſtes
  Arida ſeu dipſas, non ſuperare poteſt.
Scorpius adverſum hanc, itidem nil promovet aſpis,
  Quae in reliquis virus exitiale tenet.
Improbus ille dryas, contra hanc occurrere pugna
  Non audet, latebris ſed manet uſque ſuis.
Dryinos, necnon haemorrhun, ſanguinis expers
  Qui virus fundit, haec medicina domat.
Non hoc offendunt inimica phalangia potu,
  Quae horrifico vexant ſumpta dolore virum.

Χέρσυδρος, θανάτῳ πεπαλαγμένα χείλεα σύρων,
Ἀντόμενος, γλυκεροῦ τέρμα φέροι βιότου.
Τῇ πίσυνος λειμῶσι θέρους ἐπιτέρπεο Καῖσαρ,
Καὶ Λιβυκὴν στείχων οὐκ ἀλέγοις ψάμαθον.
Οὐδὲ μὲν ἀμφίσβαινα φέρει μόρον, οὐδέ τις ἤδη
Φρῦνος ἐνὶ ξηροῖς βοσκόμενος πεδίοις.
Ῥεῖα δὲ καὶ στομάχοιο φέροις ἄκος οἰδήναντος,
Καὶ θοὸν ἰήσαις ἆσθμα κυλινδόμενον.
Ἢ ὁπόταν περὶ γαστρὶ κυκώμενον ἔνδοθι πνεῦμα
Κυμαίνῃ, κωφὸν κῦμα βιαζόμενον.
Ἢ ὅτ' ἐνὶ στροφάλιγγι ἀπηνέϊ κυμήνειεν
Ἔντερον, ἢ ταναοῦ σφυγμὸν ἔχωσι κόλου,
Ἢ ὁπόταν χολόεντες ὅλον δέμας, ἔξοχα δ' ὄσσε,
Καὶ μερόπων χροιὴν πάμπαν ἀνηνάμενοι,
Ἴκτερον ἱλάσκωνται ἀπηνέα, μηδ' ἐπὶ θοίνας,
Εἰ καί σφιν μακρὸν Ζεὺς πετάσειε πέρας
Νεύοιεν, μοῦνον δὲ κατηφέα θυμὸν ἔχοντες,
Φεύγωσι σφετέρων ἤθεα κηδομένοιν.

Non hydrus, aut Epicherſus, aquis aut cancer oberrans,
Sub calido primum ſidere obeſſe poteſt.
Nulla tibi Amphisbaena nocet, ſiccosque ſubintrans
Campos, exitium nulla rubeta feret.
Huic fidens Caeſar, prato oblectare per aeſtum
Nec Libyae curae fiet harena tibi.
Quin ſtomachum curat medicamen, cum aeſtuat aegrum
Aſſidue vexans, inſuper aſthma velox.
Non oberit labiis cherſydrus peſtifer atris,
Qui occurrens, animam non ſinit eſſe diu.
Vel quum ventriculus turbatur flatibus, undam ut
Interius ſurdam concitet ipſe chyli.
Vel quum difficili vertuntur tormine venti
Inteſtina, colon pulſus ubi exagitat.
Vel quum jam totos confuſo felle per artus
Ut proprius nequeat eſſe colos oculis,
Regius infeſtat morbus, non ulla ciborum
Cura adſit (quamvis Juppiter annuerit

Εἰ δέ που ἢ κακόεργον ἴδοις ἐπὶ σώμασιν ὦχρον,
'Ρύσαις ὑδρηλὴν νοῦσον ἐπεσσυμένην,
Καὶ φαέων ἀμβλεῖαν ἄφαρ λάμψειεν ὀπωπὴν
Τῷ, καὶ ἀρχομένης οὐκ ἀλέγοις φθίσιος.
Οἴη καὶ τετάνοιο καὶ ἀρχομένοιο τενόντων
Σπάσματος ἦρε βυθοῦ ἄχθος ὀπισθοτόνου,
Ἦτ' ἄρα καὶ θώρακος, ὅσην ὠτρύνατο χώρην,
Λοξὸς ἀναθλίβων πνεύμονα κοῦφον ὑμήν.
Ἢ ὅτε φρικαλέην τις ἔχοι περὶ κύστιν ἀνίην
Ἕλκεος, ἢ καί που δαμναμένοιο πόρου
Οὖρον ἐπιφράσσοιτο, ὅτ' ἔσχετο πολλάκι καυλὸς
[876] 'Ορμὴν, ἢ κενεὴν σεύμενος ἐς Κυθέρην.
Νεφρῶν δ' ἡνίκα φῶτα κατ' ἰξύος ἄλγος ἐπείγοι,
Θαῤῥῶν τοιαύτην ἐξελάσεις ὀδύνην,
Καὶ μογερῶν στέρνων ἀπολύσεται ἔμπυον ἰλὺν,
Πινομένη πολλοὺς μέχρις ἐπ' ἠελίους.
'Αλθαίνει, καὶ λοιμὸν ἀηδέα, πᾶσαν ἐπ' ἠῶ
Δύσπνοον, ἐκ τοίης παρθέμενος πόσιος,

*Tempora longa) animo ſed triſtes, limina vitent
Ejus qui medicam polliceatur opem.
Si vidcas pallore malo candentia membra,
Tollet hydropa ſuis viribus Antidotum.
Et fuſcata ſtatim luſtrabit lumina, rebus
His quoque ſi incipiat, non vereare phthiſin.
Sola etiam tetanum, tendonum ſpaſma, profundi
Theriace haec adimet pondus opiſthotoni.
Vel quum ſuccingens coſtas membrana laborat,
Pulmones reprimens deſuper ipſa leves,
Vel quando horrificos patitur veſica labores
Ulceris, illius praedomitusque porus
Impedit urinam, coles et reddere eandem
Appetit, et crebro proruit in Venerem.
Quum renum ſaevit crucians injuria lumbos,
Hoc poterit potu triſtis abire dolor.
Pectoris et labem ſanioſam pellitat aegri
Multos uſque dies potus hic antidoti,*

(429) *Καὶ κυνὸς ὑδροφόβην γενύων λυσσῶσαν ἐριννὺν
Φεύξεται εὐόδμῳ γαῦρος ἐπ' ἀντιδότῳ.
Τῆς δή τοι κυάμοιο, τὸν ἔτρεφεν εὔσκιον ὕδωρ,
Τέλμασι, καὶ πολλοῖς κρυπτόμενον πετάλοις
Νειλώου κυάμοιο, διὰ βάρος ἄμμιγα χεύας,
Θερμὸν ὕδωρ τρισσῶν κιρνάμενος κυάθων.
Πίνοιεν δ' ὅτε κοῖτον ἄγοι κνέφας, ἄλλοτε δ' ἠοῦς,
Ἄλλοτε καὶ διπλῆν ἐς πόσιν ὀρνύμενοι.
Ἠοῦς μὲν κεράσαιο παρηγορέων κακοῦ ὁρμὴν,
Ὅσσοις ἀλγεινὸς λάμπεται ἠέλιος.
Νυκτὶ δ' ὁμῶς ὅσσοις περ ἐπώδυνος ἕσπεται ὄρφνη,
Εὐνάστειραν ἔχοις τειρομένων πρόποσιν.
Ἰοβόλων δ' εἴ καί τις ὑπὸ γναμπτῆρι δαμείη,
Ἢ μογερὸν κυανοῦ πῶμα λάβοι θανάτου,
Ἴσην δ' ἐντύναιο κατ' ὀρφναίην τε καὶ ἠῶ,
Δαμναμένοις ἱλαρὴν παρθέμενος κύλικα.
Καί κεν ἀεὶ πνείοντας ἄγοις ἐπὶ κοῖτον ἑτοίμως
Γηθαλέους ταύτῃ Καῖσαρ ἀνωδυνίῃ.*

*Peſtiferamque luem curat, quae tempus in omne
Spiratu gravis eſt, intima conficiens.
Atque canis rabidi virus quod morſibus indit
Laetus odorata fugeris antidoto
Hinc tu ſume fabae pondus, quam lympha creavit
Ex umbra, coeno et tecta ſimul foliis
Nempe fabae Nili, gravitatis nomine, ternis
Antidoto calidam conſocians cyathis.
Sumito quando capis ſomnum, vel luce reverſa,
Uno vel pariter pocula bina die.
Luce bibent ipſam, quibus eſt ſol triſtis, ut inde
Lenimenta mali quod furit, accipiant.
Nocte quibus tenebrae gratae minus, ordine verſo,
Ante thorum pulchre ſumpta medela facit.
Exitiale animans quos laeſit vulnere diro
Aut cui letalis potio capta fuit,
Apponens Hilares affectis pocula, eodem
Noctu et luce ſimul fac medeare modo.*

Πρῶτα μὲν ἀγρεύσαιτο κακήθεας ἐμπέραμος φὼς,
Τολμηρῇ μάρπτων χειρὶ θοοὺς ὄφιας.
Τοὺς ἤδη κρυεροῦ ἀπὸ χείματος, οὐκέτι γαίης
Κρύπτουσι στεινοὶ πάμπαν ἔνερθε μυχοὶ,
Εἰαρινὴν ἐφ᾽ ἅλωα, χυτὸν βόσκονται ἂν ἄλσος
Διζόμενοι χλωροῦ σπέρμα λαβεῖν μαράθρου.
Ὀξυτέρην τὸ τίθησιν ἐφ᾽ ἑρπυστῆρσιν ὀπωπὴν,
Πιαῖνον δειλοῖς ἄλγεα βουπελάταις.
Τῶν δ᾽ αὐτῶν οὐράς τε καὶ ἰοβόλους ἀπὸ κόρσας
Τάμνοις, καὶ κενεὰς γαστέρας ἐξερύοις.
Οὖλα γὰρ ἀμφοτέρῳ φερέει ἐπὶ τύμμασι ἄχθη,
Λυγρὸν ὑπ᾽ οὐραίην ἰὸν ἔχων φολίδα.
Τοὔνεκα οἱ τμήσαιο κατ᾽ αὐχένα, ἠδὲ κατ᾽ ἄκρα,
Ὅσσον πυγμαίης χειρὸς ἔνερθε βάθος.
Λοίγια δὲ σταλάουσι σὺν αἵματι, τῶν ἀπὸ πέζαν
Ἐκτὸς ἔχων, ἱλαρὴν δέρξεται ἀντολίην.
Ὁππότε δὴ τὰ γένοιτο, τότ᾽ ἐν κεραμηΐδι χύτρῃ
Κατθέμενος πυρσοῦ σάρκας ἐπιφλεγέτω,

Quin et perpetuo ſpiranti nocte quietem
Praebebis, Caeſar, hoc placidam antidoto.
Principio expertus vir in arte venabitur angues
Audaci, miros celeritate, manu.
Hos quum triſtis hyems abiit non amplius arctas
In terra latebras cernis habere ſuas.
Miſſis jam latebris ſubeunt nemora ampla virentis
Quaeſitum marathri ſemina grata oculis.
Haec viſum refovent ſcrpentibus, atque bubulcos
Quos metus exercet, ſaepe dolore levant.
His ipſis caudas et colla referta veneno
Praecides, vacuos ventriculosque adimes.
Quippe venenatos utraque ex parte dolores
Mittunt, nam caudis hi quoque virus habent.
Ergo ſecas ipſis cervicem, atque extima, quantum
Intus pygmaei tenditur arcta manus.
Namque cadit virus pariter cum ſanguine; motis
Extremis, Hilarem feceris Italicam.

Ὕδατι ἐγχεύσας ὅσσον ἄρκιον, καὶ ἀνήθου
Κλῶνας ἐχιδναίῃ σαρκὶ συνεψομένας.
Ἡνίκα δὲ σκολιαί γε ἀποῤῥείωσιν ἄκανθαι,
Καὶ κακὸν οἰδήνῃ νῶτον ὕπερθεν ἔχις
Ἐκτὸς ἕλοι, ζείοντα καταψύχων κυκεῶνα,
Ὄφρ' ἑκὰς ἐντύναις σάρκας ἀπεχθομένας
Ἑρπυστῶν τ' ἰόεντας ἀποῤῥίψειεν ἀκάνθας
Πάμπαν ὑπ' εὐδίφρου χειρὸς ἐλεγχομένας.
Αὐαλέου δ' ἐπὶ ταῖσι βάλοις εὐεργέος ἄρτου,
Ὅσσον τερσύναι σάρκα, δύναιτο τροχοὺς
Πλάσσασθαι δ' ὅτε μίγδα κύτει περιαγέος ὅλμου
Θλασθείη, σκιεροῦ κάτθες ὑπὲρ δαπέδου.
Αὐτίκα δὲ σκίλλην τριχώδεσιν ἄμμιγα φλοιοῖς,
Σταιτὶ περιπλάσας, θάλπε κατὰ φλογιῆς
Ὄφρα κεν ὀπταλέην τε καὶ οὐ σκληρὴν περὶ κόρσην
Ἐντείναις σποδιῆς ἠρέμα δαιομένης,
Καί ῥ' ὅτε θαλπομένη ῥῆξαι σέλας ἔκτοθι πυρσοῦ
Κάτθεο, καὶ τρισσὴν σαρκὸς ἔχεις μερίδα,

His tibi ſic factis, carnes in fictile mittens,
Una compoſitas igne parabis acri.
Lymphae quod ſatis eſt infundes, germen anethi
Cum angu na junctum carne coquens pariter.
Aſt ubi ſpina cadit coctu de carne recurva,
Deſuper atque ferae noxia terga tument,
Exime, quo fervens frigeſcat miſtio flammis,
Infeſtas carnes dimoveasque procul,
Abſtrahe ſerpentum ſpinas, virus redolentes,
Quas perſentiſcet non male docta manus.
Carnibus adjicias panis ſicci et bene piſti
Quantum paſtillos fingere ſufficiat.
Verum ubi jam iſta pilae fundo contuſa rotundae
Cuncta, ſuper nigrum tu modo funde ſolum.
Protinus hic etiam cum cortice ſquilla piloſo
Illita cui circum maſſa ſit, incaleat,
Dum ſic aſſetur, nec fiat durior inde
Cortice, nam ardeſcet leniter ille cinis;

Ὄλμοις, καὶ στρυφνοῖο βάλοις δυοῖν ὀρόβοιο,
Ἐν δ' ὑπέρῳ μίξας συνδονέων μυχόθεν
Αἴνυσο, καὶ δινήεντας ἀνάπλασσε τροχίσκους,
Τοὺς δ' ἑκὰς ἠελίου ψύχεο τερσομένους.
Τῶν δ' ἤτοι δραχμὰς μὲν ὑπὸ πλάστιγγος ἀφέλκοις
Δοιὰς, τὴν πέμπτην παρθέμενος δεκάδα,
Ἥμισυ θηρείοιο βαλὼν τροχοειδέος ἄρτου,
Καὶ δολιχὸν σταθμῷ τόσσον ἔχοι πέπερι.
[877] Ἶσα δ' ὀποῦ μήκωνος ἔχοι, καὶ μάγματος αὔτως,
Μάγματος ἡδυχρόου τόσσον ἐφελκομένου.
Δώδεκα δὲ ξηροῖο ῥόδου δραχμαῖσιν ἰσάζοις
Φύλλα, καὶ Ἰλλυρίην ἶριδα κατθέμενος,
Κυανέης μίξαιο μελιπτόρθου γλυκυρίζης
Τόσσον, καὶ γλυκερῆς σπέρματα βουνιάδος.
Σκόρδιον καὶ κεῖνον ὀπὸν μίσγοιο θυώδη,
Βαλσάμου Ἀσσυρίης ἔνδοθεν αἰνύμενος.
Τοῖς δ' ἐπὶ κιννάμωμον ἰσάζεο, μηδέ σε λήθη
Ἀγαρικὸν τούτοις ἰσοβαρὲς θέμεναι,

At poſtquam calefacta nimis diſrumpitur, ipſam
Deponis, carnis portio tripla manet.
Atque ervum gyro duplici demittis acerbum.
Piſtilloque moves, quod teris, inferius,
Aufers, et riguos paſtillos inde figuras,
Quos, ut ſiccefcant, ſole repone procul.
Fac decadas utriusque duas et quattuor aeque,
Paſtilli drachmas pondere connumeres.
Tot piperis calidi, meconis, magmatis adde,
Magmatis hedychroi par modus injicitur.
Inde quater ternas mutato pondere drachmas
Iridis, et ſiccae protinus adde roſae.
Addaturque tui radix dulciſſima ſucci,
Et dulcis tantum ſeminis inde napi.
Scordion jungas et odoribus inclyta ſemper
Balſama, qui Syrio mittitur orbe liquor.
Tum quae ſuſpendas aequata cinnama lance
Conjice, et agarici par quoque pondus eat.

Ἢ ἔτι καὶ σμύρνης καὶ εὐόδμου κόστοιο
Καὶ κρόκου, ὃν ἄντρον θρέψατο Κωρύκιον,
Καὶ κασίην, Ἰνδήν τε βάλοις εὐώδεα νάρδον,
Καὶ σχοῖνον νομάδων θαῦμα φέροις Ἀράβων,
Καὶ λίβανον μίσγοιο, καὶ ἀγλαΐην στήσαιο
Ἄμμιγα κυανέῳ κατθέμενος πεπέρει,
Δικτάμνου τε κλῶνας, ἠδὲ χλοεροῦ πρασίοιο,
Καὶ ῥῆον. στοιχὰς δ' οὐκ ἀπάνευθε μένοι,
Οὐδέ νυ πετροσέλινον. ἠδ' εὐώδης καλαμίνθη,
Δριμύ τε τερμίνθου δάκρυ λιβυστιάδος,
Ζιγγίβερι θερμὸν, κ' εὔκλωνον πενταπέτηλον,
Τὰς δοιὰς δραχμῶν πάντα φέροι τριάδας
Αὐτίκα, καὶ πολίου πίσυρας ὁλκὰς βαρυέσσας.
Ἠδὲ χαμαιζήλου πτόρθους ἄγοις πίτυος,
Καὶ στύρακος, μήου τε καὶ βοτρυόεντος ἀμώμου,
Καὶ νάρδου, Γαλάτης ἣν ἐκόμισσεν ἀνὴρ,
Λημνιάδος μίλτοιο, καὶ ἐκ Πόντοιο βάλοιο
Φοῦ, καὶ Κρηταίης σπέρμα χαμαιδρυάδος,

Hinc ſupereſt myrrham, coſtumque, ſpecuque revulſum
Corycio fragrans impoſuiſſe crocum.
Et caſiae calamos, et quam tulit India nardum,
Teque Arabi ſchoenum gloria prima ſoli.
Inde nigrum conjunge piper, thurisque nitorem,
Divite quod felix rure Sabaeus alit,
Nec tu dictamnum, nec tu quoque pontica rheon
Deſueris, ſtoechas, marrubiumque virens,
Atque apium petris quod naſceris, et calaminthe,
Afraque cum lachrimis o terebinthe tuis.
Et foliis gramen quinis, et Zingiber ardens,
Singula ſed drachmas ſex tibi quaeque trahant.
His etiam polium drachmis ſe quatuor addet,
Addet ſe polio proxima pinus humi.
Cumque racemifero Celtarum nardus amomo,
Et ſtyracis lentor, fervidaque herba meon.
Atque humilis quercus ſemen, Pontoque petita
Phu, quibus accedet Lemnia terra comes.

Μαλαβάθρου καλὰ φύλλα, καὶ ὀπταλέην χαλκῖτιν,
  Μίσγεσθαι ῥίζης οὐ δίχα γεντιάδος
Ἄνισον, χυλόν θ' ὑποκιστίδος, ἠδέ νυ καρπὸν
  Βαλσάμου, λιπαρὸν κόμμι διηνάμενος,
Καὶ μαράθρου σπέρμα, καὶ Ἰδαῖον καρδάμωμον,
  Καὶ ψαφαρὸν στήσεις παρθέμενος σέσελι.
Δάκρυον εὖ μίσγοιο βαλὼν κυανωπὸν ἀκάνθης,
  Θλάσπι σὺν τούτοις ἰσοβαρὲς τελέθοι.
Τόσσον δ' ὑπερικοῦ, τόσσον δ' ἐπιμίσγεται ἄμμι,
  Καὶ σαγαπηνὸν ἄγοις τετράδα τοσσατίην,
Δοιὰς δ' εἰσάξεις, τά περ Ἴστριος ἔκβαλε κάστωρ
  Μήδεα, καὶ λεπτὴν ῥίζαν ἀριστολόχου,
Δαύκου τε σπέρμα, καὶ αὐαλέην ἄσφαλτον
  Ἰοβόλων κοίταις ἀντία δαιομένην.
Ἶσα δ' ὀποῦ πάνακος συμμίσγεο κενταυρίῳ,
  Χαλβανίδος λιπαρῆς ἰσόμορον θέμενος.
Καὶ τὰ μὲν ἐν θυίῃ πολλῷ μαλθάσσεο οἴνῳ,
  Ὅσσα περ ὑγροτέροις δάκρυσιν ἐμφέρεται.

Nec non malabathri folium, miſcebis et aſſam
  Chalcitim, fibras gentiadasque ſimul.
Inde tenax gummi, preſſaque hypociſtide ſuccus
  Adſit, et hinc fructus balſame parva tui.
His etiam aniſum, ſeſelimque his jungere molem,
  His cardamomum, foeniculumque velis.
Atque atram lachrimam, Nili quam ſpina remittit,
  Quaeque ſuo thlaſpis ſemine nomen habet.
Hypericon rurſum, pallens miſcebis et ammin,
  Nec drachmis totidem plus ſagapenus eat.
Pondere dimidio tum quos ſibi Caſtor ad Iſtrum
  Ore ſecat teſtes, impoſuiſſe decet.
Quis nec Ariſtolochi radix, ſiccumque bitumen,
  Candida nec deſint ſemina dauce tua.
Denique cum panacis ſuccum, centaurion atque
  Addideris, finem galbanus ipſa dabit.
Antiquo primum ſolves tamen omnia vino,
  Humida quae fuerint, ut liquor et lachrimae.

Κόψαι δ' εὖ λεπτῶς, τὰ δέ κεν ξυλοειδέα πάντα
 Ἀκταίῳ μίσγοις συγκεράσας μέλιτι.
Ἱλήκοις ὃς τήνδε μάκαρ τεκτήναο Παίων,
 Εἴτε σὲ Τρικκαῖοι δαῖμον ἔχουσι λόφοι,
Ἢ Ῥόδος ἢ Βουρίννα καὶ ἀγχιάλη Ἐπίδαυρος.
 Ἱλήκοις, ἱλαρὴν δ' αἰὲν ἄνακτι δίδου
Παῖδα τεὴν Πανάκειαν. ὃ δ' εὐαγέεσσι θυηλαῖς
 Ἱλάσεται τὴν σὴν αἰὲν ἀνωδυνίην.

Κεφ. ζ'. [Ἀνδρομάχου νέου θηριακὴ δι' ἐχιδνῶν, ἡ καλουμένη Γαλήνη.] (430) Ταῦτα μὲν ὁ πρεσβύτερος Ἀνδρόμαχος ἔγραψεν· ὁ δὲ υἱὸς αὐτοῦ κατὰ τὴν φαρμακῖτιν βίβλον, ἣν τῶν ἐντὸς ἐπιγράφει, ταύτην ἐποιήσατο τὴν γραφὴν, λέξει πεζῇ χρησάμενος. ἀντίδοτος ἡ καλουμένη Γαλήνη, πρὸς πᾶν πάθος ἐντοσθίδιον, μάλιστα πρὸς τὰ τοῦ στομάχου πάθη καὶ πρὸς τὰ θανάσιμα καὶ περιόδους. ℞ Ἀρτίσκων σκιλλητικῶν < μη'. ἀρτίσκων θηριακῶν < κδ'. μάγματος ἡδυχρόου, πεπέρεως μέλανος, ἀνὰ < κδ'. ὀπίου < κδ'. ῥόδων ξηρῶν, σκορδίου Κρητικοῦ, βουνιά-

Tum quae ſicca vides, poſtquam contuſa minutim,
 Cecropio pariter jungere melle velis.
Haec qui nos primus docuiſti maxime Paean
 Adſis, ſeu Triccae te juga ſumma juvant,
Seu Burrina magis, Rhodos, aut Epidauria tellus,
 Adſis, et Regi fer tua dona meo,
Stirpe tua natam Panaceam, namque ſalutem
 Ille datam puro ſemper honore colet.

Cap. VII. [*Andromachi junioris theriaca ex viperis, Galene dicta.*] Haec quidem ſenior Andromachus literis mandavit, filius autem ipſius libro medicamentario quem de internis inſcripſit, hanc ſcripturam tradidit pedeſtri uſus oratione: *Antidotum quod vocatur Galene, ad omnem affectum interiorem, praeſertim ad ſtomachi vitia, et adverſus letalia et morborum circuitus.* ℞ Paſtillorum ſcilliticorum ʒ xlviij. paſtillorum Theriacorum drach. xxiv. magmatis hedychroi, piperis nigri, ſingulorum drach. xxiv. opii drach. xxiv. roſarum ſiccarum, ſcordii Cre-

δυς σπέρματος, ἴρεως Ἰλλυρικῆς, [878] ἀγαρικοῦ ποντικοῦ, κινναμώμου, γλυκυῤῥίζης χυλοῦ, ὀποβαλσάμου ἀνὰ < ιβ'. σμύρνης, κρόκου, ζιγγιβέρεως, ῥήου Ποντικοῦ, πενταφύλλου ῥίζης, νεπέτου, οὕτως οἱ Ῥωμαῖοι τὴν καλαμίνθην ὀνομάζουσι, πρασίου, πετροσελίνου, στοιχάδος, κόστου, πεπέρεως λευκοῦ, καὶ μακροῦ. δικτάμνου Κρητικοῦ, σχοίνου ἄνθους, λιβάνου, τερμινθίνης, κασσίας σύριγγος, νάρδου Ἰνδικῆς, ἀνὰ < στ'. πολίου Κρητικοῦ, σεσέλεως, στύρακος, θλάσπεως, ἄμμεως, χαμαίδρυος, χαμαιπίτυος, ὑποκιστίδος, χυλοῦ μαλαβάθρου, νάρδου Κελτικῆς, γεντιανῆς ῥίζης, ἀνίσου, μείου ἀθαμαντικοῦ, μαράθρου σπέρματος, Λημνίας μίλτου, χαλκίτεως ὀπτῆς, ἀμώμου, ἀκόρου, φοῦ Ποντικοῦ, βαλσάμου καρποῦ, ὑπερικοῦ, ἀκακίας, κόμμεως, καρδαμώμου, ἑκάστου < δ'. δαύκου σπέρματος, χαλβάνης, σαγαπηνοῦ, ὀποπάνακος, ἀσφάλτου, καστορίου, κενταυρίου λεπτοῦ, ἀριστολοχίας λεπτῆς, ἑκάστου < β'. μέλιτος Ἀττικοῦ < ρν'. τοῦ δὲ ὀρόβου < π'. ταῦτα γράψαντος Ἀνδρομάχου τοῦ νεωτέρου πεζῇ, πάρεστι τῷ μὴ νοοῦντι τῶν

tenſis, napi ſeminis, iridis Illyricae, agarici pontici, cinnamomi, dulcis radiculae ſucci, opobalſami, ſingulorum ʒ xij myrrhae, croci, gingiberis, Rheu pontici, quinquefolii radicis, nepitae (ſic Romani calamintham nominant) marrubii, petroſelini, ſtoechados, coſti, piperis albi, et longi, dictamni Cretenſis, junci odorati floris, thuris, terebinthinae, caſſiae fiſtulae, nardi Indicae, ſingulorum ʒ vj. polii Cretenſis, ſeſelis, ſtyracis, thlaſpi, ameos, chamaedryos, chamaepityos, hypociſtidis, ſucci malabathri, nardi Celticae, gentianae radicis, aniſi, mei athamantini, foeniculi ſeminis, terrae lemniae, chalcitidis toſtae, amomi, acori, phu pontici, balſami fructus, hyperici, acaciae, gummi, cardamomi, ſingulorum ʒ iv. dauci ſeminis, galbani, ſagapeni, opopanacis, bituminis, caſtorei, centaurii tenuis, ariſtolochiae tenuis, ſingulorum drach. ij. mellis Attici drach. cl. ervi drach. lxxx. Ex hac pedeſtri Andromachi junioris ſcriptura licet in-

εἰρημένων ὁτιοῦν ἐν τοῖς ἐλεγείοις τοῦ πρεσβυτέρου, τὴν εὕρεσιν ἐντεῦθεν ποιεῖσθαι. διὸ κἀγὼ τῶν δοκούντων ἀσαφέστερον ἐν αὐτῷ λελέχθαι τὴν ἐξήγησιν οὐ προσέθηκα τὸ μῆκος τῆς γραφῆς εὐλαβούμενος. ἐθαύμασα δὲ ἓν μόνον τοῦ νεωτέρου Ἀνδρομάχου; γράψαντος ἐν τῷ καταλόγῳ τῶν ἁπλῶν φαρμάκων, ἐξ ὧν συντίθησι τὴν ἀντίδοτον ἀντὶ καλαμίνθης τὸν νέπετον, Ῥωμαῖοι γὰρ οὕτω ὀνομάζουσι τὴν καλαμίνθην. οὐκ ἐχρῆν δ' αὐτὸν ἑλληνιστὶ πάντα γράψαντα, τοῦτο μόνον ἐνθεῖναι Ῥωμαϊκὸν ὄνομα τοῖς Ἑλληνικοῖς. ἐν ἑνὶ μέντοι διαφωνεῖ πρὸς τὴν ἔμμετρον γραφὴν τῷ τὴν ἔμμετρον < κδ'. ἔχειν τοῦ μακροῦ πεπέρεως, τὴν δὲ πεζῇ γεγραμμένην στ'. ἐπεὶ δ', ὡς ἔφην, πολλὰ τῶν ἀντιγράφων ἡμαρτημένας ἔχει τὰς ποσότητας τῶν φαρμάκων, διὰ τοῦτο α'. μὲν ὁλογραμμάτως αὐτὰς ἔγραψα, μιμησάμενος τὸν Μενεκράτην· δεύτερον δὲ ἐπὶ τῷδε καὶ διὰ τῶν ἐμμέτρως γεγραμμένων. ἀσαφέστερον δὲ συγκειμένων τῶν τοῦ Ἀνδρομάχου ἐλεγείων ἄμεινον ἔδοξέ μοι τὰ Δαμοκράτους προσθεῖναι πάνυ σαφῶς ἡρμηνευμένα.

telligere, fi quis quodcunque in elegiis fenioris dictum non affequatur; quare et ego eorum quae obfcurius ab eo dicta videbantur interpretationem non appofui, prolixitatem fcripturae devitans. Unum vero duntaxat miratus fum in juniore Andromacho, quod in fimplicium medicamentorum unde antidotum componit enumeratione, nepitam pro calamintha fcripferit. Romani enim calaminthам fic appellant; non conveniebat autem ipfum, quum omnia Graece tradidiffet, hoc folum Romanum nomen Graecis inferere. Caeterum in uno inter fe difcrepant, quoniam metrica fcriptura viginti quatuor drachmas longi piperis obtinet, pedeftris autem fex. Quia vero, ut dixi, multa exemplaria vitiatas medicamentorum quantitates habent, ideo primum quidem integris literis ipfas confcripfi, Menecratem imitatus, deinde autem poft hoc etiam numeris expreffas appofui. Porro cum Andromachi elegiaca obfcurius fint compofita, melius exiftimavi Damocratis verfus admodum manifefto interpretatos ap-

ἀλλὰ τοῦτο μὲν ὀλίγον ὕστερον ἔσται. νυνὶ δὲ ἐπειδὴ τῶν ἐμβαλλομένων εἰς τὴν ἀντίδοτον φαρμάκων ἁπλῶν εἴρηταί μοι πολλὰ, προσθεῖναι βέλτιον αὐτοῖς τὰ λείποντα.

Κεφ. η'. [Ἀρτίσκων θηριακῶν σκευασία.] Τὰς ἐχίδνας οὐχ ὥσπερ ἔνιοι μέσου θέρους, οὐ μὴν οὐδ' ἄρτι τῆς φωλεᾶς παυσαμένας θηρεύειν προσῆκεν. ἐν μὲν γὰρ τῷ θέρει διψώδης ἡ σὰρξ αὐτῶν ἐστιν, ἐπὶ δὲ τῇ φωλεᾷ ξηρὰ καὶ ψυχρὰ καὶ ἄτροφος. κάλλιστος οὖν ἐστι καιρὸς ὁ μεταξὺ τούτων, ὃν καὶ αὐτὸς ὁ Ἀνδρόμαχος ἐδήλωσεν, ἡνίκα καὶ οἱ τῷ Διονύσῳ βακχεύοντες εἰώθασι διασπᾷν τὰς ἐχίδνας, παυομένου μὲν τοῦ ἦρος, οὔπω δ' ἠργμένου θέρους, ἢ εἰ χειμέριον ἐπὶ πολὺ τὸ ἔαρ γίγνοιτο, κατὰ τὴν ἀρχὴν τοῦ θέρους, οὐ κατὰ πολὺ τῆς τῶν πλειάδων ἐπιτολῆς. ὅσαι δὲ ἐγκύμονές εἰσι τῶν ἐχιδνῶν, παραιτεῖσθαι ταύτας. ἀποτέμνειν δὲ τάς τε κεφαλὰς καὶ τὰς οὐρὰς αὐτῶν. πρὸς γὰρ τῷ δοκεῖν ἰωδέστερα ταῦτ' εἶναι τὰ μόρια καὶ τὸ σκληροῖς, καὶ ὀλιγοσάρκοις ὑπάρχειν αὐτοῖς πρόσεστιν. αὔταρκες δ' ἐπὶ τῶν μεγάλων ἐχιδ-

ponere. Sed hoc quidem paulo poſterius aggrediar, nunc quoniam multa ex ſimplicibus medicamentis quae Antidoto immittuntur expoſui, praeſtat ea quae ipſis deſunt adjicere.

Cap. VIII. [*Quomodo paſtilli theriaci praeparentur.*] Viperas non quemadmodum nonnulli media aeſtate, neque tamen quum nuper ſeceſſum terrae reliquerint, venari convenit. Etenim aeſtate caro ipſarum eſt ſitis efficax; ſeceſſus tempore ſicca, frigida, et alimenti expers. Optimum itaque tempus eſt quod haec intercedit, ut etiam Andromachus ipſe indicavit, quum qui Baccho feſta celebrant viperas ſolent diſcerpere, deſinente quidem vere, nondum autem inchoata aeſtate, vel ſi ver admodum hyemale extiterit, aeſtatis initio non longe a Pleiadum ortu. Porro foetas viperas repudiare oportet. Caeterum capita et caudas ipſis praecidere. Nam praeterquam quod hae particulae virulentiores eſſe videantur,

νῶν τὸ ἀφαιρεθησόμενον ἑκατέρωθεν, εἶναι δακτύλων δ΄. ὅλον δὲ τὸ λοιπὸν σῶμα, τῶν μὲν ἐντέρων ἐξαιρεθέντων, ἀποδαρέντος δὲ τοῦ δέρματος, ὕδατι περιπλύναντα, ἐμβάλλειν κακάβῃ προσήκει καθαρὸν ὕδωρ, καὶ ἄνηθον χλωρὸν, ἀκμάζει γὰρ τηνικαῦτα, καὶ ἕψειν ἐπ᾽ ἀνθράκων [879] διακεκαυμένων, ἢ ξύλων ξηρῶν, ἃ καλοῦσιν ἄκαπνα. βέλτιον δ᾽ αὐτὰ τὰ τῶν ἀμπέλων εἶναι κλήματα. προσεπεμβάλλειν δ᾽ ἁλῶν, ἐὰν μὲν ἐν τῷ προσήκοντι καιρῷ λάβῃς τὰς ἐχίδνας, ἐλάχιστον, ἐὰν δὲ θέρους, μηδέν. φυλάττεσθαι δὲ τὰς ἐκ παραθαλαττίων χωρίων λαμβάνειν, ἢ τινος ἁλμυρᾶς ὑδάτων συστάσεως. διψώδης γὰρ ἡ ἀντίδοτος ἡ ἐκ τῶν τοιούτων ἐχιδνῶν γίνεται. καλῶς δὲ ἑψηθεισῶν αὐτῶν, ὥσπερ εἰ καί τις ἐσθίειν ἔμελλεν, ἐξαίρειν μὲν χρὴ τοῦ ὕδατος, ἀφαιρεῖν δὲ τὰς σάρκας, ἄνευ τοῦ συναφαιρεῖν τι τῶν ἀκανθῶν, καὶ ταύτας ἀκριβῶς λειώσαντα, μιγνύειν ἄρτου καθαρωτάτου, καλῶς ἐξηρασμένου βραχύ τι. πρὸ πάντων δ᾽ εὔζυμός τε καὶ καλῶς ὠπτημένος ὁ ἄρτος ἔσται κριβανίτης, οὐκ ἰπνίτης. ἔνιοι μὲν οὖν ἥμισυ μέρος σταθμοῦ βάλλουσι

etiam durae et modicae carnis compotes exiſtunt. Sufficit autem in magnis viperis id quod auſeretur utrobique quaternos digitos aequare. Reliquum vero totum corpus inteſtinis exemptis et cute detracta aqua perlutum cacabo indere cum aqua pura viridique anetho (tunc enim viget) atque ſuper carbones peruſtos aut ligna arida, quae Graeci vocant ἄκαπνα, incoquere convenit, praeſtiterit autem vitium eſſe ſarmenta. Jam vero ſalis injici debet, ſi quidem convenienti tempore viperas ceperis, momentum, ſin autem aeſtate, nihil. At ex maritimis locis capere ipſas, aut ſalſa quadam aqua neutiquam tentabis. Quippe antidotum ex hujusmodi viperis confectum ſitim conciliat. Ubi vero diligenter ipſae incoctae fuerint, quemadmodum ſi quis comeſturus eſſet, ex aqua oportet eximere, carnes autem auferre ita, ut nihil ex ſpinis ſimul exeat. Atque his accurate detritis, panis puriſſimi probe deſiccati momentum admiſcere. Prae omnibus autem panis bene fermentatus et diligenter toſtus erit,

τοῦ ἄρτου, τινὲς δὲ τὸ τρίτον μέρος. ἐγὼ δὲ καὶ τέταρτον καὶ πέμπτον ἐνίοτε ἔβαλλον. εἰ μὴ γὰρ καλῶς ὠπτημένος εἴη, κίνδυνος ὀξύτητός τι προστρίψασθαι τῷ φαρμάκῳ. κάλλιον δὲ καὶ προεξηράνθαι τισὶν ἡμέραις ἐν οἴκῳ ξηρῷ τὸν οὕτως ὠπτημένον. μιχθέντων δὲ αὐτῶν καὶ λειωθέντων ἀκριβῶς, ὡς μηδεμίαν τῆς σαρκὸς τῶν ἐχιδνῶν ἀλείωτον ὑπολείπεσθαι, κυκλίσκους ἀναπλάττειν λεπτούς. οἱ γὰρ παχεῖς δυσξήραντοι γενόμενοι τὰς μὲν τῆς ἐχίδνης σάρκας σήπεσθαι συγχωροῦσι, τὸν δ' ἄρτον ὀξύνεσθαι. διὸ καὶ ξηρὸν λειοῦν τὸν ἄρτον ἄμεινόν ἐστιν, οὐχ ὡς οἱ πρὸ ἐμοῦ σκευάζοντες τῷ Καίσαρι συνετίθεσαν, ἐμβρέχοντες αὐτὸν τῷ τῶν ἐχιδνῶν ἀφεψήματι, κἀγὼ μέχρι πολλοῦ τοῦτ' ἐποίουν, ἀλλ' ὕστερόν μοι βέλτιον ἔδοξεν εἶναι λειώσαντι τὸν ἄρτον οὕτως ἀναμιγνύναι τῇ σαρκὶ τῶν ἐχιδνῶν ἀκριβῶς προλελειωμένῃ, θᾶττον γὰρ οὕτως οἱ κυκλίσκοι ξηραίνονται, τὸν ξηρὸν ἄρτον, οὐ τὸν ὑγρὸν ἀναμιξάντων ἡμῶν. ἔστω δὲ καὶ ὁ οἶκος ἐν ᾧ ξηραίνεσθαι μέλλουσι, πάντως μὲν ὑπερῷος, ἐστραμμένος δὲ πρὸς μεσημβρίαν, ἢ

teftuaceus, non furnaceus. Nonnulli igitur dimidiam ponderis partem ex pane injiciunt, nonnulli vero tertiam, ego etiam quartam quintamque nonnunquam indidi. Nifi enim probe fuerit toftus, periculum eft ne aliquid aciditatis medicamento obveniat. At fatius eft etiam diebus aliquot antea hoc pacto toftum in domo ficca exaruiffe. Simulatque vero ea mifta fit laevigataque adamuffim, ut nulla viperarum carnis portio non laevigata remanferit, orbiculos tenues efformabis. Nam craffi quum aegre ficcefcant viperae carnes putrefcere permittunt, panem acefcere, quare hunc ficcum laevigare potius eft, non quemadmodum qui ante me Caefari praeparantes antidotum compofuerunt, viperarum decocto ipfum irrigantes; ac ego longo tempore id factitabam, verum poftea melius effe exiftimavi, panem in laevorem detritum ita viperarum carni diligenter prius in pulverem redactae permifcere: citius enim hoc pacto orbiculi ficcefcunt, arido pane non humido illis admifto. Caeterum

πάντως γε μὴ πρὸς ἄρκτον, ὅπως δέχηται τὰς ἡλιακὰς ἀκτῖνας ἐν πολλῷ χρόνῳ τῆς ἡμέρας, ἐν τοιούτῳ γὰρ ἀλύπως ξηρανθήσονται. μετὰ τὴν ἀνάπλασιν εὐθέως ἐν ἐκείνῳ τῷ μέρει τιθέντες, ἔνθα μὴ προσβάλλουσιν αἱ ἀκτῖνες τοῦ ἡλίου. στρέφεσθαι δὲ αὐτοὺς χρὴ συνεχῶς, ὅπως ὁμαλῶς ξηραίνωνται καθ' ἑκάτερον μέρος. εἰ μὴ γὰρ τοῦτο πράττοι τις, τὸ μὲν ἕτερον μέρος ὑπερξηρανθήσεται, τὸ δὲ ἕτερον, ὑγρὸν ἕως πολλοῦ διαμένον, σηπεδόνι περιπεσεῖν κινδυνεύσει, καὶ μετὰ τὸ ξηρανθῆναι δὲ κείσθωσαν ἄλλαις ἡμέραις πλείοσι κατὰ τὸν αὐτὸν οἶκον, ἔξω τῶν ἡλιακῶν ἀκτίνων στρεφόμενοι συνεχῶς. ἀρκεῖ δ' ὁ χρόνος οὗτος ὁ πλεῖστος ἡμερῶν ιε'. μεθ' ἃς ἀποτίθεσθαί σοι (431) καιρός ἐστιν, ἕως ἂν μέλλῃς σκευάζειν τὸ φάρμακον. ἡ δ' ἀπόθεσις ἐν ἀγγείῳ καττιτερινῷ ἢ ὑαλίνῳ ἢ χρυσῷ γινέσθω. τὸ μὲν οὖν ὑάλινον καὶ τὸ χρυσοῦν οὐδεμίαν ἔχει τὴν δόλωσιν, ὁ δὲ καττιτερινὸς μίξει μολύβδου δολοῦται. τὸν τοιοῦτον οὖν φεύγειν προσήκει, οὐ μόνον ἐπὶ ταύτης, ἀλλὰ καὶ τῶν ἄλλων ἀντιδότων ἁπασῶν, ὥσπερ γε καὶ τὸν ἐξ

domus in qua ſicceſcere debent, omnino ſit ſublimis, ad meridiem converſa, vel certe non ad ſeptentrionem, ut ſolis radios bona diei parte accipiat. Siquidem in hujusmodi facile ſicceſcent, ſtatim ubi fuerint conſormati, ea domus parte locentur qua non radii ſolis erumpunt. Vertere autem eos continue expedit, ut aequabiliter utraque in parte deſicceſcant. Hoc enim niſi facias, altera pars plus (ac par eſt) ſiccabitur, altera humida diutius manens putredinem experiri periclitabitur. Simulatque jam ſiccata fuerint, aliis plurimis diebus in eadem domo extra ſolis radios condentur, ita ut continue vertantur. Abunde vero tempus hoc eſt, longiſſimum dierum quindecim, ſecundum quos reponere orbiculos tempeſtivum eſt, quousque medicamentum es praeparaturus. Repones autem vaſe ſtanneo aut vitreo aut aureo. Vitreum itaque et aureum nullum dolum experitur, ſtanneum plumbi miſtura adulteratur. Tale igitur vitare convenit non in

ἀργύρου μὴ κεκαθαρμένου, τάχιστα γὰρ καὶ οὗτος ἰὸν ἐπιτρεφόμενον ἔχει. καλοῦσι δ' οἱ Ῥωμαῖοι τὸν κεκαθαρμένον ἄργυρον κάνδιδον. ἄμεινον δὲ μὴ μετὰ πολὺν χρόνον χρῆσθαι τοῖς ἀρτίσκοις, οὐ μὴν πολύ γέ τοι βλάπτονται, κἂν μετ' ἐνιαυτὸν ἐμβληθῶσι, κἂν μετὰ πλείονα χρόνον ἔτι τοῦδε. καλῶς γὰρ ξηρανθέντες ἐν ἀρχῇ καὶ τριῶν ἐτῶν καὶ τεττάρων ἀκμαῖοι παραμένουσιν, ἐάν γε καλῶς ὦσιν ἀποκείμενοι, καὶ καθαροῖς ὀθονίοις δι' ἡμερῶν τινων ἀπομάττοιτο τὸ ἐπιτρεφόμενον αὐτοῖς κονιορτῶδες. ἐὰν γὰρ προσμείνῃ τοῦτο χρόνῳ πλέονι, διατίτρησιν αὐτούς. εὔδηλον δ' ὅτι τοῦτο παθόντες ἄχρηστοι γίνονται, ὡς πρίν γε τοῦτο παθεῖν αὐτοὺς, κἂν χρονίσωσιν ἱκανῶς διαμένουσι χρήσιμοι.

Κεφ. θ'. [880] [Ἀρτίσκων σκιλλητικῶν σκευασία.] Εἴτε σκιλλητικοὺς, εἴτε σκιλλίνους ἐθέλοι τις ὀνομάζειν τοὺς διὰ σκίλλης σκευαζομένους ἀρτίσκους, ἢ κυκλίσκους, ἢ τροχίσκους, διαφέρει οὐδέν. οὐδὲν γὰρ βλάψεις τὸ φάρμακον, ὅπως ἂν ὀνομάζῃς, ἐάν γε ἐν τῇ συνθέσει μηδὲν ἁμάρτῃς.

hoc ſolum, verum in aliis quoque omnibus antidotis, veluti et quod ex argento non purgato, celerrime enim et huic aerugo obnaſcitur. Vocant autem Romani argentum purgatum, candidum. At praeſtaret non multo tempore poſt uti paſtillis. Non tamen multum obſunt, etiamſi poſt annum injiciantur, imo poſt longius inſuper hoc tempus. Nam probe initio ſiccati et tribus annis et quatuor in vigore permanent, ſi probe fuerint repoſiti, et puris linteis diebus aliquot pulvis, qui ipſis obducitur, abſtergatur. Si namque hic longiori ſpatio adhaereſcit, ipſos perforat. Clarum vero eſt omnibus, ubi hoc fuerint experti, inutiles evadere, nam priusquam hoc ipſis accidat, etiam ſi inveterentur plurimum, utiles permanent.

Cap. IX. [*Paſtillorum ſcilliticorum compoſitio.*] Sive ſcilliticos, ſive ſcillinos malit aliquis appellare paſtillos, aut orbiculos, aut rotulas quae ex ſcilla praeparantur, nihil refert; nam quocunque nomine appelles medicamentum non offendis, modo nullum in compoſitione errorem

ἐγὼ δέ σοι φράσω καὶ ταύτην σαφῶς. σκίλλαν εὔτροφον ἀναιρήσῃ μὲν ἐκ τῆς γῆς, ὁπόταν ἀκριβῶς αὐτῆς ξηρανθῇ τά τε φύλλα καὶ ὁ καυλός. περιελὼν δὲ τὸ φλοιῶδες, εἶτα περιπλάσας τὶ πυρῶν νέων καλλίστων ὡς ὅτι μάλιστα, μετὰ ταῦτα ὄπτησον ἐν θερμῇ τέφρᾳ πολλῇ, μέχρις ἂν ἀκριβῶς ὀστρακωθῇ τὸ περιπλασθὲν σταίς. εἰ δὲ καὶ κατὰ τὸ χωρίον ἐν ᾧ σκευάζεις, ἴπνος εἴη τις, ἐν ἐκείνῳ καταθέμενος ἅμα τοῖς ἄρτοις, ὅταν ξηρανθῇ τὸ σταὶς, ἀφελὼν αὐτὸ, λείωσον τὴν σκίλλαν. αὐτάρκως δ' ὠπτῆσθαι γνώσῃ, καὶ διὰ καταθέσεως κάρφους. ἑτοίμως γὰρ αὐτὸ καταδέχεται τὸ σῶμα τῆς σκίλλης, ἐπειδὰν καλῶς ὀπτηθῇ. λειωθείσης δὲ ἀκριβῶς αὐτῆς μίγνυε τὸ τῶν λευκῶν ὀρόβων ἄλευρον, ἰσχυρῶς γάρ ἐστι τὸ τῶν μὴ λευκῶν πικρόν. εὔδηλον δ' ὅτι σεσῆσθαι τοῦτο χρὴ λεπτῷ κοσκίνῳ, καὶ μετὰ ταῦτα ἀκριβῶς λελειῶσθαι, τῷ σταθμῷ δὲ ἡμιολίαν εἶναι χρὴ τὴν σκίλλαν. λέγω δὲ ἡμιολίαν, ὡς δύο μὲν ἀλεύρου μοίρας εἶναι, τρεῖς δὲ τῆς σκίλλης. ὡς δὲ ταὐτὸν λέγων ὁ νεώτερος Ἀνδρόμαχος, οὐκ οἶδεν ὅπως π'. μὲν εἶναι δραχ-

committas. Ego vero etiam hanc tibi manifesto exponam. Scillam bonae habitudinis ex terra sumes, quum folia ipsius et caules exacte inaruerint. Cortice autem adempto, deinde tritici recentius quam licet optimi exiguo circunlitam postea in calido cinere copioso torrefacito, usque dum massa farinacea obducta in crustam omnino indurescat. Quod si etiam in loco quo praeparas fornax aliquis habeatur, in illum simul cum pane demissam, massa farinacea consiccata adempta, in laevorem cogito. At satis tostam esse deprehendes, quum festucam dimiserit, hanc enim scillae corpus quum probe fuerit tostum prompte recipit. Ubi vero exacte ipsa fuerit detrita, farinam ervi candidi immittes, nam ejus quod non album est, vehementer amara est. Caeterum liquet omnibus hanc tenui cribro esse incernendam, et deinde adamussim laevigandam. Scillam vero hujus pondere sesquialteram esse convenit, dico autem sesquialteram, ut duae quidem farinae partes, tres autem scillae existant, nam idem dicens junior An-

Ed. Chart. XIII. [889.] Ed. Baf. II. (431.)

μὰς βούλεται τοῦ ὀροβίνου ἀλεύρου, τῆς σκίλλης δὲ ρκ'. ἤρκει γὰρ εἰπεῖν ἡμιόλιον. εἶτα λεπτοὺς κυκλίσκους ἐκ τῆς μίξεως ταύτης ἀναπλάσας ἐν οἴκῳ τίθει πρὸς μεσημβρίαν ἐστραμμένῳ, καθότι προείπομεν, οὐ μὴν ἐν αὐταῖς γε ταῖς αὐγαῖς τοῦ ἡλίου ξήραινε. καὶ τὰ ἄλλα τὰ προειρημένα περὶ τῶν θηριακῶν κἀπὶ τούτων πρᾶττε.

Κεφ. ι'. [Ἡδυχρόου σκευασία.] Ἐν τῇ προγεγραμμένῃ συνθέσει τῆς θηριακῆς δυνάμεως ὁ Ἀνδρόμαχος, ὅπως μὲν χρὴ σκευάζειν τούς τε θηριακοὺς καὶ τοὺς σκιλλητικοὺς κυκλίσκους, δεδήλωκεν· ὅπως δὲ τὸ ἡδύχροον, οὐδὲν εἶπεν. καὶ ἄλλοι δὲ πολλοὶ τῶν γεγραφότων σύνθετα φάρμακα παρέλιπον εἰπεῖν τὴν σκευασίαν τοῦ ἡδυχρόου κατὰ τὴν περὶ τῆς θηριακῆς διήγησιν, ὥστε τις ἰατρὸς ἐν Ῥώμῃ τῶν μὴ τεθεαμένων σκευαζόμενον τὸ φάρμακον, ἐκ τῆς γραφῆς ἐπ' αὐτὸ παραγίνεσθαι τολμῶν, ἐζήτει παρὰ τοῖς μυροπώλαις ἡδύχροον, οἰόμενος εἶναι βοτάνην, ἤ τι τοιοῦτο τῶν ἁπλῶν φαρμάκων. ἐγὼ δὲ καὶ τοῦτο δηλώσω κατὰ

dromachus, haud novi, quomodo nonaginta drachmas ervi farinae eſſe velit, ſcillae autem centumviginti; ſatis enim erat dixiſſe ſeſcuplum. Deinde tenues orbiculos ex hac miſtura formatos in domo ad meridiem ſpectante (ſicuti praediximus) reponito, non tamen in ipſo ſolis ſplendore ſiccato, aliaque de theriacis commemorata in his etiam facito.

Cap. X. [*Hedychroi confectio.*] Superiore theriacae facultatis compoſitione Andromachus quomodo ſane tum theriacos tum ſcillinos orbiculos praeparare conveniat, indicavit; quomodo autem hedychroon conficiatur non expoſuit, ac alii plerique ex iis qui compoſita medicamenta conſcripſerunt, hedychroi confectionem in tractatione de theriaca intactam reliquerunt. Quare medicus quidam Romae ex iis qui medicamentum praeparare non viderunt, ex ſcriptura confectionem ejus aggredi auſus, quaerebat apud unguenarios hedychroon, putans herbam eſſe, aut aliquod tale ſimplex medicamentum; ego autem

Ed. Chart. XIII. [880. 881.] Ed. Baf. II. (431.)
τὴν Ἀνδρομάχου διαδοχὴν τῶν Καίσαρι σκευαζόντων αὐτὸ μέχρι νῦν, ὅπως συντιθέασιν. ἵνα δὲ καὶ αὐτὴ δυσπαραποίητος ᾖ, διὰ λέξεως ἐμμέτρου δηλωθήσεται τοῖς ὑπογεγραμμένοις.

Ἡδυχρόου δέ τι μάγμα, μάρου μὲν ἔχει δύο δραχμὰς,
Ἴσας δ' αὖ ἀσάρου τε, καὶ ἀμαράκου, ἀσπαλάθου τε
Καὶ σχοίνου, καλάμου τ' εὐώδεος, ἐκ πόντου τε
Φοῦ, ξυλοβαλσάμου τ', ὀποβαλσάμου τε δραχμὰς τρεῖς,
Καὶ κινναμώμου εἰσὶν ἴσαι, καὶ κόστου ἐπ' αὐτῷ.
Σμύρνης τ' ἓξ δραχμὰς, καὶ φύλλου μαλαβάθροιο,
Ἴσον δ' αὖ Ἰνδῆς νάρδου ξανθοῦ τε κρόκοιο.
Καὶ μὴν καὶ κασίης ἴσαι, διπλαῖ δέ τ' ἀμώμου.
Λοιπὴ δ' ἐκ κραναῆς Χίου δραχμῆς βάρος εἴη,
Μαστίχη, οἴνῳ δ' αὖ Φαλερίνῳ φυρήσασθαι.

[881] ὅταν ταῦτα μιχθῇ, κυκλίσκοι δηλονότι γίνονται παραπλήσιοι τοῖς θηριακοῖς τε καὶ σκιλλητικοῖς, καὶ ξηραίνονται

hoc quoque oſtendam ceu Andromachi ſucceſſor, inter eos qui Caeſari in hunc uſque diem id praeparant, qua ratione componant. Porro ut etiam ipſius ſcriptura aegre vitietur corrumpaturque, ligata oratione inferius ſcripta explicabitur.

Hedychroi vult magma mari binas ſibi drachmas,
Aequales et amaraci habens, aſari, aſpalatique,
Et junci teretis calami qui ſuavis odore eſt,
Phu ponti, ligni et ſucci quem balſamon edit.
Tres ſunto drachmae, totidem coſti, cinnamomi,
Myrrhae ſex alias miſces, folii malabathri.
Indorum nardi, flavique croci inſuper aequas.
Quinetiam caſiae totidem, ſed pondus amomi
Sume duplum, drachmam Chiae ſed maſtichae habebit.
Haec vino debent conſpergi cuncta Falerno.

Quum haec temperata fuerint, orbiculi nimirum finguntur et theriacis et ſcillinis perſimiles, eodemque modo

κατὰ τὸν αὐτὸν τρόπον. αὕτη μὲν ἐκ διαδοχῆς, ὡς ἔφην, εἰς ἡμᾶς ἦλθεν ἀπ' Ἀνδρομάχου σύνθεσις τοῦ ἡδυχρόου. διαφέρουσαι δ' ἄλλαι γεγραμμέναι πρός τινῶν εἰσιν, ὑπὸ μὲν τῶν ἐπιμεληθέντων ἐμπειρίας φαρμάκων ἐν τῷ σταθμῷ τῶν βαλλομένων διαλλάττουσαι. τινὲς δ' οὐδ' ὅλως ἔχουσι τὸ ἀμάρακον καὶ τὸ μάρον, ἔνιαι δὲ τὸ ἕτερον αὐτῶν ἔχουσαι μόνον. οὐδὲ γὰρ οἱ μυροπῶλαι πάντες αὐτὰ γινώσκουσι, διὰ τὸ μόνας ὠνεῖσθαι τὰς ἀπὸ Κρήτης κομιζομένας βοτάνας ἅμα τοῖς σπέρμασί τε καὶ χυλοῖς. ἐγὼ δὲ καὶ τὰς βοτάνας αὐτὰς ἠπιστάμην ἐν Ἀσίᾳ γεννωμένας, ἐν ἄλλοις μὲν χωρίοις ὀλίγας, ἐν Κυζίκῳ δὲ πλείστας, καὶ κατά γε τὴν Ἰταλίαν ὥσπερ ἄλλας τινὰς, οὕτω καὶ τὸ ἀμάρακον εἶδον γεννώμενον. ἀπολείπεται δὲ τὸ φυτὸν τοῦτο τοῦ μάρου πάμπολυ κατὰ τὴν εὐωδίαν. ἱκανῶς γὰρ εὐῶδες τὸ μάρον, καὶ τό γε καλούμενον ἀμαράκινον μύρον ἐν Κυζίκῳ σκευαζόμενον, ὅσον μὲν ἐπὶ τῇ προσηγορίᾳ, δόξειεν ἄν τις ἀμαράκου ἔχειν πλεῖστον, καὶ ἴσως οὕτως ὑπὸ τῶν παλαιῶν ἐσκευάζετο, νυνὶ δὲ τὸ μάρον ἐμβάλλουσι μόνον.

ficcantur. Haec fane haereditario, ut dixi, hedychroi compofitio ab Andromacho ad nos usque pervenit. Aliae autem diverfae a nonnullis defcriptae funt, iis nimirum qui medicamentorum experientiae ftuduerunt, pondere eorum quae injiciuntur evariantes. Nonnullae autem neutiquam habent amaracum et marum, nonnullae alterum ex eis dumtaxat obtinent. Neque enim myropolae omnes ea cognofcunt, quod videlicet folas herbas quae a Creta apportantur una cum feminibus fuccisque emant. Ego vero etiam herbas easdem in Afia generari novi, in aliis fane locis paucas, in Cyzico autem plurimas, ac in Italia ficuti alias quasdam, ita et amaracum crefcere vidi. Porro haec planta a maro permultum odore vincitur, nam marum vehementer odoratum, et quod amaracinum unguentum vocatur, in Cyzico confectum quantum ad appellationem attinet, putaverit aliquis amaraci plurimum habere, et forte hoc pacto a veteribus praeparabatur. Nunc autem marum folum immittunt. Ego vero herba guftata, et

ἐγὼ μέντοι γευσάμενος τῆς πόας, εὑρών τε πικρότητα μὲν ἐν αὐτῇ παμπόλλην, δριμύτητα δὲ οὐ πολλὴν, παρεκάλεσά τινα τῶν συνήθως ἀμαράκινον σκευαζόντων, ἐπεμβάλλειν ἀμαράκου τῇ σκευασίᾳ τοσοῦτον ὅσον καὶ τοῦ μάρου. καί μοι τὸ σκευασθὲν οὕτως ἧττον μὲν εὐῶδες ἐφάνη, χεῖρω δ' οὐδὲν ἐνήργει. ταῦτα μὲν οὖν κατὰ τὸ πάρεργον εἰρήσθω.

Κεφ. ια'. [Περὶ βασάνου τῆς ὡντινῶν δυνάμεων εἰλικρινείας.] Μεταβῶμεν δ' ἤδη πρὸς τὴν σκευασίαν ταύτης τῆς ἀντιδότου, κατὰ τὴν αὐτὴν τάξιν, ἑκάστου τῶν ἐμβαλλομένων αὐτῇ μνημονεύοντες, ἣν διὰ τῶν προγεγραμμένων ἐπῶν τῆς ἐλεγείας ὁ Ἀνδρόμαχος ἐποιήσατο, πεντήκοντα μὲν ἀξιῶν δραχμὰς δυοῖν δεούσας ἐμβάλλειν τῶν σκιλλητικῶν ἀρτίσκων, ὅπερ ταὐτόν ἐστι τῷ φάναι μη'. τούτων δ' ἡμισείας, ὅπερ ἐστὶ κδ'. δραχμὰς τῶν θηριακῶν, ὀπίου τε καὶ ἡδυχρόου καὶ μακροῦ πεπέρεως. περὶ μὲν οὖν τῶν γ'. εἴρηται. τὸ δὲ μακρὸν πέπερι πανούργως κατασκευαζόμενον ἐλέγξεις διαβρέχων ὕδατι. λύεται γὰρ τὸ σκευασθὲν, ἄλυτον δὲ μένει τὸ αὐτοφυές. ἔστι δὲ αὐτὸ

amaritudine in ipfa permulta, acrimonia autem non item multa deprehenfa, adhortatus fum aliquem ex iis qui amaricinum folent praeparare, ut tantum amaraci, quantum etiam mari, confecturae injiceret. Ac mihi praeparatum unguentum ita minus quidem odorum, nihil autem minus efficax apparuit. Haec igitur in tranfcurfu obiterque dicta fint.

Cap. XI. [*De probatione integritatis quarumdam medicinarum.*] Digrediamur igitur jam ad hujus antidoti confectionem, eodem ordine fingula quae ei immittuntur repetentes, quem Andromachus fuprafcriptis elegiacis verfibus confecit, quinquaginta fane drachmas minus duabus fcilliticorum paftillorum injiciendas cenfens, quod idem eft ac fi diceret quadraginta octo, horum dimidiatam partem, quod eft vigintiquatuor drachmas theriacorum, opiique, et hedychroi et longi piperis. De tribus itaque dictum eft. Longum autem piper fraudulenter praeparatum deprehendes aqua irrigans. Nam quod praeparatum

βοτάνη τις ξανθὴ ἀπὸ τῆς Ξένης κομιζομένη παραπλησία ἰδεῖν, οὐ μὴν τῇ γεύσει γε ἐοικυῖα, διὸ καὶ ῥᾴδιόν ἐστιν αὐτὴν διακρῖναι μακροῦ πεπέρεως. ἐλέγξεται δὲ καὶ τὸ σαγαπηνὸν καλούμενον ὕδατι βρεχόμενον, ἢ οἴνῳ. διαλύεται γὰρ εὐθὺς τὸ ἀληθινὸν, ἀτήκτου μένοντος (432) τοῦ μὴ τοιούτου. εἴτε δ', ὡς οὐδέτερον ὄνομα τὸ σαγαπηνὸν ἐθέλεις λέγειν, εἴτε δ', ὡς ἀρσενικὸν, ὅλον τοῦτο καλῶν σαγαπηνὸν ὀπὸν, ἔστι γὰρ ὄντως ὀπὸς νάρθηκός τινος ὁμοίου τῷ πάνακι, διήνεγκεν οὐδέν. ἀλλ' ὁ μὲν τοῦ πάνακος ὀπὸς οὐδὲν ἔχει παραπλήσιον τῷ ἐν τῇ χαλβάνῃ λευκοτέρῳ. ἔστι δ' αὐτῆς τὸ μὲν ὄντως εἰς σαγαπηνὸν μεταπίπτον, ὅσον ἀφρῶδές τε καὶ κοῦφόν ἐστι, τὸ δὲ τῇ καλλίστῃ χαλβάνῃ σαγαπηνιζούσῃ. πυκνὸν δ' ἐστὶ τοῦτο, καὶ πολὺ μᾶλλον ἐσφιγμένον τῆς ἄλλης χαλβάνης. κεχρῆσθαι δ' αὐτῷ προσῆκεν, ὡς ἀρίστῳ μορίῳ χαλβάνης. ἐπεὶ δὲ μεταπίπτειν εἶπον ἐκ χαλβάνης εἰς σαγαπηνὸν, ὅσον ἂν ἀφρῶδες ἐν αὐτῷ, συστὰν καὶ λευκὸν, ἑτοίμως ἐν ὑγρῷ λύεται. [882] προσθεῖναι μέντοι χρὴ τῷ λόγῳ καὶ μάλιστα διὰ τὴν

eſt ſolvitur, quod ſua ſponte provenit inſolubile permanet. Porro eſt id herba quaedam flava quae a Xene adſertur aſpectu quidem, ſed non guſtu tamen ſimilis, quare etiam facillimum eſt a longo pipere ipſam diſcernere. Jam vero et ſagapenum dictum deprehenditur, ſi aqua aut vino ſuperfundas, quippe verum ſtatim diſſolvitur, quod non tale eſt haud eliqueſcit, ſive ut neutrum nomen, ſagapenum, ſive ut maſculinum totum hoc ſagapenum liquorem appellare malis (eſt enim revera liquor ferulae cujusdam panaci ſimilis) nihil intereſt, verum panacis liquor nihil habet perſimile ei, qui in galbano albior exiſtit, altera autem ejus pars in ſagapenum degenerat, quae ſpumoſa levisque eſt, altera in optimum galbanum, ſagapenum reſipiens. Haec autem denſa eſt, et multo magis quam aliud galbanum conſtricta, uti ea convenit, ut particula galbani praeſtantiſſima. Quoniam vero tranſire dixi ex galbano in ſagapenum quod ſpumoſum in eo cohaerens albumque eſt, prompte in liquore ſolvitur. Apponere vero ſermoni oportet

Ed. Chart. XIII. [882.] Ed. Baf. II. (432.)

ὁμοιότητα τῆς μεταπτώσεως ἐκ τῆς ἀρίστης κασσίας εἰς κιννάμωμον. ἐθεασάμην γὰρ ἤδη πολλάκις ὑψηλῆς καὶ εὐθαλοῦς κασσίας ὡς εἰς θάμνου μέγεθος ἀνήκειν ἀκρέμονάς τινας ἀκριβῶς ὁμοίους κινναμώμῳ κατά τε τὴν ὄψιν καὶ τοῦ φλοιοῦ τὴν λεπτότητα, καὶ πρὸς τούτοις ἔτι τὰ βεβαιότατα γνωρίσματα κινναμώμου διά τῆς γεύσεώς τε καὶ ὀσφρήσεως γινόμενα. οὕτω δὲ καὶ κατὰ τὴν ἀρίστην σμύρναν ὀποκάλπασον εὑρίσκεται, διαφέρον σμύρνης, καὶ κατά γε τὰ τρία ταῦτα, λέγω δὲ τό τε σαγαπηνὸν καὶ τὸ ὀποκάλπασον καὶ τὴν κασσίαν, ἐν μὲν τῷ μεταξὺ γίνεταί τινα μηκέτι μένοντα, μήτε χαλβάνη, μήτε κασσία, μήτε σμύρνη, μηδέπω ἀκριβῆ τὴν ἰδέαν ἔχοντα σαγαπηνοῦ καὶ κινναμώμου καὶ ὀποκαλπάσου. διὸ καὶ πολλάκις χρὴ τεθεᾶσθαι τὸν μέλλοντα διαγιγνώσκειν καὶ διακρίνειν ἀλλήλων τὰ παραπλήσια· καθάπερ γε ἐπὶ τῶν ὁμοίων ἀλλήλοις παιδαρίων διδύμων οἱ μὲν ἀήθεις ὄντες οὐ δύνανται διακρίνειν τὸ ἕτερον ἀπὸ τοῦ ἑτέρου, ῥάστη δὲ ἡ διάγνωσις γίνεται τοῖς ὁμοδιαίτοις, οὕτως ἔχει κἀπὶ τῶν φαρμάκων

praefertim quod confimiliter optima caffia in cinnamomum degeneret. Spectavi enim jam fubinde fublimis et ramofae caffiae ut in fruticis magnitudinem erumperet, furculos quosdam adamuffim cinnamomi fimiles, tum afpectu, tum corticis tenuitate, et praeterea firmiffimis cinnamomi notis quae et guftu et olfactu deprehenduntur. Pari modo in optima myrrha opocalpafon invenitur a myrrha diverfum, ac in tribus hifce, dico fagapeno, opocalpafo et caffia medio fpatio nonnulla gignuntur, quae non amplius remanent, aut galbanum, aut caffia, aut myrrha, necdum exactam fagapeni, cinnamomi et opocalpafi fpeciem referentia. Quapropter etiam fubinde eum qui confimilia inter fe dignofcet, vidiffe oportet, quemadmodum in pueris gemellis invicem fimilibus, qui quidem non eis affuerunt, alterum ab altero nequeunt difcernere, iis autem qui una vixerunt facillima eft dignotio, ita habet in omnibus quoque medicamentis. Nam qui inter ea educatus eft et frequenter vidit ex facili parvitatis differentias et invenit et cognofcit.

ἁπάντων. ὁ γὰρ ἐντεθραμμένος αὐτοῖς καὶ πολλάκις ἑορακὼς εὑρίσκει τε καὶ γνωρίζει ῥᾳδίως τὰς παρὰ μικρὸν διαφοράς· ὁ δ' ἅπαξ ἢ δὶς ἑορακὼς ὡς ἀπαράλλακτον τεθέαται τῷ ἑτέρῳ τὸ ἕτερον, ἔχον ἐνίοτε σαφεστάτην διάκρισιν, ἐναργῶς φαινομένην τῷ πολλάκις ἑορακότι, ὥστε καὶ δι' ἑνὸς τῶν συμβεβηκότων αὐτοῖς γνωρίζεσθαι ῥᾳδίως. τὸ γοῦν ἐκ χαλβάνης σαγαπηνὸν οὐκ ἔχει τὴν ὀσμὴν τῆς ἰδιότητος τὴν αὐτὴν τῷ κυρίως ὀνομαζομένῳ σαγαπηνῷ. τὸ γὰρ ὑπὸ τῶν περὶ τὰ τοιαῦτα δεινῶν ὀνομαζόμενον ὀσμῆς εἶδος τραγίζον οὐκ ἀποτίθεται τὸ ἐκ τῆς χαλβάνης σαγαπηνόν. ἀλλὰ ἐπὶ μὲν τοῦ τοιούτου σαγαπηνοῦ καὶ τῆς χαλβάνης ταύτης οὐ μεγάλη τίς ἐστιν ἡ διαφορὰ πρὸς τὴν τοῦ φαρμάκου σύνθεσιν. ἄμφω γὰρ ἁρμόττει καὶ ἀντιτέτακται τοῖς ἰοβόλοις τε καὶ δηλητηρίοις, ἀλλ' ἧττον ἡ χαλβάνη τοῦ σαγαπηνοῦ. τὸ δὲ ὀποκάλπασον ἀναιρετικόν ἐστι, καὶ πολλοὺς κατά τινα τύχην ἐν τοῖς τῆς ἡμετέρας ζωῆς χρόνοις ἀποθανόντας οἶδα διὰ τὴν ἄγνοιαν τῆς ὀποκάλπασον ἐχούσης σμύρνης. ἐξεπίτηδες γὰρ ἔνιοι τῶν σκευα-

Qui vero ſemel aut bis conſpexerit, tanquam indifferens alterum ab altero ſpectabit, quod nonnunquam manifeſtiſſimum habet diſcrimen, ei qui frequenter intuitus eſt manifeſto apparens, ut etiam ex uno accedentium ipſis facile ſit cognoſcere. Nam ſagapenum ex galbano, non habet proprietatis odorem eundem cum eo quod proprie ſagapenum dicitur. Quod enim hujusmodi rerum periti ſic nominant, odoris ſpeciem hircinam, ſagapenum ex galbano non exuit, verum in tali ſagapeno atque hoc galbano, haud magna ad medicamenti compoſitionem differentia exiſtit. Ambo ſiquidem conveniunt adverſanturque virulentis et deleteriis, ſed galbanum minus ſagapeno. At opocalpaſon letale eſt, multosque forte fortuna noſtris temporibus propter inſcitiam myrrhae quae opocalpaſon habebat interiiſſe novimus. Nam de induſtria nonnulli ipſam praeparantium ut laudatiſſimam injecerunt, quod collyriis inditam optimum eſſe medicamentum viderent,

ζόντων αὐτὴν ὡς ἀρίστην ἔβαλον, ἐπειδὴ τοῖς κολλυρίοις ἐμβαλλομένην ὁρῶσι κάλλιστον οὖσαν φάρμακον, ἀδήκτως γὰρ διαφορεῖ τὸ πῦον. ἔστι δ' ὅτε καὶ ἀρχόμενον ὑπόχυμα λεπτὸν τῇ συστάσει, κἂν εἰς ἔμπλαστρον δὲ, κἂν εἰς κηρωτὴν, ἤ τι τῶν ἔξωθεν ἐπιτιθεμένων φαρμάκων διαφορητικῶν ἐμβάλῃς τὴν τοιαύτην σμύρναν, αὐξήσεις αὐτοῦ τὴν δύναμιν, ἀλλ' εἴσω τοῦ σώματος λαμβανομένη θανάσιμόν ἐστι φάρμακον. ταῦτα μὲν οὖν ἐπὶ πλέον εἴρηται διά τε τὴν ἀκολουθίαν τοῦ λόγου καὶ τὸ χρήσιμον τῆς θεωρίας.

Κεφ. ιβ'. [Περὶ τῶν ἐν τῇ τρίτῃ τάξει γεγραμμένων δυνάμεων.] Ἐπὶ δὲ τὴν ὑπὸ Ἀνδρομάχου τάξιν γεγραμμένην τῶν ἐμβαλλομένων ἁπλῶν φαρμάκων τῇ θηριακῇ καιρὸς ἐπανελθεῖν. γράφει οὖν τρίτην τάξιν φαρμάκων ἀνὰ < ιβ'. λαμβανόντων, ἃ προπαρασκευάσεις ἅπαντα δηλονότι κατὰ τὴν ἰδίαν ἀκμὴν ἐκλέγων, οἷον εὐθέως τὰ ῥόδα ξηραίνων μὲν, ὡς ἐπὶ τῶν ἀρτίσκων εἴρηται, τὰ κάλλιστα, λαμβάνων δ' αὐτῶν ἅπερ εὐοδμότατα πάντως ἐστὶ, καὶ μέντοι καὶ ἐρυθρότερα τῶν ἄλλων. φυλαττόμενος δὲ τοὺς

ut quae pus citra rofionem difcutiat, nonnunquam etiam fuffufionem incipientem fubftantia tenuem. Sive autem in emplaftrum, five in ceratum, aut aliquod digerens medicamentum quod intrinfecus imponitur, hujusmodi myrrham injicias, virtutem ipfius augebis, verum intra corpus affumptum letale eft medicamentum. Haec igitur fufius dicta funt, tum propter fermonem fubfequentem, tum fpeculationis utilitatem.

Cap. XII. [*De medicinis in tertio ordine pofitis.*] Praeterea vero fimplicium medicamentorum quae theriacae immittuntur ordinem ab Andromacho fcriptum perfequi tempeftivum eft. Tradit itaque tertium ordinem medicamentorum fingulorum duodecim drachmas recipientium, quae omnia praeparabis in fuo ipfa vigore deligens, exempli gratia rofas ftatim ficcans quidem, ut in paftillis expofitum eft, praeftantiffimas, capiens autem ex eis quae longe omnium fuaviffimae funt. Quin etiam aliis

καταγείους οἴκους, ὡς μηδὲν αὐτοῖς φάρμακον ἀποτίθεσθαι, καὶ μάλιστα τοὺς ὑγροὺς αὐτῶν, ἐν οἷς εὐρὼς ἐν τάχει γίνεται. ἐφεξῆς δὲ τῆς Ἰλλυρικῆς ἴρεως [883] ὁ Ἀνδρόμαχος ἀξιοῖ βάλλειν τοῖς ῥόδοις· οὗ λόγου μὴ παρέργως ἀκούσῃς, ὡς ὑπὲρ ἄλλου τινὸς φαρμάκου, περὶ ὧν ἐφεξῆς ἐρῶ, τὸ κάλλιστον ἐν ἑκάστῳ γένει διδάσκων ὁποῖόν ἐστι. πόλιον μὲν οὖν καὶ χαμαίδρυς εἰς Ῥώμην κομίζεται, βραχὺ βελτίων τῶν ἐν Ἰταλίᾳ γεννωμένων. ἔν τισι γὰρ τόποις τῶν Ἰταλικῶν οὐ πολύ τι λειπόμενα γεννᾶται κατ' ἐκεῖνα τῶν ἐτῶν, ἐν οἷς οὐκ ἐγίνετο σύμπαν τὸ ἔαρ ὑγρὸν, ὥσπερ πολλάκις γίνεται κατὰ τὸν τρόπον τοῦ θέρους. ἀλλ' ὅταν γε κατάστασις γίνηται ξηροτέρα, τοῖς πλείστοις τῶν ἀπὸ Κρήτης ὅμοια τὰ κατὰ τὴν Ἰταλίαν, ἢ οὐ πολύ γε λειπόμενα γεννᾶταί τινα, καθάπερ ἥ τε χαμαίδρυς καὶ ἡ χαμαιπίτυς καὶ τὸ ὑπερικὸν, ἥ τε γεντιανὴ, καὶ τὸ θλάσπι, καὶ ὁ μέλας ἐλλέβορος, ἕτερά τε τοιαῦτα. τὸ δὲ τῆς ἴρεως οὐχ οὕτως ἔχει. παραβαλλομένη γὰρ ἡ ἐκ τῆς μεγάλης Λιβύης, ἥπερ εἰς Ῥώμην φέρεται πλείστη, τοσοῦτον ἀπο-

rubicundiores, diligentia adhibita ne ullum medicamentum in ſubterraneis domunculis praeſertim humidis reponas, in quibus ſitus celeriter provenit. Deinde vero Illyricam iridem Andromachus roſis injiciendam cenſet, quem ſermonem ne obiter inaudias, ceu de alio quodam medicamento de quibus infra dicturus ſum, optima in unoquoque genere quale ſit edocens. Polium itaque et chamaedrys Romam apportantur paulo praeſtantiora iis quae in Italia naſcuntur. In quibusdam enim locis Italiae non multo inferiora creſcunt, illis annis quibus ver totum non humidum evaſerit, quemadmodum ſubinde fit in modum aeſtatis. Verum quum ſiccior aëris conſtitutio oboritur ea quae Italia proſert Cretenſibus ſimilia, aut non multo deteriora quaedam naſcuntur, exempli gratia chamaedrys, chamaepitys, hypericum, gentiana, thlaſpi, nigrum veratrum, aliaque ſimilia. At de iride non ita habet. Nam ſi conferas eam quae ex magna Libya Romam copioſiſſima adſertur, tantum ab Illyrica abeſt quantum mortuum

Ed. Chart. XIII. [883.] Ed. Baf. II. (432.)

λείπεται τῆς Ἰλλυρικῆς, ὅσον τὸ νεκρὸν σῶμα τοῦ ζῶντος, οὐ μὴν ἔν γε τοῖς ἄλλοις ἔθνεσιν οὕτω πολὺ φαίνεται λειπομένη. καὶ ταύτης γοῦν ἐκλέγου τὴν εὐωδεστέραν, ὥσπερ γε τῶν ἄλλων φαρμάκων. ἕκαστον γὰρ ἄριστόν ἐστι τὸ τὴν τοῦ γένους ἰδίαν ὀσμὴν ἰσχυροτάτην ἔχον, ὅπερ ἐκ τοῦ πολλὰ τεθεᾶσθαι γίνεταί δῆλον ἑκάστῳ. καὶ μέντοι καὶ περὶ τῆς κατὰ τὴν γεῦσιν ποιότητος ὁμοίως τὸ ἴδιον ἐν ἑκάστῳ γένει πρωτεῦον ἄριστον ἀποφανεῖ τὸ φάρμακον, ἀδόκιμα δὲ καὶ τὰ λεπτότερα καὶ ἀτροφώτερα τῶν ὁμογενῶν. ἀμείνω γὰρ ἐν ἅπαντι γένει τὰ μὴ ῥυσὰ μηδὲ ἄτροφα, καθάπερ γε καὶ τὰ ὑπερβάλλοντα τῶν συμμέτρων χείρω τῶν εὔτροφόν τε καὶ ἐσφιγμένην τὴν σύστασιν ἐχόντων. διόπερ, ὡς ἔφην, ἑορακέναι χρὴ πολλὰ πολλάκις, καὶ μάλιστα τὰ κάλλιστα, καὶ πολλῷ χρόνῳ πεῖραν ἐκ γενετῆς σφῶν αὐτῶν παρεσχηκότα, καὶ συμφώνως ὑπὸ τῶν ἐμπείρων ὕλης ἰατρικῆς ἐπῃνημένα. πάντες γοῦν ἔγραψαν ἶριν μὲν ἀρίστην εἶναι τὴν ἐν Ἰλλυριοῖς γεννωμένην, πετροσέλινον δὲ τὸ Μακεδονικὸν, ἄσφαλτον δὲ τὴν Ἰουδαϊκὴν,

corpus a vivo, non tamen in aliis nationibus ita multum abesse apparet. Atque in hujus genere odoratiorem deligito, quemadmodum in aliis medicamentis. Unumquodque enim praestantissimum est quod proprium generis sui odorem habet valentissimum, quod ex multa inspectione singulis innotescit. Quin etiam de gustus qualitate similiter proprietas in unoquoque genere primas obtinens optimum declarat medicamentum, ignobilia autem habentur, quae in suo genere et tenuiora et minus procera; praestant enim in quolibet genere non rugosa neque exilia, quemadmodum quae modum excedunt deteriora indicantur iis quae bene nutritam constrictamque habent consistentiam. Quamobrem, ut dixi, multa subinde spectasse convenit, praecipue optima et quae longo tempore experimenta ab origine sui ipsius exhibuerunt, unoque consensu a medicinalis materiae peritis commendata. Omnes itaque prodiderunt irim quidem esse laudatissimam quae in Illyricis nascitur, petroselinum vero

ὥσπερ γε καὶ ὀποβάλσαμον, ἐπί τε τῶν ἄλλων ὁμοίως, ὑπὲρ ὧν ἐφεξῆς κατὰ τὸν ἴδιον ἑκάστου λόγον οὐ παραλείψω τὴν ἀπὸ τῆς χώρας ἀρετήν. ἐφεξῆς δὲ γλυκυῤῥίζης τε χυλοῦ καὶ βουνιάδος αγρίας σπέρματος μνημονεύει, καλλίστων ἡμῖν ἀμφοτέρων ἐκ Κρήτης φερομένων, καὶ μάλιστα τῆς γλυκυῤῥίζης αὐτῆς τε καὶ τοῦ χυλοῦ. σκόρδιον δὲ κάλλιστον ἡμῖν ἐκ Κρήτης φέρεται. εὕροις δ' ἂν οὐ φαῦλον οὐδ' ἐν ἄλλοις τῶν ἐθνῶν. γέγραπται δ' ὑπό τινων ἀνδρῶν ἀξιολόγων, πολέμῳ νεκρῶν ἀτάφων ἡμέραις πλείοσι γενομένων, ὅσα τῶν σωμάτων ἐπὶ τοῦ σκορδίου κατὰ τύχην ἔκειτο, πολὺ τῶν ἄλλων ἀσηπτότερα διαμεῖναι, καὶ μάλιστα αὐτῶν ἐκεῖνα τὰ μόρια τοῦ σώματος, ὅσα τῆς πόας ἔψαυε τοῦ σκορδίου· καὶ δὴ καὶ πεπίστευται τοῖς σηπεδονώδεσιν ἰοῖς τῶν ζώων, καὶ φαρμάκων δηλη (433) τηρίοις ἀντιτετάχθαι. γέγραπται δὲ αὐτάρκως περὶ πάσης τῆς κατ' ἰατρικὴν ὕλης ἐν ε'. βιβλίοις Διοσκορίδου, παρ' οὗ τά τε ἄλλα καὶ τὰς ὀσφρητὰς καὶ γευστὰς ποιότητας, αἷς γνωρίζεται μάλιστα καὶ διακρίνεται τὰ δοκιμώτερα φάρμακα

Macedonicum, bitumen Judaicum, quemadmodum et opobalſamum, ac de aliis ſimiliter, de quibus deinceps in peculiari ſingulorum ſermone virtutem a regione proſiciſcentem non omittam; deinde vero dulcis radiculae ſucci et napi ſylveſtris ſeminis meminit, quae utraque ex Creta praeſtantiſſima adferuntur, potiſſimumque dulcis radicula, tum ipſa, tum ipſius liquor. Scordion optimum ex Creta nobis advehitur, quanquam non malum in aliis nationibus ſit invenire. Porro memoriae traditum eſt a viris quibusdam ſide dignis, quum bello mortui pluribus diebus inhumati jacuiſſent, corpora quae ſuper ſcordion ſorte fortuna procumberent, multo magis quam alia a putredine immunia permanſiſſe, et maxime illas corporis partes quae herbam ſcordion contingerent; ac creditum eſt putriferis animalium venenis et medicamentorum deleteriis ſuccurrere. Sed traditum eſt abunde de tota medicinali materie quinque Dioſcoridis libris, a quo praeter alia etiam olfactus guſtatusque qualitates, quibus potiſſimum proba-

τῶν φαυλοτέρων, ἔνεστί σοι μανθάνειν. ἐπ᾽ ἐνίων δὲ καὶ τὰς ὁρατὰς ποιότητας οὐ σμικρὰ συντελούσας εὑρήσεις. ἐμοὶ δ᾽ οὐ πρόκειται κατὰ τὴν ἐνεστῶσαν πραγματείαν, ὅσα καλῶς ἑτέροις γέγραπται μεταφέρειν, ἀλλ᾽ ἐξεργάσασθαι σαφῶς τὰ λείποντα.

Κεφ. ιγ΄. [Περὶ τοῦ ὀποβαλσάμου τε καὶ κινναμώμου.] Ἐφεξῆς ὀποβαλσάμου τε καὶ κινναμώμου διὰ τῶν προγεγραμμένων ἐπῶν ἐμνημόνευσεν ὁ Ἀνδρόμαχος, ἐφ᾽ ὧν ἐπὶ τοῖς γεγραμμένοις ὑπὸ τοῦ Διοσκορίδου γνωρίσμασι μέγιστόν ἐστι τεθεᾶσθαι πρότερον αὐτὰ κατὰ τί χωρίον ἕκαστον αὐτῶν ἄριστον γεννᾶται, καθάπερ ἐπειράθην ἐγὼ, γνοὺς πολυειδῶς παραποιούμενον ὀποβάλσαμον, ὡς εἶναι δυσδιάγνωστον, αὐτὸς ἰδεῖν ὀπιζόμενον αὐτὸ, καὶ σχεῖν ἐξ ἐκείνου, καθάπερ τινὰ κανόνα τῶν ἄλλων. ἔμαθον δὲ παραποιήσεις αὐτοῦ πολλὰς, ὡς καὶ τοὺς τριβακωτάτους λαθεῖν, ἃς οὐκ ἀξιῶ δημοσιεύειν τοὺς γνόντας, ὅπως μὴ κατὰ τὸ πάρεργον οἱ πονηροὶ μανθάνοντες αὐτὰς, ἐν ἔργῳ μεταφέροιεν ἐπὶ τὰς κακὰς πράξεις. οὐδὲ γὰρ οὐδὲ τὰς τῶν

tiora medicamenta a deterioribus cognofcuntur difcernunturque, licet tibi condifcere. In nonnullis etiam viforias qualitates non parum conferre reperies, fed mihi in praefenti opere inftitutum eft, non quae ab aliis recte tradita funt huc transferre, fed quae defiderantur, manifefto interpretari.

Cap. XIII. [*De opobalfamo et cinnamomo.*] Inde opobalfami et cinnamomi in praedictis verfibus Andromachus meminit, in quibus poft traditas a Diofcoride notas maximum eft ea prius infpexiffe, in qua regione unumquodque ipforum praeftantiffimum gignitur, quemadmodum ego conatus fum, fciens opobalfamum variis adulterari modis, ut aegre poffit dignofci, ipfe videre quomodo id liquorem fundat, ac inde ceu regulam quandam aliorum obtinere. Porro didici multas ipfius adulterationes, ut etiam exercitatiffimos lateant, quas publicare fcientes non dignum aeftimo, ne pravi ipfas in tranfcurfu difcentes, in opere ad malas actiones transferant. Neque enim eos

δηλητηρίων φαρμάκων γραφὰς τοὺς δημοσιεύοντας ἐπαινῶ. τὰς γοῦν ὑπὸ τοῦ Διοσκορίδου τε καὶ τῶν ἄλλων, ὅσοι περὶ ὕλης ἔγραψαν ἑκάστου τῶν φαρμάκων, δοκιμασίας ἐπιφέροντες αὐτοῖς, ὅταν προσθῆτε τὴν ἰδίαν αὐτοψίαν ἐπὶ πολλῶν, ἀκριβῶς δυνήσεσθε διακρίνειν ἀλλήλων, ὅσα γε διακρίνεσθαι δύνανται. τινῶν γὰρ, ὡς ἔφην, ἢ οὐδ' ὅλως ἐστὶν ἢ οὐκ ἀκριβὴς ἡ διάκρισις, ἀλλὰ συγκέχυται τὰ γνωρίσματα τῶν πανούργως ἐσκευασμένων. περὶ δὲ κινναμώμου τἀναντία τοῖς εἰρημένοις ἐπὶ τοῦ ὀποβαλσάμου γινώσκω. πέπεισμαι γὰρ αὐτὸ πάντων εὐδιαγνωστότατον εἶναι τοῖς ἑορακόσι πολλάκις ἄριστον κιννάμωμον. τούτου δ' οὐχ οἷόν τέ τινα τυχεῖν, εἰ μή τις θεάσοιτο τὴν παρασκευὴν τῶν αὐτοκρατόρων κινναμώμων, σχεδὸν εἰς ἓξ που διαφορὰς γενικὰς ἡκόντων. ἔστι γὰρ κἀν τούτοις αὐτοῖς ἀξιόλογος ὑπεροχὴ τοῦ καλλίστου πρὸς τὸ χείριστον, ὥσπερ κἀν ταῖς κασσίαις, ὥστε τὴν καλλίστην κασσίαν ἀπολείπεσθαι βραχὺ τοῦ φαυλοτάτου κινναμώμου, καὶ ὅτι οὐ γίνεται μακροχρόνιος ἡ κατὰ τὴν χρῆσιν ἀρετὴ τοῦ κινναμώμου. οὐδὲ γὰρ μέχρι λ'.

qui letalium medicamentorum fcripturas invulgant, probo. Si igitur probationes a Diofcoride ac aliis qui de fingulorum medicamentorum materie fcripferunt, expofitas ipfis adferatis, veftris ipfi oculis multa fpeculati, exacte invicem poteritis difcernere, quae difcerni eft poffibile. Quorundam enim (ut dixi) aut nulla prorfus, aut non exacta eft difcretio, verum notae eorum quae dolofe paratae funt, confunduntur. At de cinnamomo contraria iis quae in opobalfamo dicta funt, fentio. Perfuafum namque mihi eft, optimum cinnamomum iis qui crebro viderunt omnium facillime poffe dignofci. Hoc autem aliquem affequi non licet, nifi quis principum cinnamomorum quae in fex fere differentias generales dividuntur, praeparationem confpexerit. Eft namque in his ipfis infignis optimi ad deterrimum exceffus, quemadmodum in caffiis, ut optima caffia parum a praviffimo cinnamomo abfit. Item quia cinnamomi vis inter utendum diuturna haud efficitur. Quippe ne ad triginta quidem annos facultas ipfius, quam initio obtinebat, in-

χρόνων ὁλόκληρον αὐτοῦ τὴν ἀπ' ἀρχῆς διασώζεσθαι δύναμιν. ληροῦσι δ' ἔνιοι τῶν τοιούτων φαρμάκων τὸ κιννάμωμον ἀγήρω διαμένειν φάσκοντες. οὐδὲ γὰρ ρ'. οὐδὲ διακοσίων ἐτῶν μεταξὺ γεγενημένων, ἀλλ' ὀλίγων, ὡς πρὸς τοσοῦτον ἀριθμὸν, ἤδη τινὰ μεταβολὴν ἑόρακα τῷ παλαιοτέρῳ κινναμώμῳ γεγενημένην. Ἀντωνίνῳ γοῦν σκευάζων τὴν θηριακὴν ἐθεασάμην ἀγγεῖα πολλὰ ξύλινα, τὰ μὲν ἐπὶ Τραϊανοῦ ταῖς ἀποθήκαις ἐγκαθέντα μετὰ κινναμώμου, τὰ δὲ ἐπ' Ἀδριανοῦ, τὰ δὲ ἐπ' Ἀντωνίνου τοῦ μετὰ τὸν Ἀδριανὸν ἄρξαντος, καὶ πάντα γε τῷ ὁμογενεῖ κινναμώμῳ σαφῶς ἀλλήλων ὑπερεῖχε, κατά τε τὴν τῆς γεύσεως, καὶ τῆς ὀσφρήσεως ἀτονίαν καὶ εὐτονίαν, ὅσον καὶ τῷ χρόνῳ, καὶ μέντοι κομισθέντος ποτὲ ἐκ τῆς βαρβάρου, γλωττοκωμίου μακροῦ πηχέων δ'. καὶ ἡμίσεος, ἐν ᾧ δένδρον ὅλον ἦν κινναμώμου τοῦ πρώτου γένους, ἐξ αὐτοῦ σύνθεσίν τινα τῷ αὐτοκράτορι Μάρκῳ Ἀντωνίνῳ ποιησάμενος, ὅλην εὗρον τὴν ἀντίδοτον ἱκανῶς τῶν ἄλλων ὑπερέχουσαν, ὥστε γευσάμενον αὐτῆς τὸν αὐτοκράτορα μὴ περιμεῖναι χρόνον,

tegra conſervatur. At nonnulli nugantur, qui ex hujusmodi medicamentis cinnamomum ſenii expers permanere pronuntiant. Neque enim centum, neque ducentis annis interea delapſis, ſed paucis, ſi tantum numerum reſpicias, mutationem jam aliquam vetuſtiori cinnamomo obortam vidi. Quum itaque theriacam Antonino praepararem, vaſcula multa lignea conſpexi, alia Trajano imperante ſcriniis recondita cum cinnamomo, alia principatu Adriani, alia regnante Antonino, qui Adriano in imperio ſucceſſit, ac omnia cum congeneri cinnamomo manifeſto ſe invicem ſuperabant, tum guſtus, tum odoratus imbecillitate et vehementia, quantum et tempore evariabant. Quin etiam quum aſportatum eſſet aliquando ex barbaria ſcriniolum quatuor cubitos dimidiumque longum, ubi arbor tota cinnamomi primi generis erat condita, unde compoſitionem quandam imperatori Marco Antonino molitus, totum expertus ſum antidotum abunde aliis praecellere, ut, poſteaquam imperator ipſum deguſtaſſet, tempus non

ὥσπερ ἐπὶ τῶν ἄλλων, ἐν ᾧ πεφθήσεται τὸ φάρμακον, ἀλλ' εὐθέως χρῆσθαι, μηδὲ δύο μηνῶν ὁλοκλήρων ἐν τῷ μεταξὺ γενομένων. διαδεξαμένου δ' αὐτὸν Κομμόδου, μήτε τῆς θηριακῆς ἀντιδότου μήτε τοῦ κινναμώμου πεφροντικότος, ἐκείνου τε τοῦ δένδρου τὸ περιττὸν, ὅσον τ' ἄλλο μετὰ τοὺς Ἀδριανοῦ χρόνους ἐκομίσθη, διαπώλετο τὸ πᾶν, ὥστε τοῦ νῦν ὄντος ἡμῶν αὐτο [885] κράτορος Σεβήρου, κελεύσαντος αὐτῷ κατὰ τὸν αὐτὸν τρόπον ὃν ἐσκεύαζον Ἀντωνίνῳ συνθεῖναι τὴν ἀντίδοτον, ἠναγκάσθην ἐκ τῶν ἐπὶ Τραϊανοῦ καὶ Ἀδριανοῦ κατατεθειμένων ἐκλέγειν, καί μοι σαφῶς ἀσθενέστερα γεγονέναι νῦν ἐφαίνετο, μηδὲ λ'. πεπληρωμένων ἐτῶν τῶν μεταξύ. περὶ δ' οὖν τοῦ καλλίστου κινναμώμου προσθεῖναί τι τῷ λόγῳ βούλομαι τῶν ἀναγκαίων, εἶναι μὲν εὐωδέστατον, ἄῤῥητόν τέ τινα εὐωδίαν ὑπὲρ ἅπαντα τὰ ἄλλα ἔχειν, γευομένῳ δὲ θερμὸν ἱκανῶς, οὐ μὴν, ὥστε δάκνειν, λυπηρόν. τῇ χροιᾷ δὲ τοιοῦτον, ὡς εἴ τις μίξειε τὸ τοῦ γάλακτος χρῶμα τῷ φαιῷ, μετὰ βραχέος τοῦ κυανοῦ καλουμένου. λαβὼν δ' ὅσον ἐβουλόμην ἐξ αὐτοῦ, καθάπερ

expectaverit. Quemadmodum in aliis, in quo medicamentum concoquetur, fed ftatim ufus fit, ne duobus quidem menfibus integris interea praeteritis. Verum ubi Commodus ipfi fucceffiffet, neque Theriaces antidoti neque cinnamomi ratione ab ipfo habita tum arboris illius reliquum, tum quodcunque alius poft Adriani tempora apportatum eft, totum interiit. Quare quum hujus tempeftatis noftrae imperator Severus injunxiffet ipfum fimili modo quo Antonino praeparabam antidotum componi, coactus fum ex iis, quae Trajani Adrianique tempore erant fepofita, deligere, ac mihi evidenter imbecilliora evafiffe nunc apparebant, ne triginta quidem annis interea abfolutis. Quapropter fermoni de optimo cinnamomo habito aliquid neceffarium cogito adjicere, ut fit odoratiffimum, indicibilem quandam odoris gratiam fuper alia omnia referat, guftanti calidum admodum percipiatur, non tamen ut molefte rodat, colore autem tale, veluti fi quis lactis colorem gilvo admifcuerit cum modico caeruleo nuncupato.

ειώθειν, ἀπεθέμην ὀλίγα παρ' ἐμαυτῷ κλώνια κατὰ τὴν ἀποθήκην, ἐν ᾗ πάντα μου τὰ τιμαλφέστατα κτήματα περιείχετο. κατακαυθείσης δ' αὐτῆς, ὁπότε καὶ τὸ τῆς Εἰρήνης τέμενος ἐκαύθη, καὶ τῶν ἄλλων πέντε διαφορῶν τοῦ κινναμώμου πᾶν ὅσον ἐκεκτήμην ἀπώλετο. τῷ μὲν οὖν νῦν ἡμῶν αὐτοκράτορι Σεβήρῳ τὴν ἀντίδοτον ἐσκεύασα, τῶν Ἀδριανείων ἐκλέξας κινναμώμων, περὶ ὧν καὶ αὐτῶν χρήσιμόν τι τοῖς ἀναγνωσομένοις ἔχων προσθεῖναι, διελθεῖν οὐκ ὀκνήσω. πολλὰ μὲν οὖν ἐστιν αὐτοῦ καὶ νῦν ἔτι τὰ σωζόμενα ξύλινα σκεύη. πάντα δ' ἔχει τῶν πολυῤῥίζων, ἢ πολυκλάδων, ἢ ὅπως ἂν τις ὀνομάζειν ἐθέλῃ κινναμώμων τὰς διαφοράς. οὐδὲν δ' ὥσπερ πρέμνον εἰς πολλοὺς κλάδους σχιζόμενον εἰς μῆκος ἐκτέταται πλέον, ἀλλ' οἵα περὶ τῶν ἐλλεβόρων ἀμφοτέρων ἰδέα ἐστὶ, καὶ μᾶλλον ἔτι τοῦ καλουμένου μὲν δαμασωνίου, φερομένου δ' ἐκ Κρήτης ἡμῖν. ἕκαστον δ' αὐτῶν ἐστιν ἐξ ἑνὸς πυθμένος φυόμενον, οἷον θαμνίσκος τις, ὁ μὲν στ'. ὁ δὲ ζ'. τὰς ἐκφύσεις ἔχων, ἢ

Snmpto autem ex eo quantum volebam, ficuti confnevi, paucos ramufculos apud me repofui in fcrinium, ubi omnia quae mihi chara et in pretio erant, continebantur. At eo combufto, quando etiam Pacis delubrum incendio flagravit, cum aliis quinque cinnamomi generibus totum quod comparaveram intercidit, quam ob caufam imperatori noftro qui nunc exiftit, antidotum confeci, cinnamomis quae Adriani tempore erant apportata, ad hoc delectis, de quibus etiam ipfis quum utile quippiam lectoribus poffim adjicere, commemorare id non fubterfugiam. Multa igitur funt lignea ipfius vafcula, quae in huuc etiam diem refervantur, omnia vero continent cinnamomorum, multis radicibus, aut multis ramis, five quocunque modo libeat appellare, extantium differentias, nullum vero tanquam caudex in multos ramos fiffus in longitudinem ampliorem eft exporrectum, fed qualis utrique veratro fpecies eft, et magis adhuc ei quod damafonium quidem appellatur, ex Creta autem nobis adfertur;

βραχὺ πλείους, ἢ ἐλάττους, οὐκ ἴσων μὲν ἁπάντων κατὰ τὸ μῆκος, ἀλλὰ τὸ μέγιστον αὐτῶν οὐ μεῖόν ἐστιν ἡμίσεος ποδὸς Ῥωμαϊκοῦ. ἡ δ' ὅλη τῆς οὐσίας αὐτοῦ φύσις, παραπλησία πώς ἐστιν ἀρίστῃ κασσίᾳ, καλουμένη μὲν ὑπὸ τῶν κομιζόντων αὐτὴν ὀνόματι βαρβαρικῷ δισυλλάβῳ, τὴν μὲν πρώτην συλλαβὴν ἐκ τοῦ γ καὶ ι ἔχοντι, τὴν δὲ δευτέραν ἐκ τοῦ ζ καὶ ι. ταῦθ' ἡμῖν ἱκανὰ καὶ περὶ κινναμώμου λέλεκται.

Κεφ. ιδ'. [*Περὶ τῆς τῶν ὑπολοίπων δυνάμεων δοκιμασίας τε καὶ ἐκλέξεως.*] Γεγραμμένου δὲ ἐφεξῆς ἀγαρικοῦ δόλωσιν οὐδεμίαν ἐπιδεχομένου, τοῦτ' ἀρκέσει μόνον ἀκούειν, ὃ καὶ παρὰ τοῖς πρόσθεν εἴρηται, τὸ κουφότατον ἐν αὐτῷ κάλλιστον εἶναι· τὸ πυκνὸν δὲ καὶ βαρὺ καὶ ξυλῶδες φαυλότατον. ὅσον δ' ἐν τῷ μεταξὺ τούτων ἀφέστηκε τοῖς γνωρίσμασιν ἑκατέρου, τοσοῦτον καὶ τῇ δυνάμει. τὰ δὲ ἐφεξῆς τῶν προγεγραμμένων, ἥ τε σμύρνα καὶ ὁ κόστος, οὐ χαλεπὰ γνωρίσαι τοῖς ἤδη προεορακόσιν· εἰδέναι δὲ δεῖ

ſingula vero ipſa ex uno fundo veluti fruticulus quidam enaſcuntur: hic ſex, ille ſeptem ramorum propagines obtinens, aut paulo plures, aut pauciores, non aequales ſane omnes longitudine, ſed maximus ipſorum dimidio pede Romano minor non eſt. Porro tota ipſius ſubſtantiae natura praeſtantiſſimae caſſiae propemodum eſt conſimilis, quae ab importantibus ipſam barbarico nomine diſſyllabo nuncupatur, ita ut prima ſyllaba conſtet γ et ι, altera ex ζ et ι. Haec nobis de cinnamomo dicta ſufficiant.

Cap. XIV. [*De reliquarum medicinarum probatione et electione.*] Caeterum quoniam agaricum deinceps ſcriptum nullam adulterationem recipit, hoc ſolum intellexiſſe erit abunde, quod etiam priores tradiderunt, leviſſimum in ipſius genere eſſe laudatiſſimum; denſum autem, grave lignoſumque, deterrimum. Quantum vero in horum medio conſiſtens ab utroque notis receſſit, tantum quoque virtute deficit. Porro quae poſt commemorata habentur, nempe myrrha et coſtus, haud aegre cognoſcuntur iis qui

ἐπιτήδειον οὖσαν εἰς τὰς ἀντιδότους τὴν τρωγλοδύτιν λεγομένην σμύρναν· ἔνιοι δ' αὐτὴν ὀνομάζουσι Μιναίαν ἀπὸ χωρίου καθ' ὃ γεννᾶσθαί φασι τὴν καλλίστην. εὐοδμοτάτη δὲ ἔστω καὶ, ὡς πρόσθεν εἴρηται, μηδὲν ὀποκαλπαθίζον ἐχέτω. κρόκον δὲ τὸν κωρύκιον ἐπαινοῦσι μὲν ἅπαντες οἱ παλαιοὶ, μέχρι καὶ τῶν ποιητῶν· ἐγὼ δὲ ἀκριβῶς τό τε κωρύκιον ἄντρον ἐν ᾧ γεννᾶται, καὶ [886] τὸν κρόκον αὐτὸν ἐθεασάμην, εὐτραφῆ μὲν, οὐ μὴν ὑπὲρ (434) ἅπαντας τοὺς ἄλλους, οὔτ' ἰσχύϊ τῆς ἐν τῷ παραυτίκα ὀδμῆς οὔτ' ἐν τῷ μονίμῳ διαφέροντα. τούτοις δ' ἀξιῶ κρίνειν ὑμᾶς τὸν ἄριστον, οὐ τῷ κατὰ τὴν εὐτροφίαν ὑπερβάλλειν. πρόδηλον δ' ὅτι καὶ ξανθότατός ἐστιν, ὥσπερ εὐοδμότατος ὁ ἄριστος, καὶ χρόνῳ πλείονι παραμένων ἀκμαῖος. ἐπεὶ δὲ καὶ τούτου τίς ἐστι παραποίησις, οὐκ εὔγνωστος τοῖς μὴ πάνυ πολλάκις ἑορακόσι τὸν ἄριστον, ἄμεινον ἡμῖν ἐστιν ἐκ πολλοῦ προεωνημένοις αὐτὸν ἔχειν ἀποκείμενον ἐν ἐπιτηδείῳ τινὶ τῶν κατὰ τὴν οἰκίαν οἰκήματι, ὡς πρόσθεν εἴρηται. μέγιστον γάρ ἐστι δοκίμιον, ἐὰν παραμένῃ τοιοῦ-

jam antea viderint; fed fciendum venit myrrham troglodyten dictam antidotis recte accommodari; nonnulli eam vocant Minaeam a regione ubi praeftantiffimam gigni afféverant. Gratiffimi vero fit odoris et nullo vitiata liquore, uti a nobis antea eft commemoratum. Crocum fane omnes veteres, adeoque poëtae ipfi coryceum commendant; ego vero tum coryceum antrum in quo nafcitur, tum crocum ipfum exacte fum fpeculatus, procerum fane, non tamen fuper univerfos alios aut robore odoris praefentanei, aut diuturni differentem. His autem optimum vos judicare cenfeo, non quod proceritate excellat. Jam vero omnibus conftat optimum effe, tum flaviffimum, tum odoratiffimum, et longo tempore in vigore fuo perfiftentem. Quoniam vero et hic adulteratur, ita ut haud facile poffit dignofci, praeterquam ab iis qui faepe admodum praeftantiffimum viderint, fatius nobis eft ex longo tempore antea coemptum in apto quodam aedium receptaculo repofitum habere, ficuti prius a me dictum eft. Maxima enim eft probatio,

τος ὢν ὁποῖος ἐλήφθη. τοῦ γὰρ νενοθευμένου καὶ ἡ χρόα καὶ ὀδμὴ διὰ ταχέων ἐκλύονται. περὶ δὲ κασσίας ἀναγκαῖόν ἐστι μοι μνημονεῦσαι τοῦ γεγραμμένου κατὰ πολλὰς τῶν φαρμακιτίδων βίβλων, ὡς ἄρα τοῖς ἀποροῦσι κινναμώμου διπλάσιος ὁ τῆς κασσίας σταθμὸς ἐμβλητέος ἐστί. σκώπτων γὰρ τοῦτο Σάτυρος ὁ διδάσκαλος ἡμῶν ἔλεγεν, ὡς Κοΐντου τῶν εὐπραπέλων λόγων ἕνα καὶ τόνδε λέγοντος, ὅμοιόν τι ποιεῖν τοὺς κελεύοντας διπλασίαν ἐμβάλλειν ἡμᾶς κασσίαν, ὅταν ἀπορῶμεν κινναμώμου τοῖς ἀξιοῦσιν, ὅταν μὴ σχῶμεν οἶνον Φαλερῖνον, ποιεῖν διπλάσιον πίνειν τοῦ πιπρασκομένου κατὰ τὰ καπηλεῖα, κἂν ἄρτου ποτ' ἀπορῶμεν καθαροῦ, διπλάσιον ἐσθίειν τοῦ πιτυρίου καλουμένου. ἐμοὶ δ' ὁ λόγος οὗτος, ἢν μὲν περὶ ἑνός τινος αὐτοῦ καθ' αὑτὸ μόνου μέλλοντος εἰς χρῆσιν ἄγεσθαι, λέγηται, κατὰ πᾶν ἀληθής τε καὶ ἄμεμπτος εἶναι δοκεῖ, ἐν συνθέσει δὲ πολλῶν, οὐκέθ' ὁμοίως ἀληθής. ἓν μὲν γὰρ ὁτιοῦν εἰ δέοι προσενέγκασθαι, καθάπερ εἰ τύχοι ῥοῦν, ἢ ἀψίνθιον, ἢ ἶριν, ἢ γεντιανὴν, ἢ ὁτιοῦν ἄλλο τοιοῦτο φάρμακον, εἰ

ſi talis permaneat qualis fuerit aſſumptus, nam adulterati et color et odor celeriter evaneſcunt. At de caſſia neceſſarium eſt mihi commemorare id quod in multis medicamentoriis libris memoriae proditum eſt, nempe cinnamomi penuria duplicatam caſſiae portionem eſſe injiciendam. Quippe Satyrus praeceptor noſter hoc irridens dicebat, tanquam Quinto imperitam orationem unam etiam hanc proferente, ſimile quippiam eos facere qui caſſiam duplicatam injicere praecipiunt cinnamomi inopia, quemadmodum qui jubent vini Falerni penuria duplicatum id quod in tabernis venditur eſſe bibendum. Et ſi panis nonnunquam deſit purus, furfuracei dicti duplicationem eſſe ingerendam. Mihi vero ratio haec placet, et ſi de uno quodam ipſo quod per ſe privatim in uſum perduci debeat dictum fuerit, in totum vera et vitii expers eſſe videtur. In compoſitione autem multorum, non item vera. Unum enim quodcunque ſi aſſumere oporteat, verbi gratia Rhu, aut abſinthium, aut iridem, aut gentianam, aut aliud

διπλάσιον αὐτοῦ μοχθηρὸν ἀντὶ τοῦ καλλίστου προσφέροι τις, ἢ εἴσωθεν, ἢ ἔξωθεν ἐν τῷ σώματι, βλάψει διπλάσιον. ὅταν δὲ ἀναμίξαι δέῃ πολλοῖς τοῖς κατὰ μέρος ἕν τι κάλλιστον, αὐξήσειν τὴν τῶν ἄλλων δύναμιν ὑπισχνούμενον, ἂν ἀπορῶμεν τοῦ γενναιοτάτου, διπλασίῳ χρῆσθαι τῷ τὴν αὐτὴν ἔχοντι κατὰ γένος ἐπαγγελίαν, οὐδὲν ἂν εἴη χεῖρον, εἰ καὶ φαυλότερον φαίνοιτο τοῦ καλλίστου. ἔστι δ' ἡ κασσία πλησίον τοῦ κινναμώμου τῷ γένει. καὶ γὰρ καὶ γίνεταί ποτε κιννάμωμον ἐκ μεταβολῆς αὐτῆς, ὥστε ὅλον μὲν ὁρᾶσθαι τὸ οἷον δένδρον ἀκριβὲς κασσίαν. ἀκρέμονας δέ τινας ἐν αὐτῷ κινναμώμου, συνεχεῖς τοῖς κλάδοις τῆς κασσίας εὑρίσκεσθαι. παραπλήσιον δέ ἐστι τὸ τοιοῦτον οὐ τῷ κατὰ τοὺς οἴνους ἢ τοὺς ἄρτους, οἷα ὁ Κόϊντος ἔλεγεν, ἀλλὰ τῷ κατὰ τὰς ἐν τῷ βίῳ πράξεις, ἐν οἰκοδομίαις, ἐν ναυπηγίαις, ἐν ἄρσεσι βαρέων σωμάτων, καὶ μεταφοραῖς, ἐν πόλεσιν, ἐν ἁπάσαις ταῖς βοηθείαις, ἐν αἷς τὸ δι' ἑνὸς ἰσχυροῦ γινόμενον, ὅταν οὗτος μὴ παρῇ, διὰ δυοῖν ἀσθενεστέρων ἐπιτελεῖται. ταῦτα μὲν οὖν ἐκ τοὐναντίου ἐπι-

ejusmodi medicamentum quodlibet, fi duplum ipfius pravum loco praeftantiffimi adferas, vel extrinfecus, vel intus in corpore, duplicatum oberit, quum autem multis particularibus unum excellentiffimum mifcere convenit, aliorum virtutem augebit fimpliciter inditum, fi generofiffimi copia non datur eo quod idem genere promittit, duplicato uti, malum nullum fuerit, etiamfi optimo videatur deterius. Caffia vero cinnamomo genere proxima eft, ut quae nonnunquam ex mutatione ipfa evadat cinnamomum, ut totum quidem veluti arbor exacta caffia videatur, furculi autem nonnulli in ea cinnamomi, ramis caffiae continui reperiantur. Perfimile autem eft hujusmodi non ei quod in vinis aut pane folet accidere, quemadmodum Quintus ajebat, fed ei quod in vitae actionibus, aedificationibus, navium ftructuris, gravium corporum elevationibus, translationibusque, in urbibus, in omnibus praefidiis accidit, in quibus quod per unum validum efficitur, hoc abfente per duos imbecilliores adminiftratur. Haec

κεχειρήσθω τῷ τοῦ Κοΐντου λόγῳ, πρὸς τῷ μὴ πάντῃ δοκεῖν ἀπόβλητον εἶναι τὴν πρόσταξιν τῶν ἀξιούντων, ἀντὶ τοῦ κινναμώμου διπλάσιον ἐμβάλλειν τῆς κασσίας. ἐγὼ μέντοι διὰ παντὸς ἐνέβαλον κινναμώμου. πᾶσι γὰρ οἷς ἐσκεύασα τὸ φάρμακον, ἢ φίλοις αὐτοκράτορσιν, ἢ πλουσίοις, οὐ χαλεπὸν ἦν τοῖς μὲν αἰτῆσαι παρὰ τοῦ βασιλέως, τοῖς δὲ καὶ πρίασθαι παρά τινος. τὸ δὲ προσθεῖναι τούτῳ ὅτι μηδ' ὁσάκις ἐσκεύασα τοῖς αὐτοκράτορσιν, ἠπόρησά ποτε κινναμώμου, προφανῶς ἐστι περιττόν. περὶ μέντοι τοῦ καρπησίου τὴν Κοΐντου γνώμην, ἣν οὐ παρὰ Σατύρου μόνον, ἀλλὰ καὶ ἄλλων μαθητῶν ἤκουσα τοῦ Κοΐντου, διελθεῖν ἄμεινον. ἐνέβαλλε γὰρ ἐκεῖ [887] νος, ὥς φασιν, ὅταν ἠπόρει κινναμώμου, τὸ καρπήσιον, ὡς οὐδὲν ἀπολειπόμενον εἰς δύναμιν ἀρίστης κασσίας, καὶ πλεῖστον γοῦν αὐτοῦ κομίσας ἐγὼ διὰ τοῦτο, κατὰ τὴν γενομένην μοι τῶν ἀντολικῶν χωρίων ὁδοιπορίαν ἐπιμελῶς κατατιθέμενος, ἔχω μέχρι νῦν πάμπολυ, διασῶζον ὀσμήν τε καὶ γεῦσιν, εἰ καὶ μὴ τὴν ἴσην τῇ πρόσθεν, ἀλλ' οὐκ ἐξίτηλόν γε παντάπα-

igitur contra Quinti orationem tractata fint, ne omnino repudianda effe fententia eorum videatur, qui in vicem cinnamomi caffiae duplum injiciendum cenfent. Ego vero femper cinnamomum indidi. Nam omnibus quibus medicamentum praeparavi, aut amicis imperatoribus, aut opulentis non difficile erat: aliis quidem a rege petere, aliis etiam a quodam coemer . At huic adjicere quod nunquam quoties imperatoribus confeci medicamentum cinnamomi laboraverim inopia, plane eft fuperfluum. At vero de carpefio Quinti fententiam quam non a Satyro folum, verum etiam ex aliis quoque difcipulis Quinti audivi, praeftat commemorare. Ille fiquidem injiciebat (ut ajunt) quum cinnamomi facultas non dabatur, carpefium, ceu optima caffia viribus nihil inferius, eoque magnam ipfius copiam quum ex profectione, quam in orientalibus regionibus fubii apportatam diligenter repofuerim, in hunc ufque diem non parvam habeo, quod et odorem et guftum confervet, licet non priori aequa-

σιν. ἔστι δ᾽ ὁμοία μὲν τῷ καλουμένῳ φοῦ κατὰ γένος, ἰσχυροτέρα μέντοι, καί τι καὶ ἀρωματίζον ἔχουσα. πλεῖστον δ᾽ ἐν τῇ Σίδῃ τῆς Παμφυλίας τὸ καρπήσιον τοῦτο γεννᾶται· διὰ τοῦτο καὶ εὐωνότατόν ἐστιν, ὡς εἴ τις ὑμῶν ἐκεῖ ποτε γένοιτο, λαμβανέτω πλεῖστον, εἰδὼς ἐπὶ πλείονα χρόνον ἐξαρκοῦν αὐτῷ. λεπτὰ δέ ἐστι τὰ κάρφη, παραπλήσια τοῖς ἀκρέμοσι τοῦ κινναμώμου, καὶ καλοῦσιν οἱ ἐπιχώριοι τὸ μὲν ἕτερον αὐτῶν λαέρκινον, τὸ δὲ ἕτερον τὸ πικρὸν, ὅπερ καὶ βέλτιόν ἐστιν. ἑκατέρου δὲ ἀπὸ τοῦ ὄρους ἡ ἐπωνυμία καθ᾽ ὃ φύεται. πολὺ δ᾽ ἔχων αὐτοῦ καὶ εἰς ἄλλα πολλὰ τῶν κατὰ μέρος ἐπειράθην, εἰς ἅπερ καὶ τοῦ καλουμένου φοῦ βάλλομεν. ἔστι γὰρ αὐτὸ παραπλήσιον μὲν, ἰσχυρότερον δὲ, καὶ ὡς ἔφην, ἔχον τι ποιότητος ἀρωματιζούσης ἐν ὀσμῇ τε καὶ γεύσει. τούτων δ᾽ ἁπάντων ὧν περὶ κασσίας εἶπον ἀναγκαιότατόν ἐστι διορίσασθαι ποίαν ἐμβλητέον ἐστὶ κασσίαν, ἐπειδὴ τὴν μὲν Γιζὶ μάλιστα ἐπαινοῦσιν, ἐφεξῆς δὲ τὴν μοτὼ καλουμένην, εἰσὶ δὲ οἳ καὶ τὴν ἀρηβὼ καὶ τὴν δαφνῖτιν. ὅτι μὲν οὖν

lem, certe non omnino evanidum. Eſt autem ſimilis genere phu appellato, ſed valentior, et nonnihil etiam odoratum repraeſentans. Plurimum autem in Side Pamphyliae carpeſiun hoc gignitur, atque adeo facillime emitur, quare ſi quis veſtrum illuc quandoque contendat, copioſiſſimum exportet, ſciens diu id ſibi ſufficere. Porro tenues feſtucae ſunt perſimiles ſurculis cinnamomi, vocantque indigetes alterum ipſorum laertium, alterum amarum, quod etiam praeſtantius eſt. Utriusque autem a monte ubi naſcitur cognomentum exiſtit, cujus ſane quum copiam haberem, etiam et alia pleraque particularia ſum expertus, ad quae et pheu dictum immittimus; eſt enim ipſum conſimile quidem, ſed valentius, et ut dixi odoratae qualitatis nonnihil, et odore et guſtu repraeſentans. Caeterum ex his omnibus quae de caſſia retuli maxime eſt neceſſarium deſinire qualis caſſia ſit injicienda, quum Gizi maxime commendant. Mox appellatam moton. Sunt qui arebo et daphniten. Quod igitur Gizi cinnamomo in

ἡ Γιζὶ παραπλήσιον κινναμώμῳ κατὰ πάντα ἐστὶν εἴρηταί μοι καὶ πρόσθεν. ἡ γοῦν συνεχέστατα παρὰ τῶν περὶ τὰ τοιαῦτα δεινῶν, ὡς κιννάμωμον πιπρασκομένη, ταὐτοῦ γένους ἐστίν. ἀλλὰ τῆς γε συριγγίδος ὑπό τινων ὀνομαζομένης, ὁ νεώτερος Ἀνδρόμαχος ἐμβάλλειν ἀξιοῖ. πᾶσι δ' αὕτη γινώσκεται, καὶ γὰρ καὶ εὐωνοτάτη πάντων ἐστὶ, τὸν μὲν ἔξωθεν φλοιὸν, ὅνπερ καὶ σύριγγα καλοῦσιν, ἰσχυρὸν ἔχουσα κατ' ὀσμήν τε καὶ γεῦσιν, τὸ δ' ἔνδον ἀσθενέστατον, ὡς μηδεμίαν αὐτοῦ χρείαν ἡμῖν γίνεσθαι. διὰ μὲν οὖν τῶν προγεγραμμένων ἐλεγείων ἀδιορίστως εἴρηται τὸ τῆς κασσίας ὄνομα. κατὰ δὲ τὴν πεζῇ γεγραμμένην ὑπὸ τοῦ υἱέως αὐτοῦ πρόσκειται τῷ τῆς κασσίας ὀνόματι τὸ τῆς σύριγγος, ἥ τ' ἀπ' ἐκείνου μέχρι νῦν ἡμῖν παραδεδομένη διαδοχὴ τῶν σκευαζόντων τῷ αὐτοκράτορι, τὸ τῆς σύριγγος ὄνομα προσκείμενον ἔχει. ἐφεξῆς δὲ τῆς προγεγραμμένης ὁ Ἀνδρόμαχος Ἰνδικὴν νάρδον κελεύει βαλεῖν, ἥνπερ καὶ στάχυν ὀνομάζομεν νάρδου, καίτοι ῥίζαν οὖσαν, ἀπὸ τῆς πρὸς τοὺς ἀστάχυας ὁμοιότητος κατὰ τὴν μορφὴν, ἐφ' ἧς φυλάττεσθαι

omnibus refpondeat, dictum a me antea quoque eft. Nam quae maxime fibi continua ab hujusmodi rerum peritis ceu cinnamomum venditur, ejusdem generis exiftit. Sed fiftulam dictam ab aliquibus, junior Andromachus injiciendam cenfet. Omnibus autem haec cognofcitur, quin etiam facillime omnium comparatur, exteriorem fane corticem, quem et fiftulam dicunt fortem, tum odoratu, tum gufu obtinet, medullam vero imbecillimam, ut nullus ipfius ufus effe nobis poffit. Itaque praefcriptis elegiis indiftincte caffiae nomen prolatum eft, in pedeftri autem filii ipfius fcriptura adjectum invenias caffiae nomen fiftulae, ac ab illo in hunc usque diem tradita nobis fucceffio eorum, qui imperatori antidotum conficiunt, fiftulae nomen adjectum habet. Poft commemoratam fuperius Andromachus Indicam nardum indi jubet, quam et fpicam nardi appellamus, licet radix exiftat, a formae fimilitudine quam cum non fpicatis obtinet. In qua cavendum eft ne quis elotam dictam tradat. Eft autem illa iis qui unguenta prae-

Ed. Chart. XIII. [887. 888.] Ed. Baſ. II. (434. 435.)

χρὴ, μή πως ἀποδῷ τις ἡμῖν τὴν ἔκπλυτον ὀνομαζομένην. ἔστι δ' αὐτὴ τοῖς τὰ μύρα σκευάζουσι προϋπηρετηκυῖα κατὰ τὴν ἕψησιν αὐτῶν, ὡς εἰώθασιν, ἀκέραιος πιπρασκομένη. διὸ καὶ τὰς ὄμφας ὀνομαζομένας βαρβάρῳ γλώττῃ προσήκει λαμβάνειν, ὧν καὶ ἡ περιπεπλασμένη γῆ τῇ ῥίζῃ ἀφεψηθεῖσα τὴν ὀσμὴν ἔχει τῆς νάρδου. σχοῖνον δὲ ἐπὶ τούτοις τὴν ἐξ Ἀραβίας ἐμβάλλειν κελεύει, καλουμένην ὑπὸ τῶν πολλῶν, οὐκ οἶδ' ὅπως ἄνθος σχοίνου, καίτοι γ' ἡμῶν οὐ πάνυ τι τοῦ ἄνθους εὐπορούντων, ὅλης τῆς κομιζομένης πόας ἐπιβεβρωμένης πολλάκις ἄνωθεν ὑπὸ τῶν καμήλων· ἥδιστά τε γὰρ αὐτὴν νέμονται καὶ πλείστην ἔχουσιν ἐν ταῖς Ἀραβίαις ὁδοῖς γεννωμένην. ἔστι δ' εὔωνόν τε τὸ φάρμακον καὶ μόνῳ τῷ τῆς ὀσμῆς ἀκμαίῳ κρινόμενον, ἐπειδὴ διὰ ταχέων ἀποπνεῖ τὸ εὐῶδες αὐτῆς. ἐφεξῆς δὲ γράφοντος τοῦ Ἀνδρομάχου, καὶ λίβανον μίσγοιο καὶ ἀγλαΐην στήσαιο, τὴν ἀγλαΐην οὐ χρὴ ζητεῖν ἡμᾶς ὡς ἄλλου τινὸς φαρμάκου ὄνομα. διὰ (435) γὰρ τῆς πεζῇ γεγραμμένης τῷ νεωτέρῳ Ἀνδρο [888] μάχῳ συνθέσεως τῆς ἀντιδότου

parant in coctione ipſorum, ſicuti conſueverunt, prius in uſum miniſteriumque adhibita, quae acaerios, quod eſt pura, venundatur. Quapropter etiam omphas appellatas barbarica lingua accipere convenit, quarum et circumlita terra radici decocta nardi odorem repraeſentat. Praeterea juncum rotundum Arabicum immitti praecipit, qui a vulgo, haud ſcio quomodo, junci rotundi flos dicitur; etſi nos non adeo floris copiam habeamus, tota quae advehitur herba ſubinde ex parte ſuperiori a camelis eroſa. Libentiſſime autem eam depaſcuntur et copioſiſſimam in Arabiae viis creſcentem habent. Eſt item parvi pretii medicamentum, et ſolo odoratus vigore diſcernitur, quum gratia illius odoris celeriter evaneſcit. Jam vero quum Andromachus ſcribit, thus miſcebis et aglaiam quod eſt pulchrum ſtatues, aglaiam non diſquirendum eſt ceu alterius medicamenti nomen. Nam in compoſitione antidoti pedeſtri oratione ab Andromacho juniore ſcripta et ea traditione quae hucusque ad nos

καὶ διὰ τῆς ἄχρι νῦν εἰς ἡμᾶς καθηκούσης παραδόσεως, οὔτε φαρμάκου τινὸς ὄνομά ἐστιν ἡ ἀγλαΐα· καὶ τὰς < ιβ'. ἕλκον τῷ σταθμῷ τὸ φάρμακον πάντα συμφώνως εἴρηται τῷ τε πρεσβυτέρῳ καὶ τῷ νεωτέρῳ Ἀνδρομάχῳ, καὶ οὐδὲν ἔξωθεν ἐκείνων πρόσκειται, καθ' οὗ τὸ τῆς ἀγλαΐας ὄνομα λέγεσθαί τις ἡγήσεται, ὥστ' ἴσως τὴν ἀγλαΐαν ἐπίθετον τοῦ λιβανωτοῦ τῷ συντιθέντι τὴν ἐλεγείαν ἔδοξε προσθεῖναι. ἐφεξῆς δὲ μέλανός τε πεπέρεως καὶ δικτάμνου καὶ πρασίου καὶ ῥήου μνημονεύει, γνωρίμων ἅπασι πραγμάτων. ἡ δ' ἐκ παραδόσεως ἡμῖν δεδομένη γραφὴ προσκείμενον ἔχει τοῦ πεπέρεως τὸ βαρύσταθμον. μεῖζον δ' ἐστὶ τοῦτο τοῦ ἄλλου πεπέρεως, καὶ τὸν φλοιὸν ἔχει λεπτότερόν τε καὶ ἧττον ῥυσσόν. ἐπὶ δὲ τοῦ ῥήου καὶ αὐτοῦ παραποίησις μέν ἐστιν, ἐπειδὴ εὐθέως ἐν τοῖς χωρίοις ἐν οἷς γεννᾶται, πρόσφατον ἔνιοι λαμβάνοντες αὐτὸ καὶ ἀφέψοντες, ὡς ἀνεῖναι τὸν χυλὸν, ἐκεῖνον μὲν ἑψήσαντες πέμπουσιν ἡμῖν, ὡς εἰλικρινῆ καὶ ἄμικτον ὕδατι. τὸ δὲ ῥῆον ξηράναντες ὡς οὐδὲ αὐτὸ προαφεψημένον ἀποστέλλουσι. διὰ τοῦτ' ἐπί-

pervenit, neque medicamenti alicujus nomen eſt aglaia, et medicamentum duodecim drachmas pondere trahens omnino concordi ſententia et ſenior et junior Andromachus deſcripſit, ac nihil extra illa additur, de quo aglaiae nomen dici quis putaverit: quamobrem forte aglaia epithetum thuris auctori elegorum adjectum eſſe videtur. Deinde nigri piperis, dictamni, marrubii, rheu meminit, rerum omnibus cognitarum. At ſcriptura ex ſucceſſione nobis tradita adjectum habet piperis aequale pondus. Caeterum hoc majus eſt alio pipere, et corticem habet tenuiorem minusque rugoſum. At rheu quoque ipſum adulteratur, quandoquidem ſtatim ex regionibus ubi gignitur, recens nonnulli capientes ipſum decoquentesque, ut ſuccum demittat, ubi illum coxerint, nobis ceu purum, et aquae non mixtum transmittunt; rheon autem ſiccatum, tanquam neque id prius incoctum, ablegant; idcirco adulteratum cognoſcere oportet, iis facillimum

Ed. Chart. XIII. [888.] Ed. Baf. II. (435.)

στασθαι χρὴ γνωρίζειν τὸ πανουργηθὲν, εὐγνωστότατον ὂν τοῖς ἑορακόσι τὸ αὐτοφυὲς ῥῆον. οὔτε γὰρ τὸ διὰ τῆς ὄψεως αὐτοῦ κρινόμενον πυκνὸν καὶ συνηγμένον ἔχει τῆς ὅλης οὐσίας, ἀλλ' ἔστιν ἀραιότερον, ἐν τῇ γεύσει τε τὴν στύφουσαν ποιότητα παντάπασιν ἀμυδρὰν, ἢ οὐδ' ὅλως ἔχει, καίτοι γε ἰσχυρὰν ἔχοντος τοῦ ἀκμαίου ῥήου, τίτραται μέντοι καὶ αὐτὸ ταχέως. στοιχὰς δὲ φύεται μὲν πολλὴ πολλαχόθι τῆς γῆς. πλείστης δ' οὔσης ἐν Κρήτῃ καὶ ταῖς Κυκλάσιν ὀνομαζομέναις νήσοις, ἀφ' οὗ καὶ τοὔνομα αὐτῇ κατὰ τὴν Ἰβηρικὴν θάλασσαν κειμέναις. εὐτροφωτέρα δὲ ἐστι καὶ κρείττων ἡ ἐκ τῶν νήσων τῆς Κρητικῆς. πετροσέλινον γινώσκεται μὲν πᾶσιν ἐπῃνημένον τὸ Μακεδονικὸν, ὃ καὶ καλοῦσί τινες Ἐστρεατικὸν, ἀπὸ τοῦ χωρίου καθ' ὃ φύεται τὴν ἐπωνυμίαν αὐτῇ τιθέμενοι. παντελῶς δ' ὀλίγον ἐστὶ τὸ γεννώμενον ἐν ἐκείνῳ τῷ χωρίῳ, κρημνώδει τε ὄντι καὶ οὐ μεγάλῳ. τὸ δὲ Ἐστρεατικὸν Μακεδονικὸν ἐκ Μακεδόνων εἰς πάντα τὰ ἔθνη κομιζόμενον, ὀλίγον μὲν καὶ αὐτὸ κατὰ τὴν Μακεδόνων φύεται γῆν. ἀλλ' ὅπερ ἐπὶ τοῦ

deprehenſu, qui ſua ſponte naſcens rheon viderunt. Neque enim quod aſpectu ipſius judicatur denſum contractumque, totam ita habet ſubſtantiam, ſed rarius eſt, ac in guſtu aſtringentem qualitatem omnino obſcuram aut nullam obtinet, etſi validam occupet rheon, quum viget, perforatur autem et ipſum celeriter. Stoechas naſcitur copioſa ubique terrarum. Quum autem copioſiſſima proveniat in Creta et Cycladibus dictis inſulis, unde etiam nomen ipſi ex Hiſpanienſi mari inditum, procerior meliorque eſt quae ex Cretae inſulis petitur. Petroſelinon noſcitur quidem omnibus collaudatum Macedonicum, quod etiam nonnulli eſtreaticon a regione ubi gignitur, nomenclaturam ei imponentes, appellant. Omnino autem paucum eſt, quod in illo loco naſcitur praecipiti, neque magno. At Eſtreaticon Macedonicum a Macedonibus in omnes nationes apportatur; paucum ſane et ipſum in Macedonum terra provenit, verum quod in melle et vino Falerno, id etiam in petroſelino accidit.

μέλιτος καὶ τοῦ οἴνου τοῦ Φαλερίνου, τοῦτο καὶ ἐπὶ τοῦ πετροσελίνου συμβέβηκεν. εἰς ἅπασαν γὰρ σχεδόν γε τὴν οἰκουμένην οἱ ἔμποροι κομίζουσιν ὡς Ἀττικὸν μέλι καὶ οἶνον Φαλερῖνον, οὕτω καὶ Μακεδονικὸν πετροσέλινον, οὐ τοσούτου αὐτοῦ γεννωμένου, ὡς ἅπασι τοῖς ἔθνεσιν ἐξαρκεῖν, ἀλλ' ἐν Ἠπείρῳ πλεῖστον γεννᾶται πετροσέλινον, ὥσπερ ἐν ταῖς Κυκλάσι νήσοις τὸ μέλι. καὶ κομίζεταί γε τὸ μὲν ἐκ τῶν νήσων Ἀθήναζε, τὸ δὲ ἐξ Ἠπείρου πρότερον μὲν εἰς Μακεδονίαν, καὶ πλεῖστόν γε, καὶ σχεδὸν ἅπαν εἰς Θεσσαλονίκην, ἐκεῖθεν δ' ὡς Μακεδονικὸν ἐκφέρεται. καὶ κατὰ τὸν οἶνον δὲ τὸν Φαλερῖνον ὅμοιόν τι συμβέβηκεν. ἐν μικρῷ γάρ τινι χωρίῳ τῆς Ἰταλίας ὀλίγος γεννώμενος, ὡς δῆθεν αὐτὸς ἐκεῖνος ὢν εἰς ἅπασαν τὴν ὑπὸ Ῥωμαίοις γῆν εἰσκομίζεται, σκευαζομένων δ' ἄλλων οἴνων εἰς ὁμοίου πανουργίαν ὑπὸ τῶν περὶ ταῦτα δεινῶν. ἐὰν δ' ἀπορήσῃς ποτὲ Ἐστρεατικοῦ πετροσελίνου, μηδὲν ἡγοῦ χεῖρον ἔσεσθαί σοι τὸ τῆς θηριακῆς φάρμακον, ἐὰν ἕτερον ἐμβάλῃς. οὐ γὰρ ὡς δηλητηρίοις φαρμάκοις, ἢ ἰοβόλων θηρίων τοῖς

Nam in omnem fere terram mercatores ficut Atticum mel et vinum Falernum, ita quoque Macedonicum petrofelinum exportant; quum tamen ipfum non tantum generetur, ut univerfis gentibus fufficiat, fed in Epiro plurimum gignitur petrofelinum, quemadmodum in Cycladibus infulis mel. Atque hoc fane ex infulis Athenas importatur, illud ex Epiro prius quidem in Macedoniam, copiofiffimumque et prope totum in Theffalonicen, inde vero tanquam Macedonicum effertur. Ac in vino Falerno fimile quid accidit. Nam quum in parva quadam Italiae regione paucum generetur, ceu inde illud ipfum exiftat, in omnem Romanorum imperio fubjectam terram infertur, ita ut alia vina in fimilis adulterationem ab hujusmodi rerum peritis praeparentur. Quod fi vero eftreaticum interim defideres petrofelinum, nihilo pejus tibi fore putato theriaces medicamentum, fi alterum injicias. Non enim deleteriis medicamentis, aut virulentarum beftiarum morfibus adeo adverfatur, fed hydropicis imbecillibus, et

δήγμασιν ἐναντιοῦται, ἀλλ' ἐῤῥιμμένοις τοῖς ὑδερικοῖς, καὶ ὅσα πάθη ἄλλα τοιαῦτά ἐστιν, οὐ μὴν τῷ κυριωτάτῳ γε τῆς θηριακῆς ἐπαγγέλματι. ποιεῖ δ' αὐτὴν καὶ πικροτέραν δηλονότι τὸ Ἐστρεατικὸν πετροσέλινον, καὶ μάλιστα ἐὰν πρόσφατον ᾖ. διαφέρει γὰρ ὥσπερ δριμύτατον τῶν ἄλλων πετροσελίνων, οὕτω καὶ πικρότατον. τὴν δὲ τερμινθίνην οὐκ οἶδ' [889] ὅπως τὴν ἐκ Λιβύης ἐμβάλλειν ἐκέλευσεν ὁ Ἀνδρόμαχος, ἀτιμάσας γε τὴν ἐκ τῆς Χίου προκεκριμένην σχεδὸν ὑπὸ πάντων. ἐπαινῶ μὲν γὰρ καὶ τὴν ἐκ τῆς Λιβύης κομιζομένην ἀρίστην. οὐ γὰρ δὴ πᾶσά γέ ἐστιν ἀρίστη, καθάπερ ἡ ἐκ Χίου. γίνεται δὲ καὶ κατὰ τὴν Ποντικὴν γῆν καί τισιν ἄλλοις ἔθνεσι καλλίστη τερμινθίνη ῥητίνη, ἀλλ' ὑπερέχει πασῶν ἡ Χία κατ' ὀσμήν τε καὶ γεῦσιν. ἐφεξῆς δὲ τῶν προγεγραμμένων ὁ Ἀνδρόμαχος ἐν τῇ συνθέσει τῆς θηριακῆς ἔγραψε, ζιγγίβερι καὶ πενταπέτηλον ὅπερ ἐστὶ πεντάφυλλον πόαν ἐμβάλλομεν, οὔτε παραποιούμενα φάρμακα καὶ πᾶσι γιγνωσκόμενα. μετὰ δὲ ταῦτα πολίου μνημονεύει πᾶσι γνωρίμου καὶ μηδὲν ἔχοντος ὅμοιον, εἶτα

ſi qui ſint hujusmodi affectus, ſuccurrit, non tamen principaliſſimo theriaces promiſſo. Reddit autem ipſam amariorem indubie eſtreaticum petroſelinum, maxime ſi recens exiſtat. Differt autem ut acerrimum ab aliis petroſelinis, ita quoque amariſſimum. At terebinthinam haud ſcio quomodo Libycam Andromachus immittere praeceperit ea quae ex Chio eſt poſthabita, quum tamen ab omnibus propemodum praeponatur, quanquam et ex Libya optimam commendem; non enim quaelibet eſt optima, ſicuti quae ex Chio adſertur. Jam vero quae in Pontica terra et aliis quibusdam gentibus praeſtantiſſima terebinthina reſina naſcitur; verum Chia et odore et guſtu omnibus praecellit. Poſt commemorata deinceps Andromachus in theriaces compoſitione ſcripſit, gingiber et pentaphyllon ſeu pentapetalon herbam, quod eſt quinquefolium, injiciemus, medicamenta quae neque adulterantur et omnibus ſunt cognita. Deinde polii meminit omnibus noti et quod nihil ſimile obtinet, mox cha-

χαμαιπίτυος, ἐφ' ἧς τοσοῦτον χρὴ προσθεῖναί με κατὰ τὸν λόγον, ὡς πολλαχόθι τῆς γῆς γεννᾶται, καὶ κατ' ὀδμὴν καὶ γεῦσιν ἀκμαιότερον τῆς ἐν τῇ Κρήτῃ. φέρεται δ' ἡμῖν ἐκεῖθεν, ὡς καὶ τοὺς Καίσαρι σκευάζοντας ἀεὶ τῇ Κρητικῇ χρῆσθαι, καίτοι καὶ κατ' αὐτὴν τὴν Ῥώμην ἐν τοῖς προαστείοις καὶ τὴν χαμαιπίτυν καὶ τὴν χαμαίδρυν εὗρον εὐοσμοτέρας τῶν ἀπὸ τῆς Κρήτης, ὅταν γε μὴ πολλῷ κατακλυσθῶσιν ὄμβρῳ. ἔτι τε καὶ τοῦτο χρὴ γινώσκειν, ὡς φερομένων ἀπὸ Κρήτης τῶν βοτανῶν, ἐνειλιγμένων χαρτίοις, οἷς ἐπιγέγραπται τὸ τῆς ἑκάστης βοτάνης ὄνομα, τινὲς μὲν ἁπλῆν ἔχουσι τὴν ἐπιγραφὴν, τινὲς δὲ μετὰ προσθήκης τῆς πεδιάδος. εὑρήσεις δὲ τὴν πεδιάδα γενναιοτέραν, καίτοι τῶν πλείστων βοτανῶν ἐν τοῖς πεδίοις ἀσθενεστέρων γεννωμένων. στύρακα δὲ δῆλον ὅτι τὸν ἐν τοῖς καλάμοις φερόμενον ἐκ Παμφυλίας, ἐμβάλλειν προσῆκεν, ὀλίγιστόν τε γεννώμενον καὶ τοσούτῳ διαφέροντα τοῦ πολλοῦ τούτου στύρακος, ὅσον ὁ Φαλερῖνος οἶνος τοῦ πιπρασκομένου κατὰ τὰ καπηλεῖα. λαμβάνειν δ' αὐτοῦ χρὴ

maepityos, de qua tantum me in oratione adjicere oportet, nempe quod ubique terrarum crefcat, et odore et guftu ea quae in Creta provenit vehementior, adfertur autem nobis inde, ut etiam ii qui Caefari medicamentum conficiunt, femper Cretenfi utantur, etfi in ipfa quoque Roma, in fuburbiis, tum chamaepityn, tum chamaedryn, offenderim, iis quae ex Creta feruntur odoratiores, ubi non multo imbre fuiffent irroratae. Praeterea etiam hoc fcire expedit quod herbarum ex Creta venientium, involutarumque chartis quibus fuperfcriptum eft uniuscujusque herbae nomen, nonnullae quidem fimplicem habent defcriptionem, nonnullae vero, cum additamento, campeftris; invenies autem campeftrem generofiorem, etfi plurimae herbarum in campis generentur imbecilliores. Styracem conftat injiciendum effe, qui in arundinibus ex Pamphylia adfertur, quique pauciffimus gignitur, et tanto difcrimine a copiofo hoc ftyrace evariat, quanto Falernum vinum ab eo quod in tabernis

τὸν ὠχρότατον, εὔδηλον δ' ὅτι καὶ κατὰ ὀσμὴν οὗτός ἐστιν ἰσχυρότατος, καὶ κατὰ γεῦσιν οὐδὲν ἧττον. νάρδου δ' ἐφεξῆς ἐμνημόνευσεν ὁ Ἀνδρόμαχος, ὡς αὐτὸς προσέγραψε τῆς ἐκ Γαλατείας, ἣν συνήθως οἱ περὶ ταῦτα δεινοὶ Κελτικὴν ὀνομάζουσι. συγκέχυται γάρ πως τὰ τρία ταῦτα ὀνόματα καθ' ἑνὸς ἔθνους φερόμενα τοῦ Κελτικοῦ. καλοῦσι γοῦν αὐτοὺς ἔνιοι μὲν Γαλάτας, ἔνιοι δὲ Γάλλους, συνηθέστερον δὲ τὸ τῶν Κελτῶν ὄνομα. περὶ δὲ τῶν ἐφεξῆς γεγραμμένων τὸ μέν πού τι πρόσθεν εἴρηται, καθάπερ ἐπὶ Λημνίας γῆς καὶ μίλτου· καλεῖν δ' αὐτὴν ἄμεινον οὐ μίλτον, ἀλλὰ γῆν· ἔστι γάρ τις Λημνία μίλτος ἐν τῇ Μίλτῳ γεννωμένη, πρὸς ἄλλας χρείας ἐπιτήδειος, οὐ μὴν εἰς ἃς ἡ καλουμένη Λημνία σφραγίς. γέγραπται δὲ καὶ περὶ τούτων, ὥσπερ οὖν καὶ περὶ τῶν ἄλλων ἐν τῇ περὶ τῶν ἁπλῶν φαρμάκων πραγματείᾳ. τὰ δ' ἐφεξῆς γεγραμμένα φάρμακα σχεδὸν ἅπαντα καὶ γινώσκεται πᾶσιν ἰατροῖς, καὶ πανουργίαν οὐκ ἐπιδέχεται. τινὰ δ' αὐτῶν σαφέστερον δηλοῦται διὰ τῆς πεζῇ γεγραμμένης θηριακῆς. καὶ τὸ

venundatur. Caeterum ex ipfius genere capere oportet calidiffimum; conftat autem et odore hunc effe valentiffimum et guftu nihilo minus. Secundum haec nardi Andromachus commeminit, ut ipfe adfcripfit, ejus quae ex Galatia adfertur, quam confueto vocabulo hujusmodi rerum periti Celticam nominant; confunduntur enim quodammodo haec tria nomina de una gente Celtica prolata, vocant utique ipfos nonnulli Galatas, alii Gallos, fed familiarius nomen Celtarum eft. De fubfequentibus in fcriptura medicamentis partim fane prius dictum eft, quemadmodum in Lemnia terra et milto; praeftat autem eam vocare non milton, fed terram; eft enim aliqua Lemnia miltos in Milto proveniens, alios ad ufus idonea, non tamen ad quos Lemnia fphragis appellata. Verum de his quoque proditum eft quemadmodum de aliis in opere de fimplicibus medicamentis. Infequentia medicamenta prope univerfa et cognofcuntur omnibus medicis et dolum non recipiunt. Quaedam ipforum manifeftius indicantur in theriaca quae profa oratione fcripta eft. Item hoc

Δάκρυον εὖ μίσγοιο, βαλὼν κυανωπὸν ἀκάνθης.
δηλοῖ γὰρ τὴν ἐκ τῆς Αἰγυπτίας ἀκάνθης γεννωμένην ἀκακίαν. μόνον οὖν εἰπεῖν ἔτι περὶ θλάσπεως ἀναγκαῖόν ἐστιν, ἐπειδὴ καὶ σχεδὸν ἅπαντα ἐμβάλλουσι, τό τ' ἐκ Κρήτης φερόμενον καὶ τὸ πανταχόθι γεννώμενον, ὅπερ ἐστὶ τῇ χρόᾳ μὲν ὠχρόξανθον, τῷ σχήματι δὲ στρογγύλον πάνυ σμικρὸν, ὡς εἶναι κέγχρου (436) πολλοστὸν μόριον. ἄμεινον δὲ τὸ ἀπὸ Καππαδοκίας κομιζόμενον ἐμβάλλειν, τῇ χρόᾳ μὲν ἐπὶ τὸ μελάντερον ἀποκεχωρηκὸς πάμπολυ, τῷ σχήματι δὲ οὐκ ἀκριβῶς στρογγύλον, καὶ τῷ μεγέθει πολλῷ γε μεῖζον ἢ κατὰ τὸ προειρημένον. ἔχον δὲ κατά τι μέρος ἑαυτοῦ, [890] καὶ οἷον ἔνθλασμά τι μικρὸν, ἀφ' οὗ καὶ ὠνομάσθη θλάσπι. γεννᾶται δὲ ὥσπερ καὶ τοῦτο, οὕτω καὶ ἕτερον ἐν Καππαδοκίᾳ πάμπολυ. ὥστε οὐχ ἁπλῶς τὸ ἀπὸ Καππαδοκίας φερόμενον ἄριστόν ἐστιν, ἀλλὰ τὸ ἰδίως ἐν αὐτῷ γεννώμενον, ἀνόμοιον δὲ τῷ Κρητικῷ τε καὶ πολλαχόθι τῆς γῆς φυομένῳ. εἰ δέ τι καὶ ἄλλο μὴ σαφῶς εἴρηται διὰ τῶν ἐλεγείων μέτρων ὑπὸ τοῦ πρεσβυτέρου Ἀνδρο-

Caeruleae aſt ſpinae lacrima.
Innuit enim acaciam ex Aegyptia ſpina naſcentem. Itaque ſolum adhuc reſtat ut de thlaſpi dicamus, quoniam et fere omnia injiciunt, tum quod ex Creta adfertur, tum quod ubique naſcitur, quod colore quidem pallido flavum eſt, figura rotundum, admodum exiguum ut milii decima pars exiſtat. Satius autem eſt id quod ex Cappadocia evehitur immittere; quod colore ad nigrius permultum vergit, figura non exacte rotundum, et magnitudine multo majus quam ſupradictum. Caeterum habet in quadam ſui parte etiam veluti infractum quendam exiguum, unde etiam thlaſpi nominatum eſt. Creſcit autem ſicut et hoc, ita alterum quoque in Cappadocia copioſum. Quare non omnino id quod adfertur a Cappadocia optimum eſt, ſed quod proprie in ea naſcitur diſſimile Cretenſi, et quod diverſis terrae locis provenit. Porro ſi etiam aliud quippiam non perſpicue ſatis elegiacis numeris ab Andromacho ſeniore

μάχου, τουτέστι κεκρυμμένον, γινώσκοντί σοι τὴν ἄνευ μέτρου γραφὴν ὑπὸ τοῦ υἱέως αὐτοῦ γεγραμμένην Ἀνδρομάχου, καθάπερ καὶ τὸ,

Ἀκταίῳ μίσγοις,
Συγκεράσας μέλιτι,

τουτέστι μέλιτι τῷ Ἀττικῷ. κενταύριον γοῦν κατὰ μὲν τὴν ἔμμετρον γραφὴν οὐ προσδιώρισται ποῖον λέγει, κατὰ δὲ τὴν πεζῇ γεγραμμένην πρόσκειται τὸ λεπτὸν, διὰ τὸ καὶ ἄλλων εἶναι κενταύριον ἁδρόν. οὕτω καὶ ἀριστολοχίας εἴρηται λεπτῆς, ἔστι γὰρ καὶ ἄλλη τις ἁδρὰν ἔχουσα τὴν ῥίζαν, ὥσπερ καὶ τρίτη τίς ἐστιν ἐπὶ ταῖσδε στρογγύλη.

Κεφ. ιε'. [Περὶ τῆς σκευασίας τῆς θηριακῆς.] Εἴρηταί μοι καὶ πρόσθεν ὡς ἅπαξ μέν τις ἰδὼν σκευαζόμενον τὸ φάρμακον οὐκέτι δεήσεται θεάσασθαι δεύτερον, ἢ γ'. εἰς δὲ τὴν διάκρισιν τῶν ἀρίστων ἐν ἑκάστῳ γένει φαρμάκου οὐχ ἅπαξ καὶ δὶς καὶ τρὶς, ἀλλὰ πάνυ πολλάκις ἑωρᾶσθαι χρὴ τὰ δόξαν ἔχοντα γεννᾶσθαι κάλλιστα καθ' ἑκάστην χώραν. ἔχειν δ' οὖν χρὴ καὶ πρὸς τὴν τούτων

dictum ſit, id declaratum tibi eſt, qui ſcripturam filii ipſius Andromachi proſa expoſitam intelligas, quemadmodum et hoc:

Actaeo melle perungens
Omnia, quae miſces theriacae antidoto.

id eſt melle Attico. Centaurium itaque in ſcriptura ligata non diſtinctum eſt quale dicat, in pedeſtri vero adjectum eſt tenue, eo quod et aliud centaurium ſit amplum. Pari modo etiam ariſtolochiae tenuis dictum eſt; nam alia quoque invenitur procera radice, quemadmodum etiam tertia quaedam praeter has eſt rotunda.

Cap. XV. [*Quomodo theriace praeparetur.*] Diximus etiam antea eum qui medicamentum ſemel confici ſpectaverit, non amplius opus habiturum ut iterum aut tertio inſpiciat. Verum ut optima in ſingulis medicamenti generibus diſcernat, non ſemel biſve et ter, ſed admodum ſaepe ſpectaſſe convenit ea, quae praeſtantiſſima in unaquaque regione gigni creduntur. Habendae itaque

χρῆσιν παραγγέλματα, περὶ ὧν εἴπομεν ἤδη καὶ πρόσθεν, ἀλλὰ καὶ νῦν ἐν ὀλίγοις κεφαλαίοις περὶ πάντων ἐρῶ. τὰς μὲν ῥίζας ὧν ἂν ὦσι χρήσιμοι τεταμένον ἔχειν χρὴ τὸν φλοιὸν, οὐ ῥυσόν· ἀτρόφου γὰρ ῥίζης τοῦτο σημεῖον· τοὺς δὲ καρποὺς μετὰ τῶν ἀκρεμόνων τε καὶ βλαστημάτων ὀνομαζομένων εὐθαλεῖς, καὶ πολλοὺς ἅμα τοῖς περικαρπίοις· τὰ σπέρματα δὲ, ὥσπερ καὶ τὰς ῥίζας, εὔτροφα διὰ τοῦ τετάσθαι τὸν φλοιὸν γνωριζόμενα· τοὺς δὲ ὀποὺς καὶ τοὺς χυλοὺς μὴ κατεξηραμμένα ἐν τῷ χρόνῳ, μήτ᾽ ἀμυδρὰς ἔχοντα ἑκάστου τὰς ἑαυτῶν ποιότητας, ὀσμῇ τε καὶ γεύσει κρινομένας. οἱ μὲν οὖν καρποὶ μετὰ τῶν βλαστημάτων τε καὶ περικαρπίων, ἀνθῶν τε καὶ φύλλων, ὅσα περ τούτων εἰς τὴν θηριακὴν ἐμβάλλονται. τῶν δὲ βοτανῶν, σκορδίου, καλαμίνθης, πρασίου, στοιχάδος, δικτάμνου, πολίου, χαμαίδρυος, χαμαιπίτυος, ὑπερικοῦ, κενταυρίου. αἱ ῥίζαι δὲ τῶνδε, ζιγγιβέρεως, ἴρεως, ῥήου, πενταφύλλου, κόστου, νάρδου Ἰνδικῆς, νάρδου Κελτικῆς, γεντιανῆς, μήου, ἀκόρου, φοῦ, ἀριστολοχίας λεπτῆς. σπέρματα δὲ ἐμβάλλεται τῷ φαρμάκῳ ταυτί.

ſunt etiam ad horum uſum indicationes, de quibus jam antea quoque egimus, verum etiam nunc paucis ſummatimque de omnibus tractabo. Radices quorumcunque fuerint utiles, intentum habere corticem, non rancidum oportet; id namque macrae radicis eſt indicium; fructus autem cum ſurculis germinibusque dictis praecellentes multosque, una cum iis quae fructibus adhaereſcunt; semina quemadmodum etiam radices, plena, procerave, ex cortice intento cognoſcuntur; liquores ſuccique non exiccati tempore neque invalidas ſinguli ſuas quisque habere qualitates et guſtu et odore judicantur. Fructus itaque cum ſurculis floribusque et foliis, quae in his ſunt, in theriacen immittuntur: hujusmodi herbarum, ſcordii, nepitae, marrubii, ſtoechados, dictamni, polii, chamaedrys, chamaepityos, hyperici, centaurii. Radices autem horum, gingiberis, ireos, rheu, quinquefolii, coſti, nardi Indicae, nardi Gallicae, gentianae, meu, acori, phu, ariſtolochiae tenuis. Semina autem medicamento

βουνιάδος, πετροσελίνου, θλάσπεως, ἄμμεως, ἀνήθου, μαράθρου, δαύκου, καρδαμώμου. ταῦτα μὲν οὖν πάντα τὰ τρία γένη τοῖς Αἰγυπτίοις ὅλμοις ἐμβάλλειν προσήκει, ἐπειδὴ σκληρότατοι τυγχάνουσιν ὄντες, ὡς μηδὲν ἐν τῷ κόπτεσθαι τῆς ἑαυτῶν οὐσίας προστρίβεσθαι τοῖς κοπτομένοις. ἐμβαλλέσθω δὲ ἅμα τοῖσδε καὶ ταυτὶ, ἀρτίσκοι σκιλλητικοὶ, ἀρτίσκοι θηριακοὶ, ἡδυχρόου μάγμα, πεπέρεως τε τὸ μέλαν καὶ τὸ λευκὸν καὶ τὸ μακρὸν, καὶ ῥόδα ξηρὰ, καὶ πρὸς τούτοις ἀγαρικὸν, καὶ κρόκος ἐὰν ξηρὸς ᾖ, σφραγὶς, καὶ ἡ ὀπτὴ χαλκῖτις, ἄμωμόν τε καὶ κιννάμωμον, καὶ ἡ σῦριγξ τῆς κασσίας, ὅ τε τοῦ βαλσάμου ὀπὸς, ἥ τ᾽ ἀκακίας, πλὴν εἰ μαλακή τις εἴη καὶ ὑγρὰ, τό τε καστόριον καὶ ἡ ἄσφαλτος, ἢ ὡς τινες ἀῤῥενικῶς ὁ ἄσφαλτος. εἴρηται γὰρ πολλάκις ὡς οὐδὲν χρὴ φροντίζειν τῆς τοιαύτης λεπτολογίας. οἴνῳ δὲ διαβραχέντα λελειώσθω σμύρνα καὶ κρόκος, ἐάν γε ἀσφαλέστερον εἶναί σοι δόξῃ, μὴ κόπτειν αὐτὸν ὑγρὸν ὄντα. [891] πάντες δὲ οἱ ὀποὶ οἴνῳ διαβρεχέσθωσαν, ὥστε καὶ λυθῆναι καὶ πρὸς τὴν λείωσιν ἐπιτήδειοι γενέσθαι, ὁ τοῦ

injiciuntur haec, napi, petrofelini, thlafpi, ameos, anethi, foeniculi, dauci, cardamomi. Haec itaque omnia tria genera Aegyptiis pilis indere convenit, quoniam duriffimae exiftunt, ne quicquam inter contundendum, ex ipfarum fubftantia iis quae laevigantur, confricetur. Immittantur una cum his etiam haec: paftilli fcillini, paftilli theriaci, hedychroi magma, piper nigrum, album et longum, rofae ficcae, praeterea agaricum, crocus fi ficcus fuerit, fphragis lemnia, tofta chalcitis, amomum, cinnamomum, fiftula caffiae, balfami liquor, acaciae, praeterquam fi mollis fit et liquida, caftoreum, bitumen, quod Graecis ἄσπαλτος et mafculino et foeminino genere dicitur; fed dictum mihi fubinde eft, hujusmodi ineptiarum rationem nullam effe habendam. Porro myrrha et crocus vino macerata laevigentur, fi quidem tutius effe videatur ipfum natura liquidum non contundere. Omnes autem liquores vino debent perfundi, ut et folvantur et ad laevigationem fiant idonei, ut fagapeni, panacis, papa-

σαγαπηνοῦ, ὁ τοῦ πάνακος, ὁ τῆς μήκωνος, ὃν δὴ καὶ μηκώνειόν τε καὶ ὄπιον ὀνομάζουσιν, ἥ τε ἀκακία, ὅταν ὑγροτέρα σοι δόξῃ, καὶ δύσκοπτος ὑπάρχῃ, ὅ τε τῆς ὑποκυστίδος χυλὸς καὶ ὁ τῆς γλυκυῤῥίζης. τὸ δὲ θλάσπι καὶ τὸ τῆς γογγυλίδος σπέρμα κατὰ μὲν τὰς πρώτας σκευασίας, ὥσπερ ἑώρων τοὺς πρὸ ἐμοῦ σκευάζοντας, καὶ αὐτὸς ἐνέβαλον ἅμα τοῖς κοπτομένοις εἰς ὅλμον, εἶτά ποτε θεασάμενος ἐμπεπλασμένα διὰ γλισχρότητα τῷ κύτει τοῦ ὅλμου, κατὰ θυίαν ἐδικαίωσα μόνα προλειώσας, ἐπιχέαι οἶνον ἐπ' ἐκεῖνα, μέχρις ἂν ἀκριβῶς ὅλα διαλυθῇ, καὶ μετὰ ταῦτα μιγνύναι τοῖς ἐν τῷ οἴνῳ ἰδίᾳ βεβρεγμένοις τε καὶ λελειωμένοις. καὶ τὸν λιβανωτὸν δὲ λειοῦν ἄμεινον ἰδίᾳ καθ' ἑαυτὸν ἐν θυείᾳ κούφως, ὡς μὴ πλατύνοιτο, κἄπειτα διαττήσαντας ἔχειν ἕτοιμον ὡς ἐπιπάττειν, εἴπερ ἐθελήσειας, τοῖς μετὰ τοῦ οἴνου λελειωμένοις. τὸ δὲ κόμμι καὶ διαβρέχειν ἐν οἴνῳ ἀναγκαῖον καὶ λειοῦν αὐτό τε καθ' ἑαυτὸ καὶ μετὰ τοῦ λιβανωτοῦ. ταῦτα μὲν οὖν ἅπαντα καθ' ὃν εἴρηται τρόπον παρασκευαζέσθω, τὰ μὲν ἐν θυείᾳ μετὰ τὸ

veris, (quem et meconium et opium nominant) item acacia, quum liquidior tibi videatur, et tundi contumax ſit, ad haec hypocyſtidis ſuccus et dulcis radiculae; at thlaspi et rapae ſativae ſemen in prima confectione, quemadmodum videbam eos qui ante me praeparabant, etiam ipſe una cum iis quae contunduntur in pilam indidi; deinde aliquando conſpicatus corpori pilae interno propter viſcoſitatem adhaereſcere, volui ipſa privatim in mortario prius laevigare, ac deinde vinum eis ſuperſundere, uſque dum ad amuſſim tota diſſolverentur, inde miſcere iis quae in vino ſeorſim commaduerant detritaque erant. Ac thuris lacrimam praeſtat per ſe in mortario leviter conterere, ne dilateſcat, deinde ubi increveris, in promptu habere, ut inſpergas ſi libeat iis quae ex vino laevigata ſunt; gummi vino etiam irrigare vino oportet, idemque tum privatim tum cum thuris lachryma in pulverem redigere. Haec quidem omnia quo

εἶναι λελειωμένα, τὰ δὲ διηττημένα καὶ λελειωμένα ξηρά. κατὰ δὲ τὸν καιρὸν αὐτὸν τῆς ἁπάντων ἑνώσεως τηκέσθω μετὰ μέλιτος ἐν ἀγγείῳ διπλῷ πρώτη μὲν ἡ ῥητίνη, μετὰ ταύτην δὲ ὁ στύραξ καὶ ἡ χαλβάνη, προτεθλασμένα καὶ προκεκομμένα κατὰ τὸν ὅλμον ὑπέροις, ἢ μοχλοῖς σιδηροῖς, παρασταζομένου βραχυτάτου μέλιτος ὠμοῦ, καὶ μετὰ ταῦτα διὰ τῶν ἡμετέρων δακτύλων πλατυνόμενα, προσεμβαλλέσθω τὶ καὶ τοῦ μέλιτος τετηγμένῃ ῥητίνῃ, καὶ οὕτω πάλιν ἐπιτεθειμένου τοῦ πώματος τῷ ἀγγείῳ διαλυέσθω. βέλτιον γὰρ μηκέτι κινεῖν τὸ μέλι τούτων ἐμβληθέντων, ἀλλὰ πωμάσαντας τὸ ἐνεστηκὸς ἀγγεῖον τῷ ὕδατι τὴν ἕψησιν ποιεῖσθαι. τηκομένων δὲ τούτων ἐπεμβαλλέσθω τοῖς μετὰ τοῦ οἴνου λελειωμένοις τὰ ξηρὰ, καὶ ἀναμιγνύσθω μέχρι πάχους ἱκανοῦ, καὶ οὕτω μετὰ βραχὺ τετηγμένα χλιαρὰ παραχείσθω τοῖς ἐν τῇ θυείᾳ διὰ μεγάλου δοίδυκος, ἰσχυροῦ τινος ἀνδρὸς ἑνοῦντος. καὶ ἐπειδὰν ἑνωθῇ καλῶς ἤδη τέ πως παχὺ φαίνηται τὸ ἐξ αὐτῶν, ἐπεμβάλλειν τοῦ μέλιτος ἀφεψημένου τε μετρίως καὶ δηλονότι καὶ ἀπηφρισμένου, καὶ

dixi modo praeparari debent, alia in mortario poſtquam pertrita fuerint, alia increta laevigataque arida. Quum autem omnia uniri debent, liqueſcunt, cum melle in vaſe duplici, prima ſane reſina, mox ſtyrax galbanumque prius confracta contuſaque in pila piſtillis, aut vectibus ſerreis, ita ut mellis crudi momentum adjungatur; poſt haec digitis noſtris dilatata, injiciatur etiam mellis nonnihil reſinae liquefactae, atque ita rurſus operculo vaſi impoſito diſſolvantur. Satius enim eſt non amplius mel his injectis commovere, ſed vaſe quod aquae inſiſtit operculato coctionem moliri. His autem liqueſcentibus immittantur ex vino laevigatis arida, miſceanturque dum abunde craſſeſcant, atque ita paulo poſt liquefacta, iis quae in mortario ſunt magno cochleari tepida adſundantur, ſic ut vir aliquis robuſtus ipſa in unitatem cogat. Poſteaquam probe coierint ac jam craſſum quod ex eis oritur appareat, ſuperinjicere mel decoctum mediocriter, et nimirum etiam deſpuma-

μετὰ τοῦτο τῶν διηττημένων, εἶτ' αὖθις τοῦ μέλιτος, εἶτ' ἤδη μιγνύναι χλιαρὰ τὰ τηχθέντα, καὶ τρίβειν ἰσχυρῶς πάντα κατὰ τὴν μεγάλην θυείαν μεγάλῳ δοίδυκι, προσεμβαλλομένων ὅσα περιττὰ τῶν ξηρῶν ἐστι καὶ τοῦ μέλιτος. ὅταν δ' ὑπὸ τοῦ δοίδυκος ἑνωθῇ πάντα κατὰ τὴν θυείαν, ἐμβάλλειν ὅλμῳ τηνικαῦτα, καὶ διὰ μοχλῶν σιδηρῶν ἀκριβῶς καθαρῶν, ὡς μηδὲν ἔχειν ἰοῦ, κόπτειν συνεχῶς ἐπαλείφοντα τοὺς μοχλοὺς ὀποβαλσάμῳ, κατέχονται γὰρ ἐν τῷ γλίσχρῳ τοῦ φαρμάκου, καὶ δυσκόλως ὑπὸ τῶν κοπτόντων ἀναφέρονται. ὅπως οὖν ἑτοίμως ἀνύοιτο τὸ ἔργον, χρίειν ὀποβαλσάμῳ χρὴ τὰ τοῦ μοχλοῦ πέρατος συνεχῶς, εἰς αὐτὸ τοῦτο δαπανῶντα πᾶν αὐτό. βέλτιον δ' ἐν ἡλίῳ κόπτειν, ἑνοῦται γὰρ οὕτω θᾶττον ἅπαντα, καὶ τοῦτο πράξαντας σκεπάζειν (437) χρὴ τὸν ὅλμον ἔχοντα τὸ φάρμακον ἐν αὐτῷ, καὶ μετὰ δ' ἡμέρας ἢ ε' κόπτειν ὁμοίως ἐν ἡλίῳ, καὶ τοῦτο ποιεῖν ἐκ διαλειμμάτων αὖθις καὶ αὖθις, ἡμερῶν στ' ἢ ζ' μέχρι δύο μηνῶν, ἢ πάντως μ' ἡμερῶν. ταῦτα μὲν οὖν

tum oportet, mox increta, deinde rurfus mel, poftea jam liquefacta mifcere tepida et omnia in grandi mortario, cochleari magno valenter conterere, adjectis quae ex aridis fuperfunt, item melle. Ubi vero omnia in mortario cochleari unita fuerint, indere tunc pilae oportet, et vectibus ferreis adamuffim puris, ut nihil aeruginis obtineant, continenter tundere, illinendo vectes opobalfamo, nam lentore medicaminis detinentur et aegre a tundentibus elevantur. Quo igitur prompte opus absolvas, vectis extrema continue opobalfamo perunges, in hoc ipfum totam ejus portionem infumens. Praeftaret autem in fole contundere, nam ita citius omnia in unitatem coëunt; atque hoc ubi feceris, pilam quae medicamentum in fe continet, obtegere convenit, atque fecundum quatuor aut quinque dies, fimiliter in fole contundere, atque id ex intervallo iterum atque iterum, dierum aut feptem usque ad duos menfes, aut omnino ad quadraginta dies facere. Haec itaque ceu ad medica-

ὡς πρὸς τὴν ἀρετὴν τοῦ φαρμάκου γέγραπται πάντα. τὸ δὲ μέλαιναν αὐτὴν γίνεσθαι, τοῦτο γὰρ οὐκ οἶδ᾽ ὅπως εἴθισται, καὶ ὅστις ἀποτυγχάνει τῆς χρόας ταύτης, καταγελᾶται, φυλακτέον μὲν ἡμῖν ἐστι, γνωστέον δὲ μηδὲν ἐκ τῆς χροιᾶς ὑπαλλάττεσθαι τῆς τοῦ φαρμάκου δυνάμεως. [892] γίνεται δὲ ἡ ἀποτυχία διὰ τὴν κεκαυμένην χαλκῖτιν ξανθὴν καὶ πυῤῥὰν γινομένην. καὶ γὰρ ἐλάχιστον αὐτῆς ἐμβαλλόμενον ὅμως ἐπικρατεῖ κατὰ τὴν χροιάν. ὅπως οὖν μηδὲ κατ᾽ αὐτὸ τοῦτο δοκῇ τις σφάλλεσθαι, προσεχέτω τὸν νοῦν οἷς ἐρῶ. τέτταρας μὲν τὰς πάσας δραχμὰς ἡ ἀντίδοτος λαμβάνει τῆς χαλκίτεως, ὀπτᾶν δὲ προσῆκεν αὐτὴν πολὺ πλέονα κατὰ τόνδε τὸν τρόπον. ἔμβαλε εἰς χυτρίδιον δραχμὰς τῆς ὠμῆς χαλκίτεως οὐχ ἧττους τῶν μ΄. κἄπειτα διακεκαυμένοις ἄνθραξιν ἐντιθεὶς τὸ χυτρίδιον ἄνευ πωμάτων, ὅταν χυθῇ τὸ φάρμακον, ἐποχούμενόν τε θεάσῃ τὸ κουφότατον καὶ ἀφρωδέστατον, αἴρειν αὐτίκα, καὶ θέντα χαμαὶ μὴ καθάπερ εἰώθαμεν ἐνίοτε, παραπλησίως τοῖς τὸ πῦρ ἐξάπτουσιν, ἐμφυσᾷν αὐτῇ. θαυμαστὸν γὰρ ὅπως ἐν τῷδε τὸ πυῤῥὸν

menti virtutem fcripta funt omnia. Ut autem nigrum ipfum evadat (hoc enim haud novi quomodo confuetum eft, et qui hoc colore fruftratur rifui eft) obfervare quidem oportet, fcire autem facultatem medicamenti nihil ex colore immutari. Accidit porro coloris fruftratio propter combuftam chalcitidem flavefcentem rufefcentemque. Etenim quamvis minima ipfius portio indatur, colorem tamen aliorum fuperat. Ne igitur in hoc ipfo quoque aliquis falli videatur, animum adhibeat iis quae dicturus fum. Quatuor fane in totum drachmas chalcitidis antidotum recipit, verum toftam multo copiofiorem hoc modo capiet, indito ollae crudae chalcitidis drachmas non pauciores quadraginta; deinde peruftis carbonibus ollam imponens fine operculo, quum medicamentum fufum fuerit, videasque fupervehi id quod leviffimum et maxime fpumofum eft, ftatim tolles, et humi pofito, non quemadmodum confuevimus interdum fimiliter iis qui ignem excitant, inflare ipfi oportet. Mirum enim

τῆς χρόας ἴσχει καὶ ξανθὸν, ἀλλὰ μηδ' ἐν ἡλίῳ τιθέναι. ψυγείσης δὲ λαμβάνειν ὅσον ἀφρωδέστερον ἐποχεῖται, μηδὲν ἔχον ἐν ἑαυτῷ μήτε πυῤῥὸν μήτε ξανθὸν μήτε ὠχρὸν, εἶτ' ἐξ αὐτοῦ πείρας ἕνεκα λαβόντα βραχὺ καὶ λειώσαντα θεάσασθαι μή τι κατὰ τὴν λείωσιν ἐμφαίνοιτο τῶν εἰρημένων χρωμάτων.. ἐὰν δὲ οἷον ἐλήφθη μένῃ πρασίζον, ἢ τεφρῶδες κατὰ τὴν χρόαν, ἐκ τούτου < δ'. ἐμβάλλειν. ὀλίγον γὰρ τὸ τοιοῦτον εὑρήσεις ἐν πολλῷ τῷ κεκαυμένῳ. τὰ μὲν οὖν ἀναγκαῖα πρὸς τὴν τῆς ἀντιδότου σύνθεσίν τε καὶ κατασκευὴν ἤδη λέλεκται πάντα. διαφωνησάντων δέ τι πρὸς τὴν γραφὴν ταύτην Δαμοκράτους τε καὶ Κρίτωνος, ἄμεινον ἔδοξέ μοι καὶ τὰ πρὸς ἐκείνων γεγραμμένα παραθέσθαι, καὶ πρότερον τὰ Δαμοκράτους, ἐπειδὴ καὶ τὴν χρῆσιν αὐτῆς ὅλην ἔγραψε σαφῶς. ἔστι δὲ δι' ἐμμέτρου λέξεως, ὡς εἴωθεν, ἥτις οὐ μόνον τὸ μνημονεύεσθαι ῥᾳδίως, ἀλλὰ καὶ τὸ μὴ παραποιεῖσθαι τὰς συμμετρίας ἀγαθὸν ἔχει. ἄρχεται τοίνυν ὁ Δαμοκράτης ἐν τῷ βιβλίῳ καθ' ὃ

quam interea rufus flavusque color excellat, ſed neque in ſole ponere conſilium eſt, ſed refrigerati capere quod ſpumoſius inſidet, nihil in ſe neque rufum, neque flavum, neque pallidum, continens; deinde ex eo cauſa experientiae ſumens exiguum laevigansque, ſpectabis num inter laevigandum aliquis ex praedictis coloribus appareat. Si vero quale ſumptum eſt maneat, porraceum aut cinereum colore, ex hoc drachmas quatuor injicere convenit. Tale ſiquidem exiguum in multo combuſto reperies. Itaque neceſſaria ad antidoti compoſitionem et ſtructuram omnia jam ſunt expoſita. Verum quum in eadem ſcriptura Damocrates et Crito nonnihil diſſentiant, ſatius mihi viſum eſt etiam ab illis prodita tradere, ac prius Damocratis ſententiam, quandoquidem totum ipſius uſum manifeſto deſcripſit, idque numeris, ut aſſolet, quae non ſolum quod facile teneri memoria, ſed etiam quod pondera ac menſurae in ea adulterari nequeant, conducit. Damocrates itaque libro

Ed. Chart. XIII. [892.] Ed. Baf. II. (437.)

τὰς ἀντιδότους γράφει, τόνδε τὸν τρόπον ἀπὸ τῆς κοινῆς χρήσεως αὐτῶν, καὶ τῆς κατὰ τὴν θηριακὴν ἰδέας.

Τὰς ἀντιδότους ἔχε προπαρεσκευασμένας,
Πρὸ πάντων θ' ἁπλῶς τὰ φαῦλα δηλητήρια,
Ὧν καὶ χάριν δοκοῦσιν εὕρεσιν λαβεῖν,
Καὶ τοῖς θανασίμοις ἀντιδώσεις φαρμάκοις.
Προδιδοὺς τι τοῖς ἔχουσιν ὑπόνοιάν τινα,
Μή τις μετὰ τροφὴν φάρμακον φαῦλον λάβῃ,
Ἐπὶ τῇ τροφῇ τε. προσφέρεσθαι δ' ὅταν δοκῇ,
Ἀναιρετικόν τις, μετὰ τροφὴν εἰληφέναι,
Ἐμέσαντι πάντως τὴν προσενεχθεῖσαν τροφὴν,
Καὶ δὶς δὲ διδόναι καὶ τρὶς αὐτὰς ἐπίτρεπε,
Ὅταν μένῃ σημεῖα φαύλων φαρμάκων.
Δώσεις δὲ καὶ τοῖς ἐντυχοῦσιν ἑρπετοῖς,
Τῶν ἰοβόλων τε θηρίων τοῖς δήγμασιν,
Ὕδρων, κεραστῶν, ἀσπίδων, καὶ διψάδων,
Καὶ τῶν ἐχιδνῶν, τῶν τε λυσσώντων κυνῶν.
Καὶ γὰρ τὰ τούτων ἐστὶ φαῦλα δήγματα,

quo antidota hunc in modum tradit, a communi ipforum ufu et theriaces fpecie incipit.

Antidota confert praeparata condere
In primis ad horrenda deleteria,
Quorum videntur inventa effe nomine:
Haec pharmacis adverfantur lethalibus
Si praebeas nonnulla fufpicantibus
Ne pharmacum quis inter cibum aut poftea
Affumat; ubi vero lethale ingefferit
Cibis modo inditis, hic prorfus omnibus
Vomitu rejectis, bis, ter, imperes ea
Quum manferint maligni figna pharmaci.
Item valet antidotum ferpentibus malis
Et beftiarum virulentis morfibus
Hydri, Ceraftae, dipfadis, fic afpidis
Et viperae, et canis quem rabies occupat.
Sunt namque morfus horum valde noxii

Τῶν τ' ἐν θαλάττῃ ἰοβόλων πάντων ἁπλῶς,
Καὶ τῶν τε λεπτῶν λεγομένων θηραφίων
Σφηκῶν, μελιττῶν, σκορπίων, ἀνθηδόνων,
Φαλαγγίων τε θανασίμων, καὶ μυγαλῆς.
Τῆς ἀντιδότου μὲν πλεῖον ἢ δραχμὴν μίαν,
Τοῦ καρύου τὸ μέγεθος, καὶ μικρῷ πλέον,
Κεκραμένοιν δὲ ζωρότερον κυάθων δέκα.
Οὐκ ἀρκέσει δὲ τοῖς κακῶς δεδηγμένοις
Ἅπαξ προσενεγκεῖν, ἀλλὰ διδόναι πολλάκις
Δεῖ, τοὺς θέλοντας ἐξαλεῖψαι τοὺς φόβους.
Δίδου δὲ πρὸς πάντα τὰ πάθη καὶ τὰς νόσους,
Ὅσαι φέρουσι τῷ χρόνῳ καχεξίας,
Τοὺς περιοδικοὺς πυρετούς τε καὶ ῥίγεα,
Μάλισθ' ὅσα μένει μετὰ πόνου πολὺν χρόνον,
Ἀποστάσεις φέροντα κυρίων τόπων,
Ταῖς πνευματουμέναις τε μήτραις, ἢ κόλον,
[893] Ὅσοι τε κύστιν, ἢ νεφροὺς ἀλγήμασι
Χρονίοις ὀχλοῦνται, κἂν μεθ' ἑλκῶν, ἢ λίθων.

Et quae mari degunt, ſimpliciter omnium
Mittentium virus, eorum quae vocant
Inſecta, veſpae, ſcorpionis atque apis,
Item phalangii nocentis plurimum,
Aranei muris, ipſa drachma amplius
Prodeſt antidoti, vel nux quantum continet
Mixtis meracioribus cyathis decem.
At morſibus malignis non ſatis ſemel
Offerre antidotum, ſed dabis frequentius,
Si tu metus ex toto cures tollere.
Idem propina vitia adverſus omnia, et
Morbos qui ſpatio pravum praebent corpori
Habitum, ad febres redeuntes, item tempore
Longo rigores haerentes, doloribus
Qui conferunt locorum abſceſſus principum,
Item valet vulvis diſtorſis flatibus,
Aut qui coli, veſicae, renum, ſentiunt
Longos dolores cum ulcere aut cum calculis.

Δώσεις δὲ καὶ τοῖς ἡπατικοῖς αὐτὰς καλῶς,
Ἀνάγουσί τ' ἐκ τοῦ θώρακος αἷμα πολλάκις,
Καὶ τοῖς τρυγῶδες ἀναφέρουσι καὶ πύον,
Ὅθεν ἂν φέρηται τοῦτο, κἂν ἐκ πνεύμονος.
Δίδου δὲ καὶ τοῖς ῥήγματα, ἢ καὶ σπάσματα
Εσχηκέναι λέγουσι τῶν ἐντός τινος,
Αἴρεις γὰρ αὐτῶν τοὺς φόβους τε τοὺς πόνους.
Προσενεγκέον δὲ τὴν τροφὴν μὴ ῥᾳδίως
Πέττουσι, κἂν λάβωσιν ὀλίγην παντελῶς,
Ἀεὶ δ' ἀποξύνουσι, καὶ παραυτίκα
Ὅσοις τ' ἀνάγκη δι' ἀποδημίας μακρᾶς,
Χρῆσθαι πάνυ φαύλοις ὕδασι, καὶ τούτοις δίδου
Τῆς ἀντιδότου μὲν ὅσον ἄγειν τριώβολον,
Ὕδατος δὲ θερμοῦ τρεῖς κυάθους, ἢ τέσσαρας
Πρὸ τῆς τροφῆς, ὥραισι τρισὶν, ἢ πλείοσι.
Τοῖς δὲ περὶ κύστιν, ἐκ γλυκέος κεκραμένης,
Αἱμοπτυϊκοῖς τε καὶ στόμαχον ἡλκωμένοις.
Τοῖς ῥευματιζομένοις δὲ τὸν θώραχ' ὅλον

Et ſi jecur negotium praebet, dabis
Rite, frequenter ſanguinem educentibus
Et pectore, faeculentum et pus reddentibus
Ex qua id feratur parte, vel ex pulmonibus,
Adhaec quibus rupta aut quaedam vulſa intima
Praebebis ipſis, nam dolores et metum
Tolles etiam queis haud prompte coquitur cibus
Quantumvis exiguus, aceſcit autem protinus,
Nec non propina, quos cogit perfectio
Longinqua aquis uti longe deterrimis,
His antidoti quantum tres pendent obboli
Aquae calentis cyathos tres, aut quattuor,
Horis ante cibum ternis da, vel pluribus,
Aut qui male veſica habent, aut ſanguinem
Spuunt, aut ſtomachi langueſcunt ulceribus,
Ex paſſo antidotum temperatum praebibent.
Et pectoris quos fluxiones totius,

Δώσεις, ἀφεψῶν εἰς ὕδωρ δεσμίδιον
Πολίου, τὸ μὲν βέλτιον, ἢ τοῦ Κρητικοῦ,
Ἢ καὶ Σκυθικοῦ τὸ κρεῖσσον, τοῦ Ποντικοῦ
Θᾶττον. στελεῖς γὰρ τὰς φορὰς τῶν ῥευμάτων,
Ἐν τρισὶ δὲ κυάθοις, ὡς προεῖπον, πρόσφερε.
Τινὲς δὲ καὶ τοῖς σφόδρα πονοῦσιν ὠτίον,
Ἀνέντες αὐτὴν ἐν γλυκεῖ τῷ Κρητικῷ
Εἰς τοὺς πόρους ἐνέθεσαν ἔριον διάβροχον.
Ἐχέτω δ' ὁ ποιεῖν ἀντίδοτον θέλων καλὴν,
Πάντα μὲν ἄκρως τὰ μίγματά τ' ἐξηρασμένα,
Τὸν λεγόμενόν τε θηριακὸν πεπονημένον
Ἀρτίσκον οὕτω γεγονόθ', ὡς ὑποδείξομεν.
Ἔστιν γὰρ οὗτος τῶν καλῶν ἐκ μιγμάτων.
Λαβὼν ἐχίδνας τὰς ἀληθεῖς τοῦ θέρους
Τὰς ἀρτιθήρους, τὰς μεγάλας ὡς εἴκοσι,
Μικρῷ τε πλείους, οὐ γάρ ἐστ' αὐτῶν πολὺ,
Ὃ δεῖ λαβόντας σκευάσαι τὸ φάρμακον,
Τῶν μὲν κεφαλῶν ἀπόκοψον, ὡς τρεῖς δακτύλους,

Cruciant, fasciculum polii decoquens aqua,
Praestiterit autem Cretici, aut Scythici magis
Aut Pontici potius, nam sistes rheumata,
Ternis (ut ante dixi) cyathis offeres.
Quidam doloribus permagnis aurium
Passo subigentes Cretico, meatibus,
Per quos facultas audiendi spargitur
Lanam antidoti liquore irriguam collocant.
Porro bonum cui antidotum curae est reddere
Is cunctas habeat misturas siccas probe,
Et Theriacum elaboratum (sicut vocant)
Pastillum, ita paratum, ut indicabimus,
Nam constat hic bonis misturae pharmacis:
Aestate veras prima sumis viperas
Captas recens, notandae magnitudinis
Easque viginti aut paulo plures item;
Hoc nanque non erit nimis medicamini.
Quum praeparas, tres digitos amputa caput

Μικρῷ τε πλείους τῶν ἀπὸ τῆς οὐρᾶς μερῶν,
Πρῶτον κεφαλὰς μὲν, εἶτα τὰς οὐρὰς τότε.
Τοῦτο δὲ ποιεῖν δεῖ προσφάτων ζωσῶν τ' ἔτι,
Εἶτα περιδείρας ῥαδίως, ὡς ἐγχέλεις,
(438) Ἔκβαλλέ τ' αὐτὸς καὶ τὸ λίπος αὐτῶν ἅπαν,
Πλύνας τε καθαρῶς, εἰς λοπάδιον ἐντίθει,
Ξηροῦ τ' ἀνήθου σύμμετρον δεσμίδιον,
Ὕδατος δέ τ' ἀρκοῦν παραχέας, ἕψει μέχρι
Η σὰρξ ἀποστῇ ῥαδίως τῶν ὀστέων.
Τὸ λοπάδιόν τε βαστάσας ἀπὸ τοῦ πυρὸς,
Τῶν ὀσταρίων τὴν σάρκα καθαρὰν ἀπόβαλε,
Στήσας ἀκριβῶς ἰσοβαρῆ ταύτης σταθμὸν
Τῆς σαρκὸς, ἄρτου τοῦ καθαροῦ τοῦ πυρίνου,
Πρόσμισγε καὶ λείαινε, παραχέων βραχὺ
Τοῦ ζωμαρίου, ποιῶν τὰ λεπτὰ πέμματα,
Ξήραινε καὶ χρῶ θηριακοῖς ἀρτισκίοις.
Σκιλλητικοὺς δὲ σκευάσεις οὕτω πάλιν.
Τῷ πυραμητῷ σκίλλαν εὐμεγέθη λαβὼν,

Pauloque caudam magis, hanc poſt, illud prius.
Sed aggredi iſtud donec vivunt, convenit.
Hinc cute detracta ut anguillis facillime
Totam eximes ipſarum pinguetudinem,
Ac poſtea quam laveris, dimittito
Ollae, et mediocrem anethi faſciculum aridi,
Affuſo aquae quod ipſis ſufficit incoque,
Donec caro relinquat oſſa promptius,
Et fictili remoto ab igne, condito
Carnem oſſibus puram, pari addens pondere
Panem triticeum haud ſordidum, tritum probe,
Pauxillulum decoctionis juſculi
Fundens ſuper, paſtillos tenues fingito;
Siccato et orbiculis theriacis utitor.
At ſcillinos hoc rurſus effinges modo,
Scillam cum foliis magnitudinis bonae
Albamque ſumptam toto purga cortice,

Λευκήν τε, κάθηρον πάντα τὸν ξηρὸν φλοιὸν,
Πᾶσαν δὲ ῥίζαν τὴν ξυλώδη περίελε,
Σταιτί τε περιπλάσας ἔμβαλ᾽ αὐτὴν εἰς ἴπνον.
Ὅταν δὲ νομίσῃς πάνυ καλῶς ὀπτὴν,
Τότε στήσας αὐτῆς ὅσον ἄγει λίτρας βάρος,
Ταύτῃ κατάμισγε λεπτοτάτῃ μίαν ἥμισυ
Λίτραν, ἀλεύρου γεγονότος πεφρυγμένων
Ὀρόβων ἐπ᾽ ὀλίγον, καὶ παραχρῆμα λεοτριβῶν,
Ποίησον οὕτω λεπτὰ πάνυ κυκλίσκια,
Ξηρά τε γιγνόμενα, στῆσον ᾗ σοι φίλον·
Βαλεῖν τοιοῦτον μίγμα γεγονὸς μὴ πάνυ,
Τὴν θηριακήν τε λεγομένην, ἀπορῇς, φράσω,
Ἧι καὶ λέγουσι τὸν Μιθριδάτην χρώμενον,
[894] Ὅτ᾽ ἐγένετ᾽ αὐτῷ θανάσιμα πιεῖν φάρμακα,
Ἄπασ᾽ ἀνάγκη μετὰ τέκνων πολεμουμένων,
Αὐτὸν μὲν οὐ λαβεῖν τινος αἴσθησιν βλάβης.
Ξίφει δ᾽ ἀναιρεθέντα περιγραφῆς τυχεῖν,
Τὰς δ᾽ αὖ θυγατέρας ἀποβαλεῖν τῷ φαρμάκῳ.

Omnem eximens radicem lignoſam undique
Circumlitamque maſſa tritici, clibano
Ipſam reponas, quum vero coctam probe
Putaveris, tres ejus libras ſumito;
Huic jungito tenuiſſimae libram ſemis
Ervi farinae paululum retorridi,
Ac laevigans ſubtiliter ſtatim pilas
Effinge tenues admodum; ſiccas ubi
Libet recondes, ne talis ſit miſtio
Ignota Theriaceque dicta perſequar,
Ut uſum quoque fuiſſe Mithridatem ferunt
Quum bibere medicamenta eum neceſſitas
Omnis, nociva cum liberis bellantibus,
Nullius ipſe noxae ſenſum pertulit,
Sed enſe detruncatus vitam perdidit,
Gnatae vero potu interierunt pharmaci.
Ipſam parabis ſic: ſcillinorum orbium

Σκεύαζε δ' αὐτὴν, σκιλλίνων κυκλισκίων
Δὶς εἴκοσι δραχμὰς, χἀτέρας δὶς τέσσαρας,
Ἀρτισκίων δὲ θηριακῶν δὶς δώδεκα,
Μέλανός τε πεπέρεως καὶ ὀπίου καὶ μάγματος
Ξηροῦ, πάλαι κληθέντος ἡδυχρόου μύρου,
Τῶν τ' ἐξ ἑκάστου μίγματος δὶς δώδεκα,
Ξηροῦ γλυκυῤῥίζου χυλαρίου δραχμὰς δέκα,
Καὶ δύ' ἐπὶ ταύταις, καὶ ῥόδων ξηρῶν ἴσας,
Καὶ κινναμώμου, καὶ ὀποβαλσάμου καλοῦ,
Ἧς τ' Ἰλλυριοὶ πέμπουσιν ἴσας ἴρεως,
Λευκοῦ τ' ἀγαρικοῦ, βουνιάδος τοῦ σπέρματος,
Τούτων ἑκάστου τὰς ἴσας δυώδεκα,
Καὶ Κρητικὸν σκόρδιον ἑνὶ τούτων ἴσον,
Σμύρνης, κρόκου, ῥᾶ, πετροσελίνου, στοιχάδος,
Ξηρᾶς καλαμίνθης, πενταφύλλου ῥιζίων,
Καὶ τοῦ πρασίου σπέρματος τῶν σφαιρίων,
Λευκοῦ πεπέρεως καὶ μακροῦ, τῆς Ἰνδικῆς
Νάρδου στάχυος, λιβάνου τε καὶ τερμινθίνης,

Drachmas viginti bis (alias bis quattuor)
Sed orbium theriacorum bis duodecim,
Nigrique piperis, opii et ſicci magmatis,
Quod hedychroa quondam vocabant unguina
Bis ſingulorum duodecim denarios,
Radiculae dulcis ſucci, aridae decem
Atque inſuper duas, roſae ſiccae pares
Et cinnamomi, ad haec opobalſami boni
Atque ireos praeterea, quam dat Illyris
Aequale pondus, agarici albi, ſeminis
Napi, uniuscujusque drachmas duodecim.
Et ſcordii tantundem cretici addito.
Myrrhae, croci, rheu, petroſelini, ſtoechados,
Siccae calaminthae, quinquefolii, praeter haec
Radiculae, atque galbulorum ſeminis
Marrubii, piperis albi, et longi, et Indicae
Nardi ſpicae, thuris, nec non terebinthinae

Ed. Chart. XIII. [894.] Ed. Baſ. II. (438.)

Κόστου τε λευκοῦ, καὶ ἔτι δικτάμνου πόας,
Σχοίνου τε, μὴ τῶν καρφίων, τοῦ δ' ἄνθεος,
Ξηροῦ τ' ἀβρέκτου ζιγγιβέρεως τὰς ἴσας,
Κασίας μελαίνης τοῦ φλοιοῦ, τούτων πάλιν
Δὶς τρεῖς ἑκάστου μίγματος δραχμῆς σταθμῷ,
Πολίου τε καὶ φοῦ Ποντικοῦ, καὶ θλάσπεως,
Χαμαίδρυός τε καὶ στύρακος, καὶ κόμμεως,
Καὶ γεντιανῆς, καὶ ἀκόρου, μήου τ' ἔτι
Καὶ καρδαμώμου, καὶ μαράθρου τοῦ σπέρματος
Ὑποκυστίδος χυλοῦ τε, καὶ χαλκίτιδος
Ὀπτῆς, ὑπερικοῦ σπέρματος τοῦ Κρητικοῦ,
Χυλοῦ τ' ἀκακίας τῆς καλῆς ὑγρᾶς ἔτι,
Καθαρᾶς τε νάρδου Κελτικῆς, καὶ Λημνίας,
Χαμαιπίτυός τε καὶ ἄμμεως καὶ σεσέλεως,
Ἀνισαρίου τε σπέρματος πεφρυγμένου,
Βότρυός τ' ἀμώμου, μαλαβάθρου φύλλων ἴσας,
Πάντων δ' ἑκάστου δύο δραχμὰς ρ'. ἐπιτίθει,
Καὶ βαλσάμου, καρποῦ τε τὰς αὐτὰς δύο.

Coſtique candidi, dictamni herbae, inſuper
Junci rotundi floris, gingiberis pares
Sicci, non rigui, nigrae caſiae corticis
Bis ſingulorum ternae drachmae pondere
Poliique et pontici phu, necnon thlaſpeos,
Chamaedryos, praeterea ſtyracis, commeos
Et gentianae, et acori, meuque inſuper
Et cardamomi, ſic foeniculi ſeminis
Hypocyſtidis ſucci, toſtae chalcitidis,
Cretenſis hyperici adde ſeminis, ſimul
Succi acaciae humidae, nardique gallicae
Purae, ſphragidisque lemniae, chamaepitys,
Ameos, ſeſeleos, ſeminis retorridi
Aniſi, amomi uvae, foliorum malabathri.
Impone drachmas ſingulorum compares
Duas, et totidem balſami fructus quoque.
Sed non probe aliqui ſingulis dant quattuor.

Τινὲς δὲ τούτων οὐ καλῶς ἀνὰ τέτταρας.
Ὀποπάνακος δὲ τοῦ δακρύου, καὶ χαλβάνης,
Δαύκου τε καθαροῦ σπέρματος τοῦ Κρητικοῦ,
Καὶ καστορίου, καὶ σαγαπηνοῦ προσφάτου,
Κενταυρίου τε Κρητικοῦ, μὴ προσφάτου,
Ἀριστολοχίας τε λεπτῆς ξηρᾶς καλῶς.
Τούτων ἑκάστου πάλιν δραχμὰς β'. ἐπιτίθει
Ἴσον θ' ἑνὶ τούτων, στῆσον ἀσφάλτου καλῆς.
Τινὲς δ' ἀνὰ δύο φασὶν, ὅπερ οὐ βούλομαι.
Πολλάκι γὰρ αὐτὴν, ὡς ἔγραψ', ἐσκεύασα
Οἴνου Φαλερίνου τοῦ καλοῦ τὸ σύμμετρον,
Μέλιτος δέκα λίτρας Ἀττικοῦ τοῦ προσφάτου.
Τούτων δ', ἃ μέν ἐστι σπέρμαθ', ἃ δὲ χυλοί τινων,
Ἃ δ' ἐστὶ φύλλα καὶ δάκρυα καὶ ῥιζία,
Ἐλάχιστα δ' αὐτῶν κἂν μετάλλοις γίνεται.
Χυλοὺς μὲν οὖν δάκρυα καὶ μεταλλικὰ
Οἴνῳ λέαινε, καὶ μέλιτος ποιῶν πάχος.
Τὰ λοίπ' ἀποδίδου ξηρὰ πάντα μίγματα,

Opopanacis lachrymae, praeterea galbani
Daucique purgati Cretenſis ſeminis,
Et caſtorei, ſagapeni jungito novi
Ariſtolochiaeque tenuis ſiccae probe
Horum uniuscujusque drachmas fac duas
Aequale pondus ponito bituminis:
Sunt qui duas cuique dent, quod diſplicet.
Frequenter ipſam, veluti ſcriptum eſt, condidi,
Vini Falerni mediocrem modum, boni
Mellis recentis Attici libras decem.
Nonnulla at horum ſucci, quaedam ſemina,
Sunt ſolia quaedam, et lachrymae, aliqua radiculae,
Ipſorum minima, et in metallis invenis.
Succos itaque cum lachrymis et metallicis
Vino teras, dum craſſitudinem vides
Mellis; reliqua conjunges omnia arida,
Contuſa, tenui increta cribro protinus,

Κοπέντα καὶ σηθέντα λεπτῷ κοσκίνῳ,
Μίξας τ' ἐπιμελῶς αὐτὰ, παραχέων τότε,
Ζέσας δὶς ἢ τρὶς τὸ μέλι, καὶ δεύσας πάλιν
Ἀπόθου, φυλάττων μὴ ξυλίνοις ἀγγείοις,
Ὑαλίνοις δὲ μᾶλλον, κερατίνοις τε κἀργυροῖς,
Καὶ κασσιτερινοῖς, καὶ κεραμίοις τε πυκνοῖς.
Δίδου τε πίνειν, μήτε γεγονὸς ἀρτίως
Τὸ φάρμακον, μήτε πάλιν ἐξηρασμένον,
Ὅπερ εἰ γένοιτο διὰ τὸ μῆκος τοῦ χρόνου,
Πάλιν ζέσας πρόσβαλλε μέλιτος σύμμετρον,
[895] *Συνεκλεάνας τ' ἐφ' ἱκανὸν τοῦτο χρόνον,*
Εὔχρηστον ἕξεις τὴν ἄχρηστον τῷ χρόνῳ,
Πολλῷ δ' ἐλάττω τῆς κεκραμένης ἅπαξ.

Κεφ. ιστ'. [*Θηριακῆς ἑτέρας σκευασία.*] *Ὅτι μὲν οὖν διαφωνοῦσί τινα πρὸς τὸν Ἀνδρόμαχον, Δαμοκράτης αὐτὸς ἐδήλωσεν εἰπὼν,*

Τινὲς δὲ τούτων οὐ καλῶς ἀνὰ τέτταρας,

καὶ πάλιν.

Mixtisque exacte mel adjicias poftea
Bis terve fervefactum; ubi rurfus rigaveris,
Reponito non ligneis, verum magis
In vafis vitreis, corneis, argenteis,
Et ftanneis fervans, et denfis ollulis.
Da potioni, nec recens factum nimis,
Nec rurfus medicamentum quod peraruit:
Sin longiori hoc fuerit fpatio temporis,
Subfervefacito rurfus, addens paululum
Mellis fimulque abunde temporis terens,
Tandemque habebis utile, quod valuit nihil,
Sed inferius eo quod mifcueris femel.

Cap. XVI. [*Theriaces alterius confectio.*] Quod itaque nonnulla cum Andromacho difcordant, Damocrates ipfe indicavit his verfibus:

Sed non probe aliqui fingulis dant quattuor.

Atque iterum

Τινὲς δ' ἀνὰ δύο φασὶν, ὅπερ οὐ βούλομαι, ὅτι δὲ καὶ σαφέστερον εἴρηται τῶν ὑπὸ Δαμοκράτους γεγραμμένων, καὶ τοῦτο πρόδηλον. οὔσης δὲ καὶ ἄλλης παρ' ἡμῖν καὶ αὐτοῦ ἐμμέτρου συνθέσεως τῆς θηριακῆς, ἔδοξέ μοι κἀκείνην παραγράψαι, κατὰ τὴν ἐκ παραδόσεως τῶν ἐν αὐτῇ συμμετρίαν, διὰ τὸ σαφεστέραν τε καὶ συντομωτέραν εἶναι τῶν ἤδη γεγραμμένων.

Θηριακὴν ᾧδ' ἄν τις ἐπικεράσαιτο,
Δαύκου μὲν καρπὸς, πάνακός τ' ὀπὸς, ἀσφάλτου τε
Καὶ σαγαπηνὸν ἴσον, καὶ χαλβάνη, ἄμμι δ' αὖτις,
Λεπτὴ ἀριστολοχία, καὶ ὄρχις κάστορος εἴη,
(439) *Καὶ κενταυρίου κόμης ἶσον αὖτις ἐπ' αὐτοῖς*
Διπλάσιον, στύρακός τε καὶ ἄμμεως, ἀνίσου τε
Καὶ φοῦ, καὶ πολίοιο κόμης, μήου τ' ἀκόρου τε.
Ἠδὲ χαμαιπίτυος καὶ φύλλα μαλαβάθροιο,
Ἔστω καὶ σφραγὶς Λήμνου, ἀπὸ χαλκίτεώς τε
Χυλὸν καὶ ξανθὸν ὑποκιστίδος αὖτις ἐπ' αὐτοῖς,
Κόμμι τε καὶ νάρδου Κελτῶν, ἀπὸ θλάσπεως λεπτῆς,

Sunt qui duas cuique dent, quod difplicet.
Quod autem et manifeftius dictum fit iis quae Damocrates prodidit, hoc quoque conftat: verum quum alia ipfius theriaces compofitio numeris perfcripta apud me habeatur, vifum eft mihi et illam afcribere, juxta commoderationem medicaminum eam ingredientium, eo quod clarior compendiofiorque modo traditis exiftat.

Theriacen ratione aliquis contemperet ifta.
Dauci equidem fructus, panacis liquor, atque bitumen
Et fagapenum itidem, tum galbana rurfus, et ammi
Cum tenui terrae malo, cum caftoris ipfo
Tefticulo, atque coma centaurei pondera fument
Aequa, duplum ftyracisque, ameofque et anifi,
Phu, poliique comae pariter, meuque, acorique,
Atque chamaepityos, foliorum itidem malabathri,
Sphragidis ex Lemno, mox chalciteos, hypocifis,
Flaventis fucci, gummi, et quam Gallia donat
Nardi, praeterea tenuis thlafpi atque perinde

Καὶ σεσέλεως τὸ σπέρμα, καὶ ἐκ Κρήτης μαράθροιο,
Καὶ καρδαμώμου, ἀπὸ πάντων τέτταρες ἔστων
Δραχμαὶ, σμύρνης δ' αὖ καὶ στοιχάδος, ἠδὲ πρασίου,
Κόστου, δικτάμνου τε δραχμὰς στ'. ἔμβαλ' ἑκάστου,
Καὶ μὴν καὶ πεπέρεως μακροῦ, ἑτέρην δ' ἐπὶ τῇδε,
'Αργεννὴν, ῥῆόν τε ἴσον, ξανθοῖό τε χάλτην.
Κωρυκίου τε κρόκου, καὶ ῥίζαν πενταπετήλου,
Καὶ δέ νυ, καὶ καλάμην, ἶσα σχοίνου τ' εὐώδους.
Τερμίνθου δ' ἀπὸ ῥητίνην, νάρδοιό τε ῥίζαν
'Ινδῆς, καὶ κασίης σῦριγξ, λιβάνοιό τ' ἀμήτου
Χόνδροι, σπέρμα τε λεπτὸν ἐν οὔρεσιν ἀλδήσκοντος,
Πετροσελίνου μίσγε δραχμὰς στ'. σταθμὸν ἰσάζων.
Διπλάσιον δ' ἔστω σκορδίου, γογγυλίδος τε
Σπέρματος ἀγροτέρης, ἴριδός τε, ῥόδων τε πέτηλα
Ξηρὰ, καὶ ἀγαρικὸν, ῥίζης ἐπὶ τοῖσι γλυκείης
Χυλὸς, καὶ βαλσάμου ὀπὸς, καὶ κινναμώμου,
Καὶ δριμὺ ζιγγίβερι δραχμὰς β'. μάγματος ἔστω
Δὶς τόσον ἡδυχρόου, πεπέρεώς τε μέλανος, καὶ αὐτοὶ

Seminis ex ſeſeli, marathri quod Creta miniſtrat
Et cardamomi, drachmae cujusque parantur
Quattuor, at myrrha et praſion, cum ſtoechade, coſtus.
Dictamnus, ſenas capient haec ſingula drachmas,
Quinetiam piper oblongum, album, praeterea rheu.
Atque crocus qui corycio defertur ab antro.
Quinque ſimul folii radix et juncus odorus,
Et calamus drachmas aequales, et terebinthi
Reſina accipient, nardi ſimul Indica radix,
Fiſtula jam caſiae, inſectum thus, petroſelini
Montani tenuis ſemen, ſex ſingula drachmis
Junge, modo verum duplicato ſcordion addes
Et rapae ſemen ſylveſtris et iris odorae, et
Sicca roſae folia, agaricum, ſuccus glycyrizae,
Balſameusque liquor, cinamomum, gingiber ardens
Binas accipient drachmas, et magmatis eſto
Bis tantum hedychroi, piperisque nigri, inſuper orbes

Ἀρτίσκοι θηρίων ἶσοι, μήκωνος ὀποῖο
Σταθμῷ, δὶς δέ τι τόσσον ἐν ἀρτίσκοις βάρος εἴη,
Πικρῆς ἐκ σκίλλης μέλιτος δ' ἐπὶ πᾶσι χέασθαι.
Ἡδυχρόου δέ τι μάγμα, μάρου μὲν ἔχει δύο δραχμάς.
Ἴσας δ' αὖτ' ἀσάρου, καὶ ἀμαράκου, ἀσπαλάθου τε,
Καὶ σχοίνου καλάμου τ' εὐώδεος, ἐκ πόντου τε
Φοῦ, ξυλοβαλσάμου τ' ὀποβαλσάμου τε δραχμὰς τρεῖς.
Καὶ κιναμώμου εἰσὶν ἴσαι, καὶ κόστου ἐπ' αὐτῷ.
Σμύρνης δ' ἓξ δραχμὰς καὶ φύλλα μαλαβάθροιο,
Ἴσον δ' αὖτ' Ἰνδῆς νάρδου, ξανθοῦ τε κρόκοιο.
Καὶ μὴν καὶ κασίης ἶσαι, διπλαῖ δέ τ' ἀμώμου.
Λοιπὴ δ' ἐκ κραναῆς Χίου δραχμῆς βάρος εἴη
Μαστίχη, οἴνῳ δ' αὖ Φαλερίνῳ φυράσασθαι.

ὑπόλοιπον εἶναί μοι δοκεῖ πρὸς τὸ συμπεπληρῶσθαι τὴν περὶ τῆς θηριακῆς ἅπασαν διδασκαλίαν, ἐν οἷς ὁ Κρίτων ἤτοι διεφώνησε πρός τι τῶν πρόσθεν γεγραμμένων, ἢ προσέθηκέ τι τῶν παραλελειμμένων ὑπογράφειν.

Theriaci aequabunt opium, hos bis vincere debent
Pondere ſcillini, et cunctis mel deſuper adde,
Hedychroi vult magma mari binas ſibi drachmas,
Aequales et amaraci habens, aſari, aſpalatique
Et junci teretis, calami qui ſuavis odore eſt.
Phu ponti, ligni et ſucci quem balſamon aedit
Tres ſunto drachmae, totidem coſti, cinamomi.
Myrrhae ſex alias miſces, folii malabathri,
Indorum nardi, flavique croci inſuper aequas.
Quinetiam caſiae totidem, ſed pondus amomi
Sume duplum, drachmam chiae ſed maſtichae habebit:
Haec vino debent conſpergi cuncta Falerno.

Reliquum eſſe mihi videtur, ut tota de theriace diſciplina abſolvatur, ſubjicere in quibus Crito vel a prius deſcriptis nonnihil diſſenſit, vel aliquid ex iis quae omiſſa erant, addidit.

[896] Κεφ. ιζ. [Περὶ τῶν ὑπὸ Κρίτωνος γεγραμμένων περὶ τῆς θηριακῆς, ἐν τῷ γ΄. τῶν φαρμακιτίδων βίβλων.] Ἐν μὲν τῇ συμμετρίᾳ τῶν φαρμάκων, βάλλει καὶ αὐτὸς < κδ΄. τοῦ μέλανος πεπέρεως, ὥσπερ τοῦ μακροῦ < στ΄. βάλλει δὲ καὶ χαλκίτεως κεκαυμένης < δ΄. καὶ μέλιτος Ἀττικοῦ λίτρας ι΄. τὰ δὲ θηρία, περὶ τὰ τελευταῖα τοῦ ἔαρος κατὰ τὸ θέρος, ἢ τῷ τρυγητῷ κελεύει συλλέγειν εὐλαβούμενος δηλονότι τό τε τοῦ θέρους, μετὰ τὰ πρῶτα σύμπαντος, ἄχρι κυνὸς ἐπιτολῆς, καὶ τὸ μετὰ τοῦτο, ὃ καλοῦσί τινες ἰδίως ὀπώρας καιρὸν, ἡνίκα καὶ τοῖς ἀνθρώποις τὸ χολῶδες πλεῖστον ὑποτρέφεται. κατὰ δὲ τὸν τρυγητὸν, ὅπερ ἐστὶ τὸ μέσον τοῦ φθινοπώρου, συλλέγειν ἀξιοῖ καὶ συλλαμβάνειν ἐξ αὐτῶν τὰ μεγάλα καὶ εὔτροφα, καὶ ἕψειν μετὰ ἀνήθου μόνου. τὸ δὲ τῆς σαρκὸς αὐτῶν ἐκ δέκα θηρίων ἀθροισθὲν, μιγνύειν ἀξιοῖ σιλιγνίτου ἄρτου μίαν οὐγγίαν, καὶ οὕτως ἀναπλάττειν τοὺς καλουμένους ἀρτίσκους θηριακούς. τοὺς δὲ σκιλλητικοὺς τόνδε τὸν τρόπον σκευάζειν κελεύει. λαμβάνειν σκίλ-

Cap. XVII. [*De scriptis a Critone de theriaca in tertio medicamentorum libro.*] In medicamentorum fymmetria et ipfe nigri piperis drachmas vigintiquatuor quemadmodum longi fenas immittit. Caeterum chalcitidis uftae drachmas quatuor, mellis Attici drachmas decem imponit; feras autem vere defınente in aeftatem, aut medio autumno, quod tempus trygetum dicunt, colligere praecipit, cavens nimirum et aeftatem ab initio totam usque ad caniculae exortum. Item quod hoc tempus fubfequitur, nonnulli id proprie vocant oporam, quum fugaces fructus eduntur, et bilis hominibus copiofiffima fuboritur. In trygeto autem, quod eft autumni medio, colligendas cenfet, capiendasque ex ipfis grandes et bene habitas, quae cum anetho folum incoquantur At carnem ipfarum decem accumulatam panis filiginei unciae mifceri vult: atque ita paftillos theriacos effingi. Scillinos autem hoc modo confici jubet; fcillam quum

Ed. Chart. XIII. [896.] Ed. Baf. II. (439.)

λας ἐν τῷ πυραμητῷ, τηνικαῦτα γὰρ εἶναι μάλιστα ἀκμαίαν. εὔδηλον δ' ὅτι πυραμητὸν κέκληκε τὸν χρόνον, ἐν ᾧ τοὺς πυροὺς ἀμῶσιν, ὀπτῆσαι δ' αὐτὰς ἀποχρώντως ἐν ἴπνῳ κελεύει, περιπλασθείσας γύψῳ ἢ πηλῷ ἐγκρύπτειν πυρὶ, μέχρις ἂν αὐτάρκως ὀπτηθῶσι, εἶτα ἀνελομένους λαμβάνειν αὐτῶν τὸ ἐγκάρδιον, οὕτως γὰρ αὐτὸς ὠνόμασε, καὶ λεαίνειν τε μιγνύντας ὀρόβου μέρος ἓν τῷ διπλασίῳ τῆς σκίλλης, ἀναπλάσσειν τε μετὰ ταῦτα τροχίσκους, καὶ ψύχειν ἐν σκιᾷ. περὶ δὲ τῶν ἐν ὅλμῳ κοπτομένων φαρμάκων ἐπιμελῶς ἔγραψε, περιδεδέσθαι κελεύων δέρμα περὶ τὸν ὅλμον ἀσφαλῶς, κατὰ τὴν μεσότητα διατετρημένον τοσοῦτον, ὡς δύνασθαι μὴ μόνον τὸ κόπτον ἔλασμα διὰ τῆς ἐκτρήσεως καθίεσθαι, ἀλλὰ καὶ μετὰ τὸ ἀρθῆναι τὸ ἔλασμα, τὴν χεῖρα μετὰ τοῦ μύακος, ὥστε αἴρειν δι' αὐτοῦ τὸ κεκομμένον, καὶ ὀφεῖλον σήθεσθαι. δεήσει δὲ, φησὶ, καὶ ἄλλο δέρμα εἶναι, τὴν ἔκτρησιν ἔχον μικροτέραν, ὡς δι' αὐτῆς μόνον τὸ ἔλασμα καθίεσθαι πρὸς τὸ κόπτειν τὰ ἐν τῷ ὅλμῳ, καὶ τοῦτο ἐπιβεβλῆσθαι τῷ προτέρῳ ἄνωθεν. καὶ

triticum metunt, (tunc enim potiffimum viget) accipere confulit; deinde torrere ipfam abunde in clibano, illitamque gypfo aut luto igni condere, usque dum fatis tofta fuerit. Poftea ubi exemeris, medullam ipfius fumere ac laevigare, mifcendo ervi partem unam fcillae duplicatae, inde paftillos fingere, et in umbra refrigerare. Porro de iis quae in pila contunduntur medicamentis accurate fcripfit, dum pellem pilae tuto circumligari jubet juxta medium tantillo foramine patefcenti, ut non folum contundens lamina per id poffit demitti, fed etiam ubi lamina fuerit fublata manus cum cochleari, ut quod contufum eft et incerni defiderat, per ipfum eximatur. Oportebit autem aliam quoque pellem (inquit) circumjici, minori perviam foramine, qua fola lamina demittatur ad ea quae pilae infunt contundenda, atque haec priori ex fuperna parte injici debet. Item non ftatim ipfa detegere convenit, prius quam fuligi-

μὴ εὐθέως ἀποκαλύπτειν αὐτὰ, πρὶν ἢ τὸ χνοῶδες καταστῆναι. κατὰ ταὐτὰ δὲ καὶ διαττώντων ἡμῶν διὰ τοῦ κοσκίνου κεκαλύφθαι κελεύει τὸ διαττώμενον ἄνωθεν, ὅταν τε καταστῇ ἡ κίνησις, τότε ἀνοίγεσθαι, κἄπειτα αἰρόμενον τὸν κόσκινον ἀπομάττεσθαι πτεροῖς.

nofa portio fubfiftat, fecundum haec, ubi cribro difcrevimus, id quod cretum eft fuperne jubet obtegi, ac quum motus confliterit, tunc adaperiri, poftea cribrum fublatum pennis abftergi.

ΓΑΛΗΝΟΥ ΠΕΡΙ ΑΝΤΙΔΟΤΩΝ ΒΙΒΛΙΟΝ ΔΕΥΤΕΡΟΝ.

Ed. Chart. XIII. [897.] Ed. Baf. II. (439.)

Κεφ. α'. [Περὶ τῶν Μιθριδατείων τε καὶ ἄλλων τινῶν Ἀνδρομάχου ἀντιδότων.] Ὁ περὶ τῆς θηριακῆς λόγος εἰς ὅλον βιβλίον ἐκταθεὶς, σύντομον ἐργάζεται τὸν περὶ ἄλλων ἀντιδότων λόγον, ἃς ἐν τῷδε τῷ γράμματι πρόκειταί μοι διελθεῖν, ἀπὸ τῆς Μιθριδατείου καλουμένης ἀρξαμένῳ, πρὸς μὲν τὰ πλεῖστα τῶν δηλητηρίων φαρμάκων δραστικωτέρας ὑπαρχούσης, ἀπολειπομένης δὲ ἐν τῇ τῶν ὑπ' ἐχίδνης δηχθέντων ἰάσει τῆς θηριακῆς ὀνομαζομένης. ἐπεὶ δὲ καὶ ταύτην καὶ σχεδὸν ἁπάσας τὰς ἀρίστας ἔγραψεν

GALENI DE ANTIDOTIS LIBER SECUNDUS.

Cap. I. [*De Mithridaticis et aliis quibusdam Andromachi Antidotis.*] Expofita a nobis integro volumine theriaca, ut reliquas antidotos brevibus explicemus, efficiet, quas mihi hoc in libro recenfere propofitum eft, ab ea quam Mithridaticam vocant initio fumpto, quae quidem adverfus pleraque deleteria medicamenta efficacior eft, in viperae autem morfus curatione, theriaca dicta inferior. Quoniam vero Andromachus et hanc et

ἐφεξῆς ὁ Ἀνδρόμαχος ἐν τῇ τῶν ἐντὸς φαρμάκων διδασκαλίᾳ, διὰ τοῦτο κἀγὼ πάσας αὐτὰς, ὡς ἐκεῖνος ἔγραψεν, ἐφεξῆς παραθήσομαι.

[Ἀνδρομάχου ἀντίδοτοι.] Ἀντίδοτος Μιθριδάτειος, πρὸς τὰ θανάσιμα ἰδίως ποιοῦσα, καὶ πρὸς τὰ ἐντὸς πάθη πάντα. ℞ Γλυκυῤῥίζης < ζ' S''. καὶ τετρώβολον, ὀπίου < δ'. ὀβολοὺς β'. καστορίου < στ'. πολίου < ε'. ὀβολοὺς β'. κόστου < ε'. καὶ ὀβολοὺς β'. ναρδοστάχυος < στ'. ὀβολοὺς β'. κασίας < ε'. ὀβολοὺς β'. λιβάνου < στ'. σεσέλεως < ε'. ὀβολοὺς β'. ὑποκυστίδος χυλοῦ < στ'. ἀκόρου < β'. σκορδίου < στ'. ὀβολοὺς β'. φύλλου < δ'. γάλλου < ε'. τριώβολον. οἱ δὲ < στ'. κύφεως < στ'. (440) ὀβολοὺς β'. σμύρνης < στ'. κρόκου < ζ'. ὀβολοὺς β'. κινναμώμου < ζ'. ὀβολοὺς β'. στύρακος < ε'. ὀβολοὺς δ'. δαύκου σπέρματος < στ'. τριώβολον, ζιγγιβέρεως < ζ'. ὀβολοὺς β'. φοῦ Ποντικοῦ < β'. πετροσελίνου < δ'. ὀβολοὺς γ'. νάρδου Κελτικῆς < δ'. μαράθρου σπέρματος < δ'. νάρδου Ἰνδικῆς < δ'.

deinceps optimas quasque ferme antidotos, literarum monumentis commifit, in libro de internis medicamentis, idcirco et ipfe eas omnes, quo ordine ille confcripfit, fubjungam.

[*Andromachi antidota.*] *Antidotus Mithridatica, privatim ad lethalia praecipue faciens, et ad internas corporis affectiones efficax.* ℞ Radicis dulcis drach. vij, ß, obolos quatuor, opii drach. iv, obolos duos, caftorii drach. fex, polii drach. quinque, obolos duos, cofti ʒ v, obolos ij, fpicae nardi drach. vj, obolos ij, caffiae drach. v, obolos ij, thuris drach. fex, fefeleos ʒ v, obolos duos, fucci hypocyftidis drach. fex, acori drach. duas, fcordii drach. fex, obolos ij, folii drach. iv, gallii drach v, obolos tres, alii drach. vj, immittunt; cypheos drach. fex, obolos ij, myrrhae drach. fex, croci drach. vij, obolos duos, cinnamomi drach. vij, obolos duos, ftyracis drach. v, obolos iv, feminis dauci drach. fex, obolos tres, zingiberis drach. vij, obolos duos, phu Pontici drach. ij, petrofelini drach. iv, obolos tres, nardi Celticae drach. iv,

ὑπερικοῦ < β'. ἀκακίας < β'. Γεντιανῆς < δ'. οἱ δὲ < β'. ἀνίσου < γ'. θλάσπεως < στ'. ὀβολοὺς δ'. μήου ἀθαμαντικοῦ < δ'. οἱ δὲ < β'. ῥόδων ξηρῶν < δ'. κόμμεως < β'. καρδαμώμου < δ'. οἱ δὲ < β'. σχοίνου < στ'. ὀβολοὺς β'. ὀποπάνακος < στ'. ὀβολοὺς β'. ὀποβαλσάμου < στ'. ὀβολοὺς δ'. χαλβάνης < ζ'. σκίγκου < β'. ὀβολοὺς β'. τερμινθίνης < στ'. ὀβολοὺς β'. οἴνου Χίου τὸ ἱκανὸν, μέλιτος Ἀττικοῦ ἑφθοῦ τὸ ἱκανόν.

[898] [Ἄλλως ἡ Μιθριδάτειος ὡς Ἀντίπατρος καὶ Κλεόφαντος.] ℞ Σμύρνης < ζ' S''. ὀβολοὺς δ'. οἱ δὲ γ'. νάρδου ἴσον, κρόκου < ζ'. ὀβολοὺς γ'. ὀπίου < δ'. ὀβολοὺς β' S''. στύρακος < ε'. καστορίου < στ'. ὀβολὸν ἕνα, κινναμώμου < ζ'. ὀβολοὺς γ'. πολίου < στ'. ὀβολοὺς γ'. σκορδίου < ζ'. ὀβολοὺς γ'. ζιγγιβέρεως τὸ ἴσον, κόστου < στ'. ὀβολοὺς γ'. πεπέρεως λευκοῦ < ε'. ὀβολοὺς β'. πεπέρεως μακροῦ < στ'. ὀβολοὺς γ'. σεσέλεως < ε'. ὀβολοὺς β'. ἀβροτόνου < ε'. ὀβολοὺς β'. πετροσελίνου < ιδ'. δαύκου σπέρματος < στ'. ὀβολοὺς γ'. κασσίας < ε'. ὀβολοὺς γ'. λιβάνου <

ſeminis foeniculi drach. iv, nardi Indicae drach. iv, hyperici drach. duas, acaciae ʒ ij, gentianae ʒ iv, alii vero ʒ ij, aniſi ʒ iij, thlaſpeos ʒ vj, obolos iv, meu Athamantici ʒ iv, alii ʒ ij, roſarum ſiccarum ʒ iv, gummi ʒ ij, cardamomi ʒ iv, alii ʒ ij, junci odorati ʒ ſex, obolos duos, opopanacis ʒ vj, obolos ij, opobalſami ʒ vi, obolos iv, galbani ʒ vii, ſcinci ʒ ii, obolos ii, terebinthinae ʒ ſex, obolos ii, vini Chii quod ſatis eſt, mellis Attici cocti quod ſufficit.

[*Aliter Mithridatica ut Antipater et Cleophantus.*] ℞ Myrrhae drach. vij ß, obolos iv, alii iij, ſpicae nardi tantundem: croci drach. vij, obolos iij, opii drachmas quatuor, obolos ij ß, ſtyracis drach. v, caſtorii drach. ſex, obolos j, cinnamomi drach. vij, obolos iij, polii drach. ſex, obolos iij, ſcordii ʒ vij, obolos iij, zingiberis tantundem: coſti drach. vj, obolos iij, piperis albi drach. v, obolos ij, piperis longi drach. ſex, obolos iij, ſeſelis drach. quinque obolos ij, abrotoni drach. v, obolos duos, petroſelini drach. xiv, ſeminis dauci drach. ſex, obolos tres,

στ'. ὀβολοὺς β'. ὑποκυστίδος χυλοῦ < στ'. ὀβολὸν α' S''. νάρδου Κελτικῆς < δ'. μαράθρου σπέρματος < δ'. μαλαβάθρου φύλλων < δ'. νάρδου Ἰνδικῆς < δ'. ἀκόρου, φοῦ Ποντικοῦ, σαγαπηνοῦ, βαλσάμου καρποῦ, ὑπερικοῦ, Ἰλλυρίδος, ἀνὰ < β'. μίλτου Λημνίου < στ'. κύφεως, σκίγκου ὀσφύος, ἀνὰ < στ'. ἀκακίας, κόμμεως, καρδαμώμου, πελεκίνου, ἀνὰ < β'. θλάσπεως < στ'. ὀβολοὺς δ'. Γεντιανῆς < δ'. οἱ δὲ γ'. ἀνίσου < γ'. ῥόδων ξηρῶν < δ'. μήου ἀθαμαντικοῦ ἴσον, σχοίνου < στ'. ὀβολοὺς γ'. ὀποπάνακος < στ'. χαλβάνης < στ'. ὀβολοὺς γ'. ὀποβαλσάμου τὸ ἴσον, ἀριστολοχίας < α'. ὑσσώπου < γ'. πρασίου < α'. χαμαιπίτυος < γ'. λιβανωτίδος < ε'. τερμινθίνης < στ'. τριώβολον, μέλιτος Ἀττικοῦ τὸ ἱκανὸν, οἶνον μὴ βάλε.

[Ἀντίδοτος ἡ Ὀρβανοῦ λεγομένη τοῦ Ἰνδοῦ, πρὸς τὸ τὰ ἐντὸς βρέφη ἐκβάλλειν.] ℞ Σμύρνης < ιε'. κρόκου < ιστ'. νάρδου Ἰνδικῆς < ιστ'. κινναμώμου, κασσίας,

cassiae drach. quinque, obolos iij, thuris drach. sex, obolos duos, succi hypocystidis drach. sex, obolos j ß, nardi Celticae drach. quatuor, seminis foeniculi drach. iv, foliorum malabathri drachmas iv, nardi Indicae drach. quatuor, acori, phu Pontici, sagapeni, fructus balsami, hyperici, iridis Illyricae singulorum drachmas duas, rubricae Lemniae, cypheos, lumborum scinci, singulorum drachmas sex, acaciae, gummi, cardamomi, securidacae, singulorum drach. ij, seminis thlaspeos drach. sex, obolos iv, gentianae drach. quatuor, alii tres, anisi drach. tres, rosarum siccarum drach. quatuor, mei athamantici tantundem: junci rotundi odorati drachmas sex, obolos tres, opopanacis drach. vj, galbani drach. sex, obolos tres, opobalsami tantundem: aristolochiae drach. j, hyssopi drach. iij, marrubii drach. j, chamaepityos drach. tres, rorismarini ʒ v, terebinthinae ʒ vj, obolos tres, mellis Attici quod sufficit, vinum ne injicito.

[*Antidotus Orbani Indi dicta ad foetus ejiciendos.*] ℞ Myrrhae drach. xv, croci drachmas sexdecim, nardi Indicae drachmas sexdecim, cinnamomi, cassiae, panacis,

πάνακος, ἀνὰ < ιγ'. ἀμώμου < η'. σκορδίου < κε'. ἐν ἄλλῳ < ε'. σχοίνου ἄνθους < η'. μήου ἀθαμαντικοῦ < γ'. ῥόδων χυλοῦ < ιβ'. ὀβολοὺς γ'. φοῦ < ε'. ὀβολοὺς γ'. ὑπερικοῦ < ε'. ζιγγιβέρεως < στ'. πεπέρεως μέλανος < στ'. πεπέρεως λευκοῦ < η'. στύρακος < ε'. ὀβολοὺς γ'. μαράθρου ἀγρίου σπέρματος < γ'. ὀβολοὺς δ'. πεπέρεως μακροῦ < ε'. οἱ δὲ στ'. κόστου < ζ'. ὀβολοὺς γ'. τριφύλλου σπέρματος < ε'. Γεντιανῆς < δ'. ἀριστολοχίας στρογγύλης < δ'. πολίου < ε'. τριφύλλου ῥίζης < ε'. ὀβολοὺς γ'. καρδαμώμου < ε'. ἐχίου ῥίζης < δ'. λιβάνου δραχμὰς στ'. πετροσελίνου δραχμὰς στ'. φλόμου δραχμὰς στ'. σεσέλεως δραχμὰς ε'. κυμίνου Αἰθιοπικοῦ δραχμὰς γ'. βαλσάμου καρποῦ δραχμὰς δ'. νάρδου Κελτικῆς < ζ'. Λημνίας δραχμὰς δ'. μηκωνείου < δ'. ὀβολοὺς γ'. κάγχρυος σπέρματος δραχμὰς γ'. κύφεως δραχμὰς δ'. ἴρεως Ἰλλυρικῆς ἴσον, μανδραγόρου χυλοῦ δραχμὰς στ'. ὀβολοὺς γ'. σαγαπηνοῦ δραχμὰς δ'. ὀποπάνακος δραχμὰς γ'. ἀνίσου δραχμὰς δ'. ὑποκυστίδος

ſingulorum drachmas xiij, amomi drachmas octo, ſcordii drach. xxv, in aliis v, florum junci odorati drach. octo, mei Athamantici drach. tres, ſucci roſarum drach. duodecim, obolos tres, phu drachmas quinque, obolos tres, hyperici drach. quinque, zingiberis drachmas ſex, piperis nigri ʒ vj, piperis albi drach. octo, ſtyracis ʒ v, obolos tres, ſeminis foeniculi ſilveſtris drachmas tres, obolos iv, piperis longi drach. quinque, alii ʒ ſex, coſti ʒ vij, obolos tres, ſeminis trifolii drach. quinque, gentianae drachmas iv, ariſtolochiae rotundae drach. iv, polii drach. quinque, radicis trifolii drach. quinque, obolos tres, cardamomi drach. quinque, radicis echii drach. quatuor, thuris drach. ſex, petroſelini drach. ſex, verbaſci drach. ſex, ſeſeleos drach. quinque, cumini Aethiopici drach. tres, fructus balſami ʒ iv, nardi Celticae drach. ſeptem, terrae ſigillatae ʒ iv, opii drach. quatuor, obolos iij, ſeminis canchryos drach. tres, cypheos drach. quatuor; iridis Illyricae tantundem, ſucci mandragorae drach. ſex, obolos tres, ſagapeni drach. quatuor. opopanacis drach. tres, aniſi drach.

χυλοῦ δραχμὰς στ'. τερμινθίνης δραχμὰς ε'. ὀβολοὺς γ'. καστορίου δραχμὰς ε'. ὀποβαλσάμου δραχμὰς ιστ'. πηγάνου ἀγρίου σπέρματος δραχμὰς γ'. χαλβάνης δραχμὰς δ'. βουνιάδος σπέρματος ἴσον, ἐλαφείου μυελοῦ δραχμὰς στ'. ὀβολοὺς γ'. μύρου νάρδου δραχμὰς κ'. αἵματος ἐριφείου ξηροῦ δραχμὰς ε'. ὀβολοὺς τρεῖς, καὶ χηνείου ξηροῦ ἴσον, νήσσης αἵματος δραχμὰς γ'. τριώβολον, βουφθάλμου Αἰγυπτίου χυλοῦ δραχμὰς η'. οἴνου Χίου ἀθαμαντικοῦ τὸ ἱκανόν.

[899] [Ἀντίδοτος πανάκεια δι' αἱμάτων, ᾗ χρῶμαι, πλείστην ἐπαγγελίαν ἔχουσα ἐκ τῶν Ἀφροδᾶ.] ℞ Κινναμώμου ∠ η'. ἀμώμου ∠ δ'. κασσίας σύριγγος μελαίνης ∠ ιστ'. κρόκου ∠ ιστ'. σχοίνου ∠ ε'. λιβάνου ∠ ε'. πεπέρεως λευκοῦ ∠ δ'. ὀβολοὺς γ'. καὶ μακροῦ ∠ α'. ὀβολοὺς γ'. σμύρνης ∠ ια'. ὀβολοὺς β'. νάρδου Ἰνδικῆς ∠ ια'. τετρώβολον, Κελτικῆς ∠ ιστ'. ὀβολοὺς β'. ῥόδων ξηρῶν ∠ στ'. κόστου ∠ β'. ὀβολοὺς γ' S''. ὀποβαλσάμου ∠ δ'. ὀβολοὺς β'. ὀποῦ Κυρηναϊκοῦ ∠ γ'. ἄλλοι ∠ δ' S''. στοιχάδος ∠ ε'. ὀβο-

quatuor, ſucci hypocyſtidis drach. ſex, terebinthinae drachmas quinque, obolos tres, caſtorii drach. quinque, opobalſami drach. ſexdecim, ſeminis rutae ſylveſtris drach. iij, galbani drachmas quatuor, ſeminis napi tantundem, medullae cervinae drach. ſex, obolos tres, unguenti nardini drach. viginti, ſanguinis hoedini ſicci drach. quinque, obolos tres, ſanguinis anſerini ſicci tantundem, ſanguinis anatis drach. tres, obolos tres, ſucci buphthalmi Aegyptii drach. viij, vini Chii Athamantici, quod ſufficit.

[*Antidotus Panacea ex ſanguinibus qua utor, multa promittens ab Aphroda accepta.*] ℞ Cinnamomi drach. viij, amomi drach. iv, caſſiae fiſtulae nigrae drach. xvj, croci drach. xvj, junci rotundi odorati ʒ v, thuris drach. v, piperis albi drach. iv, obol. iij, piperis longi ʒ j, obolos iij, myrrhae drach. xj, obol. ij, nardi Indicae drach. xj, obol. iv, nardi Celticae drach. xvj, obol. ij, roſarum ſiccarum ʒ vj, coſti drach. ij, obol. iij ß, opobalſami ʒ iv, obol. ij, ſucci Cyrenaici drach. iij, alii drach. iv ß. ſtoe-

λοὺς β'. τριφύλλου ῥίζης < δ'. ἢ τοῦ σπέρματος < γ'. σκορδίου ἄνθους < ια'. ὀβολοὺς β'. πολίου Κρητικοῦ < στ'. ὀβολοὺς β'. ἀσάρου < β'. ἀκόρου < γ'. ὀβολοὺς γ' S''. δαύκου σπέρματος τὸ ἴσον, ἀνίσου σπέρματος < β'. κυμίνου Αἰθιοπικοῦ ἴσον, ῥήου Ποντικοῦ < ε'. ὀβολοὺς γ' S''. βουνιάδος σπέρματος ἀγρίας < γ'. ἢ γογγυλίδος σπέρματος ἴσον, φοῦ Ποντικοῦ < β'. μέλιτος ἑφθοῦ τὸ ἱκανόν.

[*Ἀντίδοτος ἀσύγκριτος ἣν συνέθηκα, ποιοῦσα πρὸς πάντα τὰ ἐντὸς πάθη, ὡς Νικόστρατος.*] ℞ Ῥίζης γλυκείας, μαλαβάθρου φύλλου, ὀποβαλσάμου, ἀγαρικοῦ, κινναμώμου ἀνὰ < ιγ'. ζιγγιβέρεως, τριφύλλου σπέρματος, ἀμώμου, πηγάνου ἀγρίου σπέρματος, ἀρκευθίδων μὴ πεπείρων ξηρῶν ἀνὰ < ιε'. πετροσελίνου ἀνὰ < η'. ὀποῦ μήκωνος ἴσον, καστορίου, πεπέρεως μακροῦ, ὑποκυστίδος χυλοῦ, κύφεως ἀνὰ < ιβ'. ὀβολοὺς β'. πολίου, πεπέρεως λευκοῦ, σεσέλεως, βδελλίου ἀνὰ < ιε'. ὀβολοὺς γ'. σχοίνου ἄνθους, κόστου ἀνὰ < ιβ' S''. δαύκου σπέρματος, θλάσπεως ἀνὰ

chadis drach. v, obol. ij, radicis trifolii ʒ iv, vel ejus ſeminis drach. iij, florum ſcordii drach. xj, obol. ij, polii Cretici ʒ vj, obol. ij, aſari drach. ij, acori drach. iij, obol. iij ß, ſeminis dauci tantundem: ſeminis aniſi drach. ij, cumini Aethiopici tantundem, rhei Pontici ʒ v, obol. iij ß, ſeminis napi ſylveſtris drach. iij, vel ſeminis napi ſativi tantundem, phu Pontici drach. ij, mellis cocti quod ſatis eſt.

[*Antidotus incomparabilis quam ipſe compoſui, faciens ad omnes internas corporis affectiones, ex Nicoſtrati traditione.*] ℞ Radicis dulcis, folii malabathri, opobalſami, agarici, cinnamomi, ſingulorum ʒ xiij, zingiberis, ſeminis trifolii, amomi, ſeminis rutae ſilveſtris, baccarum juniperi immaturarum et exiccatarum, ſingulorum ʒ xv, petroſelini ſingulorum ʒ viij, ſucci papaveris tantundem; caſtorii, piperis longi, ſucci hypocyſtidis, cypheos, ſingulorum drach. xij, obolos ij, polii, piperis albi, ſeſeleos, bdellii, ſingulorum drach. xv, obol. iij, florum junci odorati, coſti ſingulorum drach. xij ß, ſeminis dauci,

< ιγ'. ναρδοστάχυος < κδ'. κασσίας μελαίνης ῥίζης < ιστ'. λιβάνου, πάνακος, ὀποπάνακος, ἀνὰ < ιβ'. ἀκόρου < ε'. σκορδίου < ιζ'. μαράθρου, νάρδου Κελτικῆς, Γεντιανῆς, ῥόδων ἄνθους, κόμμεως, ὀποῦ Κυρηναϊκοῦ, καρδαμώμου, ἀμμωνιακοῦ θυμιάματος, ἐχίου ῥίζης, ἀπαρίνης χυλοῦ, ἀνὰ < η'. σαγαπηνοῦ, ὑπερικοῦ, ἀκακίας χυλοῦ, ἴρεως Ἰλλυρικῆς, ἀνὰ < ιδ'. σμύρνης στακτῆς < κ'. κρόκου δραχμὰς λ'. στύρακος δραχμὰς ια'. ὀβολοὺς β'. φοῦ, μήου, δικτάμνου, βουνιάδος σπέρματος, καλάμου ἀρωματικοῦ, ἀνὰ δραχμὰς η' ἢ ι'. ἀνίσου, ἀσάρου, ἀγαρικοῦ, σκίγκου, ἀνὰ δραχμὰς στ'. τερμινθίνης, ἀνὰ δραχμὰς ιδ'. ὀβολοὺς δ'. χαλβάνης δραχμὰς ε'. νήσσης θηλείας αἵματος, ἐριφείου αἵματος, ἀνὰ δραχμὰς ζ'. πεπέρεως μέλανος καὶ πεπέρεως μακροῦ, (441) ἀνὰ < κδ'. κροκομάγματος ἴσας, πενταφύλλου ῥίζης, ὀριγάνου ἀγρίου, πρασίου, στοιχάδος, ἄμμεως, χαμαίδρυος, χαμαιπίτυος, κενταυρίου λεπτοῦ, ἀριστολοχίας λεπτῆς, ἀνὰ < στ'. λημνίας σφραγῖδος < λ'. χηνείου αἵματος, χελώνης

thlaſpeos, ſingulorum drach. xiij; ſpicae nardi drach. xxiv, radicis caſſiae nigrae ʒ xvj, thuris, panacis, opopanacis, ſingulorum ʒ xij; acori ʒ v, ſcordii ʒ xvij, foeniculi, nardi Celticae, gentianae, florum roſarum, gummi, ſucci Cyrenaici, cardamomi, ammoniaci thymiamatis, radicis echii, ſucci aparines, ſingulorum drach. viij; ſagapeni, hyperici, ſucci acaciae, iridis Illyricae, ſingulorum drach. xiv; myrrhae ſtactae ʒ xx, croci drach. xxx, ſtyracis drach. xj, obolis ij, phu, mei, dictamni, ſeminis napi, calami odorati, ſingulorum ʒ viij aut x. aniſi, aſari, agarici, ſcinci, ſingulorum ʒ vj; terebinthinae, ſingulorum drach. xiv. obolos iv, galbani drach. v, ſanguinis anatis foeminae, ſanguinis hoedi, ſingulorum drach. vij. piperis nigri, piperis longi, ſingulorum ʒ xxiv. crocomagmatis tantundem; radicis quinqueſolii, origani ſilveſtris, marrubii, ſtoechadis, ammeos, chamaedryos, chamaepitys, centaureae minoris, ariſtolochiae tenuis, ſingulorum drachmas ſex; ſigilli Lemnii drach. xxx, ſanguinis anſerini,

θαλασσίας, ῥήου Ποντικοῦ ἀνὰ ∠ ζ΄. μέλιτος Ἀττικοῦ τὸ ἀρκοῦν· ἡ πόσις κυάμου μέγεθος ἐν ὕδατι. ποιεῖ καὶ πρὸς τεταρταῖον, πρὸς δὲ τὰ θανάσιμα, ὡς οὐκ ἄλλη. Ἀντίδοτος Αἰλίου Γάλλου, ᾗ Καῖσαρ συμφώνως, ταύτῃ καὶ Χάρμης ἐχρήσατο, ποιοῦσα πρὸς τὰ θανάσιμα καὶ ἰοβόλα, κᾂν τόπον ἑρπετῶν καταῤῥάνῃς, φυγαδεύσεις. ποιεῖ πρὸς ῥεῦμα πᾶν ὀφθαλμῶν, καὶ τῶν λοιπῶν ἀναξηραίνουσα, δυσαρεστήματα λύει, πυρετοὺς χρονίους καὶ περιοδικούς. ποιεῖ δὲ καὶ ἐπὶ τῶν δυστραπέλως καθαιρομένων γυναικῶν, ἀλύπως ἔμβρυα ἐκκρίνει, ποιεῖ καὶ πρὸς φθισικούς. ἡ δόσις καρύου Ποντικοῦ μεθ' ὕδατος κυάθων δ΄. ἐπὶ δὲ τῶν ἐχεοδήκτων σὺν οἴνῳ. [900] ℞ Σμύρνης ∠ ιβ΄. κρόκου ∠ ιδ΄. νάρδου ιδ΄. σχοίνου ιβ΄. κινναμώμου β΄. ἀμώμου δ΄. χαλβάνης ια΄. τερμινθίνης ∠ ε΄. πεπέρεως λευκοῦ ι΄, καὶ μακροῦ λβ΄. κόστου ∠ η΄. λιβάνου ιβ΄. ὀποῦ μήκωνος ἴσον, σκορδίου ∠ ν΄. ἐν ἄλλῳ η΄. πολίου δ΄. ὑποκυστίδος χυλοῦ ιβ΄. πετροσελίνου ιη΄. σεσέλεως ιδ΄. δαύκου σπέρματος ιϛ΄. ὀποβαλσάμου ιβ΄. ὀπο-

testudinis marinae, rhei Pontici, fingulorum ʒ vij. mellis Attici quod fufficit. Datur ad magnitudinem fabae ex aqua. Facit etiam ad quartanam, caeterum ad lethalia, plus aliis antidotis valet. *Antidotus Aelii Galli, qua Caefar et Charmes utebantur, ad lethalia morfuque illata venena faciens: quoque fi loca in quibus reptilia diverfantur, afperferis, ea fugabis; facit ad omnem oculorum fluxum, et reliquarum partium fluxum deficcat faftidia, et longas intermittentesque febres solvit. Mulieribus praeterea, quae difficulter purgantur, auxiliatur. Foetus fine dolore ejicit. Tabidis demum ex quatuor aquae cyathis ad nucis avellanae magnitudinem fumpta prodeft: in viperae morfibus ex vino.* ℞ Myrrhae ʒ xij, croci ʒ xiv, nardi ʒ xiv, junci rotundi odorati ʒ xij, cinnamomi ʒ ij, amomi ʒ iv, galbani ʒ xj. terebinthinae ʒ v, piperis albi ʒ x, piperis longi ʒ xxxij, cofti ʒ viij, thuris ʒ xij, fucci papaveris tantundem, fcordii ʒ l, in alio ʒ viij, polii ʒ iv, fucci hypocyftidis ʒ xij, petrofelini ʒ xviij, fefelis ʒ xiv, feminis dauci ʒ xvj, opobalfami ʒ xij, opopanacis tantundem, caftorii ʒ viij,

Ed. Chart. XIII. [900.] Ed. Baf. II. (441.)
πάνακος ἴσον, καστορίου η'. μέλιτος Ἀττικοῦ ξε. β'. Ἀντίδοτος Ζωπύριος. ℞ Κινναμώμου ∠ γ'. σμύρνης στακτῆς ∠ ε'. νάρδου ε'. δίδοται καρύου Ποντικοῦ μέγεθος σὺν ὕδατι, κυάθοις τρισὶν ἐπ' ἐνιαυτόν.

Κεφ. β'. [Περὶ τῆς Μιθριδατείου ἀντιδότου, ὡς Δαμοκράτης.] Ταύτας μὲν οὖν τὰς ἀντιδότους τὰς γεγραμμένας πάσας ὁ Ἀνδρόμαχος ἔγραψεν. ἐπεὶ δὲ τὰ διὰ μέτρων γεγραμμένα, καὶ πρὸς ἀκρίβειαν τῶν σταθμῶν τῶν φαρμάκων, καὶ πρὸς μνήμην ἐστὶ χρησιμώτατα, διὰ τοῦτο καὶ τὰς ὑπὸ Δαμοκράτους συγγεγραμμένας ἀξιολόγους ἀντιδότους ἐφεξῆς ὑπέταξα, τὴν ἀρχὴν ἀπὸ τῆς Μιθριδατείου ποιησάμενος.

[Αἱ ὑπὸ Δαμοκράτους ἀντίδοτοι γεγραμμέναι.] Ἀντίδοτος ἣν λέγουσι Μιθριδάτειόν τινες τῶν σφόδρα ἐπισήμων, δραστικὸν φάρμακον πρὸς πᾶν πάθος πᾶσάν τ' ἀντίδοτον εἶπον ποιεῖν.

Σμύρνης Ἀραβικῆς Τρωγλοδύτιδος δραχ. ι'.
Κρόκου ι'. ἀγαρικοῦ ι'. ζιγγιβέρεως

mellis Attici fextarios ij. *Antidotus Zopyria.* ℞ Cinnamomi ʒ iij, myrrhae ftactae ʒ v, nardi ʒ v. Exhibetur ad nucis avellanae magnitudinem, ex tribus aquae cyathis ad annum.

Cap. II. [*De Mithridatica antidoto ex Damocratis traditione.*] Has itaque fcriptas antidotos omnes Andromachus prodidit. Quum vero quae carminibus explicatae funt, ad ponderis finceritatem medicamentorumque memoriam maxime conducant, idcirco confcriptas quoque a Damocrate antidotos memoratu dignas fubjunximus, principio rurfus a Mithridatica fumpto.

[*Antidoti a Damocrate confcriptae.*] Antidotus quam viri quidam infignes admodum Mithridatium vocant, medicamenta ad omnes malas corporis affectiones efficax, quamque omnis antidoti vicem praeftare dixerunt.

Myrrhae Arabicae Troglodyticae drachmas decem.
Croci decem, agarici decem, zingiberis decem,

Ι'. Κινναμώμου ι'. ναρδοστάχυος
Ι'. λιβάνου ι'. θλάσπεως ι'.
Καὶ σεσέλεως, ὀποβαλσάμου, σχοίνου τε καὶ
Στοιχάδος, κόστου, χαλβάνης, τερμινθίνης,
Μακροῦ πεπέρεως, καστορίου τε Ποντικοῦ,
Ὑποκυστίδος χυλοῦ τε, καὶ στύρακος καλοῦ,
Ὀποπάνακος, καὶ μαλαβάθρου φύλλων νέου,
Πάντων ἑκάστου τὰς ἴσας δὶς δ'.
Κασίας μελαίνης ζ'. πολίου ζ'.
Λευκοῦ πεπέρεως ταὐτὸ, σκορδίου τ' ἴσον,
Τοῦ Κρητικοῦ δαύκου τε ταὐτὸν σπέρματος.
Ἴσας δ' ἑνὶ τούτων, βαλσάμου καρποῦ δραχμὰς,
Καὶ κύφεως τὸν αὐτὸν ἐνίοτε τούτων σταθμόν.
Τινὲς δὲ καὶ βδελλίου ἐπὶ τούτων ἴσον,
Νάρδου καθαρᾶς δὲ Κελτικῆς, καὶ κόμμεως,
Καὶ πετροσελίνου, καὶ ὀπίου, μηκωνείου,
Καὶ καρδαμώμου, καὶ μαράθρου τοῦ σπέρματος,
Καὶ Γεντιανῆς, καὶ ῥόδων φύλλων ἴσας,

*Cinnamomi decem, ſpicae nardi decem,
Thuris decem, et item thlaſpis decem,
At ſeſelis, et ſucci balſami, et junci odorati,
Stoechadis, coſti, galbani, terebinthinae,
Piperis longi, ac caſtorii Pontici,
Succi hypocyſtidis, ſtyracis bonae,
Opopanacis, et folii malabathri recentis,
Pares ſingulorum bis quatuor drachmas capit.
Caſiae vero nigrae ſeptem et polii ſeptem.
Piperis albi ſeptem, ſcordii tantundem;
Cretici tamen et ſeminum dauci tantum.
His pendet fructus balſami drachmas pares.
Aequale pondus cyphi praedictis dabit.
Sunt qui par velint bdelium adjicere.
Hinc nardi Celticae repurgatae, et gummi,
Et petroſelini, et opii, meconium quod vocant,
Et cardamomi, et ſeminum foeniculi,
Et gentianae, et foliorum roſae,*

Ἀνὰ ε'. δραχμὰς μικρὸν ἐπιῤῥεπέστερον.
Τοῦ Κρητικοῦ τε ταὐτὸ δικτάμνου μέρος,
Ἀνίσου τε καὶ ἀσάρου τε γ'. δραχ.
Ἀκόρου τε καὶ φοῦ, καὶ σαγαπηνοῦ τὰς ἴσας,
Ἀθαμαντικοῦ μήου τε καὶ τῆς ἀκακίας,
Σκίγκου τε γαστρὸς, ὑπερικοῦ τε σπέρματος.
Τούτων ἴσα πάντων ἀνὰ β' S''.
Ὁλκάδας, οἴνου τὸ μέτριον, καὶ μέλιτος
Τὸ σύμμετρον, ὡς τάσδ' ὁμοίως οὕτως σκεύασον.

Ἐπεὶ οὖν κύφεως ἐμνημόνευσεν ὁ Δαμοκράτης, ὃ καὶ αὐτὸς κατασκευάζεται, διὰ τοῦτο καλῶς ἐποίησε, προσγράψας αὐτοῦ τὴν κατασκευὴν, ἐφεξῆς γεγραμμένην.

Τὸ κῦφι δ' οὐδέν ἐστιν οὐδὲ μίγμ' ἁπλοῦν,
Οὐδ' αὐτὸ γῆ φέρει τις, οὐδ' ὀπίζεται.
Αἰγύπτιοι δὲ τοῦτο τῶν θεῶν τισιν
Ἐπιθυμιῶσι σκευάσαντες, ὡς φράσω.
Λευκὴν λαβόντες σταφίδα τὴν λιπαρωτάτην,
Αἴρουσι τὸν φλοιόν τε καὶ τὸ σπέρμ' ἅπαν.

Cujusque drachmas quinque, paululo amplius.
Sit Cretici dictamni aequalis portio.
Anifi et afari pariter tres drachmae
Acorique, phuque, fagapenique tres.
Meique Athamantici, et acaciae,
Et ventris fcinci, et feminum hyperici,
Singula drachmas haec pendant duas femis.
Vini et mellis adde quantum eft fatis.
Satis eft quantum haec apte jungas fimul.

Quoniam vero Damocrates cypheos mentionem facit, quod etiam ipfe componit, recte ideo illius qnoque compofitionem adfcripfit, quam deinceps fubjiciam.

Cyphi vero nec mixtum quicquam eft, nec fimplex
Ipfum fert tellus ulla, non preffus herbae fuccus.
Aegyptus quosdam hoc cum placat deos,
Incendit, et quo dicam parat modo.
Paffam et albam fumunt et pinguiffimam,

Τὴν σάρκα δ᾽ αὐτῆς λεοτριβήσαντες καλῶς
[901] Ἱστᾶσι δραχμὰς Ἀττικὰς δὶς δώδεκα,
Τερμινθίνης τε ταὐτὸ τῆς κεκαυμένης,
Σμύρνης τε ιβ'. κινναμώμου δ'.
Σχοίνου ιβ'. καὶ κρόκου μία, βδελλίου
Ὄνυχας δραχ. γ'. ἀσπαλάθου β' S''.
Ναρδοστάχυος γ'. καὶ κασίας γ'. τῆς καλῆς
Καθαρᾶς, κυπείρου γ'. δραχμὰς, ἀρκευθίδων
Ἐκ τῶν μεγίστων καὶ λιπαρῶν ταύταις ἴσας,
Θ'. δὲ καλάμου τοῦ μυρεψικοῦ δραχμὰς,
Μέλιτος τὸ μέτριον, παντελῶς οἴνου βραχὺ,
Βδέλλιον, οἶνον, σμύρναν εἰς θυΐδιον
Βαλόντες, εὖ τρίβουσιν ὡς μέλιτος πάχος
Ὑγροῦ ποιῆσαι, καὶ προσαποδόντες μέλι
Τὴν σταφίδα συντρίβουσιν, εἶτα λεῖα δὲ
Ἅπαντα καταμίξαντες ἐκ τούτου κύκλους
Βραχεῖς ποιοῦντες θυμιῶσι τοῖς θεοῖς.

Corticem demunt, eximunt vinacea.
Carnem ipſius perlaevigatam inſigniter
Bis duodecim conſtituunt drachmis Atticis.
Crematae terebinthinae pondus et idem,
Myrrhae duodecim, et cinnamomi quatuor,
Junci duodecim, et unicam ponunt croci.
Tres unguium bdellii, aſpalathi duas ſemis,
Tres ſpicae nardi, tres caſiae bonae,
Tres meri cyperi, baccas juniperi quibus
Adjungunt aequas, pingues et magnas legunt;
Accedit drachmis calamus flagrans novem,
Mellis quod ſufficit, et vini prorſus parum.
Bdellium, vinum, myrrham, in mortarium
Mittunt et terunt, quoad mellis craſſitiem
Liquentis juncta reddant. Tum mel poſtea
Affundunt, uvas miſcent; demum caetera
Imponunt, ſed contuſa. Parvos inde
Confingunt orbes, quibus deos fumigant.

Ῥοῦφος μὲν οὕτω δεῖν ἔφασκε σκευάσαι,
Ἀνὴρ ἄριστος ἰκτικός θ᾽ ἐν τῇ τέχνῃ.
Ἔνιοι δὲ κιννάμωμον οὐ σχόντες βαλεῖν
Μίσγουσι ταὐτὸ καρδαμώμου σπέρματος.
Χρῶνται δ᾽ ὁμοίως τῇ πρὸ ταύτης συνθέσει.
Τινὲς δὲ καὶ τοῖς ἧπαρ ἢ τὸν πνεύμονα,
Ἢ καί τι ἕτερον σπλάγχνον ἐξηλκωμένοις
Πίνειν διδόασιν, ὡς δραχμὴν τοῦ φαρμάκου.

Κεφ. γ΄. [Περὶ τριῶν ἀντιδότων ἀξιολόγων, δυοῖν πρὸς τὴν φθίσιν καὶ μιᾶς πρὸς τὰ δηλητήρια.] Μεμνημένου δὲ τοῦ Δαμοκράτους καὶ ἄλλων ἀντιδότων ἀξιολόγων, ἄμεινον ἔδοξέ μοι κἀκείνας διὰ τὴν αὐτὴν χρείαν ἐν μέτρῳ γεγραμμένας ὑπ᾽ αὐτοῦ παραθέσθαι. τὴν μὲν οὖν θηριακὴν ὀνομαζομένην ὅπως συντίθησιν ἐν τῷ πρὸ τούτου λόγῳ δεδήλωκα· νυνὶ δὲ τὰς ἐφεξῆς αὐτῆς γεγραμμένας παραθήσομαι.

Ἄλλη σφόδρα καλὴ πρὸς φθισικοὺς κεχρονισμένους,
Τούς θ᾽ αἷμ᾽ ἀνάγοντας, καὶ πυρέσσοντας λάθρα,

Rufus nos cyphi ſic parare docet,
Vir probus valde et peritus medicus.
Quidam ſi deſit cinnamomum ſibi,
Tantundem miſcent cardamomi ſeminum,
Et hac utuntur aeque ac priore.
Quidam, ſi pulmo, vel jecur, vel exectis
Aliud ullum, ulcus habet malum,
Hujus propinant pharmaci denarium.

Cap. III. [*De tribus Antidotis inſignibus, duabus ad Phthiſim, una ad venena.*] Quum vero Democrates aliarum quoque antidotorum inſignium meminerit, latius mihi viſum eſt illas etiam propter eundem uſum verſibus ab eo proditas exponere. Quomodo igitur theriacam quam vocant ipſe componat in praecedente libro docuimus; nunc quae deinceps ſcriptae ſunt antidoti, eas ſubjiciemus.

Antiquae phthiſi alia valde bona,
Et ſputo ſanguinis, et clam febrienti,

Καὶ τοὺς ἔχοντας ἀσθενῆ θώρηκα,
Καὶ τοὺς στομαχικοὺς, ἡπατικοὺς, νεφριτικοὺς,
Καὶ πρὸς ἃ προεῖπον πάντα. τοῖς τρυφερωτέροις
Μᾶλλον προσηνὴς, ἀλλ' ἔλαττον δραστική.
Ταύτῃ λέγουσι τὸν Σεβαστὸν ἡδέως
Χρησάμενον ὑγιᾶ γεγονέναι ἐν βραχεῖ χρόνῳ,
Πλευροῖς τε καὶ θώρακι δυσχρηστούμενον.
(442) *Ἔχει δὲ ψυλλίου τε καὶ κασίας κιῤῥᾶς,*
Ναρδοστάχυός τε, καὶ καθαρᾶς τῆς Κελτικῆς,
Καὶ κινναμώμου, καὶ κρόκου τοῦ προσφάτου,
Ἀνὰ ιβ' δραχμὰς, καὶ ὀποβαλσάμου δέκα,
Στακτῆς Ἀραβικῆς παχυτάτης ιστ'.
Σχοίνου τε λεπτῆς, Λημνίας τε τῆς καλῆς,
Ῥᾶ Ποντικοῦ τε, πηγάνου τε σπέρματος,
Τὸ δ' ἄγριόν ἐστι πήγανον κρεῖττον πολὺ,
Καλοῦ τ' ἀμώμου καὶ ῥόδων ξηρῶν ἴσον,
Λευκοῦ τε πεπέρεως, βουνιάδος τοῦ σπέρματος.
Ἔστω δ' ἀγρίας τοῦτο, μὴ τῆς ἡμέρου,

Nec non et pectus imbecille habentibus.
Stomacho, renibus, et jecori prodeſt.
Omnibus quae dixi valet, delicatis tamen
Quod poſſit minus, conveniet magis.
Libenter ſumpta hac Auguſtum ferunt
E longo morbo convaluiſſe brevi,
Pectore multum coſtisque affectum male.
Accipit et pſyllii, et ſubrubentis caſiae,
Spicaeque nardi, et purae Celticae,
Et cinnamomi, atque recentis croci,
Drachmas duodecim, opobalſami decem;
Myrrhae Arabicae ſtactae craſſiſſimae ſedecim.
Hinc junci tenuis, et ſigilli lemnii,
Rheu Pontici, et ſeminum rutae;
Silveſtris melior multo eſt ruta tamen;
Amomi quoque et ſiccae roſae tantum.
His album piper adde, ſemen napi;
Incultis locis hoc, non ſubactis lege.

Τούτων ἀνὰ δραχμὰς δ'. λιβάνου τε γ'.
Ἴσον τε λιβάνῳ προσβαλεῖς τὸ Κρητικὸν
Δίκταμνον, ἱκανῶς ξηρὸν, ἀλλὰ πρόσφατον.
Ταὐτό τε κυμίνου Θηβαϊκοῦ τοῦ σπέρματος.
Τὰ μὲν ἄλλα κόψας σῆθε λεπτῷ κοσκίνῳ,
Μόνον δὲ τὸ ψύλλιον εἰς ὅλμον βαλὼν,
Κόψον πολὺ πλέον, ἵνα λάβῃς ὅσον θέλῃς.
Ἅπαν γὰρ αὐτὸ λεπτὸν ἀδύνατον ποιεῖν.
Σκεύαζε δ' οὕτω, τὴν καλὴν στακτὴν βαλὼν
Εἰς πλατυτέραν θυείαν, οἴνου παραχέων
Λιπαροῦ Φαλερίνου τὸ μέτριον, λέαινέ τε
[902] Ἐπ' ὀλίγον αὐτὰ, καὶ ὀποβάλσαμον τότε
Μιγνὺς, διϋγρον τοῦτο δ' ἐστὶ χρήσιμον,
Παρεμπάσσων τε τὰ ξηρὰ πάντα μίγματα,
Ἄφες δ' ὀλίγον συμπιεῖν τὸ φάρμακον,
Τό, τε μέλι ζέσας, δὶς ἢ τρὶς αὐτῶν καταχέας,
Ἑνῶν τε τὴν ἀντίδοτον ἀποθήσεις τότε,
Εἰς πυξίδ' οἵαν εἶπον ἔμπροσθεν βραχὺ,

Quater haec duo drachmam, ter vero thus trahet.
Aequabit thus dictamnum Creticum, ſatis
Siccatum quidem, ſed tamen adhuc recens.
Thuri cuminum exaeques Thebaicum.
Alia cribro tuſa excerne tenui,
Immitte ſolum in mortarium pſyllium,
Multo plus tamen, ut inde quantum velis
Sumas, nam totum comminui nequit.
Conſice hoc pacto; ſtacten mitte bonam
In pilam latam, vini quantum eſt ſatis
Falerni pinguis affunde, atque dilue
Myrrham parumper; opobalſamum dein
Admiſce translucidum, nam id eſt bonum.
Hinc, ubi mixta conſperſeris cuncta arida,
Combibant ſines medicamen tantiſper,
Donec fervorem bis terve mel efferat.
Affuſo melle unies antidotum.
Repone vaſe, qualem deſcripſi modo.

Διδοὺς ὁμοίως κἀπὶ τῶν αὐτῶν παθῶν.
Ἄλλη σφόδρα καλὴ πρὸς ἃ εἶπον πάνθ' ἁπλῶς.
Φασὶν δ' ἀμείνω τήνδε πρὸς τὰ πνεύματα
Πολλοῖς χρόνοις λυποῦντα τὸν στόμαχον, ποιεῖν,
Καὶ βορβορυγμοὺς τοὺς ἐνοχλουμένους ἀεὶ,
Τῶν ἐντέρων, κώλου τε, καὶ τῆς γαστέρος.
Ποιεῖ δὲ καὶ γέρουσιν ὀξυωπίαν.
Τοῖς θηριοδήκτοις δ' ἐστὶ συμφορωτάτη.
Σκεύαζε δ' αὐτὴν, ταῦτ' ἔχων τὰ μίγματα.
Κυρηναϊκοῦ τοῦ καλοῦ δραχμὴν ὀποῦ,
Ἀκόρου τε καὶ φοῦ καστορίου τε καὶ ἀσάρου,
Καὶ καρδαμώμου σπέρματος καὶ κόμμεως,
Χυλοῦ τ' ἀκακίας, τῆς ἀρίστης ἴρεως,
Καθαροῦ σαγαπηνοῦ, ὑπερικοῦ τοῦ Κρητικοῦ,
Τούτων ἑκάστου β'. δραχμὰς ῥεπέστερον,
Ὀποβαλσάμου τε τοῦ διαυγοῦς γ'. δραχμὰς,
Ὀποβαλσάμῳ δὲ ταὐτὸ ψυλλίου βάρος,
Λευκοῦ τε πεπέρεως, πετροσελίνου, Κελτικῆς

Peraeque his ipsis in affectibus dato.
Alia, valde bona ad quae dixi omnia,
Prorsusque hanc dicunt ad flatus meliorem,
Stomachum longo qui infestarunt tempore.
Tollit rugitus, qui ventrem et colon
Perturbant, intestina discurrentes.
Acutos quoque reddit oculos senum.
Viperis morsos summa levat ope.
Ita hanc conficies, sed miscenda haec habe.
Succi Cyrenaici boni drachmam cape,
Acori, phu, castoriique et asari,
Seminis cardamomi, gummi Arabici,
Liquoris acaciae, iridis optimae,
Sagapeni puri, Cretensis hyperici,
Propensa lance drachmas injice duas.
Tres opobalsami pellucidi, parem
Mensuram psyllii opobalsamo subdes.
Tum albi piperis, petroselini, Celticae

Στάχυός τε νάρδου, μαλαβάθρου φύλλου νέου
Αἰθιοπικοῦ τε, καὶ κυμίνου σπέρματος,
Ἀθαμαντικοῦ μήου τε, κἀμώμου καλοῦ,
Μήκωνος, ὀπίου, γεντιανῆς καὶ βαλσάμου,
Στήσας ἑκάστου δραχμὰς δ'. σταθμῷ,
Στύρακος σταγόνας δὲ ε'. καὶ τριώβολον.
Κόστου δὲ λευκοῦ καὶ σεσέλεως, θλάσπεως,
Κασίας μελαίνης ε'. ἑκάστου β'. ὀβολοὺς,
Σχοίνου τε, πολίου ἀνὰ ε'. τριώβολον,
Καὶ Κρητικοῦ δὲ ταὐτὸ, δικτάμνου πόας
Ταύτης ἴσον, πρόσβαλλε σκορδίου σταθμόν.
Μακροῦ πεπέρεως καὶ λιβάνου καὶ Λημνίας
Σμύρνης, γλυκυῤῥίζης, χαλβάνης, τερμινθίνης,
Ξηροῦ τε νήσσης αἵματος, τοῦ προσφάτου,
Ὀποπάνακός τε καὶ μαράθρου τοῦ σπέρματος,
Ξηρῶν ῥόδων φύλλων, καὶ τῆς ὑποκιστίδος
Χυλοῦ καλῶς γεγονότος, ἀγαρικοῦ τ' ἴσα,
Τοῦ Κρητικοῦ δαύκου τε καθαροῦ σπέρματος,

Spicaeque nardi, malabathri folii recentis,
Aethiopicique feminum cumini;
Meique Athamantici et amomi boni,
Meconis opii, gentianae et balfami,
Cujusque pones drachmas pondere quatuor.
Styracis quinque liquidae et triobolum:
At albi cofti, thlafpeos et fefelis,
Nigraeque cafiae, cujusque duos obolos;
Schoeni, et polii, drachmas quinque tres obolos,
Item dictamni, Cretae quam tellus alit.
Pondere eodem conjicito fcordium,
Mafculum thus, Lemni terram, longum piper,
Myrrham, glycyrhizam, galbanum, terebinthinam,
Anatis recentem, fed ficcatum fanguinem,
Opopanacis, ac femen foeniculi,
Folium rofae ficcum, hypociftidis
Expreffum pulchre fuccum, dein agaricum,
Daucique femen Cretici electum adde,

Ἀνισαρίου τε σπέρματος, σκίγκου τ᾽ ἴσον,
Δὶς τρὶς ἑκάστου μίγματος βαλεῖς σταθμὸν,
Καὶ ζιγγιβέρεώς τε τοῦ ξηροῦ καλῶς,
Καὶ κινναμώμου καὶ κρόκου δὶς τέσσαρας,
Μέλιτός τε χρηστοῦ τὸν διπλοῦν πᾶσι σταθμὸν,
Οἴνου τε Χίου τοῦ καλοῦ τὸ σύμμετρον.
Ἢ τοῦ Φαλερίνου ταὐτὸ τοῦ κεχρονισμένου.
Σκεύαζε δ᾽ αὐτὴν, ὡς προεῖπον δεῖν ποιεῖν,
Τὴν θηριακὴν ἀντίδοτον ἔμπροσθεν βραχὺ,
Διδόναι θ᾽ ὁμοίως πᾶσιν, ὡς ἐκείνην ἔφην.
Ἄλλη δι᾽ αἱμάτων ἀντίδοτος, ἥν φασίν τινες
Ποιεῖν ἄμεινον πρὸς τὰ δηλητήρια.
Ἔχει δὲ χηνὸς αἵματος ξηροῦ δύο,
Καὶ τρεῖς χελώνης τῆς θαλασσίας δραχμὰς,
Τὸ δ᾽ αὐτὸ νήσσης, καὶ ἐρίφου γ΄. τὰς ἴσας.
Νήσσης δ᾽ ἄμεινον αἷμα θηλείας δοκεῖ,
Στακτῆς Ἀραβικῆς παχυτάτης δραχμὰς ι΄.
Ναρδοστάχυός τε τὰς ἴσας σμύρνης δραχμὰς,

Anisi quoque semen et scincum quoque,
Bis tres cujusque pondera denarios;
Demum zingiberis cum sicci, tum boni,
Et cinnamomi atque croci bis quatuor.
Mellis probati pondus duplex indito
Cunctis, bonique vini Chii, quod satis,
Falerni aut veteris tantundem conjungito.
At confice ipsam, uti parumper antea
Parandam antidotum Theriacen docui.
Utque illam dixi, sic hanc omnibus dabis.
Alia ex sanguinibus, quam quidam ajunt
Caeteris amplius ad venena conferre,
Continet anserini sanguinis sicci duas
Drachmas, tres marinae testudinis,
Hoedini tres, tres anserini sanguinis;
Videtur autem melior anatis foeminae,
Stactae Arabicae crassissimae drachmas decem.
Nardi spicae pares et myrrhae drachmas,

Καὶ κινναμώμου τοῦ καλοῦ δὶς τρεῖς δραχμάς.
Ῥόδων δὲ φύλλων ξηροτάτων δὶς τέσσαρας,
Σχοίνου, λιβάνου, κόστου, μία ἑκάστου δραχμὴ,
Καὶ τρεῖς ἀμώμου, πεπέρεως λευκοῦ τὰς ἴσας,
Καὶ τοῦ μακροῦ δὲ πεπέρεως μίαν ἥμισυ,
Κρόκου δὲ δώδεκα καὶ κασίας δὶς δ'.
Ῥίζης τριφύλλου ε'. πολίου τὰς ἴσας,
Ὀποβαλσάμου τρεῖς, πετροσελίνου δ'.
[903] *Ἀρκευθίδων τῶν λιπαρῶν, καὶ ἀκόρου δύο,*
Ῥᾶ Ποντικοῦ, μήου τε, δικτάμνου δύο,
Τουτέστι ἀνὰ δύο, φοῦ τε τὰς αὐτὰς β'.
Ἀμμωνιακοῦ τε ὡσαύτως θυμιάματος,
Μαράθρου δραχμὰς β'. ἀγαρικοῦ δύο ἥμισυ.
Τρεῖς τοῦ πετραίου πηγάνου, δαύκου β'.
Ἀνισαρίου τε καὶ ἀσάρου μίαν ἥμισυ,
Ἴσον δὲ τούτοις, τούτοις πάλιν
Ἴσον κυμίνου Θηβαϊκοῦ τοῦ σπέρματος,
Καὶ γ'. δραχμὰς βουνιάδος ἀγρίας σπέρματος,

Et cinnamomi drachmas bis ternas boni,
Bis quatuor foliorum ficcae rofae,
Junci rotundi, coftique, et thuris unam,
Amomi tres, piperis albi totidem,
At longi piperis unam et dimidiam,
Croci duodecim, cafiae bis quatuor,
Quinque radicum trifolii, et polii pares,
Opobalfami tres, petrofelini quatuor,
Baccarum juniperi pinguium, et acori duas,
Rha Pontici, meique, et dictamni duas,
Hoc eft cujusque binas, phu fimul duas
Ammoniacique thymiamatis fimiliter,
Duas foeniculi, agarici duas femis,
Tres rutae filveftris, dauci duas quoque,
Anifi, et afari unam cum dimidia,
Par pondus ammeos his, et his quoque,
Seminum cumini tantum Thebaici,
Tres feminum filveftris drachmas napi

Τούτοις προσαπόδος έ. σκορδίου δραχμὰς,
Τὸ Κρητικὸν δ' ἄμεινον ὡς προείπομεν,
Μέλιτος ἅπασι τοῦ καλοῦ διπλοῦν σταθμόν.
Ἅπαντα λεπτὰ λεῖα τὰ προειρημένα,
Ἑφθῷ τε τῷ μέλιτι δεύσας ἀποτίθου.

Κεφ. δ'. [Περὶ Χάρμου ἀντιδότου.] Μετὰ τὰς γεγραμμένας ἀντιδότους ἄχρι δεῦρο, τὴν Μιθριδάτειον ἔγραψεν ὁ Δαμοκράτης, ἣν ὀλίγον ἔμπροσθεν ἐγὼ παρεθέμην. ὑπερβὰς οὖν αὐτὴν, ὡς ἐφεξῆς γράφει, προσθήσω.

Ἀντίδοτος, ἥν φασιν οἱ νεώτεροι Χάρμην,
Θεραπεύει δὲ διαθέσεις κεχρονισμένας,
Ἃς οὐδὲν ὠφέλησεν ἕτερα φάρμακα.
Σμύρνης ἔχει δὲ τῆς καλῆς, ὀποβαλσάμου,
Ὑποκιστίδος χυλοῦ τε, καὶ λιβάνου καλοῦ,
Ὀποπάνακος καθαροῦ τε καὶ νέου κρόκου,
(443) Τούτων ἑκάστου μίγματος δυοκαίδεκα.
Κόστου δὲ λευκοῦ, καστορίου τε Ποντικοῦ,
Τερμινθίνης τε τῆς καθαρᾶς, σχοίνου τ' ἴσον.

Praedictis addes, quinque vero ſcordii,
Quod Creta gignit, diximus id melius.
Mellis probati duplex pondus indito.
Detrita cuncta quae praediximus nuper,
Et merſa cocto melle vaſis condito.

Cap. IV. [*De Charme Antidoto.*] Poſt antidotos hucusque deſcriptas Mithridaticam Damocrates ſcripſit, quam ego paulo ante appoſui. Ea igitur omiſſa quas deinceps conſcribit adjiciam.

Antidotus, quam recentes Charmen vocant,
Affectus ſanat, qui moleſtarunt diu,
Et quibus nullum medicamen profuit.
Myrrhae haec optimae habet, et opobalſami,
Succi hypociſtidis, et thuris boni,
Opopanacis ſinceri, et croci novi,
Drachmas duodecim, in ſingulis pares.
Albentis coſti, Pontici caſtorii,
Terebinthinae purae, junci teretis pares

Πάλιν δ' ἑκάστου μίγματος δὶς δ'.
Βότρυός τ' ἀμώμου τέσσαρας, πολίου τ' ἴσας,
Καὶ κινναμώμου δ'. πάλιν καλοῦ,
Δὶς τρεῖς δὲ δαύκου Κρητικοῦ τοῦ σπέρματος.
Τὸ δ' αὐτὸ δαύκῳ σεσέλεως τοῦ σπέρματος,
Κασσίας δὲ κιῤῥᾶς τοῦ φλοιοῦ δὶς θ'.
Καὶ πετροσελίνου σπέρματος ταύταις ἴσας,
Μακροῦ πεπέρεως προσφάτου δὶς δώδεκα,
Τὸ γὰρ παλαιὸν σητοκόπον εὑρίσκεται,
Λευκοῦ ι'. δραχμὰς, χαλβάνης καθαρᾶς ι'.
Ναρδοστάχυος δὲ τῆς καλῆς ἑκκαίδεκα,
Δὶς δ' εἴκοσιν καὶ ε'. Κρητικοῦ καλοῦ,
Καὶ προσφάτου. πρόσβαλλε σκορδίου δραχμὰς,
Τριπλοῦν δὲ μέλιτος πᾶσι τοῖς ξηροῖς βάρος.
Σκεύαζε δ' αὐτὸν, ὡς προεῖπον σκευάσαι.
Ἄλλας τε δυνάμεις καὶ διδοὺς αὕτως πάλιν.
Ταύτην ἐπώλει Χάρμης Ἀττικῶν δραχμῶν
Δὶς πεντακοσίων, οὐδ' ὅλην λίτραν διδοὺς,

Drachmas bis quatuor ſingulorum; atque
Uvaeque amomi quatuor, polii pares,
Et cinnamomi quatuor rurſus boni:
Cretenſis dauci ſeminis bis tres,
Dauco par pondus ſeminum ſeſeleos,
Rufaeque caſiae corticis bis novem,
Et petroſelini ſeminis drachmas pares.
Piperis longi et novi bis duodecim,
Abroſum carie nam vetus reperies.
Albi decem, purgati galbani decem,
At ſpicae nardi electae drachmas ſedecim,
Drachmas recentis bis viginti, et quinque
Adjunge ſcordii, quod tellus Creta parit.
Sed mellis aridis pondus triplum omnibus
Commiſce, ſicut antidotos alias
Te pridem monui, et ſimiliter dabis.
Hanc Charmes auctor bis quingentis Atticis
Vendebat drachmis, nec totam libram dabat.

Ἐδόκει δὲ χάριτα διδόναι τοῖς ὠνουμένοις.
Τῶν δ' ἀξιοπίστων Χάρμιδός τις γνωρίμων
Ταύτην ἔφασκε τὴν γραφὴν δοκιμωτάτην.
Νάρδου δὶς η'. στάχυος Ἰνδικῆς δραχμὰς,
Σμύρνης τε χρηστῆς, καὶ ὀπίου, μηκωνείου,
Ὑποκιστίδος τε χυλοῦ, καὶ ὀποβαλσάμου,
Ὀποπάνακός τε τοῦ καθαροῦ καὶ προσφάτου,
Καὶ καστορίου καὶ λιβάνου πάντων ἴσα,
Ἀνὰ ιβ'. δραχμὰς δ'. δὲ χαλβάνης,
Τερμινθίνης τε ε'. πολίου τέσσαρας,
Κασίας μελαίνης τῆς καλῆς δὶς δ'.
Λευκοῦ πεπέρεως β'. δραχμὰς, μακροῦ μίαν
Καὶ β'. ὀβολούς. κρόκου δὲ κωρυκίου ι'.
Μίαν δὲ πρὸς ταύταισι καὶ δὶς δ'.
Σχοίνου πάνυ λεπτῆς, τοῦ τ' ἀμώμου δ'.
Β'. κινναμώμου, σεσέλεως δραχμὰς δύο,
Δαύκου δραχμὰς στ'. σπέρματος τοῦ Κρητικοῦ,
[904] Καὶ πετροσελίνου σπέρματος δὶς θ'.

Dareque gratis videbatur insuper.
Quidam fide dignus Charmis discipulus,
Scripturam hanc dicebat probatissimam,
Nardi bis octo, spicae Indicae drachmas,
Myrrhaeque probatae, succi quoque papaveris,
Hypocistidis succi, succi balsami,
Opopanacis puri, recentis insuper,
Et thuris, et castorii, singulorum
Drachmas bis senas; at galbani quatuor,
Terebinthinae quinque, polii quatuor,
Bonae sed nigrae casiae bis quatuor,
Albi piperis duas, oblongi unam,
Et duos obolos, croci Coricii decem.
Unam praedictis addes et bis quatuor
Schoeni attriti, sed amomi quatuor,
Duas cinnamomi, item et seselis duas,
Sex dauci drachmas seminum Cretensis,
Petroselini seminum bis novem.

Δὶς δ'. δὲ σκορδίου κόμης δραχ. ζ'.
Βδέλλης ὄνυχός τε τῆς διαυγοῦς, ὡς δραχμὴν,
Μέλιτός τε λίτρας ε'. καὶ μικρῷ πλέον.
Σκεύαζε δ' οὕτω, προδιαλύσας τοὺς ὀποὺς
Τῷ μέλιτι θερμῷ, τήν τε ῥητίνην καλῶς,
Τὰ ξηρὰ πάντα παραπλάσσεις σεσησμένα.
Οὕτω δ' ἑνώσας πάντα, δώσεις Ποντικοῦ
Καρύου τὸ μέγεθος τοῖς ὀφείλουσιν λαβεῖν.

Κεφ. ε'. [Περί τινων ἄλλων ἀντιδότων τῶν ὑπὸ Δαμοκράτους γεγραμμένον.]

Ἐφεκτικὴν δ' ἀντίδοτον εἰ βούλει ποιεῖν,
Αἵματος ἄνω τε καὶ κάτω πολλοῦ φορᾶς,
Ταύτην ἀκριβῶς σκευάσας, ἕξεις καλὴν,
Κρόκου Κιλικίου τοῦ καλοῦ καὶ προσφάτου
Δραχμὰς δὶς η'. καὶ ὀπίου, μηκωνείου,
Λιβάνου τ' ἀτμήτου, καὶ καθαρᾶς σμύρνης ἴσον,
Πάντων ἑκάστου πάλιν δραχμας ιστ'.
Φλοιοῦ δὲ ῥίζης μανδραγόρου δὶς δ'.

*Hinc ſcordii drachmas bis quatuor, comae vii.
Bdellii unguium unam ſed pellucidi,
Mellis infunde libras quinque plus parum.
Conſice hoc pacto; Succos diſſolve prius
In melle calido, atque reſinam optime.
Cuncta aliis aſperges arida,
In unitatem ſic coactis omnibus,
Dabis rogantibus inſtar nucis Ponticae.*

Cap. V. [*De quibusdam aliis antidotis a Damocrate deſcriptis.*]

*At ſi voles tibi antidotum componere,
Quae ſanguinis ſupra infraque arcet impetum:
Hanc ſi accurate facis, habebis optimam.
Croci Cilicii tum recentis, tum boni
Drachmas bis octo, et tantundem opii;
Thurisque non ſecti, purae myrrhae pares,
Cujusque rurſus drachmas ſexdecim,
Corticum et octo radicis mandragorae,*

Ὑοσκυάμου δὲ σπέρματος τρὶς δ'.
Τρὶς β'. δραχ. μηκωναρίου τοῦ σπέρματος,
Τρεῖς κινναμώμου τοῦ καλοῦ δραχμὰς σταθμῷ.
Ῥοὸς δὲ χυλοῦ Παταρικῆς ἢ Συριακῆς
Τρὶς κε'. καὶ ἑτέρας δὶς δώδεκα.
Σκεύαζε δ' οὕτω, τὸν κρόκον κεκαθαρμένον,
Ἀπόβρεχε δ' οἴνῳ Κρητικῷ λευκῷ γλυκεῖ
Δίδου β'. τὸ πλεῖστον ἡμέρας. ὅταν ἴδῃς
Μαλακὸν ἄγαν εὔτριπτον εἰς ἴγδην βαλὼν,
Λέαινε τῷ δοίδυκι, καὶ λεῖον ποιῶν,
Πρόσβαλλε τὸν ὀπὸν τὸν λίβανον τῇ σμύρνῃ.
Χυλὸν δ' ὁμοίως κατ' ἰδίαν τὸν τῆς ῥοὸς
Διάβρεχε καὶ πρόσβαλλε τοῖς εἰρημένοις,
Καὶ πάλιν ἑνώσας λεῖα καὶ σεσησμένα,
Τὰ λοιπὰ πάντα προσαποδώσεις μίγματα,
Ἑφθοῦ τε μέλιτος Ἀττικοῦ βαλὼν βραχὺ,
Πάλιν λέανον ὡς γενέσθ' ἓν φάρμακον
Ἐκ τῆς θυΐδος εἰς ὑαλοῦν ἀγγεῖον,

Hyoſcyami ſeminum ter quatuor.
Bis ternas adde ſeminum papaveris.
Tres boni cinnamomi drachmas pondere.
Succi Pataricae aut Syriacae rhois
Ter viginti quinque, alterius bis duodecim.
Miſcebis ita. Primo ſelectum crocum
Cretico, et albo et dulci vino madeat,
Ad ſummum dies duos. Quum fracidum videris
Et mollem valde, conjice in mortarium,
Et cochleari ſubige, dum laevigatum facis,
Adjunge myrrhae thus ſimul et opium.
Seorſum rhois ſuccus madeſcat quoque,
Quem maceratum praedictis adjicies.
At unione facta laeviga et cribro
Injecta reliqua permiſcebis omnia,
Coctique mellis temperans pauxillulum
Rurſus teras ut unum fiat pharmacum.
Acervum e mortario in vas vitreum,

Καὶ κασσιτερινὸν μετακόμιζ᾽ ἡνωμένον.
Δίδου δὲ τοῖς μὲν ἐκ φάρυγγος καὶ γαστέρος
Ἀνάγουσι καὶ θώρακος, ἔτι δὲ πνεύμονος,
Τριωβόλου τὸ πλῆθος, ἢ μικρῷ πλέον
Ἐν τρισὶ κυάθοις κράματος κεκραμένου.
Οἴνου δ᾽ ἀπὸ μύρτων καὶ ὕδατος τοῦ ἀπολύτου,
Τοῖς ἀπὸ νεφρῶν οὐροῦσιν, ἢ τῆς κύστεως,
Δίδου λέον τε φαρμάκου κεκραμένου.
Ἀπὸ νήστεώς τε καταφέρει καὶ κώλου,
Λεπτῶν τε πάντων ἐντέρων τῆς θ᾽ ὑστέρας,
Τοῦ φαρμάκου δίδου μὲν ὡς δραχμὴν μίαν.
Δι᾽ ὕδατος ὀμβρίου δὲ τοῖς πυρουμένοις,
Ἀπυρέτοισι δὲ καὶ διὰ κράματος δίδου,
Ἤτοι δ᾽ ἀπὸ μύρτων ἢ γλυκέος τοῦ Κρητικοῦ.
Εἰ δέ τις ἔχειν βούλοιτο μὴ πολυμίγματον
Ἀντίδοτον, ἀλλ᾽ ἔχουσαν ὀλίγα μίγματα
Ταύτην ἀκριβῶς σκευάσας, ἕξει καλὴν
Πρὸς τοὺς ἀτόνους στομάχους τε καὶ ἀνορέκτους,

Vel ſtanno factum, transferes, et oblines.
Ex hoc iis dabis, qui ſanguinem rejiciunt
In ventre, gutture, pectore, pulmone,
Quantum tres oboli pendunt, aut plus parum
E tribus vini cyathis diluti.
Sed qui remittunt ex veſica aut renibus,
Nonnulla vino myrtorum absque aqua addita,
Iis temperatum propinato pharmacum.
Quod ſi jejunum, ſive inteſtinum aliud
Subtile, ſive colon, ſive uterus fluet,
Hujus antidoti, quantum eſt drachma, dato.
Febriat ſi quis, pluvia ex aqua;
Non ſebrienti, ex vino dabis quoque
Diluto, vel myrtaceo, vel dulci Cretico.
Si quis non multis mixtam habere velit,
Sed paucis conditam antidotum rebus,
Iſtam componat ſedulus aptiſſimam
Infirmo ſtomacho, nec appetenti cibum,

Καὶ τοὺς καχέκτας, τούς τ' ἀπεπτοῦντας ταχύ.
Πρὸς πάνθ' ἁπλῶς ἀλγήματα, κύτος
Κεχρονισμένον τε καὶ κατασκευὴν ἔχον.
Ταύτῃ Τιβέριον τὸν Σεβαστὸν χρώμενον
Λέγουσιν, ἄλλην μὴ πεπωκέναι ποτέ.
Ἔχει δὲ μέλανος πεπέρεως πέντ' οὐγγίας,
Κροκομάγματος ιε'. καὶ ῥόδων ι'.
Σεσησμένα ταῦτα πάντα μέλιτ' ἀναλάμβανε.
Ἄλλη ποιοῦσα ταυτὰ τῇ προγεγραμμένῃ.
Ἔχει δὲ ῥόδων μὲν οὐγγίας δὶς τέσσαρας,
Κεκομμένα ταῦτα πάντα καὶ σεσησμένα,
[905] *Ἀναλάμβαν' ἑφθῷ μέλιτι τῷ λίαν καλῷ,*
Δίδου καρύου τὸ μέγεθος τοῦ Ποντικοῦ,
Μετ' οἰνομέλιτος ἢ μελικράτου προσφάτου,
Ἑψημένου καλῶς τε καὶ πεφρισμένου,
Τοῖς θηριοδήκτοις, ἢ τὰ δηλητήρια
Πεπωκόσι προσένεγκε καρύου τὸ μέγεθος
Τοῦ βασιλικοῦ μεθ' ἑπτὰ κυάθων κράματος.

Squallidis, macris, tarde concoquentibus,
Dolores omnes inveteratos pectoris,
Et ventris tollit infixos jam diu.
Ferunt Augustum hac usum Tiberium,
Ullam nec unquam perbibisse aliam.
Continet nigri piperis quinque uncias,
Crocomagmatis quindecim, rosae decem,
Excussa cribro excipe melle omnia.
Alia faciens ad eadem, quae et prior
Rosarum constat unciis bis quatuor.
Contusa ea omnia et per cribrum adacta,
Melle despumato excipe valde bono.
Ad magnitudinem ex hac Ponticae nucis dabis
Cum mulso, vel recenti melicrato
Bene decocto, et spumato bene.
Percussis a serpentibus, seu venenum
Epotis, exhibe nux quantum continet
Regia, cum septem vini cyathis diluti.

Ῥοδίδος σκευή.

Αὐτὸν δ' ἐπιμελῶς δεῖ σε προδιασκευάσαι
Οὕτως ἀκριβῶς, ῥόδα λαβὼν τὰ πρόσφατα,
Τὸ φύλλον αὐτῶν ἐν σκιαῖς δυσὶ ψῦξον,
Ἢ τρισὶ τὸ πλεῖστον ἡμέραις, σήσας τε τρεῖς
(444) Λίτρας, ἀπ' αὐτῶν ὅλμῳ κόπτων συμμέτρως,
Σχοίνου τε δραχ. κ'. εὖ κεκομμένης
Σμύρνης δέκα δύο καὶ κρόκου δὶς τέσσαρας,
Προσέμπασον, καὶ κόπτε πάνθ' ὁμοῦ πάλιν
Ποιῶν κυκλίσκους εὐμεγέθεις, ψῦξον καλῶς,
Οὕτω θ' ὅσον δεῖ λάμβαν' εἰς τὸ φάρμακον.

Κροκομάγματος σκευασία.

Κροκόμαγμα δ' εἰ βούλοιο καλὸν ἔχειν ἄγαν,
Σκεύαζ' ἐπιμελῶς, Κιλικίου κρόκου δραχμὰς
Ἑκατὸν καταμίξεις, τῆς λιπαρᾶς σμύρνης ἅμα
Δὶς κε'. καὶ ῥόδων ξηρῶν ἴσον,
Ἀμύλου δὲ ν'. λευκοῦ κόμμεως
Ἴσας, ἄμυλον δὲ κόπτε σήσας ἐπιμελῶς,

Paſtilli roſacei confectio.

Hoc te oportet pulchre ſtruxiſſe prius
Quo dicam modo. Recentes carpe roſas.
Carptas ſiccato in umbra dies duos,
Vel tres ad ſummum. Tres inde libras cape,
Et tunde miſſas in pilam, quantum eſt ſatis.
Schoeni viginti bisque ſex myrrhae bene
Contuſae, drachmas bis quatuor adde croci.
Inſpergens ſimul commiſcebis omnia,
Rotulas fingens magnas ſiccatas bene.
Deſumens quantum ſatis in antidotum.

Crocomagmatis compoſitio.

Crocomagma ſi bonum nimis deſideras,
Para ſtudioſe. Cilicii drachmas croci
Centum miſcebis myrrhae pinguis ſimul
Bis xxv. tantundem ſiccatae roſae,
Sed candidi amyli l. pares gummeos:
Jam amylum contunde cribrans curioſius,

Πρόσβαλλ' ἀθάλασσον οἶνον εὐώδη βραχὺν,
Δεύσας ἐπιμελῶς κἀναπλάσας ψῦξον κύκλους
Καὶ χρῶ δεόντως ὡς καλῷ κροκομάγματι.

Ἀντίδοτος προγνωστική.

Προγνωστικὴν δ' ἀντίδοτον οὕτως σκευάσεις,
Ἣν οἱ προλαβόντες ἂν λάβωσι θανάσιμον,
Ἐμέσουσιν αὐτὸν μετὰ τροφῆς παραυτίκα.
Οἱ δ' εὐλαβῶς ἔχοντες ὡς εἰληφότες,
Ἂν ἐπιλάβωσιν, ἐξεμοῦσι τὴν τροφὴν,
Σὺν τῷ μετ' αὐτῆς καταποθέντι φαρμάκῳ.
Ὁ δὲ μηδὲν ἄτοπον, μηδὲ δηλητήριον,
Συγκαταπεπωκὼς τοῖς δοθεῖσι σιτίοις,
Οὐ ναυτιάσει, καὶ καθέξει τὴν τροφήν.
Ποιεῖ δὲ ταὐτὸ φάρμακον καὶ πρὸς πόνους
Πλευρῶν, μεταφρένων, κύστεως, καὶ τῶν νεφρῶν,
Ἐπέχει τ' ἀλύπως αἷμα φερόμενον πολὺ
Ὅθεν ἂν ἐκφέρεται τοῦτο, κἂν ἐκ πνεύμονος.
Σκεύαζε δ' οὕτω, Λημνίαν ἔχων καλὴν

Addes odori vini infulfi paululum,
Quo quum madefcant rotulas fingas, frigera.
Et quum eft neceffe, utere ut bono crocomagmate.

Antidotus Prognoftica.

Prognofticam Antidotum ita conficies.
Quam praebibentes, fi venenum fumant,
Evoment ipfum ftatim, et cibum fimul.
At qui timent ceu noxium jam ingefferint,
Hanc fi fuperbibant, cibum cum pharmaco
Quod fumpferint, reddent vomitionibus.
Quod fi nil pravum, nil noxium, inter
Dapes propofitas fumpferit, naufeam
Ne fentit quidem, atque epulum retinet.
Haec quoque medicina ad dolores facit
Lateris, dorfi, renum, et veficae. Impetum
Sanguinis cohibet abfque moleftia,
Undecunque feratur, etiam e pulmone.
Ita praeparato. Lemniam terrae bonae,

Ἀπαραχάρακτον, τὴν ὁμοίως εἰρημένην
Στήσας ἀπ' αὐτῆς δύ' ὀβολοὺς δραχμὴν μίαν,
Ἀρκευθίδων τε τῶν λιπαρῶν δραχ. β'.
Λέαιν' ἐπὶ πολὺ, παραχέων χρηστὸν βραχὺ
Ἔλαιον ἱκανῶς πρόσφατόν τε καὶ γλυκὺ,
Διὰ μελικράτου δ' ὡς καρύου τοῦ Ποντικοῦ
Μέγεθος προσοίσεις, οἷς ἐχρῆν σε προσφέρειν.
Ἐπέχειν δὲ πλεῖον αἷμα φερόμενον θέλων,
Δι' ὀξυμέλιτος σφόδρα καθέφθου πρόσφερε.

Κεφ. στ'. [Περὶ τῶν ὑπ' Ἀσκληπιάδου γεγραμμένων κατὰ τὸ ε'. τῶν ἐντὸς παθῶν, ὃ Ἄσωνος ἐπιγράφεται.] Καλεῖν μὲν οὖν ἔθος ἐστὶ τοῖς νεωτέροις ἰατροῖς ἀντιδότους οὐ μόνον ὅσα πρὸς τὰ θανάσιμα φάρμακα διδόασιν, ἀλλὰ καὶ πρὸς τὰ τῶν ἰοβόλων θηρίων δήγματα, καὶ προσέτι πάθη, καὶ μάλιστα χρόνια, κατά τι τῶν σπλαγχνῶν, ἢ ἀποστήματα. τεμὼν δὲ τριχῇ τὴν διδασκαλίαν αὐτῶν ὁ Ἀσκλη[906]πιάδης, πρῶτα μὲν ἔγραψεν ὅσα φησὶ τοῖς κατὰ περίοδον πυρέττουσιν ἁρμόττειν, ἅμα τῷ καὶ συγχρίσματά

Quae quod caret ſigno aparacharactos dicitur,
Drachmam unam atque obolos conſtitue duos.
Aequent juniperi baccae drachmas duas.
Diſſolve diu fundens olei parum,
Quod dulce, et bonum, quodque ſit recens ſatis.
E mulſa, quantum nux Pontica magna eſt,
Offeres, quibus offerre hanc erit opus.
Si profluentem ſiſtere voles ſanguinem,
E mulſo aceto quod diu ſerbuit, dabis.

Cap. VI. [*De Antidotis ab Aſclepiade conſcriptis in quinto Internarum affectionum libro, qui Aſonis inſcribitur.*] Vocare itaque conſuetudo eſt junioribus medicis antidotos, non modo remedia quae adverſus lethalia venena exhibent; ſed etiam quae ad virulentarum ferarum morſus, ac praeterea pravos affectus, praeſertimque diuturnos, alicui viſceri inſidentes, aut abſceſſus. Quum autem trifariam de ipſis Aſclepiades diſciplinam ſecuerit, prima quidem ſcripſit quae per circuitus febrien-

τινα, καλεῖ γὰρ οὕτως αὐτὸς, ἐφεξῆς προσγράψαι. ταῦτα μὲν οὖν ἅπαντα ληξιφάρμακα καὶ ληξιπύρετα καλεῖ· τὸ δὲ β'. γένος αὐτῶν θηριακὰ φάρμακα, πρὸς λυσσοδήκτους καὶ σκορπιοδήκτους, ἔτι τε τούς τε ὑπὸ φαλαγγίων δεδηγμένους καὶ ἐχιδνῶν. τὸ δὲ τρίτον γένος τῶν φαρμάκων διχῇ τεμὼν καὶ αὐτὸ, τὸ μὲν ἕτερον αὐτῶν πρὸς τοὺς τὰ θανάσιμα πεπωκότας ὀνομάζει. τὸ δ' ἕτερον προφυλακτικὸν θανασίμων φαρμάκων, οὐ κατὰ τὴν αὐτὴν τάξιν τῷ Ἀνδρομάχῳ τὴν διδασκαλίαν ποιησάμενος. ἐκεῖνος γὰρ, ὡς ἐν ἀρχῇ τοῦδε τοῦ γράμματος εἴρηταί μοι κατὰ τὴν ἐντὸς ἐπιγραφομένην τῶν βιβλίων αὐτοῦ, προτάξας ἀντίδοτα πάντα, ἐφεξῆς γράφει τὰ πινόμενα φάρμακα πρὸς ἡντιναοῦν διάθεσιν, οὐ μόνον ἀποστημάτων ἢ θανασίμων φαρμάκων ἢ θηρίων ἰοβόλων, ἀλλὰ κἂν ἔμβρυον ἐκβαλεῖν δέῃ, καὶ τοῦτο τὸ φάρμακον ἀντίδοτον ὀνομάζει, καὶ πρὸς σπάσματα καὶ ῥήγματα, καὶ συνελόντι φάναι πρὸς πάντα τὰ ἐντὸς πάθη, περὶ ὅ τι ἂν ᾖ μέρος τοῦ σώματος ἡ σύστασις αὐτῶν γε-

tibus convenire dicit, quum inunctiones quasdam (ſic enim ipſe vocat) deinceps adjicit. Atque haec omnia lexipharmaca et lexipyreta nuncupat. Secundum ipſorum genus, theriaca medicamenta adverſus rabioſorum morſus et ſcorpionum ictus, praetereaque in phalangiorum et viperarum morſus. Tertium autem medicamentorum genus, bipertito quoque id ſecuit, alterum iis qui lethalia biberunt *idoneum*, alterum ad lethalium medicamentorum praecautionem *proprium* appellat, non eodem ordine quo Andromachus diſciplinam proſequutus. Ille ſi quidem, ut per initia hujus commentarii a me dictum eſt, quum interiore librorum ipſius inſcriptione omnia antidota praepoſuiſſet, deinde medicamenta ſubjungit, quae ad quemcunque affectum, non abſceſſuum duntaxat, aut lethalium medicamentorum, aut virulentarum ferarum bibuntur; verum ſi foetum expellere oporteat, hoc quoque medicamentum antidotum nominat, item ad convulſa, rupta, et ut uno verbo dicam ad omnes affectus internos, qua-

γενημένη. τὰ δὲ πρὸς τὰ τοιαῦτα πάθη πινόμενα φάρμακα καὶ ποτίσματα κέκληκεν ὁ Ἀσκληπιάδης ἐν τῷ δ΄. τῶν Ἄσωνος κατὰ τὸ τέλος αὐτὰ γεγραφώς. ὑστάτας μὲν οὖν ἔγραψεν ἀντιδότους ὁ Ἀσκληπιάδης ἐπὶ τῇ τελευτῇ τοῦ ἐν Ἄσωνος, τὰ πρὸς τοὺς τὰ θανάσιμα πεπωκότας, ἢ προφυλακτικὰ τοῦ μηδὲν παθεῖν ὧν πίωσιν. ἐγὼ δὲ πρώτας ἐνταῦθα γράψαι τὰς τοιαύτας ἔγνωκα, διά τε τὴν πρὸς τὰς γεγραμμένας κοινωνίαν καὶ ὅτι πολύχρηστοι τυγχάνουσιν οὖσαι. καὶ γὰρ πρὸς τὰ ἀποστήματα καθ᾽ ὁτιοῦν σπλάγχνον καὶ μόριον ἐν τῷ βάθει κείμενον ἁρμόττουσι, καὶ πρὸς ἀτονίαν αὐτῶν ἔνιαι, καὶ πρὸς κακοχυμίαν, ἀνωδυνίαν τε καὶ πέψιν ἀπέπτων χυμῶν, δι᾽ ὅλης τῆς ἐπιφανείας κένωσιν ἄδηλον αἰσθήσει, καθάπερ καὶ τὰς αἰσθητὰς, δι᾽ οὔρων καὶ διαχωρημάτων καὶ πτυσμάτων, ὅσα μετὰ βηχὸς συνεκκαθαίρει πνεύμονά τε καὶ θώρακα. τὰ πλεῖστα δ᾽ αὐτῶν καὶ λεπτύνειν τοὺς παχεῖς χυμοὺς πέφυκε, καὶ τέμνειν, καὶ ἀποῤῥύπτειν τοὺς γλίσχρους, οἷς ἕπεται καὶ τὸ τὰς ἐμφρά-

cunque corporis parte conſtiterint. Quae vero ad hujusmodi affectus bibuntur medicamenta, etiam potiones appellavit Aſclepiades, in quarto Aſonis ad finem eas interpretatus. Quare poſtrema ad finem Aſonis antidota Aſclepiades conſcripſit, quae lethalibus potionibus aſſumptis auxiliantur; aut quae, ne quid mali ab iis experiatur aliquis, praeſervant. Ego vero tales antidotos primas hic deſcribere decrevi; tum quod cum deſcriptis communionem habeant, tum quod uſum praeſtent multiplicem. Etenim ad abſceſſus cujuscunque viſceris et partis in alto ſitae conducunt. Nonnulla quoque ipſorum ad imbecillitatem, vitioſos humores, indolentiam conciliandam et crudorum humorum concoctionem proſiciunt. Inſuper ad latentem ſenſui per ſumma corporis tota evacuationem, quemadmodum ad eas conferunt quae ſenſibus patent, per urinas, alvum et ſputa, quae cum tuſſi et pulmonem, et thoracem pariter expurgant. Plurima vero ex iis craſſos humores attenuare, incidere et vitioſos abſter-

ξεις ὠφελεῖν, ὅσαι συνεχῶς μὲν καθ' ἧπαρ εἰώθασι γίνεσθαι, συνίστανται δὲ καὶ κατὰ τὰ ἄλλα σπλάγχνα καὶ μόρια· σκοπὸς γὰρ ἐπ' αὐτῶν ἐστι λεπτῦναί τε καὶ ἀποῤῥύψαι τοὺς χυμοὺς, ἀναστομῶσαί τε τὰ πεφραγμένα τῶν ἀγγείων πέρατα.

Κεφ. ζ΄. [Ἀσκληπιάδου πρὸς τοὺς τὰ θανάσιμα πεπωκότας, ὡς αὐτὸς ἔγραψε κατὰ λέξιν.] [Πρὸς τὸν τῆς μήκωνος ὀπόν.] Τοῖς μὲν οὖν τὸν τῆς μήκωνος ὀπὸν πιοῦσι συνοίσει ὑδρέλαιον συνεχῶς θερμὸν διδόμενον πίνειν, καὶ ἀναγκαζόμενον ἐμεῖσθαι· ἢ θερμὸν ὕδωρ μετ' ὀξυμέλιτος διδόναι καὶ ἀναγκάζειν ἐμεῖν· ἁρμόσει δὲ καὶ διὰ κλυστῆρος τὴν κοιλίαν κενοῦν.

[Πρὸς μηκώνιον.] Τοῖς δὲ μηκώνειον πίνουσιν ἁρμόσει ἄκρατον πολὺ παραχρῆμα διδόμενον· ἢ πέπερι μετὰ οἴνου, ἢ κάρδαμον, ἢ καρδάμωμον. ἁρμόσει δὲ καὶ γάλα πίνειν ὄνειον ἢ βόειον καὶ τὰ περὶ τὴν κοιλίαν καταπλάττειν ἀλεύρῳ πυρίνῳ ἢ κριθίνῳ ἡψημένῳ μετ' οἴνου, καὶ κλύσμασι χρῆσθαι πρᾳοτέροις.

gere ſolent, eoque obſtructionibus ſuccurrere, quae frequenter in jecore oboriri conſueverunt. Fiunt etiam in aliis viſceribus et partibus, in quibus hoc conſilium dirigi debet, ut humores attenuemus, abſtergamusque et vaſorum extrema reſeremus.

Cap. VII. [*Aſclepiadis antidota, ad eos, qui lethalia biberunt, ut ipſe ad verbum ſcripſit.*] [*Adverſus papaveris ſuccum.*] Itaque qui papaveris ſuccum potaverint, iis conducet aquam cum oleo calentem ſaepius potui dare, vomitumque ciere; aut calidam aquam cum mulſo exhibere, et ad vomitum irritare; conveniet etiam alvum clyſtere vacuare.

[*Ad meconium i. e. Papaveris cocti ſuccum.*] Qui meconium potarunt, iis merum copioſius ſtatim exhibitum convenit; aut piper cum vino, aut cardamum, vel cardamomum. Conducit etiam lac aſininum bibere aut vaccinum, et ventrem farina triticea oblinere, aut hordeacea vino cocta, et clyſteribus uti mitioribus.

[907] [Πρὸς ἀκόνιτον.] Τοῖς δὲ ἀκόνιτον πεπωκόσι βοηθεῖ ποθὲν πήγανον χειροπληθὲς, λεανθὲν μὲν μετ' οἴνου ἀκράτου, καὶ ζωμὸς ὄρνιθος λιπαρᾶς.

[Πρὸς ὑοσκύαμον.] Τοῖς δὲ τὸν ὑοσκύαμον πιοῦσι συμφέρει γάλα ποθὲν, μάλιστα μὲν ὄνειον· εἰ δὲ μὴ, ἄλλο κατ' ἰδίαν, καὶ μετὰ μελικράτου θερμοῦ.

[Πρὸς κορίανον.] Τοῖς δὲ χλωρὸν κορίανον πιοῦσι βοηθεῖ οἶνος ἄκρατος ποθεὶς καὶ ζωμὸς ὄρνιθος λιπαρᾶς.

[Πρὸς λαγωὸν θαλάττιον.] Τοῖς δὲ λαγωὸν θαλάττιον εἰληφόσιν ἁρμόττει γάλα πίνειν μάλιστα μὲν ὄνειον, εἰ δὲ μή γε, βόειον ἢ αἴγειον. δοτέον δὲ καὶ καυλοὺς μαλάχης ἡψημένους ἐπιμελῶς φαγεῖν, ἢ γλήχωνος χειροπληθοῦς μετὰ γλυκέος τριβέντος πίνειν, ἢ κυκλαμίνου ῥίζαν τριβεῖσαν μετ' οἴνου· ἢ κεδρίας ὅσον ὀβολοῦ ἑνὸς, ἢ ἡμιώβολον, γλυκεῖ διεὶς πότιζε.

[Πρὸς τοξικόν.] Τοῖς δὲ τοξικὸν πιοῦσι βοηθεῖ οἶνος

[*Ad aconitum.*] Qui aconitum aſſumpſerunt, ii rutae manipulo cum vino meraciore laevigato potoque adjuvantur. Item jure pinguis gallinae.

[*Ad altercum.*] Qui altercum ſeu hyoſcyamum biberunt, iis conducit lac potum, maxime tamen aſininum, vel quodlibet aliud per ſe, et cum mulſa calida.

[*Ad coriandrum.*] Qui viride coriandrum potaverunt, iis auxiliatur vinum meracum potum et jus gallinaceum pingue.

[*Ad leporem marinum.*] Qui leporem marinum aſſumpſerint, iis prodeſt lac bibere, maxime aſininum; ſin minus, vaccinum aut caprinum. Dari autem debent eſui etiam caules malvae diligenter incocti, vel pulegii quantum manu comprehendi poteſt, cum paſſo triti, potandum; vel cyclamini radix trita cum vino; aut picis cedriae obolus, aut ſemiobolus, paſſo ſubactus potui datur.

[*Ad toxicum.*] Qui toxicum biberunt, eos vinum

πινόμενος γλυκὺς, καὶ ῥόδινον ἔλαιον, καὶ αἴγειον αἷμα, καὶ σπέρμα βουνιάδος τριβὲν μετ᾽ οἴνου.

[*Πρὸς ἐφήμερον.*] Τοῖς δ᾽ ἐφήμερον πεπωκόσι βοηθεῖ χυλὸς πολυγόνου, ἢ ἀρνογλώσσου, ἢ ὀριγάνου, (445) ἢ θύμου μέρος τι οἴνῳ διαλυθέν.

[*Πρὸς δορύκνιον.*] Τοῖς δὲ δορύκνιον πιοῦσι βοηθεῖ γάλα βόειον ποθὲν, καὶ γλυκὺ, καὶ ζωμὸς κογχυλίων.

[*Πρὸς μύκητας.*] Τοῖς δὲ μύκητας εἰληφόσι δοτέον ῥαφάνους ὠμὰς, ὥστε πλείστας ἐσθίειν· δοτέον καὶ οἶνον ἄκρατον καὶ κονίας κληματίνης ἀφέψημα, καὶ νίτρον λεανθὲν μετ᾽ ὄξους· ἢ τρύγα οἴνου καύσας, καὶ τρίψας μεθ᾽ ὕδατος δίδου πίνειν· ἢ ἀψίνθιον μετ᾽ ὄξους· ἢ πήγανον λεῖον μετ᾽ ὄξους· ποιεῖ δὲ καὶ αὐτὸ καθ᾽ αὑτὸ ἐσθιόμενον πήγανον.

[*Πρὸς ἰξίαν.*] Τοῖς δὲ τὴν ἰξίαν πεπωκόσι βοηθεῖ ἀψίνθιον πινόμενον μετ᾽ οἴνου καὶ καστορίου καὶ πηγάνου. συνοίσει δὲ καὶ ὀξύμελι ποτίζειν, καὶ ἀναγκάζειν ἐμεῖν. συνοίσει δὲ καὶ ὀρίγανον μετ᾽ οἴνου. χρηστέον δὲ καὶ τῇ τοι-

dulce adjuvat, oleum rofaceum, fanguis caprinus, femen napi contritum cum vino.

[*Ad ephemeron.*] Qui ephemeron potarunt, eos juvat fuccus polygoni aut plantaginis aut origani aut thymi pars aliqua vino foluta.

[*Ad dorycnium.*] Qui dorycnium hauferint, iis auxiliatur lac bubulum potum, et paffum, et conchyliorum jus.

[*Ad fungos.*] Fungis affumptis laborantibus dentur raphani crudi, et quamplurimi edendi; dandum quoque vinum meracum, et lixivii farmentitii decoctum; nitrum cum aceto fubactum; aut ufta vini faex, tritaque cum aqua potui datur; aut abfinthium cum aceto; aut ruta trita cum aceto. Benefacit etiam ruta ipfa per fe manducata.

[*Ad ixiam.*] Qui vero ixiam epotarunt, iis fuccurrit abfinthium potum cum vino, caftorio et ruta. Proderit etiam oxymel potare, et vomitiones ciere. Confe-

αὐτῇ σκευασίᾳ. ℞ πηγάνου < στʹ. ῥητίνης < δʹ. καστορίου < βʹ. χαμαιλέοντος κοχλιάρια γʹ. ταῦτα τρίψας καὶ ὄξει θερμῷ διαλύσας, πότιζε.

[Πρὸς βουπρήστην.] Τοῖς δὲ τὴν βουπρήστην πεπωκόσι βοηθεῖ διδόναι γλυκὺ πλεῖστον πίνειν, καὶ ἀναγκάζειν ἐμεῖν· καὶ ζωμὸν καθηψημένον κρεῶν ὑῶν, καὶ θερμὸν γάλα, καὶ οὐκ ἄπληστα φαγεῖν. καὶ ἀφέψημα σύκων δοτέον πίνειν, ἢ νίτρου ἐρυθροῦ < δʹ. λεάνας καὶ μίξας ὕδατι δίδου πίνειν.

[Πρὸς κανθαρίδας.] Τοῖς δὲ κανθαρίδας πεπωκόσι συμφέρει πίνειν γλυκὺ μετʼ ἐλαίου, καὶ στέαρ ἑφθὸν ὕδατι διηθημένον, καὶ ἀναγκάζειν ἐμεῖν. συμφέρει δὲ καὶ γάλακτι πολλῷ ποτίζειν καὶ κώνους πλείονας τρώγειν· ἢ κώνους πλείστας τρίψας μετὰ μελικράτου δίδου πίνειν· ἢ πήγανον λεάνας καὶ ἰρίνῳ μύρῳ μίξας δίδου πίνειν· ἢ τῶν κανθαρίδων τὰ πτερὰ καὶ τοὺς πόδας σὺν μέλιτι τρίψας ἐκλείχειν δίδου.

ret origanum quoque cum vino. Caeterum utendum eſt hujusmodi confectione. ℞ rutae ʒ vj, reſinae ʒ iv, caſtorii ʒ ij, chamaeleontis cochlearia iij. Haec contrita et calente aceto ſoluta propinato.

[*Ad bupreſtim.*] Bupreſti ſorpta affectis opitulatur datus paſſi plurimi potus, ac deinde irritatus vomitus. Suillarum carnium jus decoctum; lac calidum plurimum edere, et ſicuum decoctio potui data, aut nitri rubri ʒ iv, tritae mixtaeque cum aqua ac potae.

[*Ad cantharides.*] Qui cantharides deglutierunt, iis confert paſſum cum oleo bibere, et adipem coctum aqua percolatum, et ad vomitum cogere; confert etiam plurimum lactis potare, et ſtrobilos plures edere, aut ſtrobilos plurimos cum mulſa tritos potui dare, aut rutam in pulverem redactam irinoque ungnento mixtam bibendam exhibere, aut cantharidum alas pedesque cum melle tritos linctui dare.

[*Πρὸς ψίλωθρον.*] *Τοῖς δὲ ψίλωθρον πιοῦσι συμφέρει θερμῷ ἐλαίῳ ποτίζειν, καὶ ἀναγκάζειν ἐμεῖν. συνοίσει δὲ καὶ γάλα αἴγειον πίνειν, καὶ μαλάχης ἑφθῆς χυλὸν μετὰ μελικράτου θερμοῦ, ἢ μετ' ἐλαίου· ἢ ἰσχάδων ἀφέψημα μετ' ἐλαίου, ἢ σήσαμον μετ' οἴνου τρίψας δίδου πίνειν· ἢ κάρυα βασιλικὰ ε'. λεάνας μετ' ἐλαίου δίδου· ἢ τέφρας κληματίνης ἀπήθημα δίδου πίνειν.*

[*Πρὸς λιθάργυρον.*] *Τοῖς δὲ λιθάργυρον πεπωκόσι βοηθεῖ πέπερι, σέλινον, σμύρνα μετ' οἴνου λειωθέντα, καὶ πινόμενα.*

[*Πρὸς γύψον.*] *Τοῖς δὲ γύψον πιοῦσι δοτέον πίνειν τέφρας κληματίνης ἀπήθημα, καὶ θύμον μεθ' ὕδατος τριβέντα.*

[*Πρὸς τὰς τοῦ γάλακτος ἐκθρομβώσεις.*] *Πρὸς δὲ τὰς τοῦ γάλακτος ἐκθρομβώσεις συμφέρει ποτίζειν ὄξος· διδόναι δὲ χρὴ καὶ πητυὰν μεθ' ὕδατος κρηναίου ἢ σιλφίου καὶ θείου τὸ ἴσον λεανθέντα μετ' ὀξυκράτου διδόναι πίνειν.*

[*Ad pfilothrum.*] Pfilothro haufto affectis confert calidum oleum bibere, et vomitum concitare. Conferet etiam lac caprillum bibere, et malvae coctae fuccum cum mulfa calida aut cum oleo; aut caricarum decoctum ex oleo; aut fefamum ex vino tritum potui dare; aut nuces juglandes v. cum oleo tritas; aut cineris farmentitii colatum lixivii potui exhibere.

[*Ad lithargyrum.*] Abforpto lithargyro laborantibus auxiliatur piper, apium, myrrha cum vino laevigata bibitaque.

[*Ad gypfum.*] Qui gypfum ingefferint, iis dari debet potui cineris farmentitii colatura, et thymus ex aqua tritus.

[*Ad lactis grumos.*] Ad lactis grumos confert aceti potio. Dare quoque oportet coagulum cum aqua fontana, vel filphii et fulphuris par pondus, laevigatum ex pofca, potui dare.

[*Πρὸς ταύρειον αἷμα.*] Τοῖς δὲ ταύρειον αἷμα πιοῦσι συμφέρει ὄξος θερμὸν διδόναι πίνειν, καὶ ἀναγκάζειν ἐμεῖν, ἢ σιλφίου ὀβολὸν, ἢ ἡμιωβόλιον, ἢ νίτρου διώβολον, διέντας οἴνῳ διδόναι πίνειν, ἢ ἐρινεῶν καρπὸν τρίψας μετ' ὄξους δίδου. ἁρμόσει δὲ καὶ τὴν κοιλίαν κενοῦν, καὶ θερμίνῳ ἀλεύρῳ, καὶ νίτρῳ, ἡψημένοις μετ' ὀξυμέλιτος καταπλάττειν.

[*Πρὸς βδέλλας.*] Τοῖς δὲ βδέλλας καταπιοῦσιν οἱ μὲν ἅλμην παρῄνουν πίνειν, οἱ δὲ χιόνα. ὁ δὲ Ἀσκληπιάδης λούειν παρῄνει, καὶ σπόγγον ἁπαλὸν ψυχρῷ δεύσαντα καθιέναι, ὥστε τὴν βδέλλαν ἐπιβᾶσαν τῷ σπόγγῳ κομίζεσθαι, καὶ ἔπειτα φακῆς χυλὸν ἐδίδου· τοὺς δὲ ἔξωθεν τοῦ τραχήλου τόπους τοῖς ψύχουσι καταπλάττειν παρῄνει. ὁ δὲ Μῦς Ἀπολλώνιος ὄξει δριμυτάτῳ ἐπότιζε, καὶ μετὰ ἅλμης ἐχρήσατο. ὁ δὲ χιόνα θερμήνας καὶ λύσας ἐχρήσατο, καὶ τοῖς κατὰ καιρὸν τὴν κοιλίαν καθαίρουσιν, ἐδεστοῖς τε καὶ ποτοῖς, πρὸς τὴν τῶν βδελλῶν ἔκκρισιν· συγκατα-

[*Ad ſanguinem taurinum.*] Qui taurinum ſanguinem potarunt, iis confert acetum calidum propinandum exhibere, et ad vomitum cogere, vel laſerpitii obolum aut ſemiobolum, aut nitri duos obolos vino ſubactos potui dare, aut groſſorum fructum cum aceto tritum. Convenit autem et alvum ſubducere, et lupinorum farina, et nitro ex mulſo decoctis oblinere.

[*Ad hirudines.*] Qui hirudines devorarunt, eos alii muriam, alii nivem bibere hortantur. Aſclepiades autem lavare admonebat, et ſpongiam teneram frigida imbutam faucibus immittere, ut hirudo ſpongiae infixa extraheretur, ac deinde lenticulae ſuccum porrigebat. Externam colli regionem refrigerantibus obducere hortabatur. At Mus Apollonius acetum quam acerrimum propinabat, et cum muria uſus eſt. Ille nivis gleba calefacta ſolutaque utebatur, et eſculentis poculentisque alvum tempeſtive purgantibus ad hirudines excernendas,

φέρεσθαι γάρ φησι ταύτας τοῖς κατὰ τὴν κοιλίαν ἐκκρινομένοις πολλάκις.

[Πρὸς ψιμύθιον.] Τοῖς δὲ ψιμύθιον πιοῦσι συνοίσει ἐλαίῳ θερμῷ ποτίζεσθαι καὶ ἀναγκάζειν ἐμέσαι. συνοίσει δὲ καὶ γλυκὺ καὶ θερμὸν ποτίζεσθαι ὕδωρ, καὶ ἀναγκάζειν ἐμεῖν. συνοίσει δὲ καὶ γάλα ὄνειον πίνειν διδόναι, καὶ μαλάχης ἑφθῆς χυλὸν, καὶ μελίκρατον θερμὸν, μετ' ἐλαίου ἀνακόψας δίδου πίνειν· ἢ ἀφέψημα ἰσχάδων μετ' ἄλλων δίδου πίνειν, κάρυα βασιλικὰ ε'. λεάνας μετ' ἐλαίου, δίδου πίνειν· ἢ τέφρας κληματίνης ἀπήθημα δίδου. καὶ περὶ μὲν τῶν ἁπλῶν θανασίμων ἐπὶ τοσοῦτον εἰρήσθω. περὶ δὲ τῶν συνθέτων λεχθήσεται. ἐκτίθεσθαι δὲ τὰς τούτων σκευασίας μοχθηρόν μοι δοκεῖ, καίπερ πολλῶν ἐπιχειρησάντων ταῖς τούτων συγγραφαῖς, ὥς ἐστιν Ὀρφεὺς ὁ ἐπικληθεὶς Θεολόγος καὶ Ὧρος ὁ Μενδήσιος ὁ νεώτερος καὶ Ἡλιόδωρος ὁ Ἀθηναῖος τραγῳδιῶν [909] ποιητὴς, καὶ Ἄρατος, καὶ ἄλλοι τινὲς τῶν τοιούτων συγγραφεῖς. τούτους μὲν οὖν ἄν τις θαυμάσειεν ἐμμέτρως ἐπιχειρήσαν-

nam has una cum iis quae per alvum excernuntur deorfum ferri faepe afferit.

[*Ad ceruffam.*] Qui ceruffam biberint, iis ex ufu fuerit oleum calidum bibere et vomitum irritare. Confert etiam dulcem et calentem aquam affumere, atque fic ad vomitum cogere. Ad haec conduxerit lactis afinini potio data, et malvae coctae fuccum, et mulfam calidam cum oleo ceruffam bibendam porrigere; vel decoctum caricarum bibitum cum aliis, nuces juglandes quinque cum oleo tritas potui exhibere; aut cineris farmentitii excolatum lixivium. Atque hactenus de fimplicibus medicamentis lethalibus dictum efto. Nunc autem de compofitis agetur; fed flagitiofum mihi videtur horum confectiones exponere, licet eas multi confcribere fint aggreffi; inter quos eft Orpheus cognominatus Theologus et Orus Mendefius recentior et Heliodorus Athenienfis tragicus poëta, etiam Aratus, aliique nonnulli hujusmodi rerum fcriptores. Hos itaque demirari queat aliquis, quod verfibus

τας ταῖς περὶ τούτων πραγματείαις· μέμψαιτο δ' ἂν εὐλόγως διὰ τὰ πράγματα. διδάσκειν γάρ μᾶλλόν ἐστι καὶ προσάγειν τοὺς βουλομένους ἐπὶ κακῷ, τὸ πλησίον ἐπιχειρεῖν ταῖς τούτων σκευασίαις. οἱ γοῦν τῶν καλῶν τούτων ποιημάτων συγγραφεῖς τὴν παρὰ τοῖς πολλοῖς εὐλαβούμενοι καταδρομὴν, ἐναρχόμενοι τῆς τούτων παραδόσεως, τοὺς ἐντευξομένους πείθειν ἐπιχειροῦσιν ὡς οὐκ ἂν εἴησαν φαῦλοι τὸ ἦθος, οὐδὲ τῶν τοιούτων φθοροποιῶν διδάσκαλοι, ὥσπερ καὶ Ἡλιόδωρον ἐν τοῖς πρὸς Νικόμαχον ἀπολυτικοῖς ἐναρχόμενόν ἐστιν εὑρεῖν οὕτω γράφοντα.

Οὐ μὰ τὸν ἐν Τρίκκῃ πρηῢν θεὸν, οὐ μὰ τὸν ὑψοῦ
Ἠέλιον σπείροντα θεοῖς φαεσίμβροτον αἴγλην,
Οὐ μὰ θεῶν σκηπτοῦχον, ὑπερμενέα Κρονίωνα.
Οὔτε μέ τις δώροισι παρήγαγεν, οὔθ' ὑπ' ἀνάγκης,
Οὔτε χάριν φιλίης ἑτέρῳ κακὰ νεῖμαι ὑπέστην.
Ἀλλ' ὁσίας μὲν χεῖρας ἐς ἠέρα λαμπρὸν ἀείρω,
Καὶ κακίης ἀμόλυντον ἔχω κατὰ πάντα λογισμόν.

talia opera conſcribere ſint aggreſſi; merito autem damnaverit ob res ab ipſis traditas, nam docere magis eſt et allicere eos, qui nocendi proximis ſtudio horum confectionibus manum admoliri cupiunt. Pulchrorum autem horum poëmatum auctores vulgi incurſum veriti, dum haec tradere incipiunt, lectoribus perſuadere conantur, quod nullis pravis praediti moribus, neque hujusmodi exitialium venenorum praeceptores extiterint, quemadmodum et Heliodorum in Apolyticis ad Nicomachum jurantem eſt invenire, his verbis:

Non mihi per ſacram venerandae Palladis artem,
Non per luciferum ſolem mortalibus aequum,
Non per te divi cui ſubſunt, Juppiter, omnes,
Muneribus quisquam, nec vi, nec gratia amoris
Adduxit me aliis lethalia prodere verſu.
Sed palmas ſacras ſplendentia ad aethera tendo,
Nullius atque mali mens eſt ſibi conſcia noſtra.

Ἐκ τῶν λεγομένων πείθειν ἐπιχειροῦσι τοὺς ἐντευξομένους ταῖς τοιαύταις πραγματείαις, τὴν παρὰ τοῖς πολλοῖς καταδρομὴν εὐλαβούμενοι. ἀλλ' οὐδέ ἐστιν εἰπεῖν ὅτι διὰ τοῦτο χρὴ τὰς τῶν τοιούτων θανασίμων φαρμάκων σκευασίας εἰδέναι, πρὸς εὐχερῆ εὕρεσιν τοῦ βοηθηθῆναι τοῖς δυναμένοις· τοῦτο γάρ ἐστι ψεῦδος. ὁ γὰρ δυνάμενος τοῖς ὑπὸ τῶν ἁπλῶν θανασίμων βλαπτομένοις βοηθεῖν, ἕκαστον τῶν κατὰ μέρος ἐπὶ συμβαινόντων ἐποπτεύων, οὗτος ἂν εἴη ἄριστος προστάτης, καὶ τῶν ὑπὸ τῶν συνθέτων βλαπτομένων, εὐμηχάνως ἐκλαμβάνων ἕκαστον τῶν κατὰ τὴν τῶν συμπτωμάτων ἐπιπλοκὴν ἐξεχόντων. ἀντιτέον δὲ ἐπὶ τὸ προκείμενον. ἀδήλων γὰρ ὄντων τῶν βρωθέντων ἢ ποθέντων δηλητηρίων, χρὴ ὑδρέλαιον θερμὸν διδόναι, καὶ πολὺ πίνειν, καὶ ἀναγκάζειν ἐμεῖν. χρήσιμον δ' ἂν εἴη καὶ τοὺς ὕπνους περιγράφειν, οὐ μὴν ἀλλὰ καὶ εἰς τὴν τούτων φυλακὴν χρηστέον ταῖς ὑπογεγραμμέναις σκευασίαις.

Κεφ. η'. [Προφυλακτικὰ θανασίμων φαρμάκων Ἀπολλωνίου Μυός.] ℞ Πηγάνου φύλλα κ'. κάρυα βασιλικὰ β'.

Ex hujusmodi dictis perfuadere aggrediuntur iis qui in ejusmodi opera incident, vulgi infultum reveriti. Sed ne dicere quidem eft, propterea talium lethalium venenorum confectiones effe fciendas, ut qui velint opitulari, prompte remedia queant invenire; hoc enim eft mendacium: nam qui laefos a noxiis fimplicibus juvare cupit, unumquodque particulatim in accidentibus infpiciens, hic nimirum optimus falutis praefes fuerit, etiam eorum qui a compofitis offenduntur, facile fingula in accidentium complexu, ac congerie praecellentia deligens. Sed revertamur ad id quod inftituimus. Quum enim comefta aut pota deleteria non conftant, aquam cum oleo calidam dare convenit, ejusque plurimum bibere, et ad vomitum incitare. Utile fuerit etiam fomnum circumcidere; quin etiam ad horum praecautionem fubfcriptis confectionibus utendum eft.

Cap. VIII. [*Quae a lethalibus medicamentis praefervent Apollonii Muris.*] ℞ Rutae folia xx, nuces ju-

ἁλὸς χόνδρον ἕνα, ἰσχάδας β'. ταῦτα νήστει ἐσθίειν δίδου, καὶ κωλύει βλάπτεσθαι ὑπὸ τῶν θανασίμων.

(446) [*Ἀντίδοτος προφυλακτικὴ διδομένη.*] ℞ Ἀρκευθίδος < β'. Λημνίας σφραγῖδος < β'. καὶ διώβολον. ταῦτα τρίψας καὶ ἀναλαβὼν ἐλαίῳ ἀποτίθου. ἐπὶ δὲ τῆς χρήσεως καρύου Ποντικοῦ τὸ μέγεθος μεθ' ὑδρομέλιτος καὶ κυάθων β'. προπίνειν. ταύτῃ Νικομήδης ὁ βασιλεὺς ἐχρῆτο, εἴ ποτε ὑπόπτους εἶχε τοὺς κεκληκότας. τὸ μὲν οὖν φάρμακον, μηδεμιᾶς τοιαύτης δυνάμεως ὑποκειμένης, κατὰ χώραν μένει. ἐπὰν δέ τι τῶν θανασίμων δοθῇ, ναυτίαν κινεῖ, καὶ ἐμεῖν ἀναγκάζει, ὥστε τὸ δοθὲν δηλητήριον ἐκκρίνεται τῇ ἀντιδότῳ.

[*Ἀντίδοτος Κωδίου Τούκου, ῃ καὶ Κρατερὸς ἐχρήσατο.*] ℞ Πρασίου, ἱερᾶς βοτάνης, πηγάνου ἀγρίου σπέρματος, σκορδίου, ῥάμνου ῥίζης τοῦ φλοιοῦ, ἑκάστου τὸ ἴσον, μέλιτι ἀναλάμβανε καὶ δίδου, πρὸς μὲν τὰ θηρία < β'. μετ' οἴνου, πρὸς δὲ τὰ θανάσιμα μετ' οἰνομέλιτος καὶ ἐλαίου.

glandes ij, falis grumum j, caricas ij, haec jejuno manducanda dato, et oblaedi a lethalibus prohibent.

[*Antidotum ad praeservationem datum.*] ℞ Baccarum juniperi ʒ ij, lemnii figilli ʒ ij, et obolos ij, haec trita exceptaque oleo reponito. Quum ufus poftulaverit, nucis avellanae magnitudine cum hydromelitis cyathis duobus propinato. Hoc Nicomedes rex utebatur, fi quando eos quos vocaverat fufpectos haberet. Itaque medicamentum quum nulla hujusmodi vis fubeft, in loco manet. Quum autem lethale aliquod datum fuerit, naufeam movet, et vomere compellit, adeo ut deleterium exhibitum cum antidoto excernatur.

[*Antidotum Codii Tuci, quo et Craterus ufus eft.*] ℞ Marrubii, herbae facrae, feminis rutae fylveftris, fcordii, corticum radicis rhamni, fingulorum par pondus: melle excipe, daque, ad feras quidem ʒ ij, cum vino; ad lethalia autem ex mulfo et oleo.

[910] [*Ἄλλη, ὡς Ἀπελλῆς.*] ♃ *Δικτάμνου* < β΄. πολίου < γ΄. πεπέρεως μακροῦ < δ΄. πηγάνου ἀγρίου < ϛ΄. σκορδίου < γ΄. μέλιτι ἀναλάμβανε καὶ δίδου, καθάπερ εἴρηται. ἔστι δὲ καὶ πλευριτικὴ ἀγαθὴ ὀβολῶν γ΄. διδομένη. ἔμμηνά τε γυναιξὶ κατάγει ὁλκῆς μιᾶς διδομένη. *Ἀντίδοτος Μιθριδάτου*, ἀθανασία λεγομένη, πρὸς τὰ θανάσιμα τῶν φαρμάκων, καὶ παντὸς ἰοβόλου πληγήν. ποιεῖ στομαχικοῖς ἀποξύνουσιν τὴν τροφὴν, αἱμοπτυϊκοῖς, βήττουσι χρονίως, καὶ ἡπατικοῖς, καὶ σπληνικοῖς. ποιεῖ καὶ πρὸς τὰς περὶ κύστιν ἢ μήτρας διαθέσεις. τὰ δὲ τῆς σκευασίας ἔχει οὕτως. ♃ *Πεπέρεως* λευκοῦ κόκκους μ΄. κόστου, μήου, ἀσάρου, ἀκόρου, δαύκου *Κρητικοῦ* σπέρματος, πετροσελίνου, νάρδου *Ἰνδικῆς*, λίθου νηστωρίτου ἀνὰ < δ΄. κρόκου, σμύρνης ἀνὰ < η΄. κινναμώμου, κασσίας ἀνὰ < ιβ΄. μέλιτος *Ἀττικοῦ* ἑψημένου τὸ αὔταρκες. ἡ δόσις καρύου *Ποντικοῦ* τὸ μέγεθος μετ᾽ οἰνομέλιτος κεκραμένου.

[*Ἐν ἄλλαις γραφαῖς οὕτως ἔχει.*] ♃ *Ναρδοστάχυος*, πεπέρεως λευκοῦ, κόστου, μήου, ἀσάρου, ἀκόρου, ὀποβαλ-

[*Aliud, ut Apelles.*] ♃ Dictamni ʒ ij, polii ʒ iij, piperis longi ʒ iv, rutae ſylveſtris ʒ vj, ſcordii ʒ iij, melle excepta dato, quemadmodum dictum eſt. Pleuriticum quoque remedium eſt obolis iij, datum; menſesque mulieribus educit ʒ j, pondere exhibitum. *Antidotus Mithridatis, Athanaſia dicta i. e. immortalis, ad lethalia medicamenta, et omnium virulentorum ictus: benefacit ſtomachicis quibus cibus aceſcit, ſanguinem ſpuentibus, tuſſi diuturna infeſtatis, hepaticis, lienoſis: prodeſt quoque veſicae, aut uteri affectibus. Quae contineat compoſitio, ita ſe habent.* ♃ Piperis albi gr. xl. coſti, mei, aſari, acori, ſeminis dauci Cretici, petroſelini, nardi Indicae, lapidis neſtoritis an. ʒ iv, croci, myrrhae, cujusque ʒ viij, cinnamomi, caſſiae, ſingulorum drach. xij, mellis Attici cocti quod ſatis eſt. Doſis nucis avellanae magnitudine, ex mulſo temperato.

[*Haec compoſitio in aliis praeſcriptionibus ita habet.*] ♃ *Spicae nardi* piperis albi, coſti, meu, aſari, acori,

σάμου, δαύκου Κρητικοῦ σπέρματος, πετροσελίνου σπέρματος, ἑκάστου ἀνὰ < δ'. κρόκου, σμύρνης, σχοίνου ἄνθους ἀνὰ < η'. κινναμώμου, κασσίας ἀνὰ < ιβ'. μέλιτος τὸ ἀρκοῦν.

['Εν ἄλλαις ἔχει οὕτως.] ♃ Πεπέρεως λευκοῦ κόκκους μ'. κόστου, μήου, ἀκόρου, ἀγαρικοῦ, σκορδίου, δαύκου Κρητικοῦ, πετροσελίνου ἀνὰ < δ'. κρόκου, σμύρνης ἀνὰ < η'. κινναμώμου, κασσίας, σχοίνου ἄνθους ἀνὰ < ιβ'. μέλιτος τὸ αὔταρκες.

['Αμβροσία Φιλίππου Μακεδόνος, πρὸς τὰ θανάσιμα τῶν φαρμάκων, καὶ παντὸς ἰοβόλου πληγήν. ποιεῖ καὶ πρὸς τὰς ἐντὸς διαθέσεις.] ♃ Στύρακος, χαλβάνης, πεπέρεως λευκοῦ καὶ μακροῦ, καὶ κινναμώμου, ἀνὰ < β'. σελίνου σπέρματος, ἀνίσου, σχοίνου ἄνθους, κόστου, κυμίνου Αἰθιοπικοῦ, σεσέλεως, κύφεως, ῥήου Ποντικοῦ, καρδαμώμου, ἀμώμου, νάρδου, σμύρνης, κασσίας ἀνὰ < δ'. πυρήνων καθαρῶν φοινίκων, καὶ καρύων τῆς σαρκὸς ἀνὰ < στ'.

opobalfami, feminis dauci Cretici, petrofelini feminis, fingulorum an. drach. iv, croci, myrrhae, fchoenanthi an. drach. viij, cinnamomi, caffiae, an. drachmas duodecim, mellis quod fatis eft.

[*In aliis fic habet.*] ♃ Piperis albi gr. xl. cofti, meu, acori, agarici, fcordii, dauci Cretici, petrofelini, fingulorum drach. iv, croci, myrrhae, utriusque ℨ viij, cinnamomi, caffiae, fchoenanthi an. ℨ xij, mellis quantum fufficit.

[*Ambrofia Philippi Macedonis ad lethalia venena, et cujusvis virulenti ictum. Facit etiam ad internos affectus.* ♃ Styracis, galbani, piperis albi et longi; cinnamomi, an. ℨ ij, feminis apii, anifi, fchoenanthi, cofti, cumini Aethiopici, fefeleos, cypheos, rheu Pontici, cardamomi, amomi, nardi, myrrhae, caffiae, an. ℨ iv, palmularum nucleis exemptis, carnis nucum, an. ℨ vj, croci ℨ viij, uvas paffas acinis mundatas xij mellis

Ed. Chart. XIII. [910.] Ed. Baſ. II. (446.)

κρόκου < η'. σταφίδας ἐκγεγιγαρτισμένας ιβ'. μέλιτος Ἀττικοῦ τὸ αὔταρκες. συντίθει κατὰ τρόπον.

[*Ἀντίδοτος ζωπύριος. ποιεῖ πρὸς τὰ θανάσιμα τῶν φαρμάκων, καὶ παντὸς ἑρπετοῦ πληγήν.*] Ἐπὶ ταύτης τοιοῦτόν τι φέρεται, ὅτι Ζώπυρος δι' ἐπιστολῆς προτρέπει τὸν Μιθριδάτην εἰς ἐπίκρισιν τῆς ἀντιδότου, μεταπεμψάμενος ἕνα τῶν κατακρίτων, τούτῳ θανάσιμον διδόναι φάρμακον, καὶ τότε παραινεῖ ἐπιπίνειν τὴν ἀντίδοτον. ἢ πρότερον διδόναι τὴν ἀντίδοτον, καὶ τότε τὸ θανάσιμον ἐπιπίνειν. τὸ δ' αὐτὸ παρῄνει καὶ ἐπὶ ἑρπετῶν ἢ καὶ τοξικῶν πράσσειν. τούτων γὰρ οὕτω γινομένων συνέβαινε τὸν ἄνθρωπον ἀδιάπτωτον εἶναι. ποιεῖ δὲ καὶ στομαχικοῖς πρὸς ὀξυρεγμίαν, αἱμοπτυικοῖς, κοιλιακοῖς, δυσεντερικοῖς, ἡπατικοῖς, σπληνικοῖς, ἐπιληπτικοῖς, νεφριτικοῖς. ὑγιάζει δὲ καὶ τὰς περὶ μήτραν ἢ κύστιν διαθέσεις. κατάγει τὰ ἐναποθνήσκοντα τῶν ἐμβρύων, κατεχόμενα δεύτερα. τὰ δὲ τῆς σκευασίας ἔχει γε οὕτως. ℞ Ὀποβαλσάμου < δ'. νάρδου Ἰνδικῆς, σμύρνης Τρωγλοδύτιδος, σχοίνου ἄνθους, κινναμώμου, χαρα-

Attici quantum ſatis eſt; componito in modum ſuperiorem.

[*Antidotum Zopyrium valet ad lethalia medicamenta, et cujuscunque ſerpentis ictum, morſumve.*] De hoc hujusmodi quid fertur, quod Zopyrus per epiſtolam Mithridatem adhortatur ad antidoti probationem; transmittens ei unum e damnatis, ut lethale huic medicamentum daret, ac tunc antidotum potandum offerret: aut prius antidotum exhiberet, mox lethale propinaret. Id ipſum hortabatur, et in ſerpentibus vel etiam toxicis factitaret: quae quum ita fierent, contigit hominem nulli periculo implicitum fuiſſe. Valet autem ſtomachicis, ad acidos ructus, ſanguinem ſpuentibus, coeliacis, dyſentericis, hepaticis, lienoſis, comitialibus, nephriticis: jam uteri aut veſicae affectus perſanat, emortuos foetus educit, ſecundasque retentas. Confectio hunc in modum habet. ℞ Opobalſami ʒ iij, nardi Indicae, myrrhae Troglodytidis, ſchoenanthi, cinnamomi, characii, coſti

κίου, κόστου προσφάτου, πεπέρεως μακροῦ, ὑποκυστίδος, πολίου, πεπέρεως περεατικοῦ, [911] σκορδίου, μήου Κρητικοῦ, καρδαμώμου ἀνὰ < δ'. λιβάνου ἄῤῥενος, χόνδρου ὀποβαλσάμου, δικτάμνου ἀνὰ < στ'. πετροσελίνου, κασσίας κιῤῥᾶς ἀνὰ < ζ'. κρόκου κωρυκίου < η'. μέλιτος Ἀττικοῦ τὸ αὔταρκες. ἡ δόσις καρύου Ποντικοῦ τὸ μέγεθος, ἀπυρέτοις μετ' οἴνου, πυρέττουσι μεθ' ὑδρομέλιτος.

[Ἡ διὰ τῶν αἱμάτων πρὸς τὰ θανάσιμα τῶν φαρμάκων, καὶ παντὸς ἰοβόλου πληγήν.] ℞ Πεπέρεως μακροῦ καὶ λευκοῦ, κόστου, ἀκόρου, κρόκου, φοῦ, μήου, δικτάμνου Κρητικοῦ, ἀμμωνιακοῦ, ἀγαρικοῦ ἀνὰ < β'. ἀμώμου, ὀποβαλσάμου, πηγάνου ἀγρίου σπέρματος, κυμίνου Αἰθιοπικοῦ, ἀνίσου, νήσσης αἵματος, ἄῤῥενος καὶ θηλείας ξηροῦ, ἐριφείου αἵματος, χηνείου αἵματος, βουνιάδος ἀγρίας σπέρματος ἀνὰ < γ'. Γεντιανῆς, τριφυλλίου, σχοίνου ἄνθους, λιβανωτοῦ, ῥόδων ξηρῶν ἀνὰ < δ'. πετροσελίνου < ε'. πολίου Κρητικοῦ τὸ ἴσον, κινναμώμου < στ'. σκορδίου ἄνθους < η'. σμύρνης, νάρδου ἀνὰ < . κρόκου

recentis, piperis longi, hypociftidis, polii, piperis pereatici, fcordii, meu Cretici, cardamomi, an. ʒ iv, thuris mafculi, opobalfami, dictamni, fingulorum ʒ vj, petrofelini, caffiae rubentis, fingulorum ʒ vij, croci Corycii ʒ viij, mellis Attici quod fatis eft. Datur nucis avellanae magnitudine, febris expertibus ex vino; febricitantibus, cum hydromelite.

[*Ex fanguinibus antidotum ad lethalia medicamenta, et virulenti cujusvis ictum.*] ℞ Piperis longi et albi, cofti, acori, croci, phu, meu, dictamni Cretici, ammoniaci, agarici, fingulorum ʒ ij, amomi, opobalfami, feminis rutae filveftris, cumini Aethiopici, anifi, fanguinis analis mafculi et foeminae, ficci hoedini fanguinis, anferini fanguinis, napi filveftris feminis, fingulorum ʒ iij, gentianae, trifolii, fchoenanthi, lacrymae thuris, rofarum ficcarum, fingulorum ʒ iv, petrofelini ʒ v, polii Cretici tantumdem, cinnamomi drach. vi, fcordii floris drach. viij, myrrhae, nardi, utriusque ʒ x. croci drach.

< ιβ'. κασσίας < η'. κόψας καὶ σήσας ἐπιμελῶς, ἀνάκοπτε μέλιτι Ἀττικῷ ἀφηψημένῳ, καὶ ἀνελόμενος εἰς πυξίδα ἀργυρᾶν, χρῶ ὡς μεγίστῳ φαρμάκῳ.

Κεφ. θ'. [Περὶ τῆς διὰ σκίγκου ἀντιδότου, περὶ θηριακῆς, καὶ ἑκατονταμιγμάτου.] Ἀντίδοτος Μιθριδάτου Εὐπάτορος, ἡ διὰ σκίγκου λεγομένη, ποιοῦσα πρὸς τὰ θανάσιμα τῶν φαρμάκων, καὶ πρὸς πᾶσαν φθοροποιὸν ὕλην, καὶ παντὸς ἰοβόλου πληγὴν, καὶ πρὸς τὰς τῶν ἐντὸς διαθέσεις, καὶ πρὸς συλλήψεις συνεργεῖ, κατάγει ἔμμηνα· καὶ τὰ ἐναποθνήσκοντα ἔμβρυα, καὶ τὰ κατεχόμενα δεύτερα λύει, καὶ τοῖς κατὰ περίοδον πυρετοῖς βοηθεῖ, καὶ παρέτοις, τρομώδεσιν, ὀπισθοτονικοῖς, ἰσχιαδικοῖς, ποδαγρικοῖς, καὶ πρὸς πᾶσαν νευρικὴν συμπάθειαν. τὰ δὲ τῆς σκευασίας ἔχει οὕτως. ℞ Σκίγκου, σαγαπηνοῦ, ἀκόρου, φοῦ, ὑπερικοῦ, ἀκακίας, ἴρεως, μήου, κόμμεως ἀνὰ < β'. ῥόδων ξηρῶν, γεντιανῆς, καρδαμώμου ἀνὰ < δ'. μηκωναρίου σπέρματος < ε'. καὶ διώβολον, στύρακος < η'. πολίου, κασσίας μελαίνης, σεσέλεως, βδελλίου, βαλσάμου, πεπέρεως λευκοῦ

xij, caſſiae ʒ viij, contuſa, cribrataque diligenter melle Attico decocto, ſubigito; exceptis in pyxide argentea utitor, ut maximo medicamento.

Cap. IX. [*De Diaſcinco nobili antidoto, Theriaca et Centena.*] *Antidotum Mithridatis Eupatoris, quod diaſcincum dicitur, lethalibus medicamentis efficax, adverſus etiam omnem tabificam materiam, omnis virulenti ictum, interiorum affectus, inſuper conceptionem adjuvat, menſes educit, foetus emortuos, ſecundasque retentas ſolvit, nec non febribus per circuitus remeantibus auxiliatur, reſolutis, tremulis, opiſthotonicis, iſchiadicis, podagricis, et ad omnem nervorum ſympathiam. Haec confectio ita fit.* ℞ Scinci, ſagapeni, acori, phu, hyperici, acaciae, iridis, meu, gummi, ſingulorum ʒ ij, roſarum ſiccarum, gentianae, cardamomi, ſingulorum ʒ iv, papaveris ſeminis ʒ v, et obolos ij, ſtyracis ʒ viij, polii, caſſiae nigrae, ſeſeleos, bdellii, balſami, piperis albi, ſingulorum ʒ v, et obolos ij, hypociſtidis ſucci. opopanacis, myrrhae, thuris maſculi,

ἀνὰ < ε΄. καὶ διώβολον, ὑποκυστίδος χυλοῦ, ὀποπάνακος, σμύρνης, λιβάνου ἄῤῥενος, καστορίου, πεπέρεως μακροῦ, κύφεως, μαλαβάθρου φύλλων ἀνὰ < στ΄. σκορδίου, κόστου, σχοίνου ἄνθους, χαλβάνης, ῥητίνης τερμινθίνης ἀνὰ < στ΄. καὶ διώβολον, νάρδου Συριακῆς, ὀποβαλ (447) σάμου, θλάσπεως, δαύκου Κρητικοῦ ἀνὰ < στ΄. καὶ τριώβολον, κρόκου, κινναμώμου, ζιγγιβέρεως ἀνὰ < στ΄. καὶ διώβολον, γλυκυῤῥίζης χυλοῦ, ἀγαρικοῦ, ἀνὰ < ζ΄. καὶ τριώβολον, μέλιτος τὸ αὔταρκες, οἴνου καλοῦ τὸ ἀρκοῦν εἰς τὸ διαλῦσαι τοὺς χυλούς. συντίθεται δὲ τοῦτον τὸν τρόπον. κῦφι, ὑπόκιστις, σαγαπηνὸν, κόμμι, μηκώνειον, στύραξ, ὀποπάναξ ἐν οἴνῳ Χίῳ βρέχεται, μέχρι παντελῶς διαλυθῆναι, ἡμέραν καὶ νύκτα, τὰ δὲ λοιπὰ κόπτεται καὶ σήθεται λεπτῷ κοσκίνῳ, καὶ μίγνυται τοῖς ἀποβρεχθεῖσι καὶ λεανθεῖσιν. ἡ δὲ ὅλη σύνθεσις ἀναλαμβάνεται μέλιτι Ἀττικῷ ἀφηψημένῳ, ὡς πάχος ἔχειν· εἶτ᾽ ἐπὶ πᾶσι βάλλομεν ὀποβάλσαμον, εἶτ᾽ ἀνελόμενοι κατατίθεμεν εἰς ἄγγος ἀργυροῦν, καὶ ἡ χρῆσις εἰς πολλὰ, ἡ δόσις πρὸς δύναμιν. ἡμεῖς πρὸς

castorii, piperis longi, cypheos, malabathri foliorum, singulorum drach. vj, scordii, costi, schoenanthi, galbani, resinae terebinthinae, singulorum drach. vj, obolos ij, nardi Syriacae, opobalsami, thlaspeos, dauci Cretici, singulorum drach. vj, obolos iij, croci, cinnamomi, zingiberis, singulorum drach. vj, obolos ij, succi glycyrrhizae, agarici, singulorum ʒ vij, obolos iij, mellis quod sufficit, vini optimi quod satis est ad succos dissolvendos. Hunc in modum componitur. Cyphi, hypocistis, sagapenum, gummi, papaver, styrax, opopanax in vino Chio madescunt, usque dum in totum fuerint dissoluta per diem et noctem, reliqua contunduntur, et tenui cribro incernuntur miscenturque madefactis, detritisque. Tota vero compositio melle Attico decocto excipitur, ut habeat crassitiem; deinde opobalsamum omnibus superinjicitur, postea excipientes vase argenteo reponimus. Usus *antidoti* ad multa est, dosis pro viribus. Nos ad medicamenti amplificationem, ob

ἐπίτασιν τοῦ φαρμάκου, ἕνεκα τῆς τῶν ἐμμήνων ἐποχῆς, καὶ τῶν συλλημ [912] μάτων, ὥστε ἀκινδύνως φέρεσθαι, δικτάμνου Κρητικοῦ < δ'. ἀμμωνιακοῦ < γ'. πηγάνου ἀγρίου σπέρματος < γ'. κυμίνου Αἰθιοπικοῦ στ'. τριφύλλου σπέρματος δ'. βουνιάδος ἀγρίας δ'. χαμαίδρυος < δ'. ῥᾶ Ποντικοῦ γ'. ὀποῦ Κυρηναϊκοῦ < β'. τούτων προσβαλλομένων ἡ τοῦ φαρμάκου χρῆσις γίνεται πρὸς πολλὰ χρήσιμος· φθείρει γὰρ τετραμηνιαῖα, καὶ τριμηνιαῖα κατάγει.

[*Μιθριδάτου θηριακή.*] Ταύτῃ ὁ βασιλεὺς Μιθριδάτης ἀεὶ ἐχρῆτο προφυλακῆς χάριν θανασίμου. ἡνίκα γοῦν ὑπὸ Ῥωμαίων ἑάλω, δὶς πιὼν θανάσιμον, καὶ μὴ δυνηθεὶς ἀποθανεῖν, ξίφει ἑαυτὸν διεχρήσατο. πρὸς τὰ θανάσιμα δὲ τῶν φαρμάκων ποιεῖ, καὶ παντὸς ἰοβόλου πληγὴν, καὶ πρὸς τὰς τῶν ἐντὸς διαθέσεις. ταύτῃ ἐχρήσατο ὁ Ἀνδρόμαχος. τὰ δὲ τῆς σκευασίας ἔχει οὕτως. ℞ Ἀρτίσκων σκιλλητικῶν < μη'. θηριακῶν ἀρτίσκων, πεπέρεως μέλανος, ἡδυχρόου μάγματος, ὀποῦ μήκωνος Σπανοῦ, ἀνὰ < κδ'. ῥόδων ξηρῶν, σκορδίου, σπέρματος βουνιάδος, ἴρεως Ἰλλυρικῆς,

mortuorum fuppreffionem foetuum, retentionem, ut fine periculo educantur imposuimus dictamni Cretici drach. quatuor, ammoniaci drach. iij, feminis rutae filveftris drach. iij, cumini Aethiopici ʒ vi, feminis trifolii ʒ iv, napi filveftris ʒ iv, chamaedryos drach. iv, rhei Pontici drach. iij, fucci Cyrenaici drach. ij. His adjectis medicamenti ufus ad multa fit utilis: corrumpit enim foetus quadrimeftres, et trimeftres educit.

[*Mithridatis theriaca.*] Hac rex Mithridates femper utebatur, ut fe a lethali veneno praefervaret. Quum itaque a Romanis captus effet, nec bis epoto veneno interire poffet, gladio feipfum interemit. Valet ad lethalia medicamenta, et omnis virus jaculantis ictum: etiam ad internos affectus. Hac utebatur Andromachus. Confectio ipfius hunc in modum habet. ℞ Trochiscorum fcilliticorum ʒ xlviij, trochiscorum viperinorum, piperis nigri, hedychroi magmatis, fucci papaveris Hifpani, fingulorum ʒ xxiv, rofarum ficcarum, fcordii, feminis napi, iridis

Ed. Chart. XIII. [912.] Ed. Baſ. II. (447.)

ἀγαρικοῦ, κινναμώμου, γλυκυῤῥίζης χυλοῦ, ὀποβαλσάμου, ἀνὰ < ιβ'. λιβανωτίδος < η'. σμύρνης, κρόκου, ζιγγιβέρεως, ῥᾶ Ποντικοῦ, πενταφύλλου ῥίζης, καλαμίνθης ὀρεινῆς, πρασίου, πετροσελίνου, στοιχάδος, κόστου, πεπέρεως λευκοῦ, πεπέρεως μακροῦ, λιβάνου, ἀνὰ ὀβολοὺς β'. κασσίας μελαίνης < δ'. κόστου < α'. κρόκου δ'. πεπέρεως λευκοῦ μίαν, καὶ μακροῦ μίαν, Ἰλλυρίδος, σχοίνου, πολίου, σκορδίου, ῥόδων ξηρῶν, νήσσης αἵματος, ἀνὰ < γ'. μέλιτος Ἀττικοῦ ἑφθοῦ τὸ ἱκανόν.

[*Ἀντίδοτος ἑκατονταμίγματος, ᾗ χρῶμαι, ἣν ἐσκεύασα Καίσαρι πρὸς πάντα, ἰδίως δὲ πρὸς τὰ θανάσιμα.*] ♃ Ἀβροτόνου < β'. ἥμισυ, ἀριστολοχίας < κ'. ἀκακίας < δ'. ἀρκευθίδων σαρκὸς ἴσον, κρόκου < β'. ἀσάρου < δ'. ἀνίσου < γ'. ἀμώμου < στ'. ἀγαρικοῦ < γ'. καρποῦ βαλσάμου < β'. βδελλίου < γ'. ὀβολοὺς γ'. βαλαυστίου < β'. γεντιανῆς < δ'. γλυκείας χυλοῦ ἴσον, γογγυλίδος σπέρματος < δ'. ἐν ἄλλῳ < η'. γῆς Σαμίας μίαν, δαύκου σπέρματος

Illyricae, agarici, cinnamomi, ſucci glycyrrhizae, opobalſami, ſingulorum ʒ xij, roris marini ʒ viij, myrrhae, croci, zingiberis, rhei Pontici, radicis quinquefolii, calaminthae montanae, marrubii, petroſelini, ſtoechados, coſti, piperis albi et piperis longi, thuris an. obolos ij, caſſiae nigrae ʒ iv, coſti ʒ j, croci ʒ iv, piperis albi ʒ j, et longi ʒ j iridis Illyricae, junci rotundi, polii, ſcordii, roſarum ſiccarum, ſanguinis anatis, ſingulorum ʒ iij, mellis Attici cocti quantum ſufficit.

[*Antidotum hecatontamigmaton ex centum rebus conſtans, quo utor. Caeſari id praeparavi ad omnia: proprie autem ad lethalia.*] ♃ Abrotoni ʒ ij ß, ariſtolochiae drach. xx, acaciae ʒ iv, carnis baccarum juniperi tantundem, croci drach. ij, aſari ʒ iv, aniſi drach iij, amomi drach. vj, agarici ʒ iij, carpobalſami ʒ ij, bdellii drach iij, obolos ij, balauſtii drach. ij, gentianae ʒ iv, ſucci glycyrrhizae tantundem, ſeminis napi drach. quatuor, (in alio exemplari ʒ viij.) terrae Samiae drach. j, ſeminis dauci ʒ

< δ΄. δρακοντίου ῥίζης < γ΄. ὀβολοὺς γ΄. ἐρυσίμου σπέρματος < κ΄. ἴρεως Ἰλλυρικῆς < β΄. σμύρνης < ζ΄. ὀβολοὺς γ΄. ζιγγιβέρεως ἴσον, ἠρυγγίου ῥίζης < δ΄. ὀβολοὺς β΄. θλάσπεως < κ΄. κονύζης λεπτῆς < στ΄. ἀκόρου < στ΄. ὀβολοὺς γ΄. κυπέρου < στ΄. κωνείου σπέρματος ἐπτισμένου < α΄. ὀβολοὺς γ΄. ἄμμεως < δ΄. κνίκου σπέρματος < ζ΄. ὀβολοὺς β΄. κινναμώμου < ζ΄. κόστου < ζ΄. ὀβολοὺς β΄. κασσίας < ε΄. ὀβολοὺς β΄. κενταυρίου χυλοῦ < δ΄. ὀβολοὺς ε΄. καστορίου στ΄. καλάμου ἀρωματικοῦ β΄. οἱ δὲ δ΄. κόμμεως < β΄. καρδαμώμου δ΄. κάγχρυος < γ΄. ὀβολοὺς γ΄. κύφεως < στ΄. χαλβάνης < στ΄. ὀβολοὺς β΄. λιβανωτίδος φύλλων < δ΄. ἐλελισφάκου ἴσον, λογχίτιδος σπέρματος < β΄. ὀβολοὺς γ΄. λιθοσπέρμου < γ΄. λιβάνου < στ΄. τριώβολον, μαράθρου σπέρματος < στ΄. ὀποῦ μήκωνος < στ΄. μίλτου Λημνίας < α΄. μαλαβάθρου ι΄. μήου < στ΄. νήσσης αἵματος στ΄. νάρδου Συριακῆς < στ΄. ὀβολοὺς γ΄. νάρδου Κελτικῆς < η΄. ξυλοβαλσάμου < γ΄. ὀποπάνακος ἴσον, ὁρμίνου σπέρματος η΄. ὀρόβων λευκῶν ἴσον, πανακείας ῥίζης < στ΄. ὀποβαλσάμου < γ΄.

iv, radicis dracunculi ʒ iij, obolos ij, eryſimi ſeminis ʒ xx, ireos Illyricae ʒ ij, myrrhae ʒ vij, obolos iij, zingiberis tantundem, eryngii radicis drach. iiij, obolos ij, thlaſpeos ʒ xx, conyzae tenuis ʒ vj, obolos iij, cyperi drach. vj, acori ʒ vj, cicutae ſeminis decorticati drach. unam, obolos iij, ameos ʒ iv, ſeminis cnici ʒ vij, obolos ij, cinnamomi ʒ vij, coſti drach. vij, obolos ij, caſſiae ʒ v, obolos ij, centaurii ſucci ʒ iv, obolos v, caſtorii ʒ vi, calami aromatici ʒ ij, alii vero ʒ iv, gummi ʒ ij, cardamomi ʒ iv, cachryos ʒ iij, obolos iij, cypheos ʒ vj, galbani ʒ vj, obolos ij, foliorum roriſmarini ʒ iv, ſalviae tantundem, lonchitidis ſeminis ʒ ij, obolos iij, ſeminis lithoſpermi ʒ iij, thuris ʒ vj, obolos iij, ſeminum foeniculi ʒ vi, ſucci papaveris ʒ vi, terrae Lemniae ʒ i, malabathri ʒ x, mei ʒ vi, ſanguinis anatis ʒ vi, nardi Syriacae drach. vi, obolos iij, nardi Celticae drach. viij, xylobalſami drach. tres, opopanacis tantundem, ſeminis ormini drach. viij, ervorum alborum totidem, panaceae

πελεκίνου < στ'. πολίου ε. ὀβολοὺς β'. πολυγόνου φύλλων < θ'. ἑλενίου ῥίζης < ε'. ὀβολοὺς γ'. πετροσελίνου στ'. [913] ὀβολοὺς β'. πενταφύλλου < η'. ὀποῦ πευκεδάνου τὸ ἴσον, πεπέρεως μέλανος < ε'. τριώβολον, καὶ λευκοῦ δ'. ὀβολοὺς γ'. καὶ μακροῦ < α'. σκίγκου δραχμὰς γ'. τερμινθίνης β'. ῥόδων ξηρῶν < στ'. σαγαπηνοῦ δραχμὰς η'. στοιχάδος δ'. στροβίλων πεφρυγμένων < στ'. σχοίνου δραχμὰς δ'. ὀβολοὺς β'. σταφίδος σαρκὸς < δ'. σεσέλεως δραχμὰς ε'. ὀβολοὺς β'. σταφυλίνου σπέρματος < δ'. χολῆς ταυρείας < ε'. χολῆς ἀρκείας ἴσον, χαμαιπίτυος < γ'. ψυλλίου σπέρματος δ'. χαμαίδρυος ἴσον, σησάμου πεφρυγμένου < στ'. συμφύτου ῥίζης δραχμὰς β'. σκορδίου κορύμβων δραχμὴν α'. ὀβολοὺς δ'. σταφίδος ἀγρίας δραχμὰς ε'. στύρακος < ε'. ὀβολοὺς β'. τριφύλλου καρποῦ < ι'. τορδύλου σπέρματος β'. τευκρίου φύλλων, ὅ τινές φασιν εἶναι χαμαίδρυν, δραχμὴν μίαν, ὑποκυστίδος χυλοῦ δραχμὰς β' S''. ὑπερικοῦ καρποῦ β'. ὑοσκυάμου σπέρματος δραχμὰς β'. ῥοῦ Ποντικοῦ < β'.

drachmas vi, opobalſami drach. iij, ſecuridacae drach. vi, polii ʒ v, obolos ij, foliorum polygoni drach. ix, radicis helenii ʒ v, obolos iij, petroſelini ʒ vi, obolos ij, quinquefolii ʒ viij, ſucci peucedani tantundem, piperis nigri drach. v, obolos iij, et albi drach. iv, obolos iij, et longi drach. j, ſcinci drach. iij, terebinthinae drach. ij, roſarum ſiccarum drach. vj, ſagapeni drach. viij, ſtoechados drach. iv, ſtrobilorum frictorum drach. vj, junci odorati drach. iv, obolos ij, carnis uvae paſſae ʒ iv, ſeſeleos drach. v, obolos ij, ſeminum paſtinacae drach. iv, fellis taurini drach. v, fellis urſini tantundem, chamaepityos drach. iij, ſeminis pſyllii drach. iv, chamaedryos totidem, ſeſami fricti drach. vj, radicis ſymphyti drach. ij, ſummitatum ſcordii drach. j, obolos iv, ſtaphidis ſilveſtris drach. v, ſtyracis drach. v, obolos ij, fructuum trifolii drach. x, ſeminum tordyli drach. ij, foliorum teucrii (quod nonnulli dicunt eſſe chamaedryn) drach. j, ſucci hypocyſtidis drach. ij ß, fructuum hyperici drach. ij, ſeminum alterci drach. ij, rheu Pontici

φοῦ < η'. ῥοὸς τοῦ ἐπὶ τὰ ὄψα < ε'. τριώβολον· κοτυληδόνος ῥίζης < α'. ὀβολοὺς γ'. οἴνου καὶ μέλιτος τὸ ἱκανόν. ἐγὼ οἶνον οὐ βάλλω.

Κεφ. ι'. [Ποικίλαι τῶν πολλῶν ἀντίδοτοι πρὸς πολλὰ καὶ διάφορα πάθη] [Ἀντίδοτος Αἰλίου Γάλλου πρὸς ἄλλα καὶ πρὸς λυσσοδήκτους.] ♃ Νάρδου Συριακῆς < δ'. σμύρνης < η'. κινναμώμου < ιβ'. κασσίας μελαίνης ἴσον, κρόκου < η'. κόστου < δ'. δαύκου σπέρματος ἴσον, μήου ἴσον, οἱ δὲ μίαν, πετροσελίνου < δ'. πεπέρεως λευκοῦ κόκκους μ'. βαλσάμου καρποῦ < δ'. ἀκόρου, ἀσάρου ἀνὰ ἴσον, σχοίνου < η'. οἱ δὲ οὐ βάλλουσι. μέλιτος ἑφθοῦ τὸ ἱκανὸν, πλῆθος δίδοται ἐσθίειν.

[Ἄλλη ἀντίδοτος Αἰλίου Γάλλου πρὸς τὰ ἐντὸς πάθη ἐνεργής.] ♃ Κινναμώμου < στ'. κρόκου < β'. ὀβολοὺς γ'. πεπέρεως λευκοῦ < δ'. ὀβολοὺς β'. καὶ μακροῦ δὲ < γ'. ὀβολοὺς γ'. ὀπίου < γ'. νάρδου Ἰνδικῆς < δ'. σμύρνης < δ'. ὀβολοὺς β'. ἀκόρου < γ'. νάρδου Κελτικῆς < δ'. στύρακος μίαν, ὀβολοὺς β'. χαλβάνης < δ'. καστορίου <

ʒ ij, phu ʒ viij, rhus opſoniorum drach. v, obolos iij, radicis cotyledonis drach. j, obolos iij, vini et mellis quod ſatis eſt. Ego vinum non adjicio.

Cap. X. [*Variae diverſorum antidoti diverſis affectibus ſuccurrentes.*] [*Antidotum Aelii Galli ad alia, et rabioſorum morſus.*] ♃ Nardi Syriacae ʒ iv, myrrhae drach. viij, cinnamomi ʒ xij, caſſiae nigrae tantundem, croci drach. viij, coſti ʒ iv, ſeminis dauci, par pondus, mei, par pondus (quidam vero unam) petroſelini drach. iv, piperis albi g. xl, fructuum balſami ʒ iv, acori, aſari, utriusque tantundem, junci rotundi ʒ viij, alii ipſum non immittunt, mellis cocti quod ſatis eſt. Datur eſui.

[*Aliud antidotum Aelii Galli ad affectus interiores efficax.*] ♃ Cinnamomi drach. vj, croci ʒ ij, obolos iij, piperis albi drach. iv, obolos ij et longi drach. iij, obolos iij, opii ʒ iij, nardi Indicae ʒ iv, myrrhae drach. iv, obolos ij, acori ʒ iij, nardi Celticae drach. iv, ſtyracis ʒ j, obolos ij, galbani drach. iv, caſtorii ʒ iij, obolos ij, coſti

γ. ὀβολοὺς β'. κόστου < β'. ὀβολοὺς β'. μέλιτι φύρα, δίδοται καταπότια, τοῖς δὲ πότιμα. ἔστι δὲ πεπτικὴ καὶ ἀνώδυνος.

[Ἀρωματικὴ ἀρίστη Γάλλου ποιοῦσα πρὸς πάντα.] ♃ Κινναμώμου οὐγγίας ἥμισυ, κασσίας < α'. κρόκου δραχμῆς ἥμισυ, ἀμώμου < ε'. μαλαβάθρου < β'. σμύρνης < S''. οἱ δὲ < α'. σχοίνου ἄνθους α'. κόστου οὐγγίας τὸ ἥμισυ, πεπέρεως < γ'. μέλιτος Ἀττικοῦ τὸ ἀρκοῦν. ἐγὼ δὲ τοῦ κινναμώμου τὸ διπλοῦν, καὶ γίνεται καλλίων.

(448) [Ἀμβροσία Ἀρχιβίου ἱερὰ, πρὸς πάντα τὰ ἐντὸς ποιοῦσα, ᾗ χρῶμαι.] ♃ Ἀνίσου < δ'. σελίνου σπέρματος ἴσον, σμύρνης < α'. πάνακος < α'. κινναμώμου < β'. πικρολώτου σπέρματος < β'. κασσίας < β'. νάρδου < β'. κρόκου < β'. ὀβολοὺς γ'. πεπέρεως τριώβολον, ὀπίου μήκωνος < δ'. μέλιτος τὸ ἀρκοῦν. γίνεται πότιμα πρὸς δυσεντερικοὺς μετὰ μυρτίτου κοτύλης τετάρτης καὶ ὕδατος, πρὸς ἧπαρ μετὰ μελικράτου κοτύλης ἡμισείας, πρὸς ἀγρυπνίαν καὶ ὀφθαλμίαν καὶ πλευρῖτιν μετὰ μελικράτου, πρὸς

drach. ij, obolos ij, melle ſubige. Dantur pilulae, quibusdam potus; eſt autem *antidotum* concoctioni et dolori leniendo idoneum.

[*Aromaticum optimum Galli ad omnia faciens.*] ♃ Cinnamomi ℥ ß, caſſiae drach. j, croci drach ß, amomi drach. v, malabathri ʒ ij, myrrhae ʒ ß, (alii ʒ j,) ſchoenanthi drach. j, coſti ℥ ß, piperis drach. iij, mellis Attici quod ſatis eſt. Ego autem cinnamomi duplum injicio, et fit praeſtantius.

[*Ambroſia Archibii ſacra, omnibus internis faciens, qua utor.*] ♃ Aniſi drach. iv, ſeminum apii par pondus, myrrhae ʒ j, panacis drach. j, cinnamomi ʒ ij, ſeminis loti amari ʒ ij, caſſiae ʒ ij, nardi ʒ ij, croci drach. ij, obolos iij, piperis obolos iij, ſucci papaveris ʒ iv, mellis quod ſufficit. Redditur potabilis ad dyſenterias, cum ſemine myrtii quarta portione et aqua. Ad jecur cum mulſae hemina ß, ad vigilias, lippitudinem, pleuritidem cum

δὲ κακοστομάχους μετὰ ῥοΐτου οἴνου κυάθους β΄. καὶ ὕδαδος ἴσον.

[914] [Ἀντίδοτος Ἀντιπάτρου θηριακὴ, καὶ πρὸς ἀσπιδοδήκτους, προδιδομένη καὶ ἐπιδιδομένη, ᾗ χρῶμαι.] ℞ Γεντιανῆς ∠ δ΄ τριφύλλου ῥίζης ∠ δ΄. καὶ τοῦ καρποῦ ∠ β΄. πολίου ∠ δ΄. ἀριστολοχίας λεπτῆς ∠ β΄. πευκεδάνου ῥίζης ἴσον, χαλβάνης ∠ β΄. πετροσελίνου ∠ δ΄. πηγάνου ἀγρίου γ΄. πυρέθρου ∠ α΄. σταφίδος ἀγρίας ἴσον, ἀκόρου ∠ γ΄. βρυωνίας ῥίζης ∠ β΄. πεπέρεως λευκοῦ ἴσον, καὶ μακροῦ ∠ γ΄. ἀμμωνιακοῦ θυμιάματος ∠ α΄. τριώβολον, φλόμου, ἰδαίου χαμαιπίτυος, χαμελαίας, πρασίου λεπτοῦ, κονύζης λεπτῆς, κυμίνου Αἰθιοπικοῦ, ὀποῦ μήκωνος, καστορίου, μαράθρου σπέρματος, ἀγαρικοῦ, κασσίας κιῤῥᾶς, σχοίνου ἀνθοὺς, ῥήου ἀνὰ ∠ β΄. δαύκου Κρητικοῦ ∠ α΄. ὀβολοὺς γ΄. ὀποπάνακος ἴσον, σαγαπηνοῦ ∠ β΄. ὀβολοὺς γ΄. ἀβροτόνου ∠ α΄. ὀβολοὺς γ΄. δικτάμνου ἴσον, στύρακος ἴσον, κινναμώμου ∠ γ. νάρδου ∠ γ΄. σμύρνης ∠ δ΄. λιβανωτοῦ ∠ α΄. κρόκου ∠ η΄.

mulſa, ad ſtomachi vitia cum rhetis vini cyathis ij, et aquae pari menſura.

[*Antidotus Antipatri theriaca, ad aſpidum morſus, et praeſumpta, et poſtea data, qua utor.*] ℞ Gentianae ʒ iv, radicis trifolii ʒ iv, et fructus ipſius drach. ij, polii ʒ iv, ariſtolochiae tenuis drach. ij, radicis peucedani tantundem, galbani ʒ ij, petroſelini drach. iv, rutae ſilvaticae ʒ iij, pyrethri drach. j, ſtaphidos ſilveſtris tantundem, acori ʒ iij, bryoniae radicis drach. ij, piperis albi tantundem, et longi drach. iij, guttae ammoniaci drach. j, obolos iij, verbasci, idaeae chamaepityos, chamaeleae, marrubii tenuis, conyſae tenuis, cumini Aethiopici, ſucci papaveris, caſtorii, foeniculi ſeminis, agarici, caſſiae rubrae, ſchoenanthi, rheu, ſingulorum ʒ ij, dauci Cretici drach. j, obolos iij, opopanacis tantundem, ſagapeni drach. ij, obolos iij, abrotoni drach. j, obolos iij, dictamni tantundem, ſtyracis tantundem, cinnamomi drach. iij, nardi ʒ iij, myrrhae ʒ iv, thuris ʒ j, croci ʒ viij,

ἀνίσου < α΄. ὀποῦ Κυρηναϊκοῦ < α΄. πιτυᾶς νεβροῦ < γ΄. μέλι Ἀττικόν. ταύτης λαμβάνεται καρύου Ποντικοῦ μέγεθος εἰς προφυλακήν.

[Θηριακὴ Αἰλίου Γάλλου, ᾗ χρῶμαι, καλή.] ℞ Βρυωνίας ῥίζης < ιστ΄. τριφύλλου σπέρματος, ὀποπάνακος ἀνὰ < η΄. ἀριστολοχίας λεπτῆς < ιβ΄. λιβανωτίδος ῥίζης, ἴρεως Ἰλλυρικῆς, ζιγγιβέρεως, μηκωνείου ἀνὰ < η΄. πηγάνου ἀγρίου σπέρματος < ιβ΄. κυμίνου Αἰθιοπικοῦ < ιστ΄. σμύρνης, κασσίας, καστορίου, σεσέλεως, ἠρυγγίου ῥίζης, ἑρπύλλου, ὀποῦ Κυρηναϊκοῦ, ἀνὰ < στ΄. Μηδικοῦ < ιβ΄. σαγαπηνοῦ < στ΄. κρόκου < ε΄. ἀλεύρου ὀροβίνου < κδ΄. σὺν ὕδατι ἀνάπλαττε τριωβολιαίους τροχίσκους, δίδου σὺν οἴνῳ.

[Θηριακὴ ἄλλη Αἰλίου Γάλλου σφόδρα ἐνεργής.] ℞ Τριφύλλου σπέρματος < ιβ΄. ἀριστολοχίας < στ΄. ἡδυχρόου μάγματος < η΄. πενταφύλλου < δ΄. ἐχίου βοτάνης < στ΄. φιλοκράτου < ε΄. σαγαπηνοῦ < δ΄. πολίου < στ΄. καστορίου < γ΄. κρόκου < η΄. σελίνου σπέρματος, ἀνίσου,

anifi ʒ j, fucci Cyrenaici tantundem, coaguli hinnuli drach. iij, mel Atticum additur; hujus nucis avellanae magnitudo in praecautionem fumitur.

[*Theriaca Aelii Galli, qua utor, egregia.*] ℞ Bryoniae radicis drach. xvj, feminis trifolii, opopanacis, fingulorum ʒ viij, ariftolochiae tenuis drach. xij, roris marini radicis, ireos Illyricae, zingiberis, meconii, fingulorum drach. viij, rutae filvaticae feminis drach. xij, cumini Aethiopici ʒ xvj, myrrhae, caffiae, caftorii, fefeleos, eryngii radicis, ferpilli, fucci Cyrenaici, fingulorum drach. vj, medicae drach. xij, fagapeni ʒ vj, croci ʒ v, ervi farinae drach. xxiv, finguntur paftilli ex aqua triobolares, danturque cum vino.

[*Theriaca alia Aelii Galli vehementer efficax.*] ℞ Trifolii feminis drach. xij, ariftolochiae drach. vj, hedychroi magmatis ʒ viij, quinquefolii drach. iv, echii herbae ʒ vj, philocrati drach. v, fagapeni drach. iv, polii ʒ vj, caftorii drach. iij, croci ʒ viij, apii feminis, anifi, foeniculi, pe-

μαράθρου, πετροσελίνου, ἀνὰ < στ΄. ὀποπάνακος < δ΄. ὀποβαλσάμου < στ΄. σεσέλεως < δ΄. κυμίνου Αἰθιοπικοῦ ἢ Θηβαίου < ε΄. σμύρνης, σκορδίου, φοῦ, μήου ἀνὰ < στ΄. ἀλύσσου Κρητικοῦ σπέρματος < στ΄. ὀροβίνου ἀλεύρου < η΄. λεῖος οἶνος παραχεῖται Ἀριούσιος, ἀνάπλασσε τροχίσκους, ἀνὰ τετρώβολον, ἕνα δίδου σὺν οἴνῳ Χίῳ ἀθαλάσσῳ ἀκράτῳ, κοτύλῃ ἡμισείᾳ. Θηριακὴ πρὸς τοὺς ἐντὸς πόνους, Εὐκλείδου Παλατιανοῦ, ἣν ἐσκεύασεν, ὡς ἔλεγεν Εὐκλείδης, ἐπὶ ἀσπιδοδήκτων. ταῦτα καὶ πρὸς πλευριτικοὺς καὶ πρὸς τεταρταίους, προεμηκόσι, μέγεθος καρύου Ποντικοῦ· βήσσουσιν, ἀναφορικοῖς δι᾽ ὕδατος, θηριοδήκτοις, σὺν οἴνῳ· πλευριτικοῖς καὶ αἷμα ἀνάγουσι μεθ᾽ ὕδατος κυάθων β΄. καὶ ὄξους κυάθου ἑνός. ♃ Καστορίου < στ΄. ὀποπάνακος, σαγαπηνοῦ, σεσέλεως, κάγχρυος, χαμαίδρυος, χαμαιπίτυος πρασίου, ἀνὰ < ιστ΄. στύρακος, ἀσφάλτου Ἰουδαϊκῆς, σμύρνης, ἀνὰ < ζ΄. ὀποῦ μήκωνος < η΄. μέλιτος λίτραν α΄. πότιζε θηριοδήκτους, εἰ οἷόν τε ἡμεμηκότας, μετὰ χυλοῦ

trofelini, fingulorum ℨ vj, opopanacis drach. iv, opobalfami drach. vj, fefeleos ℨ iv, cumini Aethiopici aut Thebani drach. v, myrrhae, fcordii, phu, meu, fingulorum drach. vj, alyffi Cretici feminis drach. vj, ervi farinae drach. viij, vino levi Arvifio affuso paftilli formantur, qui obolos iv, pendeant, datur unus ex vino Chio marinae experti meraco, hemina dimidia. *Theriaca ad internos dolores, Euclidis Palatiani, quam, ut Euclides ajebat, praeparavit ad afpidum morfus; etiam ad pleuriticos et quartanarios, valet vomitu folicitatis, magnitudine nucis avellanae exhibita, tuffientibus, aegre excreantibus ex aqua, ferarum morfibus cum vino, pleuriticis fimulque fanguinem rejicientibus, ex aquae cyathis duobus et aceti uno cyatho.* ♃ Caftorii ℨ iv, opopanacis, fagapeni, fefeleos, canchryos, chamaedryos, chamaepityos, marrubii, fingulorum ℨ xvj, ftyracis, bituminis Judaici, myrrhae, fingulorum ℨ vij, fucci papaveris ℨ viij, mellis ℔ j. Propinato commorfis a feris, fi fieri poffit, vomitu praemiffo, cum fraxini copiofiore fucco: fin minus, cum vino ℨ j,

μελίης πλείονος· εἰ δὲ μὴ, μετ' οἴνου ∠ α'. τοῦ φαρμάκου, ἢ καὶ πλέον· τεταρταϊκοῖς, καρύου μέγεθος, χρῶ.

[Θηριακὴ Ζήνωνος Λαοδικέως, ὡς Μηνουκιανὸς λαβὼν ἔδωκεν.] ♃ Καρδαμώμου κεκαθαρμένου καὶ ἀφῃρημένου τῶν λοβῶν, ἑρπύλλου, σελίνου σπέρματος, βρυωνίας ῥίζης, τριφύλλου σπέρματος, ἀνίσου, πετροσελίνου, μαράθρου ῥίζης καὶ τοῦ σπέρματος, ἄμμεως, ἀριστολοχίας λεπτῆς, ὀροβίνου ἀλεύρου, ὀποπάνακος, ἴσον [915] ἑκάστου· κόψας ἰδίᾳ μίσγε, ἀναλάμβανε οἴνῳ αὐστηρῷ, καὶ ποίει τροχίσκους τριωβολιαίους. ὅταν ξηρανθῶσιν ἐν σκιᾷ, ἐχέτωσαν τὸ τριώβολον. πότιζε ἕνα σὺν δραχμαῖς δυσὶν ὕδατος τρὶς τῆς ἡμέρας, καὶ ἅπαξ τῆς νυκτὸς ἕνα τροχίσκον. ὁτὲ δὲ πλεονάκις, καὶ μάλιστα τοὺς συνεχῶς ἀπεμοῦντας, ποτὲ καὶ διὰ μυκτήρων ἔγχει, ἐὰν μὴ δύνηται καταπίνειν, ἤδη καταφερομένοις, καὶ ἄλλως δυσχερεῖ συμπτώματι περιπεπτωκόσι. τοὺς δὲ μετὰ φλυκταινώσεως μελανουμένους τὸ δῆγμα καὶ ἄλλως ῥέοντας σάρκας ὡς ἕλκη κακοήθη ἔχοντας θεράπευε. Ἀντίδοτος πρὸς σπάσματα ποιοῦσα, καὶ

medicamenti, vel etiam amplius: nucis magnitudinem quartanariis dato.

[*Theriaca Zenonis Laodicaei, ut Menucianus acceptam tradidit.*] ♃ Cardamomi purgati et fibris exuti, ferpilli, feminum apii, radicis bryoniae, feminum trifolii, anifi, petrofelini, feminis et radicis foeniculi, ammeos, ariftolochiae tenuis, ervi farinae, opopanacis, par pondus; contufa privatim mifce, vino auftero excipe, et confice paftillos triobolares; ubi ficcata fuerint in umbra, ternos obolos pendeant, propina unum ter die cum duabus aquae drachmis, ac femel nocte unum paftillum. At multoties et praefertim continue vomitu vexatis, nonnunquam quoque naribus infundito, fi nequeant deglutire jam fopore gravatis ac alioquin gravi fymptomate implicitis; qui vero cum puftulis in morfu nigrefcunt, et alias carnes diffluentes habent praecipue, ceu malignis ulceribus obfeffos eos curato. *Antidotum ad convulfa, rupta, fanguinem ex-*

ῥήγματα, αἱμοπτοϊκοὺς, σπληνικοὺς, ἡπατικοὺς, τοὺς περὶ κύστιν εἰλεώδεις, στομαχικοὺς, κοιλιακοὺς, πνευματώδεις, ἰκτερικούς. πρὸς πάντας ἀγαθὴ διδόναι μέγεθος ἐλαίας μετ' οἰνομέλιτος. ℞ Κινναμώμου, κόστου, ἀνὰ < στ'. νάρδου Συριακῆς < κ'. κρόκου, σμύρνης, μαλαβάθρου, ἀνὰ < η'. κασσίας < ιβ'. πεπέρεως λευκοῦ < ι'. λιβάνου < δ'. σχοίνου < ιστ'. νάρδου Ἰλλυρικῆς < ιβ'. Λημνίας < κ'. μήου, σεσέλεως, ἀνὰ < η'. σελίνου σπέρματος < δ'. στροβίλων < ιβ'. ἐρυσίμου < στ'. σικύου σπέρματος πεφωγμένου < στ'. τερμινθίνης < γ'. πετροσελίνου < δ'. ἀμώμου γ'. σκορδίου, πολίου, ὀποβαλσάμου, γεντιανῆς, κυμίνου Αἰθιοπικοῦ, ἀνὰ < ε'. πηγάνου ἀγρίου σπέρματος < γ'. ἀνίσου, τραγακάνθης, ἀνὰ < η'. φοῦ, στοιχάδος, κνεώρου, ἀνὰ < β'. τὸ ἐρύσιμον δι' ὀθονίου ἐν ὕδατι ἕψησον, ὥστε τὸ φάρμακον ἀναλαβεῖν, μῖξον πᾶσι λείοις, εἶτα ἐπέμβαλε τὴν τραγάκανθαν ὕδατι βεβρεγμένην, δίδου ἡλίκον κύαμον Αἰγύπτιον, μετὰ κυάθων δύο δι' ὕδατος, ἀπυρέτοις δι' οἰνομέλιτος. Ἀντίδοτος Μιθριδάτειος, ὡς Ξενοκράτης

puentes, lienoſos, hepaticos, ilioſos circa veſicam, ſtomachicos, coeliacos, flatulentos, ictericos. Ad omnes convenit dare magnitudinem olivae cum mulſo. ℞ Cinnamomi, coſti, an. ʒ vj, nardi Syriacae ʒ xx, croci, myrrhae, malabathri, an. ʒ viij, caſſiae ʒ xij, piperis albi ʒ x, thuris ʒ iv, junci rotundi ʒ xvj, nardi Illyricae ʒ xij, terrae Lemniae ʒ xx, mei, ſeſelcos, ſingulorum viij, ſeminis apii ʒ iv, ſtrobilorum ʒ xij, eryſimi ʒ vj, ſeminis cucumeris frixi ʒ vj, terebinthinae ʒ iij, petroſelini ʒ iv, amomi ʒ iij, ſcordii, polii, opobalſami, gentianae, cumini Aethiopici, ſingulorum ʒ v, ſeminis rutae ſilvaticae drach. iij, aniſi, tragacanthi, ſingulorum ʒ viij, phu, ſtoechados, cneori, ſingulorum ʒ ij, Eryſimum per linteum in aqua coctum, ut medicamentum excipiat, omnibus in pulverim laevigatis miſcetur. Deinde tragacanthum aqua maceratum adjicito. Datur fabae Aegyptiae inſtar, cum duobus aquae cyathis: ſi febris abſuerit, ex mulſo. *Antidotum Mithridation ut Xenocrates apud Ni-*

παρὰ Νικοστράτῳ, πρὸς πάντα θανάσιμα, καὶ πρὸς θηριοδήκτους, δυσπεψίας, πνευματώσεις, στομαχικοὺς, κοιλιακοὺς, ἡπατικοὺς, σπληνικοὺς, ἰσχιαδικοὺς, νεφριτικοὺς, πλευριτικοὺς, περιπνευμονικούς. ℞ Ὑποκιστίδος χυλοῦ < στ΄. σκορδίου < ε΄. καστορίου < δ΄. πετροσελίνου < ε΄. σεσέλεως < α΄. λιβάνου < στ΄. πολίου < β΄. δαύκου Κρητικοῦ < ι΄. πεπέρεως λευκοῦ < α΄. ὀβολοὺς γ΄. καὶ μακροῦ < α΄. κόστου < δ΄. τριώβολον, κινναμώ (449) μου β΄. κρόκου < ε΄. ὀβολοὺς γ΄. κασσίας μελαίνης < δ΄. νάρδου < η΄. σμύρνης < η΄. σχοίνου < δ΄. ἀμώμου < β΄. χαλβάνης < β΄. τερμινθίνης < α΄. ὀβολοὺς γ΄. ὀποῦ μήκωνος < κ΄. μέλιτι Ἀττικῷ δίδου, ὡς τὰς λοιπάς. Ἀντίδοτος τυραννὶς καλουμένη, ὡς Νεῖλος Ἀντιπάτρου, ποιοῦσα πρὸς λιθιῶντας, καὶ τοὺς πνιγομένους. ἐκβάλλει καὶ τὰ ἐγκατεχόμενα δεύτερα καὶ ἔμβρυα. ἐπιληπτικοῖς, ποδαγρικοῖς, ἀρθριτικοῖς, ἰσχιαδικοῖς, ἄγουσα παχέα οὖρα πλεῖστα. πότιζε κυάθου μέγεθος οἰνομέλιτι καὶ πρὸς τὰ θανάσιμα, θηριοδήκτοις οἴνῳ, ἐπιληπτικοῖς πυρέσσουσι, σὺν ὑδρομέ-

coſtratum, ad omnia lethalia, ferarum morſus, aegram concoctionem, inflationes, ſtomachicos, coeliacos, hepaticos, lienoſos, iſchiadicos, nephriticos, pleuriticos, peripneumonicos. ℞ Succi hypociſtidis ʒ vj, ſcordii ʒ v, caſtorii ʒ iv, petroſelini ʒ v, ſeſeleos ʒ j, thuris ʒ vj, polii ʒ ij, dauci Cretici ʒ x, piperis albi ʒ j, obolos iij, oblongi ʒ j, coſti ʒ iv, obolos iij, cinnamomi ʒ ij, croci ʒ v, obolos iij, caſſiae nigrae ʒ iv, nardi ʒ viij, myrrhae ʒ viij, junci rotundi ʒ iv, amomi ʒ ij, galbani ʒ ij, terebinthinae ʒ j, obolos iij, ſucci papaveris drach. xx, melle Attico datur, quemadmodum reliqua. *Antidotus Tyrannis dicta, ut Nilus Antipatri: efficax ad calculoſos et ſuffocatu periclitantes, expellit etiam ſecundas retentas foetusque; ſalutaris comitialibus, podagricis, articulariis, iſchiadicis, craſſas urinas educens copioſiſſime. Datur cyathi menſura mulſo Etiam iis, qui lethalia aſſumpſerunt: in ferarum morſibus vino, et comitiali morbo, ſi febris adeſt cum hydromelite.* ℞ Scinci ʒ viij,

λιτ. ♃ Σκίγκου ◁ η'. σμύρνης ◁ κη'. Λημνίας μίλτου ◁ δ'. νάρδου ◁ η'. σχοίνου ◁ δ'. κινναμώμου ◁ κδ'. ῥίζης γλυκείας ◁ κη'. σμύρνης ◁ κ'. ἠρυγγίου ◁ κδ'. ἀμώμου ◁ ιβ'. καρδαμώμου ◁ η'. κρόκου ◁ η'. κεδρίδων μελαινῶν ◁ ιβ'. μελιλώτου ◁ ιβ'. ὑακινθίνου σπέρματος ◁ δ'. πεπέρεως μακροῦ ◁ δ'. καὶ λευκοῦ κόκκους πε'. σφονδυλίου ◁ ιβ'. στοιχάδος ◁ ε'. πυρέθρου ◁ στ'. μαλάχης ἀγρίας σπέρματος ◁ ιβ'. λευκοΐου σπέρματος ◁ γ'. ὀποβαλσάμου δραχμὰς στ'. κόστου ◁ η'. ὀβολὸν ἕνα, ἄμμεως δραχμὰς ιβ'. κοτυληδόνος ῥίζης δραχμὰς ιδ'. δαύκου σπέρματος ◁ ιβ'. καρποβαλσάμου ◁ δ'. ξυλοβαλσάμου δραχμὰς δ'. κασσίας ◁ η'. κυμίνου Αἰθιοπικοῦ ◁ δ'. ὠκίμου σπέρματος ◁ η'. ἀκόρου ◁ η'. οἰνάνθης ◁ η'. σελίνου σπέρματος ιβ'. σαγαπηνοῦ ◁ η'. καππάρεως ῥίζης ◁ δ'. [916] γεντιανῆς ◁ ιδ'. περικλυμένου ῥίζης ◁ η'. λιβάνου ◁ η'. στύρακος ◁ α'. κέγχρου ἀγρίας ◁ κδ'. σμυρνίου ῥίζης ◁ δ'. σισάρου σπέρματος ◁ η'. ἀμμωνιακοῦ θυμιάματος ◁ ιστ'. σεσέλεως ◁ δ'. κάγχρυος ◁ δ'. οἱ δὲ ◁ α'.

myrrhae ʒ xxviij, terrae Lemniae ʒ iv, nardi drach. viij, junci rotundi ʒ iv, cinnamomi ʒ xxiv, glycyrrhizae drach. xxviij, myrrhae drach xx, eryngii ʒ xxiv, amomi ʒ xij, cardamomi ʒ viij, croci tantundem, baccarum cedri nigrarum ʒ xij, meliloti ʒ xij, feminis hyacinthini ʒ iv, piperis longi drach. iv et albi g. lxxxxv, fpondylii drach. xij, ftoechados ʒ v, pyrethri drach. vj, malvae filveftris feminis ʒ xij, albae violae feminis drach. iij, opobalfami ʒ vj, cofti ʒ viij, obolum j, ammeos ʒ xij, radicis cotyledonis ʒ xiv, feminis dauci ʒ xij, carpobalfami ʒ iv, xylobalfami ʒ iv, caffiae ʒ viij, cumini Aethiopici ʒ iv, feminis ocimi drach. viij, acori ʒ viij, oenanthae ʒ viij, feminis apii ʒ xij, fagapeni drach. viij, cappareos radicis drach. iv, gentianae ʒ xiv, radicis periclymeni ʒ viij, thuris ʒ viij, ftyracis ʒ j, milii filveftris ʒ xxiv, radicis fmyrnii drach. iv, feminis fifari drach. viij, guttae ammoniaci ʒ xvj, fefeleos drach. iv, canchryos ʒ iv, quidam

Ἰλλυρίδος ⊲ δ'. ἀνίσου ⊲ δ'. χαμαιπίτυος ⊲ ιε'. χαμαίδρυος ἴσον, σμυρνίου σπέρματος ⊲ η'. ζιγγιβέρεως ⊲ ιδ'. κενταυρίου λεπτοῦ ⊲ η'. σταφυλίνου σπέρματος, μήου ἀνὰ ⊲ η'. καλάμου ῥίζης ⊲ δ'. μύρου καλοῦ κοτύλην α'. μέλιτος Ἀττικοῦ τὸ ἱκανόν.

[*Πρὸς τεταρταίους, ὡς Ἅρπαλος.*] ♃ Σμύρνης ⊲ δ'. πεπέρεως μακροῦ ἢ λευκοῦ ⊲ β'. μηκωνείου ⊲ β'. καστορίου ὀβολοὺς γ' S''. καρδαμώμου ⊲ δ'. σαγαπηνοῦ ⊲ β'. λεῖα σὺν ὕδατι ἀνάπλασσε τροχίσκους, ἀνὰ ὀβολοὺς β'. τοῖς περιοδικοῖς σὺν οἴνου κυάθοις β'. ἀδριανοῦ, ἢ ἀμιναίου, καὶ ὕδατος πηγαίου ἀφηψημένου κυάθοις δ'. πυρέσσουσιν σὺν ὑδρομέλιτι ποιεῖ δὲ καὶ πρὸς τὰς λοιπὰς περιόδους. ἐπεὶ δὲ καὶ πρὸς τοὺς δηχθέντας ἢ νυχθέντας ὑπό τινος τῶν ἰοβόλων ζώων, ἅμα τοῖς προγεγραμμένοις φαρμάκοις, ἐπέγραψαν οἱ περὶ τὸν Ἀσκληπιάδην τε καὶ Δαμοκράτην, διὰ τοῦτο κἀμοὶ βέλτιον ἔδοξεν εἶναι κατὰ τὸ προκείμενον τοῦτο βιβλίον ἐφεξῆς αὐτὰ προσθεῖναι, καὶ πρῶτά γε τὰ τοῦ Ἀσκληπιάδου.

ʒ j, nardi Illyricae ʒ iv, anifi ʒ iv. chamaepityos ʒ xv, chamaedryos par pondus, feminis fmyrnii ʒ viij, zingiberis ʒ xiv, centaurii tenuis ʒ viij, feminis ftaphylini, mei, fingulorum ʒ viij, calami radicis ʒ iv, unguenti boni heminam, mellis Attici quod fatis eft.

[*Ad quartana laborantes, ut Harpalus.*] ♃ Myrrhae ʒ iv, piperis longi vel albi ʒ ij, meconii ʒ ij, caftorii obolos iij, ß cardamomi ʒ iv, fagapeni ʒ ij, trita cum aqua in paftillos cogantur, qui obolos ij, pendeant, quibus morbus circuitu remeat, cum vini cyathis duobus Adriani vel Aminaei, et aquae fontanae decoctae cyathis iv, fi febris urget, cum hydromelite; valet etiam ad reliquas periodos. Quoniam vero Afclepiades et Damocrates ad eos, qui virulento quodam animali morfi punctive funt, una cum praedictis medicamentis remedia adfcripferunt, mihi quoque fatius vifum eft impraefentiarum ordine ea apponere, ac prima fane quae ad Afclepiadem auctorem referuntur.

Κεφ. ια'. [*Τα ὑπὸ τοῦ Ἀσκληπιάδου γεγραμμένα κατὰ τὸ ε. τῶν Ἄσωνος, πρὸς τὰς ἐκ τῶν ἰοβόλων βλάβας.*] [*Πόμα λυσσοδήκτοις προφυλακτικὸν σφόδρα γενναῖον.*] ♃ Λυκίου Ἰνδικοῦ ὡς καλλίστου δίδου ὀβολοὺς γ'. μεθ' ὕδατος, καὶ ἱερᾶς βοτάνης μικρόν τι παραπλέκων, δίδου ἐφ' ἡμέρας ἱκανάς. δίδου δὲ καὶ χωρὶς ὕδατος εἰς ὠὸν ῥοφητὸν βαλὼν τὸ λύκιον.

[*Ἄλλη.*] ♃ Καστορίου ∠ α'. ῥοδίνου λευκοῦ κύαθον, δίδου πίνειν δεύτερον τῆς ἡμέρας καὶ διαλείπων, κενοῦ ἀψινθίου ἀφεψήματι ἁλῶν ἐπεμβεβλημένων τοσούτων, ὥστε τὸ ἐνειμένον σφοδρότερον εἶναι. *Ἀντωνίνου Κώου.* Ἄλυσσον βοτάνην κόψας καὶ σήσας, ἀπόθου, ἐν τῇ χρήσει δίδου κοχλιάριον λυσσοδήκτοις, μεθ' ὕδατος καὶ ὑδρομέλιτος κυάθων γ'. ἀπὸ α'. ἡμέρας, καλὸν μὲν εἰ ἐπὶ ἡμέρας μ'. εἰ δὲ μή γε, ἐπὶ τὰς πρώτας ἡμέρας ζ'. ἄλυσσος δέ ἐστι βοτάνη τῷ πρασίῳ παρεμφέρουσα, τραχυτέρα δὲ, καὶ μᾶλλον ἀκανθώδης περὶ τὰ σφαιρία, ἄνθος δὲ φέρει κυανίζον. ταύτην χρὴ συλλέγειν ἐν τοῖς ὑπὸ κύνα καύμασι, καὶ ξηράναντας

Cap. XI. [*Quae Aſclepiades in quinto Aſonis tradiderit ad virulentorum animalium noxas.*] [*Potio a rabioſorum morſu praeſervans admodum generoſa.*] ♃ Lycii Indici quam optimi obolos iij, cum aqua propinato; item herbae ſacrae exiguum implicatum diebus ſat multis dato. Jam et ſine aqua lycium ovo ſorbili inditum porrigitur.

[*Alia.*] ♃ Caſtorii ʒ j, roſacei albi cyathum da potui, ſecundo die etiam intermiſſo, immittes abſinthio decocto ſale injecto tantiſper, ut quod diluitur, ſit vehementius. *Antonini Coi* Alyſſon herbam contuſam cribratamque reponito; in uſu, dato cochleare a rabioſo morſis, cum aquae et hydromelitis cyathis iij, ab uno die; praeſtat ad xl usque, ſin minus ad primos dies ſeptem exhiberi. Alyſſus autem herba eſt marrubio perſimilis, aſperior autem et magis ſpinoſa eſt circa galbulos, florem fert ad caeruleum ſpectantem. Haec legenda eſt ſub aeſtu caniculae; ſiccata, contundi, cribrari, ſervarique

κόπτειν, καὶ σήθειν, καὶ φυλάττειν ἀδιάπνευστον. Ἄλλη ἔνδοξος πάνυ. ♃ Μιθρέου καρκίνων ποταμίων ἐπὶ κλημάτων λευκῆς ἀμπέλου κεκαυμένων καὶ τετριμμένων μύστρα ί. ῥίζης γεντιανῆς μύστρα γ'. τερμινθίνης μύστρα β'. δίδου δηχθεῖσιν εὐθέως μετ' οἴνου ἀκράτου παλαιοῦ κυάθων γ'. ἢ ὀλίγῳ πλέονος, ἢ ἐλάττονος. δεῖ γὰρ παραμετρεῖν ταῖς ἡλικίαις καὶ τὴν δύναμιν τῶν δηχθέντων· δίδου ἐπὶ ἡμέρας γ'. τοῖς δὲ ὕστερον τῆς α'. ἡμέρας, ἢ τῆς β'. ἢ καὶ τῆς γ'. μέλλουσι λαμβάνειν τὸ φάρμακον, ἐπιμηχανητέον, ὥστε τὸ ἅπαξ διδόμενον τῆς ἡμέρας, τοῦτο τριπλοῦν, καὶ διπλοῦν τοῦ φαρμάκου διδόναι, ὁ γὰρ οἶνος αὐτάρκης. ἐκπληρώσαντα δὲ τὸ ἐλλεῖπον τῶν ἡμερῶν, διδόναι καρκίνων ποταμίων μύστρον ἓν, καὶ γεντιανῆς μύστρα β'. ἐπ' ἄλλας ἡμέρας γ'. μετ' οἴνου κυάθων γ'. τὸ δὲ λεγόμενόν ἐστι τοιοῦτον. τοῖς μὲν εὐθέως δηχθεῖσι διδόναι καρκίνων μύστρον, καὶ γεντιανῆς μύστρα β'. καὶ οἴνου ἀκράτου κυάθους γ'. [917] καθ' ἑκάστην ἐπὶ ἡμέρας ϛ'. εἰ δέ τις ἀφυστερήσει τῆς θεραπείας, εἰ μὲν δευτεραῖος εἴη, λαμβάνειν τοῦ φαρ-

debet, ne diffletur. *Alia celebris admodum.* ♃ Tegminis cancrorum fluviatilium in ſarmentis albae vitis uſtorum tritorumque myſtra x, radicis gentianae myſtra iij, terebinthinae myſtra ij, dato morſis ſtatim cum vini meracioris vetuſti cyathis iij, vel paulo ampliori vel pauciori; nam pro aetate et viribus morſorum metiri convenit; propinato ad triduum; qui autem poſt primum aut ſecundum aut etiam tertium diem medicamentum ſunt aſſumpturi, in iis conandum eſt, ut quod ſemel die exhibetur, id triplicatum duplicatumque ex medicamento exhibeatur; etenim vinum ſufficit. Expletis autem qui reſtant diebus, cancrorum fluviatilium myſtrum j, dabitur; gentianae myſtra ij, ad alios dies iij, cum tribus vini cyathis. Quod autem dicitur ejusmodi eſt. Statim commorſis dato cancrorum myſtrum, gentianae myſtra ij, et vini meraci cyathos iij, quotidie ad dies ſex. At ſi quis curationem procraſtinaverit, ſiquidem ſecundus dies eſt, duplum medicamenti capere oportet, nam vinum abunde

μάκου τὸ διπλοῦν, ὁ γὰρ οινος αὐτάρκης. εἰ δὲ τριταῖος, λαμβανέτω τριπλοῦν. μετὰ δὲ ταῦτα τρὶς ἐπ᾽ ἄλλας ἡμέρας λαμβανέτω, ὅπερ ἔθος ἔχει, καθ᾽ ἑκάστην ἡμέραν λαμβάνειν. τὸ φάρμακον ποθὲν, ἱκανὴν ἀσφάλειαν ποιεῖ, ὥστε μὴ περιπεσεῖν τῷ ὑδροφόβῳ.

[*Κρατίππου ἀνδρὸς, καὶ ἐπισήμου καὶ κυνοτρόφου.*] ℞ *Καρκίνων* ∢ κ'. σμύρνης ∢ β'. κρόκου ∢ α' S''. γεντιανῆς ∢ α'. πεπέρεως λευκοῦ κόκκους ι'. οἴνου ὅσον ἐξαρκεῖ εἰς ἀνάληψιν. ἡ δόσις ∢ α'. μετ᾽ οἴνου κυάθων γ'. κεκραμένου.

[*Ἄλλη, ᾗ ἐχρήσατο Ηρας ὁ Καππαδόκης.*] ℞ *Σκορδίου* ∢ β'. πεπέρεως λευκοῦ ∢ β' S''. ὀπίου ∢ γ'. ὀποῦ Κυρηναϊκοῦ ∢ γ' S''. κάγχρυος ∢ δ'. γεντιανῆς, πηγάνου ἀγρίου σπέρματος, μίλτου Λημνίας, ἀνὰ ∢ ε'. σμύρνης ∢ ζ'· ὀποβαλσάμου ∢ η'. σκεύαζε οἴνῳ, καὶ ἀναλάμβανε μέλιτι ἑφθῷ, ὕστερον ἐπιβαλὼν τὸ ὀποβάλσαμον, καὶ δίδου εὐτονωτέροις κυάμου Αἰγυπτίου. τὸ διπλοῦν, καὶ ὕδατος θερμοῦ κυάθους γ'.

[*Ἄλλη Αἰλίου Γάλλου, ὡς Βελχιόνιος ἔφη παρὰ Καί-*

eft; fi tertius, triplum. Posthaec ter ad alios dies capiat, quae confuetudo eft fingulis diebus affumere. Medicamentum potum, magnam fecuritatem concilial, ne in hydrophobiam i. e. *aquae metum* incidant.

[*Cratippi viri et celebris, et canum altoris.*] ℞ Cancrorum ʒ xx, myrrhae ʒ ij, croci ʒ j ß, gentianae ʒ j, piperis albi gr. x, vini quod ad excipiendum fatis eft. Dofis ʒ j, cum vini cyathis tribus temperati.

[*Aliud, quo ufus eft Heras Cappadox.*] ℞ Scordii ʒ ij, piperis albi ʒ ij ß, opii ʒ iij, fucci Cyrenaici ʒ iij ß, canchryos ʒ iv, gentianae, feminis rutae filvaticae, minii Lemnii, fingulorum ʒ v, myrrhae drach. vij, opobalfami drach. viij. Praepara haec vino, et excipe melle cocto; poftea opobalfamum adjicito; dato valentioribus fabae Aegyptiae duplum, et aquae calidae cyathos iij.

[*Aliud Aelii Galli, ut Belchionius ajebat, a Caefare*

σαρος εἰληφέναι.] ℞ Πολίου, ὀποῦ Κυρηναϊκοῦ, ἀνὰ < γ' S''. κάγχρυος, πηγάνου ἀγρίου σπέρματος, ἀνὰ < δ'. γεντιανῆς, μίλτου Λημνίας, ἀνὰ < ε'. σμύρνης < στ'. ἢ ζ'. ὀποβαλσάμου < η'. σκορδίου, πεπέρεως, ἀνὰ < ιβ'. μέλιτι ἀναλάμβανε.

[Ζήνωνος Λαοδικέως λυσσοδήκτοις. Ἔστι δὲ καὶ θηριακὴ ἀγαθή.] (450) ℞ Πετροσελίνου σπέρματος, ἄμμεως, ἀνίσου, ἑρπύλλου, βρυωνίας ῥίζης, μαράθρου σπέρματος, ὀροβίνου ἀλεύρου, ἀριστολοχίας μακρᾶς, τριφύλλου σπέρματος, ὀποπάνακος, καρδαμώμου τῶν λοβῶν χωρὶς τῆς ἐντεριώνης, ἀνὰ < δ'. τὸν ὀποπάνακα οἴνῳ διαλύσας, ἔχε ἐν ἑτοίμῳ· τὰ δὲ ξηρὰ κόψας καὶ σήσας λεπτῷ κοσκίνῳ, φυράσας καὶ τῷ ὀποπάνακι μίξας, ἀνάπλασσε τροχίσκους, καὶ ξήραινε ἐν σκιᾷ, καὶ δίδου λυσσοδήκτοις < α'. μετ' οἴνου ἀκράτου κυάθων γ'. ἐπὶ ἡμέρας γ' τοῖς δὲ ἤδη κατισχομένοις δίδου μετὰ ὕδατος ψυχροῦ. τὸ φάρμακον εἰς Διόνυσον ἀναφέρεται τὸν Μιλήσιον.

[Κλαυδίου Ἀπολλωνίου φάρμακον ἐπιτετευγμένον λυσ-

acceptum.] ℞ Polii, fucci Cyrenaici, utriusque ʒ iij ß, canchryos, rutae filveftris feminis, fingulorum ʒ iv, gentianae, minii Lemnii, fingulorum ʒ v, myrrhae ʒ vj vel vij, opobalfami ʒ viii, fcordii, piperis, fingulorum ʒ xii, melle excipito.

[*Antidotus Zenonis Laodicaei ad rabioforum morfus, eft etiam bona theriaca.*] ℞ Seminis petrofelini, ammeos, anifi, ferpilli, bryoniae radicis, feminis foeniculi, ervi farinae, ariftolochiae longae, feminis trifolii, opopanacis, fibrarum cardamomi fine medulla, fingulorum ʒ iv, opopanax vino folutus in promptu habeatur; arida contufa, et tenui cribro increta, confperguntur, et opopanaci mifcentur, inde paftilli finguntur, ficcanturque in umbra. Dato morfis a rabiofo ʒ j, cum ternis vini meraci cyathis ad triduum; iis autem qui jam detinentur, cum aqua frigida propinatur. Medicamentum ad Dionyfium Milefium refertur.

[*Claudii Apollonii medicamentum ad rabioforum mor-*

σοδήκτοις. εστι καὶ θηριακή.] ℞ Τριφύλλου σπέρματος, μαράθρου ῥίζης, ἀνὰ ∠ στ΄. σκίλλης τῶν φύλλων ξηρῶν, ἀριστολοχίας μακρᾶς, ἀνὰ ∠ ε΄. σκίγκου, ἑρπύλλου κλάδων, ἀνὰ ∠ δ΄. καρδαμώμου κεκαθαρμένου, γλυκυῤῥίζης, ἀνὰ ∠ γ΄. ἄμμεως, πηγάνου ῥίζης, ἀνὰ ∠ β΄. ὀποπάνακος, ὀποῦ Κυρηναϊκοῦ, ἀνὰ ∠ α΄. οἴνου Φαλερίνου ξέστας γ΄. καὶ καρκίνων θαλασσίων κεκαυμένων λίτρας γ΄. εἰς τὸν οἶνον ἔα βρέχεσθαι, καὶ ὅταν συμπίωσι, λεάνας ἐπιμελῶς, ἔχε ἐν ἑτοίμῳ. τὰ δὲ ξηρὰ κόψας, καὶ σήσας λεπτῷ κοσκίνῳ, μίξας τοῖς καρκίνοις, ἀνάπλασσε τροχίσκους, καὶ δίδου τριώβολον μετ᾽ οἴνου ἀκράτου κυάθου α΄ S″. ἐπὶ ἡμέρας γ΄. καὶ περὶ μὲν τούτων ἐπὶ τοσοῦτον. συναπτέον δὴ τούτοις καὶ τὰς τῶν ἔξωθεν ἐπιτιθεμένας σκευασίας.

[*Μενίππου πρὸς λυσσοδήκτους, ᾗ ἐχρήσατο Πέλοψ.*] ℞ Πίσσης Βρυττίας λίτραν α΄. ὀποπάνακος γο δ΄. ὄξους ξέστην ἕνα. διάλυε τὸν ὀποπάνακα καὶ ὄξους κυάθοις δ΄. καὶ τὸ λειπόμενον ὑγρὸν μετὰ τῆς πίσσης ἕψε, καὶ ὅταν ἀναλωθῇ [918] ἐπίβαλλε τὸν ὀποπάνακα, καὶ τήρει μὴ ἀναζέσῃ· καὶ

fus idoneum, eft etiam theriaca.] ℞ Seminum trifolii, radicis foeniculi utriusque ʒ vj, foliorum ficcorum fcillae, ariftolochiae longae, fingulorum ʒ v, fcinci, ramorum ferpilli, an. ʒ iv, cardamomi purgati, glychyrrhizae, fingulorum ʒ iij, ammeos, radicis rutae, fingulorum ʒ ij, opopanacis, fucci Cyrenaici, fingulorum ʒ j, vini Falerni fextarios iij, cancrorum marinorum crematorum lib. iij. In vino madefcere finito, ac ubi combiberint, trita diligenter in procinctu habeto, arida vero tunfa et tenui cribro increta, mixtaque cancris, in paftillos redigito: ac tres obolos cum vini meraci fesquicyatho ad dies tres propinabis. Atque de his tantum. Porro connectendae iis funt confectiones quae extrinfecus imponuntur.

[*Menippi ad rabioforum morfus, quo ufus eft Pelops.*] ℞ Picis Brutiae lib. i, opopanacis ℥ quatuor, aceti fextarium i, opopanacem etiam diluito in aceti cyathos quatuor, quod reftat liquidum, cum pice incoquito, et ubi confumpta *fuerint*, opopanacem addito, cura adhibita ne

ὅταν εὖ ἔχῃ, ἐμπλάσας ποίει σπλήνια εὐμεγέθη, καὶ κατὰ τοῦ δήγματος ἐπιτίθει. δεῖ δὲ τὸ ἕλκος παραφυλάττειν ἐπὶ ἡμέρας μ'.

[*Μενελάου λυσσοδήκτοις, ποιεῖ καὶ πρὸς αἰγίλωπας καὶ παντὸς ἑρπετοῦ πληγήν.*] ℞ Νίτρου ἐρυθροῦ ◁ β'. τρυγὸς οἴνου κεκαυμένης ◁ ζ'. ἀμμωνιακοῦ θυμιάματος ◁ ζ'. στέατος αἰγείου λίτραν α'. ἐλαίου λίτραν α' S''. κηροῦ λίτρας β'. ὕδατος ξέστην ἕνα. τρῖβε ἀμμωνιακὸν μεθ' ὕδατος, ὥστε γλοιοῦ σχεῖν τὸ πάθος· τὸ δ' ὑπολειπόμενον τοῦ ὕδατος ἕψε μετὰ νίτρου καὶ τῆς τρυγός. καὶ ὅταν συστῇ, ἐπίβαλλε τὰ τηκτά. καὶ ὅταν διαλυθῇ, ἄρας ἀπὸ τοῦ πυρὸς, ἐπίβαλλε ἀμμωνιακὸν, καὶ ἑκάτερα εἰς θυείαν, καὶ καταμαλάξας ἐπιμελῶς ἀνελόμενος χρῶ. *Λευκὴ Βαφούλλου, ἢ Ἥρα πρὸς λυσσοδήκτους ἔξωθεν ἐπιτιθεμένη, δίδοται καὶ καταπότιον ἐξ αὐτῆς καρύου Ποντικοῦ τὸ μέγεθος, καὶ καταπίνεται ἐπὶ ἡμέρας μ'. καὶ μάλιστα τοῖς κεκρατημένοις, ῥύεται γὰρ τοῦ κινδύνου. ἐπιτίθεται δὲ τῷ τραύματι, καὶ παρὰ μίαν ἡ λύσις γίνεται, καὶ διὰ τοῦτο*

efferveſcat; quum bene habuerit, emplaſtri modo ſplenia bonae magnitudinis ſingito, ac morſui imponito; oportet autem ulcus ad xl, dies apertum ſervare.

[*Menelai ad rabioſorum morſus remedium efficax. Item ad aegilopas, et omnis ſerpentis ictum.*] ℞ Nitri rubri ℨ ij, faecis vini uſtae ℨ vij, guttae ammoniaci drach. vij, ſevi caprilli ℔ j, olei ℔ j ß, cerae ℔ ij, aquae ſextarium j, ammoniacum cum aqua terito, ut ſtrigmenti habeat craſſitudinem; quod reſtat aquae cum nitro, et faece incoquito. Ubi conſtiterint, ea quae liquari poſſunt indito; poſtquam diſſolveris, ab igne ſublatis, ammoniacum injicito ac in mortarium defuſa, emollitaque diligenter, excipiens in uſum ducito *Album Baphulli vel Herae, quod ad rabioſorum morſus extrinſecus imponitur; datur etiam catapotium ex eo nucis avellanae magnitudine, et deglutitur ad dies xl. praeſertim ab his, qui malo jam victi ſunt; liberat enim a periculo. Imponitur autem vulneri, et die interpoſito ſolvitur, ac pro-*

Ed. Chart. XIII. [918.] Ed. Baf. II. (450.)

δεῖ λύειν παρὰ μίαν, καὶ ἀποσπογγίζειν τὴν ἀπὸ τοῦ ἕλκους μελανίαν, καὶ τοῦτο ποιεῖν, ἄχρις οὗ λευκὸν παραμείνῃ τὸ φάρμακον. ἔχει δὲ οὕτως. ℞ Κηροῦ Ποντικοῦ λίτρας β'. λιθαργύρου, ψιμυθίου, ἀνὰ λίτραν μίαν, ἐλαίου παλαιοῦ ξέστην ἕνα, σμύρνης, μυελοῦ ἐλαφείου, ἀνὰ ∠ β'. λιβάνου ἄῤῥενος ∠ α'. ἕψε τὴν λιθάργυρον ἐλαίῳ, καὶ ὅταν μεταβάλλῃ, κατάπασσε τὸ ψιμύθιον, καὶ ἐπίβαλλε κηρόν· καὶ ὅταν ἀμόλυντος γένηται, ὑφελὼν τὸ πῦρ, ἀποδίδου τὸν μυελὸν, ἐπιπάσσων σμύρναν, καὶ λιβανωτὸν, καὶ μαλάσσων χρῶ. ἐν ἄλλαις γραφαῖς οὕτως ἔχει. ℞ Κηροῦ λίτρας β'. ψιμυθίου, λιθαργύρου, ἀνὰ λίτραν μίαν, ἐλαίου παλαιοῦ ξέστην ἕνα, σμύρνης, λιβανωτοῦ, μυελοῦ ἐλαφείου, ἀνὰ ∠ α'. ἐλαίου παλαιοῦ κοτύλην α'.

[Ἐν ἄλλαις οὕτως ἔχει.] ℞ Κηροῦ Ποντικοῦ λίτραν α'. ψιμυθίου, λιθαργύρου, ἀνὰ ∠ γ'. λιβάνου, σμύρνης, μυελοῦ ἐλαφείου, ἀνὰ γο S''. ∠ α'. ἐλαίου παλαιοῦ ∠ δ'.

[Βασιλικὴ πρὸς λυσσοδήκτους, φάρμακον ἐπιτετευγμέ-

pterea diei intervallo solvendum est, ac nigrities ab ulcere per spongiam detergenda, idque faciendum est, usque dum medicamentum album permaneat; sic autem habet. ℞ Cerae Ponticae ℔ ij, spumae lithargyri, cerusae, singulorum ℔ i, olei veteris sextarium j, myrrhae, medullae cervinae, utriusque ʒ ij, thuris masculi ʒ i. Lithargyrum oleo coquitur, et quum mutatum fuerit, cerusa inspergitur, ac cera injicitur. Ubi tam spissum evaserit, ut manus non inquinet, ab igne sublato, medulla injicitur, myrrha et thus, emolliens utitor. *In aliis scripturis sic habet.* ℞ Cerae ℔ ij, cerusae, lithargyri, singulorum lib. j, olei veteris sextarium j, myrrhae, thuris, medullae cervinae an. drach. j, olei veteris heminam j.

[*In aliis ad hunc modum.*] ℞ Cerae Ponticae lib. j, cerusae, lithargyri, singulorum drach. iij, thuris, myrrhae, medullae cervinae, singulorum ℥ ß ʒ, unam, olei veteris drach. quatuor.

[*Basilice, ad rabiosorum morsus medicamentum ac-*

νον, ὃ κωλύει περιπεσεῖν τῷ λεγομένῳ ὑδροφόβῳ. ταύτην Σεβαστὴ ἔσχε συγκειμένην ἀεί.] ℞ Ἁλὸς ἀμμωνιακοῦ, ὀποῦ Κυρηναϊκοῦ, ἀνὰ < β'. ἐὰν δὲ μὴ παρῇ Κυρηναϊκὸς, τοῦ Συριακοῦ τὸ διπλοῦν. πιτυᾶς βάλλε λαγωοῦ < δ'. ἴρεως Ἰλλυρικῆς, καστορίου Ποντικοῦ, ἀνὰ < ε'. σύκων ὀλύνθων ὀποῦ πεπηγότος ξηροῦ, τὸ ἴσον. εἰ δὲ μὴ, ὑγροῦ τὸ διπλοῦν· στέατος ὑαίνης < η'. ῥητίνης τερμινθίνης < θ'. κυνὸς μελαίνης, ὑαίνης, ἀνὰ < ια'. κηροῦ Ποντικοῦ < λστ'. ἐλαίου παλαιοῦ κυάθους δύο, ὄξους σκιλλητικοῦ κυάθους γ'. τὰ ξηρὰ τρῖβε μετ' ὄξους, τὰ δὲ τηκτὰ τήκεται, εἶτα ἐπιβάλλεται τοῖς τετριμμένοις, καὶ εἰς χρῆσιν ἐπιτήδειον γίνεται.

Κεφ. ιβ'. [Τὰ τῶν ἐντός τε καὶ τῶν ἐκτὸς πρὸς σκορπιοδήκτους φάρμακ.] [Πρὸς δὲ τὰς τῶν σκορπίων πληγὰς χρηστέον ταῖς ὑπογεγραμμέναις σκευασίαις. σκορπιοδήκτοις καὶ πρὸς φαλαγγίων δήγματα ἐχρήσατο Διόφαντος.] ℞ Ἀριστολοχίας < δ'. πεπέρεως < β'. ὀπίου < α'. πυρέθρου < δ'. ἀνάπλαττε τροχίσκους κυάμου

commodatum, quod ab aquae metu asserit; hoc Augusta semper habebat compositum.] ℞ Salis ammoniaci, succi Cyrenaici, an. ʒ ij, si Cyrenaicus desideretur, Syriaci duplum, coaguli leporis ʒ iv, ireos Illyricae, castorii Pontici, utriusque ʒ v, ficuum silvestrium succi coacti aridi tantundem; si desit, humoris duplum, adipis Hyaenae ʒ viij, resinae terebinthinae ʒ ix, canis nigrae, Hyaenae, utriusque ʒ xj, cerae Ponticae ʒ xxxvj, olei veteris cyathos ij, aceti scillitici cyathos iij, arida cum aceto teruntur; quae liquefieri possunt, liquantur. Deinde contritis immittuntur; et in usu redditur idoneum medicamentum.

Cap. XII. *Remedia ad scorpiones sumenda et admovenda.*] [*Ad scorpionum ictus utendum est subscriptis confectionibus. Diophantus etiam ad scorpionum ictus et phalangiorum morsus usus est.*] Aristolochiae ʒ iv, piperis ʒ ij, opii ʒ j, pyrethri ʒ iv, finguntur pastilli fabae

[919] *Αἰγυπτίου τὸ μέγεθος, καὶ δίδου καταπίνειν β'. καὶ οἴνου ἀκράτου κυάθους β'.*

[*Ἄλλο πρὸς σκορπίους καὶ τὰ δηκτά.*] ℞ *Ἀριστολοχίας, ζιγγιβέρεως, ἀνὰ* ◁ *η'. καλαμίνθης, πηγάνου ἀγρίου καρποῦ, ἀνὰ τριώβολον, πεπέρεως διώβολον. φύρα αἵματι χελώνης, καὶ ἀνάπλασσε τροχίσκους τριωβολιαίους, καὶ δίδου μετ' οἴνου ἀκράτου.*

[*Ἄλλο.*] ℞ *Κυμίνου Αἰθιοπικοῦ, θείου ἀπύρου, πεπέρεως λευκοῦ, ἀνὰ* ◁ *β'. καστορίου, σιλφίου, τριφύλλου, ἀνὰ* ◁ *α'. οἴνῳ ἀνάπλασσε καὶ δίδου μετ' οἴνου ἀκράτου.*

[*Πρὸς τοὺς ἐπικινδύνως πεπληγμένους ὑπὸ σκορπίων, ἢ φαλαγγίων, καὶ παντὸς ἑρπετοῦ.*] ℞ *Πηγάνου ἀγρίου καρποῦ, εὐζώμου καρποῦ, πυρέθρου, στύρακος, θείου ἀπύρου, ἀνὰ* ◁ *στ'. καστορίου* ◁ *β'. ἀνάπλασσε αἵματι χελώνης, καὶ δίδου τετρώβολον μετ' οἴνου ἀκράτου, ἢ ὄξους ἡμικοτυλίου.*

[*Ἀνώδυνον φάρμακον ἐπιτετευγμένον πρὸς σκορπίων καὶ φαλαγγίων, καὶ παντὸς ἑρπετοῦ πληγὰς, ποιεῖ καὶ ταῖς*

Aegyptiae magnitudine, danturque duo deglutiendi, et vini meraci cyathi ij.

[*Aliud ad ſcorpiones, et venenoſa animalia.*] ℞ Ariſtolochiae, zingiberis, utriusque ʒ viij, calaminthae fructus, rutae ſilveſtris, ſingulorum tres obolos, piperis obolos ij, conſpergito teſtudinis ſanguine et in paſtillos trium obolorum cogito, datoque cum vino meraco.

[*Aliud.*] ℞ Cumini Aethiopici, ſulphuris vivi, piperis albi, ſingulorum ʒ ij, caſtorii, laſeris, trifolii, an. ʒ j, vino formantur, et ex vino meraco offeruntur.

[*Ad eos qui periculose icti ſunt a ſcorpionibus, aut phalangiis, aut quolibet ſerpente.*] ℞ Rutae ſilveſtris fructus, ſeminis erucae, pyrethri, ſtyracis, ſulphuris vivi, ſingulorum ʒ vj, caſtorii ʒ ij, ſanguine teſtudinis ſingito, ac ternos obolos ex vino meraco, aut aceti ſemi-hemina exhibeto.

[*Medicamentum anodynum ad ſcorpionum, phalangiorum, omnisque ſerpentis ictus efficax; benefacit etiam*

δυστοκούσαις. ἐπιγράφεται δὲ Καλλίστη.] ℞ Σμύρνης, καστορίου, στύρακος, ἀνὰ < α΄. ὀπίου < β΄. χαλβάνης < γ΄. σελίνου σπέρματος ὀξύφαβον, ἀνίσου τὸ ἴσον, πεπέρεως κόκκους λ΄ ἀνάπλαττε δι' οἴνου, καὶ δίδου < α΄. μετ' οἴνου κοτύλης μιᾶς. τὸ φάρμακον ἄγαν ἐστὶ καλόν.

[Ἀβασκάντου ἰατρεύοντος ἐν Λουγδούνῳ.] ℞ Πεπέρεως λευκοῦ, κόκκους κ΄. καστορίου, ὀπίου, κρόκου, σμύρνης, ἴρεως Ἰλλυρικῆς, σταφίδος ἀγρίας, χαμαίδρυος, βρυωνίας ῥίζης, πυρέθρου, ἑκάστου τὸ ἴσον, οἴνῳ ἀνάπλαττε, καὶ δίδου < α΄. μετ' οἴνου ἀκράτου κυάθους γ΄. (451) Ἀντίδοτος σκορπιακὴ, καὶ ἀδιάπτωτος, μετὰ σπουδῆς ἡμῖν δοθεῖσα, ὑπό τινος τῶν τὴν Λιβύην οἰκούντων ταύτῃ χρωμένου· ἀπήλλαττε παντὸς κινδύνου τοὺς σκορπιοδήκτους. ἔστι δὲ προφυλακτικὴ ἀγαθή. πίνεται δὲ ὑπὸ τῶν μηδέπω πεπληγότων πρὸς ἀσφάλειαν τῶν ἐσομένων. ℞ Θείου ἀπύρου, θείου ὀρυκτοῦ, ἀνὰ λίτρας β΄. πεπέρεως λευκοῦ < δ΄. ὀποπάνακος, βράθυος, λιβάνου ἄῤῥενος ἀνὰ < γ΄. ἀριστολοχίας στρογγύλης, πευκεδάνου, σμύρνης, κενταυρίου, ἐρ-

aegre parturientibus; inscribitur autem Calliste i. e. optimum.] ℞ Myrrhae, castorii, styracis, an. ʒ unam, opii ʒ ij. galbani ʒ iij, seminis apii acetabulum, anisi tantundem, piperis g. xxx, forma ex vino datoque ʒ j, ex vini hemina j, medicamentum est praestantissimum.

[*Abascanti medicinam facientis Lugduni.*] ℞ Piperis albi g. xx, castorii, opii, croci, myrrhae, ireos Illyricae, staphidos silvestris, chamaedryos, radicis bryoniae, pyrethri, singulorum par pondus, vino formantur, ʒ j, ex eis datur, cum tribus vini meraci cyathis. *Antidotum ad scorpiones et minime fallax, nobis datum cum sedulitate a quodam in Libya degente; qui hoc utens omni periculo a scorpionum ictibus laesos liberabat. At ad praecautionem bonum est; bibitur autem ab iis, qui nondum icti sunt ad futurorum securitatem.* ℞ Sulphuris ignem non experti, sulphuris fossilis, utriusque lib. ij, piperis albi ʒ iv, opopanacis, sabinae, thuris masculi, singulorum ʒ iij. aristolochiae rotundae, peucedani, myrrhae,

πύλλου, χαμαίδρυος, χαμαιπίτυος, σκορπιακῆς βοτανης, ἀναγαλλίδος, ἀσφάλτου ἀνὰ ⊲ β'. γέγραπται δὲ ἐν τῇ γραφῇ, καὶ Ῥωμαϊστὶ ἑρβανικάτου κέστρου ⊲ β'. τουτέστι βετονικῆς, μυελοῦ ἐλαφείου, κροκοδείλου χερσαίου τῆς σαρκὸς, ἢ τοῦ λεγομένου σκίγκου, ἀνὰ ⊲ α'. ἕκαστον δὲ τῶν εἰρημένων κόπτεται καὶ σήθεται λεπτοτάτῳ κοσκίνῳ, εἶθ' ὁμοῦ μίγνυται καὶ ἀδιάπνευστον φυλάττεται. ἐν δὲ τῇ χρήσει δίδου τοῖς πεπονθόσι κοχλιάριον, καὶ οἴνου ἀκράτου κυάθους β'. προφυλακτικῆς δὲ χάριν ἐπ' ἐνιαυτὸν πινέτωσαν, ὥστε ἀκινδύνως διάγειν τοὺς παθησομένους. δεῖ δὲ τοὺς ἀρχῇ πίνοντας τοῦτο τὸ φάρμακον ἕνεκεν προφυλακῆς ἐν ἐκείνῃ τῇ ἡμέρᾳ μήτε λούσασθαι μήτε συνουσιάζειν.

[Παρὰ Ζωΐλου, ᾗ ἐχρήσατο Ἐπαφρόδιτος ὁ Καρχηδόνιος. ἄπονον ποιεῖ παραχρῆμα, ἔστι δὲ καὶ προφυλακτικὴ ἀγαθὴ, ἐνιαυτὸν πινομένη.] ℞ Θείου ἀπύρου λίτρας δ'. λιβάνου λίτραν α'. βράθυος, στοιχάδος, ἀριστολοχίας ἀνὰ ⊲ στ'. σμύρνης ⊲ ε'. μυελοῦ ἐλα [920] φείου, ὀποπάνακος ἀνὰ ⊲ δ'. δικτάμνου Κρητικοῦ ⊲ γ'. ἀσφάλτου, ἑρπύλλου,

centaurii, ferpilli, chamaedryos, chamaepityos, fcorpiacae herbae, anagallidis, bituminis, fingulorum ʒ ij. Scriptum autem eft in libro etiam Romane, herbanicati ceftri ʒ ij, hoc eft, betonicae, medullae cervinae, carnis crocodili terreftris vel fcinci dicti, fingulorum ʒ j, unumquodque praedictorum contunditur et tenuiffimo cribro incernitur, deinde una mifcetur et ne diffletur, refervatur. Quum ufus exigit, dato affectis cochleare et vini meraci cyathos ij. Praecautionis autem gratia ad annum bibant, ut qui afficientur, tuto tranfeant. Oportet autem initio bibentes hoc medicamentum ad praefervationem illo die neque lavare, neque venerem exercere.

[*Zoili medicamentum, quo ufus eft Epaphroditus Carthaginenfis, levat protinus dolorem; eft etiam ad praecautionem accommodatum ad annum epotum.*] ℞ Sulphuris vivi lib. iv, thuris lib. j, fabinae, ftoechados, ariftolochiae, an. ʒ vj, myrrhae ʒ v, medullae cervinae, opopanacis, fingulorum ʒ iv, dictamni Cretici ʒ iij, bi-

σκορδίου, ῥοῦ, τριφύλλου, κενταυρίου, χαμαίδρυος, πεπέρεως λευκοῦ, ἀβροτόνου, κέστρου, πολίου, πιτυῶν ἐριφείων, ἀναγαλλίδος ἀνὰ < β'. κροκοδείλου χερσαίου < ι'. σκεύαζε καθάπερ εἴρηται, καὶ δίδου τοῖς πεπονθόσι κοχλιάριον, καὶ οἴνου ἀκράτου κύαθον. ποιεῖ δὲ καὶ πρὸς φυλακὴν, ἐνιαυτοῦ ἅπαξ δοθεῖσα.

[*Ἐπίθεμα σκορπιοπλήκτων.*] ℞ Δάφνης φύλλα ἑψήσας μετ' οἴνου, καὶ τρίψας ἐπιτίθει, ἢ κρίνων τὰς ῥίζας τρίψας μετ' ὄξους, ἐπιτίθει.

[*Ἄλλο.*] ℞ Ἀριστολοχίας ἐν οἴνῳ ἡψημένης, καὶ πηγάνου ἀκρεμόνων, καὶ νίτρου τὸ ἴσον τρίψας μετ' οἴνου, ἐπιτίθει.

[*Ἄλλο.*] ℞ Καρκίνων ποταμίων, κάγχρυος, σταφίδος ἀγρίας, πηγάνου τὸ ἴσον μετ' οἴνου, ἐπιτίθει.

[*Ἄλλο.*] ℞ Χαμαιμήλων, καὶ μελανθίου, καὶ νίτρου ἐρυθροῦ τὸ ἴσον, τρίψας μετ' ὄξους, ἐπιτίθει.

[*Ἀραβᾶ Θηβαίου, ἐπιτετευγμένον φάρμακον, πρὸς σκορπίου πληγάς.*] ℞ Χαλβάνης, τερμινθίνης ἀνὰ < β'.

tuminis, ferpilli, fcordii, rheu, trifolii, centaurii, chamaedryos, piperis albi, abrotoni, ceftri, polii, coaguli hoedini, anagallidis, fingulorum ʒ ij, crocodili terreftris ʒ x. Praeparato quemadmodum dictum eft, affectis cochleare et vini meraci cyathum propinato: benefacit etiam ad praefervationem femel anno exhibitum.

[*Epithema ad fcorpionum ictus.*] Lauri folia cum vino cocta tritaque imponito; vel liliorum radices tritas cum aceto impone.

[*Aliud.*] Ariftolochiae in vino coctae et rutae furculorum, nitrique aequalem portionem tritam ex vino impone.

[*Aliud.*] ℞ Cancrorum fluviatilium, canchryos, ftaphidos filveftris, rutae, par modus, cum vino admove.

[*Aliud.*] ℞ Chamaemeli, nigellae, nitri rubri, paria pondera, detrita ex aceto impone.

[*Arabae Thebani medicamentum ad fcorpionis ictus admovendum.*] ℞ Galbani, refinae terebinthinae, utriusque

σταφίδος ἀγρίας, πυρέθρου, θείου ἀπύρου, ἀνὰ ∠ α΄. σμύρνης, πεπέρεως, ἀνὰ ∠ α΄ S″. πίσσης ὑγρᾶς τὸ αὔταρκες.

Κεφ. ιγ΄. [Διάφορα πρὸς τὰ τῶν φαλαγγίων δήγματα φάρμακα.] [Πρὸς φαλαγγίων δήγματα Χαρίτωνος ὀχλαγωγοῦ.] ♃ Σπονδυλίου καρποῦ, καλαμινθίνης τὸ ἴσον, τρίψας ὁμοῦ, δίδου ὅσον ∠ α΄. μετ᾽ οἴνου κυάθων β΄. πλεονάκις τῆς ἡμέρας. ταύτῃ Χαρίτων χρώμενος περιήκει τὰς πανηγύρεις, ἀρήγειν βουλόμενος τοῖς δακνομένοις.

[Ἄλλο. Σιμμία τοῦ Μηδίου.] ♃ Ὀποῦ κυρηναικοῦ, δαύκου Κρητικοῦ σπέρματος, ἡδυόσμου ξηροῦ, νάρδου Ἰνδικῆς, ἑκάστου τὸ ἴσον, ἀνάπλασσε δι᾽ ὄξους, καὶ δίδου ∠ α΄. μετ᾽ ὄξους κυάθων δ΄. καὶ πιόντα εἰς θερμὸν ὕδωρ κάθιε.

[Ἀνδρέου, πρὸς φαλαγγιοδήκτους.] ♃ Ἀσταφίδος ἀγρίας, πυρέθρου, σμύρνης, ὀπίου, βρυωνίας, χαλβάνης ἴσον ἑκάστου, ἀνάπλασσε μετ᾽ οἴνου εὐώδους, καὶ διδοὺς ∠ α΄. μετὰ γλυκέος κοτύλης μίας.

ʒ ij, ſtaphidos ſilveſtris, pyrethri, ſulphuris vivi an. ʒ j, myrrhae, piperis, utriusque ʒ j ß, picis liquidae, quod ſatis eſt.

Cap. XIII. [*Diverſa ad phalangiorum morſus remedia.*] [*Ad phalangiorum morſus Charitonis circulatoris antidotus.*] ♃ Fructus ſpondylii, calaminthae par pondus, trita ſimul drachmae unius pondere, cum duobus vini cyathis, ſaepe in die propinato. Hoc Chariton utens, comitia circumibat, cupiens commorſis auxiliari.

[*Aliud Simmiae Medi.*] ♃ Succi Cyrenaici, ſeminum dauci Cretici, mentae ſiccae, nardi Indicae, cujusque par pondus, forma antidotum ex aceto, daque ʒ j, cum iv, aceti cyathis; at qui biberit eum in aquam calidam demitte.

[*Andreae ad phalangiorum morſus.*] ♃ Staphidos ſilveſtris, pyrethri, myrrhae, opii, bryoniae, galbani, ſingulorum par pondus. Forma antidotum ex vino odoro, et ʒ j, cum paſſi hemina una exhibe.

["Αλλο, σφόδρα γενναῖον.] ℞ Κάγχρυος, πηγάνου ἀγρίου καρποῦ, πεπέρεως λευκοῦ, ἀσταφίδος ἀγρίας, σμύρνης, ἑκάστου < α'. κυπρίου ῥίζης < β'. ἀνάπλαττε μετ' οἴνου εὐώδους κυάθων δ'. καὶ μέλιτος κύαθον α'.

[Πρὸς φαλάγγια, καὶ σκορπίους, καὶ παντὸς ἑρπετοῦ πληγὰς, ὡς ἐχρήσατο Διόφαντος.] ℞ Καστορίου, πεπέρεως λευκοῦ, σμύρνης, ὀποῦ μήκωνος, ἑκάστου τὸ ἴσον, οἴνῳ διαλύσας ἀνάπλαττε τροχίσκους καὶ διδοὺς τριώβολον μετ' οἴνου ἀκράτου κυάθων γ'. ὡς Διόφαντος.

[921] ["Αλλη.] ℞ Μανδραγόρου φλοιοῦ ῥίζης, πεπέρεως λευκοῦ, καστορίου, ὀποῦ μήκωνος, ἑκάστου τὸ ἴσον, σκεύαζε, καὶ δίδου καθὰ προείρηται. "Αλλη ἐκ τῶν 'Απολλοδώρου, ἣν καὶ ὁ Ταραντῖνος ἐν τῷ πρὸς 'Αστυδάμαντα ἀναγράφει, πρὸς παντὸς θηρίου πληγὴν, καὶ τὰ σφοδρότατα τῶν ἀλγημάτων, καὶ πνίγας ὑστερικάς. ℞ Κωνείου χυλοῦ, ὑοσκυάμου, ἀνὰ < δ'. καστορίου, πεπέρεως λευκοῦ, κόστου, σμύρνης, ὀπίου, ἀνὰ < α'. ταῦτα λεάνας καὶ ἐπιβαλὼν κυάθους β'. γλυκέος, τρῖβε ἡλιάζων, ἕως συστραφῇ

[*Aliud valde generosum.*] ℞ Canchryos, seminum rutae silvaticae, piperis albi, staphidos silvestris, myrrhae, singulorum ʒ j, radicis cyperi ʒ ij, formantur ex vini odorati cyathis iv et mellis cyatho j.

[*Ad phalangia, scorpiones, et omnis serpentis ictus, ut usus est Diophantus.*] ℞ Castorii, piperis albi, myrrhae, succi papaveris, singulorum aequale pondus; vino dissoluta, in pastillos cogito, ac iij obolos cum tribus vini meraci cyathis propinato, ut Diophantus.

[*Aliud.*] ℞ Corticis mandragorae radicis, piperis albi, castorii, succi papaveris, singulorum pares portiones. Praeparato, exhibetoque quemadmodum praedictum est. *Aliud ex commentariis Apollodori, quod etiam Tarentinus in opere ad Astydamantem inscribit ad omnis ferae ictum et vehementissimos dolores, uterique strangulatus.* ℞ Succi cicutae, hyoscyami, utriusque ʒ iv, castorii, piperis albi, costi, myrrhae, opii. an. ʒ j. Haec laevigata ex duobus passi cyathis, terito in sole, donec coie-

καὶ ἀνάπλαττε τροχίσκους κυάμου Ἑλληνικοῦ τὸ μέγεθος, καὶ δίδου μετ' οἴνου κυάθων β'.

[Ἄλλη Ἡρακλείδου Ταραντίνου πρὸς φαλάγγια, καὶ παντὸς ἑρπετοῦ πληγὰς, τὸ δ' αὐτὸ πινόμενον βοηθεῖ.] ℞ Κάγχρυος, πηγάνου ἀγρίου σπέρματος, πεπέρεως λευκοῦ, σμύρνης, κόκκου κνιδίου, κόστου, πυρέθρου, ἀσταφίδος ἀγρίας, ἑκάστου τὸ ἴσον, κυπέρου διπλοῦν, ὄξει διαλύσας καὶ μέλιτι ἀναλαβὼν, ἐπιτίθει.

[Ἄλλη πρὸς φαλάγγια, καὶ παντὸς ἰοβόλου ἑρπετοῦ πληγήν.] ℞ Ἀσταφίδος ἀγρίας, πυρέθρου, σμύρνης, ὀποῦ Λιβυκοῦ, ἀνὰ < δ'. βρυωνίας ῥίζης, χαλβάνης ἴσον, ὄξει διαλύσας, καὶ μέλιτι ἀναλαβὼν ἐπιτίθει. τὸ δ' αὐτὸ καὶ πινόμενον σφόδρα βοηθεῖ. ἐπίθεμα πρὸς φαλαγγίων πληγὰς καὶ παντὸς ἑρπετοῦ. τὸ δ' αὐτὸ καὶ πινόμενον βοηθεῖ. τούτῳ Σιμμίας ὁ ὀχλαγωγὸς ἐχρήσατο. ℞ Θείου ἀπύρου, χαλβάνης ἀνὰ < δ'. ὀποῦ Λιβυκοῦ, καρύων Ποντικῶν κεκαθαρμένων, ἀνὰ < β'. οἴνῳ διαλύσας καὶ μέλιτι ἀναλαβὼν ἐπιτίθει.

rint, ac effingito paſtillos ad fabae Graecae magnitudinem; dato cum vini cyathis ij.

[*Aliud Heraclidis Tarentini ad phalangia et omnis virulenti ſerpentis ictus; idem potum auxiliatur.*] ℞ Canchryos, ſeminum rutae ſilveſtris, piperis albi, myrrhae, cocci Gnidii, coſti, pyrethri, ſtaphidis ſilveſtris, ſingulorum aequale pondus, cyperi duplum, aceto diſſoluta melleque excepta imponito.

[*Aliud ad phalangia et omnis venenoſi ſerpentis ictum.*] ℞ Herbae ſtaphidos agriae, pyrethri, myrrhae, ſucci Libyci, ſingulorum ʒ iv, radicis bryoniae, galbani, par pondus; aceto diſſoluta et melle excepta admove. Idem etiam potum valde auxiliatur. *Epithema ad phalangiorum ictus et omnis ſerpentis: idem quoque in potu auxiliatur. Hoc Simmias circulator uſus eſt.* ℞ Sulphuris vivi, galbani, utriusque ʒ iv, ſucci Libyci, nucum avellanarum purgatarum, ſingulorum ʒ ij, vino diſſoluta et melle excepta imponuntur.

["Αλλη.] ℞ Πηγάνου ἀγρίου σπέρματος, ἀγρίας ἀσταφίδος, εὐζώμου σπέρματος, κάγ (452) χρυος, ἄγνου καρποῦ, κυπαρίσσου τῶν σφαιρίων, ἀνὰ ὀξύβαφον. ὄξει διαλύσας καὶ μέλιτι ἀναλαβὼν, ἐπίθες. τὸ δ' αὐτὸ καὶ πινόμενον βοηθεῖ.

Κεφ. ιδ'. [Φάρμακα πρὸς ἐχιοδήκτους, ἐν οἷς καὶ ἡ Ἀντιόχου θηριακὴ περιέχεται, ἣν Πλίνιός φησι παρὰ πυλῶν Ἀσκληπιοῦ ἀναγεγράφθαι.] Καὶ ταῦτα μὲν ἐπὶ τοσοῦτον. ἐπὶ δὲ τῶν ἐχιοδήκτων χρηστέον ταῖς ὑπογεγραμμέναις σκευασίαις.

[Πρὸς ἐχιοδήκτους Δωροθέου Ἡλίου.] Λέγει δὲ οὕτως. ποτήμασι μὲν οὖν ἐχρησάμην ἁπλοῖς τοῖς δι' ὄξους· ὄξος γὰρ ὅσον ἡμικοτύλιον θερμανθὲν καὶ ποθὲν ὠφελεῖ. ℞ Ἀριστολοχίας ὅσον < β'. τοῦ φλοιοῦ ἐν οἴνῳ, ἢ ὄξει κοτύλας ἡμισείας. καὶ ℞ Τριφύλλου καρποῦ ὅσον τριώβολον ἐν οἴνῳ κυάθου ἥμισυ. καὶ πάνακος τοῦ χειρωνείου < β'. ἐν ὄξει. καὶ πιτυᾶς νεβρείας < α'. ἐν οἴνῳ. καὶ χελώνης θαλασσίας ἐξηραμμένου αἵματος < β'. ἐν ὄξει.

[*Aliud.*] ℞ Seminum rutae ſilveſtris, ſtaphidis ſilveſtris, ſeminum erucae, canchryos, ſeminis viticis, galbulorum cupreſſi, ſingulorum acetabulum j, vino ſoluta et melle excepta applicato. Idem quoque in potu proficit.

Cap. XIV. [*Remedia ad viperas, in quibus Antiochi theriaca continetur, quam Plinius in foribus aedis Aeſculapii deſcriptam fuiſſe tradit.*] Et haec quidem hactenus. At in viperarum morſibus, iis quae ſubſcribuntur confectionibus, utendum eſt.

[*Ad viperarum morſus Dorothei Helii.*] Dicit itaque hunc in modum; potionibus quidem uſus ſum ſimplicibus ex aceto; acetum namque ad dimidiam heminam calefactum potumque prodeſt. ℞ corticis ariſtolochiae ʒ ij, in vino aut aceto heminam dimidiam. Item ℞ trifolii ſeminis obolos iij, in dimidio vini cyatho, panacis chironii ʒ ij, in aceto, coaguli hinnuli ʒ j, ex vino ſanguinis teſtudinis marinae exiccati ʒ ij ex aceto.

[Τῶν δὲ συνθέτων, ἡ μὲν παρ' Ἀπολλοδώρου τεθειμένη, καὶ ὑπὸ Σωστράτου ἐπαινουμένη, καὶ πάντων δὲ τῶν μετενεγκόντων παρ' αὐτοῦ, ἡ διὰ τοῦ αἵματος τοῦ χελώνης ἐστὶν ἥδε.] ℞ Κυμίνου ἀγρίου σπέρματος ὀξύβαφον, χελώνης θαλασσίας αἵματος ξηροῦ < δ'. στατῆρας β'. πιτυᾶς νεβροῦ, εἰ δὲ μὴ, λαγωοῦ < γ'. ἐριφείου αἵματος < δ'. πάντα μίξας, [922] καὶ οἴνῳ βελτίστῳ ἀναλαβὼν, ἀπόθου. ἐν δὲ τῇ χρήσει λαβὼν ἐλαίας τὸ μέγεθος, τρίψας μετ' οἴνου, ὡς βελτίστου, κυάθου ἥμισυ δίδου πίνειν. ἐὰν δὲ ἀπεμέσει τὸ φάρμακον, πάλιν δίδου ἐλαίας τὸ ἥμισυ, καθὰ προείρηται, καὶ πάλιν εἰ ἀποβάλλειν, ἐκ τρίτου δίδου κυάμου Αἰγυπτίου τὸ μέγεθος, καθὰ προείρηται.

[Ἡ τοῦ ἀγροίκου ἐχιοδήκτου.] ℞ Τριφύλλου, στάχυος, ὀρόβου ἡλεσμένου, πηγάνου ἀγρίου σπέρματος, ἀριστολοχίας στρογγύλης, ἀνὰ < η'. οἴνῳ διαλύσας ἀνάπλαττε τροχίσκους, καὶ δίδου < α'. μετ' οἴνου κυάθων γ'. δὶς καὶ τρὶς τῆς ἡμέρας.

[*Inter compoſita, quod ab Apollodoro compoſitum eſt, et a Soſtrato commendatum, ac omnibus qui ab eo acceperunt. Quod ex ſanguine teſtudinis conſtat, ita habet.*] ℞ Seminum cumini ſilveſtris acetabulum, ſanguinis teſtudinis marinae aridi drach. iv, ſtateres ij, coaguli hinnuli; ſin minus, leporini drach. iij, hoedini ſanguinis ʒ iv, omnia mixta, vinoque optimo excepta reponito. In uſu magnitudinem olivae ſumens, conterito, ex vino quam praeſtantiſſimo cyathi dimidium potui dato. Si medicamentum evomat, rurſus olivae dimidium, ſicuti praedictum eſt, exhibeto; ac rurſus ſi ejicit, tertio fabae Aegyptiae magnitudine porrigito, quemadmodum a me dictum eſt prius.

[*Medicamentum Ruſtici a vipera morſi.*] ℞ Trifolii, ſpicae, ervi inſolati, ſeminum rutae ſilveſtris, ariſtolochiae rotundae, ſingulorum drach. viij. Vino ſoluta in paſtillos redigito, datoque ʒ j, cum tribus vini cyathis, bis terque die.

[Ἄλλη τῶν παρ᾽ Εὐδήμου ἐμμέτρως ἀναγεγραμμένη, θηριακὴ Ἀντιόχου τοῦ Φιλομήτορος, ἧς ἡ ἀρχὴ ἥδε.]

Ἴησιν μάθε τήνδε πρὸς ἑρπετὰ, ἣν Φιλομήτωρ
Νικήσας, πείρᾳ κέκρικεν Ἀντίοχος.

Τὰ δὲ τῆς σκευασίας ἔχει οὕτως.

Μήου ἀπὸ ῥίζης ὁλκὴν διδραχμίαν ὀρύξας,
Σὺν τῷ δ᾽ ἑρπύλλου κλῶνας ἰσοῤῥεπέας.
Σὺν δ᾽ ὀπὸν ἐκ πάνακος στήσας ἴσον ἠδὲ τριφύλλου
Καρπὸν, ὅσον δραχμῆς σταθμὸν ἄγοντα δίδου,
Ἀνίσου, μαράθρου τε καὶ ἄμμιος, ἠδὲ σελίνου
Ἐξ ἑνὸς, ἓν πληρῶν σπέρματος ὀξύβαφον.
Σὺν δ᾽ ὀρόβου λείου δύο ὀξύβαφ᾽ ἔμπασ᾽ ἀλεύρου,
Πάντα δ᾽ ὁμοῦ Χίῳ νέκταρι συγκεράσας,
Κυκλοτερεῖς ἀνάπλασσε τροχοὺς, ἰσότητι μερίζων,
Ἡμιδραχμοῖο ῥοπῆς, ὄφρ᾽ ἂν ἕκαστος ἔχῃ.
Χίῳ δ᾽ ἐγκεράσας τάδε μίγματα, πικρὸν ἐχίδνης,
Ἡμίσεως δραχμὴν, ἰὸν ἀποσκεδάσεις.

[*Alia ab Eudemo verſibus conſcripta, theriaca Antiochi Philometoris, cujus initium ita ſonat.*]

Hoc cape praeſidium ad ſerpentia, quod Philometor
Uſu praecipuum repperit Antiochus.

His miſtura conſtat.

Meu drachmas binas radicis ponito, tantum
Germina ſerpilli ponderis accipiant,
Et panacis totidem drachmas liquor aſſerit aeque
Triffolii, quantum drachmula fructus habet,
Oxybaphum marathri, nec non ammeos et aniſi,
Atque apii; ſument ſemina quaeque ſuum.
Aſt ervi pones acetabula bina farinae;
Omnia cum Chio nectare conſocians,
Orbiculos finges, juſto qui ſinguli in illis
Drachmae dimidium pondere conſtituant.
Irrigans Chio medicamina, viperae amarum
Aequali virus aſſociato modo.

Τῷ δὲ ποτῷ καὶ δεινὰ φαλάγγια, καὶ σκολιοῖο
Σκορπίου ἐκφεύξῃ κέντρα φέροντ᾽ ὀδύνας.

Τὰ δὲ κατὰ μέρος ἐστὶ ταῦτα. ℞ Μήου ῥίζης, ἑρπύλλου, ὀποπάνακος, ἀνὰ < β΄. τριφύλλου σπέρματος < α΄. ἀνίσου, μαράθρου, ἄμμεως, σελίνου σπέρματος, ἀνὰ ὀξύβαφον, ἀλεύρου ὀροβίνου λεπτοτάτου ὀξύβαφα β΄. οἴνου παλαιοῦ εἰς ἀνάληψιν ὅσον ἐξαρκεῖ, ἀνάπλασσε τροχίσκους, καὶ ξήραινε ἐν σκιᾷ, καὶ δίδου τριώβολον μετ᾽ οἴνου κυάθων γ΄.

[Ἡρακλείδου Ταραντίνου ἐννεαφάρμακος· ταύτην ἔθηκεν ἐν τῇ περὶ θηρίων αὐτοῦ πραγματείᾳ. ἔχει δὲ οὕτως.] ℞ Σμύρνης τρωγλοδύτιδος, ὀποπάνακος, ὀποῦ μήκωνος, ἀνὰ < β΄. βρυωνίας ῥίζης < δ΄. ταύτην οἱ μὲν ψίλωθρον, οἱ δὲ ἄμπελον ἀγρίαν, οἱ δὲ μάδον, οἱ δὲ χειρωνείαν, οἱ δὲ κερκίδα καλοῦσιν. ἀριστολοχίας μακρᾶς τοῦ φλοιοῦ < δ΄. καθόλου γὰρ τῶν ῥιζῶν χρησιμώτεροί εἰσιν οἱ φλοιοὶ μᾶλλον, ἤπερ ἐντεριῶναι. πυρέθρου ῥίζης < δ΄. πηγάνου ἀγρίου σπέρματος, κυμίνου Αἰθιοπικοῦ, τριφύλλου σπέρμα-

Hoc autem effugies horrenda phalangia potu.
Scorpi etiam ſtimulum non vereare gravem.

At in particulari haec ſunt. ℞ radicis meu, ſerpilli, opopanacis, ſingulorum ʒ ij, ſeminis triſolii ʒ j, aniſi, foeniculi, ammeos, ſeminis apii, ſingulorum acetabulum j, farinae ervi tenuiſſimae acetabula ij, vini veteris quantum ad excipiendum ſufficit. Paſtillos ſingito ſiccatoque in umbra et tres obolos cum vini tribus cyathis dato.

[*Heraclidis Tarentini enneapharmacum; hoc in opere ipſius de feris deſcripſit; habet autem in hunc modum.*] ℞ Myrrhae Troglodytidis, opopanacis, ſucci papaveris, ſingulorum ʒ ij, bryoniae radicis ʒ iv, (hanc alii pſilethron, alii vitem ſilvaticam, alii madon, alii chironiam, alii cercida vocant) corticis ariſtolochiae longae drach. iv, (in totum enim radicum cortices multo utiliores ſunt, quam medullae) pyrethri radicis ʒ iv, ſeminum rutae ſilveſtris, cumini Aethiopici, ſeminis triſolii, ſingulorum

τος, ἀνὰ ὀξύβαφον, πάντα κόψας καὶ σήσας, αναλάμβανε ὄξει, ἐναποβεβρεγμένου κόμμεως, ὥστ᾽ ἔχειν τι κολλῶδες, καὶ ἀνάπλασσε τροχίσκους, καὶ ξήραινε ἐν σκιᾷ. ἐν δὲ τῇ χρήσει δίδου τροχίσκου ἥμισυ, ἤτοι μετ᾽ οἴνου, ἢ μετ᾽ ὄξους ἐναφηψημένων πηγάνου φύλλων. ποίει τοῦτο πολλάκις τῆς ἡμέρας, ὥστε εἶναι τὴν τελείαν δόσιν τοῦ φαρμάκου < β΄. πλεῖον γὰρ διδόμενον ἔμετον κινεῖ, ὥστε μὴ πλέον διδόναι παραινοῦμεν. ἐμέτου δὲ γενομένου πάλιν δοτέον πολλάκις τὸ φάρμακον τῆς ἡμέρας. δεῖ δὲ καὶ τρέφειν τὸν πεπονθότα, καὶ οἴνῳ κεκραμένῳ ποτίζειν, καὶ πολλάκις τοῦτο ποιεῖν. ἀλλὰ καὶ πυριᾷν ὕδατι πολλῷ, καὶ καταντλεῖν τοῖς ὠφελεῖν δυναμένοις. ἡ δὲ κατάκλυσις ἔστω τοῦ πεπονθότος τόπου κατάῤῥοπος.

[923] [Δωροθέου φάρμακον ἐπιτετευγμένον πρὸς παντὸς ἑρπετοῦ πληγήν.] ♃ Ῥίζης φλόμου θήλεως τοῦ φλοιοῦ, τριφύλλου καρποῦ, ἀνὰ < α΄. ὀποπάνακος, ἑρπύλλου, μήου, νεβροῦ πιτυᾶς, ἀνὰ < β΄. σελίνου σπέρματος, ἄμμεως, μαράθρου σπέρματος, ἀνίσου σπέρματος, ἀνὰ ὀξύβαφον,

acetabulum. Omnia contufa cribrataque aceto excipiuntur, gummi prius macerato, ut glutinofum aliquid habeat, paftillique finguntur, in umbra ficcantur; in ufu, datur paftilli dimidium, vel cum vino, vel cum aceto, foliis rutae incoctis; idque frequenter die fiat, ut plurimum ʒ ij, medicamenti exiftant; nam plus exhibitum vomitum proritat. Quare non amplius exhibere adhortantur; vomitu autem oborto rurfus dari debet crebro medicamentum die. Quin etiam affectum nutrire convenit et vino temperato recreare, ac id multoties facere; imo etiam aqua calida fovere et ea quae juvare poffunt, fuperfundere. Caeterum affecti loci decubitus declivis efto.

[*Dorothei medicamentum, cujuslibet ferpentis ictui accommodatum.*] ♃ Corticis radicis verbafci foemellae, feminis trifolii, fingulorum ʒ j, opopanacis, ferpilli, meu, coaguli hinnuli, fingulorum ʒ ij, feminis apii, ammeos, feminis foeniculi, feminis anifi, fingulorum acetabulum,

Ed. Chart. XIII. [923.] Ed. Baſ. II. (452.)

ὀρόβων ἡλεσμένων < β'. τὰ ξηρὰ κόψας καὶ σήσας ἀναλάμβανε οἴνῳ Ἀριουσίῳ· ἐν τούτῳ διαλυθείσης τῆς πιτυᾶς καὶ τοῦ ὀποπάνακος, ἀνάπλαττε τροχίσκους, καὶ δίδου πρὸς δύναμιν· τοῖς μὲν ἤδη συντόνως κατεχομένοις < α'. καὶ οἴνου κοτύλην α'. τοῖς δὲ ἄλλοις τριώβολον. ἐχρήσατο δὲ τῷ φαρμάκῳ καὶ πρὸς τὰς περὶ ἔντερα διαθέσεις, καὶ ὧν ἐβούλετο τὴν κύστιν ῥευματίζειν, καὶ πρὸς βῆχας, καὶ ἄλλας περιστάσεις, ὡς σφόδρα γενναίῳ. ἡ χρῆσις ἐπὶ μὲν τῶν ἰοβόλων μετ' οἴνου, ἐπὶ δὲ τῶν ἄλλων μεθ' ὕδατος. Ἄλλη Ὑβριστοῦ Ὀξυῤῥυγχίτου, φάρμακον ἐπιτετευγμένον πρὸς παντὸς ἰοβόλου πληγήν. ἀνεγράφη ὑπὸ Ἀπολλωνίου τοῦ Μεμφίτου. τὰ δὲ τῆς σκευασίας ἔχει οὕτως. ♃ Ἀριστολοχίας, πάνακος, ἄγνου σπέρματος, ἀνὰ < δ'. κάγχρυος καὶ σμύρνης, πεπέρεως, σεσέλεως Μασσαλεωτικοῦ, νάρδου Ἰνδικῆς, καστορίου, κινναμώμου μέλανος, ὡς λεπτοτάτου, πεπέρεως μακροῦ, Κυρηναϊκοῦ ὀποῦ, ἴριδος, πηγάνου ἀγρίου σπέρματος, ἀνὰ < β'. ὑπερικοῦ < α'. πάντα κόψας, καὶ σήσας λεπτοτάτῳ κοσκίνῳ, ἀνάπλασσε τροχίσκους,

ervorum inſolatorum ʒ ij, arida contuſa, cribrataque, vino Ariuſio excipiuntur, diſſoluto in eo coagulo et opopanace, paſtilli fiunt; danturque pro virium ratione; iis qui jam valide detinentur, ʒ j, et vini hemina; aliis autem, oboli iij. Uſus eſt etiam medicamento ad inteſtinorum affectus et quorum volebat aſſluxionem perducere, item ad tuſſes et ad alios caſus, ceu vehementer generoſo uſus eſt, in virulentis quidem ex vino, in aliis autem ex aqua. *Aliud Hybriſti Oxyrrhynchiti medicamentum ad omnis venenati ictum utile; inſcriptum ab Apollonio Memphite. Hoc modo conficitur.* ♃ Ariſtolochiae, panacis, ſeminis viticis, ſingulorum ʒ iv, canchryos, myrrhae, piperis, ſeſeleos Maſſaleotici, nardi Indicae, caſtorii, cinnamomi nigri quam tenuiſſimi, piperis longi, ſucci Cyrenaici, iridis, ſeminum rutae ſilveſtris, ſingulorum ʒ ij, hyperici ʒ j. Omnia contuſa et tenuiſſimo cribro increta in paſtillos coguntur; vino marinae experti imbuti ſic-

οἴνῳ ἀθαλάσσῳ φυράσας, ξήραινε ἐν σκιᾷ, καὶ δίδου < α΄. ἐν οἴνῳ ἀκράτῳ κοτύλης α΄. καὶ ὕδατος δ΄. ἐπιτίθει δὲ καὶ ἐπὶ τὸ δῆγμα θλάσας ἕνα τῶν τροχίσκων, καὶ οἴνῳ διαλύσας, καὶ προσβαλὼν ἀριστολοχίας τῆς καλῆς λείας, ὅσον < β΄. καὶ ἀλφίτου πάλιν < δ΄. ταῦτα συλλεάνας καὶ τρίψας ἐπιμελῶς, ἐπιτίθει ἔξωθεν σκεπάσας συκῆς φύλλῳ, καὶ ταινιδίῳ καταδήσας. (453) Ἀντίδοτος θηριακὴ ἐχιοδήκτοις. ποιεῖ δὲ καὶ πρὸς παντὸς ἑρπετοῦ πληγήν. ταύτην Γάλλος παραγενόμενος ἐκ τῆς Ἀραβίας ἔδωκε Καίσαρι, πολλοὺς τῶν συστρατευσαμένων αὐτῷ πληγέντας ἀπό τε λυσσοδήκτων καὶ σκορπίων, καὶ φαλαγγίων, καὶ τῶν ἄλλων ἑρπετῶν διασώσας. ἔχει δὲ οὕτως. ℞ Ὀρόβων ἠλεσμένων < κε΄. βρυωνίας ῥίζας < ιστ΄. πηγάνου ἀγρίου σπέρματος < ιβ΄. τριφύλλου καρποῦ, ἴρεως Καρχηδονίας, ὀποπάνακος, ἀριστολοχίας μακρᾶς, ὀποῦ μήκωνος, ζιγγιβέρεως, ἑκάστου < η΄. κυμίνου Αἰθιοπικοῦ, σμύρνης, ἠρυγγίου, ὀποῦ Κυρηναϊκοῦ, κρόκου, ἑρπύλλου, κόστου, σαγαπηνοῦ, ἑκάστου < στ΄. οἴνῳ Ἀμιναίῳ φυράσας, ἀνάπλαττε τρο-

cantur in umbra, ac datur ʒ j, in vini meraci hemina j, et aquae iv. Item morſui conſractus unus ex paſtillis vinoque ſolutus imponitur. Jam adjectis ariſtolochiae bonae laevigatae ʒ ij et polentae rurſus drach. iv, haec laevigata, tritaque diligenter, imponito, ſici ſolio extrinſecus cooperiens et ſasciola deligans. *Antidotus Theriaca ad viperae morſus; facit etiam ad cujusvis ſerpentis ictum; hanc Gallus profectus ex Arabia donavit Caeſari, quum multos commilitonum ipſius ictos a rabioſis, ſcorpionibus, phalangiis, aliisque ſerpentibus conſervaſſet; habet autem hunc in modum.* ℞ Ervi in farinam redacti ʒ xxv, radicis bryoniae ʒ xvj, ſeminum rutae ſilveſtris ʒ xij, ſeminum triſolii, iridis Carthaginenſis, opopanacis, ariſtolochiae longae, ſucci papaveris, zingiberis, ſingulorum ʒ viij, cumini Aethiopici, myrrhae, eryngii, ſucci Cyrenaici, croci, ſerpilli, coſti, ſagapeni, ſingulorum ʒ vi. Vino Aminaeo conſperſo, forma paſtillos, ac pro viribus

χίσκους, καὶ δίδου πρὸς δύναμιν. ἔστω δὲ ἡ τελεία δόσις τριώβολον ἐξ οἴνου κοτύλης α΄. πρὸς δὲ τὰς λοιπὰς διαθέσεις μετ᾽ οἰνομέλιτος.

[Ἐπίθεμα ἐχιοδήκτοις.] ℞ Σαγαπηνοῦ, πεπέρεως, ὀποῦ Κυρηναϊκοῦ, ὀποπάνακος ἀνὰ μέρος ἕν, χαλβάνης, θείου ἀπύρου, ἀνὰ < β΄. τὰ ξηρὰ κόπτε καὶ σῆθε λεπτοτάτῳ κοσκίνῳ, τοὺς δ᾽ ὀποὺς διαλύσας, ἐπίβαλλε τοῖς ξηροῖς, καὶ ποίει ἐμπλάστρου τὸ πάχος, καὶ ἐπιτίθει κατὰ τῶν πληγῶν, ἔξωθεν δὲ τούτων φύλλα συκῆς ἢ κνίδης.

["Αλλο.] ℞ Καρδαμώμου, ἠρυγγίου ῥίζης, θείου ἀπύρου, πεπέρεως, ἑκάστου μέρος ἕν, σμύρνης, χαλβάνης, ἀνὰ β΄. μέρη, σκεύαζε καθὰ προείρηται.

["Αλλο.] ℞ Κενταυρίου, ἀριστολοχίας, πευκεδανοῦ ῥίζης, ἴσον ἑκάστου, κόψας, καὶ σήσας, καὶ ὄξει φυράσας, ἀναλάμβανε χαλβάνῃ, καὶ χρῶ καθὰ προείρηται.

[924] ["Αλλο.] Κάγχρυος, σταφίδος ἀγρίας, βρυωνίας ῥίζης, ἀριστολοχίας, ἑκάστου μέρος ἕν, σμύρνης, ὀποπάνακος, ἀνὰ μέρη β΄. ὄξει φυράσας ἀναλάμβανε, καθὰ προείρηται.

dato, ſit autem ex tribus obolis perfecta doſis ex vini hemina una; ad reliquos autem aſſectus ex mulſo.

[*Epithema ad viperarum morſus.*] ♃ Sagapeni, piperis, ſucci Cyrenaici, opopanacis, ſingulorum partem unam, galbani, ſulphuri vivi, ſingulorum ʒ ij, arida tundito et tenuiſſimo cribro incernito. Succos autem ſolutos aridis injicito, fiatque emplaſtri craſſities atque vulneribus admove; extrinſecus autem folia fici, vel urticae.

[*Aliud.*] ♃ Cardamomi, radicis eryngii, ſulphuris vivi, piperis, ſingulorum partem unam, myrrhae, galbani, ſingulorum partes ij, praeparato, ut praedictum eſt.

[*Aliud.*] ♃ Centaurii, ariſtolochiae, radicis peucedani, ſingulorum par pondus; contuſaque, cribrata, aceto ſuperfuſa, galbano excipito et utitor ſicut praedictum eſt.

[*Aliud.*] ♃ Canchryos, ſtaphidis ſilveſtris, radicis bryoniae, ariſtolochiae, ſingulorum partem unam, myrrhae, opopanacis, ſingulorum partes ij, aceto conſperſa excipito, ut praedictum eſt.

Κεφ. ιε'. [Ἀντίδοτοι Δαμοκράτους πρὸς ἑρπετὰ καὶ λυσσοδήκτους.] Ἐπεὶ δὲ τὰ ἔμμετρα τό τ' εὐμνημόνευτον ἔχει καὶ τὸ ἀναμάρτητον ἐν τῇ συμμετρίᾳ τῶν φαρμάκων, ἄμεινον ἔδοξεν εἶναί μοι καὶ τὰ Δαμοκράτους ἐνταῦθα γράψαι μέτρα, τόνδε τὸν τρόπον ἔχοντα.

Νυνὶ δ' ἀποδοῦναι βούλομαι τὰς δυνάμεις,
Μόνον θεραπεύειν ἰοβόλων δήγματα,
Ἔχεων, κεραστῶν, ἀσπίδων, καὶ χερσύδρων,
Πληγάς τε θηρίων, καὶ δήγματα
Σφηκῶν, μελιττῶν, σκορπίων, φαλαγγίων.
Σκεύαζε δ' οὕτως. ἴρεως δὶς δ'.
Τῆς Ἰλλυρικῆς. τὸ δ' ἀπὸ ζιγγιβέρεως
Ὀποπάνακός τε καὶ ὀπίου, μηκωνίου,
Λιβανωτίδος ῥίζης τε, καὶ τοῦ Κρητικοῦ
Παντὸς τριφύλλου σπέρματος δὶς δ'.
Ἀριστολοχίας τῆς μακρᾶς, καὶ πηγάνου
Σπέρματος ἀγρίου τε, τὰς ἴσας ἀνὰ δώδεκα,
Ἑκκαίδεκα ῥίζης λευκοτάτης βρυωνίας.

Cap. XV. [*Damocratis ad venenoſorum ac rabioſorum morſus antidoti.*] Quum autem verſibus conſcripta facile memoria contineantur et ponderis medicamentorum ſymmetriam inculpatam ſortiantur, ſatius mihi viſum eſt etiam Damocratis verſus hic adſcribere, qui hoc modo ſe habent.

Nunc autem tradere medicinas volo,
Quae morſus tantum venenatos ſanent,
Cornutae, viperarum, aſpidum et cherſydrum;
Ictus ferarum et puncturas quoque
Apium, veſparum, ſcorpii, phalangii.
Sic praeparato, drachmae Illyricae octo iridis,
Opopanacis, zingiberis et meconii
Roris marini radicis, tum Cretici
Omnis trifolii ſeminis, bis quatuor,
Ariſtolochiae praelongae, atque ſeminis
Silvaticae rutae, utriusque duodecim,
Albiſſimae radicis ſexdecim bryoniae,

Ἑρπυλλαρίου δὲ τῆς πόας καὶ σμυρνίου,
Καστορίοιό τε Ποντικοῦ πάντων ἴσα.
Ἠρυγγίου δὲ καὶ σελίνου σπέρματος
Αἰθιοπικοῦ μάλιστα, καί τι ἐπὶ προσφάτου
Δραχμὰς ἑκάστου γ΄. δύο ἐκ πάντων σταθμῶν,
Ὀρόβου τε λευκοῦ, τοῦ καθαροῦ δύο δώδεκα.
Ἅπαντα ταῦτα ξηρὰ καὶ σεσησμένα,
Ἀναλάμβαν᾽ οἴνῳ καὶ ποιήσας σφαιρία,
Ἢ καὶ τροχίσκους, δὸς δραχμὴν πιεῖν μίαν,
Τοῦ φαρμάκου κοτύλην τε μὴ κεκραμένην,
Οἴνου λιπαροῦ, καλοῦ τε καὶ μὴ προσφάτου.
Ποιεῖ δὲ καὶ δι᾽ ὕδατος ἀνεθὲν ἥμισυ
Τοῖς πνευματουμένοισι κῶλον, ἢ γαστέρα,
Δίχ᾽ αἰτίας φανερᾶς τε τοῖς πονοῦσί τι.

Ἄλλη.

Σφόδρα ἀγαθὴ δύναμις, ᾗ καὶ χρωμένους
Πίνοντας αὐτοὺς οἶδα, δηχθέντας κακῶς

At herbulae ſerpilli, nec non ſmyrnii,
Caſtoriique Pontici, pares trium modi,
Eryngii vero, ad haec apii ſeminis
Aethiopici recentis maxime inſuper,
Drachmae bis ternae ſingulorum erunt,
Ervique candidi purgati bis duodecim.
Haec omnia arida et cribro increta, excipe
Vino pilulas, vel orbiculos effingito,
Drachmam unam propinato medicaminis,
Et heminam, non commixtam vini optimi,
Pinguis, vetuſti. Jam ſubactum aqua,' facit
Drachmae dimidio, coli, aut ventris flatibus,
Et citra manifeſtam cauſam dolentibus.

Aliud.

Valde bonum remedium, quo uſos etiam
Ipſos bibendo novi commorſos male

Τοῖς ἀρτιθήροις ἔχεσι, τοῖς καλουμένοις
Ψυλλίοις. ἔθνος δέ φασι τοῦτο δυσπαθὲς
Φύσει νενομίσθαι πρὸς τῶν δακετῶν φόβους.
Ἑτέροις δὲ δόντας, σφόδρα κακῶς δεδηγμένοις.
Μελισσόφυλλον μαλακὸν ἐν σκιᾷ ψυγὲν,
Ξηρὸν γενόμενον κόψον, ἐκ τούτου λαβὼν
Δραχμὰς δὶς ὀκτὼ, πρόσβαλ' αὐτῷ στρογγύλης
Ἀριστολοχίας, ἢ μακρᾶς, δραχμὰς δέκα
Ξηρᾶς, χαμαίδρυος δὲ τὰς αὐτὰς δέκα,
Σμύρνης τε χρηστῆς Τρωγλοδύτιδος δραχμὰς δέκα.
Ταῦτ' ὁλμοκοπήσας, σῆθε λεπτῷ κοσκίνῳ,
Μέλιτός τε μέτριον προσβαλὼν αὐτοῖς, ἑνοῦ.
Δίδου τε δραχμῆς πλῆθος, ἢ μικρῷ πλέον
Ἐν ζωροτέροις κυάθοισι κράματα δέκα.
Τινὲς δὲ φύλλων τῶν μακρῶν καὶ προσφάτων
Τὸν χυλὸν ἀποθλίψαντες, ἴσον αὖ καλῷ
Οἴνῳ κατέμιξαν, καὶ ἔδοσαν πιεῖν αὐτίκα.
Πλῆθος τὸ πᾶν δὶς ε'. κυάθους, ἢ βραχὺ

A viperis nuper captis, quos vocant
Pſyllos (gens haec natura non ferme ſolet
Pati ſerpentes, neque aſſueta timet)
Dediſſeque aliis valde commorſis male.
Mollem ſiccabis umbra meliſſophyllon:
Siccatum tunde, moxque drachmas accipe
Inde bis octo. Tum longae vel rotundae
Ariſtolochiae drachmas adde decem,
Siccae tamen: chamaedryos decem quoque,
Myrrhae et bonae, et Troglodyticae item decem.
Iſtaec contuſa ſubtili cribro excute:
Mellis quod ſatis dulcis adde et unias.
Dato quod pendet drachmam vel plus parum,
E vini purioris cyathis decem.
Quidam e longo atque recenti folio
Exprimunt ſuccum, ſicque menſura pari
Vinum conjungunt, utque bibatur jubent.
Menſura utriusque ſint cyathi decem,

Ἐλαττόνων, βραχύ τε δαψιλέστερον,
Τά τε φύλλα λεῖα κατέπλασαν τοῖς δήγμασι.

Ἄλλη.

[925] *Πρὸς θηρίων μὲν πάντων ἰὸν ἑρπετῶν*
Μάλιστα δ᾽ ἐχεων φάρμακον δραστήριον.
Ἔχε δὲ διὰ παντὸς πιτυὰν ἀποκειμένην
Νεβρῶν ἐλάφου, καὶ μὲν ἂν τὴν πρόσφατον.
Τῆς γὰρ παλαιᾶς ἐστὶν εὐστομαχωτέρα,
Ταύτης δραχμῶν τὸ πλῆθος ἐν κυάθοις δυσὶν
Οἴνου Φαλερίνου καὶ ὕδατος τοῦ συμμέτρου
Κεράσας, προσένεγκε τοῖς σφόδρα δεδηγμένοις,
Κέλευε τούτοις γρηγορεῖν, καὶ περιπατεῖν.
Ἂν ἐπιτρέπωσιν οἱ δεδηγμένοι τόποι,
Εἰς τὰ βαλανεῖά τ᾽ εἰσιέναι χρόνους τινὰς
Μένοντας ἐν τούτοισι, καὶ μετ᾽ οὐ πολὺ
Πάλιν ὡς προεῖπον, λαμβάνειν τὴν πιτυάν.
Ἐκ τοῦ γένους τε τῶν πρὸς τοὺς θανασίμους.

Parum vel minus, aut parumper amplius.
Impoſitum quoque folium attritum prodeſt.

Alia.

Ad omnium venena pharmacum efficax
Serpentium, ſed viperae potiſſimum.
At ſemper habeas coagulum recentium
Cervi hinnulorum, idemque praecellit recens,
Hoc nanque ſtomacho vetuſto gratum magis,
Denarium iſtius, cyathis binis cape
Vini phalerni et mediocris, aquae et temperans,
Animalium ferorum morſibus applica.
Laeſis obambulare et vigilare impera.
Quod ſi locus commorſus hoc admiſerit,
Et balnea ingredi, atque in his aliquandiu
Manere, necnon rurſus paulo poſtea,
Quemadmodum praedixi, ſumere coagulum,
Quod noxiis lethalibusve ſit efficax.

"Αλλη.

Ἀντίδοτός ἐστι πρὸς τὰ τῶν λυσσώντων κυνῶν,
Δήγματα φέροντα παρακοπὰς ὑλακτικὰς,
Φόβους ἀλόγους τε παντὸς ὑγροῦ καὶ ποτοῦ,
Ὡς κἂν ἴδωσι παντελῶς ὕδωρ βραχὺ,
Τρόμοισι καὶ σπασμοῖσι κατέχοντ' αὐτίκα,
Ἐν ἀγρυπνίαις τε καὶ παρακοπαῖς συνεχέσι
Διάγοντες, ἀποθνήσκουσι συντομώτατα.
Κἂν τῷ παραχρῆμα δ' ἐκφύγωσι τοὺς φόβους,
Μένει τὰ τοιαῦτα κατὰ χρόνους συμπτώματα
Ἄφνω γενόμενα τοῖς πάλαι δεδηγμένοις.
Πρὸς τοὺς φόβους οὖν τῶν τοιούτων δηγμάτων
Ἱερὰν ἔχε πάντως ἀντίδοτον παρακειμένην.
Οἱ γὰρ πιόντες, ὡς ἐρῶ, ταύτην ἐγὼ,
Εἰς οὐδὲν ἄτοπον ἐμπεσοῦνται ῥᾳδίως.
Σκεύαζε δ' αὐτὴν, καρκίνους τοὺς ποταμίους
(454) Ἐπὶ κληματίδων κατάκαιε λευκῆς ἀμπέλου,
Τήρει τε λειῶν ἐπιμελῶς ἐν πυξίδι,

Alia.

*Antidotus ad rabioſorum morſus canum.
Qui mentem alienantes vexant latratibus,
Metuque cujuſvis liquoris, maxime
Potus, idque ſine ratione, ut ſi viderint
Vel paululum prorſus aquae, protinus
Tremore crucientur, convulſionibus,
Pervigiliis continuis et deliriis
Vitam peragentes, moriuntur citiſſime;
Et ſi repente effugerint diros metus,
Ejusmodi manent diu ſymptomata,
Quae ſunt oborta confeſtim morſus nuper.
Proinde ejusmodi ut morſu te vindices,
Omnino antidotum ſacrum habeas repoſitum.
Nam hoc qui biberint, ſicut nos percenſebimus,
In nullum facile concident incommodum.
Ipſum parato. Cancros fluviatiles
In candidae vitis ſarmentis urito.*

Καὶ γεντιανῆς τὴν ῥίζαν εὖ σεσησμένην
Ἐν πυξίδι δ' ἑτέρᾳ τῆς δὲ χρείας γενομένης
Κατάπασον οἴνου τρισὶ κυάθοις ἡδέος,
Μύστρα δὲ β'. μακρὰ τῆς σποδοῦ τῶν καρκίνων,
Τῆς γεντιανῆς δ', ὡς ἔφην, λελεασμένης
Ἓν μύστρον, οὕτως ἐκπιεῖν κέλευ' ἄθρουν
Τρισὶν καθεξῆς ἡμέρας νήστει διδούς.
Πρώτην κατὰ τύχην δ' ὑστερήσας ἡμέραν,
Ἄλλαις δυσίν τε προσφέρων ἁπλοῦν μέτρον
Διπλοῦν προσοίσεις δεύτερον τῷ φαρμάκῳ,
Εἰς τρεῖς δὲ κυάθους, ὡς ἔφην, οἴνου βαλὼν
Ἢ κᾀν τρισίν γε τοῖς σφοδρῶς δεδηγμένοις,
Τῆς γεντιανῆς δ' αὖ μόνοις τρισὶν δοκεῖ
Τριωβόλου τὸ πλῆθος ὁλκῆς προσφέρειν
Λείας ἐπιμελῶς ἡμέραις δυσὶν εἴκοσιν
Ἐν ζωροτέροις κυάθοις τρισίν, ἢ μικρῷ πλέον.

Ἄλλη.

Καὶ τοῦτο πρὸς τοὺς ὑδροφόβους δεδοικότας

Servaque diligenter tritum in pyxide,
Et gentianae radicem incretam probe.
Altera fed in pyxide, quum uti velis,
Infpergito fuavis vini cyathis tribus,
At myftra cineris magna cancrorum duo,
Sed gentianae laevigatae, veluti diximus,
Myftrum unicum, fic bibere totum praecipe,
Per tres dies deinceps, jejuno porrigens.
Sin forte primum praetergreffus eft diem,
Et fimplicem duobus aliis adferens
Modum, duplum fecundo addes medicamini
In vini cyathos tres mittens, ut diximus,
Vel in tribus fi morfus fuerit grandior.
At gentianae laevigatae tres placet
Nonnullis obolos folum viginti dies
Offerre, in cyathis cumulatis vel plus parum

Alia.

Tritoque id ufu comperiffe Niceratus

Ἔλεγε διὰ πείρας γεγονέναι Νικήρατος.
Αὐτῷ τε καὶ φίλοις κρίνειν δυναμένοις,
Τὰ τῶν παραδόξων φαρμάκων ἰδιώματα.
Λυκίου κρατίστου Παταρικοῦ τριώβολον,
Τοῦ δ' Ἰνδικοῦ βέλτιστον ἂν ᾖ σοι παρὸν,
Διδόναι προσέταττεν ἡμέρας δυσὶν εἴκοσι,
Νήστεσι δι' ὕδατος, ὥσπερ εἶπον ἀρτίως.
Λέγεται δὲ ποιεῖν ταῦτα καὶ Βρεττανικῆς
Δοθεὶς ὁμοίως χυλὸς, ὥσπερ τὸ Λύκιον.
Καὶ τοῦτο δ' ἱκανῶς παρ' ἐνίοις θαυμάζεται,
Ἄρκτου χολῆς β'. μύστρα καταμίξας δυσὶν
Ὕδατος κυάθοις, πρόσφερ' ἐπὶ τρεῖς ἡμέρας,
Μήπω λαβοῦσι τὴν τροφὴν, ὄρθρον τ' ἄγαν.
Πρὸς λυσσοδήκτους ἔχε μάλισθ' ὅπου πολὺς
Εἰς τὸ πάθος ἐμπίπτει καὶ λυσσᾷ κύων.
[926] Ἔμπλαστρος ᾗ χρῶμαι πρὸς τὸν τῶν δηγμάτων
Ἰχῶρ', ἀρέσκει τὶ πέλιόν τ', ἢ καὶ μέλαν
Τοῖς τραύμασιν πρόσεστι, τοῦτο περικνίσας

Adverſum aquae metum, recenſuit,
Ipſi atque amicis qui norunt medicaminum
Inſignium proprietates diſcernere.
Lycii Patarici ternos obolos optimi,
Sed Indici praeſtaret, ſi copia datur,
Jubebit offerre dies viginti duos
Jejuno, ex aqua, ſicut vobus dictum eſt nuper.
Narratur haec praeſtare quoque Britannicae
Potus ſimiliter ſuccus, veluti Lycium.
Atque hoc apud nonnullos eſt miraculum,
Fellis myſtra duo urſini, binis temperans
Aquae cyathis et ſummo ad tres dies dato,
Nondum datis cibariis diluculo
Ad morſus rabioſorum. Sed quum plurimi
Magis laborant affectu, rabiunt canes,
Emplaſtrum habeto quo utor contra morſuum
Tergendam ſaniem, ſi quid lividum aut nigrum
Vulneribus adhaeret; quo affricto pluribus

Ἐπίβαλλε τὴν ἔμπλαστρον ἐπὶ χρόνον πολὺν,
Δι' ἡμερῶν τὸ τραῦμα πλατύτερον ποιῶν,
Ἑλκοῦν δυναμένῳ φαρμάκῳ ἐσχαρωτικῷ,
Ποιοῦσαν ἀμέλει καὶ πρὸς ἄλλων θηρίων
Τῶν ἰοβόλων πληγάς τε καὶ τὰ δήγματα,
Ἀκίδων τε φαύλοις φαρμάκοις βεβλαμμένων,
Καὶ πρὸς κακοήθη πάντα ἐξηλκωμένα,
Τῆς γῆς μελαίνης ἀμπελίτιδος δραχμὰς
Δὶς κέ. καὶ λιθαργύρου καλῆς
Σταθμὸν τὸν αὐτὸν, ταὐτό τ' ἀσφάλτου βάρος
Ἴσας τ' ἐλαίου. τοῖς τρισὶν τούτοις δραχμὰς
Τῆς Ἀττικῆς τε προπόλεως δὶς εἴκοσι,
Ἀριστολοχίας, συμφύτου τ' ἀνὰ τέσσαρας,
Δὶς δύο πρασίου, καὶ ἑλενίου τὰς ἴσας,
Χαμαιλέοντος τέσσαρας, τρεῖς σμυρνίου.
Τὸ δ' αὐτὸ λευκῆς ἴρεως ξηρᾶς καλῆς.
Τρεῖς δ' ὀμφακίνης κηκίδος, ἓξ στυπτηρίας,
Πολίου τε ταὐτὸ, χαλβάνης τ' ὀβολοῦ πλέον,

Diebus emplaſtrum injectum permittito,
Latius efficiendo vulnus, medicamine,
Quod ducere poſſit cruſtam; confert inſuper
Ferarum reliquarum virus jaculantium
Ad ictus, itidem morſus, atque ſpicula
Pravis medicamentis infecta et omnia
Maligna corporis totius ulcera,
Terrae nigrae ampelitidis et bituminis,
Spumae bonae argenti atque olei denarios
Fac ſingulorum quinquaginta horum trium.
Verum propoleos bis vigenos, Atticae
Ariſtolochiae et ſymphyti ana quatuor.
Bis duo praſſii et helenii pares
Chamaeleonis quatuor, tres ſmyrnii,
Tot candidae iris aridae drachmas bonae,
Tres omphacinae gallae, ſex aluminis,
Poliique totidem, galbani obolo largius,
Thuris duodecim non ſecti drachmam ſemis,

Λιβάνου τ' ἀτμήτου ιβ'. ὁλκῆς ἥμισυ,
Χαλκίτεως ὀπτῆς τε τέσσαρας δραχμὰς,
Κενταυρίου λεπτοῦ τε δραχμὰς τρὶς β'.
Δὶς πέντε καὶ δέκα μέλιτος Ἀττικοῦ νέου.
Σκεύαζε δ' αὐτὴν ἐπιμελῶς αὐτὸς παρών.
Καὶ γὰρ σφόδρ' εἰ καὶ κατακαίεται ταχὺ,
Τὴν ἀμπελῖτιν καὶ λιθάργυρον βαλὼν,
Εἰς λοπάδα καινὴν εὐμεγέθη προσέμβαλε,
Λεῖον ἔλαιον ἕψε μαλθακῷ πυρὶ,
Ὅταν δ' ἴδῃς ῥυπῶδες, ἔμπασον τότε
Στυπτηρίαν, χαλκῖτιν, ἑτέραν δῆτ' ἔχων
Χύτραν τε, τῆκε τὸ μέλι καὶ τὴν χαλβάνην,
Πρόπολίν τε καὶ τὰ λοιπὰ τηκτὰ μίγματα
Κατάχει μετρίως ζέοντα τῆς λιθαργύρου,
Καὶ συζέσας ἐπ' ὀλίγον, ὅταν ἴδῃς ὅτι
Ἔμπλαστρος ἔσται ἀμόλυντος, ἐμπάσσεις τότε
Τὰς πόας τε καὶ τὰ λοιπὰ ῥιζία,
Ἄρας τε ταχέως τὴν χύτραν ἀπὸ τοῦ πυρὸς,

Chalcitis autem teſtae drachmas quatuor,
Centaurii tenuis drachmas ſex, mellis Attici
Denarios quinos denos mittes novi.
Sed fac diligenter ipſe praeſens praepares.
Siquidem ocyus etiam valde comburitur,
Terram ampelitidem mittens et lithargyron
In fictile novum magnitudinis bonae
Adjunge laeve oleum, mollique igne incoquas.
Quum ſordidum videbis, tunc inſpergito
Calcitem, alumen, alia rurſus ollula
Mel, galbanum, propolim, reliquaque liquida
Liquato, modice fervida ſuperfundito
Lithargyro, calefaciens pauxillulum,
Quum videris manus ceu emplaſtro haud infici,
Tunc herbulas adde et reliquas radiculas.
Sublato ab igne confeſtim jam fictili:
Refrigera parum, medicamen commovens,
Palmis valentioribus permolliens

Ψῦξον, διακινῶν ἐπ᾽ ὀλίγον τὸ φάρμακον,
Συνεκμαλάσσων χερσὶν εὐτονωτέραις,
Ἀπόθου, φυλάττων δέρματ᾽ ἐσκεπασμένην,
Καὶ τῶν ἀκίδων τῶν πεφαρμακευμένων,
Τὰ τραύματ᾽ ἔγνω ταὐτὰ ποιεῖν ἑρπετοῖς
Τῶν ἰοβόλων τε θηρίων τοῖς δήγμασι.
Διὸ καὶ θεραπείας ἐστὶν ὁμογενὴς τρόπος,
Καὶ γὰρ ἐπὶ τούτοις σάρκα τὴν τετρωμένην
Ταχίως περικόπτειν σμιλίῳ δεῖ, καὶ πυρὶ
Συκίας τ᾽ ἐπιβάλλειν εἰ δυνατὸν τοῖς τραύμασι,
Τοῖς δριμέσιν τε φαρμάκοις καὶ καυστικοῖς,
Τηρεῖν τὸ τραῦμα πλείονας χρόνους πλατὺ,
Ὥσπερ ὑπέδειξα θᾶττον ἐν συντάγματι
Ἑτέρῳ, γραφέντι τοῖς θέλουσι φάρμακα
Ποιεῖν ὅσα καύσοις σμιλίῳ τε γίγνεται.
Χρῆσθαι δὲ καὶ ταῖς ἀντιδότοις ποτήμασι
Τοῖς ἐχιοδήκτοις, ἃς ἐκέλευσα προσφέρειν,
Καὶ πητύας δὲ τῶν νεβρῶν αὐτοῖς δίδου,
Καὶ γεντιανῆς, ὡς ἔφην, δεῖ προσφέρειν

Reponito, conservans pelle conditum.
Valet sagittarum infectarum pharmaco
Vulneribus, veluti morsibus serpentium,
Item jaculantium virus animalium.
Quare medendi existit consimilis modus.
In his enim carnem oblaesam scalpro statim
Circoncidere necesse est et cucurbitas
Si liceat, admoveri flammis vulneri,
Acribus et medicamentis ac urentibus,
Id longiore servans latum tempore.
Quod indicavi prius in commentario
Alio, iis qui medicamina tradita desiderent
Efficere, quae scalpro fiunt, urentibus.
Sunt utiles antidoti in potionibus,
Quas viperae applicari jussi morsibus.
Item coagulum ipsis offer hinnuli,
Et gentianae, ut rabiosorum morsibus

Τοῖς λυσσοδήκτοις, καὶ τὰ λοίφ', ὡς εἴπομεν
Ποεῖν ἐπ' ἐκείνων ταῦτα, καὶ τοῖς δ' ἁρμόττει
Ὀπόν τε Κυρηναῖον αὐτοῖς προσφέρειν.
Οὗ μὴ παρόντος δὲ, διδόναι καὶ Μηδικὸν
Ὀβολοῦ τὸ πλῆθος μεθ' ὕδατος κυάθων δυοῖν,
Τῆς γεντιανῆς δ' ὅσον ἄγει τριώβολον,
Χυλὸς δ' ἀμείνων ἐστὶ τῆς ῥίζης πολύ.

[927] Κεφ. ιζ'. [*Αἱ ὑφ' Ἥρα γεγραμμέναι ἀντίδοτοι θηριακαὶ, ὧν καὶ ἡμεῖς πεπειράμεθα.*] Θηριακὴ ᾗ ἐχρήσατο Μάρκος ὁ αὐτοκράτωρ. ℞ Τριφύλλου ἀσφαλτώδους σπέρματος μέρος ἓν, ἀριστολοχίας στρογγύλης μέρος ἓν, πηγάνου ἀγρίου μέρος ἓν, ὀρόβου ἠλεσμένου μέρος ἓν, οἴνῳ ἀναλάμβανε καὶ ποίει τροχίσκους < δ'. δίδου ἕνα μετ' οἴνου καὶ ἐλαίου.

[*Ἀντίδοτος ἄλλη ποιοῦσα πρὸς τὰ αὐτὰ, λίαν καλῶς.*]
Ἴησιν μάθε τήνδε πρὸς ἑρπετὰ, ἣν Φιλομήτωρ
Νικήσας πείρᾳ κέκρικεν Ἀντίοχος.

Adferre oportet reliqua, ficut docuimus
In illis facere: quippe haec iftis congruunt.
Succumque Cyrenaeum iftis fac temperes:
Sin copia negetur, des etiam medicum,
Aquae duobus cyathis oboli pondere,
At gentianae, quantum oboli tres pendeant,
Eft autem melior fuccus, quam radicula.

Cap. XVII. [*Antidoti ab Hera confcriptae theriacae, quas etiam nos experti fumus.*] Theriaca qua ufus eft Marcus Imperator. ℞ Seminis trifolii bituminofi partem unam, ariftolochiae rotundae partem unam, rutae filveftris partem unam, ervi moliti partem unam, vino excipe et confice paftillos drachmarum iv, dato unum ex vino et oleo.

[*Antidotum aliud ad eadem vehementer efficax.*]
Hoc cape praefidium ad ferpentia, quod Philometor
Ufu praecipuum repperit Antiochus.

Ed. Chart. XIII. [927.] Ed. Baf. II. (454. 455.)

Μήου ἀπὸ ῥίζης ὁλκὴν διδραχμίαν ὀρύξας,
(455) Σὺν τῷ δ᾽ ἑρπύλλου κλῶνας ἰσοῤῥεπέας.
Σὺν δ᾽ ὀπὸν ἐκ πάνακος στήσας, ἴσον ἠδὲ τριφύλλου
Καρπὸν, ὅσον δραχμῆς σταθμὸν ἄγοντα δίδου,
Ἀνίσου, μαράθρου τε καὶ ἄμμιος, ἠδὲ σελίνου
Ἓξ ἑνὸς, ἓν πληρῶν σπέρματος ὀξύβαφον.
Σὺν δ᾽ ὀρόβου λείου δύο ὀξύβαφ᾽ ἔμπασ᾽ ἀλεύρου,
Πάντα δ᾽ ὁμοῦ Χίῳ νέκταρι συγκεράσας,
Κυκλοτερεῖς ἀνάπλασσε τροχοὺς, ἰσότητι μερίζων,
Ἡμιδραχμοῖο ῥοπῆς, ὄφρ᾽ ἂν ἕκαστος ἔχῃ.
Χίῳ δ᾽ ἐγκεράσας τάδε μίγματα, πικρὸν ἐχίδνης,
Ἡμίσεως δραχμὴν, ἰὸν ἀποσκεδάσεις.
Τῷ δὲ ποτῷ καὶ δεινὰ φαλάγγια, καὶ σκολιοῖο
Σκορπίου ἐκφεύξῃ κέντρα φέροντ᾽ ὀδύνας.

Ἡ αὐτὴ ἠκριβωμένη ταῖς συσταθμίαις. ℞ Μήου Κρητικοῦ < β΄. τριφύλλου σπέρματος < β΄. ἑρπύλλου ξηροῦ < δ΄. μαράθρου < δ΄. ἄμμεως < δ΄. σελίνου σπέρματος < δ΄. ὀροβίνου ἀλεύρου < η΄. λεῖα ποιήσας, ἀναλάμβανε

Meu drachmas binas radicis ponito, tantum
Germina ſerpilli ponderis accipiant,
Et panacis totidem drachmas liquor aſſerit aeque
Triffolii, quantum drachmula fructus habet,
Oxybaphum marathri, necnon ameos et aniſi,
Atque apii; ſument ſemina quaeque ſuum.
Aſt ervi pones acetabula bina farinae;
Omnia cum Chio nectare conſocians,
Orbiculos finges, juſto qui ſinguli in illis
Drachmae dimidium pondere conſtituant.
Irrorans Chio medicamina, viperae amarum
Aequali virus aſſociato modo.
Hoc autem effugies horrenda phalangia potu.
Scorpi etiam ſtimulum non vereare gravem.

Eadem exacte ſcripta ponderibus. ℞ Meu Cretici drach. ij, ſeminis trifolii drach. ij, ſerpilli ſicci drach. iv, foeniculi drach. iv, ammeos ʒ iv, ſeminis apii drach. iv, ervi farinae ʒ viij, trita excipito vino Chio et ſingito paſtillos

οἴνῳ Χίῳ, καὶ ποίει τροχίσκους τριωβολιαίους, καὶ δίδου ἕνα μετ᾽ οἴνου. Ἄλλη θηριακὴ πρὸς σκορπίων πληγὰς, καὶ ὅσα τῶν δακνόντων, ἰοῦ ἕνα ἀφιέναι δοκεῖ, καὶ πρὸς ῥήγματα καὶ σπάσματα, ἐμπνευματώσεις κώλου, καὶ πρὸς πολλὰ τῶν ὁμοίων. ταύτην τὴν δύναμιν Γάλλος ἐκ τῆς Ἀραβίας παραγενόμενος Καίσαρι ἔδωκε, πολλοὺς αὐτῇ τῶν συστρατευσαμένων διασώσας. ♃ Βρυωνίας λευκῆς ῥίζης < η'. τριφύλλου σπέρματος < δ'. ἴρεως, χαλκίτιδος ἀνὰ < δ'. ἀριστολοχίας λεπτῆς < δ'. λιβανωτίδος ῥίζης < δ'. ὀποῦ μήκωνος < δ'. ζιγγιβέρεως < δ'. πηγάνου ἀγρίου σπέρματος < στ'. ἑρπύλλου < γ'. κυμίνου Αἰθιοπικοῦ < γ'. ἠρυγγίου ῥίζης < γ'. ὀρόβου ἀλεύρου λευκοῦ < ι'. οἴνου Χίου ἀθαλάσσου τὸ ἱκανὸν, ἀνάπλασσε τροχίσκους, ἀνὰ δραχμιαίους, καὶ δίδου μετ᾽ οἴνου ἀκράτου κοτύλης.

[Ἄλλη πρὸς ἐχιοδήκτους.] Μελίας φύλλα κόψας, καὶ ἐκθλίψας τὸν χυλὸν, δίδου μετ᾽ οἴνου πίνειν, καὶ τοῖς φύλλοις τοῖς ἀποτεθλιμμένοις τὸ τραῦμα κατάπλασσε.

[Ἄλλη πρὸς φαλαγγιοδήκτους.] Ἑνὶ τροχίσκῳ τῆς

triobolares, ac dato unum ex vino. *Aliud antidotum, theriaca ad ſcorpionum ictus et quae morſu virus emittere videntur, ad rupta et convulſiones; inflationes coli et multa ſimilia; hanc medicinam Gallus ex Arabia profectus Caeſari donavit, multis ea commilitonibus ſervatis.* ℞. Radicis bryoniae albae drach. viij, trifolii ſeminis drach. iv, ireos, chalcitidis, utriusque drach. iv, ariſtolochiae tenuis drach. iv, roriſmarini radicis drach. iv, ſucci papaveris drach. iv, zingiberis drach. iv, ſeminum rutae ſilveſtris ʒ vj, ſerpilli drach. iij, cumini Aethiopici drach. iij, radicis eryngii drach. iij, ervi farinae albae drach. x, vini Chii marinae expertis quod ſatis eſt; paſtillos ſingito qui pendent ʒ ſinguli et ex vini meraci hemina dato.

[*Aliud ad viperarum morſus.*] ℞. Fraxini ſoliis contuſis expreſſisque ſuccum ex vino potui dato, ſoliiſque contractis vulnus obducito.

[*Aliud ad phalangiorum morſus.*] Uni paſtillo try-

τρυγόνος μίσγε πεπέρεως κόκκους ιγ'. σπέρματος φύλλου κόκκους μ'. ἐξ οἴνου κράματος πότιζε θερμοῦ ἐπὶ ἡμέρας γ'.

["Αλλη ὁμοίως ποιοῦσα.] ℞ Ἀριστολοχίας Κρητικῆς μακρᾶς < α'. κυμίνου Αἰγυπτίου τριώβολον, πηγάνου ἀγρίου σπέρματος < στ'. ὀποῦ Κυρηναϊκοῦ < γ' S''. μίλτου Λημνίας < ι'. σμύρνης < ζ'. ὀποβαλσάμου < η'. πεπέρεως λευκοῦ < β' S''. κάγχρυος [928] < δ'. κόψας καὶ σήσας, φύρα μέλιτι, καὶ δίδου δι' ὕδατος θερμοῦ κυάμου Αἰγυπτίου τὸ μέγεθος. ἐὰν δ' εὐτονώτερον θελήσῃ χρήσασθαι, διπλοῦν δίδου.

["Αλλη μετὰ τὰς πρώτας γεγραμμένας ἀντιδότους θηριακή.] Οὐκ οἶδ' ὅπως ἀτάκτως πρὸς ἰσχιαδικοὺς ποτήματα γράψας β'. μετὰ ταῦτα πάλιν ἔγραψεν ἀντιδότους, τὴν Ζωπύριον ὀνομαζομένην, καὶ ἄλλην θινὰ πολυμίγματον ἅπασι τοῖς θανασίμοις ἁρμόττουσαν, ὥς φησι, προλαμβανομένην τε καὶ ἐπιλαμβανομένην. ἁρμόττει δὲ καὶ λυσσοδήκτοις, καὶ πλευριτικοῖς, καὶ τοῖς ἐντὸς ἀλγήμασιν ἅπασιν, ὥσπερ γε καὶ τοῖς γυναικείοις πάθεσι, καὶ μετὰ ταύτην

gonis miſceto, piperis gr. xiij, ſeminis phylli gr. xl, ex diluta vini potione calida ad triduum propinato.

[*Aliud idem faciens.*] ℞. Ariſtolochiae Creticae longae drach. j, cumini Aegyptii obolos iij, rutae ſilveſtris ſeminis drach. vj, ſucci Cyrenaici drach. iij ß, minii Lemnii drach. x, myrrhae drach. viij, opobalſami drach. viij, piperis albi drach. ij ß, canchryos ʒ iv, contuſa cribrataque, melle conſpergito et ad ſabae Aegyptiae magnitudinem ex aqua calida propinato; quod ſi valentiori uti velis, duplum exhibeto.

[*Alia poſt commemorata prima antidota theriace.*] Haud novi quomodo potionibus ad coxendicum dolores duabus citra ordinem conſcriptis, poſtea rurſus antidota addiderit, Zopyrion dictum; ac aliud quoddam ex variis mixturis conſtans, omnibus (ut inquit) lethalibus accommodatum: ſive antea, ſive poſt aſſumatur. Caeterum congruit etiam ad rabioſorum morſus, pleuriticos et internos dolores univerſos, quemadmodum et ad mulierum affe-

πάλιν ἑτέραν πολύχρηστον ἔγραψεν ἐξ ρ'. συγκειμένην, ἐξαιρέτως δὲ, ὥς φησι, πρὸς τὰ θανάσιμα καὶ τοὺς πνιγομένους ὑπὸ ψιμμυθίου. εἶτα μετὰ ταύτας τὴν διὰ τῆς Λημνίας μίλτου, περὶ ἧς ἤδη καὶ πρόσθεν ἔγραψα, παραγράψας τὰ Δαμοκράτους ἔπη. τὴν ἄλλην οὖν παραλιπὼν, τὴν ἐξ ρ'. συγκειμένην, ἀρκεσθήσομαι τῇ τε Ζωπυρίῳ καὶ τῇ μετ' αὐτὴν γεγραμμένῃ. καὶ προσέτι τὴν διὰ τῆς Λη- (456) μνίας μίλτου παραλιπὼν τὴν ἑκατονταμίγματον. ἡ αὐτὴ γὰρ ἐστὶ τῇ ὑπ' Ἀνδρομάχου γεγραμμένῃ Ζωπύριος ἀντίδοτος, ποιοῦσα πρὸς ἅπαντα, ἰδιαίτερον δὲ πρὸς τὰ θανάσιμα καὶ πρὸς ἡπατικοὺς, καὶ τὰς ἐμπνευματώσεις τῆς κοιλίας, καὶ τὰς ἀρχομένας παρεγχύσεις, καὶ μάλιστ' ἐφ' ὧν ἐστι πλέον πνεῦμα, τὸ παρακείμενον. ℞ Σμύρνης < ε'. νάρδου Συριακῆς < ε'. S''. κρόκου < δ' S''. σχοίνου ἄνθους < β' S''. κασσίας < δ'. κινναμώμου < γ'. πεπέρεως λευκοῦ < α' S''. λιβάνου < α'. ὀβολὸν α'. κόστου < α'. μέλιτι Ἀττικῷ ἀναλάμβανε, καὶ ποιῶν τροχίσκους καρύου Ποντικοῦ τὸ μέγεθος, δίδου μετ' οἰνομέλιτος ἢ μεθ' ὕδα-

ctiones confert. Poſt hoc rurſus aliud multiplicis uſus tradidit ex centum rebus compoſitum, eximium vero, ut ait, ad lethalia et a ceruſſa ſuffocatos. Deinde poſt haec illud quod Lemnia terra conſtat appoſuit, de quo jam prius etiam egi, Damocratis carminibus adſcriptis; itaque alio quod ex centenis medicamentis conficitur praetermiſſo, ſatis mihi erit Zopyrion et poſt id ſcriptum adjicere. Praeterea eo quod ex Lemnia terra conſtat omiſſo, quod centum ſimplicia recipit. Reſpondet enim Zopyrion antidotum cum eo quod Andromachus tradidit, ad omnia efficax: ſed peculiarius ad lethalia, hepaticos, inſlationes ventris et incipientes ſuffuſiones, praeſertim in quibus id quod inſidet largior eſt ſpiritus. ℞ Myrrhae drach. v, Syriacae nardi ʒ v ß, croci ʒ iv ß, ſchoenanti ʒ ij ß, caſſiae ʒ iv, cinnamomi ʒ iij, piperis albi drach. j ß, thuris drach. j et obolum j, coſti drach. j, melle Attico excipe, ac finge trochiscos nucis avellanae magnitudine, dantur ex mulſo vel aqua. *Aliud antidotum omnibus*

τος. Ἄλλη ἀντίδοτος, ποιοῦσα πρὸς πάντα τὰ θανάσιμα, καὶ προλαμβανομένη, καὶ ἐπιλαμβανομένη. ποιεῖ καὶ πρὸς λυσσοδήκτους. ποιεῖ δὲ καὶ πρὸς πλευριτικοὺς, καὶ τὰ ἐκτὸς ἀλγήματα· εὐθετεῖ δὲ καὶ πρὸς τὰ γυναικεῖα ἀλγήματα καὶ πάθη. ♃ Γλυκυῤῥίζης < στ'. καὶ ὀβολὸν α' S''. δαύκου Κρητικοῦ σπέρματος < στ'. ὀβολὸν α' S''. ὀπίου < δ'. ὀβολοὺς β'. καστορίου < β'. ὀβολὸν ἕνα, πεπέρεως μακροῦ < στ'. τετρώβολον, κόστου < στ'. ὀβολοὺς β'. ναρδοστάχυος < στ'. ὀβολὸν α' S''. κασσίας μελαίνης < ε'. ὀβολοὺς β'. λιβάνου ἄῤῥενος < α' S''. σεσέλεως < ε'. ὀβολοὺς β'. σκορδίου < στ'. ὀβολοὺς β' S''. ὑποκυστίδος χυλοῦ < στ'. ἀκόρου < β'. μαλαβάθρου φύλλων < στ'. ὀβολὸν ἕνα, σαγαπηνοῦ < β'. βαλσάμου καρποῦ < ε'. ὀβολοὺς β'. σμύρνης < στ'. κρόκου < ζ'. ὀβολοὺς β'. στύρακος < στ'. κινναμώμου < ζ'. ὀβολοὺς β'. ζιγγιβέρεως < ζ'. ὀβολοὺς β'. πεπέρεως λευκοῦ < ε'. ὀβολοὺς β'. φοῦ < ε'. πετροσελίνου < δ'. νάρδου Κελτικῆς < δ'. ὀβολοὺς β' S''. ὑπερικοῦ < β'. ἀκακίας χυλοῦ < β'. γεντιανῆς < δ'. Ἰλλυρι-

lethalibus faciens et praeſumptum et poſtea datum; valet etiam ad rabioſorum morſus; facit et ad pleuriticos, internosque dolores; accommodatur etiam mulierum doloribus et affectionibus. ♃ Glycyrrhizae drach. vj et obolum j ß, dauci Cretici ſeminis drach. vj, obolum j ß, opii ʒ iv, obolos ij, caſtorii drach. ij, obolum j, piperis longi drach. vj, obolos iv, coſti drach. vj, obolos ij, ſpicae nardi drach. vj, ſesquiobolum, caſſiae nigrae drach. v, obolos ij, thuris masculi drach j ß, ſeſeleos ʒ v, obolos ij, ſcordii drach. vj, obolos ij ß, ſucci hypocyſtidis drach. vj, acori drach. ij, foliorum malabathri drach. vj, obolum j, ſagapeni drach. ij, fructus balſami drach. v, obolos ij, myrrhae ʒ vj, croci drach. vij, obolos ij, ſtyracis drach. vj, cinnamomi drach. vij, obolos ij, zingiberis drach. vij, obolos ij, piperis albi drach. v, obolos ij, phu ʒ v, petroſelini drach. iv, nardi Celticae drach. iv, obolos ij ß, hyperici drach. ij, acaciae ſucci drach. ij, gentianae drach. iv, iris Illyricae drach. ij, aniſi ʒ iij, thlaſpeos drach. vj,

κῆς < β΄. ἀνίσου < γ΄. θλάσπεως < στ΄. ὀβολοὺς β΄ S″. ῥόδων ξηρῶν < δ΄. μήου < β΄. κόμμεως < β΄. καρδαμώμου < δ΄. σχοίνου ἄνθους < στ΄. ὀβολοὺς β΄. ὀποπάνακος < ζ΄. ὀποβαλσάμου < στ΄ S″. χαλβάνης < γ΄. ὀβολοὺς β΄. τερμινθίνης < στ΄. ὀβολοὺς β΄. ἀγαρικοῦ < ζ΄ S″. κύφεως < στ΄. βδελλίου < στ΄. σκίγκου < β΄. ἀμώμου < γ΄. πολίου < ε΄. ὀβολοὺς β΄. δικτάμνου < στ΄. πηγάνου ἀγρίου σπέρματος < δ΄. σφραγῖδος Λημνίας < β΄ S″. ἐρυσίμου < δ΄. οἴνῳ Φαλερίνῳ ἀναλάμβανε, καὶ μέλιτι Ἀττικῷ.

[929] [*Ἄλλη ἀντίδοτος· ποιεῖ καὶ πρὸς θανάσιμα, προδιδομένη καὶ ἐπιδιδομένη, καὶ οὐδὲν ἐμποδίζουσα πρὸς τὰ λοιπὰ διδόμενα φάρμακα· ὅταν δὲ δοθῇ, ναυτίαν κινεῖ, ὥστε ἀναβάλλεσθαι πᾶν τὸ φθαρτικόν.*] ℞ *Μίλτου σφραγῖδος Λημνίας* < α΄. ὀβολοὺς β΄. ἀρκευθίδων < β΄. λεῖα τρίψας, ἀναλάμβανε ἐλαίῳ καλλίστῳ, καὶ δίδου καρύου Ποντικοῦ τὸ μέγεθος σὺν οἰνομέλιτι.

[*Ἐκ τῶν Ἀφροδᾶ πρὸς ὑδροφόβους.*] ℞ *Λαθυρίδος*

obolos ij ß, rofarum ficcarum drach. iv, mei drach. ij, gummi drach. ij, cardamomi drach. iv, fchoenanti drach. vj, obolos ij, opopanacis drach. vij, opobalfami drach. vj ß, galbani drach. iij, obolos ij, refinae terebinthinae drach. vj, obolos ij, agarici drach. vij ß, cypheos drach. vj, bdellii drach. vj, fcinci drach. ij, amomi drach. iij, polii drach. v, obolos ij, dictamni ʒ vj, rutae filveftris feminis drach. iv, figilli Lemnii drach. ij ß, eryfimi drach. iv, vino Phalerno et Attico melle excipiantur.

[*Aliud antidotum; valet ad lethalia praefumptum, et poftea datum, nihilque reliqua medicamenta exhibita impedit; quum vero datum fuerit, naufeam movet, quoad totum quod perniciofum eft, expellatur.*] ℞ Minii figilli Lemnii ʒ j, obolos ij, baccarum juniperi ʒ ij, oleo quam optimo trita excipe, daque nucis avellanae magnitudine cum mulfo.

[*Ex commentariis Aphrodae ad aquae metum.*] ℞ La-

οὐγγίας α'. καστορίου < γ'. λειώσας, δίδου μετὰ κοτύλης δραχμῆς ῥοδίνου πίνειν.

[*Καταπότιον τοῦ αὐτοῦ ὑδροφοβικόν.*] ℞ *Καστορίου* < α' S''. λαθυρίδων κόκκους θ'. δίδου.

[*Ἄλλως, παρὰ Νικοστράτου.*] ℞ *Καστορίου* < η'. λυκίου Ἰνδικοῦ < δ'. γεντιανῆς < β'. καρκίνων κεκαυμένων < α' S''. μέλιτι μίξας δίδου.

[*Πρὸς δὲ ὑδροφόβον, θαυμαζόμενον.*] *Εἰ* ὕδωρ εἰς ὃ ἀποκαταῤῥίπτουσιν οἱ σιδηρουργοὶ τὰ σιδηρᾶ, ἀγνοοῦντος τοῦ τεχνίτου δίδοται, λίαν θαυμάζεται. τοῖς δὲ ἤδη φοβουμένοις τὸ ὕδωρ, ἵνα πίῃ, ὑπόθες τῷ ποτηρίῳ ῥάκος ἀπὸ ἀφέδρου, καὶ πίεται. ποιεῖ δὲ καὶ γεντιανὴ καθ' ἑαυτὴν, κοχλιάρια γ'. σὺν ὕδατι.

[*Ἀμαράντου Γραμματικοῦ πρὸς ποδαλγικοὺς, ᾧ καὶ αὐτὸς ἐχρῆτο.*] ℞ *Ῥήου Ποντικοῦ* < ι'. πεπέρεως λευκοῦ < η'. πετροσελίνου, ἀγαρικοῦ, ὑπερικοῦ, ἀκόρου, ἠρυγγίου, ἀνὰ < ιστ'. καρδαμώμου, θλάσπεως, ἀκακίας, γλυκείας χυλοῦ < β'. ῥόδων ξηρῶν, ἀνὰ < ιδ'. μαράθρου σπέρματος

thyridis ℥ j, castorii ʒ iij, laevigata cum hemina rosacei dantur potui.

[*Pilula ejusdem ad aquae metum.*] ℞ Castorii ʒ j ß, lathyridum g. ix, dato.

[*Aliter, a Nicostrato.*] ℞ Castorii ʒ viij, lycii Indici ʒ iv, gentianae ʒ ij, cancrorum crematorum ʒ j ß, melle mixta dato.

[*Ad aquae metum admirabile.*] Si aqua in qua fabri ferrumen abstergunt, inscio artifice, exhibeatur, mirum in modum perficit: at iis qui jam aquam extimescunt, ut bibant, poculo panniculum ex sella supponito et bibitur. Confert etiam gentiana per se, tribus cochleariis cum aqua.

[*Amaranti Grammatici ad pedum dolores, quo etiam ipse usus est.*] ℞ Rhei Pontici drach. x, piperis albi drach. viij, petroselini, agarici, hyperici, acori, eryngii, singulorum drach. xvj, cardamomi, thlaspeos, acaciae, succi glycyrrhizae drach. ij, rosarum siccarum, singulorum

< β΄. ἀριστολοχίας μακρᾶς < β΄. καὶ στρογγύλης, ὀξυμυρσίνης καρποῦ, ἀνὰ < γ΄. σελίνου σπέρματος < γ΄. βουνιάδος ἀγρίας σπέρματος < γ΄. ζιγγιβέρεως < γ΄. γεντιανῆς < στ΄. σκίγκου < β΄. λιβανωτοῦ < ε΄. φοῦ Ποντικοῦ < γ΄. ἐρυσίμου < στ΄. ἴρεως Ἰλλυρικῆς < ιγ΄. κασσίας, λιγυστικοῦ, σχοίνου ἄνθους, ναρδοστάχυος, σίου, σκορπιούρου, ἀνὰ < στ΄. μέλιτος τὸ ἱκανόν. δίδου μέγεθος Ποντικοῦ καρύου ἐπ' ἐνιαυτόν.

[*Ἄλλο, ᾧ ἐγὼ χρῶμαι.*] ♃ Χαμαίδρυος < οδ΄. σκορδίου < γ΄. πετροσελίνου < γ΄. καρδαμώμου < γ΄. πρασίου, γεντιανῆς ἀνὰ < δ΄. κενταυρίου < δ΄ S″. ἀριστολοχίας στρογγύλης ἴσον, μέλιτος τὸ ἱκανόν. δίδου Ποντικοῦ καρύου μέγεθος σὺν ὕδατι ἐπ' ἐνιαυτόν.

drach. xiv, feminis foeniculi drach. ij, ariftolochiae longae drach. ij et rotundae, baccarum rufci, utriusque drach. iij, feminis apii drach. iij, feminis napi filveftris drach. iij, zingiberis drach. iij, gentianae drach. vj, fcinci drach. ij. thuris drach. v, phu Pontici drach. iij, irionis drach. vj, iridis Illyricae drach. xiij, caffiae, liguftici, fchoenanthi, fpicae nardi, fii, fcorpiuri, fingulorum drach. vj, mellis quod fatis eft: datur nucis avellanae magnitudo ad annum.

[*Aliud, quo ego utor.*] ♃ Chamaedryos drach. lxxxiv, fcordii drach. iij, petrofelini drach. iij, cardamomi drach. iij, marrubii, gentianae, utriusque drach. iv, centaurii drach iv ß, ariftolochiae rotundae tantundem, mellis quod fufficit: datur ad nucis avellanae magnitudinem cum aqua ad annum.

ΓΑΛΗΝΟΥ ΠΡΟΣ ΠΙΣΩΝΑ ΠΕΡΙ ΤΗΣ ΘΗΡΙΑΚΗΣ ΒΙΒΛΙΟΝ.

Ed. Chart. XIII. [930.] Ed. Baf. II. (456.)

[930] *Κεφ. α'. [Πίσωνι τὸν λόγον ἀνατίθησιν, Ἀνδρόμαχον ἐπαινεῖ, καὶ τῆς γραφθησομένης πραγματείας τὸ αἴτιον ἐκδηλοῖ ὁ Γαληνός.]* Καὶ τοῦτόν σοι τὸν περὶ τῆς θηριακῆς λόγον ἀκριβῶς ἐξετάσας ἅπαντα, ἄριστε Πίσων, σπουδαίως ἐποίησα, καὶ μάλιστα ἐπεί σε κατεῖδον περὶ τὴν γνῶσιν αὐτῆς μὴ παρέργως ἔχοντα. εἰσελθὼν γάρ ποτε πρός σε κατὰ τὸ ἔθος, πολλὰ μὲν καὶ ἄλλα τῶν συνήθων σοι παρακείμενα βιβλία εὗρον. καὶ γὰρ καὶ ἄλλως ἐστί σοι φίλον, μετὰ τὰς δημοτικὰς τῶν πράξεων ἀσχολίας, τοῖς

GALENI AD PISONEM DE THERIACA LIBER.

Cap. I. *[Librum dicat Pifoni, Andromachum commendat, et caufam operis confcribendi aperit Galenus.]* Librum hunc de Theriaca tibi (optime Pifo) omnibus accurate perpenfis ftudiofe conftruxi, quum potiffimum te ad ejus cognitionem haud frigide affectum perfpexerim. Profectus enim interdum ad te pro more, multos fane et diverfos a confuetis libros tibi propofitos offendi. Etenim tibi gratum eft, ac praefertim a publicis negotiorum

παλαιοῖς τῶν φιλοσόφων ἀνδρῶν ὁμιλεῖν. γενόμενον δέ τι σύγγραμμα περὶ τῆς ἀντιδότου ταύτης οὐκ ἀηδῶς ἀνεγίνωσκες τότε, καί μοι παραστάντι σοι εὐθέως μὲν φιλικοῖς ἐνεῖδες τοῖς ὄμμασι, δεξιῶς δὲ καὶ προσηγόρευσας, καὶ μετὰ ταῦτα πάλιν ἀνεγίνωσκες τὸ βιβλίον, ἀκροατὴν ἔχων ἐμέ. ἤκουον δὲ καὶ αὐτὸς, οὐκ ἀμελῶς γὰρ ἦν τὸ σύγγραμμα συντεταγμένον ὑπό τινος Ἀνδρομάχου καλουμένου, ἐντελῶς πεπαιδευμένου τὴν τέχνην, μὴ μόνον τῇ πείρᾳ τῶν ἔργων, ἀλλὰ καὶ τοῖς λόγοις, τὸν ἐπ᾽ αὐτοῖς λογισμὸν ἀκριβῶς ἠσκημένου. τὸ γοῦν ἄρχειν ἡμῶν, διὰ τὴν ἐν τούτοις ὑπεροχὴν, ὑπὸ τῶν κατ᾽ ἐκεῖνον καιρὸν βασιλέων ἦν πεπιστευμένος, ὥς ἔμοιγε δοκεῖ, τάχα τι καὶ τῆς πατρίδος αὐτῷ εἰς τὸ ἀκριβῶς ἐκμαθεῖν τὴν ἰατρικὴν συναραμένης. Κρὴς γὰρ τὸ γένος ἦν, καὶ εἰκὸς ἦν τὴν Κρήτην, ὡς ἄλλα (457) πολλὰ τῶν βοτανῶν, οὕτω καὶ εἴς τι φάρμακον ἀγαθὸν τοῖς ἀνθρώποις ἐνεγκεῖν τὸν τοιοῦτον ἄνδρα. ἀναγινώσκοντος δέ σου τὰ γεγραμμένα, πάνυ γε ἐγὼ ἔχαιρον, ὅτι οὕτως ἀκριβῶς προσεῖχες τοῖς ὑπὸ τοῦ ἀνδρὸς λεγομένοις, καὶ ἀλη-

occupationibus cum veteribus philoſophis viris conſuetudinem habere. Imo commentarium quendam de Antidoto hac conſcriptum, tunc non ſine voluptate legebas; et me tibi aſtantem, ilico amicis intuitus oculis, comiter etiam alloquebaris; ac deinde iterum, me audiente, librum relegebas. Auſcultabam vero et ipſe, quoniam commentarius non oſcitanter erat compoſitus a quodam Andromacho vocato, qui artem non modo rerum experientia perfecte calluerit, ſed etiam ſermonibus ratiocinationem in ipſis prorſus exercuerit. Itaque praecellere ipſum noſtralibus, quod his in rebus praevaleret, illius tempeſtatis reges, meo quidem judicio, crediderunt, forſan patria quoque nonnihil ad medicinam exquiſite diſcendam ipſi opitulante. Cretenſis ſiquidem erat natione; ac veriſimile eſt Cretam, ut diverſas pleraſque herbas, ita etiam ad quoddam medicamentum ſalutare hominibus talem virum tuliſſe Quum autem illius ſcripta perlegeres, admodum ego gaviſus ſum, quod ita accurate mentem iis quae ab illo dicebantur.

θῶς μέγα με θαῦμα κατεῖχε, καὶ τῇ καθ' ἡμᾶς τύχῃ πολλὴν τὴν χάριν εἶχον, ὅτι σε φιλοπόνως οὕτως ἔχοντα περὶ τὴν τέχνην ἔβλεπον. οἱ μὲν γὰρ πολλοὶ τῶν ἄλλων ἀνθρώπων μόνην τὴν ἀκοὴν ὑπὸ τῶν ταύτης λόγων εὐφραίνεσθαι θέλουσι. σὺ δὲ οὐ μόνον τῶν λεγομένων ἡδέως ἀκούεις, ἀλλὰ καὶ πολλὰ τῶν μὴ λεγομένων ἐξ ἐμφύτου συνέσεως εὑρίσκεις εὐφυῶς. ἔνια δὲ καὶ τῶν ἔργων οὕτως ἀκριβῶς ἐπίστασαι καὶ βλέπεις, ὡς οἱ φιλοπόνως μαθόντες ἡμεῖς. ὅπερ ὡς ἀληθῶς ἐγὼ θεασάμενος ἐπὶ σοῦ καὶ πάνυ κατεπλάγην. ὁπότε γάρ σου τῶν παίδων ὁ φίλτατος τὴν περὶ τὸ περιτόναιον διάθεσιν ἔσχεν ἔκ τινος τοῦ [931] ἱππεύειν ἀνάγκης, ἐπειδή τις καὶ δημοτελὴς ἦν μυστηρίων ἱερουργὸς, διὰ θρησκείαν, τὴν ὑπὲρ Ῥωμαίων θεῶν ἀναγκαίως ἀγομένην τότε, ἐφ' ᾧ δὴ καὶ τοὺς εὐγενεστάτους παῖδας ἱππεύοντας εὐρύθμως, καὶ χορεύοντας, ὥσπερ τοῖς ἵπποις, ἔδει τινὰ τῶν μυστηρίων καὶ αὐτοὺς ἐπιτελεῖν. ὅτε δὴ καὶ τοῦ παιδὸς τοῦ σοῦ ἁπαλοῦ τυγχάνοντος πάνυ, ὁ τόπος οὗτος περιθλασθεὶς, βιαίως ἀπέστη τε τῶν ὑποκει-

intenderes vereque magna me admiratio detinuit, atque noſtrae fortunae multam gratiam habui, quod te tanto artis ſtudio teneri conſpexerim. Siquidem plerique aliorum hominum ſolas aures hujus ſententiis oblectari deſiderant; tu vero non ſolum ea quae dicuntur, cum oblectatione audis, verum etiam multa quae non exprimuntur, inſita prudentia ingenioſe invenis; nonnulla opera quoque tam accurate pernoviſti et perſpicis, ut nos qui ſtudioſo labore didicimus. Quod quam veriſſime ego in te contemplatus et magnopere ſum admiratus. Nam quum liberorum tuorum cariſſimus ex quadam equitandi neceſſitate peritonaei affectu laboraret; ut qui ſacris adminiſtrandis publice eſſet praefectus, ceremoniarum gratia, quae diis Romanorum neceſſario tunc fiebant; quamobrem et generoſiſſimos pueros concinne equitantes, ſaltantesque, tanquam equis ſacra quaedam et ipſos obire oportebat. Quum igitur filii tui natura admodum teneri, locus hic undequaque contuſus violenter, a ſubjectis partibus ab-

μένων, καὶ μετ' αὐτὸ πῦον συναγαγὼν, ἐδεήθη καὶ τομῆς, καὶ ὁ μὲν παῖς, ὥσπερ τὶς ἀνὴρ ἤδη, τλημόνως ἁπάντων ἀνεχόμενος, ἐπιεικῶς ἐθεραπεύετο, καθάπερ ἔκ τινος τοῦ φιλοσοφίας λόγου, καρτερίᾳ τε καὶ ἀνδρείᾳ πρὸς τὰ παρόντα εὐφυῶς συνησκημένος. σὺ δὲ ἐφεστὼς ἀκριβῶς οὕτως ἔβλεπες, καὶ τοῖς γιγνομένοις ὑφ' ἡμῶν ἅπασι προσεῖχες, ὡς εἴ ποτέ τι καὶ παρέργως ἐγίγνετο, εὐθέως ἐφεστάναι, καὶ παραινεῖν κατὰ τὸν Ἱπποκράτην, μηδὲν εἰκῆ ποιεῖν. ἐγὼ δέ τι καὶ φιλοτιμότερον θεώμενος, περιεργότερον τὸ ὑπὸ σοῦ γιγνόμενον ἔβλεπον. εἴ ποτε γάρ τι καὶ τῶν ἐπιθετιμένων ὑπὸ τοῦ θεραπεύοντος φαρμάκων ἀτόπως ἔκειτο, τοῦτο τοῖς σαυτοῦ δακτύλοις μετετίθεις τε καὶ δεόντως ἥρμοττες τῷ τραύματι, ὡς θαυμαστὸν εἶναι δοκεῖν, ἐκ τῆς περὶ τὸν υἱόν σου στοργῆς καὶ τῆς φυσικῆς ἐντρεχείας, αἰφνίδιόν σοι οὕτω τῶν χειρῶν ἐνδεικνυμένων ἀκριβῆ τέχνην, καὶ τοῦτ' ἄρ' ἦν ἰδεῖν ἐπὶ σοῦ φαινόμενον ἐκεῖνο, ὥσπερ δὴ καὶ ὁ σοφώτατος Πλάτων, ὡς εἰκὸς ἐπὶ πολλῶν πολλάκις ἰδὼν, καὶ χαίρων τῇ τῆς ἀληθείας ἀνάγκῃ, καὶ τὰς μαθή-

fcederet, ac deinde pure collecto, incifione etiam opus haberet; puer fane tanquam vir quidam jam patienter omnia fuftinens praeter expectationem curabatur, ceu ex quodam philofophiae ftudio, fortitudine ac magnanimitate ad praefens malum probe inftructus exercitatusque. Tu vero adftans diligenter infpiciebas, animumque omnibus quae a nobis fiebant, intendebas; ut fi quando nonnihil etiam ofcitanter fieret, ftatim inftares, admoneresque fecundum Hippocratem, nihil temere agendum. Sed ego aliquid etiam laudabilius fpectans difficilius a te fieri animadverti, nempe fi quando medicamentum quoddam a medente impofitum fuo in loco minus recte haerebat, id tuifmet digitis transpofitum, apte vulneri applicabas, ut miraculum effe videretur, te tam repente manibus ex tuo erga filium amore et naturali dexteritate, abfolutam artem oftendiffe. Atque id ipfum tibi ufu venire comperio, quemadmodum etiam Plato fapientiffimus in multis, ut eft confentaneum, frequenter fpeculatus et veritatis gau-

σεις ἀναμνήσεις εἶναι λέγει, καὶ τὴν ψυχὴν, πάντων τὰς ἐννοίας ἔχειν δοκεῖν, ἐμφαίνεσθαι δὲ αὐτὰς τότε, ὅτε ἡ χρεία καλεῖ. ὥσπερ δὲ δὴ καὶ ἐπὶ σοῦ, διὰ τὴν περὶ τὸν παῖδα φροντίδα, ἀπροσδόκητος ἡμῖν ἡ παροῦσά σοι τῆς τέχνης ἐμπειρία κατεφαίνετο, καὶ εἰκότως φιλόκαλός τε ὢν, οὕτω καὶ εὐφυής. οὐδὲ περὶ τὸ φάρμακον τοῦτο τὴν θηριακὴν ἔσχες ἀμελῶς, ἀλλ' ἐσπούδασας αὐτοῦ εἰδέναι τήν τε δύναμιν καὶ τὴν κρᾶσιν, τόν τε καιρὸν καὶ τὸ μέτρον τῆς χρήσεως ἀκριβῶς ἐκμαθεῖν.

Κεφ. β'. [Θηριακῆς ἔπαινος καὶ διάγνωσις, καὶ τῶν περὶ ταύτην ἀρχόντων Ῥωμαίων σπουδή.] Καὶ γὰρ ἐστὶν ὡς ἀληθῶς, παρὰ τοῖς ἀνθρώποις ἅπασιν ἐνδοξότατον, διά τε τὸ ἄπταιστον τῆς ἐπαγγελίας καὶ διὰ τὸ δυνατὸν τῆς ἐνεργείας· οὔτε γάρ τις δηχθείς ποτε ὑπὸ τῶν ἀναιρεῖν εἰωθότων θηρίων εὐθὺς πιὼν τὴν ἀντίδοτον ἀποθανὼν ἱστόρηται, οὔτ' ἂν προπιών τις, εἶτ' οὐ μετὰ πολὺ δηχθεὶς ἰσχυρότερον πρὸς τὸ ἀποκτεῖναι τὸν ἰὸν ἔσχε τοῦ θηρίου, ὅπερ πολλάκις καὶ τῶν ἀρχόντων τινὲς, ἐξουσίαν θανάτου

dens necefſitate et diſciplinas, inquit, rerum eſſe recordationes et animum omnium habere videri notitias; quae tunc nimirum apparent, quum uſus poſtulat. Ita in te quoque ob filii ſolicitudinem praeſens tibi artis experientia praeter noſtram opinionem apparebat. Nec id ſane immerito, quum ſis adeo honeſti amans atque ingenioſus. Neque in hoc medicamento theriacam neglexiſti; verum et facultatem ipſius et temperamentum ſcire ſtuduiſti, ad haec, tempus, menſuramque uſus adamuſſim perdiſcere.

Cap. II. [*Theriacae commendatio et dignotio, principumque Romanorum hac in re ſtudium.*] Etenim hoc eſt, ut revera, apud univerſos homines celebratiſſimum, tum ob pollicitationis certitudinem, tum ob ipſius actionis facultatem. Nullus enim unquam a feris quae interimere conſueverunt, commorſus narratur, qui hac ſtatim epota antidoto interierit. Nullus eadem praeſumpta, haud multo poſt morſu impetitus, ferae veneno ceu illam ſuperante occubuit; quod ſaepe nonnulli praetores etiam,

καὶ ζωῆς ἔχοντες. εἶτα τὸ κρῖναι τὸ φάρμακον θέλοντες, εἰ τοῦθ' ὅπερ ἐπαγγέλλεται, καὶ δρᾷν δύναται, ἐπὶ τῶν ἤδη διά τινας πονηρὰς καὶ παρανόμους πράξεις κατακριθέντων ἀποθανεῖν δοκιμάζουσιν αὐτὸ, ἡμεῖς μὲν ἐπ' ἀνθρώπων τὴν κρίσιν αὐτοῦ ποιεῖσθαι μὴ δυνάμενοι, ἐπί τινων ἄλλων ζώων τὸ αὐτὸ δρῶντες, τὴν ἀληθῆ τοῦ φαρμάκου κρίσιν εὑρίσκειν πειρώμεθα. ἀλεκτρυόνας γὰρ λαβόντες, τοὺς μὴ ὅσοι γέ τινες οἰκοδίαιτοί τέ εἰσιν, καὶ ἡμῖν ὁμορόφιοι, ἄγριοι δὲ μᾶλλον τυγχάνουσιν ὄντες, καὶ ξηρότερον κεκραμένοι τὸ σῶμα, οὕτως αὐτοῖς προβάλλομεν τὰ θηρία, καὶ τὰ μὲν εὐθέως ἀποθνήσκει τὰ μὴ πιόντα, ὅσα δὲ πέπωκεν, ἰσχύει καὶ μετὰ τὸ δῆγμα τὴν ζωὴν ἔχει. [932] δοκιμάζειν δ' ἐνίοτε χρὴ τὸ φάρμακον, εἰ μή ἐστι δεδολωμένον. καὶ τούτῳ τῷ τρόπῳ. διδόντες γάρ τι τῶν διὰ γαστρὸς καθαίρειν δυναμένων φαρμάκων, προδίδομεν τῆς θηριακῆς, καὶ ὅταν δοθείσης αὐτῆς μὴ καθαίρηται ὁ λαβὼν τὸ καθαρτικὸν φάρμακον. αὐτῷ δοκιμάζομεν τὴν ἀντίδοτον ἀρίστην οὖσαν, ἐπειδὴ ἐκώλυσε τὴν κάθαρσιν γενέσθαι τῷ

penes quos vitae et necis poteſtas eſt, experiuntur, atque medicamentum probare volentes, an quod promittat, praeſtare quoque poſſit, in reis jam ob prava quaedam et illegitima facinora ad mortem judicatis id explorarunt. Nos autem quum in hominibus hujus rei explorationem facere non poſſimus, in aliis quibusdam animantibus idem facientes, veram medicamenti probationem invenire conamur; gallis namque domi non enutritis, neque nobis ſunt contubernales, ſed potius agreſtibus et ſicciore praeditis corporis temperamento captis, ſic feras objicimus, et qui inter illos non biberint ex medicamento, protinus intereunt; qui vero biberint, convaleſcunt et a morſu vitam retinent. Interdum vero medicamentum num adulteratum ſit, hoc quoque modo probare convenit. Dantes enim portionem eorum quae per ventrem purgare queant medicamentorum, prius theriacam exhibemus; quicunque data ipſa non purgetur, qui purgans ſumpſit medicamentum, hoc ipſo judicamus antidotum eſſe praeſtantiſſimam,

λαβόντι τὸ καθαρτικὸν φάρμακον, ὡς διὰ τὴν τοιαύτην κρίσιν, μή ποτ᾽ ἂν ἡμᾶς σφαλῆναι περὶ τὴν τοῦ ἀληθοῦς φαρμάκου εὕρεσιν. πολλὴ γάρ ἐστιν ὑπὸ τῶν πανουργούντων καὶ ἡ περὶ αὐτὸ γινομένη πανουργία, καὶ οἱ πολλοὶ τῇ δόξῃ μόνῃ τῆς ἀντιδότου ἀπατώμενοι, παρὰ τῶν καπηλικῶς χρωμένων τῇ τέχνῃ, πλείστῳ ἀργυρίῳ, κἂν μὴ καλῶς ἐσκευασμένον ᾖ, ὠνοῦνται τὸ φάρμακον. εἰσὶ γὰρ καὶ τῶν ὑγιαινόντων τινὲς οἳ ἐν ὅλῳ καὶ παντὶ τῷ ἑαυτῶν βίῳ ἀδιαλείπτως χρῶνται τῷ φαρμάκῳ, μάλιστα ὅσοι διὰ τὸ σκαιὸν, καὶ ἀνελεύθερον τοῦ τρόπου μὴ ζῶσιν ἀμερίμνως, ἀλλ᾽ ἀεὶ πρὸς τὸ ἐπιβουλεύεσθαι τὴν ὑποψίαν τοῦ ῥᾳδίως ὑπὸ τῶν ἐχθρῶν ἀποθανεῖν ἔχουσιν. ἔνιοι δὲ δι᾽ ὠφέλειαν τοῦ σώματος καθ᾽ ἑκάστην ἡμέραν προσφέρονται τοῦ φαρμάκου, ὥσπερ δὴ τὸν θεῖον Μάρκον καὶ ἡμεῖς οἴδαμεν ἐνθέσμως ποτὲ βασιλεύσαντα, καὶ ἀκριβῶς ἑαυτοῦ διὰ τὴν σύνεσιν τῇ συγκράσει τοῦ σώματος παρακολουθήσαντα, κατακόρως τε, καὶ ὥς τινι τροφῇ χρησάμενον τῷ φαρμάκῳ. ἐξ ἐκείνου γὰρ καὶ μᾶλλον δεδόξασται τὸ φάρμακον, καὶ

quandoquidem purgationem ei qui medicamento ufus fit purgante prohibuit ut tali probatione a veri medicamenti inventione nunquam aberraverimus. Multae fiquidem a fraudulentis in hoc quoque fraudes fiunt; ac vulgus fola antidoti opinione deceptum ab iis, quibus ars eft mercenaria, plurimo argento medicamentum etiam prave confectum redimit. Sunt enim et ex fanis qui tota omnique ipforum vita affidue medicamento utantur, praefertim qui ob inhumanos illiberalesque mores non citra folicitudinem degunt, fed perpetuo fufpicionem habent, facile ab inimicis fibi ftrui mortis infidias. Nonnulli vero corporis juvandi gratia quotidie medicamentum affumunt, quemadmodum fane divum Marcum nos quoque novimus, qui legitime aliquando imperium geffit et adamuffim, ut erat vir prudens, corporis fuis temperamentum intellexit, abunde et veluti alimento quodam medicamento effe ufum. Ab illo namque viro potius medicamentum bonae exiftimationis cepit initium et facultas

εἰς τὸ φανερὸν αὐτοῦ τοῖς ἀνθρώποις ἡ δύναμις τῆς ἐνεργείας ἐλήλυθε. τῇ γὰρ ἐπὶ τὸν βασιλέα γενομένῃ ὑγιεινῇ καταστάσει τὴν πίστιν τῆς ὠφελείας ἡ ἀντίδοτος μᾶλλον προσείληφεν. ἀλλ᾽ ἐπὶ μὲν ἐκείνου τοῦ βασιλέως μόνον αὐτῆς τὸ ἔργον εἰς τὴν γνῶσιν τῶν εἰδότων κοινὸν ἦν, ἐπὶ δὲ τῶν νῦν μεγίστων αὐτοκρατόρων ἡ χρῆσις εἰς τὸ κοινὸν ἔφθασε. πᾶσι γὰρ ἡμῖν ἔξεστι τοῖς παρ᾽ αὐτῶν κεχρῆσθαι καλῶς καὶ θεραπεύεσθαι ἀφθόνως, ἄλλου παρ᾽ ἄλλου λαμβάνοντος τὸ φάρμακον, ἐπεὶ μὴ μόνον τῷ παρὰ θεῶν ἔχειν τὸ βασιλεύειν ὑπερέχουσιν ἁπάντων, ἀλλὰ καὶ τῷ τῶν ἀγαθῶν ἁπάντων ἅπασι μεταδιδόναι ἡδέως, ὥσπερ καὶ αὐτοὶ οἱ θεοὶ, ἐν τῷ ἴσῳ καὶ τοσούτῳ τὴν εὐφροσύνην ἔχοντες, ἐν ὅσῳ περ καὶ οἱ ἀπ᾽ αὐτῶν διασωζόμενοι διατίθενται, καὶ νομίζοντες τὸ μέγιστον εἶναι τῆς βασιλείας μέρος τὴν τοῦ κοινοῦ σωτηρίαν, ὅπερ δὴ καὶ μᾶλλον ἐπ᾽ αὐτῶν τεθαύμακα. οὐ γὰρ περὶ τοῦτο τὸ φάρμακον μόνον τὴν σπουδὴν ἔχουσιν, ἀλλ᾽ οὕτως εἰσὶ περὶ πάντα φιλότιμοι, ὡς εἴ ποτέ τινι τῶν φίλων αὐτοῦ χρεία γένοιτο, θαυμαστὸν ὅπως

ipſius actionis hominibus innotuit; ex contracta namque imperatoris ſana conſtitutione fidem utilitatis antidotus majorem conſequuta eſt. Verum illius principis tempore ad eorum duntaxat cognitionem, qui viderant, theriacae opus perveniebat; ſub hujus autem ſeculi maximis imperatoribus uſus ejus prodiit in publicum. Omnibus enim licet nobis ipſorum bonis probe uti et liberaliter curare, alio ab alio medicamentum capiente; quoniam non ſolum hoc nomine caeteris omnibus praecellunt, quod imperium a diis ſint adepti, ſed etiam quod univerſa bona univerſis libenter impartiant, ſicut et dii ipſi tantum ex aequo gaudii concipiunt, quantus eorum numerus extiterit, qui ab ipſis redduntur incolumes, cenſentque maximam regni eſſe partem communem omnium ſalutem; quod ſane in ipſis etiam magis ſum admiratus. Non enim in hoc duntaxat medicamento conſiciendo ponunt induſtriam, ſed ita ſunt in omnibus erga commune benigni magnificique, ut ſi quando amicis aliquibus uſus venerit, mirum ſit quam

ἐξ ἑτοίμου, καὶ μετὰ πολλῆς τῆς προθυμίας κοινωνοῦσι τῶν φαρμάκων. οὐ γὰρ περιμένοντες τὴν ἀνάγκην τῆς χρήσεως, τότε καὶ σκευάζουσιν αὐτὰ, ἀλλὰ πρὸς τὸ τάχος τῆς τῶν καιρῶν ὀξύτητος ἑτοίμην καὶ τὴν παρασκευὴν αὐτῶν φιλοκάλως ἔχουσιν. (458) ὁπότε γοῦν Ἀντίπατρος, ὁ τὰς Ἑλληνικὰς ἐπιστολὰς αὐτῶν πράττειν πεπιστευμένος, καὶ διὰ τὸ σεμνὸν τοῦ ἤθους καὶ διὰ τὴν ἐν τοῖς ῥητορικοῖς λόγοις ἐντελῆ παιδείαν μεγάλως ὑπ' αὐτῶν τιμώμενος, τῇ νεφριτικῇ διαθέσει περιπεσὼν, δεινὰ καὶ ἀνήκεστα ὑπὸ τοῦ πάθους ἔπασχεν, ἀξιέπαινον αὐτῶν εἶδον τὴν περὶ τοὺς φίλους εἰς τὸ σώζεσθαι σπουδὴν, καὶ θαυμαστὴν τὴν περὶ τὴν ἰατρικὴν φιλοτιμίαν. οὕτω γὰρ πρὸς τὸ ποικίλον καὶ διάφορον τῶν συμπτωμάτων ἐνιστάμενοι ἀντηγωνίζοντο τῷ πάθει διὰ τῶν καλλίστων φαρμάκων, ὡς τῶν ἰατρῶν οἱ ἄριστοι, καὶ τὸν πάντα βίον περὶ τὴν ἄσκησιν αὐτῆς ἠσχολημένοι. τὴν δὲ πάντα μοι φιλτάτην Ἀῤῥίαν, καὶ αὐτὴν ὑπ' αὐτῶν ἐξόχως ἐπαινουμένην, [933] διὰ τὸ φιλοσοφεῖν ἀκριβῶς, καὶ τοῖς Πλάτωνος μάλιστα χαίρειν λόγοις, ἀνέσωσάν

prompte ac quanta alacritate medicamenta communicent. Non enim ea ubi ufus neceffitas ingruit, tunc conficiunt, fed ad ipfum temporis articulum exprompiam quoque illorum compofitionem egregie poffident. Quum igitur Antipater, qui Graecas ipforum epiftolas facere creditus eft, et propter morum gravitatem et abfolutam in dicendo facultatem magno in pretio habitus, nephritico infeftaretur affectu, gravemque ex eo et intolerabilem dolorem conciperet, ftudium ipforum amicis fervandis quavis laude digniffimum cognovi, mirificamque circa medicinam animi contentionem. Ita namque variis differentibusque fymptomatis obfiftentes cum morbo longe pulcherrimis medicamentis certabant, praeftantiffimorum medicorum inftar, qui vel omnem vitam in ipfius exercitatione contriverint. Jam vero Arriam multo omnium mihi cariffimam, quae et ipfa fupra modum ab eis commendabatur, quod diligentem philofophiae navaret operam et Platonis maxime libris gauderet, aegrotantem quandoque graviter fanarunt,

ποτε νοσήσασαν οὐ παρέργως καὶ τὸν στόμαχον ἐκλελυμένον ἔχουσαν, καὶ κειμένην οὕτως ὑπτίαν, ὡς μηδὲ τὰς τροφὰς δύνασθαι λαμβάνειν, καὶ διὰ τοῦτο εἰς τὸν τῆς ἀτροφίας κίνδυνον ἐλθεῖν· ὅτε δὴ καὶ ὡς οἱ ἐμπειρότατοι τῶν ἰατρῶν ἐθεράπευσαν τὴν γυναῖκα, ὑποδείξαντος ἐμοῦ, τὸν ἀψινθίτην οἶον παρασχόντες αὐτῇ πιεῖν· πιοῦσα γὰρ εὐθέως ἀνεῤῥώσθη τε τὸν στόμαχον, καὶ ταχέως ἀπείληφε τῆς ὀρέξεως τὸ ἔργον. τὸ δὲ ἐπὶ τοῦ σοῦ παιδὸς γενόμενον εἰκὸς ὅτι καὶ μνημονεύεις ἔτι· ὁπότε γὰρ γενομένης τῆς ἀποστάσεως σὺ μὲν, ὡς χρηστὸς πατὴρ, ὀκνηρότερον εἶχες πρὸς τὴν τομὴν, ἤπειγε δὲ ὁ καιρὸς ἀποκριθῆναι τὸ ἐγκείμενον ὑγρὸν, δόντες αὐτοὶ τὸ φάρμακον ἀπήλλαξαν ἡμᾶς τῆς μεγάλης ἐπ' αὐτῷ φροντίδος· ἐπιτεθεῖσα γὰρ ἡ ἔμπλαστρος διεῖλε μὲν τὸ ἐπικείμενον σῶμα ὀξύτερον τῆς τομῆς, ἐκένωσε δὲ πᾶν τὸ ὑγρὸν τὸ ὑποκείμενον, ὡς μηκέτ' ἔχειν διὰ τοῦτο τὸ παιδίον τὰς ἀλγηδόνας.

Κεφ. γ'. [*Τίνος ἕνεκα ἐκ πολλῶν σύγκειται ἡ ἀντίδοτος· ἔμφυτον δὲ πᾶσιν δύναμιν ὑπάρχειν, ἣν λόγῳ τε καὶ*

ſtomachique diſſolutione affectam, jacentemque adeo ſupinam, ut ne cibos quidem potuerit capere, atque ideo in atrophiae periculum veniret; non aliter quam medici expertiſſimi mulierem curaverunt, propinantes ei vinum, meo conſilio, ex abſinthio confectum. Hujus ſiquidem potu illico ſtomachum ab imbecillitate vindicavit et ſine mora appetentiae opus recuperavit. Ceterum quid in filio tuo evenerit, nimirum adhuc in memoria retines. Quum enim facto abſceſſu tu quidem, ut benignus pater, tardior ad ſectionem eſſes, tempus autem humorem contentum excerni poſtulaſſet, ipſi medicamento exhibito magna nos ipſius ſolicitudine liberarunt. Applicatum namque emplaſtrum locum quidem incumbentem celerius quam ſcalpellum diviſit, totum vero humorem ſubjectum evacuavit, ut puer hinc non amplius dolorem perſentiſceret.

Cap. III. [*Cur e multis antidotus componatur, inſitamque rebus omnibus eſſe facultatem, quam ratione*

αἰσθήσει ἰσχνεύομεν.] Ταύτην οὖν ἔχοντες περὶ ταῦτα τὰ φάρμακα, ὡς ὁρᾷς, τὴν βασιλικὴν φιλοκαλίαν, εἰκότως καὶ τὴν θηριακὴν σκευάζουσιν ἐπιμελῶς, καὶ ἓν ἕκαστον ὧν μιγνύουσιν ἀκριβῶς δοκιμάζοντες αὐτοὶ, ὡς μηδὲν παρορᾷν, καὶ διὰ τοῦτο θαυμαστῶς τὴν ἀντίδοτον ἀποτελεῖν τὰ ἔργα· καὶ γάρ ἐστιν, ὡς οἶδας, ποικιλίαν ἔχουσα τοῖς μίγμασι καὶ πολυειδῆ τὴν χρῆσιν ἐν τοῖς ἔργοις. τεθαύμακα γοῦν ἐγὼ τὸν πρῶτον ποιησάμενον αὐτῆς τὴν σκευασίαν. καί μοι δοκεῖ μήτ' ἀλόγως, ἀλλ' ἀκριβεῖ τινι λογισμῷ, καὶ βεβασανισμένῃ πάνυ τῇ φροντίδι πεποιῆσθαι αὐτῆς τὴν σύνθεσιν· οὐ γὰρ ὥσπερ οἱ ἀπὸ τῆς ἐμπειρίας ἰατροὶ ἄνευ λόγου κατὰ τὰς φύσεις ἕκαστον ἀτέχνως ἰατρεύοντες αἰσχρῶς τὰ μὲν ἐξ ὀνειράτων, τὰ δὲ καὶ παρ' αὐτῆς τῆς τύχης λαβεῖν φασιν εἰς τὴν τέχνην τὰ φάρμακα, οὕτω καὶ ἡμεῖς περὶ τὴν ἰατρικὴν σπουδάζομεν, ἀλλ' ὅσα μὲν ὁ λόγος αὐτὸς πρῶτος καὶ μόνος ἐξευρίσκειν δύναται, ταῦτα ἀκριβῶς παντὶ τῷ λογισμῷ ζητοῦντες φιλοπόνως εὑρίσκομεν, ὅσα δὲ εὑρεῖν ἀδυνατεῖ, ταῦτα διὰ τῶν αἰσθήσεων τῇ πείρᾳ κρί-

ſenſibusque inveſtigamus.] Hac igitur circa iſta medicamenta, uti vides, honeſtate regia praediti haud immerito quoque theriacen diligenter praeparant, ſingula quae miſcent accuratius probantes ipſi, quo nihil praetereant, atque hanc ob cauſam mirifica antidotum opera edere. Etenim varia eſt, ut noſti, miſtura et multiplicem in operibus uſum exhibet; quo nomine ego illum qui primus confecturam ipſius molitus eſt admiror. Quippe mihi videtur non temere, ſed exacta quadam ratione, atque explorata admodum cura compoſitionem ipſius inveniſſe. Non enim ſicuti medici, qui ſe ab unica experientia empiricos appellaverunt, neglecta naturarum ratione unumquemque ſine artificio curant, turpiter quaedam ex inſomniis, quaedam vero ab ipſa fortuna ad ipſam artem medicamenta capere ſe pronunciantes, ita nos quoque medicinam tractamus: verum quae ratio ipſa prima ſolaque poteſt invenire, eadem exacte omni conſideratione disquirentes magno ſtudio comperimus. At quae invenire ne-

νομεν, πολλάκις μηδ' αὐτῇ μόνῃ καὶ μιᾷ τῇ αἰσθήσει πιστεύοντες αὐτῶν ποιεῖσθαι τὴν κρίσιν· οὔτε γὰρ τὴν τίτανον, ὅτι λευκή ἐστιν ὥσπερ ἡ χιὼν, τῇ ὄψει μόνον ὡς ψύχουσαν κρίνειν αὔταρκες εἶναι νομίζομεν· οὐθ' ὅτι τὸ ῥόδον, διὰ τὸ ἐρυθρὸν εἶναι, διὰ τοῦτο καὶ θερμαίνειν αὐτὸ εὐθέως πεπείσμεθα, ἀλλ' ἅμα τῇ ὄψει καὶ τὴν αἴσθησιν τῆς ἁφῆς προσπαραλαμβάνοντες τὴν μὲν, ὅτι θερμαίνειν μέχρι τοῦ καίειν ἀδιαψεύστως εὑρίσκομεν, τὸ δὲ ῥόδον ἀντιπαραλαμβανόμενοι τῆς ἐπ' αὐτοῦ ψύξεως, ὅτι τῶν ἐμψυχόντων ἐστὶν, ἀκριβῶς ἐπιστεύσαμεν. καὶ οὕτω λοιπὸν ἀκριβῶς ἑκάστου τῶν φαρμάκων τὴν δυνάμιν διὰ τῆς αὐτῆς αἰσθήσεως κρίνοντες εὑρίσκομεν, τὸ μὲν ὅτι τόδε ἐστὶν ἁλμυρὸν, ἢ ὀξὺ, τὸ δ', ὅτι πικρὸν, ἢ γλυκὺ, τῇ γεύσει δοκιμάζοντες αὐτά· τὸ δ' ὅτι τὸ μὲν θερμαίνει, τὸ δὲ ψύχει, καὶ ἄλλο ὑγραίνει, ἕτερον δὲ ξηραίνει, ἡ διὰ τῆς ἁφῆς ἀντίληψις γνωρίζειν ἡμῖν παρέσχε. πολλὰ δ' αὐτῶν διὰ τῆς ὀδμῆς κρίνειν ἐπινοοῦμεν, καὶ τὸ μὲν εὔτονον τῆς δυνάμεως ἐκ τοῦ πληκτικοῦ τῆς ἀποφορᾶς εὑρίσκομεν, τὸ

quit, ea ſenſuum experimento judicamus; plerumque ne ipſi quidem ſoli ac unico ſenſui judicium de eis concredentes. Neque enim calcem quod candida ſit, quemadmodum nix, viſu duntaxat frigidam judicare ſatis eſſe cenſemus; neque roſam, quod rubra ſit, ideo etiam calefacere ipſam illico perſuademur; ſed una cum viſu ſenſum quoque tactus adhibentes illam quidem calefacere, adeo ut urat, certo invenimus; hanc vero roſam, quod frigiditatem e contrario in ea tactu percipiamus, ex refrigerantium numero eſſe firmiter credidimus. Atque hoc pacto reliquorum adamuſſim medicamentorum ſingulorum facultatem ipſo ſenſu judicantes invenimus aliud eſſe ſalſum vel acidum, aliud amarum vel dulce, guſtu ipſa explorantes. Quod autem aliud calefaciat, aliud refrigeret, aliud humectet, aliud exiccet, tactus objectio condiſcere nobis efficit. Eorum vero multa ipſo odoratu explorare ſtatuimus et facultatis robur ex vehementi exhalatione deprehendimus, imbecillitatem virtutis ex odoris

δ' ἄτονον τῆς ἰσχύος διὰ τῆς ἐκλύσεως [934] τοῦ ὀσφραντοῦ. γνωρίζωμεν δ' εἰ δόκιμόν τε καὶ μὴ, κριτήριον τῶν ἁπλῶν φαρμάκων τὰς ἑαυτῶν αἰσθήσεις ποιησάμενοι, καὶ ταύταις αὐτὰ πειράσαντες τὸ πρῶτον, καὶ διὰ τῆς χρήσεώς τε καὶ αἰσθήσεως τὸ πιστὸν αὐταῖς ἐργασάμενοι, οὕτω λοιπὸν προσάγοντες τῇ πείρᾳ τὸν λόγον, καὶ εἰς πάντα ὁδηγῷ χρώμενοι, καὶ τοῖς ἁπλοῖς φαρμάκοις δεόντως χρώμεθα, καὶ τὴν σύνθεσιν αὐτῶν τῇ τοῦ λόγου τέχνῃ ἀρίστην ποιούμεθα. ἐκμαθόντες γὰρ ἑκάστου τῶν παθῶν τὴν φύσιν, καὶ τὸ πολὺ καὶ διάφορον τῆς τῶν ἁπλῶν κράσεως εἰδότες, οὕτω σκευάζομεν τὰ σύνθετα τῶν φαρμάκων ἑκάστῳ τῶν νοσημάτων, τὸ συμφέρον διὰ τῆς ποικίλης αὐτῶν σκευασίας ποιούμενοι, καὶ πρὸς ἕκαστον τῶν ἀνθρώπων, ὅπως αὐτῷ κατεσκεύασται τὸ σῶμα, διὰ τοῦ τρόπου τῆς φαρμακείας ἐντέχνως ἁρμοσάμενοι· πολλὴ γάρ ἐστιν, ὡς οὐκ ἀγνοεῖς, παροῦσα ἡμῖν εἰς τὴν χρῆσιν ἡ τῶν φαρμάκων περιουσία, καὶ οὕτως διάφορος, ὡς μὴ μόνον αὐτῆς ἐν τῇ συνθέσει τὸ ποικίλον τῆς δυνάμεως ὁρᾶσθαι δύνασθαι, ἀλλὰ καὶ τῶν

remiſſione. At probatumne ſit an minus quodlibet medicamentum ſimplex, ſenſus ipſius judices ſtatuentes cognoſcimus; atque his primum illa experti et fide ex uſu ſenſuque aſtructa; ita deinceps experimento rationem adjungentes, ac in omnibus veluti ducem ipſam ſequentes tum ſimplicibus medicamentis congrue utimur, tum compoſitionem ipſorum rationis artificio praeſtantiſſimam reddimus. Nam morbi cujusque natura comperta, ac varietate differentiaque temperamenti ſimplicium medicamentorum cognita, ſic compoſita praeparamus, unicuique morbo quod congruum eſt, varia ipſorum compoſitione diſtribuentes, ſingulisque hominibus pro corporis ipſorum ſtatu, ut pharmacia praecipit, artificioſe adaptantes. Multa namque, uti non ignoras, penes nos eſt ad uſum parata medicamentorum copia, adeoque diverſa, ut non ſolum in compoſitione facultatis diverſitas videri queat, ſed etiam ſimplicium medicamentorum alia ex tota ipſorum ſubſtantia unam quandam et ſimplicem facultatem indicent, quem-

ἁπλῶν φαρμάκων, τὰ μὲν ἐξ ὅλης αὐτῶν τῆς οὐσίας, μίαν τινὰ καὶ ἁπλῆν ἐπιδείκνυται τὴν δύναμιν, ὥσπερ ἡ σκαμμωνία ξανθὴν χολὴν ἕλκουσα φαίνεται. τὸ δὲ ἀπὸ τῆς Ἀττικῆς ἐπίθυμον, τὸν τῆς μελαίνης χυμὸν διὰ τῆς κοιλίας καθαῖρον ὁρᾶται, καὶ ὁ κνίδιος κόκκος τοῦ φλέγματος, καὶ παντὸς τοῦ ὑδατώδους περιφανῶς ἄγωγός ἐστι. ταῦτα γὰρ τὰ φάρμακα ἐκ παντὸς αὐτῶν τοῦ μέρους καὶ ἐξ ὅλης ἑαυτῶν τῆς οὐσίας τὴν ὁλκὴν τῶν χυμῶν τούτων ποιεῖσθαι φαίνεται. μὴ γὰρ πιστεύομεν Ἀσκληπιάδῃ τῷ ἀπὸ τῆς Βιθυνίας ἰατρῷ, παρὰ τὸν καιρὸν ἐκεῖνον λέγοντι, ὅτε ἤδη καὶ ὁ ἄνθρωπος καθαίρεται, τότε καὶ τοὺς χυμοὺς τούτους εὐθέως κατά τινα μεταβολὴν γίγνεσθαι· διὰ τὴν γὰρ τῶν ὄγκων τε καὶ πόρων ἐξ ἀρχῆς αὐτῷ γενομένην τοῦ σώματος ὑπόθεσιν, τούτῳ ἀνάγκην ἔχοντι τῆς φύσεως ἀναιρεῖν τὰ ἔργα, ἀκόλουθον ἦν καὶ τοῦτον περὶ τῶν χυμῶν λέγειν τὸν λόγον, ὡς ἀλόγου καὶ παντάπασιν ἀδυνάτου ὄντος τοῦ ὑπ' αὐτοῦ λεγομένου. τίς γὰρ ἂν πιστεύσειε νοῦν ἔχων ἐν τοσούτῳ τάχει ἅμα τῷ προσάγειν τοῦ σώματος

admodum fcammonium bilem flavam trahere apparet; epithymum Atticum atrae bilis humorem ex ventriculo purgare cernitur; granum gnidium pituitam et totum aquofum humorem evidenter educit. Haec fiquidem medicamenta ex tota ipforum parte totaque fua fubftantia hujusmodi humorum eductionem moliri confpiciuntur. Non enim fidem Afclepiadi Bithyno medico adhibemus, data occafione dicenti, quum homo jam purgatur, tunc etiam humores hos ftatim aliquam fubire mutationem. Quippe quoniam auctor fuit de corpore hypothefeos atomorum coacervatione et meatibus contentae, naturae opera de medio tollens neceffario, confentaneum erat et hunc de humoribus fermonem ipfum dicere, tanquam id quod ab eo adducitur a ratione fit alienum et omnino fieri nequeat. Quis enim fanae mentis crediderit tam fubito quam medicamentum corpori adhibeatur, humoris qui excernetur, fubftantiam generari? Quis contra non facile fibi perfuaferit humores hosce prius quoque fecundum

τὸ φάρμακον εὐθέως καὶ τοῦ μέλλοντος ἐκκρίνεσθαι χυμοῦ γίγνεσθαι τὴν οὐσίαν; τίς δ' οὐκ ἂν πεισθείη ῥᾳδίως τοὺς χυμοὺς τούτους, καὶ πρότερον κατὰ φύσιν εἶναι τοῖς σώμασιν, ὁρῶν τὸν μὲν ἰκτεριῶντα παρὰ τὸν καιρὸν τοῦ λαβεῖν τὸ χολαγωγὸν φάρμακον, ταχέως τε καθαιρόμενον τὴν τοσαύτην χολὴν, καὶ τοῦ πάθους εὐκόλως ἀπαλλασσόμενον; τὸν δὲ ὑδεριῶντα οὐδαμῶς τινι φαρμάκῳ, πᾶν τὸ ἐγκείμενον ὕδωρ τῇ γαστρὶ, ἅμα τῷ λαβεῖν αὐτίκα μάλα κενούμενον, καὶ ἐκ τῆς τοσαύτης παραχρῆμα κενώσεως, μηδ' ὁτιοῦν, ἢ ὀλίγιστόν γε πάνυ τὸ ὑγρὸν ἐγκείμενον τοῖς σώμασιν ἔχοντα. ἀλλὰ ταῦτα ὁ μὲν Ἀσκληπιάδης παιδαριωδῶς τῇ ἀνάγκῃ τοῦ δόγματος δουλεύων, ὡς ἔφην, διὰ τὸ φιλόδοξον, οὐ προσποιεῖται βλέπειν, καὶ πάντα μᾶλλον πιθανῶς πλαττόμενος εὑρίσκειν βούλεται, ἤπερ ἑκάστου τῶν φαρμάκων τὸ οἰκεῖον (459) τῆς δυνάμεως φιλαλήθως ὁμολογεῖν. ἡμεῖς δὲ ταῦθ' ὁρῶντες, καὶ τῷ λόγῳ τῆς ἑκάστου φύσεως τῶν φαρμάκων, τὸ οἰκεῖον τῆς δυνάμεως φιλαλήθως ὁμολογεῖν τὸ δυνατὸν εἰδότες, κἀνταῦθ' ὅτι φάρμακα φυσικῇ τινι

naturam corporibus ineſſe? quum videat ictero laborantem, eo tempore quo medicamentum bilioſum humorem purgans cepit et bilem ſubito copioſam excernere et affectu expedite liberari? Eum vero qui hydrope laborat, neutiquam medicamento quodam ſimul ac fuerit aſſumptum, omnem aquam ventriculo inſidentem cito admodum vacuare, atque ex tam ſubita vacuatione nullum ſane humorem, aut certe pauciſſimum in partibus inſarctum habere. Verum haec Aſclepiades, pueriliter dogmatis neceſſitati inſerviens, ambitionis ſtudio, ut dixi, videre ſe diſſimulat, omniaque probabilibus potius figmentis conatur invenire quam propriam cujusque medicamenti facultatem vere confiteri. Nos autem quum haec videamus, ſciamusque id quod poſſit ratione uniuscujusque medicamentorum naturae facultatis proprietatem vere agnoſcere, hic quoque medicamenta nativa quadam facultate familiarem ſibi ſuccum attrahere, accurate didicimus; quemadmodum

δυνάμει ἕλκειν τὰ οἰκεῖα πέφυκεν ἀκριβῶς ἐπιστάμεθα, ὥσπερ καὶ ἐν τῷ τὴν Μαγνῆτιν λίθον ἕλκειν τὸν σίδηρον εἰς ἑαυτὴν, δύναμίν τινα ἑλκτικὴν εἶναι αὐτῇ, τὴν ἔμφυτον δύναμιν εὐλόγως ἑαυτοὺς ἐπείσαμεν. Θεὸς γὰρ οὖσα ὥσπερ ἡ ἐν ἡμῖν φύσις, κατὰ τὸν Ὅμηρον, καὶ ἄγουσα τὰ ὅμοια πρὸς τὰ ὅμοια, οὕτω τὰς θείας δυνάμεις ἑαυτῆς ἐπιδείκνυται.

[935] Κεφ. δ'. [*Τὰ ἁπλᾶ τῶν φαρμάκων συνθέτους ὡς ἐπὶ τὸ πολὺ ἔχειν δυνάμεις καὶ διάφορα τοῦ σώματος μόρια βλάπτειν τε καὶ ὠφελεῖν, καὶ διαφόροις διάφορα προσήκειν.*] *Καὶ τῶν ἄλλων δὲ ἁπάντων τὴν φύσιν φιλοτίμως ἐξετάζομεν, ἵνα καὶ τὴν δύναμιν αὐτῶν καθ' ἣν ἐνεργεῖ ἀκριβῶς μάθωμεν. εὑρίσκομεν γοῦν ἐν τῇ ἐξετάσει αὐτῶν γενόμενοι τὰ μὲν, ὡς ἔφην, καθ' ὅλας ἑαυτῶν ἐνεργοῦντα τὰς οὐσίας, τὰ δὲ καὶ μικτὸν ἐν τῇ οὐσίᾳ τὴν δύναμιν ἔχοντα καὶ διπλῆν ἀποτελοῦντα τὴν ἐνέργειαν οὕτω φανερῶς πολλάκις, ὡς καὶ τὰ ἐναντιώτατα ὑπ' αὐτῶν ἐπὶ τοῦ σώματος γιγνόμενα ἡμᾶς βλέπειν, καὶ θαῦμα τοῖς*

etiam ex eo quod Magnes lapis ferrum ad fe attrahat, facultatem quandam attractricem ei ineffe, nativam facultatem merito nobis ipfis perfuafimus. Deus enim quum fit, quemadmodum natura in nobis, fecundum Homerum, fimilia fimilibus adjungens, ita divinas ipfius facultates oftendit.

Cap. IV. [*Simplicia medicamenta plerumque compofitas facultates obtinere, diverfas corporis partes et laedere et juvare, diverfisque diverfa convenire.*] Ac reliquorum omnium naturam pari ftudio examinamus, ut facultatem quoque ipforum per quam operantur exquifite perdiscamus. Nam dum examen illorum molimur, alia, quemadmodum dixi, per totas ipforum fubftantias functionem obire deprehendimus, alia mixtam quoque in fubftantia facultatem habere et duplici fungi actione tam manifefto faepe, ut etiam quam maxime contraria ab eis fieri in corpore confpiciamus, atque id miraculum effe

ὁρῶσι τὸ τοιοῦτον εἶναι δοκεῖν. λαπάθου γοῦν εἴ τις μὲν τὰ φύλλα φάγοι, τὴν κοιλίαν ἐκταράσσεται· εἰ δέ τις τὸ σπέρμα λάβοι, ἐπεχομένην αὐτὴν ἔχει. ὁμοίως δ' οὖν καὶ ὁ τῆς κράμβης χυλὸς καὶ τῶν γερόντων ἀλεκτρυόνων ὁ ζωμὸς καὶ τῶν ἀπὸ τῆς θαλάττης κοχλιῶν οἱ χυμοὶ ληφθέντες ἐκταράσσουσι τὴν κοιλίαν. τὸ δὲ λάχανον αὐτὸ ἡ κράμβη, καὶ τούτων αἱ σάρκες ἐσθιόμεναι, ἐπέχουσιν αὐτάς. ἡ δὲ ἀλόη καὶ ἡ τοῦ χαλκοῦ λεπὶς στύφει τε τὰς ὑπὸ τῶν ἑλκῶν ὑπεραυξανομένας σάρκας, καὶ ἐπιξηραίνει πολλάκις τὰ ὑπ' αὐτοῖς γιγνόμενα ῥεύματα, ληφθέντα δὲ διὰ τοῦ στόματος καθαρτικὰ τοῦ ὅλου σώματος γίνονται. τὸ δὲ γάλα διαιρούμενον ὑφ' ἡμῶν ἐναντίας ἐν τῇ χρείᾳ δυνάμεις ἐπιδείκνυται. ὁ μὲν γὰρ ὀῤῥὸς αὐτοῦ πινόμενος ἐκλύει τὴν γαστέρα, ἐσθιόμενος δὲ ὁ τυρὸς ἐπέχει αὐτὴν ἀκριβῶς. ἔνια δὲ οὕτως τι παράδοξον ἐργάζεται ἐν τῇ μίξει τῶν ἐν αὐτῇ μιγνυμένων δυνάμεων, ὡς καὶ ἀδύνατον εἶναι γενέσθαι τοῖς ἀκούουσι δοκεῖν, εἰ μὴ τὴν παρὰ τὴν γινομένην διὰ τῆς ὄψεως πίστιν παρὰ τοῦ γινομένου λάβωσι. τὸ γοῦν τρίφυλλον ἡ βοτάνη, ἥτις ὑακίνθῳ ὡμοίω-

videntibus appareat. Lapathi igitur folia ſi quis edat, alvum ſubducet; ſi quis ſemen aſſumat, ipſam aſtrictam habebit. Similiter et braſſicae ſuccus et vetulorum gallorum jus et cochlearum marinarum ſucci aſſumpti alvum movent. Olus autem ipſum braſſicae et illarum carnes comeſtae ventrem comprimunt. Aloë ſquamaque aeris ſupercrescentes ulcerum carnes aſtringunt; et qui fluxus ſub ipſis fiunt, eos ſubinde exiccant; aſſumpta vero per os univerſum corpus purgant. Lac ubi a nobis dividitur, contrarias in uſu facultates demonſtrat; nam ſerum ipſius bibitum ventrem ſolvit; caſeus ingeſtus exacte ipſum cohibet. Nonnulla vero tam inopinabile quippiam in mixtione facultatum quae commiſcentur efficiunt, ut auditoribus quoque nullo fieri modo poſſe videatur, niſi ſuis ipſi oculis id quod accidit contueantur. Trifolium itaque herba, quae hyacintho ſimilis eſt, quum vere parturit et

ται, ὁπόταν τοῦ ἔαρος ἐγκύμων γένηται, καὶ τὸ σπέρμα ὅμοιον ἔχῃ τῇ ἀγρίᾳ κνίκῳ, ὅταν τις ἀφεψήσῃ πάνυ, εἶτα τῷ δήγματι τοῦ φαλαγγίου ἢ καὶ τοῦ ἔχεως τῷ ὕδατι ἐπαντλήσει, ἰᾶται αὐτὸ καὶ εὐθέως ἀνώδυνον ἐργάζεται. εἰ δέ τις ἐπ' ἄλλου μὴ δεδηγμένου τὸν ὑγιῆ τόπον τῷ αὐτῷ ἐπαντλήσει καταντλήματι, τὴν αὐτὴν αἴσθησιν καὶ τὰς αὐτὰς ὀδύνας ὁμοίας τῷ δεδηγμένῳ πάσας ἀποτελεῖ, ὡς εἶναι τὸ γινόμενον ἀληθῶς θαύματος ἄξιον, τὴν αὐτὴν βοτάνην καὶ ἰᾶσθαι τὸ δῆγμα καὶ ὁμοίως τοῖς θηρίοις διατιθέναι τὸν ὑγιῆ τόπον πονηρῶς. τινὰ δὲ τῶν φαρμάκων τὴν ἀρχὴν οὐδὲ ὅλως ἐστὶ τοῖς ἀνθρώποις σύντροφα. τὸ γοῦν κώνειον τοὺς μὲν ψάρους τρέφει καὶ τὴν θανατικὴν δύναμιν ἐπ' αὐτῶν οὐκ ἔχει, ἡμᾶς δὲ, ὡς οὐκ ἀγνοεῖς, ἀναιρεῖ. καὶ ὁ ἐλλέβορος τῶν μὲν ὀρτύγων ἐστὶ τροφὴ, τοὺς δὲ ἀνθρώπους διαφθείρει κακῶς. ἔνια δὲ εὑρίσκομεν καὶ μερῶν τινων ἐν τῷ σώματι τὴν κάκωσιν ἰδίως ποιούμενα. ὁ γοῦν θαλάττιος λαγωὸς ἑλκοῖ τὸν πνεύμονα καὶ ἡ καν-

femen agrefti cnico perfimile obtinet; decocta admodum, deinde morfibus aranei, vel viperae quoque ex aquae fotu adhibita ipfis medetur et dolores ftatim fedat. Sin autem in alio non commorfo fanum locum eodem fotu circumdederis, fimilem fenfum fimilesque dolores iis quos morfus invehit, omnes conciliat; ut revera miraculo dignum opus effe videatur eandem herbam et morfum fanare et ferarum pari modo fanam partem prave afficere. Jam vero ex medicamentis quaedam hominum nutritioni per initia minime conveniunt. Cicuta enim fturnos quidem nutrit et letalem in ipfis vim non exercet, nos autem, quemadmodum probe nofti, interimit. Veratrum etiam coturnicum cibus eft, homines vero male corrumpit. Nonnulla quoque reperimus quae partes quasdam corporis privatim vitiant. Nam lepus marinus pulmonem exulcerat; cantharis veficam peculiariter afficit. E contrario pleraque medicamenta quibusdam corporis partibus eximie curandis funt idonea. Patienti igitur jecinori faepe eupatoria herba

θαρὶς ἰδίως τὴν κύστιν κακοῖ. πολλὰ δὲ τῶν φαρμάκων πάλιν ἐξαιρέτως τινὰ τῶν μερῶν τοῦ σώματος ὠφελεῖν πέφυκε. πάσχον γοῦν τὸ ἧπαρ πολλάκις εὐπατόριος ἡ βοτάνη ἀγωνιστικῶς ὠφέλησε, καὶ ἡ μυροβάλανος τὸν σπλῆνα ὤνησε. τὸ δὲ σαρξιφαγὲς καὶ ἡ βετονίκη τοὺς νεφροὺς διέθηκε καλῶς, καὶ ὁμοίως ἄλλα ἐστὶν ἄλλων, ὡς τῇ πείρᾳ τετηρήκαμεν, οἰκεῖα φάρμακα, ἅπερ ἡμεῖς, ὡς ἔφην, ἀκριβῶς ἐξετάζοντες οὕτως ἑκάστῳ τῶν παθῶν τὴν κατάλληλον προσφορὰν ποιούμεθα, διδασκάλῳ καὶ τούτων, ὥσπερ καὶ τῶν ἄλλων ἁπάντων, Ἱπποκράτει τῷ ἀρίστῳ χρώμενοι. ὅτι γὰρ ἀκριβεστάτην τὴν περὶ τῶν φαρμάκων τέχνην πεποίηται καὶ ἐξ ἄλλων πλείστων ὑπ᾿ αὐτοῦ λεγομένων ἔστιν ἰδεῖν, μάλιστα δὲ ἐξ ὧν φησιν ἐν τῷ β' τῶν ἐπιδημιῶν οὕτω· [936] φαρμάκων δὲ τρόπους ἴσμεν ἐξ ὧν γεγένηται ὁκοῖα ἄττα. οὐ γὰρ πάντες ὁμοίως, ἀλλ᾿ ἄλλοι ἄλλως σύγκεινται, καὶ ἄλλα ὅσα πρωϊαίτερον, ἢ ὀψιαίτερον ληφθέντα, καὶ οἱ διαχειρισμοὶ, οἷον ξηρᾶναι, ἢ κόψαι, ἢ ἑψῆσαι, καὶ τὰ τοιαῦτα, ἔως τὰ πλεῖστα μειώσει πλείω

perſtrenue auxiliata eſt; et myrobalanus lienem adjuvat; ſaxifragia et betonica renibus probe faciunt; et ſimiliter alia aliorum, ut experientia obſervavimus, propria ſunt medicamenta, quae nos, ut dixi, diligenter perſcrutati ita cuilibet morbo, ut conveniunt, admolimur, Hippocratem magiſtrum longe optimum in his quoque, ut in aliis omnibus, aemulantes. Quod enim exactiſſimam de medicamentis artem fecerit cum ex aliis plerisque ab ipſo conſcriptis eſt cernere, tum maxime ex iis quae ſecundo Epidemiorum libro in hunc modum prodita reliquit: *Medicamentorum modos ſcire convenit, ex quibus alia quaedam conficiantur; non enim omnes ſimiliter, ſed alii aliter conſtituuntur; et alia medicamenta maturius, vel tardius capta, poſſunt praeparari; nempe ſiccari, vel tundi, vel concoqui et hujusmodi, donec plerunque plurima minuantur. Huc accedit explicandum quae ſingulis conveniant, in quibus morbis, quo morbi tempore, qua*

Ed. Chart. XIII. [936.] Ed. Baf. II. (459.)
καὶ ὁκοῖα ἑκάστῳ καὶ ἐφ᾽ οἷσι νοσήμασι, καὶ ἐφ᾽ ᾗ τε τοῦ νοσήματος ἡλικίᾳ, ἰδέᾳ, καὶ διαίτῃ ὁκοίᾳ, ἢ ὥρῃ ἔτεος, ὁκοίως ἄγωμεν, καὶ τὰ τοιαῦτα. διὰ γὰρ τούτων, ὡς ὁρᾷς, καθολικώτερον ἡμᾶς διδάσκει, παραινῶν καὶ τὰς φύσεις τῶν φαρμάκων εἰδέναι, καὶ τὸν καιρὸν ἐξετάζειν, ἐν ᾧ τις τὸ φάρμακον μέλλει λαμβάνειν, καὶ τὰς κράσεις τῶν λαμβανόντων ἐπιβλέπειν. εἰσὶ γὰρ ὡς ἀληθῶς οἱ μὲν εὐκόλως λαμβάνειν δυνάμενοι, ὡς καὶ πέπτειν αὐτὰ πολλάκις, ἢ κατὰ μηδὲν ὑπ᾽ αὐτῶν κακοῦσθαι, ἀλλ᾽ ἐνίοτε καὶ τροφὴν αὐτοῖς γίνεσθαι αὐτὸ τὸ φάρμακον. ἔνιοι δὲ ἀφυῶς οὕτως ἔχουσι πρὸς τὰς φαρμακείας ὡς μηδὲ τὴν ἀρχὴν αὐταῖς χρῆσθαι δύνασθαι, ἀποστρέφεσθαί τε αὐτοῖς τὸν στόμαχον καὶ πρὸ τῆς χρήσεως ἐκλύεσθαι ῥᾳδίως.

Κεφ. ε΄. [Τί ποτ᾽ ἐπήγαγε τοὺς ἰατροὺς πρὸς τὴν σύγκρασιν πολλῶν ἁπλῶν. καὶ τίς ὁ πρῶτος ἐπιβαλὼν τῇ θηριακῇ τὰς ἐχίδνας.] Ταῦτα γοῦν, ὡς ἔγωγε νομίζω, καὶ τῶν παλαιῶν ἰατρῶν οἱ ἄριστοι παρ᾽ αὐτοῦ μαθόντες οὕτως ἀρίστας καὶ τὰς συνθέσεις ἐποιοῦντο τῶν φαρμάκων,

ſpecie, quali victu, vel anni tempore, quomodo tractemus et id genus alia. His enim, uti vides, generalius nos docet, ut qui et medicamentorum naturas diſcere nos adhortetur et tempus exquirere, quo medicamenta debent aſſumi, et eorum qui aſſumunt temperaturas inſpicere. Sunt enim nonnulli procul dubio qui tam facile ea poſſunt capere ut etiam multoties concoquant, vel nihil ab ipſis incommodi, ſed aliquando ipſis nutrimento eſſe medicamentum experiantur. Quidam tam inepti medicamentis aſſumendis exiſtunt, ut nequaquam uti ipſis poſſint et ſtomachus averſetur, ac ante uſum facile diſſolvatur.

Cap. V. [*Quid medicos induxerit ut plura ſimplicia commiſcerent; quique primus viperas theriacae impoſuit.*] Haec igitur, ut ego arbitror, et veterum medicorum praeſtantiſſimi ab ipſo edocti, optimas ſic medicamentorum compoſitiones effecerunt, ex ſingulorum natura

ἐκ τῆς ἑκάστου φύσεως αὐτῶν τὴν τέχνην τῆς συνθέσεως ποιούμενοι, καὶ τὰ μὲν ἐπιτεταμένα ταῖς ποιότησιν αὐταῖς, τῇ τῶν ἄλλων μίξει καθαιροῦντες, ὁμοίως δὲ καὶ ἀμβλύνοντες τὰ δριμέα, καὶ ὅλως πρὸς τὴν ἑκάστου λοιπὸν τῶν παθῶν διαφορὰν καὶ τῶν ἀνθρώπων τὴν σύγκρισιν ἐντέχνως τοῖς φαρμάκοις χρώμενοι. διόπερ οἶμαι καὶ ταύτην τὴν θηριακὴν, περὶ ἧς ἡμῖν ὁ πᾶς οὗτος λόγος φιλοτίμως τετεχνολόγηται, ἐκ πλείστων καὶ τῶν καλλίστων φαρμάκων ἐσκεύασαν. λογισάμενοι γὰρ τῶν πονηρῶν θηρίων τὰ δήγματα ὅτι ἐστὶν ἄφυκτα, καὶ τῶν δηλητηρίων φαρμάκων τὰ συμπτώματα ὅτι ἐστὶ θανατικὰ, προσεπιλογισάμενοι δὲ καὶ τὴν τῶν ἀνθρώπων ἐν ταῖς φύσεσι πολλὴν οὖσαν διαφορὰν, καὶ ὅτι ἄλλο φάρμακον ἄλλῳ ἁρμόζειν πέφυκεν, εἰκότως αὐτῆς ἀκριβῆ τε καὶ ποικίλην ἐποιήσαντο τὴν σκευασίαν, ὡς διὰ τοῦτο καὶ ἀπταίστως αὐτὴν ἐπὶ τούτων ἁπάντων τυγχάνειν τοῦ τέλους, καὶ διὰ τὸ ἀναγκαῖον τῆς χρείας, καὶ περισπούδαστον πάνυ τοῖς ἀνθρώποις γενέσθαι. οὐδὲν γὰρ ἐμοὶ τῶν ἐν τῷ βίῳ χαλεπώτερον εἶναι δοκεῖ τῶν

compositionis artificium invenientes, quaeque intensa sunt ipsis qualitatibus aliorum mixtione remittentes, simili ratione acria hebetantes et, ut summatim comprehendam, pro reliqua cujusque affectus differentia et hominum temperie medicamentis cum artificio utentes. Quare puto, hanc quoque theriacen, de qua totus hic liber ampliter differit, ex plurimis optimisque medicamentis praepararunt. Quum enim considerarent morsus noxiarum ferarum esse inevitabiles et venenosorum medicamentorum symptomata letalia, ad haec quum perpenderent hominum naturas permultum invicem differre et aliud alii medicamentum idoneum, merito exactam ipsius et variam fecerunt confectionem, ut hujus rei gratia certo ipsa in his omnibus finem assequeretur, atque ob usus necessitatem magno studio ab hominibus affectaretur. Nihil siquidem inter vitae mala difficilius esse mihi videtur viru-

δηλητηρίων φαρμάκων καὶ τῶν δακετῶν θηρίων. τὰ μὲν γὰρ ἄλλα τῶν δεινοτάτων καὶ φυλακὴν ἔχει τὴν ἀπ' αὐτῶν φυγὴν, ταῦτα δὲ τὴν μεγίστην τοῖς ἀνθρώποις ἐπιβουλὴν ἐργάζεται. διὰ γὰρ τὸ ἀφύλακτον τὶς οὐκ εἰδὼς ἑαυτῷ πολλάκις προσφέρει τὸ φάρμακον, καὶ ἄλλως ἀγνοῶν, εἶτα δηχθεὶς ὑπό τινος θηρίου αἰφνίδιον τελευτᾷ. ἐμοὶ δὲ καὶ ἐξ ἱστορίας τὶς ἐμήνυσε λόγος ὡς ἄρα πολεμεῖν Ῥωμαίοις τὶς ἐθέλων καὶ τὸ δυνατὸν ἐκ τῆς στρατιωτικῆς τάξεως οὐκ ἔχων, ἄνθρωπος δὲ, φησὶ, Καρχηδόνιος οὗτος, ἐμπλήσας (460) πολλὰς χύτρας θηρίων τῶν ἀναιρεῖν ὀξέως δυναμένων, οὕτως αὐτὰ προσέβαλε πρὸς τοὺς πολεμίους. οἱ δὲ τὸ πεμπόμενον οὐ νοοῦντες καὶ διὰ τοῦτ' ἀφύλακτοι μένοντες, οὐ γὰρ ἦν τοιαῦτα εἰθισμένα ἐν τοῖς πολεμίοις πέμπεσθαι βέλη, ταχέως πίπτοντες ἀπέθνησκον· καὶ διὰ τοῦτο πολλάκις ὁ ἄνθρωπος οὗτος τῇ τοιαύτῃ πρὸς τὸ πολεμεῖν πανουργίᾳ, ὥσπερ τι καὶ αὐτὸς θηρίον ὑπάρχων, διέφυγε τῶν ἐναντίων τὰς χεῖρας. διόπερ οἶμαι, καὶ εἰς τὰς τοιαύτας χρείας ὑμῖν τοῖς ὑπερέχουσι καὶ τοῖς τῶν

lentis medicamentis et feris noxiis. Etenim ab aliis etiam graviſſimis fuga nos praeſervamus, illa maxime hominibus imponunt, quod videlicet aliquis nulla praemunitione adhibita frequenter venenum neſciens imprudensque aſſumit, deinde commorſus a fera quadam ſubito interit. Ego autem ex quodam hiſtoriae libro accepi, quomodo aliquis bellum contra Romanos gerere voluerit nulla militaris ordinis potentia munitus. Homo vero hic (inquit) Carchedonius, complures ollas feris, quae repente poſſunt occidere, reſertas adverſus hoſtes projecit. Illi autem non intelligentes quid mitteret eoque neutiquam ſibi caventes, quippe tales emitti ſagittae inter hoſtes non ſolebant, protinus collapſi perierunt; atque propterea homo ille frequenter ejusmodi aſtutia, tanquam et ipſe fera quaedam exiſteret, inimicorum manus effugit. Quamobrem putaverim et vobis primatibus et exercituum ducibus ad tales uſus hoc eſſe habendum medicamentum; quod non-

στρατοπέδων ἄρχουσιν, ἀναγκαῖον [937] ἔχειν καὶ τοῦτο τὸ φάρμακον, διὰ τὴν τοῦ πολεμεῖν ἐνίοτε γινομένην ἀνάγκην. πάλαι μὲν οὖν καὶ ἄνευ τῆς τῶν θηρίων μίξεως σκευαζόμενον τὸ φάρμακον ὁμοίως ἐποίει πρὸς τὰ τοιαῦτα καρτερῶς. ἀεὶ δὲ τῶν ἰατρῶν φιλοτίμως πρὸς τὴν κατασκευὴν αὐτῆς ἐχόντων καὶ ἄλλο συμμίσγειν ἐπινοούντων, οὕτως τὶς προσεπενόησε καὶ ἔμιξεν αὐτῇ τὰ θηρία. Ἀνδρόμαχος δὲ, φασὶν, οὗτος ἀνὴρ ἦν ἀξιόλογος ἰατρὸς, καὶ οὐ πολὺ πρὸ ἡμῶν γεγενημένος. συνῆν γὰρ τῷ Νέρωνι, ᾧ καὶ προσεφώνησε, γράψας αὐτὴν ἔπεσι, καὶ τὴν ἐπαγγελίαν καὶ τὴν σκευασίαν. καὶ παραθήσομαί γέ σοι αὐτὰ τὰ ἔπη, ἵνα μηδὲ τούτων ἀνίστορος ἦς, οὕτω φιλόκαλος ὢν, ἐκεῖνο πρότερον εἰπὼν, ὅτι διὰ τὸ τὸν ἐπινοήσαντα μῖξαι τῷ φαρμάκῳ τὰ θηρία εἰκότως, οὐχ ὅτι μόνον πρὸς τὰ ἀπ' αὐτῶν δήγματα ἁρμόζει καλῶς, θηριακὴ ἂν λεχθείη πρὸς ἡμῶν, ἀλλ' ὅτι καὶ αὐτὰ τὰ θηρία λοιπὸν ἐν τῇ σκευασίᾳ μιγνύμενα ἔχει, προσηκόντως ἐξ ἀμφοτέρων τῶν σημαινομένων ἑτοίμως ἂν θηριακὴ λέγοιτο. ἔστι δὲ τὰ ἔπη ταῦτα.

nunquam bellandi incidat neceſſitas. Olim itaque citra ferarum quoque mixtionem confectum medicamentum, ſimiliter ad hujusmodi ſtrenue faciebat. Quum autem medici ſemper in hujus praeparationem certatim incumberent, ac aliud commiſcere cogitarent, in hunc modum quidam conſideravit, miscuitque ipſe beluas. Ajunt autem Andromachum hunc virum ſuiſſe, medicum mehercule memoria dignum, haud multo ante nos natum. Quippe Neroni convixit, cui etiam ipſam dedicavit, tum vires tum confectionem carmine complexus. Quod tibi hic ſubjungam, ne ipſius hiſtoria careas, tam ſtudioſus alioqui et cupidus literarum. Illud tamen praefabor, theriacen non ſolum quod ferarum morſibus probe conveniat, ſed etiam quod ferae ipſae deinceps in confectione miſceantur, congrue ex utroque ſignificato eſſe nominandam. Verſus autem hi ſunt.

Κεφ. στ' καὶ ζ'. [Ἀνδρομάχου πρεσβυτέρου, Νέρωνος ἀρχιάτρου θηριακὴ δι' ἐχιδνῶν ἡ καλουμένη Γαλήνη.]

(Cum haec jam ſuperius libro de antidotis I. p. 428. ſſq. ed. Baſ. ſine ulla lectionis varietate exhibita fuerint, ea h. l. omittere viſum eſt.)

[940] *Κεφ.* η'. [Διὰ τί ὁ Ἀνδρόμαχος τὴν ἔχιδναν μᾶλλον ἢ ἄλλον τινὰ ὄφιν τῇ θηριακῇ ἐπέμιξε; καὶ περὶ Κλεοπάτρας θανάτου ἀκριβὴς ἱστορία.] Τούτων οὖν τῶν ἐπῶν οὐκ ἀφυῶς ὑπὸ τοῦ ἀνδρὸς γενομένων σκέψασθαι ἀναγκαῖον ἔμοιγε δοκεῖ, τί δή ποτε πολλῶν ὄντων τῶν τοιούτων θηρίων οὐχὶ τῶν ἄλλων τινὸς, ἀλλὰ τῶν ἐχιδνῶν τὰς σάρκας ἐπιτηδείους εἰς τὴν μίξιν εἶναι νομίζομεν. αὐτὸς μὲν γὰρ, ὡς ὁρᾷς, περὶ τούτων οὐδὲν ἔγραψεν· ἐμοὶ δὲ δοκοῦσι τῶν ἄλλων θηρίων αὗται μὴ τοσαύτην ἐν τοῖς σώμασι τὴν φθοροποιὸν δύναμιν ἔχειν. ὁ μὲν γὰρ βασιλίσκος, ἔστι γὰρ τὸ θηρίον ὑπόξανθον, καὶ ἐπὶ τῇ κεφαλῇ τρεῖς ὑπεροχὰς ἔχον, ὥς φασιν, ὅτι καὶ ὁραθεὶς μόνον καὶ συρίττων ἀκουσθεὶς ἀναιρεῖ τοὺς ἀκούσαντας καὶ τοὺς ἰδόντας αὐτόν· καὶ ὅτι τῶν ἄλλων ζώων, εἴ τι καὶ ἅψαιτο τοῦ

Cap. VI. et VII. [*Andromachi ſenioris, Neronis archiatri, ex viperis theriace, appellata Galene.*]

Cap. VIII. [*Cur Andromachus viperam potius quam ſerpentem alium theriacae admiſcuerit; deque Cleopatrae morte diligens hiſtoria.*] His itaque verſibus non inepte a viro compoſitis neceſſarium mihi videtur inſpicere cur tandem, quum multae ſint ejusmodi ferae, non alterius quam viperae carnes in miſturam eſſe idoneas cenſeamus. Ipſe enim nihil de his, uti vides, ſcriptum reliquit. Ego vero has minus aliis feris corrumpendi facultatem obtinere autumo. Nam baſiliscus, bellua ſufflava et triplici frontis apice munita, ut ajunt, viſus etiam ſolum conſpectusque et ſibilo auditus homines qui ipſum viderint et audierint momento perimit; etiam ex aliis animantibus ſi quod illum jam extinctum jacentemque attigerit, et ipſum ſubito interimit; quare omne aliarum ferarum ge-

ζώου ἀνῃρημένου, καὶ αὐτὸ τελευτᾷ εὐθέως, καὶ διὰ τοῦτο πᾶν αὐτοῦ τὸ γένος τῶν ἄλλων θηρίων ἐγγὺς εἶναι φυλάττεται. ὁ δὲ δρυϊνος ὄφις ἐν ταῖς τῶν δρυῶν ῥίζαις τὸν βίον ποιούμενος οὕτως πονηρός ἐστι πρὸς τὸ διαφθεῖραι κακῶς, ὥστε εἴ τις, φασὶν, αὐτοῦ ἐπιβαίη, ἐκδέρεσθαι αὐτοῦ τοὺς πόδας, καὶ οἴδημα πολὺ γίνεσθαι καθ' ὅλων τῶν σκελῶν. καὶ ἔτι τὸ θαυμασιώτερόν φασιν, ὅτι καὶ εἰ θεραπεύειν τις ἐθέλοι, τούτων τὰς χεῖρας ἐκδέρεσθαι. εἰ δέ τις καὶ ἁμιλλώμενος αὐτὸ ἀποκτεῖναι βούλοιτο τὸ θηρίον, λέγουσιν αὐτὸν μοχθηρὸν νομίζειν εἶναι πᾶν τὸ εὔφραντον καὶ μηδενὸς ἄλλου ὀσφραίνεσθαι δυνάσθαι. ὁ δὲ αἱμόῤῥους καὶ ἡ αἱμοῤῥοῒς τοῖς ἑαυτῶν ὀνόμασιν ὁμοίαν ποιοῦνται τῶν ἀνθρώπων τὴν διαφθοράν. αἱμοῤῥαγοῦντες γὰρ διὰ τοῦ στόματος καὶ τῶν μυκτήρων καὶ τοῦ παντὸς σώματος οὕτως ἀπόλλυνται. ὥσπερ γε καὶ οἱ ἀπὸ τῆς διψάδος ὑπὸ τοῦ καύσου διαφθειρόμενοι κακῶς, καὶ γὰρ οὗτοι διψῶντες πάνυ καὶ διακαιόμενοι σφοδρῶς, ἐνίοτε καὶ διαῤῥηγνύμενοι, τελευτῶσιν. ὁ δὲ ἀκοντίας ἐκτείνας ἑαυτὸν πάνυ καὶ ὥσπερ τι ἀκόντιον ἐφαλλόμενος τοῖς σώμα-

nus propinquitatem ipſius devitat. Dryinus ſerpens ſic nominatus, quod in radicibus quercuum vitam vivat, tam malignus ad perdendum proditur, ut ejus qui ſupergreditur imprudens cutis a pedibus excorietur, tota crura multum intumeſcant et quod magis mirificum proferunt, manus quoque ipſas curantium excorientur. Si autem quis aggrediatur hanc feram perimere, olfactu mulctatur adeo, ut quemlibet gratum odorem pravum eſſe exiſtimet, nec rem alteram praeterea queat odorari. Haemorrhus et haemorrhois ſuis ipſorum nominibus ſimilem hominibus perniciem inferunt; quippe percuſſi, ſanguine per os et nares totoque corpore effuso, intereunt; quemadmodum a dipſade commorſi cauſo febre male conficiuntur. Nam et multa ſiti et aeſtu vehementi, interdum ſtomachi motu vexati, diem obeunt. Acontias ſerpens, ubi ſe multum extenderit, ceu jaculum quoddam corpo-

σιν οὕτως ἀναιρεῖ. καὶ τῶν ἀσπίδων ἡ λεγομένη πτυὰς ἐπανατείνασα τὸν τράχηλον καὶ συμμετρησαμένη τὸ τοῦ διαστήματος μῆκος, ὥσπερ τότε λογικὸν γιγνόμενον τὸ θηρίον εὐστόχως ἐμπτύει τοῖς σώμασι τὸν ἰόν. τούτων γοῦν φασι τῶν θηρίων τινὶ, τριπλοῦν γάρ ἐστι τὸ εἶδος τῶν ἀσπίδων, ταύτης τε καὶ τῆς μὲν χερσαίας λεγομένης, τῆς τε χελιδονίας καλουμένης, τὴν βασιλίδα Κλεωπάτραν βουληθεῖσαν λαθεῖν τοὺς φυλάττοντας, ταχέως τε καὶ ἀνυπόπτως ἀποθανεῖν. ἐπεὶ γὰρ αὐτὴν ὁ Αὔγουστος νικήσας τὸν Ἀντώνιον ζῶσαν λαβεῖν ἠβούλετο, καὶ ζῆν, καὶ διὰ σπουδῆς φυλάττειν ὡς εἰκὸς, ἵνα δείξῃ Ῥωμαίοις ἐν τῷ θριάμβῳ τὴν οὕτω διάσημον γυναῖκα. ἡ δὲ συνεῖσα, φασὶ, τοῦτο, καὶ ἑλομένη μᾶλλον ἔτι βασίλισσα οὖσα ἐξ ἀνθρώπων γενέσθαι ἤπερ ἰδιώτης Ῥωμαίοις φανῆναι, τότε ἐμηχανήσατο τῷ θηρίῳ τούτῳ τὸν θάνατον αὐτῆς. καὶ φασὶν αὐτὴν καλέσαι τὰς πιστοτάτας δύο γυναῖκας, αὗται δὲ ἦσαν αἱ πρὸς τὸ κάλλος αὐτῆς εἰς τὸν κόσμον τοῦ σώματος ὑπηρετεῖν ἡρμοσμέναι καὶ τοῖς ὀνόμασι λεγόμεναι Νάειρα καὶ Καρ-

ribus infiliens fic perimit. Inter afpides nominata ptyas cervicem exporrigens et intervalli longitudinem metita rationalis cujusdam animalis modo venenum corporibus infpuit. Harum igitur ferarum una (nam triplex afpidum fpecies eft, haec videlicet et cherfaea i. e. *terreftris*, et chelidonia) perhibent reginam Cleopatram quum vellet latere cuftodes, ftatim et citra fufpicionem mortem fibi confciviffe. Quum enim Auguftus devicto Antonio eam capere incolumem vellet ac vivere, ftudiofiusque, ficut par erat, fervare, ut Romanis tam infignem mulierem in triumpho oftenderet, haec, ajunt, re intellecta optavit regina adhuc ex humanis potius decedere quam privata Romanis videri. Et tunc molita eft fibi hac beftia mortem confcifcere. Praeterea memoriae produnt ipfam duas omnium fidiffimas mulieres ad fe vocaffe, quae ad pulchritudinem corporis mundo fubminiftrando erant accommodatae; nominabantur Naera et Carmione; haec comam

μιόνη. ἡ μὲν ἀναπλέκουσα τὰς τρίχας εὐπρεπῶς, ἡ δὲ ἀποτέμνουσα τὰς ὑπεροχὰς τῶν ὀνύχων εὐφυῶς, εἶτα κελεύσασα σταφυλαῖς τε καὶ σύκοις κεκρυμμένον εἰσκομισθῆναι τὸ θηρίον, ἵνα, ὡς ἔφην, τοὺς φυλάττοντας λάθῃ, προπειρασαμένη αὐτὸ πρότερον ἐπὶ τούτων τῶν γυναικῶν, εἰ ὀξέως ἀναιρεῖν δύναται, καὶ μετὰ τὸ ταύτας ταχέως ἀνελεῖν λοιπὸν αὐτῇ, [941] ἐφ' ᾧ δὴ καὶ τὸν Αὔγουστον πάνυ καταπλαγῆναι λέγουσι, τῶν μὲν μέχρι τοῦ συναποθανεῖν αὐτῇ τοσαύτην φιλοστοργίαν, τῆς δὲ τὸ μὴ βουληθῆναι ζῆν δουλικῶς, ἀλλ' ἑλέσθαι μᾶλλον ἀποθανεῖν εὐγενῶς. καὶ γὰρ λέγουσιν αὐτῆς εὑρεθῆναι τὴν χεῖρα τὴν δεξιὰν ἐπὶ τὴν κεφαλὴν κειμένην καὶ κρατοῦσαν τὸ διάδημα, ὡς εἰκὸς, ἵνα καὶ μέχρι τότε τοῖς ὁρῶσι βασίλισσα οὖσα βλέπηται· ὥσπερ καὶ ὁ τραγικὸς ποιητὴς ἡμῖν λέγει τὴν Πολυξένην, ὅτι καὶ αὕτη ἀποθνήσκουσα ὅμως πολλὴν πρόνοιαν εἶχεν εὐσχημόνως πεσεῖν. οἱ δὲ τὸ μὲν τῆς γυναικὸς πρὸς τὸ λαθεῖν εὐμήχανον, τοῦ δὲ θηρίου πρὸς τὸ ἀποκτεῖναι τάχος βουλόμενοι ἡμῖν δεῖξαι τῷ λόγῳ, λέγουσιν αὐτὴν μὲν ἐνδα-

decenter implicabat; illa extremos ungues dextre praecidebat; deinde juffiffe ut feram uvis ficubusque tectam importarent, quo, ut dixi, cuftodes falleret, prius expertura in ipfis mulieribus, an fubito poffet perimere; et hae quum actutum periiffent, deinde ipfam fibi admoviffe. Ob quam rem Auguftum vehementer fuiffe attonitum commemorant, partim ob harum erga reginam amorem, ut cum ea mori non dubitarint; partim quod illa generofam potius mortem oppetere maluerit quam in fervitute vivere. Etenim ajunt ipfam manu dextra capiti admota et diadema, ficut eft confentaneum, tenente, fuiffe inventam, ut vel eousque fpectatoribus regina effe videretur; quemadmodum et tragicus poëta fcribit nobis Polyxenam et ipfam mortuam, quae tamen accurate praenoviffet cum decoro fe occafuram. Porro qui mulieris profperum ut falleret cuftodes conatum, ferae autem ad occidendum pernicitatem fermone volunt oftendere, refe-

Ed. Chart. XIII. [941.] Ed. Baf. II. (460. 461.)
κεῖν τὸν ἑαυτῆς βραχίονα μεγάλῳ πάνυ καὶ βαθεῖ τῷ δήγματι. ἐργασαμένην δὲ εἴς τι σκεῦος εἰσκομισθῆναι αὐτῇ τὸν ἰὸν τοῦ θηρίου ἐγχέαι τῷ τραύματι, καὶ οὕτω διαδοθέντος αὐτοῦ μετ' οὐ πολὺ λαθοῦσαν τοὺς φυλάσσοντας εὐκόλως ἀποθανεῖν. ἀλλὰ τοῦτο μὲν οὐκ ἀτερπῶς ἱστορείσθω, διὰ τὴν σὴν ἐν πᾶσι τοῖς λόγοις φιλοτιμίαν, καὶ ἵνα διὰ τούτου τὴν ὀξύτητα πρὸς τὸ ἀποκτεῖναι τούτων τῶν θηρίων ὦμεν εἰδότες. ὀξέα γάρ ἐστιν ἀληθῶς πρὸς τὸ ἀναιρεῖν ταῦτα τὰ θηρία. καὶ πολλάκις γὰρ ἐθεασάμην ἐγὼ ἐν τῇ μεγάλῃ Ἀλεξανδρείᾳ τὸ τάχος τοῦ ὑπ' αὐτῶν γιγνομένου θανάτου. ὅταν γάρ τινα τούτῳ τῷ νόμῳ τῆς κολάσεως κατακριθέντα φιλανθρώπως καὶ ταχέως ἀποκτεῖναι θέλωσι, προσβάλλοντες αὐτοῦ τοῖς στέρνοις τὸ θηρίον καὶ ποιήσαντες ὀλίγον περιπατῆ- (461) σαι, οὕτω ταχέως ἀναιροῦσι τὸν ἄνθρωπον. ὁρᾷς οὖν ὅπως ἡμεῖς δεόντως οὐδὲν τῶν τοιούτων θηρίων ἐγκαταμίγνυμεν τῷ φαρμάκῳ, διὰ τὴν τοσαύτην ἐν τοῖς σώμασιν αὐτῶν φθοροποιὸν δύναμιν.

Κεφ. θ'. [*Τί δή ποτε τῇ θηριακῇ ὁλόκληρος ἡ ἔχιδνα*

runt ipfam fuummet brachium magno morfu eoque alto vulneraffe et belluae virus in vafe quodam ipfi allatum vulneri infudiffe, quo fic transmiffo, haud multo poft nefciis cuftodibus prompte interiiffe. Verum hanc hiftoriam animi gratia commemorare vifum eft, quod te in omnibus difciplinis diligentem dextrumque videam; ad haec, ut intelligamus quam fubitam hae ferae necem concilient; etenim exitio inferendo haud dubie funt praecipites. Ac in magna Alexandria fubinde fum contemplatus quam celeriter perimerent. Quum enim quendam hac poenae lege damnatum humaniter citoque volunt occidere, adjicientes ipfius pectori feram jubentesque paululum obambulare, ita fine mora hominem tollunt e medio. Vides igitur quam nos decenter nullam ex hujusmodi feris, quod tantam habeant in ipforum corporibus vim noxiam, medicamento admifcemus.

Cap. IX. [*Cur vipera theriacae integra non pona-*

οὐκ ἐπιτίθεται· πολλάς τε ἐκ τῶν ζώων ἡμᾶς λαμβάνειν τὰς θεραπείας.] *Καὶ αὐτῶν δὲ τῶν ἐχιδνῶν οὐχ ὅλα τὰ ζῶα εἰς ἀντίδοτον πέμπομεν, ἀλλ' ἀποτεμόντες τὰς κεφαλὰς καὶ τὰς οὐρὰς οὕτω τοῖς ἄλλοις αὐτῶν σώμασιν εἰς τὴν μίξιν χρώμεθα, καὶ τοῦτο οὐ παρέργως οὐδ' ἄνευ λόγου τινὸς ποιούμενοι, ἀλλ' ἐπειδὴ αἱ κεφαλαὶ τὸν κάκιστον τῶν χυμῶν, αὐτὸν τὸν ἰὸν, ἐν αὑταῖς ἔχουσι, διὰ ταῦτ' ἀποκόπτειν αὐτὰς πειρώμεθα, ἵν' ὀλιγώτερον τῆς ἀπ' αὐτῶν δυνάμεως ἔχῃ τὸ φάρμακον, τῆς τούτων φύσεως μεταβλητικήν τινα δύναμιν εἰς τὸν ἰὸν ἐχούσης· ὥσπερ δὴ καὶ ἐν τοῖς παραστάταις τὸ σπέρμα καὶ ἐν τοῖς μαζοῖς τὸ γάλα μεταβαλλόμενον γίνεται. ἡ δὲ ἔχιδνα τῶν ἄλλων ἁπάντων τὴν κεφαλὴν πρὸς τὸ διαφθεῖραι κακῶς ἐπιτηδειοτέραν ἔχει. φασὶ γὰρ αὐτὴν ἀνοίγουσαν τὸ στόμα πρὸς τὸ δέξασθαι τοῦ ἄῤῥενος τὸν θορὸν μετὰ τὸ λαβεῖν ἀποκόπτειν αὐτοῦ τὴν κεφαλήν· καὶ τοῦτον αὐταῖς εἶναι τῆς πονηρᾶς συμπλοκῆς τὸν τρόπον. εἶτα ἀπὸ τοῦ σπέρματος τὰ ζῶα γενόμενα κατά τινα φυσικὴν ἄμυναν ἀναβιβρώσκειν μὲν τῆς μητρὸς τὴν γαστέρα, ἐκθρώσκειν δὲ εἰς τὰ ἔξω· καὶ οὕτως αὐτὰ*

tur, multaque ex animalibus remedia haberi.] Atque ipſarum viperarum corpora non integra in antidotum immittimus, ſed amputatis capitibus caudisque ita reliquis ipſarum partibus in mixtione utimur, idque non obiter nec ſine ulla facientes ratione, ſed quoniam capita peſſimum humorem, *nempe* ipſum virus, in ſe continent, ideo ipſa praecidere conamur, ut minus ex ipſorum facultate medicamentum recipiat, quum natura eorundem facultatem quandam mutatricem in virus obtineat; quemadmodum et in paraſtatis ſemen fit, in mammis lac dum mutatur. Vipera autem inter omnes alias feras ad prave corrumpendum caput habet opportunius. Siquidem aiunt ipſam os aperire ad ſuſcipiendam maris genituram; qua accepta caput illius amputare. Atque hunc ipſis eſſe pravi complexus modum. Deinde foetus ex ſemine prognati naturali quadam ultione parentis ventrem erodere

εἰς ἐκδικίαν τοῦ πατρὸς ἀναιρεῖν τὴν μητέρα. ὅπερ ἡμῖν ὁ καλὸς Νίκανδρος ἐν τοῖς ἔπεσιν αὐτοῦ οὐκ ἀφυῶς γράφει, καὶ ἔστι τὰ ἔπη ταῦτα·

Μὴ σύ γ' ἐνὶ τριόδοισι τύχῃς ὅτε δῆγμα πεφυγὼς
Περκνὸς ἔχις θύῃσι, τυπὴν χολόεσσαν ἐχίδνης.
Ἡνίκα θορνυμένου ἔχιος θολερῷ κυνόδοντι,
Θουρὰς ὀδὰξ ἐμφῦσα κάρην ἀπέκοψεν ὁμεύνου·
Οἱ δὲ πατρὸς λώβην μετεκίαθον αὐτίκα τυτθοὶ
Γεινόμενοι ἐχιῆες, ἐπεὶ διὰ μητρὸς ἀραιὴν
Γαστέρ' ἀναῤῥήξαντες ἀμήτορες ἐξεγένοντο.

[942] *Τὰς δὲ οὐρὰς καὶ αὐτὰ ἀφαιροῦμεν τὰ ἔσχατα τοῦ σώματος, ὥσπερ οὐρᾶς ὄντα μέρη καὶ, ὡς οἶμαι, τὸ ῥυπαρώτερον τῆς οὐσίας ἕλκοντα μᾶλλον, καὶ πλείονά γε τὴν ὁλκὴν διὰ τὴν κίνησιν ποιούμενα, ὥσπερ τὰ πρὸς ταῖς οὐραῖς τῶν ἰχθύων μέρη διὰ τὴν πολλὴν κίνησιν τροφιμώτερα εἶναι λέγουσι. μὴ θαυμάζῃς δὲ, εἰ μετὰ τὴν τούτων ἀποκοπὴν τὰ λοιπὰ σώματα τῶν ζώων ἰσχυρότερον ποιεῖ τὸ φάρμακον τῆς ἐμφύτου πρὸς τὸ σώζειν δυνάμεως καὶ*

et foras prorumpere feruntur, ac ita ipſos patris vindices matrem perimere. Quod nobis egregius Nicander verſibus ſuis ingeniose ſcribit. Sunt autem hi verſus

Ne ſis in triviis quum morſus vipera conjunx
Foemellae fugiens agitatae vulnera abhorret;
Et quum dente caput magno maris amputat atri
Foemina dira nimis, labiis et mordicus haerens.
Sed catuli ultores patris ſunt protinus, ut qui
Perrumpant latera occiſae jam rara parentis.

Caudas atque ipſa extrema corporis tollimus, tanquam caudae partes et, ut arbitror, ſordidiorem ſubſtantiae portionem magis trahentes; adeoque crebrius motus gratia trahentes, quemadmodum partes quae proximae ſunt caudis piſcium, magis nutrire ob frequentem motum dicuntur. Ne mireris ſi his amputatis reliquae animantium partes efficacius reddant medicamentum, nativa ad ſalutem

ἐν αὐταῖς ταῖς σαρξὶν αὐτῶν καταμεμιγμένης. ὥσπερ δὴ καὶ ἐπ' ἄλλων ζώων πολλὰ τῶν μερῶν οὐκ ὀλίγα τῶν παθῶν ἀγωνιστικῶς θεραπεύεσθαι οἴδαμεν. ἐνίοις γοῦν βοηθοῦσιν αἱ κεφαλαὶ τῶν μυῶν, καυθεῖσαι γὰρ καὶ μετὰ μέλιτος χριόμεναι, τὰς ἀλωπεκίας ἰᾶσθαι δύνανται. καὶ τοῦ ἰκτίνου τὴν κεφαλὴν, φασὶν, ὁμοίως τοὺς ποδαγριῶντας ὠφελεῖν, εἴ τις αὐτῆς ξηρανθείσης ἄνευ τῶν πτερῶν ὅσον ὑπὸ τοῖς τρισὶ δακτύλοις ἐπιπάσας ὕδατι πίνειν ἐθέλοι. καὶ τῶν μερῶν δὲ πολλάκις αὐτὰ μόνα τὰ μόρια τινὰ τῶν παθῶν ἰᾶσθαι δύνανται. ὁ γοῦν τῆς καμήλου ἐγκέφαλος ξηρανθεὶς καὶ μετ' ὄξους πινόμενος ἐπιληπτικοὺς ἰᾶται καὶ ὁ τῆς γαλῆς ὁμοίως. ὁ δὲ τῆς χελιδόνος μετὰ μέλιτος πρὸς ὑποχύσεις ποιεῖ. καὶ ὁ τῶν προβάτων σκευασθεὶς ὁμοίως ταῖς τῶν παίδων ὀδοντοφυΐαις ἄκρως βοηθεῖ. τοῦ δὲ ταυρείου κέρατος τὸ ξύσμα μεθ' ὕδατος πινόμενον αἱμοῤῥαγίας ἐπέχει. καὶ οἱ μηροὶ δὲ καιόμενοι ἐπέχουσι τὸ αἷμα. πολλάκις δὲ καὶ τὴν γαστέρα λελυμένην τὸ αὐτὸ τοῦτο ἵστησι. τὸ δὲ τοῦ ἐλάφου κέρατος ῥίνημα καιόμενον

facultate etiam carnibus ipſarum indita; veluti in aliis animantibus pleraſque partes non paucos affectus ſtrenue ſanare novimus. Nonnullis igitur capita murium cremata ex melle illita alopeciam ſanare poſſunt. Et milvi caput ajunt ſimiliter podagricis auxiliari, ſi quis ex eo uſto ſine plumis quantum ſub tribus digitis inſpergere poſſit cum aqua volet bibere. Et partium nonnunquam ſolae particulae aliquos morbos ſanare poſſunt. Itaque cameli cerebrum areſactum potumque ex aceto comitialibus morbis medetur, et muſtelae ſimiliter. Item hirundinis cerebrum ex melle ad ſuffuſiones oculorum facit; et ovillum ſimili modo confectum ad dentitionem inſantium eſt utiliſſimum. Taurini cornu raſura cum aqua pota ſanguinis eruptionem cohibet, femoraque uſta ſanguinem ſtringunt et ſaepenumero ſolutam alvum ea ipſa ſiſtunt. Cervini cornu ramentum aduſtum et cum vino tritum, deinde circumlitum, vacillantes dentes conſirmat, ſicut et

καὶ μετ' οἴνου λειούμενον, εἶτα περιπλασσόμενον, τοὺς σειομένους ὀδόντας πήγνυσιν, ὥσπερ δὴ καὶ τὸν ἀστράγαλον τῆς βοὸς τοῦτο ποιεῖν δύνασθαι λέγουσιν· ἐξάγει δὲ καὶ στρογγύλην ἕλμινθα μετὰ μέλιτος πινόμενος, καὶ μετ' ὀξυμέλιτος σπλῆνα τήκει, καὶ τὰς λεύκας καταχριόμενος, συμμέτρως δὲ ἀφροδισιαστικός ἐστιν. οἱ δὲ τοῦ κάστορος ὄρχεις ὁμοίως πινόμενοι σπασμοὺς ἰῶνται. πολλὰ δὲ τῶν ζώων καὶ τὰς χολὰς ἑαυτῶν ἔχει βοηθεῖν τῷ ἀνθρώπῳ δυναμένας, καὶ τὰ στέατα, καὶ τοὺς μυελοὺς, καὶ τὸ γάλα, καὶ τὸ δέρμα, καὶ τὸ αἷμα αὐτὸ, καὶ τῶν ὄφεων τὸ γῆρας. ἤδη δὲ καὶ τὰς ἀφόδους αὐτῶν ὠφελούσας τινὰς εἴδομεν. ἡ γοῦν τῆς βοὸς ἄφοδος ξηρὰ κεκαυμένη τρισὶ κοχλιαρίοις ὑδρωπικῷ βοηθεῖ. καὶ ἡ τῶν μυῶν ἄφοδος λεία μετ' ὄξους ἀλωπεκίας θεραπεύει· ἐν ποτῷ δὲ λαμβανομένη τοὺς ἐν κύστει θρύπτει λίθους· τὸ δὲ τοῦ χηνὸς στέαρ τὰς φλεγμονὰς μετὰ ῥοδίνου ἰᾶται· καὶ ὁ τοῦ ἐλάφου μυελὸς παρηγορικώτατόν ἐστι φάρμακον. τὸ δὲ τῆς βοὸς γάλα πινόμενον δυσεντερικοῖς βοηθεῖ. τῆς δὲ ὑαίνης ἡ χολὴ μετὰ μέλιτος πρὸς ὀξυδερκίαν ποιεῖ, καὶ τὰς ὑποχύσεις διαφορεῖ ἐγχριομένη. τοῦ δ' ἱπποποτάμου τὸ δέρμα

bovis talus idem poſſe traditur; idem educit rotundos lumbricos cum lacte potus, ex oxymelite lienem conſumit et leucas tollit illitus; ad haec mediocriter venereus eſt. Et caſtoris teſticuli ſimiliter poti convulſionibus medentur. Multa autem ſunt animalia, quorum fel homines poteſt juvare, adeps, medulla, lac, cutis, ſanguis ipſe et ſerpentis ſenectus; quin et aliquando ſtercora ipſorum quibusdam auxiliata vidimus. Bovis itaque ſtercus aridum uſtum tribus cochleariis hydropicum juvat; murium ſtercus cum aceto tritum alopecias curat; in potu autem ſumptum veſicae calculos comminuit; adeps anſerinus inflammationibus ex roſaceo medetur; et cervi medulla blandiſſimum eſt medicamentum; vaccini lactis potus dyſentericos adjuvat; fel hyaenae cum melle viſum exacuit, illitum, ſuffuſiones diſcutit; Hippopotami cutis uſta et ex aqua laevigata, ſi corpori admovetur, tubercula diſcutit, quemadmodum et viperae cutis in pulverem redacta, im-

καιόμενον, καὶ μεθ' ὕδατος λεῖον ἐπιτιθέμενον, φυμάτων σκορπιστικὸν γίνεται, ὥσπερ δὴ καὶ τὸ ἔχεως δέρμα, λεῖον ἐπιτιθέμενον ταῖς ἀλωπεκίαις, θαυμαστῶς ἀναφύει τὰς τρίχας. τὸ δὲ τῆς ἀσπίδος γῆρας τριφθὲν μετὰ μέλιτος καὶ ὑπαλειφόμενον ὀξυδερκέστατόν ἐστιν. καὶ ὅλως πολλή τίς ἐστιν ἡ τῶν τοιούτων ὕλη, ἣν οὐκ εὔκαιρον εἶναι νομίζω νῦν ἀναγράφειν, ἵνα μὴ μακρὸς ὑμῖν ὁ λόγος γένηται, ἀρκούντων εἰς τὴν ἀπόδειξιν τοῦ λεγομένου καὶ μόνων μοι τῶν προειρημένων. ἐκεῖνο δὲ ἀναγκαῖόν ἐστιν εἰδέναι, ὅτι τῶν ζώων αὐτῶν ὅλα τὰ σώματα πολλάκις τοῖς ἀνθρώποις βοηθεῖ. καρκίνος γοῦν ὁ ἀπὸ τῶν ποταμῶν λειωθεὶς καὶ καταπλασθεὶς ἀνεκβάλλει τοὺς σκόλοπας καὶ τὰς ἀκίδας. καὶ ἡ καρὶς ὁμοίως λειωθεῖσα μετὰ βρυωνίας ῥίζης πινομένη ἕλμινθας ἐξάγει. ὁ δὲ σκορπίος σὺν ἄρτῳ ἐσθιόμενος ὀπτὸς θρύπτει τοὺς ἐν τῇ κύστει λίθους. ὁμοίως δὲ καὶ τὸ γῆς ἔντερον μετ' οἴνου πινόμενον τὸ αὐτὸ ποιεῖ. εἰ δέ τις αὐτὰ τρίβων ἐν μελικράτῳ λάβοι ἰκτεριῶν εὐθέως καθαρθεὶς ἀπαλλάσσεται. πολλάκις δὲ καὶ σὺν ῥοδίνῃ κηρωτῇ ἐπιτιθέντα τῶν ποδαγρῶν ταῖς φλεγμοναῖς ἥρμοσαν, ὁ δὲ

pofitaque alopeciis, mirifice pilos regenerat; afpidis fenile exuvium ex melle tritum et illitum, acutiffimum vifum conciliat. In fumma, multa eft talium materia, quam nunc refcribere tempeftivum non effe judico, ne liber vobis fiat prolixior, quum etiam fola quae nos praediximus ad fermonis demonftrationem fufficiant Illud vero fcitu eft neceffarium, tota ipforum animalium corpora frequenter hominibus auxiliari. Cancer enim fluviatilis tritus illitusque fpicula et furculos extrahit. Caris, i. e. fquilla pifcis, fimiliter laevigata cum bryoniae radice pota lumbricos educit. Scorpius fi affus cum pane comedatur, conterit veficae calculos. Terrae quoque inteftinum ex vino affumptum idem facit; fi autem ea in melicrato contrita quis regio morbo laborans fumat, ftatim purgatus liberatur; faepe etiam cum rofaceo cerato impofita podagricorum inflammationibus convenerunt. Accipiter in fufino unguento decoctus hebetudini oculorum medetur.

ἱέραξ ἑψηθεὶς μετὰ μύρου [943] σουσίνου ἀμβλυωπίας ἰᾶται. καὶ ὁ κάνθαρος δὲ θεραπεύει τὰς ὠταλγίας ἀποζεσθεὶς ἐλαίῳ καὶ ἐνσταζόμενος εἰς τὸ οὖς. ὁ δὲ κορυδαλὸς ὀπτὸς τρωγόμενος θαυμασίως τοὺς κωλικοὺς πολλάκις ὠφέλησε, καὶ ἵνα μᾶλλον τὴν ἐν τοῖς σώμασιν αὐτῶν δύναμιν θαυμάσῃς, ἐκεῖνό σοι φιλοτιμότερον διηγήσομαι. πολλὰ γὰρ καὶ ὁραθέντα μόνον τὴν ἑαυτῶν ἰσχὺν ἐπιδείκνυνται. ὁ οὖν ἀσκαλαβώτης ὁραθεὶς ὑπὸ τῶν σκορπίων ὑποπήγνυσιν αὐτοὺς, καὶ οὕτως ἀναιρεῖ. ἡ δὲ ἀμφίσβαινα, ἔστι δὲ τὸ ζῶον ἀμφικέφαλον, ὥσπερ δὴ καὶ τῶν πλοίων τὰ ἀμφίπρωρα, τῆς φύσεως τῷ περιττῷ τῆς οὐσίας δύο κεφαλὰς ἔχειν αὐτῇ χαρισαμένης, τοῦτο δή φασι τὸ ζῶον εἰ ὑπερβάλῃ γυνὴ κατὰ γαστρὸς ἔχουσα, ἐκτιτρώσκει τὸ παιδίον κακῶς, ὥστε οὐδὲν θαυμαστὸν, εἰ καὶ τὰ τῶν ἐχιδνῶν σώματα ἀποκοπέντων τοῖς τῶν μερῶν ἐκείνων ὁμοίως ἔτι πρὸς τὸ βοηθεῖν τὴν ἰσχὺν ἔχει. ἐπέδειξα γὰρ, ὡς οἶμαι, φιλοπόνως ὅτι καὶ ὅλα μὲν τὰ ζῶα τοῖς ἀνθρώποις βοηθεῖ ποτε, ἔσθ᾽ (462) ὅτε δὲ καὶ αὐτὰ μόνα τὰ μέρη. ἐνίοτε δὲ καὶ τῶν μερῶν αὐτῶν τὰ οὕτω μικρὰ μόρια.

Scarabaeus in oleo decoctus, ſi in aurem ſtilletur, dolores ipſius medicatur. Alauda uſta ſi edatur, mirifice colicos ſubinde juvat; et quo magis facultatem in ipſorum corporibus admireris, illud tibi ſtudioſius percenſebo; multa namque et viſa ſolum robur ſuum oſtendunt. Stellio ſcorpiones viſos ſuſtringit frigore atque ita perimit. Amphiſbaena (eſt autem animal biceps, quemadmodum ſane et navigia utrinque proram habentia, cui natura ex ſuperfluo ſubſtantiae bina capita eſt largita) hoc inquam animal, ajunt, ſi mulier gravida ſupergreſſa fuerit, male abortum facit. Quare non eſt mirabile, ſi etiam viperarum corpora amputatis illis partibus adhuc auxiliandi robur obtineant. Nam oſtendi, ut puto, diligenter et tota animalium corpora nonnunquam hominibus auxiliari; interdum etiam ſolas ipſas partes; aliquando partium quoque ipſarum particulas minimas.

Κεφ. ί. [*Πῶς τὰ βλαβερὰ ἐνίοτε ἔχουσιν ὠφελεῖν· μίαν τε ἐκ πολλῶν γίγνεσθαι ποιότητα ἐν τοῖς μικτοῖς φαρμάκοις.*] Ἐκεῖνο δὲ ἀναζητῆσαι τῷ λόγῳ μᾶλλόν ἐστιν ἀναγκαῖον, ὅπερ καὶ τοῖς πολλοῖς θαυμασίας ἄξιον εἶναι δοκεῖ. αὐτὰ γὰρ τὰ θηρία ὄντα τοῖς σώμασι πολέμια καὶ οὕτω τὸν ἄνθρωπον ἀναιροῦντα ὀξέως, πῶς πάλιν αὐτὰ τοῖς ὑπ᾽ αὐτῶν γενομένοις δήγμασι βοηθεῖν δύναται, καὶ μόνα διασώζειν ἐκ τοῦ τοιούτου κακοῦ τὸν ἄνθρωπον; καί φησί τις ἀρχαῖος λόγος ὅτι τινὰ τῶν ζώων ὁμιλήσαντα μὲν ἐν τῷ δάκνειν τῷ ἐκ τοῦ δήγματος ἀποκρινομένῳ ἀνθρωπείῳ αἵματι ἀναιρεῖ τοὺς δακνομένους. μὴ γευσάμενα δὲ τοῦ αἵματος, ἀλλ᾽ οὕτως ἐσθιόμενα, τοὺς δηχθέντας διασώζειν πέφυκεν. ὥσπερ καὶ ἐπὶ τοῦ ἑλενίου μὲν ὑπὸ τῶν Ἑλλήνων, ὑπὸ δὲ τῶν ἐπιχωρίων νίκου ἢ νίνου καλουμένου, τὸ αὐτὸ ἱστορεῖσθαι λέγουσι. φασὶ γὰρ τοὺς Δάκας καὶ τοὺς Δαλμάτας περιπάττειν αὐτὸ ταῖς ἀκίσι τῶν βελῶν, καὶ οὕτως ὁμιλῆσαν μὲν τῷ αἵματι τῶν τιτρωσκομένων ἀναιρεῖν δύνασθαι, ἐσθιόμενον δὲ ὑπ᾽ αὐτῶν ἀβλαβὲς εἶναι, καὶ

Cap. X. [*Quomodo noxia interdum prodeſſe queant; unamque in compoſitis medicamentis qualitatem ex omnibus reſultare.*] Illud autem ratione perſcrutari magis eſt neceſſarium, quod et multis admiratione dignum eſſe videtur. Siquidem ipſae ferae quum ſint corporibus inimicae et tam ſubito hominem perimant, quomodo e contrario morſibus ab ipſis factis poſſint ſuccurrere et ſolae hominem ex tali periculo perſervare. Vetus quidam ſermo eſt, quaedam animalia ubi inter mordendum ſanguinem humanum ex vulnere manantem contigerint, commorſos occidere; ubi vero ſanguinem non guſtaverint, ſed ita vorantur, morſos ſervare incolumes poſſe; ſicut etiam de helenio a Graecis quidem, ab indigenis vero nico vel nino appellato, idem memoriae proditum eſſe dicunt. Nam Dacas inquiunt et Dalmatas id telorum cuspidibus circumſpergere, atque ſic poſtquam ſanguinem vulneratorum attigerit, poſſe necare; eſum vero ab ipſis eſſe innocuum, neque mali quicquam ipſis facere. Ad haec cer-

μηδὲ κακὸν αὐτοὺς ἐργάζεσθαι, καὶ τὰς ὑπ' αὐτῶν γε ἀναιρουμένας ἐλάφους ἐν τῷ κατατοξεύεσθαι μηδ' αὐτὰς ἐσθιομένας κακόν τι τοὺς ἐσθίοντας διατιθέναι λέγουσιν. ἀλλ' οὗτος ὁ λόγος οὐ δοκεῖ μοι αὐτάρκης εἶναι πρὸς τὴν εὕρεσιν τοῦ ὑφ' ἡμῶν ζητουμένου, ἐμπειρικός τις ὢν καὶ μόνον τὸ γενόμενον διηγούμενος. καὶ γὰρ αὐτοὺς τοὺς ἐμπειρικοὺς οὐκ ἀποδέχομαι, ὅτι καὶ αὐτοὶ, ὥσπερ ἰδιῶται μόνον ὁρῶντες τὸ βλεπόμενον, θαυμάζουσι μὲν τὸ γιγνόμενον, τοῦ δὲ γιγνομένου τὴν αἰτίαν ἀγνοοῦσιν. οἱ μὲν μηδὲ τὴν ἀρχὴν ἐπιζητοῦντες μαθεῖν, ἀλλ' ἀποκνοῦντες αὐτὴν εὑρεῖν τῷ λόγῳ, καὶ μόνον τῶν γιγνομένων ἀποπειρώμενοι, καὶ τὴν τῶν πολλάκις ὁρωμένων ἐμπειρίαν ἀρκεῖν αὐτοῖς εἰς τὸ ἰατρεύειν λέγοντες, τὸν αὐτὸν ἔχουσιν, ὡς ὁρᾷς, τοῖς ἰδιώταις τοῦ θαύματος τρόπον. οἱ δὲ τούτων φιλοτιμότεροι ὁμολογοῦσι μὲν ὅτι χρή τι ἐπιστημονικώτερον τῶν ἰδιωτῶν εἰς τὰ τοιαῦτα ἔχειν τοὺς ἰατροὺς, εὑρεῖν δὲ ἀδυνατοῦντες, καὶ τὸ ζητεῖν περιττὸν εἶναι νομίζουσιν. ἀλλ' ἡμεῖς πλέον εἶναι τούτων τὸ φιλότιμον εἰς τὴν τέχνην ἔχοντες, καὶ τὰ γιγνό-

vos ab ipsis sagittarum ictu trucidatos, neque ipsos comestos, mali quid edentibus afferre perhibent. Verum haec ratio non mihi videtur sufficere, ut quod quaerimus possit inveniri, quum experientia nitatur et solum quod accidit commemoret. Etenim empiricos non recipio, quoniam et ipsi idiotarum modo propositum speculantes rem quidem admirantur, caeterum causam ipsius ignorant. Hi neque principium id requirunt discere, imo detrectant ipsum ratione invenire, ac solum facta probantes experientiam multoties visorum satis esse ipsis ad medendum affirmant, eundem admirationis modum cum idiotis, uti vides, obtinent. His autem diligentiores fatentur quidem medicos eruditius aliquid idiotis merito habere, sed nequeunt invenire et inquirere supervacuum esse arbitrantur. At nos multo accuratius in medicinam incumbentes ac quae fiunt vulgi duntaxat more nolentes inspicere neque experientiam repudiamus, sed ei rationem consociantes,

μενα μόνον βλέπειν ἰδιωτικῶς μὴ θέλοντες, οὔτε τὴν ἐμπειρίαν ἐκβάλλομεν καὶ συναρμόζοντες αὐτῇ τὸν λόγον ὅταν ἐνδέχηται, τελείαν οὕτω καὶ λογικὴν ἀναγκαίως ἔχομεν [944] τὴν τέχνην, οὐχ ἵνα μόνον εὕροιμεν, ὅπως γίνεται φιλοπονοῦντες εὑρεῖν, ἀλλ᾽ ἵνα τι καὶ εἰς τὴν θεραπείαν εὔχρηστον ἐκ τοῦ εὑρεθέντος μάθωμεν. κἀνταῦθα οὖν ἐπαγωνισώμεθα τῷ λόγῳ, ἵνα εὕρωμεν τοῦ γιγνομένου τὴν αἰτίαν. θαυμαστὸν γὰρ ὡς εἴ γε ἐκ τῆς περὶ τὸ ζητεῖν αὐτὸ φιλοτιμίας, ἐξ ἑτοίμου καὶ αὐτὸ, ὥσπερ ἀμειβόμενον, ταχέως εὑρίσκεται· καὶ ἵνα σοι πιστότερον ποιήσω τὸν λόγον, ἀπ᾽ ἄλλων τινῶν ἐν τοῖς ἔργοις σαφῶς ὁρωμένων τὴν ἀπόδειξιν ποιήσομαι καὶ ἔξωθέν γε ἐπιτιθεμένων μόνον καὶ διὰ τοῦ στόματος λαμβανομένων. τοὺς γὰρ ὑπὸ τῶν κροκοδείλων βρωθέντας ὑπ᾽ αὐτοῖ τοῦ στέατος ἐπιτιθεμένου τοῖς τραύμασιν ἄκρως βοηθουμένους οἴδαμεν· καὶ τῆς μυγαλῆς τὰ δήγματα καὶ αὐτὰ ἀναιροῦντα ὑπ᾽ αὐτῆς πάλιν τῆς μυγαλῆς τριβομένης καὶ ἐπιτιθεμένης ἀνωδύνως θεραπεύεται. ὁμοίως δὲ αὐτοὶ οἱ ἐχιόδηκτοι ἀπαλλάττονται τοῦ κινδύνου, εἴ τις αὐτῶν λειώσας τὰ σώματα ἐπιθείη αὐτοῖς τοῖς τραύ-

quum datur occafio, abfolutam ita et rationalem necessario habemus artem, non ut folum disquirendi ftudio quomodo fiat, affequamur, verum ut etiam aliquid ad utilem curationem ex invento condiscamus. At hic ideo infiftemus rationi, ut rei, quae fit, caufam inveniamus. Miraculum enim videri queat, quod fi ex inquirendi ipfius ftudio prompte et ipfa tanquam refpondens fubito reperiatur. Et ut magis fermoni fidem adhibeas, ex aliis quibusdam, quae manifefto ex operibus apparent, demonftrationem producam; infuper ex iis quae foris imponuntur duntaxat et per os fumuntur. Nam a crocodilo laefis ipfius adipem vulneribus impofitam fummo effe praefidio novimus. Item muris aranei morfus aeque letales ab ipfo rurfus in pulverem redacto fuperpofitoque citra dolorem curari. Similiter qui a vipera funt percuffi periculum effugiunt, fi trita ipfarum corpora vulneribus ipfis applicuerint. Nec talia citra rationem in ipfis, ut dixi,

μασιν, οὐκ ἀλόγως καθ' ἡμᾶς, ὡς ἔφην, καὶ τῶν τοιούτων γιγνομένων, μήτε τοσαύτην δύναμιν ἐχόντων, ὡς καὶ ἀποκτεῖναι δύνασθαι, κατὰ διάδοσίν τε τῆς δυνάμεως χωρούσης εἰς βάθος τῶν σωμάτων. ὥσπερ δὴ καὶ ἐπὶ τῶν καταπλασμάτων καὶ αὐτὸ γιγνόμενον ὁρῶμεν, τῆς ἐν τοῖς σώμασιν αὐτῶν δυνάμεως συμμέτρου γιγνομένης καὶ θεραπεύειν λοιπὸν, ἀλλ' οὐκ ἀναιρεῖν δυναμένης. τὸ δὲ ἐπὶ τῆς θηριακῆς γιγνόμενον φανερώτερον ἔχει τὸν λογισμόν. φημὶ γὰρ ὅτι διὰ τοῦτο ταῦτα ἀναιροῦντα τὰ θηρία βοηθεῖ τοῖς ὑπ' αὐτῶν δακνομένοις, ἐπειδὴ πλείων ἐν τούτοις ἐνοῦσα ἡ φθοροποιὸς δύναμις, ταῖς κεφαλαῖς ἀφαιρουμέναις συναποκόπτεται. καὶ ἐπεὶ τὴν ἐν τοῖς ἄλλοις μέρεσιν αὐτῶν ὑπολειπομένην δύναμιν ταῖς σκευασίαις ἡμεῖς ἀπαμβλύνομεν ἕψοντες αὐτὰς, καὶ τῶν ἁλῶν καὶ τοῦ ἀνήθου οὐκ ὀλίγα τῷ ὕδατι μιγνύντες, οὐχ ἡδύσματος μόνου χάριν τὴν μίξιν τῶν τοιούτων ποιούμενοι, ἀλλ' ἵνα ἐκτήξωμεν τὰ σώματα, καὶ οὕτως αὐτὰ ὀλίγον τὸν ἰὸν, ἢ μηδ' ὅλως ἔχειν ἐργασώμεθα. τὸ δὲ πλεῖστον αὐτῇ τῆς δυνάμεως εἰς τὸ βοηθεῖν ἡ σκευασία παρέχεται. τοσούτοις οὖν καὶ τοιούτοις μιγνύμενα φαρμά-

eveniunt, nec tantam obtinent facultatem, ut poſſint perimere, ſi reſpicias diſtributionem facultatis in altum corporum penetrantis; quemadmodum ſane in cataplasmatis idem quoque fieri cernimus, facultate in corporibus ipſorum moderata, quae mederi deinceps queat, non autem occidere. Verum quod in theriaca accidit, maniſeſtiorem habet rationem. Dico enim, propterea feras has noxias ab ipſis commorſos juvare, quod copioſior vis tabiſica quae in illis eſt, ſimul cum capitibus amputatis tollatur. Ad haec vim in aliis partibus reliquam conſectionibus nos obtundimus, dum ipſas coquimus, et ſalis anethique non parum aquae miſcentes, nec condimenti ſolius gratia talia contemperantes, ſed ut corpora eliqueſcant; atque hoc modo ipſa paucum virus, aut nullum prorſus habere facimus; plurimum autem facultatis auxiliatricis praeparatio exhibet. Quomodo igitur ferae tot et talibus miſtae medicamentis amplius queant perimere,

κοις τὰ θηρία, πῶς ἂν ἔτι καὶ ἀναιρεῖν δύναιτο, ἐκλυομένης τῆς οὔσης ἐν αὐτοῖς πρὸς τὸ διαφθεῖραι πονηρίας; ἔτι δὲ καὶ ἀληθέστερος ὁ λόγος φανήσεται, εἰ καὶ ἐπί τινων ὁμοίων τὴν ἀπόδειξιν αὐτοῦ ποιησόμεθα. ἥ γάρ τοι κανθαρὶς μόνη μὲν διδομένη τὴν κύστιν ἑλκοῖ, καὶ πολέμιον αὐτῆς ἐστι τὸ φάρμακον, καὶ ἀναιρεῖ τῇ ἰσχυρᾷ δυνάμει τὸν ἄνθρωπον πολλάκις. μιχθεῖσα δ' ἄλλοις τισὶ πάλιν αὐτῆς τῆς κύστεως γίνεται βοήθημα, καὶ ἔστι διουρητικὴ πάνυ. ὁ δὲ ὀπὸς τῆς μήκωνος ὅτι μέν ἐστιν ἀναιρετικὸς μόνος ποθεὶς οὐδεὶς ἀγνοεῖν μοι δοκεῖ. οὗτος δὲ μετ' ἄλλων τινῶν σκευασθεὶς τοῖς νοσοῦσι βοηθεῖ πολλάκις, ὡς σωτηριωδέστατον αὐτοῖς εἶναι φάρμακον. τὰς γοῦν τῶν νεφριτικῶν παρακοπὰς οὐκ ὀλιγάκις ἀγωνιστικῶς ἰάσατο, καὶ τοὺς ἐξ ἀγρυπνιῶν τὴν δύναμιν ἀφῃρημένους, ὕπνον ἐργασάμενον, θαυμασίως ἀνεκτήσατο. τοῖς δὲ φαλαγγιοδήκτοις αὐτὰ τὰ φαλάγγια λειωθέντα καὶ μετ' οἴνου πινόμενα ἀπαλλακτικὰ τοῦ κακοῦ γίνεται, ὡς ἐκ τούτου μάλιστά σε πιστεύειν δύνασθαι τῷ ὑπ' ἐμοῦ λεγομένῳ. εἰ γὰρ καὶ μόνος

quum malitia ipforum corruptrix fit exoluta? Infuper verior ratio videbitur, fi in quibusdam quoque fimilibus hujus rei demonftrationem afferamus. Cantharis namque fola exhibita veficam ulcerat et inimicum eft ipfi medicamentum et valida faepenumero facultate hominem jugulat; mixta vero aliis quibusdam e contrario, ipfius veficae fit auxilium et vehementer urinam provocat. Succus autem papaveris quod per fe potus exitialis fit neminem latere exiftimo; hic autem cum aliis nonnullis praeparatus aegrotos ita faepe juvat ut maxime falutiferum ipfis medicamentum effe videatur; itaque phreniticorum deliria haud raro ftrenue curavit, ex pervigiliis viribus privatos fomno reconciliato mirifice reftituit. Jam ab araneis commorfos ipfi aranei triti et cum vino poti malo liberant; ut hinc maxime poffis quod a me dicitur credere. Si namque vel folum vinum feris mixtum a periculo reddit fecuros, nimirum et theriaca ex tot tali-

ὁ οἶνος μιχθεὶς τοῖς θηρίοις τὸν ἀπ᾽ αὐτῶν τῶν θηρίων κίνδυνον ἐκφεύγειν ποιεῖ, δηλονότι καὶ ἡ θηριακὴ ἐκ τοσούτων καὶ τοιούτων τὴν σκευασίαν ἔχουσα παιώνιόν τι φάρμακον μᾶλλον, ἀλλ᾽ οὐκ ἀναιρετικὸν τῶν ἀνθρώπων γίνεται. ἐκεῖνο γὰρ ἐν ταῖς μίξεσι τῶν φαρμάκων γιγνόμενον εἰδέναι χρὴ, ὅτι μηκέτι ἀποσώζεται ἡ ἑκάστου τῶν μιγνυμένων δύναμις, ἡ αὐτὴ μένουσα καὶ ἄτρεπτος, εἰς τὸ μηδὲν ἀλλοιουμένη, ἀλλ᾽ ἕνωσίς τις ἀποτελεῖται τῶν ἁπάντων, ὅλης δι᾽ ὅλων τῆς κράσεως αὐτῶν μιγνυμένης [945] καὶ μιᾶς τινος δυνάμεως ἄλλης ἐξ αὐτῶν γινομένης, ὅνπερ τρόπον ἐστὶν ἰδεῖν καὶ ἐπὶ τοῦ οἰνομέλιτος γιγνόμενον. ὅταν γὰρ ἡ κρᾶσις ἀμφοῖν ἀκριβὴς γένηται, οὔτε τὴν τοῦ μέλιτος γεῦσιν τὸ μέλι μιχθὲν ὅλως ἔχει καὶ ὁ οἶνος οὐκέτ᾽ ὢν οἶνος ἐν τῇ μίξει φαίνεται, ἀλλὰ παρ᾽ ἑκάτερον τῶν συνελθόντων ἄλλο τι, αὐτὸ δὴ τοῦτο οἰνόμελι, γιγνόμενον ἐκ τῆς κράσεως ἀποτελεῖται. τὸ αὐτὸ δή μοι νόμιζε γίγνεσθαι ἐπὶ τῶν ἄλλων μὲν ἁπάντων φαρμάκων, καὶ ἐπὶ τῆς θηριακῆς δὲ μάλιστα αὐτῆς, μηκέτι τὴν ἑνὸς ἑκάστου τῶν μιγνυμένων δύναμίν τε καὶ ποιότητα αὐτὴν μένειν, ἀλλὰ συγκρινομένων

busque confecta falutiferum quoddam medicamentum potius quam hominibus exitiale redditur. Illud enim in medicamentorum mixtionibus fieri fciendum eft, puta fingulorum quae mifcentur facultatem non magis confervari, ita ut eadem maneat, nec mutetur, nec in ullam qualitatem tranfeat, fed aliquam omnium unionem effici, tota ipforum temperie per tota mixta et una quadam alia ex illis facultate profecta, quomodo etiam in mulfo fieri confpicimus. Quum enim exacta utriusque temperatura facta fuerit, neque mellis guftum, mel mixtum omnino repraefentat; neque vinum amplius vinum effe in mixtura apparet; verum ftatim duobus congreffis diverfum quiddam, id jam ipfum mulfi naturam induens ex temperatura perficitur. Hoc utique cum in aliis omnibus medicamentis tum maxime in ipfa theriaca fieri arbitrator; non adhuc uniuscujusque mixtorum facultatem et qualitatem eandem manere, fed univerfis omnibus confufis

πᾶσι πάντων καὶ ἕνωσίν τινα φυσικὴν λαμβανόντων μίαν μὲν καὶ λοιπὴν ἄλλην ἐξ ἁπάντων τῶν μιγνυμένων τοῦ φαρμάκου γίνεσθαι τὴν φύσιν.

Κεφ. ια΄. [Ἀσκληπιάδου τε καὶ Ἐπικούρου ἀντίῤῥησις, τῶν τὴν ἀλλοίωσιν ἀποφασκόντων καὶ τὰ τῆς φύσεως ἔργα πρὸς τοὺς ἀτόμους τε καὶ ὄγκους ἀναφερόντων.] Εἰ μὲν γὰρ ἐξ ἀτόμου καὶ τοῦ κενοῦ κατὰ τὸν Ἐπικούρου τε καὶ Δημοκρίτου λόγον συνειστήκει τὰ πάντα, ἢ ἔκ τινων ὄγκων καὶ (463) πόρων κατὰ τὸν ἰατρὸν Ἀσκληπιάδην· καὶ γὰρ οὕτως ἀλλάξας τὰ ὀνόματα μόνον καὶ ἀντὶ μὲν τῶν ἀτόμων τοὺς ὄγκους, ἀντὶ δὲ τοῦ κενοῦ τοὺς πόρους λέγων τὴν αὐτὴν ἐκείνοις τῶν ὄντων οὐσίαν εἶναι βουλόμενος· εἰκότως ἂν ἔμενεν ἀναλλοίωτα τὰ φάρμακα, κατὰ μηδὲν τρέπεσθαι μηδ᾽ ὅλως ἐξίστασθαι τῆς αὐτῶν ποιότητος δυνάμενα. ἐπεὶ δ᾽ οὐκ ἔστιν ἀληθὴς ὁ λόγος οὗτος, ὡς δείξομεν, ἀλλ᾽ ἀλλοιοῦται, ὡς ἔφην, τὰ πάντα καὶ τρέπεται ῥᾳδίως καὶ εἰς ἄλληλα τὴν κρᾶσιν λαμβάνει, ἀνάγκη τῆς κράσεως δι᾽ ὅλων τῶν κιρναμένων γιγνομένης τὸ ἰσχυρότερον τοῦ ἥττονος

bus confufis et in unitatem quandam nativam coëuntibus unam et fuperftitem diverfam ex omnibus permixtis medicamenti naturam procreari.

Cap. XI. [*Afclepiadis Epicurique refutatio, qui alterationem negabant et opera naturae in atomos et moles referebant.*] Si etenim ex atomis et vacuo fecundum Epicuri et Democriti opinionem conftant omnia, vel ex quibusdam molibus et meatibus fecundum medicum Afclepiadem (nam ita permutatis folum nominibus pro individuis *vel atomis* corpufcula, pro vacuo meatus dicens fimilem illis rerum effentiam effe voluit), merito medicamenta manerent inalterabilia quae in nihil mutari neque omnino fuam ipforum qualitatem exuere poffent. Quum autem hic fermo verus non fit, ut oftendemus, imo omnia, ut dixi, alterentur mutenturque facile et mutuam inter fe temperaturam fufcipiant, necesse eft omnibus quae mifcentur per tota contemperatis validius imbecilliori praepollere, cujus rei gratia nos artificialibus

κρατεῖν, καὶ διὰ τοῦτο ἡμεῖς ταῖς ἐντέχνοις μίξεσι πρὸς τὴν χρείαν τῆς ἐνεργείας τὰς ποιότητας τῶν φαρμάκων ἐναλλάσσομεν, οὐκ ἂν δυναμένου τούτου γενέσθαι, εἰ μικρά τινα ἦν καὶ ἀπαθῆ καὶ ἄτρεπτα τῆς οὐσίας τὰ σώματα. διόπερ δὴ καὶ πολλάκις ἐγὼ τεθαύμακα πῶς ὁρῶντες ἐπὶ τοῦ παντὸς οὕτω γενομένας ταχείας τροπὰς καὶ τὴν τοσαύτην ἐν ταῖς κράσεσι μεταβολὴν, εἶθ' ὑπομένουσιν ἀρχὰς τῶν ὅλων τὰς τοιαύτας τίθεσθαι, καὶ μάλισθ' ὁ νῦν εἰρημένος ἰατρὸς Ἀσκληπιάδης· πρὸς τοῦτον γὰρ οἰκείως μᾶλλον ποιήσομαι τὸν λόγον, ἐπεὶ καὶ φανερωτέρας ἐν τῷ σώματι τροπάς τε καὶ μεταβολὰς οὐκ ἐνδείκνυται. τί γάρ ἐστιν εἰπεῖν, ὅταν μόνου τοῦ δακτύλου εἰς ψυχρὸν ὕδωρ κατατεθέντος ὅλου τοῦ σώματος ἐν τάχει ἡ τροπὴ γίνηται; ἢ ὅταν ταῖς τῶν ἀνέμων μεταβολαῖς συμμεταβάλληται ἡμῶν τὰ σώματα; ἔγωγ' οὖν οἶδα τῶν μὲν ἑταίρων τινὰ ἐπὶ τοῦ σκίμποδος ἔτι κατακείμενον ἐκ τῆς περὶ τὴν κεφαλὴν ἑαυτοῦ συναισθήσεως διαγινώσκοντα τοῦ ἀνέμου τὴν πνοήν. εἴ ποτε γὰρ ἐκαρηβάρει, εὐθέως ἐγίνωσκεν ὅτι νότος ὁ

mixtionibus, quum ufus poftulat, qualitates medicamentorum inalteramus; quod fieri non poffet, fi exigua quaedam et impatibilia immutabiliaque fubftantiae corpora effent. Atque ideo jam faepe ego fum demiratus, quomodo, quum in quocunque tam fubitas fieri converfiones tantamque temperamentorum mutationem viderent, fuftineant deinde talia rerum univerfarum principia ftatuere et praecipue jam citatus medicus Afclepiades; ad hunc enim peculiariter verba potius habeo, quoniam manifeftiores etiam in corpore converfiones mutationesque non indicat. Quid namque dicendum eft, quum folo digito in frigidam impofito totius corporis mutatio actutum oriatur? vel quum pro ventorum variatione corpora noftra fimul mutentur? Ego itaque ex familiaribus quendam novi in lecto adhuc decumbentem, ex capitis ipfius confenfu venti flatum cognoviffe. Quum enim capitis gravitate laboraret, ftatim ventum qui fpirabat auftrum effe

πνέων ἄνεμος ἦν. καὶ ἀκούσασα μόνον βροντῆς γυνὴ ἐγκύμων καὶ θεασαμένη φοβερόν τι θέαμα, ἐξέβαλε τὸ παιδίον. ἔσθ' ὅτε δὲ καὶ βοηθεῖν ὀξέως θέλοντες καὶ ταχεῖαν τῷ νοσοῦντι τοῦ βοηθήματος τὴν αἴσθησιν γενέσθαι, ταχίστην ὁρῶμεν γιγνομένην τῶν σωμάτων τὴν τροπήν. ἐπὶ γοῦν τινων ἐκλελυμένων σφόδρα ὀξυθυμίαν τινὰ τῷ ἀῤῥώστῳ ὁ θαυμάσιος Ἱπποκράτης γίνεσθαι συμβουλεύει, ἵνα τῷ εὐτόνῳ τῆς ὁρμῆς τὸ ἄτονον τῆς ἐκλύσεως ἰασώμεθα. πολλάκις δὲ καὶ ὀλίγη τις αὐτοῖς προσενεχθεῖσα τροφὴ εὐθέως ἀνέῤῥωσε καὶ τὴν δύναμιν αὐτῶν εὐτόνωσε, τῆς τροφῆς τοῦ σώματος, [946] ὡς οἶμαι, ταχέως ἐπὶ τὸ κρεῖττον γιγνομένης, ἀλλ' οὐχὶ τῶν ὄγκων ἀπαθῶν ὑπαρχόντων, καὶ διὰ τοῦτο τὴν αἴσθησιν ἡμῖν τῶν τοιούτων παρέχειν μὴ δυναμένων. τίς γὰρ ἐν τοσούτῳ τάχει τοὺς ὄγκους συντιθέναι δυνήσεται; ἢ τίς οὕτως ἐξ ἀπαθῶν τῶν ὄγκων συγκείμενος ταχέως τῶν προσπιπτόντων αἰσθήσεται; ἡ γὰρ ποιὰ τῶν ὄγκων μετατιθεμένων σύνθεσις τοῦ μὲν σχήματος ἀλλαγὴν μόνην ἐργάζεται, ἀλλοίωσιν δὲ καὶ ποιότητα ἄλλην ἐξ ἄλλης

deprehendebat. Jam mulier gravida folo tonitru exaudito et horribili quodam fpectaculo vifo infantem ejecit. Interdum quum repente volumus auxiliari et velocem praefidii fenfum aegro moliri, celerrimam in corporibus mutationem fieri videmus. In quibusdam igitur admodum exolutis admirandus Hippocrates infirmo excandefcentiam concitari confulit ut concitationis robore exolutionis imbecillitati medeamur; faepe etiam paucum aliquod oblatum ipfis alimentum ftatim refocillat viresque eorum reftituit, corporis mutatione, ut opinor, ftatim vergente in melius, non autem corpusculorum impatibilium, eoque talium nobis fenfus nequeunt imprimere. Quis enim in tantillo temporis momento corpuscula compofuerit? aut quis fic ex impatibilibus corpufculis conftructus repente occurrentia perceperit? Etenim certa corpufculorum tranfpofitorum compofitio figurae quidem folam efficit mutationem, caeterum alterationem qualitatemque aliam ex alia generare neutiquam poteft. Atque hujus rei gratia

γεννῆσαι ἀδυνατεῖ. καὶ διὰ τοῦτο ἐδόκει μοι τὸν ἄνδρα μὴ μόνον τὸ ἐπὶ τῶν φαρμάκων γιγνόμενον ἀκολούθοις ἀναιρεῖν διὰ τὴν ἀκολουθίαν τοῦ δόγματος, ἀλλὰ καὶ τὴν φύσιν αὐτὴν τὴν διοικοῦσαν ἐν ἡμῖν τὰ πάντα μηδὲν εἶναι οἴεσθαι. ἕκαστα γὰρ τῶν γιγνομένων ἐκ τῆς τῶν ὄγκων συνθέσεως καὶ συμπλοκῆς γίγνεσθαι βούλεται. διόπερ καὶ θαυμάζειν ἐπέρχεταί μοι, ὅταν αὐτὸν ὁρῶ τὰ οὕτω θαυμαστὰ τῆς φύσεως ἔργα μὴ βλέποντα, καὶ μάλιστα τὰς ἐξ ἀρχῆς ἐν αὐτῇ τῇ γενέσει τοῦ ἀνθρώπου γιγνομένας τέχνας, ὅπως μὲν διαπλάττεται τὸ ἔμβρυον ἐν τῷ τῆς μήτρας τόπῳ, ὅπως δ᾽ ἂν καὶ διαπλασθὲν εὐμηχάνως τρέφεται, ὅσοις δὲ καὶ οἵοις αὐτὸ τοῖς ἁπαλωτάτοις δεσμοῖς ἄχρι τοῦ ὡραίου τόκου ἔνδον κρατεῖ, οἵᾳ δέ τινι θείᾳ τέχνῃ καὶ ὁμοιότητι τύπον ἐν τοῖς γεννωμένοις ἐργάζεται, ἐφ᾽ οὗ μάλιστα καὶ ἡ τῶν ὄγκων ὑπόθεσις αὐτοῦ ἀσχημόνως ἐλέγχεται. οὐ γὰρ μόνοις τοῖς γεννῶσιν, ἀλλὰ καὶ προγόνοις τισὶ τὰ τικτόμενα ὅμοια γίνεται. ἐμοὶ δὲ καὶ λόγος τὶς ἀρχαῖος ἐμήνυσεν ὅτι τῶν ἀμόρφων τὶς δυνατὸς εὔμορφον θέλων γεννῆ-

putabam virum non modo quod in medicamentis fieri apparet, congruenter ob placiti rationem tollere; fed naturam quoque ipfam omnia in nobis difpenfantem nihil effe arbitrari. Singula enim quae nafcuntur ex corpusculorum compofitione et complexu fieri autumat. Quamobrem etiam mirari mihi fubit, quoties ad ipfum mentem dirigo, qui tam mirifica naturae opera, potiffimumque artes quae in ipfius hominis generandi initio fiunt, non videat quomodo quidem infans in uteri loco formetur, quomodo formatus jam apte nutriatur, quot et qualibus vinculis tenerrimis ipfum ad maturum usque partum intus contineat, quali vero divina arte et fimilitudine imaginem in generatis efficiat, in qua re praefertim corpusculorum quoque hypothefis ipfius non citra dedecus coarguitur. Non enim folis parentibus, fed proavis etiam quibusdam foetus redduntur fimiles. Porro mihi vetus quaedam hiftoria indicavit, quod quum deformis quidam opibus potens formofum vellet procreare puerum,

σαι παῖδα, ἐποίησε γράψαι ἐν πλατεῖ ξύλῳ εὐειδὲς ἄλλο παιδίον, καὶ ἔλεγε τῇ γυναικὶ συμπλεκόμενος ἐκείνῳ τῷ τύπῳ τῆς γραφῆς ἐμβλέπειν. ἡ δὲ ἀτενὲς βλέπουσα καὶ ὡς ἔστιν εἰπεῖν ὅλον τὸν νοῦν ἔχουσα οὐχὶ τῷ γεννήσαντι, ἀλλὰ τῷ γεγραμμένῳ ὁμοίως ἀπέτεκε τὸ παιδίον, τῆς ὄψεως, οἶμαι, διαπεμπούσης τῇ φύσει, ἀλλ' οὐκ ὄγκοις τισὶ τοῦ γεγραμμένου τοὺς τύπους. ἐπεὶ δὲ ἀμύητος τῶν τοιούτων τῆς φύσεως μυστηρίων ὁ ἀνὴρ εἶναι διὰ τοὺς ὄγκους ὑπομένει καὶ διὰ τὸ ἀφανές τε καὶ ἄδηλον τῆς ὄψεως τοὺς ἑαυτοῦ μαθητὰς πιστεύειν τοῖς οὕτω θαυμασίοις ἔργοις οὐκ ἐᾷ, ἐπὶ τὰ ἔξωθεν αὐτὸν καὶ παντάπασι φαινόμενα μεταβάλλειν βούλομαι. τίς γὰρ τὰς ὑπὸ τοῦ ζώου τῆς ἀράχνης γιγνομένας τέχνας βλέπων απιστεῖ καὶ τὴν διὰ τῶν οὕτω διαφανῶν τε καὶ λεπτῶν νημάτων γιγνομένην ὑπ' αὐτῆς ὑφὴν, ὡς καί τινας λέγειν τὴν ὑφαντικὴν τοὺς ἀνθρώπους λαβόντας τὸ πρῶτον παρ' αὐτῆς ἔχειν; τίνα δ' οὐ πείθει λέγειν θαυμάσιόν τι χρῆμα τὴν φύσιν ὑπάρχειν ὁρῶντα τὸ ὑπὸ τῆς ἄρκτου γιγνόμενον ἔργον; ἀποτίκτει μὲν γὰρ ἡ ἄρκτος

depinxit in lato ligno elegantem alium puellum dicebatque mulieri inter coëundum ut illam picturae figuram inſpiceret. Haec autem deſixis intuens oculis et, ut ita dicam, totam illuc mentem advertens, infantem non quidem patri, ſed picto ſimilem peperit, viſu opinor, naturae, non corpusculis quibusdam picti imaginem transmittente. Quoniam autem vir hujusmodi naturae myſteriorum imperitus eſſe corpusculorum gratia ſuſtinet et propter viſus obſcuritatem incertitudinemque, ſuos ipſius discipulos tam mirificis operibus fidem accommodare non ſinit, ad externa ipſum omninoque apparentia traducere cogito. Quis namque artes ab animalculo araneo factas inſpiciens non credit etiam telam per dilucida adeo tenuiaque fila parari? ut etiam aliqui dicant texendi artem homines primum ipſi referre acceptam. Quis non adducitur ut mirabilem quandam rem naturam eſſe pronunciet, ſi opus videat quod ab urſa efficitur? Etenim urſa omnibus quae

ἅπασι τοῖς γεννωμένοις ὁμοίως ζώοις. ἔστι δὲ σὰρξ μόνη γεννωμένη ἄπλαστός τε καὶ ἀδιάρθρωτος, μορφὴν μὲν οὐδεμίαν ἔχουσα, εὐθὺς δὲ ὑπὸ τῆς γεννώσης τῇ φυσικῇ τέχνῃ διατυπουμένη. τῇ γὰρ γλώττῃ ὥσπερ χειρί τινι χρωμένη ἡ τεκοῦσα οὕτω μεμορφωμένον ζῶον τὸ τεχθὲν ἀποτελεῖν ἀλλὰ πρὸς μὲν τούτους παύσομαι λέγων. καὶ γὰρ εἴωθα ἐν τοῖς φιλοτίμοις λόγοις ὥσπερ τινὶ χαλινῷ, καθάπερ ἵππου τινὸς γαύρου τρέχοντος τῷ μέτρῳ, τοῦ λόγου αὐτοῦ εὐτόνως κρατεῖν.

[947] Κεφ. ιβ'. [Ἕκαστα τὰ τὴν θηριακὴν συντιθέμενα ἀκριβῶς ἐξεταστέον. καὶ τὴν Ἀνδρομάχου γραφὴν προκριτέον.] Ἐπιδείξας δὲ, ὡς οἶμαι, σαφῶς μηκέτι εἶναί σοι θαυμαστὸν τὰ θηρία αὐτὰ καὶ ἀναιρεῖν καὶ βοηθεῖν δύνασθαι, διὰ τὴν ποικίλην σκευασίαν τε καὶ μίξιν τῶν συμμιγνυμένων αὐτοῖς φαρμάκων, μετὰ τοῦτο λοιπὸν τὴν ἀντίδοτον σκευάζειν ἄρξομαι. οὐ γάρ ἐστιν ὀλίγη καὶ ἡ ἐν τῇ σκευασίᾳ αὐτῆς γιγνομένη ὑφ' ἡμῶν τέχνη. ἥ τε γὰρ ἐν τοῖς θηρίοις πολλάκις ὑπὸ τῶν θηρευόντων αὐτὰ γιγνομένη πανουργία καὶ ἡ

generant animantibus fimiliter parit; caro autem fola generata informis et inarticulata eft, nullam obtinens figuram; ftatim vero a parente naturali arte figuratur; nam lingua veluti manu quadam utens editum foetum effigiatum reddit. Verum contra hos fermonem finiam; quippe confuevi in contentiofis orationibus ceu freno quodam equum folito ferocius currentem, menfura fermonem ipfum valide coërcere.

Cap. XII. [*Singula quae theriacam ingrediuntur diligenter exploranda effe: Andromachique defcriptionem caeteris praeferendam.*] At quum manifefto, ut auguror, demonftraverim, ne mirum amplius tibi fit, easdem feras et perimere et auxiliari poffe, propter variam tum confectionem tum mixturam medicamentorum quae ipfis contemperantur, deinceps antidotum praeparare aggrediar. Non enim ars eft exigua qua confectionem ipfius molimur; siquidem et dolus quem in feris faepe venatores

ἐν τοῖς ἄλλοις μίγμασι τῶν σκευαζόντων ἀπειρία ἄχρηστον πολλάκις ἐποίησε τὸ φάρμακον. πολλοὶ γὰρ αὐτῶν τὴν περὶ τὸ θηρεύειν τέχνην ἐπιδείκνυσθαι βουλόμενοι, καὶ μάλισθ' ὅσοι καὶ φάρμακά τινα πρὸς τὰ τοιαῦτα εὑρίσκειν ἐπαγγέλλονται, τὸ μὲν ἔχειν τὰ φάρμακα ψεύδονται. οὐ γὰρ εὕρομέν ποτε ἡμεῖς αὐτοὺς ἔχοντας, διὰ δὲ τοῦ πανουργεῖν τὰ θηρία τοὺς ὁρῶντας πλανῶσι, πρῶτον μὲν αὐτὰ θηρεύοντες οὐ τῷ δέοντι καιρῷ, ἀλλὰ μετὰ πολὺν τῆς φωλειᾶς τὸν χρόνον, ὅτε μηκέτ' ἐστὶν ἀκμαῖα. λαβόντες δὲ αὐτὰ καὶ προεθίζουσιν ἑαυτοῖς πολλάκις καὶ τρέφουσιν οὐ ταῖς εἰθισμέναις τροφαῖς, ἀλλὰ σάρκας αὐτοῖς ἐπιδιδόντες καὶ συνεχῶς ἐνδάκνειν ἀναγκάζοντες, οὕτως ἐκ τοῦ στόματος αὐτῶν κενοῦσθαι ποιοῦσι τὸν ἰὸν καὶ δὴ καὶ μάζας τινὰς ἐπιδιδόντες ἐμφραττούσας τῶν ὀδόντων τὰ τρήματα καὶ οὕτω τούτων ἀσθενῆ γίνεται τὰ δήγματα, ὡς θαυμάζειν πάνυ τοὺς ὁρῶντας τὴν τοιαύτην αὐτῶν εἰς τὸ πανουργεῖν τέχνην οὐκ εἰδότας· ὁμοίως δ' αὖ καὶ ἡ περὶ τὰ φάρμακα τῶν μιγνυμένων, ὡς ἔφην, ἀπειρία οὐκ ἔστιν (464) ὀλίγη.

ipfarum machinantur et in aliis mixturis praeparantium imperitia, inutile frequenter medicamentum effecerunt. Plerique enim ipforum venandi artem volentes oftendere et praefertim qui etiam medicamenta quaedam ad res hujusmodi invenire profitentur, habere quidem fe medicamenta mentiuntur; haud enim unquam nos ipfos habentes invenimus; dolo autem in belluis, videntibus imponunt, primum ipfas haud congruo tempore venantes, fed multo poft vernationem, quum non amplius vigent. Captas autem ipfas crebro fibi ipfis affuefaciunt et cibis non folitis enutriunt, imo carnes ipfis permittentes et continue mordere cogentes fic ut virus ex earum ore vacuetur efficiunt. Quin etiam mazas quasdam objiciunt, quae dentium foramina obftruant; atque hac ratione morfus fiunt imbecilles, ut videntibus magnum fit miraculum, talis ipforum ad fraudem parandam artificii imperitis. Simili modo etiam in medicamentis mixtorum haud mediocris, ut dixi, eft infcitia. Quid multis opus eft, in optimis quae

αὐτίκα γέ τοι περὶ τὰ κάλλιστα τῶν ἐμβαλλομένων, κασσίαν λέγω καὶ τὸ κιννάμωμον αὐτὸ, οὐκ ὀλίγη τίς ἐστι διαφορὰ, καὶ πολλοὺς τῶν σκευαζόντων εἴωθε πλανᾷν. τό τε γὰρ καλούμενον ψευδοκιννάμωμον ὅμοιόν ἐστι τῷ ἀληθεῖ, κατὰ δὲ τὴν γεῦσιν καὶ τὴν ὀσμὴν πολὺ ἐνδεέστερον εὑρίσκεται. τὸ δὲ ξυλοκιννάμωμον διαφέρει τῷ ξυλῶδες εἶναι καὶ ἰσχυρὰς τὰς ῥάβδους ἔχειν καὶ οὐχ ὁμοίαν τὴν εὐωδίαν. καὶ αὐτοῦ δὲ τοῦ ἀληθινοῦ κινναμώμου τὸ μὲν ἐν τοῖς ὄρεσι γιγνόμενον, οὐκ ὂν λεπτὸν οὐδὲ μακρὸν, μᾶλλον κιῤῥόν ἐστι τῇ χροιᾷ. ἕτερον δέ ἐστι ποσῶς μέλαν καὶ ὥσπερ ἶνας ἔχον τινάς. ἄλλο τι λευκὸν εὑρίσκεται ἀκριβῶς καὶ οὐ σκληρὸν, ῥᾳδίως θραυόμενον καὶ μικρὰν ἔχον τὴν ῥίζαν. ἔστι δέ τι καὶ τῇ κιῤῥᾷ κασσίᾳ ὅμοιον ἕτερον λεῖον καὶ εὐῶδες. τὸ δὲ πάντων κάλλιστόν ἐστι τὸ μόσυλλον ὑπὸ τῶν ἐγχωρίων οὕτω καλούμενον, τεφρῶδες τῇ χροιᾷ καὶ λεπτὰ ἔχον τὰ ῥαβδία καὶ τοὺς ὄζους πυκνοὺς, σφόδρα εὐῶδες, ὃ καὶ μάλιστα προκρίνειν ἡμεῖς εἰώθαμεν. ἔστι γὰρ πάνυ τῇ ὀδμῇ κάλλιστόν τε καὶ ἥδιστον καὶ τῇ γεύσει δριμὺ ἡμῖν κατα-

immittuntur, caſſia dico et cinnamomo ipſo haud modica exiſtit differentia et multos ex iis qui praeparant, ſolet decipere. Nam quod vocatur pſeudo-cinnamomum, veroſimile eſt, niſi quod guſtu et odore longe reperiatur inferius. Atqui xylocinnamomum hac re differt, quod lignoſum ſit, valida habeat virgulta, nec ſimilem ſuaveolentiam prae ſe ferat. Porro inter ipſius veri cinnamomi genera aliud in montibus naſcitur, non tenue, nec longum, magis gilvum colore. Aliud aliquantulum nigricat et tanquam fibris quibusdam intertextum. Aliud adamuſſim album reperitur, non durum, ex facili fragile, parva radice. Eſt et aliud quoddam caſſiae gilvae ſimile, laeve et odoratum. Praeſtantiſſimum omnium eſt quod ab indigenis moſyllon dicitur, cinereum colore, virgultis gracilibus, ramusculis frequentibus, vehementerque odoratum, quod etiam potiſſimum nos praeponere conſuevimus. Eſt enim odore longe optimum ſuaviſſimumque et guſtu acre nobis apparet, mordax admodum; manſum rutam prae

φαίνεται καὶ δηκτικὸν λίαν, καὶ διαμασώμενον πηγανίζειν δοκεῖ. ἔστι δὲ καὶ λεῖον καὶ ῥᾳδίως θραύεσθαι δυνάμενον. ἡ δὲ κασσία καὶ αὐτὴ, εἰ μή τις ἔμπειρος εἴη περὶ τὴν κρίσιν, πλανᾷν εἴωθε πολλάκις. ἔστι γάρ τις καὶ ψευδοκασσία πάνυ μὲν ἐμφερὴς τῇ ἀληθινῇ κασσίᾳ, οὐκ ἔχουσα δὲ τὴν τοιαύτην εὐωδίαν, ἀλλὰ καὶ ὁ φλοιὸς αὐτῆς συνηνωμένος τῇ ἐντεριώνῃ εὑρίσκεται, ὡς ἥ γε καλλίστη κιῤῥά τε καὶ ῥοδίζουσα, ὥσπερ καὶ ἡδὺ τὸ γευστικὸν ἐν τῇ γεύσει ποιουμένη, συριγγώδης τε οὖσα καὶ οἰνίζουσα καὶ πολὺ τὸ ἀρωματίζον ἔχουσα, ζιγγίβερ ὑπὸ τῶν ἐπιχωρίων οὕτω λεγο- [948] μένη. εἰκὸς δέ σε καὶ τὴν περὶ τὸ μακρὸν πέπερι γιγνομένην πανουργίαν μὴ ἀγνοεῖν. ἀναπλάσσοντες γάρ τινες αὐτὸ ἴσον τῷ ἀληθεῖ ἔχον τὸ μῆκος καὶ ἐνθέντες αὐτῷ τοῦ πυρέθρου ἢ τοῦ νάπυος ὀλίγον, οὕτω τῷ δηκτικῷ τῆς γεύσεως πλανῶσι τὸν γευόμενον. ἀλλ' ὁ περὶ ταῦτα τριβακὸς ὢν καὶ τὸ ἥδιόν τε καὶ δριμὺ ἐν τῇ γεύσει μὴ ἀγνοῶν, ἔτι τε καὶ τὴν ἀπὸ τοῦ δένδρου ῥίζαν προσκειμένην αὐτῷ περιεργότερον βλέπων, εὑρίσκει τὸ ἀληθινὸν πέπερι καὶ πλανᾶσθαι ὑπ'

ſe ferre videtur; ad haec laeve eſt et facile poteſt confringi. Caſſia vero itidem niſi in dijudicando fueris expertus, frequenter ſolet imponere. Eſt enim et pſeudocaſſia, mirum quam germanae ſimilis, ſed odore minus grato coarguitur, corticem medullae adhaerentem obtinens. Quare optima gilva eſt et roſam expirat, ſicut etiam dulcem guſtum praeſert, fiſtulis plena et vinum naribus obolens et aromatum modo vehementer odorata, atque haec zingiber ab indigenis ſic nominatur. Jam vero in pipere oblongo dolos fieri te ignorare haud eſt veriſimile. Siquidem nonnulli adulterantes ipſum aequale cum vero pondus habens, pyrethri vel ſinapi modico indito, ita guſtus mordacitate guſtantem fallunt. Verum in his exercitatus et qui gratius in cibis acriusque guſtu novit deprehendere, necnon arboris radicem ei adhaerentem curioſius inſpicit, germanum piper invenit et falli ab ipſis nequit. Porro quum multa in aliis quoque univerſis ſit

αὐτῶν οὐ δύναται. πολλῆς δ' οὔσης καὶ ἐν τοῖς ἄλλοις ἅπασιν ἀκριβείας, ὥσπερ καὶ ἐν τούτοις ἱστόρησά σοι, ἐγὼ μὲν καὶ ταῦτα πρὸς τὴν τοῦ λόγου ὑπόμνησιν ἀρκεῖν νομίζω, ἵνα μὴ μακρὸν τὸ βιβλίον ἡμῖν γένηται. συμβουλεύω δὲ, ἕκαστον αὐτῶν ἀκριβῶς δοκιμάζοντα οὕτω σκευάζειν τὸ φάρμακον. ἡ γὰρ ἑνός τινος κακία πολλάκις διαφθείρει τὰ πάντα. ἔστι δὲ αὐτοῦ καὶ γραφὴ, ἵνα μηδὲ τοῦτο ἀγνοῆς, διαφόρως ὑπὸ τῶν ἰατρῶν γινομένη. ὁ μὲν γὰρ Ἀνδρόμαχος, ἀκριβὴς περὶ τὰ φάρμακα γενόμενος, οὗπερ καὶ πρότερον ἐμνημόνευσα, κατὰ ταύτην τὴν γραφὴν ἐσκεύαζε τὸ φάρμακον. ℞ Ἀρτίσκων θηριακῶν < κδ'. ἀρτίσκων σκιλλητικῶν < μη'. πεπέρεως μακροῦ < κδ'. ὀποῦ μήκωνος < κδ'. ἡδυχρόου μάγματος < κδ'. ῥόδων ξηρῶν < ιβ'. ἴρεως Ἰλλυρικῆς, γλυκυῤῥίζης, βουνιάδος ἀγρίας σπέρματος, σκορδίου, ὀποβαλσάμου, κινναμώμου, ἀγαρικοῦ ἀνὰ < ιβ'. σμύρνης, κόστου, κρόκου, κασσίας, νάρδου, σχοίνου ἄνθους, λιβάνου, πεπέρεως λευκοῦ καὶ μέλανος, δικτάμνου, πρασίου, ῥήου, στοιχάδος, πετροσελίνου Μακεδονικοῦ, καλα-

accurata examinatio, quemadmodum in his pariter tibi percenfui, ego fane vel haec ad libri commentationem fufficere exiftimo, ne fermo nobis fiat prolixior. Caeterum confulo fingulis ipfis accurate exploratis medicamentum praeparari. Nam unius cujusdam vitium omnia faepe corrumpit. Defcriptio autem ipfius, ne hoc etiam ignores, varie apud medicos invenitur. Etenim Andromachus, qui in medicamentis accuratus eft, cujus etiam prius mentionem feci, fecundum hanc defcriptionem medicamentum praeparabat. ℞ Paftillorum theriaces ʒ xxiv, paftillorum fcilliticorum ʒ xlviij, piperis longi ʒ xxiv, fucci papaveris ʒ xxiv, paftilli hedychroi ʒ xxiv, rofarum ficcarum ʒ xij, ireos Illyricae, glycyrrhizae, feminis napi filveftris, fcordii, opobalfami, cinnamomi, agarici, fingulorum drach. xij, myrrhae, cofti, croci, caffiae, nardi, fchoenanthi, thuris, piperis albi et nigri, dictamni, marrubii, rheu, ftoechados, petrofelini Macedonici, calaminthae, terebinthinae, zingiberis, quinquefolii radicis, fin-

μίνθης, τερμινθίνης, ζιγγιβέρεως, πενταφύλλου ῥίζης, ἀνὰ < στ'. πολίου < δ'. χαμαιπίτυος < δ'. στύρακος < δ'. ἀμώμου βότρυος, μήου, νάρδου Κελτικῆς, Λημνίας σφραγῖδος, φοῦ Ποντικοῦ, χαμαίδρυος Κρητικῆς, φύλλων μαλαβάθρου, χαλκίτεως ὀπτῆς, γεντιανῆς, ἀνίσου, ὑποκιστίδος χυλοῦ, βαλσάμου καρποῦ, κόμμεως, μαράθρου σπέρματος, καρδαμώμου, σεσέλεως, ἀκακίας, θλάσπεως, ὑπερικοῦ, σαγαπηνοῦ, ἄμμεως, ἀνὰ < δ'. καστορίου, ἀριστολοχίας λεπτῆς, δαύκου σπέρματος, ἀσφάλτου Ἰουδαϊκῆς, ὀποπάνακος, κενταυρίου λεπτοῦ, χαλβάνου, ἀνὰ < β'. μέλιτος λίτρας ι'. οἴνου Φαλερίνου τὸ ἀρκοῦν. Ξενοκράτης δὲ καὶ αὐτὸς σπουδὴν οὐκ ὀλίγην περὶ τὰ τοιαῦτα ποιησάμενος ὁμοίως μὲν τὰ ἄλλα τῷ Ἀνδρομάχῳ ἐσκεύαζε τὴν ἀντίδοτον, μόνον δὲ ἀντὶ τῶν < δ'. τοῦ σαγαπηνοῦ αὐτὸς < β'. ἔμισγε τῷ φαρμάκῳ. ὁ δὲ Δαμοκράτης, ἄριστος ἰατρὸς καὶ αὐτὸς γενόμενος καὶ ὅλον βιβλίον φιλοτίμως συντάξας καὶ αὐτὸς ἔπεσι περὶ τῆς τῶν ἀντιδότων σκευασίας, πάντα μὲν τὰ μίγματα τούτοις ὁμοίως μίγνυσι ἐν τῇ σκευασίᾳ τοῦ φαρ-

gulorum ʒ vj, polii ʒ iv, chamaepityos ʒ iv, ſtyracis ʒ iv, amomi, uvae, meu, nardi Celticae, ſigilli Lemnii, phu Pontici, chamaedryos Creticae, foliorum malabathri, chalcitidis toſtae, gentianae, aniſi hypociſtidis ſucci, balſami fructus, gummi, feniculi ſeminis, cardamomi, ſeſelis, acaciae, thlaſpis, hyperici, ſagapeni, ammeos, ſingulorum drach. iv, caſtorii, ariſtolochiae tenuis, dauci ſeminis, bituminis Judaici, opopanacis. centaurii tenuis, galbani, ſingulorum ʒ ij, mellis libras x, vini Phalerni quod ſatis eſt. Porro Xenocrates et ipſe non mediocri ſtudio in hujusmodi verſatus in reliquis ſane Andromacho ſimiliter antidotum praeparabat, ſolum vero pro quatuor ſagapeni drachmis duas ipſe medicamento oommiſcebat. At Damocrates, praeſtantiſſimus ipſe quoque medicus factus, integrum librum de antidotorum confectione verſibus eleganter complexus, omnes quidem mixturas his ſimiliter in medicamenti praeparatione temperat: ſed in *ſimplicium* mixtorum menſuris ab ipſis diſcrepat. Nam quae illi ſin-

μάκου, διαφωνεῖ δὲ αὐτοῖς ἐν τοῖς τῶν μεμιγμένων μέτροις. τινὰ γὰρ ὧν ἐκεῖνοι πέμπουσι τῷ φαρμάκῳ, ἀνὰ < δ'. ἔχοντα, οὗτος ἀνὰ < β'. μίγνυσι τῷ φαρμάκῳ, καὶ πάλιν τῶν ἀνὰ < β'. τὴν συσταθμίαν ἐχόντων, αὐτὸς ταῦθ' ἵστησιν ἀνὰ < α'. ἔχοντα. Μάγνος δὲ, ὁ καθ' ἡμᾶς ἀρχίατρος γενόμενος, τὰ ἄλλα πάντα ὁμοίως τοῖς ἀνδράσι τούτοις ἐν τῇ σκευασίᾳ φυλάττων, ἐν τῷ κινναμώμῳ μόνον αὐτοῖς διαφωνεῖ. τὸ γὰρ διπλοῦν τῆς περὶ τούτων συσταθμίας μίγνυσιν αὐτὸς τῷ φαρμάκῳ, οὕτως δὲ καὶ περὶ τῆς χαλκίτεως, οὕτως δὲ καὶ περὶ τοῦ σαγαπηνοῦ τῷ Ἀνδρομάχῳ διαφωνεῖ. τὰς γὰρ < β'. ὁμοίως τῷ Ξενοκράτει μίγνυσιν εἰς τὸ φάρμακον, τοῦ Ἀνδρομάχου < δ'. βάλλοντος· κατὰ δὲ τὸ σαγαπηνὸν καὶ τῷ Δαμοκράτει. μίαν μὲν γὰρ δραχμὴν ὁ Δαμοκράτης μίγνυσι τῷ φαρμάκῳ, ὁ δὲ Μάγνος β'. προστίθησι δὲ καὶ τῷ μιγνυμένῳ οἴνῳ ὁ Μάγνος τὸ μέτρον. δύο γὰρ ξέστας τοῦ βαλλομένου εἶναι βούλεται, τῶν ἄλλων, ὡς εἰκὸς πρὸς τὴν χρείαν, [949] ὁπόσῳ μέτρῳ τοῦ οἴνου χρωμένων. Δημήτριος δὲ, καὶ αὐτὸς καθ' ἡμᾶς ἀρχίατρος γενόμενος, τῷ μὲν Ἀνδρομάχῳ ὁμοίως κατὰ πάντα τὰ ἄλλα

gula drachmis quatuor medicamento injiciunt, hic drach. ij, sigillatim miscet, contra quibus binas drachmas singulis temperant, ipse unam drachmam immittit. Magnus autem, qui nostro tempore archiatros evasit, alia omnia sicut hi viri in confectione servans, solo cinnamomo ab ipsis evariat. Nam duplicatum hujus pondus medicamento ipse adjungit, ita vero in chalcitide, ita quoque in sagapeno, ab Andromachi sententia discordat; quippe duas drachmas veluti Xenocrates in medicamentum conjicit, quum Andromachus drachmas quatuor mittat. Verum in sagapeno Damocrati etiam refragatur. Etenim hic unam drachmam, Magnus duas medicamento injicit, praetereaque immixto vino addit mensuram Magnus; quippe duos sextarios infundendum censet, aliis ut usus postulat, qualicunque vini mensura utentibus. Demetrius, qui et ipse nostra tempestate primarius medicus constitutus est, in omnibus aliis juxta Andromachi sententiam medicamentum praepa-

συμφώνως σκευάζει τὸ φάρμακον, μόνῃ δὲ τῇ τῶν σκιλλητικῶν ἀρτίσκων συσταθμίᾳ τῷ Ἀνδρομάχῳ διαφωνεῖ καὶ τοῖς ἄλλοις πᾶσιν. ἐκείνων γὰρ μη'. δραχμὰς βαλλόντων μέτρον, οὗτος μόνος μστ'. δραχμὰς μόνας μίγνυσι τῇ ἀντιδότῳ. τοσαύτης γὰρ οὔσης τῆς περὶ τὰς γραφὰς διαφορᾶς, ἡμεῖς τῇ Ἀνδρομάχου ὡς ἀρίστῃ χρώμεθα, καὶ εἰς γε τὰς βασιλικὰς χρείας οὕτως σκευάζομεν. γίνεται δὲ αὐτῆς ἡ σκευασία τὸν τρόπον τοῦτον. καὶ γὰρ εὔχρηστον νομίζω σκευάσαι σοι αὐτὴν τῷ λόγῳ, ἵνα ἤν ποτε καὶ μὴ παρόντος ἰατροῦ εὐφυὴς ὢν σκευάζειν αὐτὴν ἐθέλῃς, ὡς ἄριστα σκευάσῃς, διδάσκαλον τῆς σκευασίας ἔχων αὐτὸν τὸν λόγον.

Κεφ. ιγ'. [Πῶς κατασκευαστέοι οἵ τε ἡδύχροοι, σκιλλητικοὶ καὶ θηριακοὶ ἀρτίσκοι.] Πρὸ δὲ τῆς κατασκευῆς αὐτῆς ἐχρῆν σε καὶ τὴν ἐμβαλλομένου εἰς αὐτὴν ἡδυχρόου μάγματος γραφὴν εἰδέναι. ἔστιν οὖν ἡ ἀρίστη σκευασία ἡ παρὰ Μάγνῳ, ἧς ἡ γραφὴ αὕτη. ℞ Ἀσπαλάθου ῥίζης φλοιοῦ, καλάμου ἀρωματικοῦ, σχοίνου ἄνθους, φοῦ, κόστου, ἀσάρου, ξυλοβαλσάμου, ἀσίας, ἀνὰ < στ'. κινναμώμου

rat, folo fcilliticorum paftillorum pondere ab eo difcrepat et aliis univerfis fcriptoribus. Siquidem illi cum drachmis xlviij, menfuram complectantur, folus hic xlvj, drachmas duntaxat antidoto admifcet. Nam quum tanta in defcriptionibus fit differentia, nos Andromachi tanquam praeftantiffima utimur et in regios ufus ita praeparamus. Porro confectio ipfius hunc in modum fit. Etenim utilem tibi ac dexteram ratione praeparandam cenfeo, ut fi quando medici inopia, dexteritate ingenii praeditus voles conficere, quam optime conficias, loco magiftri praeparationis, ipfo rationis adminiculo fretus.

Cap. XIII. [*Quo pacto componendi fint paftilli hedychroi, fcillini et viperini.*] Caeterum ante illam confectionem conveniebat etiam paftilli hedychroi, quae ei inditur, praefcriptionem pernoviffe. Eft igitur laudatiffima praeparatio apud Magnum hifce verbis expreffa. ℞ Afpalathi radiculae corticis, calami aromatici, fchoeni floris, phu, cofti, afari, xylobalfami, afiae, fingulorum ʒ vj,

< κδ'. ἀμώμου < κδ'. ἀμαράκου < κ'. νάρδου Ἰνδικῆς < ιστ'. μαλαβάθρου φύλλων < στ'. σμύρνης < κδ'. μαστίχης < στ'. κρόκου < ιθ'. οἴνῳ Φαλερίνῳ ἀναλάμβανε, ὀποβαλσάμου παραπτόμενος ἐν τῷ ἀναλαμβάνειν, καὶ ψῦχε τοὺς τροχίσκους ἐν σκιᾷ. ὁμοίως δὲ καὶ τοὺς σκιλλητικοὺς ἀρτίσκους σκεύαζε οὕτως. λαβόντα χρὴ σκίλλαν νεαρὰν καὶ μὴ πάνυ μεγάλην περιπλάττειν, μὴ ὥς τινες πηλῷ, ῥυ-(465) παρὸν γάρ εἶναί μοι δοκεῖ, ἀλλὰ ζύμῃ, ὀπτᾶται γὰρ ῥαδίως τῇ ἁπαλωτάτῃ, ἵνα ἐν τῇ ὀπτήσει καὶ αὐτοῦ τι μεταλαμβάνῃ. εἶτα ὅταν ὀπτήσῃ καλῶς ἐν τῷ καλουμένῳ ἴπνῳ, ἢ ἐν τοῖς κλιβάνοις, ἢ κακάβοις ἐν οἷς οἱ ἄρτοι ὀπτῶνται, ἵνα ὁμαλὴ ἡ ὄπτησις γένηται, λαβόντα χρὴ τὰ ἔνδον αὐτῆς μέρη τὰ ἁπαλώτατα λειοῦν ἐπιμελῶς, μίσγοντα καὶ ὀροβίνου ἀλεύρου καλλίστου καὶ νεαρωτάτου τὸ ἴσον, ὡς ὁ Δαμοκράτης βούλεται. ὁ γὰρ Μάγνος τὸ ἥμισυ πέμπων ὀλίγον μοι μιγνύναι δοκεῖ, καὶ ὁ Ἀνδρόμαχος δὲ δύο πέμπων μέρη πολύ μοι πέμπειν δοκεῖ. τὸ δ' ἴσον ἐστὶ τὸ πρὸς ἀνάπλασιν σύμμετρον, καὶ οὕτως συλλειώσαντα αὐτῷ

cinnamomi ʒ xxiv, amomi ʒ xxiv, amaraci ʒ xx, nardi Indicae ʒ xvj, foliorum malabathri ʒ vj, myrrhae ʒ xxiv, maſtiches ʒ vj, croci ʒ xix, excipe vino Phalerno, opobalſami contactu ſinge paſtillos et in umbra deſicca. Simili modo ſcilliticos quoque orbiculos praepara. Sumitur ſcilla recens, parvae magnitudinis, oblinitur non, ut quidam volunt, luto, nam id ſordidum eſſe mihi apparet, ſed fermento, nam facile tenerrimo torrentur, ut interea nonnihil etiam ipſius aſſumat. Deinde ubi probe in furno, vel in patinis ubi panes coquuntur, ut aequalis ſiat toſtio, incaluerit, ſumptis interioribus ipſius partibus tenerrimis, laevigare diligenter oportet; ervi quoque farina laudatiſſima recentiſſimaque pari portione admiſcebitur, ut Damocrates praecipit. Nam Magnus dimidiam partem immittens parum mihi admiſcere videtur; Andromachus autem duas injiciens portiones multum mittere mihi videtur. Aequalis autem modus ſingendis paſtillis optimus eſt, atque hac ratione trita cum ervo ſcilla orbiculos

τοσοῦτον, ἀναπλάττειν τροχίσκους συμμέτρους χρὴ, καὶ ἐν σκιᾷ ἀποτιθεμένους εἰς τὴν χρῆσιν φυλάττειν, εἶτα μετὰ ταῦτα χρὴ λαμβάνειν αὐτὰς τὰς ἐχίδνας πρὸς τὸ πλῆθος τῆς ὅλης σκευασίας αὐτάρκεις, μὴ ἐν παντὶ καιρῷ τεθηραμένας, ἀλλὰ μάλιστα περὶ τὴν ἀρχὴν τοῦ ἔαρος, ὅταν τῆς μὲν φωλείας παύονται, προέρχονται δὲ λοιπὸν ἔξω εἰς τοὺς ὑπαίθρους τόπους, καὶ οὐκέθ᾽ οὕτως ἔχουσι πονηρὸν τὸν ἰόν. ἔνδον γὰρ φωλεύοντα, καὶ κατὰ μηδὲν διαφορούμενα πονηροτέραν συνάγει καὶ τὴν ἐν αὐτοῖς φθοροποιὸν δύναμιν, ὅτε καὶ τὸ καλούμενον γῆρας συλλέγειν εἴωθε πᾶς ὄφις, ὅπερ ἐστὶν ἐπίπαγός τις παχύτατος, συναγόμενος ἐν τῷ τῆς φωλείας χρόνῳ, καὶ τῷ χρόνῳ τῆς φωλείας μᾶλλον ἤπερ τῆς ἡλικίας τοῦ ζώου γῆρας τυγχάνον. διόπερ χρὴ μὴ εὐθέως αὐτὰ λαμβάνειν, ἀλλὰ ἐᾷν τινα χρόνον ἀπολαῦσαί τε τοῦ ἀέρος καὶ τραφῆναι τὴν συνήθη νομήν. νέμεται δὲ ταῦτα τὰ θηρία καὶ βοτάνης μέν τινας καὶ ζῶα καὶ τὰ συνήθως αὐτὰ τρέφειν δυνάμενα, ὥσπερ τὰς βουπρήστεις καὶ κανθαρίδας [950] καὶ τὰς καλουμένας πιτυοκάμπας. αὗται γὰρ αὐτῶν εἰσιν αἱ κατάλληλοι τροφαί. ἔστω δὲ καὶ

formabis mediocres et in umbra repoſitos in uſum ſervabis; deinde poſt haec viperae ipſae, quae ad totius confectionis copiam ſufficiant, ſumendae ſunt, non quovis tempore, ſed potiſſimum veris initio captae, quum latebris relictis foras in apricum prodeunt et non adhuc virus tam pravum occupant. Intus enim delitescentes, cum nulla ex parte digeruntur, maligniorem etiam vim tabificam in ſe contrahunt; quando etiam ſenium dictum ſolent, ſicut omnis ſerpens, colligere, quod eſt craſſiſſimum quoddam integumentum, tempore quo delituerunt contractum, atque tunc magis quam animantis aetate ſenium exiſtens. Quapropter non ſtatim ipſas capere oportet, ſed permittere aliquamdiu et aëre frui et conſueto cibo veſci. Porro veſcuntur hae ferae tum herbis quibusdam tum animalibus et quibus aſſuetae ſolent nutriri, cujusmodi ſunt bupreſtes, cantharides et quas vocant pityocampas; haec enim idonea ipſarum ſunt alimenta. Sint

ὑπόξανθα τὰ ζῶα καὶ εὐκίνητα σφόδρα, καὶ μάλιστα ἐπανατείνοντα τὸν τράχηλον, καὶ τοὺς ὀφθαλμοὺς ὑπερύθρους ἔχοντα, καὶ ἀναιδεῖς καὶ θηριῶδες βλέποντα, καὶ τὰς κεφαλὰς πλατυτέρας καὶ τὸ πᾶν σῶμα, καὶ τὴν γαστέρα προκολπότερον, καὶ τὸν πόρον πρὸς ἄκρᾳ μᾶλλον τῇ οὐρᾷ ἔχοντα, καὶ τὴν οὐρὰν μὴ περιειλημένην, ἀλλὰ μᾶλλον συστρέφοντα, καὶ ἠρεμαῖον τὸν περίπατον ποιούμενα. τούτῳ γὰρ τοῦ ἄῤῥενος ἡ ἔχιδνα διήνεγκε καὶ τῷ πλέονας τῶν δύο κυνοδόντων ἔχειν, ὥσπερ δὴ καὶ Νίκανδρος διὰ τῶν ἐπῶν τούτων λέγει

Τοῦ μὲν ὑπὲρ κυνόδοντε δύο χροΐ τεκμαίρονται,
ἰὸν ἐρευγόμενοι, πλέονες δέ τοι αἰὲν ἐχίδνης.

καὶ δὴ λαβόντα αὐτὰ τῷ καιρῷ τούτῳ πρῶτον μὲν αὐτῶν χρὴ ἀποκόπτειν τὰς κεφαλάς τε καὶ τὰς οὐρὰς, τοσοῦτον ἀποκόπτοντας, ὡς εἶναι τὸ μέτρον τῆς ἀποκοπῆς τεσσάρων δακτύλων. ἐπιβλέπειν δὲ καὶ ἐν τῷ ἀποκόπτειν τὰ μέρη ταῦτα ἀκριβῶς παραινῶ, εἰ μετὰ τὴν ἀποκοπὴν ἄναιμά τε εὐθέως καὶ ἀκίνητα καὶ πάντῃ νεκρὰ τὰ ζῶα εἶναι φαί-

autem animalia colore fufflava, admodum motu facilia, collum praecipue extollentia, oculis fubrubentibus, afperis, ferinum cernentibus, capite latiore, corpore et ventre craffiora, meatu magis ad extrema caudae, quae non involuta eft, fed potius converfa, inceffu quieti proximo. Hac enim re foemina a mafculo differt, ad haec quod caninos dentes duobus plures habeat, quemadmodum fane et Nicander hifce verfibus dicit

Sunt gemini dentes maribus, fua figna, canini
Virus fundentes: habet hos fed foemina plures.

Et fane hoc tempore captis primum capita et caudas amputare convenit, ita ut amputatio fiat pro quatuor digitorum menfura. Dum autem partes has abfcindis, infpicere confilium eft num his amputatis exanguia protinus, immobilia, prorfufque emortua effe animalia videantur. Nam fi tales offenderis beftias, nihil ad medi-

νοιτο. εἰ γὰρ τοιαῦτα εὑρίσκοιτο τὰ θηρία, ἄχρηστα αὐτὰ πρὸς τὴν τοῦ φαρμάκου μῖξιν εἶναι νόμιζε. εἰ δὲ βλέποις ἐν αὐτοῖς ἀποκοπέντων τῶν μερῶν ὑπολειπομένην κίνησίν τινα καὶ τὸ ἔναιμον ἐπί τινα χρόνον ἀποσώζειν δυνάμενα, ταῦτα ὡς ἄριστα ὄντα, μιγνύναι τῇ σκευασίᾳ τῆς ἀντιδότου, οὐ γὰρ ἐξίτηλον, ἀλλὰ ἰσχυρὰν πρὸς τὸ σώζειν ἔχοντα δύναμιν φαίνεται. εἶτα μετὰ τοῦτο ἀποδέρειν αὐτῶν ὅλον ἀκριβῶς τὸ δέρμα, ἐξαίρειν δὲ καὶ τὸ στέαρ ὡς ἄχρηστον καὶ τὰ ἐντόσθια ἅπαντα, ἔστι γὰρ τῶν περιττωμάτων δοχεῖα. καὶ μετὰ τοῦτο ἐμβάλλειν αὐτὰ λοιπὸν εἴς τι κεραμοῦν ἀγγεῖον, ὡς κάλλιστα κατασκευασθὲν, ἢ εἰς λέβητα γεγανωμένον καλῶς, καὶ τοῖς ἄνθραξιν ἀνακεκαυμένοις ἐπικείμενον, ἵνα ἀκνίσως ἡ ἕψησις αὐτῶν γένηται. ἑψήσθωσαν δὲ ἐν ὕδατι πηγαίῳ καὶ προσεμβαλέσθωσαν ἅλες νεαροὶ, καὶ ἀνήθου μὴ ξηροῦ κλῶνες σύμμετροι. εἶθ' ὅταν ἑψηθῶσιν αἱ σάρκες καλῶς, τὸ μέτρον δὲ τῆς ἑψήσεως ἔστω σοι, ὅταν αἱ ἄκανθαι χωρισθῶσι τῆς σαρκὸς τῶν θηρίων, τότε ἀνελόμενος τὸν λέβητα ἀπὸ τοῦ πυρὸς ἀκριβῶς χώριζε τὰς

camenti mixtionem conducere ipſas cenſeto. At ſi motum quendam in ipſis partibus reſiduum conſpicias et ſanguinem conſervare aliquamdiu poſſe, has ceu praeſtantiſſimas antidoto praeparando immittes, ut quae haud ignavam exoleſcentemque, ſed validam ad ſervandum vim habere appareant. Deinde tota adamuſſim cute ipſis detracta, adeps ceu nullius momenti, omniaque interanea, tanquam excrementorum receptacula eximentur; mox reliquum corpus in vas quoddam fictile quam elegantiſſime conſtructum, vel in lebetem probe exterſum ſplendidumque indetur, ac prunae impoſitum, ut citra nidorem ac fumum illius concoctio ſiat; incoquatur autem ex aqua fontis ſale recenti, cum mediocribus anethi non aridi virgultis adjecto; deinde carnibus jam bene coctis, quod nimirum cognoſces quum ſpinae a viperarum carne ſeparantur, et lebete ab igne depoſito, diligenter carnes a ſpinis ſegrega, tritisque ipſis panis quam maxime puri et ex ſincera facti

σάρκας τῶν ἀκανθῶν, καὶ λειώσας αὐτὰς, ἄρτου ὡς μάλιστα τοῦ καθαρωτάτου καὶ ἀπὸ σεμιδάλεως τῆς καθαρωτάτης γενομένου μίσγε τὸ σύμμετρον πρὸς τὴν ἀνάπλασιν, ὥσπερ καὶ ὁ Ἀνδρόμαχος βούλεται. ὁ γὰρ Μάγνος, καὶ ὁ Δαμοκράτης καὶ μέτρον τὶ ὡρισμένον αὐτοῖς μίγνυσθαι θέλουσιν· ἴσον γὰρ τοῦ ἄρτου πρὸς ἴσον τῶν σαρκῶν ἀποστήσαντες, οὕτως αὐτὰς συλλειοῦσι τῷ ἄρτῳ· εἶτα παραχέας τὸ αὔταρκες τοῦ ζωμοῦ, οὕτως ἀνάπλασσε συμμέτρους τροχίσκους, παραπτόμενος ἐν τῇ ἀναπλάσει, ὀποβαλσάμου ὀλίγου, καὶ ἐν σκιᾷ ἀποτιθέμενος εἰς τὴν τοῦ ὅλου φαρμάκου σκευασίαν φύλαττε.

Κεφ. ιδ'. [Θηριακῆς σκευασία, ἀποθήκη, ἡλικία, κρίσις, δόσις.] Καὶ λοιπὸν τῶν ἄλλων ὅσα καὶ κόπτεσθαι καὶ σήθεσθαι χρὴ, κοσκινέειν κοσκίνῳ, ὡς ἔνι μάλιστα λεπτοτρήτῳ γενομένῳ. πάνυ γὰρ τὸ λεῖον πρὸς τὴν ὠφέλειαν εἶναί μοι δοκεῖ χρήσιμον, διὰ τὸ μᾶλλον εὐπρόσθετον εἶναι τοῖς σώμασιν. ὅσα δὲ διαβρέχειν τε καὶ λειοῦν χρὴ, καὶ ταῦτα λείου καὶ τῷ οἴνῳ βρέχε. ἔστω δὲ ὁ οἶνος κάλλιστος, οἷος ὁ Φαλερῖνος γλυκὺς, ὁ * μὴ Φαυστιανὸς, ἀλλ'

ſimilagine, quantum paſtillis formandis ſufficiat, admiſceto, quemadmodum etiam Andromachus autumat. Nam Magnus et Damocrates definitam quandam hujus menſuram ipſis adjungi volunt, aequali ſiquidem panis modo aequalem carnium adjungentes, ita ipſas cum pane ſimul conterunt; poſtea juſculi quod ſatis eſt affuſo, paſtillos mediocres confinges, atque opobalſami modico ſubactos in umbraque repoſitos ad totius medicamenti confectionem reſervabis.

Cap. XIV. [*Theriacae compoſitio, repoſitio, aetas, probatio, doſis.*] Reliqua contundi et cribro quam licet ſubtiliſſimo concerni expedit; nam laevia admodum inſigniter juvare mihi videntur, quod corporibus facilius apponantur. Porro quae conſpergenda ſunt laevigandaque, haec conteres et vino conſperges; ſit autem vinum laudatiſſimum Phalernum; non dulce Fauſtianum, ſed acre et quod omnibus vocatur Actum; deinde omnibus hunc

ὁ δριμύς τε καὶ πᾶσι καλούμενος ἄκτος. εἶθ' οὕτως πάντα λειώσας πρόσβαλε τὸ αὔταρκες μέλι· [951] ἔστω δὲ τὸ αὔταρκες, ὥσπερ αἱ γραφαὶ ἔχουσι, λίτραι δέκα ἀφηψημέναι μετρίως, ὥστε ἐν τῇ ἑψήσει πᾶν αὐτοῦ τὸ κηρῶδες καὶ πνευματῶδες χωρισθῆναι. ἔστω δὲ καὶ τὸ μέλι τὸ καλούμενον Ὑμήττιον. τὸν γὰρ θύμον τὸν ἐν τούτῳ τῷ ὄρει τῷ καλουμένῳ Ὑμηττῷ γινόμενον νέμονται αἱ μέλισσαι, καὶ οὕτω κάλλιστον ποιοῦσι τὸ μέλι. πειρῶ δὲ καὶ τὴν ῥητίνην καὶ χαλβάνην προαποτήξας ἰδίᾳ, οὕτω πρὸς τὴν θυείαν ἐπιβάλλειν τῷ φαρμάκῳ, καὶ λοιπὸν ἑνώσας τὰ πάντα καὶ λειώσας ἐπιμελῶς, πάλιν παραπτόμενος τοῦ ὀποβαλσάμου συμμέτρως, οὕτως ἀποτίθεσο τὴν ἀντίδοτον εἰς ὑάλινα ἢ ἀργυρᾶ σκεύη, μὴ πάνυ πληρῶν αὐτὰ, ἀλλὰ καταλιπών τινα τόπον εἰς διαπνοὴν τῷ φαρμάκῳ, καὶ συνεχῶς γε ἀποπωμάτιζε αὐτὰ, ἵνα μᾶλλον διαπνέηται, καὶ ταχυτέρα σοι αὐτῆς ἡ χρῆσις γενήσεται. χρόνου γὰρ εἰς πέψιν οὐκ ὀλίγου χρείαν ἔχει, ἵνα πρὸς τὴν χρῆσιν ἡ ἀντίδοτος πεφθῇ καλῶς. πέσσεται δὲ ὡς ἐπὶ τὸ πλεῖστον τῷ μὲν ιβ'. ἐτῶν χρόνῳ. οἱ δὲ ἀ-

in modum contritis, mellis quantum ſatis eſt adjicitur: erit autem ſatis, quemadmodum deſcriptiones continent, librae decem diſcoctae mediocriter, ut quicquid in eo cereum eſt flatulentumque in coctione ſeparetur; deligendum autem mel Hymettion nuncupatum, quod apes probatiſſimum efficiunt, thymum hoc in monte, cui nomen Hymetto, naſcentem depaſtae. Jam vero reſinam galbanumque ſeorſum prius eliquata medicamento in mortario ſic adjunges, ac deinde omnibus in unitatem redactis tritisque diligenter, rurſus manu in opobalſami modicum intincta, ita antidotum in vitreis aut argenteis vaſis repones, non vehementer ipſa replens, ſed relicto quodam ſpatio, quo medicamentum perſpiret; ad haec aſſidue operculum detrahes, ut et liberius exhalet et maturior uſus tibi ipſius contingat. Quippe haud modico tempore ad concoctionem indiget, ut quando uſus poſtulat, antidotum probe ſit concoctum; concoquitur autem ut plurimum duodecim annorum ſpatio. Qui vigentiore

κμαιοτέρᾳ τε αὐτῇ καὶ ἰσχυροτέρᾳ χρῆσθαι θέλοντες, καὶ ἐτῶν που πέντε καὶ ἑπτὰ τὸν χρόνον ἐχούσῃ, οὕτως ἐχρήσαντο, καὶ μάλιστα ἐπὶ τῶν θηριοδήκτων τε καὶ λυσσοδήκτων καὶ τῶν φαρμάκων τῶν δηλητηρίων. ἰσχυρὰν γὰρ οὗτοι τὴν ἀπὸ τῶν τοιούτων βλάβην ἔχοντες, δυνατωτέρας καὶ τῆς ἀπὸ τοῦ φαρμάκου βοηθείας χρείαν ἔχουσιν. ἔστι δὲ δυνατὸν τὸ φάρμακον ἕως ἐτῶν τριάκοντα. ὡς ἐπί γε τῶν ἄλλων παθῶν, ὅπου μὴ τηλικαύτη ἐστὶν ἡ τοῦ βλάπτειν αἰτία, αὐτάρκης εἶναι δοκεῖ καὶ ἐτῶν ἑξήκοντα χρόνος εἰς τὴν χρῆσιν τοῦ φαρμάκου. πάνυ γὰρ τὸ πέρας τοῦ τοσούτου διαστήματος ἐξίτηλόν τε καὶ ἄτονον πρὸς τὸ βοηθῆσαι ποιεῖ τὸ φάρμακον. πολλοὶ γοῦν τινες αὐτῆς τὴν δύναμιν κρῖναι θέλοντες πρῶτον διδόντες τὶ τῶν καθαρτικῶν φαρμάκων, εἶτα ἐπιδιδόντες τὶ τῆς ἀντιδότου πιεῖν, οὕτως αὐτῆς ποιοῦνται τὴν κρίσιν. εἰ μὲν γὰρ εὔτονος καὶ ἀκμαία εἴη, οὐδ᾽ ὅλως ἀφίησι τὴν κάθαρσιν γενέσθαι, ἐκνικῶσα τῷ ἑαυτῆς δυνατῷ (466) τοῦ καθαρτικοῦ φαρμάκου τὴν ἰσχύν. εἰ δὲ οὕτως καθαρθείη, ὡς μηδὲ τὴν ἀντίδοτον

ipfa validioreque uti volunt, etiam quinto anno et feptimo exhibuerunt, praefertim in his qui a virulentis feris et a cane rabido commorfi funt, praeterea in medicamentis letalibus; hi enim quum gravem ab ejusmodi noxam acceperint, potentiore etiam medicamenti praefidio indigent. Eft autem potens medicamentum adusque triginta annos, ut in aliis affectibus, ubi tanta noxae caufa non eft, fufficere videtur, quum ufus exigit, fexagenarium: nam in tanti intervalli fine vehementer exolefcit et ut juvare queat, imbecillum eft medicamentum. Plerique igitur dum vim ipfius volunt experiri, primum medicamentum quoddam purgans exhibentes, deinde nonnihil ex antidoto propinantes, fic de ipfa faciunt judicium. Si namque valida vigensque fuerit, neutiquam purgationem fieri permittit, fua ipfius potentia medicamenti purgantis efficaciam evincens. Quod fi ita fuerit purgatus, ut qui antidotum non affumpfiffet, liquido conftat vires effe in-

λαβὼν, κατάδηλος γίγνεται ὅτι ἄτονός τε καὶ ἐξίτηλός ἐστιν ἡ ἰσχὺς, ὡς μηδὲ κρατῆσαι τῆς τοῦ φαρμάκου δυνάμεως. ἔστι δὲ αὐτῆς τὸ μέτρον τῆς πόσεως οὐκ ἐπὶ πάντων τὸ αὐτὸ, ὥσπερ οὐδὲ τὸ ὑγρὸν, ᾧ διαλύοντες αὐτὴν δίδομεν. ἐπὶ μὲν γὰρ τῶν προειρημένων Ποντικοῦ καρύου τὸ μέγεθος ἀνιέντες μετ' οἴνου κυάθων τριῶν οὕτως αὐτὴν διδόναι πίνειν τοῖς λαμβάνουσιν εἰώθαμεν. ἐπὶ δὲ τῶν ἄλλων παθῶν καὶ τῷ μέτρῳ καὶ τῷ ὑγρῷ διαφόρως χρώμεθα. πρὸς γὰρ τὴν τῶν παθῶν διαφορὰν ἁρμοζόμενοι καὶ τὴν ποσότητα τοῦ φαρμάκου μετροῦμεν καὶ τὸ κατάλληλον ὑγρὸν τῆς μίξεως κρίνομεν. οὐ γὰρ μόνον πρὸς τὰ τῶν θηρίων δήγματα καὶ τὰ δηλητήρια φάρμακα βοηθεῖν ἡ ἀντίδοτος πέφυκεν, ἀλλὰ καὶ πρὸς τὰ μέγιστα τῶν ἄλλων παθῶν ἀλεξητήριον φάρμακον ἐκ τῆς ἐν πείρᾳ χρήσεως ὑφ' ὑμῶν οὖσα εὑρέθη.

Κεφ. ιε'. [*Πρὸς πόσας νόσους βοηθεῖν πέφυκεν ἡ θηριακή.*] Γαλήνην γοῦν αὐτὴν ἐν τοῖς προκειμένοις ἔπεσιν ὁ Ἀνδρόμαχος διὰ τοῦτο, οἶμαι, κέκληκεν, ἐπειδὴ ὥσπερ

validas et exoletas, ut ne quidem medicamenti facultatem ſuperare potuerit. Caeterum menſura ipſius potus in omnibus eadem non eſt, quemadmodum neque liquor, quo ipſum exhibituri diluimus. Siquidem in praedictis avellanae nucis magnitudine ex tribus vini cyathis dilutam propinare affectis conſuevimus; in aliis autem affectibus et menſura et liquore varie utimur. Nam ad affectuum differentiam ea adaptantes, tum medicamenti quantitatem metimur, tum congruum mixtionis humorem judicamus. Non enim ſolum ad ferarum morſus et letalia medicamenta auxiliari ſolet antidotum, verum ad maximas etiam alias affectiones praeſentaneum eſſe remedium experientia ac uſu a nobis compertum eſt.

Cap. XV. [*Quot et quantis morbis auxiliatur theriaca.*] Itaque galenen ipſam in propoſitis verſibus Andromachus ideo, arbitror, vocavit, quoniam ceu ex qua-

ἔκ τινος τοῦ κατὰ τὰ πάθη χειμῶνος καθάπερ τινὰ γαλήνην τὴν ὑγείαν τοῖς σώμασιν ἐργάζεται. κεφαλαίας γοῦν τὰς χρονίας καὶ τὰ σκοτώματα ἰᾶσθαι πέφυκε καὶ δυσηκοΐας καὶ ἀμβλυωπίας παύειν. ἐνίοτε δὲ καὶ τὸ τῆς γεύσεως ὄργανον ἀσθενοῦν κα στησι. πολλάκις δὲ καὶ τὰς ἐπὶ τῶν φρενιτικῶν παρακοπὰς γενναίως [952] ἔπαυσεν, ὕπνον ἐπιφέρουσα· ἀπ' αὐτοῦ δὲ καὶ τὰς τῆς γνώμης ταραχάς τε καὶ τὰς περιπλοκὰς φαντασίας παύουσα τοῖς ὕπνοις. καὶ ταῖς ἐπιληψίαις δὲ αὐταῖς ἀγωνιστικῶς εἴωθε βοηθεῖν, ἀναπίνουσα τὴν πολλὴν ἐκ τῆς κεφαλῆς ὑγρασίαν καὶ ἀνεμπόδιστον ποιοῦσα τὴν ὁδὸν τῷ πνεύματι. βοηθεῖ δὲ καὶ τοῖς δυσπνοοῦσιν, ὅταν ἐγκείμενά τινα παχέα φλέγματα εἰς τὰς σήραγγας τοῦ πνεύμονος, ἀναπνεῖν κωλύωνται τὸν ἄνθρωπον, εὐκόλως τέμνουσα καὶ εὐανάγωγα ποιοῦσα καὶ λεπτύνουσα τὰ συνεστῶτα, καὶ γλίσχρα τῶν ὑγρῶν. καὶ τοὺς αἷμα δὲ ἀνάγοντας πάνυ ὠφελεῖ, εἴ τις αὐτὴν σύμφυτον ἑφεψήσας καὶ ἀνιεὶς τῷ ὕδατι οὕτως ἐπιδῴη. πολλάκις δὲ καὶ τὰς περὶ τὸν στόμαχον κακώσεις θερα-

dam affectuum tempeftate tranquillitatem quandam, ipfam nempe fanitatem corporibus conciliat. Capitis igitur dolores diuturnos et tenebricofas vertigines fanare, ad haec auditus difficultatem et oculorum hebetudinem fedare poteft. Nonnunquam vero et guftus inftrumentum laborans reficit; faepe in phreniticis deliria, generofe fomnum inducens fedavit; infuper animi perturbationes et implexas imagines fomnis abigit. Comitialibus quoque ipfis vehementer folet auxiliari, copiofam ex capite humiditatem abforbens et liberas fpiritui vias efficiens. Jam et fufpiriofos juvat, quum craffae quaedam pituitae in pulmonis fiftulas impactae refpirare hominem prohibent, prompte incidens, ut facile educantur, attenuansque fixos viscofosque humores. Sanguinem rejicientes admodum juvat, fi quis ipfam cum fymphyto decoctam dilutamque aqua exhibuerit. Saepe ftomachi vitiis mederi folet et naufea laborantem cibumque non capientem fuaviter re-

πεύειν εἴωθε καὶ ἀνόρεκτον αὐτὸν ὄντα καὶ τὰς τροφὰς λαμβάνειν μὴ δυνάμενον εἰς τὸ προσίεσθαι αὐτὰς ἡδέως κατέστησεν. ἐνίοτε δὲ καὶ τὴν ἐπιτεταμένην ἀλόγως ὄρεξιν ἔκ τινος παρακειμένης αὐτῷ δριμυτέρας καὶ δακνώδους οὐσίας ἀγωνιστικῶς ἔπαυσε, καὶ ἑλμίνθων τοῖς ἐντέροις ἐγκειμένων, καὶ διὰ τοῦτο αὐτοῦ τοῦ στομάχου ἀπλήστως τῆς τροφῆς ὀρεγομένου πνῖγον τὰ θηρία τὸ φάρμακον τῆς πολλῆς πείνης γενναίως ἀπήλλαξεν. ἔτι καὶ τὴν μεγίστην, καὶ πλατεῖαν ἕλμινθα γενομένην καὶ πᾶσαν τὴν εἰσφερομένην τροφὴν ἐκνεμομένην, καὶ διὰ τοῦτ' ἐκτήκουσαν τὸ ἄλλο πᾶν σῶμα, θαυμασίως ἐξάγει τῶν ἐντέρων. καὶ τὰς ἡπατικὰς καὶ σπληνικὰς διαθέσει ἰᾶται πολλάκις, ἐκλύουσα τὰς ἐμφράξεις καὶ τὰς περὶ τὸ ἧπαρ διαθέσεις καὶ σπλῆνα ἰωμένη. καὶ τὸν ἴκτερον διά τινα παρὰ τὸ ἧπαρ διάθεσιν γιγνόμενον γενναίως θεραπεύει, ἀποκαθαίρουσα τὴν χολὴν καὶ ὥσπερ ἀπομάττουσα καὶ ποιοῦσα τὸ ἧπαρ διακρίνειν αὐτὴν ἀκριβῶς ἀπὸ τοῦ αἵματος. τήκει δὲ ἐνίοτε καὶ τοὺς σπλῆνας τοῖς ἐσκιῤῥωμένους, κατ' ὀλίγον ἀναλίσκουσα τὴν ἐν αὐτοῖς ῥυ-

ftituit; interdum etiam appetitum fine ratione intenfum ex mordaci quadam et aeri fubftantia ipfum infeftante, certatim repreffit. Infuper lumbricis inteftina occupantibus, eoque ftomacho infatiabiliter cibum appetente, medicamentum hoc propemodum enecatos magna fame feliciter liberavit. Praeterea maximum latumque helminthem, i e. *taeniam*, generatum, qui omnem affumptum cibum depafcitur, eoque reliquum totum corpus emaciat, mirabiliter ab inteftinis educit. Hepaticos quoque et lienofos affectus faepe fanat, obftructiones aperiens et jecoris lienisque affectibus medetur. Item arquatum ex aliquo jecoris vitio oborientem ftrenue curat, bilem expurgans et veluti abftergens, tum ut jecur bilem a fanguine examuffim fegreget, efficiens. Aliquando lienes fcirrho induratos folvit, paulatim fordidam fuperfluamque in eis fubftantiam abfumens. Conterit et renum calculos et quicquid terreum fordidumque in eis continetur facile expurgat. In vefica difficultatem urinae fedat et exulce-

παρίαν καὶ περιττὴν οὐσίαν. θρύπτει δὲ καὶ τοὺς ἐν νεφροῖς λίθους, καὶ πᾶν τὸ γεῶδες ἐν αὐτοῖς καὶ ῥυπαρὸν ἀποκαθαίρει ῥᾳδίως, καὶ τὰς τῆς κύστεως δυσουρίας παύει, καὶ τὰς ἐν αὐτῇ ἑλκώσεις ἰᾶται πολλάκις, καὶ τὰς περὶ τὴν κοιλίαν δυσπεψίας τε καὶ ἀτονίας θεραπεύει, θερμαίνουσα καὶ τονοῦσα τῆς γαστρὸς τὸ σῶμα, καὶ τῶν ἐντέρων τὰς ἑλκώσεις καὶ τὰς δυσεντερίας αὐτὰς καὶ τὰς λειεντερίας ἀπαλλάττειν εἴωθε. ὠφελεῖ δὲ καὶ τοὺς εἰλεωδῶς τὰ ἔντερα διατιθεμένους καὶ τοὺς χρονίως τῇ κωλικῇ διαθέσει περιπεπτωκότας, μάλιστα ὅταν ἀφλέγμαντα ᾖ τὰ ἔντερα, ἐξαναλίσκουσα τὰς ἐν αὐτοῖς δριμύτητας τῶν ὑγρῶν καὶ διατμίζουσα τὰς πνευματώσεις τῶν ἐντέρων. ἐνίοτε δὲ καὶ τοῖς χολεριῶσι γενναίως βοηθεῖ, τονοῦσα τὴν σύγκρισιν καὶ ἐπέχουσα τὰ πολλὰ τῶν ῥευμάτων. τὸ μέγιστον δ' αὐτῆς ἔργον πολλάκις ἐπὶ τῶν καρδιακῶν φαίνεται. ῥεομένου γὰρ τοῖς πολλοῖς καὶ συνεχέσιν ἱδρῶσι τοῦ σώματος καὶ τῶν τόνων λελυμένων, μηδὲ τοῦ οἴνου πολλάκις κρατεῖν τοῦ πάθους δυναμένου, ἡ ἀντίδοτος πινομένη καὶ τοὺς ἱδρῶτας ἵστησι καὶ τὴν δύναμιν πίπτουσαν ὥσπερ ἐξανίστησι καὶ

rationibus in ea plerumque eſt praeſidio et difficilem ventriculi concoctionem imbecillitatemque reficit, ventris corpus calſaciens confirmansque. Inteſtinorum ulcera ipſasque dyſenterias et lienterias tollere conſuevit: ileoſis quoque inteſtinorum torminibus affectis ac diu in colicum affectum collapſis prodeſt, praeſertim quum inteſtina vacant inflammationibus, acres ipſorum humores conſumens et inteſtinorum flatus per vaporem discutiens. Interdum quoque cholera laborantibus egregie conducit, *corporis* coagmentum corroborans multasque fluxiones ſiſtens. Porro maximum ipſius opus ſaepe in cardiacis innoteſcit; quippe dum corpus multis continuisque ſudoribus diffluit et robur ipſius diſſolutum eſt, neque vinum frequenter continere morbus poteſt, antidoti potio et ſudores ſiſtit et facultatem collapſam veluti erigit validamque efficit. Jam vero in mulieribus etiam menſes educit et uteri ſedisque

ἰσχυρὰν ἀπεργάζεται. ἔστι δὲ ἐπὶ τῶν γυναικῶν καὶ τῶν καταμηνίων αἱμάτων ἀγωγὸς καὶ τὰς ἐν τῇ μήτρᾳ καὶ ἕδρᾳ γιγνομένας αἱμοῤῥοΐδας ἐπισχεθείσας πολλάκις ἀναστομοῖ. θαυμασίως δὲ καὶ τὰς αμέτρους τῶν αἱμάτων αποκρίσεις εἴωθεν ἐπέχειν. μέμνησαι γὰρ ὅτι μικτὴν καὶ ποικίλην τὴν δύναμιν αὐτῆς ἐν τοῖς ἔμπροσθεν εἴπομεν καὶ διὰ τοῦτο τὰ μὲν διαχέουσα καὶ λεπτύνουσα ἐκκρίνεσθαι ποιεῖ, τὰ δὲ δι' ἀτονίαν τῆς ἐμφύτου δυνάμεως ἀποκρινόμενα περιττῶς, ταῦτα τονοῦσα τὴν δύναμιν τῶν σωμάτων εἴωθεν ἐπέχειν. καὶ τοὺς ποδαγριῶντας δὲ καὶ τοὺς πάντα τὰ ἄρθρα ῥευματιζομένους ὠφελεῖ μάλιστα τότε, ὅταν ὁ τῆς ἐπιδόσεως καιρὸς παρέλθῃ καὶ ἡ στάσις τῆς ἀκμῆς γένηται. παραμυθούμενον γὰρ τὰ ἀλγήματα τοῖς παρηγορεῖν δυναμένοις ἐπιθέμασι διδόναι πίνειν χρὴ τοῦ φαρ- [953] μάκου, ἵνα ἐπέχηται τὰ ῥεύματα. ἐξαναλίσκει γὰρ ἡ ἀντίδοτος τὰ ἤδη ἐπενεχθέντα καὶ ἄλλα κωλύει φέρεσθαι. μάλιστα δὲ ὀνίνησιν ὅταν τις αὐτὴν καὶ ὑγιαίνων συνεχῶς λαμβάνῃ, ἐκδαπανᾶται γὰρ τὰ περιττὰ τῶν ὑγρῶν καὶ τὴν ὅλην ἀλλοιοῖ σύγκρισιν. τὰ μὲν γὰρ ἄλλα τῶν φαρμάκων, ὅσα εἰς ἀπαλ-

haemorrhoidas fuppreffas multoties aperit. Mirifice vero et immoderatas fanguinis excretiones cohibere confuevit. Succurrat enim memoriae quod mixta variaque ipfius facultas, quam in fuperioribus fumus interpretati, ideo alia diffundens extenuansque cogat excerni, alia ob nativae facultatis imbecillitatem fuperflue excreta, viribus partium confirmatis foleat inhibere. Quin etiam podagricos omnesque articulorum fluxionibus tentatos tunc potiffimum adjuvat, quum augmenti tempus praeterierit et vigoris ftatus accefferit. Nam dolores epithematis lenientibus mitigans medicamentum propinabis, ut fluxiones cohibeat; quippe hoc antidotum jam infarctas digerit et alias invehi prohibet. Maxime vero prodeft quum quis fanus frequenter id affumit, nam humorum fuperflua confumit et totam compagem alterat. Alia vero medicamenta, quae podagrici in morbi propulfionem bibunt, ad pedes quidem

Ed. Chart. XIII. [953.] Ed. Baf. II. (466.)

λαγὴν τοῦ νοσήματος οἱ ποδαγριῶντες πίνουσι, τὴν μὲν ἐπὶ τοὺς πόδας τοῦ ῥεύματος φορὰν κωλύει γίγνεσθαι, οὐκ ἐξαναλίσκοντα δὲ τὴν περιττὴν τούτων ὑγρασίαν ἄλλου τινὸς μείζονος νοσήματος γένεσιν ἐργάζεται. πλανωμένου γὰρ ἐν τῷ σώματι τοῦ ῥεύματος ὁ πνεύμων ἀεὶ κινούμενος διὰ τὴν τῆς ἀναπνοῆς ἀνάγκην, καὶ διὰ τὸ μανὸν τοῦ σώματος δέξασθαι τὸ ῥεῦμα ῥαδίως δυνάμενος, τὸ πᾶν αὐτὸς ἐφ᾽ ἑαυτὸν ἕλκων, οὕτω πνίγει τὸν ἄνθρωπον, ὅπερ ἱστορικῶς ἐπὶ πολλῶν ἐγὼ τῇ πείρᾳ κατέμαθον, καὶ διὰ τοῦτο ἀποσυμβουλεύω μηδ᾽ ὅλως πίνειν ταῦτα τὰ φάρμακα. τῇ δὲ θηριακῇ ἐν τοῖς τοιούτοις χρῆσθαι καὶ πάνυ παραινῶ· καὶ γὰρ ξηραίνουσα τὰ περιττὰ τῶν ὑγρῶν ὠφελεῖ καὶ ἕτερα συλλέγεσθαι οὐκ ἐᾷ. πολλοὶ γοῦν ἐν ἀρχῇ συνεχῶς πίνειν ἀρξάμενοι ἀπηλλάγησαν τελέως τοῦ πάθους, καὶ τούτῳ γε οἶμαι τῷ λόγῳ καὶ τοὺς ὑδεριῶντας πολλάκις μεγάλως ὠφέλησεν, ἐκδαπανῶσα τὸ ἐν αὐτοῖς ὑγρὸν καὶ κατεψυγμένον, τὸ ἔμφυτον θερμὸν ἀναθερμαίνειν δυναμένη, καὶ μάλιστα τοὺς ἀνασάρκας καὶ λευκοφλεγματίας λεγομένους ὕδρω-

fluxionem ferri vetant, fed hujus fuperfluitatem non discutientia majorem quendam morbum faciunt. Nam fluxione per corpus oberrante, pulmo qui femper ob refpirandi neceffitatem movetur, ac propter corporis fui raritatem ad illam excipiendam facilis, totam ipfe ad fe trahens, ita hominem fuffocat, quod ego in multis contemplatus experientia didici, atque hujus rei gratia omnino ab hisce medicamentis bibendis abftinere confuluerim. Theriaca vero in talibus uti etiam vehementer adhortor; etenim humorum fuperfluitates exiccans juvat et alias colligi non permittit. Plerique igitur initio affidue hac ufi potione in totum ab affectu liberati funt; atque hac, opinor, ratione etiam hydero laborantes multum faepe adjuvit, dum fupervacaneum humorem abfumeret et infitum calorem perfrigeratum facultate calefaceret, praefertim hydropas, quos anafarcas et leucophlegmatias appellant, infigniter adjuvare confuevit, in totum fefe corpus diftri-

πας γενναίως εἴωθεν ὠφελεῖν, εἰς ὅλον τὸ σῶμα ἀναδιδομένη καὶ πολλαχόθι ἐκθλίβουσα τῶν σαρκῶν τὴν ὑγρασίαν. διόπερ καὶ τῆς καχεξίας λεγομένης ἄριστόν ἐστι φάρμακον, μετασυγκρίνουσα τὴν ἕξιν τοῦ σώματος, καὶ τὰ μὲν περιττὰ διαφοροῦσα, τὴν δὲ φύσιν ἐνεργεῖν εὐτόνως τὰς φυσικὰς ἐνεργείας παρασκευάζειν δυναμένη. τούτῳ δὲ τῷ τρόπῳ (467) τῆς βοηθείας καὶ τοῖς ἐλεφαντιῶσι πολλάκις ἐπικουρεῖν πέφυκε. πολλοῦ γὰρ ὄντος τοῦ διεφθορότος ῥεύματος καὶ σηποίσης τῆς τούτου δυνάμεως τὴν ὅλην σύγκρισιν, ἐκνικᾷν εἴωθεν ἡ ἀντίδοτος τὸ νόσημα, ἐπέχουσα μὲν τοὺς ῥευματισμοὺς, κωλύουσα δὲ τὴν διαφθορὰν γίγνεσθαι τοῦ αἵματος. τοὺς δὲ τετανικῶς σπωμένους καὶ αὐτοὺς πολλάκις ἐθεράπευσε, θερμαίνουσα τὰ νεῦρα καὶ τὰς τάσεις αὐτῶν χαλῶσα, ὥσπερ δὴ καὶ τὰς παραλύσεις τῶν μερῶν ἐξιωμένη πολλάκις καὶ ἀναζωπυρεῖν ποιοῦσα τὸ πνεῦμα εἰς τὸ κατὰ φύσιν ἤγαγε καὶ τὰς κινήσεις τοῖς μέρεσιν ἐνεργεῖν ἀπέδωκε. θαυμάζειν δὲ ἔστι τὴν ἀντίδοτον, ὅταν μὴ μόνον αὐτὴν πάσχον θεραπεύουσαν βλέπωμεν, ἀλλὰ καὶ αὐτὴν τὴν ψυχὴν πολλάκις ὑπὸ τῶν παθῶν διατιθεμένην

buens et undequaque carnium humiditatem exprimens. Quapropter etiam pravo corporis habitui, cachexiam dicunt, optimum est remedium, ut quae corporis habitum coagmentet, superflua discutiat, naturam ad naturales functiones fortiter obeundas praeparet Hoc auxilii modo etiam elephanticis crebro succurrimus, nam quum multus rheumaticus humor sit corruptus, cujus vis totam corporis molem putrefaciat, antidotum morbum solet evincere dum rheumatismos sistit et sanguinis fieri corruptionem prohibet. Ad haec tetanicos convulsos haud raro persanavit, nervos calefaciens et tensiones ipsorum laxans; quemadmodum etiam partium paralyses saepe curans, spiritu recreato, in naturalem statum reduxit et motus obeundos partibus reddidit. Mirari vero antidotum licet, quum non modo ipsum corpus aegrotum sanare conspiciamus, sed etiam animo saepe affectibus obnoxio posse auxiliari; quippe vitia ex melancholia oborta feda hoc

κακῶς ὠφελεῖν δυναμένην. τὰς γοῦν ἐκ τῆς μελαγχολίας γινομένας αὐτῇ κακώσεις παύει διδόμενον συνεχῶς τὸ φάρμακον, ὥσπερ ἐκπῖνον καὶ ἐξαναλίσκον ἐκ τῶν ἀγγείων καὶ ἐκ τοῦ σπληνὸς τὴν μέλαιναν χολὴν, καθάπερ καὶ τὸν ἰὸν τῶν θηρίων, διόπερ καὶ πρὸς τὸν πυρετὸν τὸν τεταρταῖον μάλιστα ἁρμόζει καλῶς. ὑπὸ γὰρ τῆς μελαίνης χολῆς γενόμενος ὁ πυρετὸς οὗτος εὐκόλως ὑπὸ τῆς ἀντιδότου ἀπαλλάττεται, μάλισθ' ὅταν τὶς αὐτῇ τεχνικῶς ᾖ χρώμενος. ἔγωγ' οὖν πολλοὺς τῶν τεταρταιζόντων τῇ ἀγωγῇ ταύτῃ χρησάμενος ἀπήλλαξα ῥᾳδίως τοῦ νοσήματος, προκενώσας αὐτοὺς τῷ ἀπὸ δείπνου ἐμέτῳ, εἶτα τῇ ἑξῆς ἐπιδοὺς τὸν χυλὸν τοῦ ἀψινθίου, ἵνα ἐπιγλυκάνω καὶ κατακεράσω τὴν χολὴν, οὕτως πρὸ ὡρῶν δύο τῆς ἐπισημασίας τὴν ἀντίδοτον δίδωμι. καὶ θαυμαστῶς οἶδα πολλάκις ἐπιτυχοῦσαν αὐτὴν, ὡς ταχέως ἀνεπισήμαντον μεῖναι τὸν λαμβάνοντα.

[954] Κεφ. ιϛ'. [*Μεθοδικῶν ἔλεγχος ἄχρηστον εἶναι νομιζόντων τὸ εἰδέναι τὰς τῶν νόσων αἰτίας· καὶ πάλιν τὰ χρήσιμα τῆς θηριακῆς διεξίησι.*] *Καὶ τὸν ὑδροφόβον δὲ, τὸν κάκιστον τῶν νοσημάτων, τοῦτο τὸ φάρμακον πολλάκις*

medicamentum continuo exhibitum, ceu exhauriens exugensque atram ex vafis et liene bilem, ficut et beftiarum virus; quare ad febrem quartanam potiffimum pulchre convenit. Siquidem febris haec ab atra bile oborta prompte antidoto tollitur, praefertim fi quis artificiose ipfo utatur. Ego igitur multos quartana laborautes hoc praefidio ufus facile a morbo vindicavi; nam vomitu prius a ientaculo ipfos vacuans, deinde fequenti die abfinthii fuccum exhibens, ut bilis edulcefcat contempereturque, ita horis duabus ante acceffionem antidotum exhibeo, ac mirifice ipfum frequenter vidi proficere, ut protinus qui caperet, fine morbi acceffione maneret.

Cap. XVI. [*Methodicorum reprehenfio, qui morborum caufas nofcere fupervacaum arbitrantur: et inde reliqua theriacae remedia.*] Hydrophobiam, id eft *aquae metum*, morborum peffimum, hoc medicamentum faepe

Ed. Chart. XIII. [954.] Ed. Baf. II. (467.)

ἀπαλλάττειν εἴωθε καὶ θαυμασίως ἀνταγωνίζεσθαι τῇ τῶν τοσούτων κακῶν συνδρομῇ. οὐ γὰρ μόνον αὐτοῖς τὸ σῶμα ξηραίνεται καὶ σπώμενον γίνεται ἐνίοτε καὶ πυρετὸν δριμέως ἔνδοθεν καίεται, ἀλλὰ καὶ γνώμῃ παρανοεῖ καὶ τὸ χαλεπώτατον αὐτοῖς φέρει σύμπτωμα. τὸ γὰρ ὕδωρ φοβοῦνται καὶ διὰ μὲν τὴν πολλὴν ξηρότητα τοῦ ὑγροῦ ἐπιθυμίαν ἔχουσι καὶ τοῦ πιεῖν ἀπέχονται, διὰ δὲ τὴν παρακοπὴν τὸ ὠφελῆσαι δυνάμενον οὐκ ἐπινοοῦσι. φεύγοντες γὰρ τὸ ὕδωρ καὶ φοβούμενοι τῷ οἰκτίστῳ θανάτῳ ἀποθνήσκουσι κακῶς, ἐφ᾽ ὧν μάλιστα ἐγὼ καὶ τοὺς μεθοδικοὺς τεθαύμακα, ἀχρήστους γὰρ αἰτίας πρὸς τὰς θεραπείας εἶναι λέγοντες οὐκ οἶδ᾽ ὅπως καὶ θεραπεύειν ποτὲ τούτους δύνανται, ἁπλοῦ τοῦ δήγματος ὄντος καὶ ὁμοίου φαινομένου τῷ ὑπὸ τοῦ μὴ λυσσῶντος δεδηγμένῳ κυνός. τίνα γὰρ καὶ θεραπείας τρόπον αὐτοῖς ἐνδείξεται, ἀπερισκέπτως ὁρώμενον τὸ τραῦμα τοῦ σώματος, μὴ ἐξεταζομένης ὑπ᾽ αὐτῶν τῆς ἔνδον αἰτίας οὔσης καὶ τοῖς μὲν ὀφθαλμοῖς τοῦ μεθοδικοῦ μὴ ὁρωμένης, ὑπὸ δὲ τοῦ λογικοῦ ἰατροῦ μόνῳ τῷ λογισμῷ καὶ τῇ ἐξε-

tollere confuevit et mirabiliter tantorum malorum concurfui refiftere. Non enim corpus duntaxat ipfis inarescit et convellitur interdum febreque acri intus uritur, fed animus etiam delirat et graviffimum ipfis adfert fymptoma. Quippe aquam timent ac propter multam ficcitatem humidi tenentur defiderio et a potu abftinent, quia mente alienati id quod auxiliari poffit confiderare nequeunt; fugientes enim aquam paventesque miferrimo mortis genere intereunt, in quibus potiffimum methodicos fum demiratus, qui caufas ad curationem effe inutiles dicunt; haud enim fcio quomodo his queant mederi, quum fimplex morfus exiftit et fimilis a non rabiofo cane illato apparet; quem enim curationis modum ipfis indicabit vulnus corporis obiter infpectum, nec interiore caufa ab eis examinata nec ipforum oculis animadverfa, a rationali autem medico fola ratione et diligenti examine adinventa? Quamobrem qui in methodicum male curantem

Ed. Chart. XIII. [954.] Ed. Baf. II. (467.)
τάσει ἀκριβῶς ἐξευρισκομένης; διὸ καὶ ὁ μεθοδικῷ θεραπεύοντι κακῶς ἐμπεσὼν ἄθλιος, ὥσπερ ἀλόγῳ τινὶ καὶ αὐτῷ ὄντι θηρίῳ, πάντως τεθνήξεται, ἀκολούθως ἀπολλύμενος αὐτοῦ τῇ αἱρέσει, ἐπεὶ διὰ τὴν ἀκολουθίαν τοῦ δόγματος ἐξετάζειν τὴν αἰτίαν οὐ βούλεται. ὁ δὲ εὐτυχῶς τῷ μετὰ λόγου θεραπεύοντι προσελθὼν οὔτε τοῖς οὕτω πονηροῖς συμπτώμασιν ἁλώσεται ῥᾳδίως καὶ τὸν θάνατον ἐκφεύξεται διὰ τὴν τοῦ λογικοῦ ἰατροῦ τέχνην. παραλαβὼν γὰρ αὐτὸν ὁ τοιοῦτος ἰατρὸς εὐθέως ἀκριβῶς ἐξετάσει ὁποῖός τις ἦν αὐτὸν ὁ κατεδηδοκὼς κύων. εἰ γὰρ ἀκούσεις ὅτι ἰσχνὸς μὲν καὶ κατάξηρος τῷ σώματι, καὶ τοῖς ὄμμασιν ἐξέρυθρος, καὶ τὴν οὐρὰν παρειμένος καὶ τὸν ἀφρὸν ἐκ τοῦ στόματος ἔχων ῥέοντα, μάθοις δὲ ὅτι καὶ τὴν γλῶτταν ἔξω εἶχε προβεβλημένην καὶ ὥσπερ χολὴν κεχρωσμένην, ἐμπίπτων τε τοῖς ἐντυγχάνουσι καὶ ἀλόγως τρέχων, εἶτα πάλιν αἰφνίδιον ἑστάναι θέλων καὶ δάκνων μετ' ὀργῆς τινος μανικωτέρας ἀπροοράτους αὐτοῦ γενομένους, εἰ ταῦτα ἀκούσῃς οὕτως ἔχοντα, εὐθέως μὲν συνήσεις λυττῶντα γεγονέναι τὸν κύνα. θερα-

inciderit miser, ceu irrationalem quandam et ipsum bestiam existentem, omnino moriturus est, merito per illius sectam occumbens, quoniam ob dogmatis sequelam causam inquirere non dignatur. Qui vero in rationalem medicum feliciter inciderit, neque tam pravis symptomatis facile corripietur et mortem propter rationalis medici artificium evadet. Nam hujusmodi medicus eo qui commorsus est suscepto, statim accurate perquiret qualisnam canis fuerit qui ipsum momordit. Si enim audieris gracilem corpore, siccum, oculis rubentibus, cauda demissa, spuma ex ore fluente, praeterea lingua foras porrecta et tanquam bile colorata, obvium quemque insiliisse citraque rationem cucurrisse, deinde rursus subito consistentem cum ira quadam magis furenti non ipsi praevisos momordisse; haec, inquam, si in eo sic habere audieris, statim rabidum canem fuisse intelliges. Itaque vulnus haud simpliciter quemadmodum methodicus curabis. sed con-

πεύσεις δὲ οὐχ ἁπλῶς οὕτως ὥσπερ ὁ μεθοδικὸς τὸ τραῦμα, ἀλλ' εὐθέως μὲν αὐτὸ καὶ μεῖζον ἐργάσῃ, περιτεμὼν τὴν σάρκα, ἐκ πολλοῦ τοῦ διαστήματος καὶ κυκλοτερὲς αὐτοῦ τὸ σχῆμα ποιῶν, ἵνα μὴ ῥαδίως ἐπουλοῦσθαι δύναται, ἀλλ' ἔχοι ἀνεῳγότα τὸν πόρον, εἰς πολὺ τοῦ χρόνου τὸ μῆκος τοὐλάχιστον εἰς τὰς τετταράκοντα ἡμέρας, καὶ ἐξέλθοι διὰ τούτου ἰὸς τοῦ κυνός. καυτηρίοις γοῦν εἰώθαμεν πάνυ πεπυρακτωμένοις ἐπικαίειν τὸν τόπον καὶ κεχρῆσθαι τοῖς ἄλλοις φαρμάκοις ὅσα ἐπισπαστικά ἐστι, καὶ ἔνδον τῆς σαρκὸς τὸν ἰὸν μένειν οὐκ ἐᾷ. ἐγὼ δὲ ἐπινοήσας ποτὲ, καὶ τὴν ἀντίδοτον αὐτὴν ἀνῆκα τῷ ἀπὸ τῶν ῥόδων σκευαζομένῳ ἐλαίῳ, καὶ ὥς τι φάρμακον ἔμμοτον ἐπέθηκα τῷ τραύματι, ἵνα ὥσπερ τὶς σικύα ἐκμυζήσῃ καὶ ἐκ τοῦ βάθους ἐπισπάσηται τὸ διαφθεῖραι δυνάμενον· καὶ ὅλως καθάπερ τι παιώνειον φάρμακον ἡ θηριακὴ καὶ ἔξωθεν ἐπιτιθεμένη καὶ πινομένη τοῖς λυσσοδήκτοις ἀκριβῶς βοηθεῖ. ἐφάνη δὲ ἡμῖν ἡ [955] ἀντίδοτος αὕτη καὶ ἐν ταῖς λοιμικαῖς καταστάσεσι μόνη τοῖς ἁλισκομένοις βοηθεῖν δυναμένη, μηδενὸς

festim ipsum etiam amplius efficies, carne multo intervallo orbiculari figura praecisa, ne facile ad cicatricem perveniat; sed foramen diu, minimum quadraginta diebus patescat, ut per hoc canis virus emanet. Cauteriis igitur admodum candentibus locum adurere solemus et aliis uti medicamentis, quae extrahendi vim obtinent, nec virus intra carnem manere sinunt. Ego autem considerans aliquando antidotum ipsum oleo ex rosis confecto dilui et ceu medicamentum, *linteolis concerptis excipitur* (emmotum, id est *linamentum*) in vulnus indidi, ut cucurbitulae cujusdam modo exugeret et ex alto quod corrumpendo corpori erat extraheret. In summa theriace et extrinsecus imposita et epota rabiosorum morsibus praesentanei medicamenti cujusdam instar exacte opitulatur. Caeterum nobis etiam in pestifera lue solum hoc antidotum malo correptis prodesse adeo visum est, ut nullum aliud praesidium tanto malo resistere fuerit idoneum. Nan-

ἄλλου βοηθήματος τῷ μεγέθει τοῦ κακοῦ ἀντιστῆναι οὕτως πεφυκότος. ὥσπερ γάρ τι θηρίον καὶ αὐτὸς ὁ λοιμὸς οὐκ ὀλίγους τινὰς, ἀλλὰ καὶ πόλεις ὅλας ἐπινεμόμενος διαφθείρει κακῶς, τροπῆς τινος μοχθηρᾶς εἰς τὸ διαφθείρειν δύνασθαι περὶ τὸν ἀέρα γιγνομένης, καὶ τῶν ἀνθρώπων τῇ τῆς ἀναπνοῆς ἀνάγκῃ τὸ δεινὸν φεύγειν μὴ δυναμένων, ἀλλὰ αὐτὸν εἰς αὑτοὺς ὥσπερ τι δηλητήριον διὰ στόματος ἑλκόντων τὸν ἀέρα. διόπερ ἐπαινῶ καὶ τὸν θαυμασιώτατον Ἱπποκράτην, ὅτι τὸν λοιμὸν ἐκεῖνον τὸν ἐκ τῆς Αἰθιοπίας εἰς τοὺς Ἕλληνας φθάσαντα οὐκ ἄλλως ἐθεράπευσεν ἀλλ' ἢ τρέψας τὸν ἀέρα καὶ ἀλλοιώσας, ἵνα μηκέτι τοιοῦτος ὢν ἀναπνέηται. κελεύσας οὖν ἀνὰ τὴν πόλιν ὅλην ἐξάπτεσθαι τὸ πῦρ, οὐχ ἁπλῆν τῆς ἀνάψεως τὴν ὕλην ἔχον, ἀλλὰ στεφάνων τε καὶ τῶν ἀνθῶν τὰ εὐωδέστατα, τοιαῦτα συνεβούλευσεν εἶναι τοῦ πυρὸς τὴν τροφὴν, καὶ ἐπισπένδειν αὐτῷ τῶν μύρων τὰ λιπαρώτατα, καὶ ἡδεῖαν τὴν ὀδμὴν ἔχοντα, ἵν' οὕτω καθαρὸν γενόμενον οἱ ἄνθρωποι ἀναπνεύσωσιν εἰς τὴν ἀπαλλαγὴν τὸν ἀέρα. τὸν αὐτὸν τρόπον νομίζω καὶ

que peſtis tanquam et ipſa exiſtat quaedam bellua, haud paucos aliquos, verum civitates quoque totas depaſcens male conſicit. Quippe prava quaedam aëris ad corruptionem prompta mutatio efficitur et homines quum reſpirationis neceſſitate periculum evitare nequeant, ipſum aërem veluti venenum quoddam ad ſe per os attrahunt. Quamobrem etiam Hippocratem illum multis modis admirandum laudo, qui peſtem illam ex Aethiopia Graecos invadentem non aliter curaverit quam aëris mutatione alterationeque, ne talis amplius inſpiraretur. Quum igitur ignem per totam *Athenarum* urbem incendi juſſiſſet, non ſimplicem accenſionis materiam, verum ſerta floresque ſuaviſſimos alimentum ipſius eſſe conſuluit, unguentaque pinguiſſima et odoriſera ipſis ſuperſundi, ut aërem purum hoc modo redditum homines in mali ſubſidium reſpirarent. Simili ratione theriacen, ceu ipſa quoque ignis quidam purgatorius exiſtat, praeſumentes in peſtiſero *aëris*

Ed. Chart. XIII. [955.] Ed. Baſ. II. (467. 468.)
τὴν θηριακὴν, ὥσπερ τι καὶ αὐτὴν οὖσαν πῦρ καθάρσιον, τοὺς μὲν προπίνοντας αὐτὴν ἐν τῇ λοιμικῇ καταστάσει μηδ' ὅλως ἐᾷν ἁλίσκεσθαι τῷ κακῷ, τοὺς δὲ ἤδη φθάσαντας παθεῖν ἐξιᾶσθαι δύνασθαι, ἀλλοιοῦσαν καὶ τρέπουσαν τὴν τοῦ ἀναπνευσθέντος ἀέρος πονηρίαν καὶ μηκέτ' ἐῶσαν διαφθείρειν τὴν σύγκρισιν. διόπερ ἐγὼ συμβουλεύω σοι καὶ διὰ ταύτας μὲν τὰς οὕτω γιγνομένας αἰφνιδίους περὶ τὸν ἀέρα καταστάσεις, καὶ διὰ τὰς ἄλλας τῶν βλαπτόντων αἰτίας λαμβάνειν τῆς ἀντιδότου συνεχῶς καὶ ὑγιαίνοντι ἵνα καὶ τοῖς ἔξωθεν προσπίπτουσιν ἀνθιστῆταί σοι τὸ σῶμα καὶ ὅταν ἤδη πάθῃ, εὐίατον εὕρῃς. αὕτη γὰρ ὡς εὐκρασίαν τινὰ καὶ ὑγιεινὴν κατάστασιν περιποιεῖ τοῖς σώμασιν, ἀναλίσκουσα τὰ περιττώματα τῶν ὑγρῶν καὶ ἀναθερμαίνουσα τὰ κατεψυγμένα τῶν μερῶν, καὶ τὴν ἔμφυτον δύναμιν τονοῦσα πρὸς τὸ τὰς φυσικὰς ἐνεργείας ἐκτελεῖσθαι (468) καλῶς. ὅταν γὰρ ἡ φύσις εὐρώστως ἔχῃ, τότε καὶ ἀνεκποδίστως ἡ κοιλία πέσσει τὰς τροφὰς, καὶ αἱ φλέβες ἐξαιματοῦσιν αὐτὰς εὐχερῶς, καὶ τὸ ἧπαρ ῥαδίως διακρίνει τὴν χολὴν, καὶ καθαρὸν παραλαβοῦσα ἡ καρδία τὸ αἷμα, ὅλῳ

ſtatu, neutiquam malo corripi ſinere novimus, corruptis jam poſſe mederi, aëris inſpirati malitiam inalterantem mutantemque, ut quae compagem inſici magis prohibeat. Quapropter conſilium tibi do ut ob has tam repentinas aëris conſtitutiones aliasque noxarum cauſas oborientes in proſpera quoque valetudine crebro antidotum aſſumas, quo et externis accidentibus corpus reſiſtat, ac ubi jam fuerit affectum, illud invenias propitium. Hoc enim veluti bonam quandam temperiem ſalubremque ſtatum corporibus inducit, dum humorum ſuperfluitates abſumit, partes perfrictionibus emortuas recalefacit et inſitam facultatem naturae functionibus probe obeundis corroborat. Quum enim natura valida eſt, tunc etiam ſine impedimento ventriculus cibos concoquit, ac venae ipſos prompte in ſanguinem redigunt, jecur bilem ex facili ſecernit, cor purum ſanguinem ſuſcipiens univerſo deinde, ut jam nutrire queat, corpori transmittit, excretiones ipſas moderate mo-

Ed. Chart. XIII. [955.] Ed. Baf. II. (468.)
λοιπὸν, ὡς ἤδη τρέψαι δυνάμενον, ἐπιπέμπει τῷ σώματι, τάς τε ἀποκρίσεις καὶ αὐτὰς ἀποδίδοσθαι συμμέτρως ποιεῖ, καὶ τὰ περιττὰ τῷ σώματι δι᾽ ὅλης τῆς ἀναπνοῆς ὑγιεινῶς διαφορεῖ. μάλιστα δὲ ἐν ταῖς ὁδοιπορίαις συμβουλεύω σοι τῆς ἀντιδότου λαμβάνειν, ὁπότε ψυχροῦ ὄντος τοῦ ἀέρος χειμῶνος ὁδεύῃς. ἔσται γὰρ ὥσπερ τι τῶν σπλάγχνων ἀγαθὸν ἔνδυμα καὶ πολλὴν τὴν θερμότητα αὐτοῖς παρέχειν δυνάμενον. οἶδα δ᾽ αὐτὴν καὶ εἰς τὴν τῆς ψυχῆς σύνεσίν τε καὶ ὀξύτητα μὴ οὖσαν ἀσύμβολον. τάς τε γὰρ αἰσθήσεις ἐνεργεῖν εὐτόνως ἀπεργάζεται καὶ καθαρὸν τῶν ἀναθυμιάσεων ἀποφαίνουσα τὸν νοῦν ἀκριβέστερον αὐτὸν διακεῖσθαι ποιεῖ. συνελόντι δ᾽ εἰπεῖν, ὅλον δυσπαθὲς εἶναι τὸ σῶμα κατασκευάζει, ὡς μηδὲ ὑπὸ δηλητηρίου τινὸς διαφθείρεσθαι. ἡ γὰρ ποικίλη καὶ τοσαύτη τῆς μίξεως τοῦ φαρμάκου δύναμις τὴν τοιαύτην δυσπάθειαν ἀποτελεῖ, καὶ μάλιστα ἐπεὶ τὸ τῶν θηρίων ἔχει μίγμα. φασὶ γὰρ καὶ τὸν Μιθριδάτην ἐκεῖνον τὸν μέγαν πολεμιστὴν, τὴν μὲν θηριακὴν μὴ λαμβάνοντα, οὐδέπω γὰρ ἦν, ἄλλην δ᾽ ἀντίδοτον λαμβάνοντα πολυμίγματόν τινα, καὶ αὐτὴν τῷ ἐκείνου ὀνόματι οὕτω

derate molitur, recrementa corporis per totam reſpirationem ſalubriter diſcutit. Maxime vero in peregrinationibus antidoti potionem conſuluerim, quum in frigido aëre per hiemem iter aggrederis. Erit enim ceu ſalubre quoddam viſcerum indumentum et multum calorem praebere ipſis idoneum. Jam vero ad animi prudentiam aciemque non eſſe ineſſicacem pernovi; quippe ſenſus valide ſuo fungi munere efficit mentemque vaporibus liberatam ſubtiliorem reddit. Breviter totum corpus ita ab injuriis ſecurum facit, ut ne a deleterio quodam poſſit infici. Nam varia et tantae mixtionis medicamenti facultas ejusmodi firmitatem producit, praeſertim quum beſtiarum mixtura conſtat. Proditur enim Mithridatem magnum illum bellatorem non theriacam, ut quae necdum eſſet, ſed aliud antidotum variis quoque mixtionibus compoſitum, ipſiusque dictum nomine (Mithridatium enim appellatur) prae-

καλουμένην, Μιθριδάτειος γὰρ ὀνομάζεται, διὰ τὴν ἐξ αὐτῆς κατεσκευσμένην τῷ σώματι δυσπάθειαν μὴ δυνηθῆναι λαβόντα τὸ φάρμακον ἀποθανεῖν. ὁπότε γὰρ πολεμῶν πρὸς τοὺς Ῥωμαίους ὑπὸ τοῦ Πομπηΐου [956] νικώμενος καὶ ἐν τοῖς ἐσχάτοις ὢν ὑπὸ τοῦ φαρμάκου τοῦ ἰοῦ ἄνοσος ἀποθανεῖν ἠπείγετο, πιὼν τὸ φάρμακον καὶ πολύ γε αὐτοῦ λαβὼν αὐτὸς μὲν οὐκ ἀπέθνησκε, τὰς δὲ θυγατέρας πάνυ βουληθείσας αὐτῷ διὰ τὴν φιλοστοργίαν συναποθανεῖν πιούσας τὸ αὐτὸ φάρμακον ταχέως ἀποκτανῆναι, εἶθ᾽ ὡς ἐβράδυνε μὴ ἀποθνήσκων, τοῦ φαρμάκου δι᾽ ἣν προέπινεν ἀντίδοτον μηδὲν ἰσχῦσαι δυναμένου, καλέσας Βιστόκον τοὔνομα τῶν φίλων αὐτοῦ τινα, ἐκέλευσεν αὐτὸν ἀποσφάξαι, καὶ οὕτω ποιήσας τῷ σιδήρῳ τοῦ φαρμάκου γενέσθαι τὸ ἔργον, ἀποθανεῖν αὐτὸν βιαίως ἠνάγκασεν.

Κεφ. ιζ'. [*Πόσον καὶ πότε καὶ ὑφ᾽ ὧν ληπτέον τὴν θηριακήν.*] Ὁρᾷς οὖν ὅπως τὰ πολυμιγῆ τῶν φαρμάκων πολλὴν τὴν ἰσχὺν πρὸς τὸ ποιῆσαι τὴν δυσπάθειαν ἔχει, καὶ μάλιστα ἡ θηριακὴ, διὰ τὴν τοσαύτην δύναμιν, ὡς

ſumentem, ob ſirmam corporis conſtitutionem ex illo praeparatum, non potuiſſe veneno poto interire. Quum enim bellum adverſus Romanos gerens a Pompejo victus in extremis medicamenti veneno ſanus mori cogeretur, medicamento epoto eoque copioſo ipſe quidem non interiit, ſiliae autem ob eximium erga patrem amorem cum eo mortem volentes oppetere ejusdem medicamenti potu ſubito conciderunt; deinde quum mortem ille obire ſtatim non poſſet, veneno propter antidotum praeſumptum inefficace, vocato quodam ipſius amico nomine Biſtoco injunxit ipſum jugularet; atque ſic medicamenti opus ſerro abſolvens mori ipſum violenter coëgit.

Cap. XVII. [*Quantum et quando et a quibus theriaca ſit accipienda.*] Vides igitur quantum efficaciae ad ſirmam corporis habitudinem conciliandam variae mixtionis medicamenta obtineant et potiſſimum theriace, ob

ἔφην, τῶν θηρίων. λαμβάνειν δέ σοι τὸ φάρμακον συμβουλεύω, ὅτε εὔπεπτος εἶ καὶ σιτίων μὴ πλήρης, καὶ τῷ μέτρῳ δὲ ἄλλοτε ἄλλως χρώμενος εὖ ποιήσεις. ποτὲ μὲν γὰρ κυάμου τοῦ Αἰγυπτίου τὸ μέγεθος μετὰ κυάθων δύο ὕδατος λάμβανε, ὅταν ὀλίγον ᾖ τὸ μέλλον αὐτῆς πρὸς τὴν πέψιν γίνεσθαι διάστημα· ποτὲ δὲ καρύου Ποντικοῦ τὸ μέγεθος πίῃς, καὶ ἀνιεὶς κυάθοις τρισὶν οὕτως αὐτὸ πῖνε, ὅταν πλείονα πρὸς τὴν διοίκησιν τοῦ φαρμάκου τὸν χρόνον ἔχῃς. ἐπίβλεπε δὲ ἅμα καὶ τὴν ὥραν καὶ τὴν χώραν, ἐν αἷς μέλλεις λαμβάνειν τοῦ φαρμάκου. θέρους μὲν γὰρ ὅταν ᾖ, οὐδ᾽ ὅλως αὐτοῦ σοι συμβουλεύω λαμβάνειν. θερμοῦ γὰρ ὄντος τοῦ καταστήματος, ἔτι καὶ μᾶλλον θερμότερον γιγνόμενον βλάπτεται τὸ σῶμα, καὶ τοῦτό γε συνιδὼν ὁ θαυμασιώτατος Ἱπποκράτης τὰς πρὸ κυνὸς καὶ κατὰ κύνα φαρμακίας ἐργώδεας εἶναι λέγει. πυρετὸν γὰρ ὁ καιρὸς ὡς ἐπὶ τὸ πλεῖστον οὗτος τοῖς ἀνθρώποις φέρει. διόπερ καὶ τοῖς ἀκμάζουσι τὴν ἡλικίαν καὶ πολλὴν ἔχουσι τὴν φυσικὴν θερμότητα μὴ πολὺ μηδὲ πολλάκις προσφέρεσθαι τὸ φάρ-

tantam, ut dixi, ferarum facultatem. Caeterum medicamentum hoc meo conſilio ſumes proba fruitus concoctione nec cibis repletus; menſuraque alias alia utens recte facies. Interdum enim fabae Aegyptiacae magnitudinem cum duobus aquae cyathis capies, ubi exiguum ad concoctionem ipſius intervallum erit; interdum vero avellanae nucis magnitudine bibes tribus cyathis temperatum, quum plus temporis ad medicamenti diſtributionem habiturus es. Porro inſpice et anni tempus et regionem ubi medicamentum aſſumes. Nam per aeſtatem neutiquam id capere conſuluerim, quippe ſtatu aëris calido etiam ex antidoto corpus longe calidius evadens laeditur, atque hoc mirabilis ille Hippocrates conſiderans *medicamenti exhibitiones ante caniculae ortum et ſub ea difficiles eſſe tradit*, quoniam febrem hoc potiſſimum tempus hominibus advehit. Quapropter et aetate ſlorentibus et multo naturali calore praeditis neque multum neque ſaepe exhiberi

μακον παραινῶ· ὥσπερ γε τοῖς ἤδη τοῦ βίου τὴν παρακμὴν ἔχουσι καὶ πλεῖστον καὶ μὴ ὀλιγάκις οὐ μεθ' ὕδατος, ἀλλὰ μετ' οἴνου μᾶλλον συμβουλεύω λαμβάνειν, ἵνα τὸ μαραινόμενον ἤδη τοῦ σώματος καὶ τὸ ἀπεσβεσμένον τοῦ ἐμφύτου θερμοῦ ἀναζωπυρεῖν καὶ ἀνάπτεσθαι ὑπ' αὐτοῦ δύνηται. ἐπὶ δὲ τῶν παιδίων παντάπασι δεῖ φυλάττεσθαι τὸ φάρμακον. μεῖζον γάρ ἐστιν αὐτῆς τῆς δυνάμεως τὸ μέγεθος τοῦ φαρμάκου, καὶ διαλύει ῥᾳδίως τὸ σῶμα καὶ τὸ ἔμφυτον πνεῦμα ταχέως σβέννυσιν· ὥσπερ δὴ καὶ τὴν λυχνιαίαν φλόγα τὸ ἔλαιον τοῦ πυρὸς πλέον γενόμενον εὐκόλως ἀποσβέννυσιν. ἐγὼ γοῦν ἱστόρησα διαλυθέν ποτε παιδίον ὑπὸ τῆς ἀκαίρου τῆς ἀντιδότου χρήσεως. τὸ μὲν γὰρ ἐπύρεττε χρονίως καὶ ἦν ἰσχνὸν αὐτῷ πάνυ τὸ σῶμα καὶ τὴν δύναμιν ἀσθενές, μόλις δὲ καὶ διὰ πολλῆς ἐπιμελείας διαζῆν δυνάμενον, ἅπερ ἐγὼ συνορῶν ἐκ τοῦ ἰατρικοῦ λογισμοῦ καὶ πάνυ διεκώλυον αὐτῷ δίδοσθαι τοῦ φαρμάκου. κηδόμενος γάρ τις αὐτοῦ καὶ πατὴρ εἶναι δῆθεν λέγων καὶ τυραννικὴν ἐξουσίαν τοῦ κελεύειν ἔχων μᾶλλον ἤπερ τὴν

medicamentum eſt conſilium; quemadmodum iis qui jam vita declinant et plurimum et crebro non ex aqua, ſed vino magis aſſumi profuerit, ut corporis virtus jam emarceſcens et genuinus calor extinctus refocillari accendique ipſius poſſit beneficio. At in pueris omnino medicamentum eſt vitandum; quippe cujus magnitudo illorum virtute major ſit et corpus ex facili diſſolvat, nativum ſpiritum cito extinguat; quemadmodum ſane et lucernae flammam oleum igne copioſius adhibitum prompte extinguit. Ego itaque ex hiſtoria memini puellum aliquando ex intempeſtivo antidoti uſu diſſolutum. Etenim diuturna febre laborabat, gracilis admodum corpore et viribus imbecillis, ut qui vix multa diligentia poſſet ſupereſſe; quae quum ego ex medica ratione conſpicerem, etiam vehementer ipſi medicamentum dari prohibebam. Nam quidam ejus curationi praefectus, qui videlicet patrem ſe eſſe diceret et tyrannicam imperandi facultatem potius haberet quam ex ratione conſilium audiret, temere et vio-

Ed. Chart. XIII. [956. 957.] Ed. Baf. II. (468.)

ἐκ τοῦ λόγου συμβουλίαν ἀκούων ἀλόγως καὶ μετὰ πολλῆς ἀνάγκης ἐξηνάγκασέ με τοῦ φαρμάκου διδόναι τῷ παιδίῳ. τὸ δὲ ληφθὲν μὲν οὐκ ἠδυνήθη πεφθῆναι· κρεῖττον γὰρ ἦν τῆς ἰσχύος τοῦ λαμβάνοντος· διέλυσε δὲ αὐτοῦ τὴν σύμπασαν ἕξιν [957] καὶ τὴν γαστέρα ῥεῖν ἐποίησε, καὶ οὕτω διὰ τὴν ἄλογον τοῦ φαρμάκου χρῆσιν νύκτωρ ἀπώλετο τὸ παιδίον. εἰ δέ ποτε καὶ ἐν θερμοτέρᾳ χώρᾳ διατρίβων εἴης, φυλάττου χρῆσθαι τῷ φαρμάκῳ, ἀρκούσης σοι τῆς ἐκεῖ τοῦ ἀέρος θερμότητος, διόπερ καὶ τοῖς ὑπὸ τῆς πρώτης ἀνατολῆς τοῦ ἡλίου ἀνθρώποις θερμοτάτοις οὖσι καὶ πολλὴν ἔχουσι τὴν ἐκεῖθεν ξηρότητα ἀκατάλληλον εἶναί μοι δοκεῖ τὸ φάρμακον.

Κεφ. ιη'. [Περὶ ἁλῶν θηριακῶν.] Σκευάζονται δέ τινες διὰ τῶν θηρίων τούτων καὶ ἅλες. ἀναγκαῖον γὰρ ἔδοξέ μοι καὶ τῶν ἁλῶν μνημονεῦσαι, ἵνα τελειότατος ὁ περὶ τούτων σοι λόγος γένηται, ποιοῦσι καὶ αὐτοὶ πρὸς πάντα τὰ προειρημένα, μετρίως μὲν καὶ χρόνῳ πολλῷ τὸ χρήσιμον παρασχεῖν δυνάμενοι, τὸ δὲ συνεχὲς τῆς χρήσεως

lenter admodum me compulit, ut infanti medicamentum exhiberem; quod jam aſſumptum concoqui non potuit, fortius videlicet ejus virtute qui ceperat, verum totum ipſius habitum diſſolvit alvumque fecit profluentem, atque ita propter irrationalem medicamenti uſum noctu infans periit. Porro ſi in calidiore nonnunquam verſeris regione, cave medicamento utaris, aëris caliditate illic ſufficiente, qua de cauſa etiam hominibus ſub primo ſolis ortu calidiſſimis et multa inde ſiccitate praeditis medicamentum eſſe mihi videtur diſſentaneum.

Cap. XVIII. [*De ſalibus theriacis.*] Praeparantur et ſales quidam ex his feris. Nam illorum etiam meminiſſe neceſſarium mihi viſum eſt, ut abſolutiſſimus hisce de rebus tibi ſermo ſiat. Faciunt iidem ad omnia praedicta, modice quidem longoque temporis ſpatio praeſidium praebere habiles, frequenti autem uſu paulatim adjuvan-

κατ᾽ ὀλίγον τὴν ὠφέλειαν ποιούμενοι. διόπερ δὴ καὶ πολλοὶ τῶν χρωμένων τὴν συναίσθησιν τῆς ἀπ᾽ αὐτῶν βοηθείας ταχεῖαν οὐκ ἔχοντες τὴν ἀρχὴν οὐδ᾽ ὅλως βοηθεῖν δύνασθαι νομίζουσι, μάλιστα ἐπειδὴ καὶ τῷ πυρὶ σποδὸς αὐτῶν τὸ σῶμα γίγνεται, ἐξαφανίζεσθαι λέγοντες τῇ καύσει τὴν πρὸς τὸ ἐπικουρεῖν δύναμιν αὐτῶν. ἐγὼ μέν φημι τὴν μὲν δύναμιν αὐτὴν τῇ θηριακῇ μὴ ἔχειν τοὺς ἅλας, μὴ μέντοι τελέως αὐτῶν ἐξαφανίζεσθαι τὴν ἐπίκουρον ἰσχύν. πολλὰ γὰρ τὸ πυρὶ ὁμιλεῖν ἀποφαίνει κρείττονα, καὶ ποτὲ μὲν καὶ κρυπτομένην αὐτῶν τὴν φύσιν εἰς τὸ φανερὸν ἄγει, τινὰ δὲ καὶ πρὸς ἣν βουλόμεθα χρείαν εὐαρμόστως ἔχειν παρασκευάζει. ὁ γοῦν χρυσὸς ὑφ᾽ ἡμῶν δι᾽ αὐτοῦ κρίνεται, καὶ ὁ μὲν κίβδηλος πυρωθεὶς ἐλέγχεται, ὁ δὲ ἐν τῷ πυροῦσθαι καθαρθεὶς ἀκριβῶς δόκιμος εἶναι φαίνεται. καὶ ὁ σίδηρος πυῤῥούμενος μαλάττεται καὶ καμπτόμενος ὑφ᾽ ἡμῶν εὔχρηστος εἶναι πρὸς πολλὰ τῶν ἐν τῷ βίῳ φαίνεται. οὐχὶ δὲ καὶ τῶν προσφερομένων τὰ πλεῖστα πρὸς τὸ θρέψειν ἡμᾶς διὰ τὸ πῦρ κατάλληλα γίγνεται; ἄρτος γέ τοι καὶ

tes; quocirca plerique ex iis qui utuntur, ubi non velox ab eis praeſidium ſentiunt, nequaquam poſſe opitulari arbitrantur, maxime quia igne corpus ipſorum in cinerem redigitur, dicentes auxiliatrices eorum facultates per uſtionem evaneſcere. Ego quidem aſſirmo ſales, etſi vim theriacae imparem habeant, non tamen omnino robur auxiliarium in eis obliterari. Multa ſiquidem ignis commercio redduntur meliora; interdum latentem ipſorum naturam in apertum edunt, nonnulla vero ad quem volumus uſum accommoda eſſiciuntur. Aurum itaque ipſo igne exploratur et adulterum, igne ſi accendatur, arguitur, atque flamma exacte purgatum germanum eſſe apparet. Jam ferrum igne mollescit et flexum nobis ad multos vitae uſus habile eſſe videtur. Nunquid etiam plurima quae in corpus ingeruntur nutriendis nobis ignis beneſicio redduntur idonea? Panis ſiquidem et reliquorum animalium et piſcium carnes crudae adhuc appetitus uſui ſunt in-

Ed. Chart. XIII. [957.] Ed. Baf. II. (468. 469.)

τῶν κρεῶν καὶ τῶν ἰχθύων αἱ σάρκες ὠμὰ μὲν ὄντα πρὸς τὴν χρείαν τῆς ὀρέξεως ἄχρηστά ἐστιν, ὀπτηθέντα δὲ τότε γίγνονται καὶ τῶν σωμάτων τροφαί. ὁ δὲ οἶνος καὶ αὐτὸς εὐθέως μὲν καὶ ἀπὸ τῶν βοτρύων ἐκθλιβεὶς ὠμὸς καὶ ἄπεπτός ἐστι, πεφθεὶς δὲ τῷ τοῦ ἡλίου πυρὶ τότε καὶ ἥδιστος καὶ ποτι- (469) μώτατος γίγνεται. ὅτι δὲ πολλὰ καὶ τῶν ἐν τῇ τέχνῃ φαρμάκων τὴν ἀρχαίαν ἑαυτῶν φύσιν ἔχοντα δριμύτατά τέ ἐστι καὶ πολέμια τοῖς σώμασιν ἡ πεῖρα διδάσκει· κολασθέντα δὲ τῇ τοῦ πυρὸς ἀνάγκῃ εὔχρηστα πρὸς θεραπείαν γίνεται. ἡ γοῦν χαλκῖτις ὠμὴ μὲν καίει τὰ σώματα καὶ ῥᾳδίως τὰς ἐσχάρας ἀπεργάζεται, ὀπτηθεῖσα δὲ ἐπουλοῖ τὰ ἕλκη· καὶ ὁ ἀπὸ τῆς Φρυγίας λίθος ὠμὸς μὲν ὢν δριμύτατός ἐστιν, ἀνθρακούμενος δὲ καὶ λειούμενος μετ' ἄλλων τινῶν ἀγαθὸν γίνεται τῶν ὀφθαλμῶν φάρμακον. ἡ δὲ ἀπὸ τοῦ καιομένου σπόγγου γιγνομένη σποδιὰ καρτερῶς τὰς αἱμοῤῥαγίας εἴωθεν ἐπέχειν. τὸ αὐτό μοι δοκεῖ καὶ ἐπὶ τῶν θηριακῶν ἀλῶν γίγνεσθαι νομίζειν. πάντα γὰρ ὁμοῦ καιόμενα καὶ ὁλόκληρα συναπτόμενα τὰ θηρία τὴν μὲν ὑπερτεταμένην καὶ πονηρὰν τοῖς σώμασι

utiles, coctae, tunc etiam corporum alimenta fiunt. Jam vinum ipfum ftatim ab uvis expreffum crudum incoctumque eft, folis autem aeftu coctum tunc et fuaviffimum et maxime potabile redditur. Porro multa in arte medicamenta quamdiu veterem ipforum naturam retinent, acerrima effe et corporibus inimica experientia docet; domita vero ignis neceffitate curationi fiunt congrua. Itaque chalcitis cruda quidem corpora contingens facile cruftas excitat tofta vero cicatricem ulceribus inducit. Item lapis Phrygius crudus acerrimus eft, ignitus autem et cum aliis quibusdam tritus praefens fit oculorum remedium. Spongiae uftae cinis fanguinis fluxionem potenter inhibet; idem mihi etiam in theriacis falibus fieri apparet. Omnia enim fimul ufta ac integrae accenfae beftiae pravam vim corporibus inditam ex uftione deponunt et ab igne auxilii fymmetriam fortiuntur. Pe-

δύναμιν διὰ τῆς καύσεως ἀποτίθεται, τὴν δὲ ἀπὸ τοῦ πυρὸς πρὸς τὸ βοηθεῖν συμμετρίαν λαμβάνει. ἰδίως δὲ καὶ ἅλες θεραπεύουσι μάλιστα τὰ περὶ τὴν ἐπιφάνειαν γιγνόμενα πάθη, λεύκας λέγω καὶ λέπρας καὶ λειχῆνας τοὺς ἀγρίους· τά τε γὰρ ὑπὸ τῷ δέρματι περιττὰ καὶ δριμέα μάλιστα διαφοροῦσιν. ἐσθίοντες γοῦν αὐτοὺς οἱ πλεῖστοι ἱδρωτικώτεροι γίγνονται καὶ τὴν διεφθαρμένην κενοῦσιν οὐσίαν, ὡς καὶ τοὺς καλουμένους φθεῖρας ἐκβάλλειν τινὰς, ἐκ δια- [958] φθορᾶς ἰδίαν γένεσιν ἐχούσας, καὶ διὰ τοῦθ', ὡς οἶμαι, φθεῖρας καλουμένας. σμήχουσι δὲ καὶ ἄριστα τοὺς ὀδόντας, καὶ τὰ πλαδαρὰ τῶν σωμάτων πυκνοῦσι, καὶ τὸ ἐπ' αὐτοῖς ἐπιφερόμενον ἀναστέλλουσι ῥεῦμα, ἀσήπτους τε τοὺς ὀδόντας φυλάττουσι, τιτρώσκεσθαι ἢ βιβρώσκεσθαι αὐτοὺς οὐκ ἐῶντες.

Κεφ. ιθ'. [Περὶ ἁλῶν θηριακῶν κατασκευῆς.] Γίνεται δ' αὐτῶν ἡ σκευασία τοῦτον τὸν τρόπον. πειράσομαι γάρ σοι πάλιν καὶ τούτους σκευάζειν τῇ ὑπογραφῇ τοῦ λόγου χρώμενος. λαβόντα γὰρ χρὴ ἐχίδνας ταῖς προειρημέναις ὁμοίας καὶ τῷ αὐτῷ χρόνῳ τεθηραμένας, ἔστωσαν δὲ

culiariter autem et maxime fales medentur affectibus fumma in cute obortis, leucis dico, lepris impetiginique agrefti; nam fuperfluitates cutis fubditas acresque potiffimum difcutiunt. Plurimi igitur ipfos manducantes fudoribus largiter diffluentes corruptam vacuant fubftantiam, ut pediculos quoque vocatos quosdam ejiciant, ex corruptione proprie nafcentes; quos ideo, ut autumo, phthiras appellant. Dentes optime abftergunt et flaccidas partes denfant, fluorem ipfis illabentem reprimunt, imputres fervant, perforari aut erodi ipfos non finunt.

Cap. XIX. [*De falium theriacorum compofitione.*] Hunc in modum ipfi praeparantur; conabor enim tibi rurfus horum quoque confectionem fermone defcribere. 24 Viperas praedictis fimiles et eodem tempore captas, numero quatuor, non biduo plus poft venationem, verum

τὸν ἀριθμὸν δ'. καὶ μὴ πλεῖον δύο ἡμερῶν μετὰ τὴν θήραν ἐχούσας, ἀλλ' εἰ δυνατὸν, αὐτῆς τῆς ἡμέρας ἧς εἰσιν εἰλημμέναι. εἶτα τῶν ἁλῶν καλὸν μὲν εἰ τῶν ἀμμωνιακῶν, εἰ δὲ μή γε, τῶν κοινῶν καὶ τῇ χρόᾳ λευκῶν καὶ ἐξηθριασμένων ἠρέμα μόδιον Ἰταλικὸν, εἶτα καὶ σὺν αὐτοῖς κόψας ἁδρομερῶς γεντιανῆς Κρητικῆς λίτραν α' S''. ἀριστολοχίας στρογγύλης λίτραν α' S''. κενταυρίου λεπτοῦ κόμης λίτρας β'. καρδαμώμου Ἀρμενιακοῦ, πρασίου, ἀνὰ γο. στ'. σκορδίου ὀρεινοῦ, σελίνου, χαμαίδρυος Κρητικῆς λίτραν α'. πηγάνου ἡμέρου σπέρματος λίτραν α'. μέλιτι Ἀττικῷ ἑνώσας αὐτὰ, καὶ ἥμισυ λίτραν μέρος αὐτῶν εἰς χύτραν ἐξ ὀστράκου γενομένην καινὴν βαλὼν, εἶτα δ'. ἐχίδνας ζώσας προεπιβαλὼν, σὺν αὐταῖς καὶ σκίλλας ἁπαλὰς καὶ πάνυ νεαρὰς ε'. εἰς λεπτὰ κατατεμὼν, οὕτως ἐπίβαλε τὸ λοιπὸν ἥμισυ τῶν ἄλλων μέρος, καὶ πωματίσας καὶ πηλώσας ἐπιμελῶς τρῆσον τέσσαρσί που τρήμασιν αὐτῆς τὸ σῶμα, ἵνα δι' αὐτῶν ὁ ἀτμὸς διασημήνῃ σοι τὸ μέτρον τῆς ὀπτήσεως. τὸ μὲν γὰρ πρῶτον φανήσεται καπνὸς ἐξιὼν, πολὺς, ζοφώδης καὶ τε-

ſi fieri poſſit, eodem die quo ſunt captae; deinde ſalis ammoniaci, ſin minus, communis colore albi et leniter ſplendeſcentis modium Italicum; mox cum ipſis tunde minutatim gentianae Creticae libram unam ß, ariſtolochiae rotundae libram unam ß, centaurii tenuis comae libras ij, cardamomi Armeniaci, marrubii, ſingulorum ℥ vj, ſcordii montani, apii, chamaedryos Creticae libram unam, rutae ſativae ſeminis libram j, melle Attico haec unita excipe et libram ß, mediam ipſorum portionem in ollam ex argilla factam vacuam praemitte et cum ipſis conjice; deinde quatuor viperas vivas, mox ſcillas teneras et recentiſſimas quinque in tenues partes concide; ita reliquam aliorum partem dimidiam adjice, ac ubi cooperueris ollam, lutoque diligenter obliveris, quatuor ipſam foraminibus aperies, ut per ea vapor coctionis modum indicet. Nam primum fumus exire videbitur copioſus, obſcurus admodumque turbidus, notans ignem jam feras invaſiſſe; quando te animum quoque diligenter advertere

θολωμένος πάνυ, σημαίνων ὅτι τὸ πῦρ ἤδη ἅπτεται τῶν θηρίων, ὅτε σε καὶ προσέχειν ἀκριβῶς παραινῶ, μήποτε ἀναπνεύσῃς τούτου καπνοῦ, κεκακωμένου τοῦ ἀέρος ὑπὸ τῆς ἀναθυμιάσεως τῶν ἐχιδνῶν. εἶθ' ὅταν παύσηται ὁ ἀτμὸς, ἀναβαλλομένην δέ τινα φλόγα λεπτὴν διὰ τῶν τρημάτων βλέπῃς, τότε νόμιζε ὡς ἄριστα αὐτὰ ἡψῆσθαι καὶ οὕτω βάσταζε ἀπὸ τοῦ πυρὸς τὴν χύτραν, ψύξας ὅλην ἡμέραν τε καὶ νύκτα, εἶτα ἀνοίξας καὶ ἀνελόμενος τοὺς ἄνθρακας, ἐπιμελῶς κόπτε καὶ σῆθε μετὰ τούτων τῶν μιγμάτων, πηγάνου ἀγρίου σπέρματος γο. θ'. ὑσσώπου Κρητικοῦ γο. θ'. μαράθρου σπέρματος ἀγριου γο. στ'. νάρδου Κελτικῆς, στάχυος Σκυθικοῦ, ἀνὰ γο. στ'. πετροσελίνου Μακεδονικοῦ γο. δ'. ἀμώμου βότρυος γο. γ'. ὀριγάνου Ἡρακλεωτικοῦ κορύμβων γο. θ'. ὁρμίνου σπέρματος πεφρυγμένου γο. γ' θύμου κορύμβων Ἀττικοῦ γο. θ'. μαλαβάθρου φύλλων Ἰνδικοῦ γο. δ'. ἀρκευθίδων Λακωνικῶν σαρκὸς λίτρας β'. κορίου σπέρματος ἡμέρου γο. στ'. πεπέρεως λευκοῦ λίτρας β'. πεπέρεως μέλανος λίτρας β'. σιλφίου ῥίζης γο. ι'. ζιγγιβέρεως ἀτρήτου λίτρας β'.

moneo, ne tandem hujus fumi aërem ex viperarum exhalatione infectum inſpires. Poſtea ubi vapor ceſſaverit et tenuem quandam flammam per foramina ejici conſpexeris, tunc ipſa cocta eſſe quam optime cenſeto, atque ita ollam de igne tollito, tota die et nocte refrigerans. Deinde apertos exemptosque carbones diligenter tundito et cum hisce mixturis cribrato, rutae agreſtis ſeminis ℥ ix, hyſſopi Cretici uncias novem, foeniculi ſeminis agreſtis ℥ vj, nardi Celticae, ſpicae Scythicae, ſingulorum uncias ſex, petroſelini Macedonici uncias quatuor, amomi uvae uncias tres, origani Heracleotici ſummitatum uncias novem, hormini ſeminis torrefacti uncias tres, thymi Attici ſummitatum uncias novem, malabathri Indici foliorum uncias quatuor, baccarum juniperi Laconici carnis libras duas, adianti ſativi ſeminis uncias vj, piperis albi libr. ij, piperis nigri libras duas, laſeris radicis uncias decem, zingiberis non forati libras duas, ſatyrii ſeminis

σατυρίου σπέρματος, ἢ ῥίζης οὐγγίας στ'. γλήχωνος ὀρεινοῦ γο. στ'. σεσέλεως Μασσαλεωτικοῦ πυῤῥοειδοῦς γο. στ'. τορδύλου ὀρεινοῦ σπέρματος γο. στ'. ἡδυόσμου γο. στ'. κασσίας τῆς καλλίστης γο. β'. κινναμώμου γο. α'. πυρῶ δ' αὐτὰ κόψας, καὶ σήσας, πάλιν ἐπικόπτειν καὶ διακοσκινεύειν πολλάκις, ἵνα ἀκριβῶς λεῖα γένωνται, καὶ οὕτως ἐν ὑελίνοις σκεύεσιν ἀποτιθέμενος χρῆσθαι μὴ εὐθέως, ἀλλὰ μεθ' ἡμέρας που δέκα. ἐσκεύασα δ' αὐτοὺς ἐγὼ, μὴ καύσας τὰ θηρία, ἀλλὰ τοὺς ἐξ αὐτῶν ἀρτίσκους, [959] ὥσπερ ἐπὶ τῆς θηριακῆς ὑπέδειξα σκευάζεσθαι, ἀναμίξας τοῖς μετὰ τῶν θηρίων καιομένοις καὶ αὐτοὺς, ἵνα ἥν περ ἔχῃ πικρότητα ἐν αὐτοῖς, ἐν τῇ καύσει ταύτην ἀποβάλῃ, τοσοῦτον μέτρον τῶν ἀρτίσκων προσβάλλων, ὅσον περ ἐτεκμηράμην ἔχειν τὸν ἀριθμὸν τῶν τεσσάρων ἐχιδνῶν, καὶ ἀπέβησαν ὡς ἀληθῶς ἄριστοι, οὔτε τὸ ἐκ τῆς καύσεως σποδῶδες ἐν τῇ γεύσει ἔχοντες οὔτε μέλανες ὄντες τὴν χροιὰν, ἀλλὰ καὶ τὴν ποιότητα ἐν τῇ χρήσει ἥδιστοι γενόμενοι, καὶ τὴν δύναμιν πρὸς ἅπερ εἶπον αὐτοὺς ἰδίως ποιεῖν, ἐνεργεστέραν ἔχοντες.

vel radicis ℥ vj, pulegii montani ℥ vj, feſelis Maſſaliotici rufi ℥ vj, tordyli montani ſeminis ℥ ſex, mentae ℥ ſex, caſſiae optimae uncias duas, cinnamomi unciam unam. Conare autem ipſa contuſa cribrataque rurſus contundere et cribro frequenter incernere, ut adamuſſim fiant laevia; atque ſic in vaſis vitreis repoſita non ſtatim uſurpare convenit, ſed poſt decem fere dies. Porro ego ipſos praeparavi beſtiis non uſtis, ſed ipſarum paſtillis quemadmodum in theriaca oſtendi confici, miſcens ipſos quoque iis quae cum belluis comburuntur, ut quam habeant in ſe amarulentiam, eam in uſtione deponant, tanta paſtillorum menſura adjecta, quantam quatuor viperarum numerum habere conjecturabam, et facti ſunt longe praeſtantiſſimi, nec cinereum ex uſtione guſtu referentes, nec colore nigri, ſed etiam qualitate in uſu ſuaviſſimi redditi et vires, ad quae dixi peculiariter ipſos facere, evidentiores obtinentes. Hic eſt de theriaca et ſalibus theriacis liber, diligenter, ut judico, a me examinatus, hac maxime

Ed. Chart. XIII. [959.] Ed. Baſ. II. (469.)

οὗτός ἐστιν ὁ περὶ τῆς θηριακῆς καὶ τῶν θηριακῶν ἄλων λόγος, φιλοπόνως, ὡς οἶμαι, ἐξετασθεὶς ὑπ' ἐμοῦ μάλιστα, ἐπεὶ καὶ σὺ περὶ πάντας τοὺς λόγους φιλοτίμως ἔχεις. μέμνημαι γάρ σε, ὁπότε τοῖς λόγοις ἐνδόξως ἔτι δημοσιεύων ἐσχόλαζες, ἤ τι λέγων πρόβλημα, κρῖναι τοὺς λέγοντας διαλιπεῖν ποτε, πολλὰς ἀφορμὰς εὑρίσκειν σε φιλοτιμούντων εἰς τόδε διαλεγομένων. ἔλεγες γὰρ ὅτι καὶ οἱ θεοὶ μὴ χρῶντες οὐ λαλοῦσιν. ἐνίοτε δὲ καὶ τὰ χρηστήρια σιωπᾷ, ποτὲ καὶ ἡ θάλασσα τοῖς χειμῶσι τὸ πλεῖσθαι οὐκ ἔχει. τὰ δὲ ῥεῖθρα τῶν ποταμῶν παύεται ῥέοντα καὶ μετὰ χρόνον ἐπιῤῥεῖν πάλιν ἄρχεται καὶ ἡ γῆ τοὺς καρποὺς οὐκ ἀναφύει πάντοτε. μιμησάμενος οὖν σε κἀγὼ οὐδὲν τῶν περὶ τῆς θηριακῆς ζητουμένων παρέλιπον, ἅμα καὶ σοι προτρεψάμενος ἡδέως χρῆσθαι τῷ φαρμάκῳ, ἐπεὶ καὶ πολυετῆ τῆς ζωῆς τὸν χρόνον ἡ χρῆσις αὐτοῦ παρέχεσθαι τετήρηται, ὅν περ εἰκότως ἐγὼ τῶν παρὰ θεῶν γενέσθαι σοι εὔχομαι.

cauſa, quoniam et tu in omnes diſciplinas ſtudioſe incumbis. Memini enim te, quum literarum ſtudiis egregie inter civilia adhuc negotia vacares, vel legeres quoddam problema judicare oratores nonnunquam ut deſinant multas conari occaſiones invenire, atque hoc agitare. Etenim deos ajebas, dum non vaticinantur, nihil eloqui; interdum vero etiam oracula ſilent. Eſt quum et mare tempeſtatibus navigari non poteſt, agmina fluviorum ſiſtuntur et paulo poſt rurſus fluere incipiunt. Item terra fructus non ſemper producit. Quare tuum ego exemplum imitatus, nihil ex his quae de theriaca quaeruntur omiſi; ſimulque te adhortor ut libenter medicamento utaris, quoniam longaevum vitae uſum ipſius exhibere obſervatum eſt; quod merito ut tibi a diis contingat exopto.

ΓΑΛΗΝΟΥ ΠΕΡΙ ΘΗΡΙΑΚΗΣ ΠΡΟΣ ΠΑΜΦΙΛΙΑΝΟΝ.

Ed. Chart. XIII. [960.] Ed. Baf. II. (469.)

[960] Πολλάκις ἐπιζητοῦντί σοι, κράτιστε Παμφιλιανὲ, την μέθοδον τῆς θηριακῆς ἀντιδότου καὶ τὴν χρῆσιν παρ᾽ ἡμῶν ἀκοῦσαι τὰ μὲν ἐκ τοῦ παραστάντος ἡμῖν ῥηθέντα οὔτε σε νομίζω διαμνημονεύειν οὔτε ἐμαυτὸν ἀποχρώντως εἰρηκέναι. νυνὶ δὲ ἐπὶ σχολῆς γενόμενος καὶ διὰ τῆς μνήμης ἀνακαλεσάμενος ὅσα κατὰ τὴν περιοδίαν εἶδον ἐν Ῥώμῃ, παρά τε τοῖς ὑφηγησαμένοις ἡμῖν κατορθούμενα διὰ τοῦ

GALENI DE THERIACA AD PAMPHILIANUM.

Tibi multoties efflagitanti, clariffime Pamphiliane, theriacae antidoti methodum ac ufum ex nobis audire, quae ex tempore a me dicta funt, ea neque te in memoriam revocare neque me ipfum fatis explicaffe arbitror. Nunc vero otium nactus et in memoriam revocans quaecunque dum Romae verfarer didici, tum ab iis qui nobis enarrarunt eo medicamento pro-

φαρμάκου τούτου καὶ ὅσα χρησάμενος αὐτὸς ἐπιτυχὼν κατώρθωσα, ταῦτ᾽ ᾠήθην δεῖν σοι προσφωνῆσαι συναγαγὼν, μετὰ τοῦ καὶ τοὺς τρόπους τῆς χρήσεως ὑπογράφειν, καὶ τὰς διαφορὰς τῶν παθῶν, καὶ τοὺς καιροὺς ἐφ᾽ ὧν τινων, καὶ πότε χρώ- (470) μενος αὐτῇ τις οὐκ ἂν διαμαρτάνοι. κομιδῇ γὰρ ἀκούσου τινὸς εἶναι δοκεῖ μοι τὸ ἀποκρύπτεσθαί τι τῶν εἰς σωτηρίαν διαφερόντων, ὑπὲρ ἧς ἅπαντες οἱ κατὰ τὴν μητρόπολιν εὔχονται δικαίως, ἅτε δὴ κατ᾽ ἰδίαν εὐεργετούμενοι καὶ κοινῇ κοσμούμενοι, διὰ τῶν ὑπὲρ τῆς προνοίας τῇ πόλει πάσῃ κατασκευαζομένων κοινωφελῶν ἔργων. οἶδα δὲ καὶ τὰς ἄλλας πόλεις ἁπάσας ὅσαι Κρητικαὶ τῆς σῆς γνώμης τὸ περὶ πάντας δεξιὸν καὶ ἐπιεικὲς οὐ τιμώσας μόνον, ἀλλὰ καὶ ἀγαπώσας. εἰσὶ δὲ καὶ ἐπὶ τῆς Αἰγύπτου καὶ ἐπὶ τῆς βασιλίδος πόλεως τοσοῦτοι τὸ πλῆθος φίλοι σοὶ μόνῳ Κρητῶν, ὅσοι τοῖς ἄλλοις ἅπασιν οὐκ εἰσὶν, ὥστ᾽ εὐλόγως ἄν τινα θαυμάσαι καὶ τὴν τύχην οἰκείως σοι θεμένην πρὸς τὴν φύσιν τοῦ τρόπου καὶ τοῦ ὀνόματος τὸ ἐπίσημον, ὡς ἂν προγινώσκουσαν ὅτι μέλλεις ὑπὸ πάντων

ſperrime effici, quaeque ex uſu ipſe probe facta conſequutus ſum, ea collecta tibi conſecranda eſſe duxi, ſimulque praeſcribere utendi modum, morborum differentias ac tempora, in quibus et quando aliquis ea utens non aberraverit. Ad modum enim ruſtici cujusdam eſſe mihi videtur aliquid occultare quod ad ſalutem conferat, pro qua omnes in urbe principe merito vota faciunt; quippe quod privatim beneficiis et publice ornamentis afficiantur ex operibus, quae ut toti civitati provideant, ad communem utilitatem praeparantur. Novi autem tum alias urbes omnes Creticas tum tui ingenii dexteritatem in omnibus et manſuetudinem non ſolum venerari, ſed etiam diligere. Sunt vero tum in Aegypto tum in regia urbe Alexandria tot multitudine amici tibi ſoli Cretenſium, qui caeteris omnibus non ſunt. Quamobrem jure quiſpiam fortunam quoque miraretur cum naturae tum tuis moribus conſentaneum nomen inſigne perinde impoſuiſſe, ac ſi praeſagiret te cunctis amabilem fore. Itaque compara-

φιλεῖσθαι. ἡ μὲν οὖν κτῆσίς σοι τῆς ἀντιδότου δαψιλὴς καὶ παρὰ πολλῶν, ἡ δ' ἔντεχνος χρῆσις παρ' ἡμῶν καὶ τῆς ἡμετέρας περὶ σὲ σπουδῆς καὶ εὐνοίας ὑπόμνημα. ὅνπερ γὰρ τρόπον αὐλοῦ καὶ λύρας καὶ τῶν ἄλλων μουσικῶν ὀργάνων οὐδὲν πλέον τοῖς κεκτημένοις μὲν, μὴ χρωμένοις δὲ, τὸν αὐτὸν τρόπον καὶ ἐπὶ τῶν ἀντιδότων ἔχει, οἷον καὶ ἐπὶ τῶν ἄλλων ἰατρικῶν φαρμάκων οὐδὲν ὀνίνησιν ἡ κτῆσις αὐτῶν, τῆς χρήσεως [961] ὑστεριζούσης. εἰ μὲν γὰρ, ὡς ἡ παρὰ τοῖς πολλοῖς ἐπικρατοῦσα φήμη, πρὸς μόνα τὰ δήγματα τῶν ἰοβόλων καὶ πρὸς τὰς τῶν δηλητηρίων φαρμάκων ἐποίει πόσεις, ἔδει καθάπερ τι κειμήλιον οἴκοι κατακείμενον περιορᾷν τὸ φάρμακον, ὑπὸ τοῦ χρόνου δαπανώμενον, τῆς χρείας οὐ καλούσης. ἐπεὶ δὲ πρὸς τούτοις καὶ εὐγηρίαν ὑπισχνεῖται καὶ μακροβιότητα καὶ ἀκρίβειαν αἰσθήσεως, καὶ διαμονὴν ὑγείας, καὶ οὐ μόνον τῶν παρόντων νοσημάτων λύσιν, ἀλλὰ καὶ τῶν ἔσεσθαι μελλόντων κώλυσιν, εὔλογον οἴομαι καὶ ἐν ὑγείᾳ οὐκ ἀποστρέφεσθαι τὴν χρῆσιν αὐτῆς, τῆς ἀπαλλαγῆς τῶν ἐνοχλούντων παθῶν τὸ τὴν

tio quidem copiofae hujus antidoti tibi et a multis, artificialis vero ufus a nobis noftri in te ftudii, benevolentiaeque monumentum erit. Quo namque modo qui fiftulam, lyram et caetera mufica inftrumenta compararunt, nec his uti queunt, hi plus non habent, eodem modo et in antidotis *fe res habet*, ut et in caeteris medicis medicamentis, nihil juvat eorum comparatio, fi intempeftivus fit ufus. Si namque, ut apud plerosque fama praevalefcit, adverfus folos virulentorum ferpentum morfus et deleteriorum medicamentorum pocula vim habeat antidotus, oportebat feu pretiofum aliquod domi repofitum circumfpicere medicamentum tempore, ufu non poftulante, evanescere. Quum vero ad haec et profperam fenectutem et vitae diuturnitatem et fenfuum integritatem et fanitatis perpetuitatem polliceatur, neque folum praefentium morborum folutionem, verum etiam imminentium futurorumque fore obftaculum; par, arbitror, et in fanitate eum hujus ufum haud negligere, qui pluris aeftimat per initia in morbos

ἀρχὴν μὴ παθεῖν προτιμῶντα. πολλοὶ γοῦν τῶν ἐν Ῥώμῃ μεγάλα δυναμένων κατὰ νεομηνίαν τοῦ φαρμάκου προσφέρονται. οἱ δὲ ἀπολεξάμενοι τὴν τετάρτην τῆς σελήνης ἐπὶ τρεῖς κατὰ τὰς ἑξῆς ἡμέρας προευπεπτηκότες καὶ τῆς κοιλίας ἠρέμα προεπιμεληθέντες, περὶ τὴν τρίτην ὥραν προσφέρονται τοῦ Ἑλληνικοῦ κυάμου μέγεθος, σὺν μέλιτος κοχλιαρίῳ ἑνὶ καὶ ὕδατος θερμοῦ κυάθοις δυσὶν, οὐχ ἵνα τι διοχλοῦν νόσημα ἀποστρέψωνται, ἀλλ' ἵνα παντὸς νοσήματος ἀπερίπτωτοι μένωσι καὶ τῆς προθέσεως οὐκ ἀποτυγχάνωσι. χρηστὸν γὰρ αὐτοῖς ἀποφαίνει τὸ αἷμα, οὐ τὴν φερομένην ἐν αὐτῷ φαυλότητα ἀποκρίνουσα, ἀλλ' ἐξοικειοῦσα τὴν ἀτοπίαν καὶ κρατοῦσα τῆς παρὰ φύσιν ποιότητος. κατὰ δὲ τὰς ἀποδημίας, ὅταν ὑπονοήσωσι χώρας τινὰς νοσώδεις, ἢ μοχθηρίας ὑδάτων, τὸν αὐτὸν τρόπον προσφερόμενοι ἐξασφαλίζονται τὴν ἕξιν τοῦ σώματος, ὥσπερ ὅπλῳ τινὶ σωτηρίῳ τῷ φαρμάκῳ χρώμενοι, καὶ διαμένουσιν ἀπήμονες. τῶν δ' ἐμῶν διδασκάλων ὁ πρεσβύτατος ἀνὴρ, εἰ καί τις

non incidere quam vexantium morborum propulſationem moliri. Proinde multi Romae ſummates primo lunae die hoc medicamentum aſſumunt, quidam quartum lunae diem eligunt, quum prius tribus ſubſequentibus diebus *interjectis* coctioni incubuerint ac ante alvi leviter *ſolvendae* curam dederint, circiter horam tertiam id capiunt Graecae fabae magnitudine, cum mellis cochleari uno et aquae calidae cyathis duobus, non quo morbum aliquem inſeſtantem avertant, ſed ut a quocunque morbo immunes tutique permaneant et a propoſiti ſpe non decidant. Bonum enim ipſis theriaca conciliat ſanguinem, non quod eam quae in eo fertur pravitatem excernat, ſed ejus contumaciam qualitate praeter naturam domita in familiaritatem adducat. Caeterum in profectionibus quum ſuſpicantur regiones *quas adeunt* aliquas inſalubres et aquas eſſe pravas, ea ratione theriacam conſerunt, eoque medicamento utentes corporis habitum tanquam armatura quadam ſalutari muniunt ac illaeſi permanent. At meo-

ἄλλος ἐμπειρίᾳ τέχνης καὶ ἐπιεικείᾳ γνώμης διαφέρων, Αἰλιανὸς Μέκκιος, ἔφη ποτὲ τὴν Ἰταλιῶτιν χώραν ὑπὸ λοιμοῦ πιεσθεῖσαν, ὀξεῖς θανάτους καὶ φθορὰν ἀνθρώπων πολλὴν παθεῖν, ἐν δέει δὲ πάντων ὁμοίως, καὶ τῶν ἰατρῶν καὶ ἡγουμένων ἀνδρῶν ὑπαρχόντων, εἰσηγήσασθαι μόνῃ χρῆσθαι τῇ θηριακῇ, τῶν ἄλλων ἁπάντων ἀπρακτούντων βοηθημάτων, καὶ τῶν μὲν ἤδη νοσούντων λαβόντων τινὰς ἀνασφῆλαι, τινὰς δὲ καὶ διαφθαρῆναι. τοὺς δὲ πρὸ τοῦ νοσῆσαι προσενεγκαμένους πάντας οὐ μόνον τὸν κίνδυνον, ἀλλὰ καὶ τὴν πεῖραν τοῦ πάθους διαφυγεῖν, καὶ θαυμαστὸν οὐδέν· εἰ γὰρ καὶ θανασίμων φαρμάκων πινομένη δύναται κρατεῖν, νικήσει καὶ φθορὰν ἀέρος ἀδικοῦσαν τὸν ἄνθρωπον, ὅπερ δὴ καὶ τοὺς πολλοὺς τῶν ἰατρῶν καὶ τοὺς ἰδιώτας ἅπαντας κοινῇ διαλανθάνειν μὴ θαυμάσαις. ὁποῖ γάρ εἰσι καὶ χυλοὶ καὶ φλοιοὶ καὶ ῥίζαι καὶ ἄνθη καὶ σπέρματα καὶ σαρκία ἐξ ὧν συνέστηκεν. ὥσπερ οὖν καθ' ἓν τούτων ἕκαστον ἱκανὸς ὁ χρόνος ἐξίτηλον ἀποφῆναι, οὕτω καὶ τὴν

rum praeceptorum vetuſtiſſimus, artis ſi quis alius experientia et animi aequitate praeſtans, Aelianus Meccius, aſſirmavit aliquando Italam regionem a peſte divexatam acutas mortes et jacturam hominum multam ſubiiſſe, in aequali vero omnium metu, tum medicorum tum optimatum virorum et principum, ſe auctorem fuiſſe ut ſola theriaca uterentur, caeteris omnibus auxiliis nihil quicquam proficientibus; ac tum aegrotantium qui eam aſſumpſerant quosdam convaluiſſe, nonnullos quoque interiiſſe, qui vero hanc priusquam aegrotarent aſſumpſiſſent, eos omnes non ſolum vitae periculum eſſugiſſe, verum etiam minime morbum expertos fuiſſe. Nam ſi et letale venenum epota theriaca poſſit evincere, evincet quoque contagioſam aëris corruptionem, quae tantam homini vim infert. Quod certe et plerosque medicos et privatos omnes vulgo latere ne mireris. Succi namque ſunt et liquores et cortices et radices et flores et ſemina et carnes ex quibus conficitur. Quemadmodum igitur unum

ὅλην τοῦ φαρμάκου σύνθεσιν, τοῦτό τε ὑφορώμενοι τῶν ὑλικῶν ἰατρῶν οἱ χαριέστατοι πωλοῦσιν ἢ δωροῦνταί τισι τὴν ἄγαν παλαιουμένην. αὐτοὶ δὲ τῆς χρείας καλούσης ἐνεργεστάτῳ καὶ ὡραιοτάτῳ χρῶνται τῷ φαρμάκῳ, οὐ γὰρ ἔξεστιν ἑαυτοῖς βοηθοῦσιν ἀποτυγχάνειν. ὁριῶ δέ σοι καὶ τὰς ἄλλας προθεσμίας τῶν χρόνων καὶ τὰς διαφορὰς τῶν νοσημάτων, πρὸς ἅστινας καὶ ὁπότε χρώμενος αὐτῇ τις οὐκ ἀποτεύξεται. ἐπὶ μὲν γὰρ τῶν ἐχεοδήκτων καὶ ὀφιοδήκτων καὶ ἀσπιδοδήκτων καὶ λυσσοδήκτων καὶ καθόλου τῶν ὑπό τινος τῶν ἰοβόλων δηχθέντων, ἢ νυγέντων, ἢ ψυγέντων, ἱκανῶς ἄγαν ἡ πρόσφατος δύναται βοηθεῖν· ἔστι δὲ πρόσφα- [962] τος μέχρις ἐτῶν λϛʹ· καὶ πρὸς τὰ θανάσιμα πάντα. μετὰ δὲ τὸν χρόνον τοῦτον κατάλληλος ἅπασι τοῖς ἄλλοις πάθεσι, περὶ ὧν ὑπόμνημα γράψομεν, πολλῶν πλειόνων ὄντων ἄλλων εἰς ἀριθμὸν τῶν προειρημένων. δοκίμιον οὖν τοῦτο ἐνεργοῦς καὶ ἀπράκτου φαρμάκου· φάρμακον ὑπήλατον, ἢ ἐμετήριον, ἢ ἐλλέβορον, ἢ σκαμμωνίαν, ἢ ἄλλο ὅ τι βούληταί τις ἀν-

horum quodque evanidum efficere tempus poteſt, ſic et totam medicamenti compoſitionem: idque deprehendentes materiales medici praeſtantiſſimi hanc admodum inveteratam quibusdam vendunt, aut dono largiuntur. Hi autem, uſu poſtulante, efficaciſſimo et pulcherrimo utuntur medicamento, non enim his opem ferentibus aberrare licet. Sed tibi definiam tum alias temporum praeſcriptiones, tum morborum differentias, in quibus et quum aliquis ipſa uti voluerit, non fruſtrabitur. Nam viperarum, ſerpentum, aſpidum et rabidorum canum morſibus, ac univerſe ab aliquo venenoſo animali commorſis aut punctis, aut vehementer admodum refrigeratis, recens poteſt auxiliari, eſt autem recens ad annum usque xxxvj, etiam adverſus letalia univerſa. At poſt id tempus idonea eſt caeteris omnibus affectibus, de quibus commentarium ſcribemus, quum multi ac praedictis numero plures exiſtant. Haec ſit itaque efficacis ac inutilis medicamenti probatio. Medicamentum alvum ſubducens, aut

δρικώτατον, ὡς μέλλον καθαίρειν, ἐπιδώσει, προσεπιδοὺς τῆς ἀντιδότου, κυάμου Ἑλληνικοῦ τὸ μέγεθος, καὶ οὐ καθαρθήσεται, οὐδ᾽ ἔν τινι συναισθήσει καθάρσεως ὁ λαβὼν ἔσται. γενόμενος δὲ ἐξελέγχει τῆς ἀντιδότου τὴν διὰ χρόνου ἀπραξίαν· δίδοται δὲ πρὸς τὰς τῶν θανασίμων φαρμάκων πόσεις καὶ πρὸς τὰς τῶν ἰοβόλων πληγὰς μετ᾽ οἴνου κυάθους γ΄. τοῦ φαρμάκου καρύου Ποντικοῦ τὸ μέγεθος, καὶ ἐπιδιδομένη καὶ προσλαμβανομένη, εἰ δι᾽ ὑφοράσεώς τις ἔχει φαρμακείας· ὁμοίως καὶ πρὸς τοὺς ὑπό τινος αἰτίας ἀδήλου κινδυνεύοντας, τῆς ἐν τῷ σώματι διαφθορᾶς μιμησαμένης θανασίμου φαρμάκου ποιότητα. βοηθεῖ καὶ ταῖς προσφάτοις καὶ χρονίαις βηξὶ, καὶ ἐφ᾽ ὧν ἄλγημά τι τοῦ θώρακος, ἢ πλευρᾶς, ἀπυρέτοις μετ᾽ οἰνομέλιτος, πυρέσσουσι δὲ μεθ᾽ ὑδρομέλιτος εἰς νύκτα, κυάμου τὸ μέγεθος Αἰγυπτίου. ὁμοίως καὶ πρὸς τοὺς ἐμπνευματουμένους στομάχους ἢ στροφουμένους, ἔντερον ἢ κῶλον ὀδυνωμένους, ἐπὶ τούτων ἡ πόσις γενέσθω δι᾽ ὕδατος, τὸ δ᾽ αὐτὸ φάρ-

vomitum concitans, vel elleborum, vel ſcammonium, vel aliud quod quispiam voluerit validius, ſeu purgaturum porriget, moxque antidotum ſabae Graecae magnitudine exhibeat; qui aſſumpſerit, is neque purgabitur, neque ullum purgationis ſenſum percipiet. Secus contingens convincit antidoti vires tempore concidiſſe. Datur autem medicamentum ad letalium venenorum pocula et ad virus ejaculantium animalium ictus, ex vini cyathis tribus nucis Ponticae magnitudine, idque poſt exhibetur, etiam ante aſſumitur, ſi quis veneni ſuſpicionem habeat. Eodem pacto his praeſcribitur, qui ab aliqua cauſa abdita, ut corporis corruptela periclitantur, letalis veneni qualitatem imitante. Auxiliatur quoque tum recenti tum diuturnae tuſſi et hinc ſuccedenti thoracis, aut pleurae dolori non febricitantibus ex mulſo et febricitantibus ex mulſa aqua, noctu fabae Aegyptiae magnitudine, exhibeatur. Similiter prodeſt ſtomachi inſlationibus et ventris torminibus, inteſtinum vel colum dolore cruciantibus, in his potus ſiat ex aqua; id vero medicamentum detur ſa-

μακον διδόσθω κυάμου τὸ μέγεθος ἕωθεν. δύναται καὶ ὄρεξιν ἐπιτεταμένην ἀναστεῖλαι, καὶ ὑπτιωμένην ἀναγεῖραι, τὸ οἰκεῖον ἑκάστῳ τῶν τῆς φύσεως ἔργων μέτρον ἀποκαθιστᾶσα. ἡ δὲ πόσις καὶ ἐπὶ τούτων ἰσομεγέθης τῇ προειρημένῃ δι' ὕδατος, ἢ κράματος, μήτε πλείων κυάθων γ'. μήτε ἐλάσσων δύο· ἀγαθὴ καὶ παντὸς τύπου ῥῖγος ἀπαλλάξαι, καὶ περίψυξιν, καὶ χολημεσίαν τὴν ἐν ταῖς ἐπιβολαῖς ἔσθ' ὅτε συνεδρεύουσαν τῶν παροξυσμῶν, κατὰ ταὐτὰ τοῖς προειρημένοις διδομένη εἰ δέ τις αὐτῇ πρὸ τῶν ἐπισημασιῶν τρὶς ἢ τὸ πλέον τετράκις χρήσεται, περιγράφει τέλεον τοὺς πυρετοὺς, μετὰ τοῦ καὶ τὴν δίαιταν τῇ ὠφελείᾳ τῇ ἀπὸ τοῦ φαρμάκου μὴ ἀντιπράσσειν. οὐδὲν γὰρ οὕτως ἐστὶν ἰσχυρὸν ἐν ἰατρικῇ βοήθημα, ὃ τὴν ἐξ αὐτοῦ γινομένην ὄνησιν δύναται ἐπαγαγεῖν, ἢ ἀντιπρασσόμενον ὑπὸ τῶν κατὰ δίαιταν, ἢ μὴ συνεργούμενον. πεπίστευται δὲ καὶ ταῖς γυναιξὶ τὰς ἐπιμηνίους καθάρσεις κινεῖν, καὶ τὰ νεκρὰ τῶν ἐμβρύων ἐκβάλλειν, ἃ δι' ἀσθένειαν οὐ δύναται ἡ φύσις ἀποτρίψασθαι πολλάκις θέλουσα. δίδοται δὲ ἐπὶ τού-

bae magnitudine ſtatim ab aurora. Poteſt et intenſam orexin, i. e. *cibi appetentiam,* coërcere, projectamque excitare, proprium ſingulis naturae functionibus modum inſtaurans. Potio autem adhaec praedictae aequalis magnitudine, ex aqua aut diluto vino, neque amplius tribus neque minus duobus cyathis. Data quoque vim habet propellendi rigorem, partium extremarum frigus, bilioſamque vomitionem in febrilibus acceſſionibus paroxysmis aſſidentem. Si quis vero ipſa ante febrium ſignificationes ter aut quater utatur, febres penitus obliterat, modo ſervata victus ratio medicamenti utilitati non repugnet. Nullum enim eſt tam potens in medicina remedium quod manantem ex eo utilitatem inducere queat, ſi victus ratio ei repugnet, aut niſi mutuas det operas. Creditur etiam mulieribus menſtruales purgationes ciere et mortuos foetus ejicere, quos ob imbecillitatem non poteſt natura, licet ſaepe foras protrudere tentaverit. Datur autem his

των διὰ γλυκέος, ἢ μελικράτου προεψηψημένου, (471) δικτάμνου, ἢ πηγάνου, κυάμου Αἰγυπτίου τὸ μέγεθος, ὅ τινες ἐπιχωρίως κίθη καὶ κιβώριον καλοῦσι. χρήσιμος δὲ καὶ ὑδρωπικοῖς καὶ ἰκτερικοῖς μετὰ ἀσάρου ἀφεψήματος. ἐπὶ μὲν τῶν ὑδρωπικῶν οἱ μὲν αὐτὸ καταπίνειν διδόασι τὸ φάρμακον πρὸ τῶν σιτίων, οἱ δὲ καὶ ἀνιέντες ὀξυκράτου κυάθῳ ἑνὶ, τότε γὰρ δίψους ἄκος μέγα γίνεται, καὶ τὴν ὅλην ἕξιν εὐτονωτέραν ἀποδείκνυσι, καὶ τὴν πλεονεξίαν τῶν ὑγρῶν μετὰ τοῦ μειοῦν καὶ ξηροτέραν ἀποφαίνει τῇ φύσει. ποιεῖ καὶ πρὸς τὰς τῆς φωνῆς ἀποκοπὰς, καὶ κατ' ἰδίαν πινομένη καὶ ἐν τῷ στόματι κατεχομένη, μιγνυμένης τραγακάνθου διπλῆς τῷ ποτῷ, μετ' οἰνομέλιτος, ἢ γλυκέος. τοὺς δὲ ὑπὸ τῆς γλώττης κατέχοντας, ἀποτήκειν δεῖ τὸ φάρμακον κατ' ὀλίγον, ὅνπερ εἰώθαμεν χρῆσθαι τρόπον κἀν ταῖς καλουμέναις ἀρτηριακαῖς. ἁρμόζει καὶ τοῖς αἱμοπτοϊκοῖς, ἐάν τε ἀπὸ θώρακος ἐάν τε ἀπὸ πνεύμονος ἡ ἀναγωγὴ γίγνεται, προσφάτου μὲν οὔσης τῆς ἀναφορᾶς, μετ' ὀξυκράτου διδομένη, κεχρονισμένης δὲ, μεθ' ὕδατος κυά-

ex paſſo, aut mulſa, in quibus ſerbuerit dictamnum, aut ruta, fabae Aegyptiae magnitudine, quidam patrio vocabulo cithe et ciborium vocitant. Utilis eſt hydropicis et ictericis ex aſari decocto. Hydropicis quidam id ſolum medicamentum deglutiendum ante cibum exhibent; nonnulli oxycrati cyatho uno diluunt; tunc enim ſitis magnum ſit remedium, totum corporis habitum robuſtiorem efficit, humorum redundantiam minuit et naturae ſtatum ſicciorem reddit. Facit et ad vocis interceptionem cum ſeorſum pota tum in ore retenta; admixto tragacanthi duplo potui ex paſſo, vel mulſa datur; ſub lingua vero retinentibus medicamentum paulatim eliquandum, quomodo etiam in arteriacis vocatis uti conſuevimus. Convenit quoque haemoptoicis ſanguinem expuentibus ſive a thorace, ſive a pulmonibus ſanguinis ſiat eductio; quum recens eſt ſanguinis rejectio, ex oxycrato exhibetur, quum vero inveterata, ex aquae cyathis tribus. Multo tamen

θων γ'. πολλῷ δ' ἄμεινον, εἰ προαφεψήσεις τὶ τῷ ὕδατι, τοῦ καλουμένου συμφύτου τῆς πόας. ἡ δὲ πόσις εἰς νύκτα καὶ πρωῒ κυάμου [963] Αἰγυπτίου τὸ μέγεθος. ἐπὶ δὲ τῆς Ῥώμης οἶδα τοὺς καθηγησαμένους ἡμῶν ἐπὶ τῶν τοιούτων χρωμένους καὶ τῇ διὰ φελλῶν δυνάμει, ἧς τὴν πλοκὴν ἂν οὕτω δέῃ εὐκαιροτέραν σοι παραθήσομαι, καὶ ἐν κύκλῳ δὲ καὶ ἔμπροσθεν, καὶ ὄπισθεν περιθάλποντας δαψιλεῖ τῷ φαρμάκῳ τὸν θώρακα, καὶ τὰ πολλὰ ἐκράτουν τὸ πάθος διὰ τῆς τοιαύτης ἀγωγῆς. ἁρμόζει δὲ καὶ τοῖς νεφριτικοῖς καὶ δυσεντερικοῖς καὶ τοῖς λιθιῶσι καὶ δυσπνοϊκοῖς καὶ τοῖς περὶ τὸ ἧπαρ καὶ σπλῆνα καὶ σκιῤῥώδη τινὰ πεῖσιν, ἢ ἄλλως κεχρονισμένην ἔχουσι, δι' ὀξυμέλιτος διδομένη ἐπὶ τῶν σκιῤῥωδῶν· ὀξύμελι δὲ ἀπὸ τῶν μελικηρίδων ληπτέον, τοῦτο γὰρ εὔθετον, καὶ Ἱπποκράτης ἐν τῷ περὶ διαίτης λέγει· ὁποῦ δὲ δι' ὄξους σκιλλητικοῦ κυάθου ἑνὸς ἥμισυ, ἐπὶ τῶν δυσπνοϊκῶν· ἐπὶ δὲ τῶν λιθιώντων μετὰ ἀφεψήματος σελίνου, ἢ πετροσελίνου· ἐπὶ δὲ τῶν νεφριτικῶν μετὰ οἰνομέλιτος· ἐπὶ δὲ τῶν δυσεντερικῶν μετὰ Συριακοῦ

praeftantius remedium fiet, fi aliquam fymphyti herbae appellatae portionem praecoxeris; fed potio vesperi et in aurora fabae Aegyptiae magnitudine. Romae novi meos praeceptores in talibus affectibus confecto ex fubere medicamento uti confueviffe, cujus texturam, fi ita oporteat, opportuniori tempore tibi apponemus, eoque copiofo medicamento thoracem et in circuitu et ante et poft circumfoventes, ut plurimum hac arte morbum fuperaffe. Convenit vero nephriticis et dyfentericis et calculo laborantibus et aegre fpirantibus, fcirrhofis hepatis et lienis affectibus, aut alias inveteratum morbum habentibus, quod ex aceto mulfo in fcirrhofis affectibus datur; acetum autem mulfum ex favis fumendum; id enim idoneum eft, quod et Hippocrates in libro de diaeta acutorum profert; aegre vero fpirantibus ex aceti fcillitici cyatho uno et dimidio; calculo laborantibus cum petrofelini, aut apii decocto; nephriticis ex mulfo; dyfentericis ex rhu Syriaci decocto; comitialibus, fi per habitum fanguinis fit

ῥοῦς ἀφεψήματος. ἐπὶ δὲ τῶν ἐπιληπτικῶν, ὀλιγαιμίας μὲν περὶ τὴν ἕξιν οὔσης, μελικράτῳ, πολυαιμίας δὲ καὶ πάχους, ἐν ὀξυμέλιτι· τινὲς δὲ τῶν δοκίμων ἰατρῶν ἐπὶ τούτων νᾶπυ διδόασι προαναγαργαρίζεσθαι, ἔπειθ' οὕτως τοῦ φαρμάκου προσφέρουσιν εἰς νύκτα μεθ' ὕδατος, ὅσον Ἑλληνικοῦ κυάμου τὸ μέγεθος. καθόλου δ' εἰπεῖν, ὅπου τὰ ἄλλα πάντα βοηθήματα μηδὲν ἰσχύσει, ἀλλ' ἡττᾶται πρὸς τῶν νοσημάτων, ἐπὶ τούτων ἡ ἀντίδοτος πινομένη παραδόξως κατορθοῖ. ἤδη γοῦν καὶ ἐπὶ τῶν χολερικῶν ἀπαυδώντων καὶ ἐπὶ καρδιακῶν ἐν ἐσχάτοις ὄντων ἐπιδοθεῖσα παλιγγενεσίαν ὥσπερ τοῖς λαβοῦσιν ἐπεδωρήσατο. ἀλλ' οὔτε δυνατὸν οὔτε ἁρμόζον περὶ πάντων γράφειν. ἀπὸ γὰρ τῶν γεγραμμένων τὶς ὁρμώμενος, δυνήσεται τοὺς λογισμοὺς μετατιθεὶς καὶ ἐπὶ τῶν λοιπῶν ἐπιτυχῶς αὐτῇ χρῆσθαι. τοὺς δὲ ἐπὶ πλέον ἤδη σπουδάζοντας ἐπαινεῖν τὸ φάρμακον παραμεμπτέον, οὐχ ὡς ἰατρικὴν, ὀχλαγωγικὴν δὲ μᾶλλον ὑπόσχεσιν αὐτῷ προσάπτοντας, οἳ καὶ πρὸς ὠταλγίαν αὐτό φασι ποιεῖν καὶ δυσηκοΐας καὶ ἀμβλυωπίας καὶ κιονίδας καὶ τὰς καλουμένας

inopia; ex aqua mulſa, ſi vero copia ſanguinis et corpulentia, ex aceto mulſo; his prius quidem illuſtres medici ex ſinapi gargarismos praeſcribunt, deinde ſub noctem tantum medicamenti ex aqua exhibent, quantum Graecae fabae complectitur magnitudo. Atque ut in univerſum dicam, ubi caetera omnia nihil valuerint, imo vi morborum ſuperata fuerint, his antidotus propinata praeter vulgi opinionem ſummas promit vires. Quamobrem cholericis deficientibus et cardiacis in extremis degentibus exhibita, tanquam novum vitae ortum nactis reſtituit. Sed de omnibus ſcribere neque poſſibile neque idoneum eſt. Quicunque enim ab iis quae *a nobis* ſcripta ſunt concitatur, deducta ratione et in reliquis affectibus ipſa proſpero ſucceſſu uti poterit. Jam vero qui magis id medicamentum laudare ſtudent, improbandi ſunt, quod ipſi non medicas, ſed potius circulatorias pollicitationes attribuunt; quique ad aurium dolorem, audiendi difficultatem, amblyopias, *oculorum hebetudines,* cionidas et voca-

ἄφθας. ὁ γὰρ τοιοῦτος ἔπαινος διαβολὴν ἔοικε φέρειν μᾶλλον τῷ φαρμάκῳ ἢ σύστασιν. εἰ γάρ ἐστι δι' εὐτελοῦς ὕλης ἄμεινον ἰᾶσθαι τὰ τοιαῦτα τῶν παθῶν, ἄπρακτον τὸ μετὰ πολυτελείας ἔλαττον περιγιγνόμενον τοῦ τέλους. ὑπὲρ δὲ τῆς σκευασίας εἰπεῖν τι ἀναγκαῖον, ἐπεὶ καὶ αὐτὴ δεῖταί τινος ἐντρεχείας. ὁ μὲν γὰρ Μενεκράτης οὐδὲν ὑπὲρ αὐτῆς διέσταλκε. ἐπεὶ δὲ λαμβάνειν ἡδυχρόου τὸ φάρμακον, καὶ ἑτέρων ἀρτίσκων, σκιλλητικῶν καὶ θηριακῶν, πρότερον περὶ τῆς σκευασίας τούτων λεκτέον. Ἡδυχρόου σκευασία. ♃ Ἀσπαλάθου ῥίζης φλοιοῦ, καλάμου ἀρωματικοῦ, κόστου, ἀσάρου, ξυλοβαλσάμου, φοῦ, ἀμαράκου, μαστίχης, ἀνὰ < στ'. σχοίνου ἄνθους < ιβ'. οἱ δὲ < κδ'. κινναμώμου < ιβ'. ἀμώμου, κασσίας, ῥᾶ Ποντικοῦ, ἀνὰ < ιε'. νάρδου Ἰνδικῆς, μαλαβάθρου φύλλων, ἀνὰ < * ιστ', σμύρνης, κρόκου, ἀνὰ < ιβ'. οἴνῳ Φαλερίνῳ ἀναλάμβανε, ὀποβαλσάμῳ παραπτόμενος ἐν τῷ ἀναπλάττειν καὶ ἔα ξηραίνεσθαι ἐν σκιᾷ. Περὶ ἀρτίσκων σκιλλητικῶν. Τροχίσκους

tas aphthas id conducere proferunt. Ejusmodi namque laus calumniam potius medicamento quam commendationem adferre videtur. Si enim vili materia, aut remedio tales morbi melius fanari queant, cum profufione minus ipfi finem confequi fupervacaneum eft. At de *theriacae* compofitione aliquid dicere neceffe eft, quum etiam ipfa narrationis quadam fedulitate indigeat. Menecrates fiquidem de ea nihil diftincte differuit. Quum autem haec hedychroi medicamentum affumat, aliosque trochiscos, fcilliticos et theriacos, prius horum confectio proferenda eft. *Hedychroi confectio.* ♃ Radicis afpalathi corticis, calami aromatici, cofti, afari, xylobalfami, phu, amaraci, maftiches, fingulorum ʒ vj, fchoenanthi ʒ xij, (quidam ʒ xxiv,) cinnamomi ʒ vij, amomi, caffiae, rha Pontici, fingulorum ʒ xv, nardi Indicae, foliorum malabathri, fingulorum ʒ xvj, myrrhae, croci, fingulorum ʒ xij, excipe haec Falerno vino et infingendo inunge opobalfamo et ficcentur in umbra. *De paftillis fcillicitis.* Orbiculos fcilliticos fic

τοὺς σκιλλητικοὺς οὕτω σκευάζομεν. σκίλλαν περίπλασσε πηλῷ καὶ βάλλε εἰς κάμινον βαλανείου καιομένην, τῇ δ' ἐπιούσῃ ἡμέρᾳ τοῦ ἐντὸς λαβὼν < ρκ'. καὶ ὀροβίνου ἀλεύρου < ξ'. λειώσας ὁμοῦ ποίει τροχίσκους. Ἀρτίσκοι θηριακοί. Ἀρτίσκοι δὲ θηριακοὶ οὕτω σκευάζονται, λαβὼν ἔχεις δ'. ἢ πέντε πυῤῥὰς, ἄμεινον δὲ εἶναι νεοθηράτους, αἱ γὰρ πολλῷ χρόνῳ καθειργμέναι ἰωδέστεραι τὴν ἕξιν εἰσίν. ἔστι δὲ τοῦτο τεκμήρασθαι ἀπὸ τοῦ νηστεύσαντος ἀνθρώπου, ἔπειτα τοῦ πρὸς κεφαλὴν μέρους καὶ τοῦ πρὸς οὐρὰν ἀφαιρεῖν ἀνὰ τετραδάκτυλον καὶ τὴν φολίδα πᾶσαν ἀποδέρειν, [964] καὶ πᾶν τὸ ἔντερον ἐκβάλλειν· τὰ δὲ λοιπὰ ἕψειν ἐν καινῇ χύτρᾳ μετ' ἀνήθου· ἑψηθεισῶν δὲ τῶν σαρκῶν καθαίρειν τὰς ἀκάνθας, ἐπιμελῶς δὲ τὰς σάρκας ἱστᾶν δεῖ, ἵνα μὴ διαλάθῃ ἄκανθα, καὶ ῥῖψαι καὶ ἄρτου καθαροῦ ξηροῦ τὸ ἴσον προσβάλλειν, καὶ συλλειοῦν, ἔπειτα προσαπτόμενος ὀποβαλσάμῳ τροχίσκον ἀνάπλασσε καὶ ψῦχε ἐν σκιᾷ. αὐτὴ δὲ ἀντίδοτος κατὰ Ἀνδρόμαχον τὸν πεποιηκότα αὐτὴν συντίθεται τρόπῳ τοιῷδε. ὠνομάσθη δὲ παρ' Ἀνδρομάχου

conficias. Scillam luto circumline et in flagrantem balnei caminum mitte, poſtridie quod intus eſt hujus accipe ʒ cxx, ervi farinae ʒ lxxx, atque ex his ſimul tritis orbiculos confice. *Orbiculi theriaci.* Orbiculi theriaci ſic conficiuntur. Viperas flavas iv, aut quinque accipe, eſſe recenter captas melius: nam incluſae multo tempore virulentiores habitu ſunt; hoc autem de jejuno homine licet conjicere; deinde partis ad caput et ad caudam cujusque quatuor digitos exime, ſquamoſam cutem detrahe et tota interanea abjice; reliqua coquantur in ollo nova cum anetho; coctae carnes, ſpinis expurgandae; accurate vero carnes ponderandae ſunt, ne ſpina delituerit, ac examinandae: tum panis puri et aridi par pondus accipiendum et conterendum et adjecto opobalſamo orbiculos forma et ſicca in umbra. Haec autem antidotus ex Andromacho ejus auctore hoc modo componitur et ab Andromacho nominata eſt galene. Qui vero hanc ab eo acceperunt, ut Crito et ejus coaetanei, quod viperarum carnem con-

γαλήνη. οἱ μετ᾽ αὐτὸν δὲ παραλαβόντες, οἷον Κρίτων καὶ οἱ κατ᾽ αὐτὸν, διὰ τὸ ἔχειν αὐτὴν τῆς σαρκὸς τῶν ἐχιδνῶν, ὠνόμασαν αὐτὴν θηριακήν. ♃ Ἀρτίσκων σκιλλητικῶν < μδ΄. ἀρτίσκων θηριακῶν < κδ΄. ἀρτίσκων ἡδυχρόου < κδ΄. κινναμώμου, πεπέρεως μέλανος, ὀποῦ μήκωνος, ἀνὰ < κδ΄. ἴρεως Ἰλλυρικῆς, γλυκυῤῥίζης, ὀποβαλσάμου, ῥόδων ξηρῶν, σκορδίου Κρητικοῦ, βουνιάδος σπέρματος, γογγυλίδος ἀγρίας, ἀγαρικοῦ, ἀνὰ < ιβ΄. κρόκου, σμύρνης, ζιγγιβέρεως, ῥᾶ Ποντικοῦ, πενταφύλλου ῥίζης, καλαμίνθης, πρασίου, πετροσελίνου, στοιχάδος, κόστου, πεπέρεως λευκοῦ, ἀνὰ < στ΄. δικτάμνου Κρητικοῦ, σχοίνου ἄνθους, λιβάνου ἄῤῥενος, τερμινθίνης Χίας, κασσίας σύριγγος μελαίνης, νάρδου Ἰνδικῆς, ἀνὰ < στ΄. πολίου ἄνθους Κρητικοῦ, στύρακος, σελίνου σπέρματος, σεσέλεως, θλάσπεως, ἄμμεως, χαμαίδρυος, χαμαιπίτυος, ὑποκιστίδος χυλοῦ, μαλαβάθρου, νάρδου Κελτικῆς, γεντιανῆς ῥίζης, ἀνίσου, μήου, μαράθρου σπέρματος, Λημνίας μίλτου σφραγῖδος, χαλκίτεως ὀπτῆς, ἀμώμου, ἀκόρου, καρποβαλσάμου, φοῦ Ποντικοῦ, ὑπερικοῦ, ἀκακίας, καρδαμώμου, κόμμεως, ἀνὰ < δ΄. δαύκου

tineat, ipſam theriacam nominarunt. *Confectio antidoti.* ♃ Orbiculorum ſcilliticorum ʒ xlviij, paſtillorum theriacalium ʒ xxiv, orbiculorum hedychroi ʒ xxiv, cinnamomi, piperis nigri, opii, ſingulorum ʒ xxiv, iridis Illyricae, glycyrrhizae, opobalſami, roſarum aridarum, ſcordii Cretici, ſeminis rapae agreſtis, agarici ann. ʒ xij, croci, myrrhae, zingiberis, rha Pontici, radicis quinqueſolii, calaminthes, marrubii, petroſelini, ſtoechados, coſti, piperis albi, ſingulorum ʒ vj, dictamni Cretici, ſchoenanthi, thuris maſculi, terebinthinae Chiae, caſſiae fiſtulae nigrae, nardi Indicae, ſingulorum ʒ vj, florum polii Cretici, ſtyracis, ſeminum apii, ſeſeleos, thlaspeos, ammeos, chamaedryos, chamaepityos, ſucci hypociſtidos, malabathri, nardi Celticae, radicis gentianae, aniſi, mei, ſeminum foeniculi, lemnii minii ſigillati, chalciteos uſtae, amomi, acori, fructuum balſami, phu Pontici, hyperici, acaciae, cardamomi, gummi ſingulorum ʒ iv, ſeminum

σπέρματος, χαλβάνου, σαγαπηνοῦ, ἀσφάλτου, ὀποπάνακος, καστορίου, κενταυρίου λεπτοῦ, ἀριστολοχίας κληματίτιδος, ἀνὰ < β΄. μέλιτος Ἀττικοῦ λίτραν ι΄. οἱ δὲ στ΄. οἱ δὲ δ΄. οἴνου Φαλερίνου ξε. β΄. βαλὼν εἰς ὅλμον ὀπὸν ὑποκιστίδος, σμύρναν, σαγαπηνὸν, γλυκύῤῥιζον, στύρακα, ἀκακίαν, ὀποπάνακα, παραστάζων κατὰ μικρὸν μέλι καθ᾽ ἓν, κόπτε καὶ διάλυε καὶ πρόσβαλε τοῦ οἴνου, ὥστε ὑπερέχειν, καὶ ἔμβρεχε ἐπὶ ἡμέρας τρεῖς, εἶτα κιννάμωμον, κρόκον, κασσίαν, στάχυν, θλάσπι, μαλάβαθρον, Λημνίαν σφραγῖδα, χαλκῖτιν κεκαυ- (472) μένην, (αὕτη γὰρ καὶ τὸ μέλαν χρῶμα χαρίζεται τῷ φαρμάκῳ καυθεῖσα ἐντέχνως) ἄμωμον, ἄσφαλτον, καστόριον κεκομμένον, καὶ σεσησμένον βαλὼν εἰς θυείαν καὶ παραχέων οἶνον, λειοτρίβει, ὡς κολλύριον, ἔπειτ᾽ ἐκ τοῦ ὅλμου προσβαλὼν τοῖς ἐν τῇ θυείᾳ, λειοτριβήσας καὶ παρεγχέας οἶνον πρόσμισγε τὰ ξηρὰ πάντα καὶ ἀνάπλαττε. μετὰ δὲ ταῦτα τὸ μέλι καὶ τὴν ῥητίνην καὶ χαλβάνην καὶ ὀποβάλσαμον χλιάνας ἐν κακκάβῃ, κατάχει τῶν ἐν τῇ θυείᾳ, καὶ ἑνώσας ἀπόθου εἰς ἀγγεῖον κασσιτερινὸν ἢ ἀργυροῦν καὶ

dauci, galbani, fagapeni, bituminis, opopanacis, caftorii, centaurii minoris, ariftolochiae clematitidis, fingulorum ʒ ij, mellis Attici lib. x, fed alii malunt vj, alii iv, vini Phalerni fextarios ij. In pilam conjice fuccum hypociftidos, myrrham, fagapenum, glycyrrhizam, ftyracem, acaciam, opopanacem, et paulatim inftilla mel; omnia contunde, diffolve; tum vinum adjice, ut fupereemineat, et macerato dies tres; poftea cinnamomum, crocum, caffiam, fpicam, thlafpi, malabathrum, figillum Lemnium, chalcitim uftam, (ipfa namque artificiose ufta, nigrum colorem medicamento conciliat) amomum, bitumen, caftorium incifum et cribratum in pilam conjice, vinum affunde et ficut fit collyrium, contere; deinde *remota* ex mortario his adjice quae in pila funt tritis et vino affufo arida omnia commifce et maffam finge; poftea mel, refinam, galbanum et opobalfamum in caccabo tepefacta offunde his quae in pila funt et unum forma corpus et in vafe ftan-

χρῶ. Κρίτων δ' ἔγραψε περὶ αὐτῆς οὕτως, ὅτι τὰ θηρία περὶ τὰ τελευταῖα τοῦ ἦρος, ἢ τῷ τρυγητῷ συλλέγειν δεῖ, καὶ λαμβάνειν ἐξ αὐτῶν τὰ μεγάλα καὶ εὔτροφα καὶ ἕψειν μετ' ἀνήθου μόνου. τῷ δὲ τῆς σαρκὸς αὐτῶν ἐκ δέκα θηρίων ἀθροισθέντι μιγνύειν ἀξιοῖ σιλιγνίτου ἄρτου μίαν οὐγγίαν, καὶ οὕτως ἀναπλάττειν τοὺς καλουμένους ἄρτους· τὰς δὲ σκίλλας ἐν τῷ πυρῶν ἀμήτῳ, τηνικαῦτα γάρ εἰσι μάλιστα ἀκμαῖαι.

neo aut argenteo repone et utere. Crito vero de ea ita fcripfit, viperas in veris fine aut vindemia colligendas et ex his grandiusculas et corpulentas et cum anetho folo effe coquendas, carnibus autem viperarum decem admifcendam cenfet filiginei panis unciam unam ficque fingendos paftillos appellatos; fcillas denique meffis tempore colligendas; tunc enim maxime vigent.

ΓΑΛΗΝΟΥ ΠΕΡΙ ΕΥΠΟΡΙΣΤΩΝ ΒΙΒΛΙΟΝ ΠΡΩΤΟΝ.

Ed. Chart. X. [574.]

Προοίμιον. [*Τοῖς ἔξω πόλεων παραμένουσι καὶ τοῖς κατ' ἀγροὺς καὶ τοὺς ἐρήμους τόπους διατρίβουσι τῶν εὐπορίστων χρῆσιν προσήκουσαν εἶναι.*] *Τὴν ἰατρικὴν τέχνην, οὐ πόλεσιν οὐδὲ δημοσίοις τόποις, ἢ ἀνδράσι πλουσίοις καὶ εὐγενέσιν ἄρχουσί τε καὶ μεγάλως δυναμένοις ὁριζομένην, διὰ δὲ τὸ φιλάνθρωπον καὶ πολύχρηστον αὐτῆς ποικίλως ἐπὶ πάντας ἀνθρώπους διήκουσαν καὶ ἄχρις ἀγροικίας καὶ ἐρήμων τόπων φθάνουσαν μὲν ὁρῶν τῇ δυνάμει, ἐλλείπουσαν δὲ τῇ ἐνεργείᾳ διὰ τὸν ἀμελέτητον τῆς περὶ*

GALENI DE REMEDIIS PARABILIBUS LIBER PRIMUS.

Prooemium. [*Extra urbes, rura et ſolitaria loca incolentibus parabilium medicamentorum uſum eſſe neceſſarium.*] Medicam artem, quae non civitatibus, non publicis locis, non opulentis hominibus, nobilibus, principibus et potentibus circumſcribitur, imo ob amplissimam erga homines hujusce benevolentiam atque utilitatem ad univerſos mortales longe lateque propagatur, etiam adusque rura et ſolitaria loca ſuos fines poteſtate proro-

αὐτὴν φιλοτιμίας, δίκαιον ᾠήθην κατ᾽ ἐμὴν δύναμιν εἰσενέγκασθαι ἐπικουρίαν τοῖς ἐν ὁδοῖς, μάλιστα καὶ κατ᾽ ἀγροὺς καὶ κατά τινας ἐρήμους τόπους διατρίβουσιν, ἐφ᾽ ὧν τὰ μὲν πάθη ῥᾳδίαν καὶ ἀπροσδόκητον ἔχει τὴν κατὰ τῶν σωμάτων φορὰν καὶ δύναμιν, οὐκ ἔτι δὲ καὶ τὴν ἐκ τῶν ἰαμάτων ἐπικουρίαν εὔπορον. οὔτε γὰρ φαρμάκων πολυτελῶν ἐν παντὶ τόπῳ ῥᾴδιον εὐπορεῖν οὔτε τοὺς χρησομένους αὐτοῖς ἰατροὺς ἀφθόνως ἔχειν ἐπιτηδείους, οὔτε μὴν τὰς περιστάσεις παρεῖναι τῆς ὑποπροσθέσεως καὶ ἀναβολῆς καιροὺς διδούσας, οἷον ἐπὶ συνάγχης καὶ δηλητηρίων φαρμάκων καὶ τῶν ἰοβόλων, αἱμοῤῥαγίας τε καὶ χολέρας καὶ τῶν [575] τούτοις παραπλησίων. διὰ ταῦτ᾽ οὖν οὐκ ἀκριβῶς καὶ ἐπιστημονικῶς θεραπείαν καὶ πάντη τοῖς οἰκείοις θεωρήμασι συνεκπληρουμένην ἐνθάδε λέγειν προυθέμην, ἀλλ᾽ ὅπως ἄν τις καὶ ἰδιώτης ἐκ τοῦ παραχρῆμα βοηθεῖν ἔχῃ τοῖς κινδυνεύουσιν ἢ ἄλλως πάσχουσι κατὰ τὸ ἐνδεχόμενον ἐκ τῶν ὡς οἷόν τε ἐπ᾽ ἀπόροις εὐπορουμένων βοηθημάτων, ὑποθέσθαι δίκαιον ᾠή-

gat, ſed operibus, ob ſummam eorum qui illi operam navant, negligentiam, e ſuo ſplendore decidit, aequum eſſe duxi pro meis viribus ad eorum ſubſidium traducere, tum quia vias moliuntur, tum maxime qui ruri et in locis quibusdam deſertis verſantur, ubi morbis quidem faciles ac repentini in corpora ſunt impetus ac imperia, nequaquam vero etiam facilia ex officinis remedia ſuppetunt. Neque enim profuſis in omni loco medicamentis abundare, neque idoneos qui ipſis uti noverint, affluenter habere medicos facile eſt; neque certe circumſtantias adeſſe, quae et incrementi et dilationis tempus concedant, ut in angina, venenoſis medicamentis, animalibus virus ejaculantibus, haemorrhagia, cholera et his ſimilibus. Quas ob res non accuratam et ſcientificam curandi rationem et omnibus ſuis praeceptis abſolutam hic explicare mihi propoſui, ſed ut quisque etiam plebejus ſolis ardore, aut alia quacunque cauſa male affectis *hominibus* opem illico ferat illis ſane uſus remediis, quae in paratorum inopia paratu facilia ſuppetant. Supponi juſtum arbitror, accu-

Ed. Chart. X. [575.]
θην τὸ μὲν ἀκριβὲς ἄγαν τῆς κατὰ τὴν τέχνην ὕλης καὶ τῆς ἐπιστημονικῆς χρήσεως τῶν βοηθημάτων, ἐν οἷς φαρμάκων καὶ ἰατρῶν εὐπορία καὶ τὰ πάθη συγχωρεῖ, ἀναγκαῖον εἶναι κρίνει, ὅπου δὲ ὀξὺς ὁ καιρὸς καὶ οὐκ εὔπορος ἡ τῶν βοηθημάτων εὐπορία καὶ ἀφθονία, τὴν ἐκ τῶν εὐπορίστων φαρμάκων δύναμιν ἀναγκαιοτάτην εἶναι λογιζόμενος τοῖς ὁτιοῦν μέρος τοῦ σώματος πάσχουσιν. ἀναγράψω τοιγαροῦν εὐπορίστων βοηθημάτων ὕλης σπανίως που πολυτελεστέρων μὲν, συνήθων δὲ τοῖς πολλοῖς, καὶ διὰ τοῦτο εὐπορουμένων φαρμάκων μνημονεύσομεν, ἀπὸ κεφαλῆς ἀρξάμενοι. αὕτη γὰρ καθάπερ τις ἀκρόπολίς ἐστι τοῦ σώματος καὶ τῶν τιμιωτάτων καὶ ἀναγκαιοτάτων ἀνθρώποις αἰσθήσεων οἰκητήριον, διὸ καὶ τὴν ἀρχὴν τῶν βοηθημάτων ἀπ' αὐτῆς ποιησόμεθα τοῦ δυνατοῦ μάλιστα καὶ σαφῶς στοχαζόμενοι. πάσχει δὲ αὕτη ποικίλως, ἐγκαιομένη τε καὶ ψυχομένη, καὶ ὑπὸ ἀναθυμιάσεων τῶν ἐκ τῆς κοιλίας πληρουμένη, καὶ ἀπὸ τῶν ἔξωθεν, τῶν καρωδῶν καὶ δυσωδῶν, καὶ διὰ πολλὰ ἕτερα.

ratiſſimam ex arte materiae, atque etiam e ſcientia prodeuntis uſus remediorum, quo tempore tum medicamentorum et medicorum copia eſt, tum morbi poſtulant, administrationem judicari ac neceſſariam At ubi praeceps occaſio eſt, nec ſuppetit copioſa remediorum multitudo et ubertas, medicamentorum parabilium facultatem quacunque corporis parte laborantibus neceſſariam eſſe mente conjeci. Deſcribam itaque parabilium remediorum materiam, quibusdam etiam in locis, quanquam raro exquiſitiorum, permultis conſuetorum, proindeque facile ſuppetentium medicamentorum mentionem faciam, a capite ducto exordio. Ipſum enim tanquam arx quaedam corporis eſt ac domicilium ſenſuum, qui hominibus pretioſi maximeque neceſſarii ſunt; proindeque ab ipſo remediorum principium faciemus, idonea et maniſeſta potiſſimum aggredientes. Caput varie afficitur, ab aeſtu aeſtuat, a frigore frigescit, ac vaporibus e ventriculo ſublatis repletur; et ab externis gravitatem ſoporoſam efficientibus, foetidis

ἐξ ἐπιμέτρου καὶ ταῖς κατὰ τὸ δέρμα καὶ τὰς τρίχας ἀπρεπείαις ἁλισκομένη, ἀλωπεκίαις, ὀφιάσεσι, διαφόροις ἑλκώσεσιν. ἐγκαύσεως μὲν οὖν καὶ ψύξεως καὶ τῆς ἀπὸ τῶν ἔξωθεν ἀναθυμιάσεως ἱκανὰ σημεῖα ταῦτα προκατάρχοντα αἴτια. ἤδη δὲ τοῖς ἐξ ἐγκαύσεων ἄλγημα παρακολουθεῖ σφυγματῶδες ὅλης σφακελιζούσης δοκεῖν τῆς κεφαλῆς μετὰ πυρώδους αἰσθήσεως καὶ διάτασις τῶν περὶ τὸ μέτωπον ἀγγείων καὶ ὀφθαλμῶν ἔρευθος, τὰ πολλὰ καὶ ἀγρύπνια· τοῖς δὲ ἀπὸ ψύξεως ναρκῶδες βάρος καὶ πῆξις καὶ τῶν μετὰ τὸ μέτωπον ἀγγείων σύμπτωσις· εἰ δὲ μεθ' ὑγρότητος καταψύχοιντο, καὶ καταφορώδης ὕπνος· τοῖς δ' ἐξ ἀναθυμιάσεων ἄλγημα νυγματῶδες καὶ σφυγμὸς τῶν περὶ τὸ μέτωπον ἀρτηριῶν, ἴλιγγοί τε καὶ παροράσεις καὶ ὤτων ἦχοι. ὁμοίως καὶ τοῖς ἀπὸ τῶν ἐντὸς ἀναθυμιάσεων πληρουμένοις τὰ αὐτὰ ταῦτα συμπίπτειν εἴωθεν.

Κεφ. α'. [Πρὸς τὰ ἐντὸς τῆς κεφαλῆς πάθη, καὶ πρῶτον (472) περὶ τῆς ἐξ ἐγκαύσεως κεφαλαλγίας.] Ἁρμόσει δὲ τοῖς μὲν ἐξ ἐγκαύσεως ἐμβροχὴ ἐλαίου ὀμφακίνου ψυχροῦ·

et caeteris multis. Praeterea vero cutis et capillorum deformitatibus obfidetur, alopecia, ophiafi, diverfisque ulceribus. Aeftus itaque, frigoris et vaporis ab externis rebus exurgentis idonea figna funt hae caufae evidentes. Jam vero ab aeftu laborantes comitatur dolor pulfatorius totius capitis, quod fiderari videtur, cum ignei caloris fenfu, vaforum frontis diftenfio, oculorum rubor, plerumque etiam vigilia; frigore vero laborantes ftupefaciens gravitas, congelatio, vafa fecundum frontem collapfa, fi cum humiditate frigeant, etiam vehementior fomnus; at vaporibus male affectos dolor punctorius, pulfus arteriarum quae circa frontem funt, vertigines, hallucinationes, aurium fonitus. Peraeque quibus ab internis vaporibus repletur caput, haec ipfa accidere confuescunt.

Cap. I. [*Ad internos capitis affectus, ac primum pro capitis dolore ab aeftu folis.*] Dolore capitis ab aeftu folis *laborantibus* idonea erit embroche ex oleo omphacino

εἰ δ' ἐπιτείνοιτο, δι' ὀξυῤῥοδίνου, μὴ παρόντος δὲ τοῦ ῥοδίνου ἐλαίου, χρηστέον ὀμφακίνῳ, τέτρασι μέρεσι τοῦ ἐλαίου συμπλέκοντας ὄξους μέρος ἓν, εἰ συμμέτρως ψύχειν βούλοιντο, εἰ δὲ μὴ, πλεῖον ἔτι ὄξους. διακαιομένης δὲ σφοδρῶς τῆς κεφαλῆς, συμπλέκειν χρὴ τῷ ὄξει πολυγόνου χυλὸν, ἢ ἀρνογλώσσου, ἢ ἀνδράχνης, ἢ θριδακίνης, ἢ ὄμφακος σταφυλῆς, ἢ τῶν τοιούτων τινός. δῆλον δὲ ὡς τὸ μᾶλλόν τε καὶ ἧττον τῆς εὔξεως αὐτῶν δηλώσει τὸ μέγεθος τῆς ἐγκαύσεως καὶ ἡ τοῦ σώματος κατασκευή. ἀνακλίνειν δὲ αὐτοὺς ἄμεινον καὶ ἐν ψυχροτέροις οἴκοις εἰσφέροντας ἀμπέλου φύλλα καὶ [576] βάτου, μήλων τε καὶ τῶν τούτοις παραπλησίων, ὅσα χωρὶς τοῦ κάρου ψύχειν δυνήσεται. παραπλήσιαι δὲ ταύτῃ διαθέσεις καὶ αἱ ἀπὸ τῶν δυσκρασιῶν συμβαινόμεναι. ἀλλ' αἱ μὲν ἀπὸ θερμοτέρας καὶ ξηροτέρας, ἔτι τε ψυχροτέρας καὶ ξηροτέρας δυσκρασίας, ὀδύναι μεγάλαι γίγνονται, ἥκιστα δ' ἐν τῇ ὑγρᾷ δυσκρασίᾳ πόνοι συμβαίνουσι, θεραπεύονται κατὰ ἐναντίωσιν τῶν διαθέσεων.

frigido; ſi adaugeatur dolor, ex roſaceo et aceto; at ſi non adſit roſaceum oleum, omphacino utendum. Olei partibus quatuor aceti unam commiſceant, ſi mediocriter refrigerare velint, alioqui plus aceti adjiciendum. Aeſtuante vero vehementer capite commiscendus aceto ſuccus ſanguinariae, aut arnogloſſi, aut portulacae, aut lactucae, aut uvae acerbae, aut alicujus ejusmodi facultatis. Conſtat autem quod et liberaliorem et parciorem eorum uſum tum ardoris magnitudo, tum corporis praeparatio indicabit. Sed praeſtat etiam ipſos aegrotos in frigidiore domo decumbere, ſtrata foliis vitis et rubi et pomi et aliis horum ſimilibus, quae citra veternum refrigerare valuerint. Conſimiles ipſi ſunt affectus qui ab intemperie oboriuntur. Verum ab intemperie tum calidiore quidem et ſicciore, tum etiamnum a frigidioreet ſicciore dolores maximi nascuntur, ſed minime ab humida intemperie dolores contingunt. Curantur vero etiam ipſi dolores eodem modo, quo qui ab externis cauſis ortum ducunt per remedia affectibus contraria.

[*Περὶ τῆς ἀπὸ ψύξεως κεφαλαλγίας.*] *Τοῖς δὲ ἀπὸ ψύξεως ἁρμόζουσιν αἱ θερμότεραι τῶν ἐμβροχῶν, ὅτε μὲν συμμέτρως εἴη ἡ ψύξις, ἀρκουμένοις ἀνηθίνῳ καὶ πηγανίνῳ ἐλαίῳ θερμῷ· εἰ δὲ ἐπιτείνοιτο μεγάλης τῆς ψύξεως ὑπαρχούσης, σικύου ἀγρίου ῥίζαν ἐμβαλεῖν δεῖ, ποτὲ δὲ καὶ εὐφορβίου βραχύ. χρῆσθαι δὲ καὶ ἰρίνῳ ἐλαίῳ, ἤ τινι τῶν τοιούτων λεπτῶν εἰρημένων τινὰ τούτοις ἐμβαλόντα· ἐλάττω δὲ ἢ πλείω κατὰ τὴν ἐπικρατοῦσαν ψύξιν σκοποῦντα καὶ συμμετρούμενον.*

[*Περὶ τῆς ἐξ ἀναθυμιάσεως κεφαλαλγίας.*] *Ὅσοις δὲ ἀπὸ ἀναθυμιάσεων αἱ κεφαλαλγίαι γίγνονται, ὑπάγειν τε τὴν γαστέρα καὶ ἄγειν αὐτοὺς εἰς εὐπνουστέρους οἴκους καὶ λεπτὸν ἀέρα ἔχοντας, ἐπιτηδεύειν τε καὶ πταρμοὺς, μάλιστα εἰ ἀπύρετοι εἶεν, ἐμβαλόντας τοῖς πόροις ἢ στρούθιον λεῖον, ἢ πέπερι, καὶ ἀνέλκειν κελεύοντας. κενουμένων γὰρ τῶν ἀτμῶν ῥᾷον διαφορηθήσεται ἡ κεφαλή. ἐμβρέχειν δ᾽ αὐτοὺς καὶ ἐλαίῳ, βραχὺ ὄξους παραχέοντας. ἥ τε γὰρ ἄμετρος ἐπὶ τὴν κεφαλὴν τῶν ἀτμῶν φορὰ ἀποκρουσθήσεται καὶ τὸ*

[*Pro capitis dolore a frigore.*] A frigore vero caput dolentibus medentur embrochae calidiores. Quod fi moderatum fuerit frigus, anethino et rutaceo oleo calido uti fatis erit; fi autem intendatur ex vehementi graffante frigore, cucumeris agreftis radicem infundere oportet, ac interdum euphorbii pauxillum. Utendum quoque irino oleo, aut talium tenuium enarratorum aliquo, quaedam his inferendo; fed pauciora aut plura pro ratione exuperantis frigoris obfervando ac commetiendo.

[*Pro capitis dolore a vaporibus.*] Quibus dolores capitis a vaporibus excitantur, fubducenda eft alvus, iique in domos quae ventis magis perflentur, tum tenui aëre gaudeant, ducendi funt; fternutamenta cienda, praefertim fi febre vacent, injecto et ex praefcriptis attracto per narium meatus aut ftruthio trito, aut pipere. Vacuatis enim vaporibus facilius difcutietur capitis dolor. Irrigandum autem eorum caput eft etiam oleo, cui aceti nonnihil effundatur; immoderatus namque ad caput vaporum afcen-

ἐνιζάνον ταῖς κοιλίαις τοῦ ἐγκεφάλου διαφορηθήσεται, μὴ ἐᾶν καθεύδειν, καὶ μάλιστα μεθ' ἡμέρας.

[*Περὶ τῆς ἐξ ἀπέπτων βρωμάτων κεφαλαλγίας.*] Εἰ δ' ἀπέπτων ἐγκειμένων τῇ γαστρὶ συμπάσχοι τι ἡ κεφαλὴ, διδόντας πιεῖν ὕδατος χλιαροῦ συχνῶς ἐμεῖν κελεύειν. γίγνονται δὲ πολλοῖς τῶν στομαχικῶν ἐξ ἀναστάσεως κεφαλαλγίαι, ἐφ' ὧν αἱ παραθέσεις τῆς τροφῆς αὐτίκα κουφίζειν εἰώθασιν. εἰ δ' ἀπὸ μεγάλης ποτὲ ἀλγηδόνος τῆς κεφαλῆς ἄφωνοι γίνονται ἄφνω, μηδὲ τῆς αἰτίας καταλαμβανομένης, καταντλεῖν προσήκει τὴν κεφαλὴν ὕδατι θερμῷ δαψιλεῖ, ἐγχέοντας τοῖς ὠσὶν ἔλαιον καὶ ἔριον ἐμβάλλοντας.

[*Περὶ τῆς ἐξ οἴνου κεφαλαλγίας.*] Ὅτι μὲν οἱ θερμότεροι τῶν οἴνων τὰς κεφαλαλγίας γεννῶσιν, ἀτμῶν πληροῦντες ῥᾳδίως τὴν κεφαλὴν, ἔσθ' ὅτε δὲ καὶ χυμῶν, καὶ ὅτε χωρὶς οἴνου πόσεως πρὸς τὴν κεφαλὴν ἑτοίμως οὗτοι ἀναφέρονται, καὶ μάλιστα οἷς φύσει θερμότεραι τὴν κρᾶσιν αἱ κεφαλαὶ τυγχάνουσιν, ἅπασιν οἶμαι φανερὸν εἶναι. σκοπὸς

ſus reprimetur et quae portio cerebri ventriculis inſedit, diſcutietur. At dormire non ſinendum eſt, ac potiſſimum interdiu.

[*Pro dolore capitis ab eduliis crudis ventriculi.*] Quod ſi ab eduliis crudis ventriculo incumbentibus per conſenſum doleat caput, aqua tepida liberalius potui exhibenda eſt vomitusque imperandus. Multis autem ſtomachicis a ſurrectione capitis dolores oriuntur, quos ſtatim ciborum aſſumptiones levare conſueverunt. Quod ſi a vehementi aliquando dolore capitis derepente quidam obtumeſcunt, neque cauſa deprehendatur, caput aqua calida liberalius perſundere convenit et auribus oleum inſundere et lanam inſerere.

[*Pro capitis dolore ex vino.*] Quod vina calidiora capitis dolores procreent, facileque caput oppleant vaporibus, interdum etiam humoribus, quodque citra vini potum ad caput hi prompte efferantur, iisque potiſſimum qui calidiora temperamento capita ſortiuntur, omnibus maniſeſtum eſſe arbitror. Proinde ſcopus curationis ipſo-

τοίνυν τῆς ἰάσεως ἡ κένωσις αὐτῶν. ἐπειδὴ δὲ θερμότεροι τυγχάνουσιν ὄντες οἱ πεπληρωκότες τὴν κεφαλὴν ἀτμοὶ, καὶ τῆς ἐντυχούσης αὐτοῖς βοηθείας δέονται. ἔλαιον οὖν ῥόδινον καὶ πάνυ ψυχρὸν προσφερόμενον, ὕπνος τε καὶ ἡσυχία, καὶ μετὰ ταῦτα εἰς ἑσπέραν λουτρὸν καὶ τροφαὶ εὔχυμοι, οὐ μέντοι θερμαίνουσαι. τοιαῦται δ' εἰσὶν ὁ πτισάνης χυλὸς, καὶ τὰ ὑγρὰ τῶν ᾠῶν ἄνευ γάρου καὶ ἐξ ὕδατος ἄρτος, θριδακίνη τε ὡς ἐμψύχουσα καὶ κράμβη ὡς ἀτμῶν ξηραντική. ποτῷ δὲ ὕδατι χρηστέον. ἀλλ' ἐπί τινων ὁ στόμαχος ἐπὶ ταῖς ὑδροποσίαις ἀνατρέπεται, ῥοιὰν οὖν αὐτοῖς ἐπιδοτέον, ἢ μῆλον, ἢ ἄπιον [577] ἡψημένα. χρὴ δὲ ἕψειν οὕτως αὐτά· πρῶτον ἐν χύτρᾳ ὕδωρ ἐγχέοντας θερμὸν, εἶτα κρεμάσαντας ἐν ἀγγείῳ τὰς ὀπώρας ὑποκαίειν τὴν χύτραν, ὅπως ὁ ἀναφερόμενος (473) ἐκ τοῦ ὕδατος ἀτμὸς ἕψειν οἷός τε εἴη. καὶ σταφίδες δὲ ῥωννύουσι τὸν στόμαχον. φοινίκων δὲ παντελῶς ἀπέχεσθαι. ἔχουσι γάρ τινα ἰδιότητα κεφαλαλγίας ποιητικήν. εἰ δ' ἐπὶ τούτοις ὑπνῶσαι καλῶς δυνηθεῖεν, ἐπὶ λουτρὸν μὲν ἄγειν αὐτοὺς κατὰ τὴν ὑστε-

rum eſt vacuatio. Quoniam vero hi vapores calidiores ſunt caputque repleverunt, egent remedio ipſos refrigerante. Oleum itaque roſaceum admotum frigidum admovendum eſt, ſomnus quoque congruit et quies, et poſtea ſub veſperam balneum et cibi boni ſucci, qui tamen non calefaciant. Ejusmodi ſunt hordei cremor, ova ſorbilia absque garo, panis aqua maceratus, lactuca et braſſica, quae vapores exiccando diſcutit, aquae potu utendum. Caeterum quorum os ventriculi aquae potu ſubvertitur, iis granatum offerendum, ſeu malum Punicum, aut pyrum, eaque cocta exhibenda ſunt. Haec autem ita coquenda. Primum inſuſa in ollam aqua fervida, deinde ſuſpenſis in vaſe his fructibus autumnalibus, ſub olla ignem ſuccendemus, quoad vapor elevetur, qui hosce fructus coquere queat. Quin et uvae paſſae ſtomachum corroborant. A palmulis prorſus abſtinendum, quod proprietate quadam polleant dolores capitis effectrice. Si his peractis

ραίαν, καὶ καταχεῖν ἐν τῷ βαλανείῳ θερμὸν ὕδωρ πολλάκις, εἶτα μικρὸν ἠρεμήσαντας αὖθις παραπλησίως λούειν, εἶθ' οὕτως τρέφειν ὡς πρόσθεν εἴρηται. εἰ δέ ποτέ τι τῶν ἀνελθόντων ἐπὶ τὴν κεφαλὴν ἀτμῶν τε καὶ χυμῶν ὑπολείποιτο τι λείψανον ἐσφηνωμένον πόροις λεπτοῖς, καὶ διὰ τοῦτο παραμένει τι τῆς κεφαλαλγίας, ἀφίστασθαι μὲν τοῦ ῥοδίνου, ἐμβρέχειν δὲ τῷ χαμαιμηλίνῳ συμμέτρως θερμῷ, καὶ μετὰ ταῦτα ἰρίνῳ μεγάλως ὠφελοῦντι τὰς τοιαύτας διαθέσεις· μηδενὸς δὲ τούτων ὄντος, οἴνῳ χρῆσθαι.

[*Περὶ τῆς ἐκ πληγῶν καὶ συμπτωμάτων κεφαλαλγίας.*] Ἐπεὶ δὲ καὶ διά τινα συμπτώματα καὶ πληγὰς γίνονται κεφαλαλγίαι, χρήσιμον βραχέα καὶ πρὸς ταῦτα ὑποσχέσθαι. ἁρμόζει τοίνυν ἡ διὰ σπόγγων πυρία καὶ μαλακῶν ἐρίων ἐλαίῳ θερμῷ δεδευμένων. πρὸς δὲ τούτοις ἡσυχία, ὑποστολὴ τροφῆς, κένωσις τοῦ κάτω γαστρός. φυλακτέον δὲ ἥλιον, λουτρὸν, οἰνοποσίαν, κραυγὴν καὶ διάτασιν, καὶ τῶν ἐν τροφῇ προσφερομένων τὰ δριμέα καὶ ὀξέα καὶ ἁλικά· δῆλον δ' ὡς

aegri probe dormire nequeant, ad balnea ipfi poftridie ducendi funt et in balneo aqua calida faepe perfundendi, poftea pauxillo temporis interjecto denuo fimiliter lavandi, ac tandem, ut prius dictum eft, cibandi. Si vero aliquando elatorum ad caput et vaporum et humorum nonnihil relinquatur exilibus meatibus impactum, ob idque doloris capitis refiduum quidpiam permaneat, rofaceo parcendum et caput perfundendum chamaemelino moderate calido et poftea irino, quod ejusmodi affectibus magnopere confert; fed eorum nulli vino uti concedatur.

[*Pro dolore capitis ex ictu et cafu ab alto.*] Quoniam vero et ob cafus quosdam ab alto et ictus dolores capitis obveniunt, utile quoque eft ad ea pauca proferre. Conveniet igitur fotus fpongia aut molliori lana oleo calido inebriata, praeterea quies, alimenti fubtractio, ventris inferioris vacuatio. Vitanda funt fol, balneum, vini potus, clamor et contentio, etiam edulia acria, acida, falfa. Liquet

σκοποὶ πλείονες ἔσονται τῆς τῶν ἰαμάτων εὑρέσεως κατὰ τὰς ποιούσας τὰ πάθη αἰτίας.

[*Περὶ τῆς ἐκ θλασμάτων κεφαλαλγίας.*] *Καὶ γὰρ κεφαλὴν καὶ θλᾶσθαι συμβαίνει, καὶ ποτὲ μὲν μετὰ τραύματος, ποτὲ δὲ καὶ χωρὶς τραύματος γίνεσθει τὴν θλάσιν, ὡς κᾀκ τούτων ἐπιπλέκεσθαι σκοποὺς θεραπείας. θλάσει μὲν οὖν οἰκεῖα τὰ παρηγορικὰ τῶν βοηθημάτων οἷον θερμοῦ κατάχυσις ὕδατος καὶ ἐπίβλημα ἐλαιοβρεχές. τὴν δὲ διαίρεσιν περίστασις παροῦσα εἰ μὴ κωλύει κολληθήσεσθαι, σιδηρίτην βοτάνην λειώσας καὶ ἀπυσπογγίσας οἴνῳ ἐπιδέσμει. Ἄλλο. ῥητίνην φρυκτὴν καταπλάσας τὸ ἕλκος ἐπιδέσμει. Ἄλλο. ἀλόην λειώσας καὶ μέλι προσμίξας ἐπιτίθει. Ἄλλο. γῆς ἔντερα κόψας ἐπιτίθει. Ἄλλο. πτελέας φύλλα χλωρὰ κόψας ἐπιτίθει, πρότερον τρίψας. καὶ ὁ φλοιὸς δὲ τοῦ αὐτοῦ δένδρου περιειληθεὶς ὡς ἐπίδεσμος τὸ αὐτὸ ποιεῖ.*

[*Πρὸς καταφοράν.*] *Πιτύαν ἐρίφων βάλε εἰς ἄκρατον οἶνον Αἰγύπτιον καὶ δὸς ἴσον καὶ δίδου πίνειν νηστικῷ ἐπὶ ἡμέρας γ'.*

autem pro diverfis morborum caufis efficientibus plures fore inveniendorum remediorum indicationes.

[*Pro dolore capitis a contufione.*] Caput etenim etiam contundi accidit, interdum cum vulnere, interdum fine vulnere contufionem fieri, adeo ut ex his curationis fcopi implicentur. Enimvero contufioni propria remedia funt mitigantia, cujus generis funt aquae calidae affufio et panniculus oleo inebriatus. At divifioni nifi cafus aliquis conglutinari prohibeat, prius fpongia vino madente deterfae fideritim herbam alligabis. *Aliud.* Refinam frictam ut cataplasma vulneri alligato. *Aliud.* Aloëm tritam et melli admixtam admove. *Aliud.* Terrae inteftina concifa ac trita impone. *Aliud.* Ulmi folia virentia contufa ac trita applicato. Quin etiam ulmi cortex pro vinculo vulneri circumvolutus idem praeftat.

[*Ad cataphoram.*] Coagulum hoedi conjice in meracum vinum Aegyptium, daque par pondus et exhibe potui jejuno per tres dies.

[Πρὸς τὰς ἐκ μέθης καὶ ἐγκαύσεως κεφαλαλγίας.] Ἐπεὶ δὲ τὰ περίαπτα ἔγραψεν ὁ Ἀρχιγένης τοῖς κεφαλαλγοῦσιν, οὐκ ἄτοπον ᾠήθην καὶ ταῦτα ἀναγράψαι πρὸς τὰς ἐκ μέθης καὶ ἐγκαύσεως κεφαλαλγίας, πολυγόνου δύο κλωνία πλέξας στεφάνωσον. ἄλλο. πολύγονον τρίψας μετὰ κορυφῆς γάλακτος καὶ ἀλείψας τὴν κεφαλὴν τῷ βάθει τῆς ἑσπέρας καὶ ἐπάνω λαγωοῦ δέρμα βαλὼν, ἕως πρωῒ, ἆρον τὸ δέρμα καὶ ἰαθήσῃ. ἄλλο. κιχώριον τὸ Ῥωμαϊστὶ λεγόμενον ἰντυβολάχανον, ἐπιτίθει τοῦ πάσχοντος τὴν κεφαλήν. ἄλλο. ῥόδινον στέφανον ἐπιτίθει τῇ κεφαλῇ, νέα ἄνθη ῥόδου ἐκ νεαρῶν ῥόδων. ἄλλο. καλλιτρίχῳ στέφε τὴν κεφαλὴν, ὃ τινὲς καλοῦσιν ἀδίαντον, ἔνιοι δὲ τριχομανές. ἄλλο. ἄκρως δὲ ἀπάλλασσειν τῆς κεφαλαλγίας φησὶν Ἀρχιγένης [578] περιστερεῶνα, ἥν τινες ἱερὰν βοτάνην καλοῦσι, καὶ στεφομένην καὶ καταχριομένην μετ' ὄξους καὶ ῥοδίνου. ἄλλο. χελώνης λιμναίας ἥν τινες ἀμύδα καλοῦσιν, αἷμα ἐπίσταζε ἐπὶ τὸ βρέγμα.

Κεφ. β'. [Περὶ εὐπορίστων πρὸς τὰ ἐκτὸς τῆς κε-

[*Ad capitis dolores ex ebrietate et folis aeftu.*] Quandoquidem Archigenes capitis doloribus amuleta fcripfit, haud abfurdum duxi haec etiam ad capitis dolores ab ebrietate et folis aeftu obortos adfcribere. Duos polygoni ramulos coronae inftar connexos admove. *Aliud.* Polygono trito cum lactis cremore caput fub vefperam inunge ac leporis pellem fuperponito adusque auroram, tumque pellem tolle et fanatus comperietur. *Aliud.* Cichorium Romane intybum olus dicitur, laborantis capiti impone. *Aliud.* Rofarum coronam capiti admove, ex recentibus rofarum floribus recenter factam. *Aliud.* Corona caput callitricho, quod quidam adiantum vocant, nonnullique trichomanes. *Aliud.* Summopere conferre capitis dolori narrat Archigenes verbenam, quam quidam herbam facram vocitant, tum coronae modo impofitam tum ex aceto et rofaceo inunctam. *Aliud.* Teftudinis lacuftris, quam amyda quidam vocitant, fanguinem inftilla fincipiti.

Cap. II. [*De parabilibus ad externos capitis affe-*

φαλῆς πάθη, καὶ πρῶτον πρὸς ῥεούσας τρίχας.] Λάδανον ἀποβρέχων οἴνῳ εὐώδει καὶ στύφῳ λαίου, παραχέων καὶ μύρσινον, καὶ γλοιῶδες ποιήσας κατάχριε. ἄλλο. κάρυα χλωρὰ, ἀκμάζειν ἀρξάμενα, θλάσας ρ'. μίξας τε ἐλαίου ξέστας β'. στυπτηρίας ὑγρᾶς λίτρας γ'. καὶ βαλὼν εἰς σκεῦος καινὸν ὀστρακινὸν προβραχὲν, ὡς μὴ ἀναποθῆναι τὸ ἐμβληθὲν ὑγρὸν, ἐπιμελέστατα περίχρισον, καὶ καταθέμενος ἐν εὐαέρῳ οἴκῳ ἐπὶ ἡμέρας μ'. καὶ μετὰ τοῦτο ἀνελόμενος, χρῶ τῷ ἐλαίῳ. ἄλλο. λάδανον καὶ ἀψίνθιον καὶ ἀρκευθίδας λειώσας, εἰς ὀθόνην ἔνδησον, καὶ ἔμβαλε εἰς ἔλαιον καὶ μετὰ ἡμέρας ε'. χρῶ. ἢ μυρσίνης μελαίνης, ἢ κηκίδος μέρη β'. μετ' ἐλαίου. τὸ αὐτὸ δὲ πιτυρίασιν ἰᾶται. ἄλλο. λάδανον λειώσας μετὰ γλυκέος οἴνου γλοιῶδες ποιήσας χρῖε. ἄλλο. ἀνεμώνης τὸ ἄνθος λειώσας μετ' ἐλαίου κατάχριε, τὸ αὐτὸ καὶ μελαίνει. ἄλλο. περιστερεῶνα τὸ ὀρθὸν σὺν ταῖς ῥίζαις ξηράνας καὶ εὖ μάλα λειώσας μῖξον ἐλαίου, ὡς πάχος ἔχειν γλοιοῦ καὶ ἐάσας σαπῆναι κατάχριε.

ctus; primumque ad defluentes capillos.] Ladanum inebriatum vino odorato ac aſtringenti laevigato, aſſundens myrteum et lentitiam factam illine. *Aliud.* Recipe nuces virides adoleſcere incipientes conſractas centum, olei ſextarios ij, aluminis liquidi lib. iij, miſce ac injice in novum vas teſtaceum prius irrigatum, ne conjectum humorem combibat, quod poſtea accuratiſſime oblitum reponitur in domum ſalubris aëris diebus xl, et poſtea auſer et oleo utere. *Aliud.* Recipe ladanum et abſinthium et juniperi baccas, contere, linteoque illigata in oleum conjice et poſt dies v utitor. *Vel.* Recipe myrti nigrae, aut gallae partes ij, ex oleo. Id autem medetur etiam capitis furfuribus. *Aliud.* Ladanum laevigatum ex vino dulci lentitiam conſequutum illine. *Aliud.* Anemones florem laevigatum ex oleo illine, id quoque capillos denigrat. *Aliud.* Verbenam rectam cum radicibus deſiccatam, deinde exacte admodum laevigatam miſceto oleo, quoad luti craſſitiem conſequatur, ſinitoque putreſieri; illine.

[*Περὶ πιτυριάσεως.*] *Προσμήξας τὴν κεφαλὴν σεύτλου χυλῷ καὶ τηλίνοις ἀλεύροις, καὶ νίτρῳ λείοις ἴσοις σμῆχε. ἄλλο. Κιμωλία γῆ ὄξει καὶ βοείᾳ χολῇ φυραθεῖσα, χρῖε. ἄλλο. ἀμυγδάλοις πικροῖς μετ' ὀξυκράτου ἀπόσμηχε. ἄλλο. ἀφρόνιτρον καὶ χάλκανθον ἴσα λειώσας μετ' οἴνου χρῶ. ἄλλο. βολβοῖς ὀπτοῖς καὶ νίτρῳ λείοις ἴσοις σμῆχε.*

[*Περὶ φθειριάσεως.*] *Σταφίδος ἀγρίας μέρη β'. σανδαράχης μέρος α'. νίτρου μέρος α'. σὺν ὄξει καὶ ἐλαίῳ ἄλειφε τὴν κεφαλήν. ἄλλο. στυπτηρίῳ σχιστῇ μετ' ἐλαίου χρῶ.*

[*Περὶ ἀχώρων καὶ κηρίων.*] *Ἀχῶρες συνίστανται περὶ τὸ τῆς κεφαλῆς δέρμα. ὠνόμασται δὲ ἀπὸ τοῦ συμπτώματος, λεπτὰς γὰρ ἔχει κατατρήσεις, δι' ὧν ἀποῤῥέει ἰχὼρ γλίσχρος. ὅμοιον δ' αὐτῷ πάθος ἐστὶ καὶ τὸ καλούμενον κηρίον, τὰς κατατρήσεις μείζονας ἔχον, ὑγρὸν ἐχούσας μελιτῶδες· ἐστὶ δ' ἑκατέροις ἡ γένεσις ἐξ ὑγρότητος περιττωματικῆς. συμβαίνει δ' αὐτοῖς τὸ πρῶτον κνησμὸς, μετὰ ταῦτα δὲ καὶ εἰς ὄγκον ἐπανάστασις. θεραπεία δὲ, μεγάλης οὔσης τῆς διαθέ-*

[*Pro capitis furfuribus.*] Praefricatum caput betae fucco, foenigraeci farina et nitro aequa portione contritis deterge. *Aliud.* Terra Cimolia aceto et bubulo felle macerata, illinatur. *Aliud.* Amygdalis amaris cum oxycrato deterge. *Aliud.* Aphronitri et chalcanthi aequis portionibus tritis ex vino utere. *Aliud.* Bulbis coctis et cum nitro tritis aequis partibus deterge.

[*Pro capitis pediculis.*] Recipe ftaphidos agreftis partes ij, fandarachae partem j, nitri partem j, ex aceto et oleo caput illine. *Aliud.* Alumine fciffili ex oleo utere.

[*Pro achoribus et favis.*] Achores manantia cutis capitis ulcera funt; ab ipfo autem fymptomate nomen ducunt, tenuia fiquidem foramina prae fe ferunt, per quae lenta fanies effluit. Similis ipfi affectus eft favus appellatus, majora habens foramina melleum humorem continentia. Utriusque ortus ab excrementofo humore ducitur. His autem accidit primum pruritus, poftea etiam in tumorem eruptio. Curatio fit, quum magnus eft affectus,

σιως προηγουμένη μὲν κάθαρσις τῶν καταποτίων διὰ σκαμμωνίας καὶ ἀλόης, καὶ κολοκυνθίδος, ἑκάστου δ' αὐτῶν ἴσον, λειωθέντα δὲ ἀναλαμβάνεται χυλῷ κράμβης, καὶ ἀναπλάσσεται καταπότια ὀρόβου μέγεθος ἔχοντα. δίδοται δὲ τοῖς ἰσχυροτέροις ἑπτακαίδεκα τῆς τελείας δόσεως, τοῖς ἄλλοις πρὸς ἀναλογίαν τοῦ σώματος. ἐπὶ δὲ τῶν μικρῶν διαθέσεων ἀρκεῖ καὶ τὰ τοπικὰ τῶν βοηθημάτων. ἔστι δὲ ταῦτα κιμωλία μετὰ ὄξους δριμυτάτου καταχριομένη. ἄλλο. κρήταν μετὰ ὄξους δριμυτάτου κατάχριε. ὁμοίως δὲ καὶ Σαμία γῆ καὶ πομφόλυξ. ἄλλο. λιθαργύρου [579] καὶ χάρτης κεκαυμένης λύχνῳ, χρῶ μετ' ὄξους. ἐφ' ὧν μέντοι ἕλκωσίς ἐστιν ὀδυνώδης, ὕδατι ἀπαντλεῖν αὐτοὺς θερμῷ προσήκει ἑκάστης ἡμέρας, ἀφηψημένης ἐν αὐτῷ μυρσίνης, βάτου, συκαμίνου, ἢ ἀσπαράγου ῥίζης, καὶ κατάχριε. ἄλλο. ἰτέας φύλλοις μεθ' ὕδατος, ἢ φακῷ μετὰ μέλιτος, ἢ ἀσπαράγου ῥίζῃ ἑφθῇ ἀπόσμηχε, ἢ σεῦτλον χυλῷ ἔχοντι τήλινον ἄλευρον. φάρμακα δ' ἐπιτήδεια πίτυος φλοιὸς μετὰ κηρωτῆς, ἢ καδμεία μετ' ἐλαίου, ἢ λιθάργυρος, ἢ ψιμύθιον. σμήχειν δὲ ἐν βαλα-

purgatio quae praecedat, catapotiis ex fcamonio, aloë et colocynthide, fingulorum pari pondere, contrita brafficae fucco excipiuntur, ac formantur in pilulas ervi magnitudinem aemulantes. Dantur autem robuftioribus feptemdecim pro integra dofi; caeteris vero ad corporis analogiam. Sed in parvis affectibus topica remedia fufficiunt. Haec autem funt cimolia ex acerrimo aceto illita. *Aliud.* Cretam cum aceto acerrimo illine. Similiter quoque Samia terra et pompholyx admoventur. *Aliud.* Lithargyri et chartae uftae lychno ex aceto utere. At quibus ulceratio dolorem excitat, eos aqua calida quotidie fovere convenit, in qua decocta fit aut myrtus, aut rubus, aut morus, aut afparagi radix, atque illine. *Aliud.* Salicis foliis ex aqua, aut lente ex melle, aut decocta afparagi radice etiam deline, aut betae fucco foenigraeci farina excepto. Idonea praeterea medicamenta funt pini cortex cum cera vel cadmia ex oleo, aut lithargyrus, aut ceruffa. Proderit

νείῳ τεῦτλον χυλῷ μετὰ κιμωλίας. δῆλον δὲ ὡς ἐπὶ τῶν ἁπαλοσάρκων γυναικῶν φυλάττεσθαι μὲν δεῖ τὸ ὄξος, οἴνῳ δὲ καταχρίειν τὰ φάρμακα.

(474) [Περὶ ἀλωπεκίας καὶ ὀφιάσεως.] Συμβαίνει διττὸν πάθος περὶ τὰς ἐν κεφαλῇ τρίχας, ὁτὲ μὲν ἔκλειψις αὐτῶν, ὁτὲ δὲ εἰς ἑτέραν χροιὰν μεταβολή. ἔκλειψις μὲν ἐν ταῖς φαλακρώσεσιν, ἑτεροχροία δὲ ἐν ταῖς ἀλωπεκίαις τε καὶ ὀφιάσεσιν, ἀπρεπεστάτη βλάβη τῶν τριχῶν. ἔστι δ' αὐτοῖς ἡ βλάβη παραπλησία τοῖς φυτοῖς. καθάπερ γὰρ ἐκεῖνα παραπλησίαν τῷ τρέφοντι ὑγρῷ τὴν γένεσιν ἔχει· ὁμοίως δὲ ταῖς τριξὶν ἡ παθητικὴ κατασκευή. ὁτὲ μὲν ἐνδείᾳ τοῦ τρέφοντος ὑγροῦ ἀφαιρούμενα φθείρεται, ἢ ἀλλοτριώσει τὴν κατὰ φύσιν ὑπαλλάττει διάθεσιν. ἔστι δὲ ἀλωπεκία καὶ ὀφίασις ἑκάτεραι μὲν διαθέσεις παρὰ φύσιν τὴν αὐτὴν αἰτίαν ἔχουσαι τῆς γενέσεως, κοινὴν δὲ καὶ τὴν ἴασιν, ὀνόμασι δὲ διαφόροις ὠνομασμέναι κατὰ τὸ σχῆμα. ἐπί τε γὰρ τῆς ὀφιάσεως παραπλήσιον ὄφει τὸ σχῆμα ἐπὶ τῆς κεφαλῆς φαίνεται, ἡ δ' ἀλωπεκία, ὥς φασιν, ὠνόμασται διὰ τὸ συνεχὲς ταῖς ἀλώπεξι συμβαίνειν τὴν διάθεσιν, ψίλωσιν

etiam abftergere in balneo cimolia ex betae fucco. Conftat autem mollioris carnis mulieribus haec remedia non aceto, fed vino illinenda.

[*Pro alopecia et ophiafi, i. e. areis.*] Duplex affectio pilis capitis accidit, altera quidem eorum defectus, altera vero in alienum colorem mutatio. Defectus in calvitie, alienus color in alopecia et ophiafi, quae inhoneftiffima eft pilorum laefio. Eft autem ipfis et ftirpibus laefio confimilis. Quemadmodum enim illae fimilem nutrienti humido generationem habent; fimiliter quoque capillis pathetica conftitutio. Interdum enim illae nutrientis humoris penuria corrumpuntur et intereunt; aut alienatione eum qui fecundum naturam eft affectum immutant exuuntque. At alopecia et ophiafis utraque affectiones praeter naturam funt, tum quae eandem caufam fortiuntur, tum communem curationem, diverfis ex figura nominibus appellatae. Etenim in ophiafi perfimilis ferpenti figura in

οὖσαν τριχῶν, μετὰ τοῦ ἀναιμόχρουν φαίνεσθαι τὸν πεπονθότα τόπον. ἡμεῖς δὲ διὰ τί οὕτως ὠνόμασται οὐ πολυπραγμονοῦμεν. μοχθηρὸν δὲ πλῆθος ὑγρῶν αἴτιον τῆς γενέσεως εὑρόντες τῷ φυσικῷ λόγῳ ἑξῆς ἐπὶ τὰς θεραπείας χωρήσομεν. εἰσὶ δ' αὐτῷ διαφοραὶ πλείους κατὰ τὴν χρόαν. αἱ μὲν γὰρ λευκότεραι, αἱ δὲ ὠχρότεραι, ἕτεραι δὲ μελάντεραι. δῆλον δὲ ὡς κακοχυμίας ἐστὶν ἅπαντα ἔγγονα τοιαῦτα. αἱ μὲν οὖν λευκότεραι ὑπὸ τῆς τοῦ φλέγματος κακοχυμίας γίγνονται, καὶ ἰῶνται τοῖς φλεγμαγωγοῖς τῶν καθαρτηρίων καὶ τοῖς ἀποφλεγματισμοῖς, αἱ δὲ ὠχρότεραι τοῖς τὴν τοιαύτην καθαίρουσι χολὴν, αἱ δὲ μελάντεραι τοῖς τὸν μελαγχολικὸν καθαίρουσι χυμόν. χρὴ γὰρ πρὸ τῆς τοῦ πεπονθότος μορίου θεραπείας ἅπαν προκαθαίρειν τὸ σῶμα, ὡς μηκέτι ἐπιῤῥεῖν ἐξ αὐτοῦ τὴν κακοχυμίαν τῷ πεπονθότι μέρει, καὶ εἶθ' οὕτως ἑξῆς ἐπὶ τὸ πεπονθὸς μόριον παραγίγνεσθαι. ἔστι δὲ ἀποφλεγματικὰ μὲν πύρεθρον καὶ σταφὶς ἀγρία· θάτερον δ' αὐτῶν ἢ καὶ ἄμφω μετὰ μαστίχης

capite confpicitur. Sed alopecia, ut afferunt, appellata eft, quod haec affectio vulpibus frequenter accidat, quae pilorum eft denudatio, qua locus affectus exanguis apparet. At nos cur ita nominata fit curiofius non inquirimus, fed pravam humorum multitudinem naturali ratiocinatione generationis caufam indagatam fortiti, deinceps ad curationes progrediemur. Sunt autem ipfarum differentiae colore plures. Aliae namque albidiores, aliae pallidiores, aliae nigriores. Liquet haec omnia vitiofi humoris effe propagines. Albidiores fiquidem affectiones a vitiofa pituita fiunt et medicamentis pituitam purgantibus et apophlegmatismis curantur; pallidiores ipfam pallidam bilem purgantibus et nigriores melancholicum humorem purgantibus. Nam ante partis affectae curationem univerfum corpus purgandum eft, ne poftea ex ipfo in affectam partem pravus humor defluat, atque ita deinceps in partem affectam decumbat. Medicamenta autem e capite per os pituitam educentia funt pyrethrum et ftaphis agria; ipforum alterum aut etiam utrumque cum maftiche mi-

μαλασσόμενα καὶ ἅλας βωλικὸν μετὰ γλήχωνος, ἢ νᾶπυ λελειωμένον μετ' ὀξυμέλιτος καὶ διακρατούμενον ἐπὶ πλέον καὶ ἀναγαργαριζόμενον. ἰδίως μὲν οὖν ἕκαστον τῶν καθαρτηρίων φαρμάκων ἕλκει καὶ καθαίρει τὸν οἰκεῖον ἑαυτῷ χυμόν· τὰ μὲν φλέγμα, τὰ δὲ ξανθὴν, τὰ δὲ μέλαιναν χολήν. καὶ μακρὸν ἂν εἴη ἕκαστον κατ' εἶδος διεξιέναι, ἑτέρας ὄντα πραγματείας. κοινῶς δὲ ἐπί τε τῶν ἄλλων ἀλωπεκιῶν καὶ ὀφιάσεων ὠφελεῖν εἴωθε πρῶτα μὲν τὰ διὰ τῆς ἀλόης καταπότια· ἔχει δὲ ταῦτα κολοκυνθίδος ἐντεριώνης μέρος α'. ἀλόης τε καὶ σκαμμωνίας μέρη δύο, χυλοῦ ἀψινθίου μέρος α'. ἀναλάμβανε χυλῷ μήλων, δίδου πρὸς τὴν δύναμιν. μικρὸν δ' ἐπ' αὐτοῖς διαλείποντα ἡμερῶν που ζ'. χρῆσθαι τῇ ἱερᾷ τῇ διὰ κολοκυνθίδων· ἔστι δ' αὐτῆς ἡ σύνθεσις [580] ὧδε. ℞ κολοκυνθίδος ἐντεριώνου τοῦ ἐντὸς ἁπαλοῦ γο. ιστ'. χαμαιπίτυος γο. στ'. σχοίνου ἄνθος γο. στ'. κασσίας, κινναμώμου ἀνὰ γο. στ'. ναρδοστάχυος, σμύρνης ἀνὰ γο. δ'. κρόκου ἑξάγια ζ'. ὀποπάνακος γο. γ'. πεπέρεως μακροῦ καὶ μέλανος ἀνὰ γο. γ'. πρασίου, στοιχάδος, ἀνὰ γο. ζ'. γεντιανῆς, ἀγα-

ſticatur; et ſal globoſum cum pulegio aut ſinapi contritum ex oxymelite et diutius ore contentum ac gargariſatum. Enimvero purgantium medicamentorum quodque proprie peculiarem ſibi humorem trahit educitque: illud pituitam, hoc flavam bilem, aliud atram bilem. Atque longum eſſet unum quodque ſigillatim recenſere, quum alterius id ſit inſtituti. At vulgo alopeciae et ophiaſi prodeſſe conſueverunt, primo pilulae ex aloë; hae vero recipiunt colocynthidis medullae partem j, aloes et ſcamonii partes duas, ſucci abſinthii partem j, excipe ſucco pomorum; dato pro viribus. Deinde paucis, ut ſeptem fere interjectis diebus, utendum hiera diacolocynthidi: ipſius autem compoſitio ita ſe habet. Recipe medullae interioris colcoynthidos fragilis unc. xvj, chamaepityos unc. vj, ſchoenanthi unc. vj, caſſiae, cinnamomi ana unc. vj, ſpicae nardi, myrrhae ana unc. iv, croci ſextulas vij, opopanacis unc. iij, piperis longi et nigri ana unc. iij, marrubii, ſtoechados ana unc. vij, gentianae, agarici

ρικοῦ, ἀνὰ γο. ε΄. σαγαπηνοῦ γο. ι΄. κοπτὰ, λεῖα μέλιτι Ἀττικῷ ἀναλάμβανε, καὶ δίδου καρύου Ποντικοῦ τὸ μέγεθος, εἰς ὕδωρ εἰ πυρέττοιεν, εἰ δὲ μὴ, μετὰ οἰνομέλιτος. ὁ μὲν οὖν κατ᾽ ἀρχὰς τῆς θεραπείας τρόπος τοιόσδε, ἀρκῶν πολλάκις μόνος πρὸς θεραπείαν. ἐπὶ γὰρ τῶν χρονίων δυσίατον ἤδη γίγνεται τὸ πάθος καὶ τοπικῶν δεόμενον φαρμάκων· ὅταν οὖν, ὡς ἐνὶ μάλιστα καθάπερ προείρηται, ἀπέριττον ἐκ τῆς καθάρσεως ἅπαν γένηται τὸ σῶμα, τότε ἤδη θαῤῥοῦντα καὶ τῇ τοῦ βεβλαμμένου μέρους ἐγχειρεῖν θεραπείᾳ, τοῖς τοπικοῖς χρώμενον βοηθήμασι. ἔστι δ᾽ ἅπαντα τῷ γένει θερμὰ καὶ διαφορητικά. ταύτῃ γὰρ τῇ δυνάμει καὶ τὴν κακοχυμίαν κενοῦντα διαφορεῖν πέφυκεν. ἔστι δὲ τάδε, θαψίας χυλὸς μετὰ κηρωτῆς καταχριόμενος. ἄλλο. εὐφόρβιον λεῖον μετὰ ἐλαίου καταχριόμενον. ἄλλο. θεῖον ἄπυρον καὶ νίτρον Ἀλεξανδρινὸν σκευάσας ὄξει κατάχριε. ἄλλο. δάφνινον ἀλειφόμενον, καρδάμου σπέρμα μετ᾽ ἐλαίου. ἄλλο. εὐζώμου σπέρμα λειώσας μετὰ στέατος ἀρνείου κατάχριε. ἄλλο. ἀλκυόνιον τραχὺ καύσας καὶ λειώσας ὄξει, ἢ κεδρίᾳ,

ana unc. v, ſagapeni unc. x, tuſa, trita melle Attico excipe, ac nucis Ponticae magnitudine exhibe, in aqua, ſi ſebricitent; ſi non, in vino mulſo. Per *morbi* initia haec curandi ratio plerumque ſola ſatis eſt ad perfectam curationem; nam diuturnitate curatu jam difficilis affectus redditur, topicisque medicamentis opus habet. Quum igitur, ut ſemel potiſſimum ante dictum eſt, purgatione fuerit jam corpus univerſum vacuum excrementis, tum jam audacter partis affectae curationem aggredieris topicorum remediorum uſu. Sunt autem omnia genere calida et diſcutientia, hac enim facultate cacochymiam tum vacuant tum diſcutiunt; cujusmodi ſunt quae ſequuntur; thapſiae ſuccus cum cerato illitus. *Aliud.* Euphorbium detritum ex oleo inunctum. *Aliud.* Sulphur vivum et nitrum Alexandrinum praeparata ex aceto illine. *Aliud.* Laurinum illitum; cardami ſemen ex oleo. *Aliud.* Erucae ſemen tritum cum ſevo agnino illine. *Aliud.* Alcyonium aſperum uſtum ac laevigatum ex aceto, aut cedrino liquore

κατάχριε. ἄλλο. καλάμου ῥίζαν, ἢ φλοιὸν καύσας μετὰ κέδρου χρῶ, ἢ μετὰ ὑγροπίσσης. ἄλλο. μυῶν κόπρον λειώσας ὄξει κατάχριε. ἄλλο. ἀμύγδαλα ὁλόκληρα καύσας, κατάβρεχε ὄξει δριμεῖ. ἄλλο. ἐχίνου χερσαίου τὸ δέρμα μετὰ τῆς κεφαλῆς κατάκαυσον, καὶ λειώσας μέλιτι κατάχριε. ἄλλο. κρομμύῳ παλαιῷ συνεχῶς ἀπότριβε τὸν τόπον, ὀθόνῃ προανατρίψας, ἕως οὗ ἐρυθρὸν γένηται. ἄλλο. ῥαφάνου φλοιὸν λειώσας μετὰ μέλιτος κατάχριε. ἄλλο. σιδήρῃ στομώματος λεπίδα ὀξελαίῳ τρίψας ἄλειφε, ἕως οὗ ἐρυθρὸν γένηται. ἄλλο. κριθῶν κεκαυμένων καὶ μυοχόδων ἴσον μετὰ ὄξους κατάχριε. ἁπάντων δὲ τῶν εἰρημένων φαρμάκων, τῶν μὲν θερμοτάτων ὄντων, τῶν δ' ἀσθενεστέραν ἐχόντων τὴν θερμασίαν, δῆλον ὡς τοῖς μὲν ἰσχυροῖς φαρμάκοις ἐπὶ σκληρῶν σωμάτων καὶ τῶν κεχρονισμένων διαθέσεων χρηστέον, τοῖς δ' ἀσθενεστέροις ἐπί τε προσφάτων διαθέσεων καὶ παίδων καὶ γυναικῶν καὶ μαλακωτέρων. κοινὸς ἔστω ὁ τοιόσδε λόγος ἐπὶ πάντων βοηθημάτων. προανατρίβειν χρὴ τὸ πεπονθὸς

illine. *Aliud.* Calami radix uſta, aut cortex uſtus ex oleo cedrino, aut pice liquida delinitur. *Aliud.* Murium ſtercus contritum ex aceto inunge. *Aliud.* Integra amygdala uſta acri aceto imbue. *Aliud.* Erinacei terreſtris pellem cum ipſius capite toſtam et in pulverem tuſam ex melle inunge. *Aliud.* Caepam vetuſtam affecto loco, ſed praefricato panno lineo, donec rubescat, frequenter infrica. *Aliud.* Raphani corticem contritum ex melle illinito. *Aliud.* Laevigatam ferri ſquamam ex oleo et aceto tritam inducito, infricans donec locus rubescat. *Aliud.* Hordeum toſtum et mucerdam aequali pondere ex aceto illine. Quum autem omnium dictorum medicamentorum quaedam calidiora ſint, quaedam vero imbecilliorem calorem ſortiantur, manifeſtum eſt validis medicamentis in duris corporibus et inveteratis affectibus utendum eſſe, imbecillioribus vero tum in recentibus affectibus, tum in pueris, mulieribus et molliori carne donatis. Eſto id commune praeceptum in omnibus remediis. Praefricanda eſt

μέρος ὀθόνῃ μήτ' ἄγαν σκληρῶς, ὡς ἀναδέρεσθαι τὰ σώματα, μήτ' ἄγαν μαλακῶς, ὑπὲρ τοῦ ἐρυθραίνεσθαι συμμέτρως πρὸ τῆς χρήσεως τῶν φαρμάκων. χρὴ δὲ καὶ αὐτὸ τὸ δέρμα ξυρᾶν συνεχῶς· εἰ δέ ποτε ἑλκωθείη τὸ μέρος ὑπὸ τῶν φαρμάκων, ἰᾶσθαι χοιρείῳ στέατι ἢ χηνείῳ ὑπαλείφοντα, ἢ ῥοδίνῳ.

Κεφ. γ'. [Πρὸς τὰ τῶν ὤτων πάθη, καὶ πρῶτον πρὸς τὰς ὠταλγίας.] Ὤτων πονοι γίνονται κατὰ ψύχωσιν ὑπὸ ἀνέμων ψυχρῶν, ἢ λουτροῦ ψυχροῦ, καὶ ὑδάτων φαρμακωδῶν εἰσρυέντων, ἢ διὰ φλεγμονὴν, ποτὲ μὲν αὐτοῦ μόνου [581] κατὰ τὸν πόρον τοῦ δέρματος, ποτὲ δὲ καὶ διὰ βάθους τοῦ ἀκουστικοῦ πόρου ἢ μέρους φλεγμήναντος καὶ διατείναντος τὰ μόρια, ἔσθ' ὅτε δὲ καὶ διὰ πνεύματος φυσώδους οὐκ ἔχοντας διέξοδον ὀδυνηρὸν γίνεται. ὀδυνῶσι δὲ καὶ οἱ ἐν αὐτοῖς τοῖς ὠσὶ διά τινα πρόφασιν γεννηθέντες ἰχῶρες. τὰς μὲν οὖν ἀπὸ ψύξεως μόνης γινομένας ὀδύνας τὰ θερμαίνοντα θεραπεύει τάχιστα· ἔστι δὲ ταῦτα κρόμμυον ἐλαίῳ ζέσας ἔγχει τοῖς ὠσίν. ἄλλο. πέπερι εὖ μάλα

pars affecta panno lineo, neque adeo aſpere, ut corpora excorientur, neque adeo leniter, ut non mediocriter rubescant ante medicamentorum localium uſum. Cutis autem ipſa frequenter radenda eſt; quod ſi pars interdum his medicamentis ulceretur, aut ſuillo adipe aut anſerino, aut roſaceo illinenda.

Cap. III. [*Ad aurium affectus, ac primum ad aurium dolores.*] Dolores aurium oboriuntur a frigoribus, a ventis frigidis, aut balneo frigido et aquis medicatis in aurem incidentibus; aut propter inflammationem, interdum ipſius ſolius meatus auditorii cute, interdum una auditorii meatus parte inflammata atque partes diſtendente proximas; interdum etiam a ſpiritu flatulento exitum non habente dolor accidit. Dolores etiam efficit in ipſis auribus quavis occaſione procreata ſanies. Itaque dolores a ſolo frigore obortos celerrime curant caleſacientia. Sunt autem haec. Caepam in oleo elixatam in aures infunde. *Aliud.* Piper curioſe admodum tritum ex oleo.

λελειωμένον μετ' ἐλαίου. ἄλλο. νάρδος ἐγχεομένη θερμη. ἄλλο. πήγανον ἐνεψημένον ἐλαίῳ.

[Πρὸς τὰς ἐκ τῶν ὑδάτων βλάβας τῶν ὤτων.] Ἔλαιον ἐγχέων συνεχῶς θερμὸν δι' ἐρίου μαλακοῦ σπόγγιζε, εἶτ' αὖθις ἔγχει. ἄλλο. ὠοῦ τὸ λευκὸν, ᾧ καὶ πρὸς τὰς ὀφθαλμίας χρώμεθα, ἢ γάλα γυναικεῖον χλιάνας χρῶ. ἄλλο. στέαρ χήνειον, ἢ ἀλωπέκειον, ἢ ὀρνίθειον.

[Πρὸς τὰς ἐν ὠσὶ φλεγμονάς.] Νάρδος μετὰ βασιλικοῦ φαρμάκου ἐγχεομένη· εἰ δ' ἀνύποιστος εἴη ὀδυνη, καστόριον γάλακτι γυναικείῳ, ἢ ὠοῦ τὸ λευκὸν χλιάνας χρῶ. ἄλλο. ὄπιον ἐλάχιστον μετὰ ἑψήματος. οὐ χρὴ δὲ ἐνοχλεῖν τῷ πόρῳ κατὰ τὸν καιρὸν τῆς ὀδύνης, ἀλλὰ καὶ διὰ μηλωτίδος περικείμενον ἐχούσης ἔριον μαλακὸν ἐκμάσσειν· καὶ πυριᾶν δὲ σπόγγοις τρυφεροῖς ἐν ὕδατι (475) ἡψημένην ἔχοντι ἀλθαίαν, ἣν καὶ δενδρομαλάχην καλοῦσιν, ἢ πιτύροις ἐλαφροῖς. εἰ δὲ φυσῶδες εἴη τὸ ἀπολειφθὲν, καὶ ἔμφραξις μᾶλλον ἢ

Aliud. Nardinum calidum auri infuſum. *Aliud.* Ruta in oleo decocta.

[*Ad aurium dolores ex aqua.*] Oleum frequenter infunde calidum, ac molli lana detergendo exuge et iterum atque iterum infunde. *Aliud.* Ovi albo, quo etiam ad oculorum inflammationes utimur, aut lacte muliebri tepido utere. *Aliud.* Adeps anſerinus, aut vulpinus, aut gallinaceus.

[*Ad aurium inflammationes.*] Nardus cum baſilico medicamento infuſa. Quod ſi intolerabilis ſit dolor, caſtorio ex lacte muliebri, aut ovi albo tepido utere. *Aliud.* Exigua opii portio cum ſapa. Cave vero ne auditorio meatui noxa inferatur pro doloris occaſione; ſed is ſpecillo molli lana circumvoluto extergendus; atque fovenda eſt auris ſpongiis mollibus ex aqua cui incocta ſit althaea, quam arboreſcentem malvam vocitant; aut furfuribus lenibus. Quod ſi quod incluſum eſt flatulentum fuerit et obſtructio magis quam dolor obſideat, aphronitro ex ace-

πόνος, ἀφρονίτρῳ μετ' ὄξους χρῶ, ἢ δρακοντίου βοτάνης χυλῷ, ἢ κενταυρίου, ἢ πολίου.

[Περὶ πυρώσεως τῶν ὤτων.] Ἐν δὲ ταῖς ἀρχαῖς πυρώδους αἰσθήσεως περὶ τὸν ἀκουστικὸν πόρον γινομένης, χωρὶς σφυγματώδους ὀδύνης, ὄξος μετὰ ῥοδίνου ὠφελεῖν εἴωθεν.

[Περὶ τῶν ἐν τοῖς ὠσὶ ἑλκῶν.] Γλαύκιον μετ' ὄξους ἀποτρίψας ἔγχει. εἰ δὲ ὑγρὰ πάμπολλα φέροιτο χωρὶς πόνων, σκωρίαν σιδήρου ὄξει λειώσας ἐπιμελῶς ἐν ἡλίῳ χρῶ.

[Πρὸς δυσηκοίας καὶ ἤχους.] Ἐπὶ τῶν ἐξαίφνης ἤχων ὄξος μετὰ ναρδίνου ἔγχει. ἄλλο. κύμινον καὶ ἔλαιον ὡς μέλιτος πάχος ποιήσας ἔγχει. ἐπὶ δὲ τῶν ἐκ νόσου ἤχων ἀψινθίου ἀφεψήματι πυριάσας τὸ ὄξος καὶ τὸ ῥόδινον ἔγχει, ἢ ῥαφάνου χυλὸν μετὰ ῥοδίνου, ἢ ἐλλέβορον μέλαν μετ' ὄξους, ἢ ὄξος δριμὺ καθ' ἑαυτὸ χλιαίνων ἔνσταζε, ἢ μέλι καθ ἑαυτὸ, ἢ ὀξύμελι, ἢ ὀξέλαιον. ἄλλο. πράσου χυλὸν μετὰ γάλακτος γυναικείου ἢ ῥοδίνου ἐγχυμάτιζε. ἄλλο. ἀμυγδάλων

to utitor, aut dracontii herbae ſucco, aut centaurii, aut polii.

[*Pro aurium incendio.*] Per initia ignei ardoris in auditorio meatu oborto ſenſu citra pulſatorium dolorem, hunc acetum cum roſaceo juvare conſuevit.

[*Pro aurium ulceribus.*] Glaucium ex aceto contritum inſtillato. Quod ſi permulta ab his defluat humiditas citra dolores, ſcoriam ferri ex aceto accurate laevigato in ſole utitor.

[*Ad gravem auditum et iteratos aurium ſonitus.*] Ad aurium ſonitus repente obortos acetum cum nardino infunde. *Aliud.* Cuminum et oleum ceu mellis craſſitudinem adepta infunde. Ad ſibilos morbi reliquias ex abſinthii decocto facto fotu, acetum et roſaceum inſtilla; aut raphani ſuccum cum roſaceo, aut veratrum nigrum cum aceto; vel acetum acre per ſe inſtilla tepidum; aut mel per ſe; aut aqua mulſa; aut oxelaeum. *Aliud.* Porri ſuccum cum lacte muliebri aut roſaceo inſtilla. *Aliud.* Amygdarum amararum oleum oleo

πικρῶν ἔλαιον μίξας ἐλαίῳ ἔμβαλε εἰς φλοιὸν κρομμύου, καὶ χλιάνας ἔνσταζε. ἄλλο. κρόμμυον καὶ σκόροδον καὶ στέαρ χήνειον ἴσα τρίψας καὶ διηθήσας ἔγχει. ἄλλο. φακοῦ ἀφέψημα μετὰ μέλιτος ἔγχει. ἄλλο. μυρσίνην ἀφηψημένην ἐν οἴνῳ γλυκεῖ ἔνσταζε, ἢ ἐλαίας φύλλα χυλώσας καὶ μέλιτι μίξας συνέψησον καὶ τούτῳ χρῶ. ἄλλο. κρομμύων χυλίσματι μετὰ μέλιτος χρῶ. ἄλλο. κάρδαμον τρίψας ῥοδίνῳ διεὶς χρῶ. ἢ ἔντερα γῆς ἑψήσας τῷ ἰχῶρι ἐγχυμάτιζε.

[Πρὸς δυσηκοΐας.] Χρῶ μὲν περὶ τὰς ἀρχὰς ἀποφλεγματισμῷ διὰ πυρέθρου καὶ μαστίχης, καὶ τὴν γαστέρα ὕπαγε διὰ τῆς κολυκινθίδος καταποτίοις. εἰς αὐτὸ δὲ τὸ οὖς [582] χρῶ πυρίᾳ διὰ καλάμου, ἀψίνθιον μετὰ ὕδατος ἑψήσας χρῶ. κλύζε δὲ μετὰ τὴν πυρίαν τὸ οὖς ὄξει λευκῷ καὶ ὕδατι ἴσοις, ἐμβληθέντος νίτρου συμβρασθέντος. ἄλλο. δάφνης φύλλα, ἢ δαφνίδας ὁμοίως ἑψήσας χρῶ.

[Ἐγχύματα εἰς τὰ ὦτα.] Πράσου χυλὸν καὶ ἴρινον μύρον μίξας ἐγχυμάτιζε. ἄλλο. χολὴν βοείαν, ἢ αἰγείαν

miſceto, ac in caepae corticem injice, ac tepefactum inſtilla. *Aliud.* Caepam, allium et adipem anſerinum aequa portione trita et colata infundito. *Aliud.* Lentis decoctum cum melle infunde. *Aliud.* Myrtinum decoctum ex vino dulci immittito. *Vel.* Expreſſum ex olivae foliis ſuccum et melli mixtum incoque ac eo utere. Caeparum ſucco expreſſo cum melle utere. *Aliud.* Naſturtium tritum roſaceo diſſolve ac utere. *Vel.* Inteſtina terrae ichori incoque et inſtilla.

[*Ad gravem auditum ſeu audiendi difficultatem.*] Per initia ventrem pilulis ex colocynthide ſubducito, deinde apophlegmatismo utere ex pyrethro et maſtiche. Ad ipſam autem aurem ſotu utere per calamum, abſinthio ex aqua decocto utere. Poſt fotum vero aurem elue aceto albo et aqua pari menſura, injecto nitro ſimul fervefacto. *Aliud.* Lauri foliis vel baccis ſimiliter coctis utitor.

[*Inſtillationes in aures.*] Porri ſuccum et irinum unguentum mixta inſtillato. *Aliud.* Fel bubulum vel ca-

μετὰ ῥοδίνου μίξας ἔνσταζε. ἄλλο. φλοιοῦ τοῦ ῥαφάνου τὸν χυλὸν σὺν τῷ ῥοδίνῳ λεάνας ἔνσταζε.

[Πρὸς τοὺς ἐν ὠσὶ σκώληκας.] Ἐφ' ὧν δὲ σκώληκές εἰσι, βοείου κρέατος παρωπτημένου τὸν ἰχῶρα λαβὼν ἔνσταζε, ἢ ἀριστολοχίαν λειώσας ἔμπλαττε· ἢ καλαμίνθην ἔνσταζε, ἢ βάτου χυλόν. ὁμοίως δὲ καὶ ἀψινθίου χυλὸν ἔνσταζε.

[Περὶ παρωτίδων.] Αἱ ἐκ νόσων συμβαίνουσαι παρωτίδες διαφέρουσι τῶν ἄλλως γινομένων φλεγμονῶν· διάφορον δὲ καὶ τὴν θεραπείαν ἀπαιτοῦσιν. ἐπὶ μὲν γὰρ τῶν διὰ ῥεύματος ἐπιφορὰν γιγνομένων, εἰ μήτε πολὺ εἴη τὸ ἐπιῤῥέον, μήτε κακόηθες, μήτε πληθωρικοῦ τοῦ ὅλου σώματος ὑπάρχοντος, σπόγγος μόνος ἐπιτεθεὶς ὀξυκράτῳ καταστέλλει τὰς ἀρχομένας φλεγμονάς. ἐπὶ δὲ τῶν παρωτίδων τῶν ἄλλου νοσήματος ἐκγόνων πᾶν τοὐναντίον ἐργαζόμεθα, φαρμάκοις ἑλκτικοῖς χρώμενοι καὶ σικύαν προσφέροντες. βουλόμεθα γὰρ ἐκ τοῦ βάθους ἐπὶ τὸ δέρμα τὸν λυποῦντα χυμὸν ἐπισπάσασθαι. ὅταν μέντοι σφοδρὰν ὁρμὴν ἐξ ἑαυτοῦ ἔχῃ τὸ ἐπιῤ-

prinum cum roſaceo mixtum inſtillato. *Aliud.* Corticis raphani ſuccum ex roſaceo ſubigendo impone.

[*Ad aurium vermes.*] In quibus autem ſunt vermes, bubulae carnis inter aſſandum deſluentem liquorem inſtilla. *Vel.* Ariſtolochiam tritam ceu emplaſtrum admove. *Aut.* Calaminthem inſtilla, vel rubi ſuccum. Eodem modo abſinthii ſuccum inſtilla.

[*Pro parotidibus.*] Quae ex morbis oriuntur parotides ab inflammationibus alio modo procreatis differunt, proinde diverſam etiam curationem poſtulant. In iis enim quae ob defluxionis decubitum nascuntur, ſi neque copioſus qui defluit humor fuerit, neque malignus; etiam ſi neque totum corpus plethoricum existat, ſola ſpongia ex poſca impoſita incipientes inflammationes ſiſtit. In parotidibus autem ex alio morbo productis contrarium molimur, attrahentibus utentes *remediis* etiam cucurbitulam admovemus. Volumus enim ab alto ad cutim noxium humorem attrahere. Quum tamen vehementem ex ſe impetum de-

ῥέον, οὐδὲν ἡμεῖς τηνικαῦτα προσπεριεργαζόμεθα τῇ φύσει. ἐν τούτῳ γὰρ, ἐὰν ἤτοι σικύαν ἢ φάρμακον ἕλκον ἐκ τοῦ βάθους ἐπὶ τὸ δέρμα τοὺς χυμοὺς ἐπενέγκωμεν, ὀδύνη σφοδρὰ καταλαμβάνει τὸν ἄνθρωπον, ὡς δι' αὐτὴν ἀγρυπνίας τε γίνεσθαι καὶ πυρετοὺς ἐπιγίνεσθαι καὶ τὴν δύναμιν καταλύεσθαι. παρηγορεῖν οὖν τηνικαῦτα μᾶλλον, οὐ συμπράττειν τῇ ῥοπῇ τῶν χυμῶν προσήκει, καταπλάσμασι χρωμένους παρηγορητικωτάτοις· ἔστι δὲ τάδε.

[*Πρὸς ἐπωδύνους παρωτίδας.*] Ἄρτον μετ' ἐλαίου κατάπλασσε. ἄλλο. πύρινον ἄλευρον μετ' ἐλαίου κατάπλασσε. ἄλλο. κρίθινον ἄλευρον μετὰ ἀξουγγίου κατάπλασσε. ἄλλο. ὑοσκύαμον βοτάνην μετὰ βουτύρου κατάπλασσε. ἐὰν δὲ ἐκπυήσωσι, διὰ τομῆς ἐκκρῖναι χρὴ τὸ πῦον, καὶ ἰᾶσθαι τὸ ἕλκος κοινῶς, ἢ πειρᾶσθαι διαφορεῖν αὐτὸ φαρμάκοις ἑλκτικήν τε ἅμα καὶ λεπτομερῆ δύναμιν ἔχουσιν, ἀφαιροῦντας δὶς τῆς ἡμέρας αὐτὰ, καὶ πυριᾷν, μέχρις ἂν ἐνδῶσιν αἱ ὀδύναι. ἔστι δὲ παυσαμένης τῆς ὀδύνης διαφορητικὰ τάδε.

fluens humor habet, tum nihil eorum nos molimur quod naturae opituletur. Tunc enim fi aut cucurbitulam, aut medicamentum quod ex alto ad cutim humores attrahat admoverimus, dolor adeo ingens hominem prehendit, ut eo et vigiliae concitentur et febres fuccedant et vires profternantur. Proinde hic lenientibus potiffimum medicamentis opus eft, non iis quae humorum fluxum juvant; cataplasmatis, inquam, utendum eft, maxime lenientibus, quae fubfequuntur.

[*Ad dolorem inferentes parotidas.*] Panem cum oleo ad formam cataplafmatis admove. *Aliud.* Triticeam farinam cum oleo cataplasma admove. *Aliud.* Ex hordeacea farina et axungia cataplasma admove. *Aliud.* Hyoscyamum herbam cum butyro admove. Quod fi fuppurent parotides, incifione pus excernendum eft et ulcus vulgari methodo curandum, aut medicamentis ipfum difcutere tentandum, attrahendi fimulque attenuandi facultate praeditis, iisque bis diebus fingulis renovandis; atque foven-

ἀρνογλώσσῳ λείῳ μεθ' ἁλῶν κατάπλασσε, ἢ λαπάθου ῥίζης ἡψημένης ἐν οἴνῳ, ἢ θείῳ ἀπύρῳ καὶ κιμωλίᾳ μετ' ὄξους, ἢ σύκων ἐν ἅλμῃ ἡψημένων καὶ ἐπιτιθεμένων λείων, ἢ πράσιον μεθ' ἁλῶν· ἢ ἅλας λεῖον μετὰ βουτύρου οἰσυπηρῷ ἐρίῳ ἐπιθέντος, μάλιστα πρὸς τὰς ἀρχομένας παρωτίδας, καὶ μάλιστα ἐπὶ τῶν ἁπαλοσάρκων· ἐπὶ δὲ τῶν ἀνωδύνων καὶ ἐσκιῤῥωμένων κόπρος αἰγεία μετ' ὄξους καταπλασσομένη. ἐφ' ὧν μέντοι ἐκπυῆσαι ταχέως βουλόμεθα, ἀπαντλήσομεν ὕδατι θερμῷ συνεχῶς καὶ κριθίνοις ἀλεύροις καταπλάσομεν.

[583] Κεφ. δ'. [Περὶ τῶν ἐν τῇ ῥινὶ παθῶν, καὶ πρῶτον ὀζαινῶν καὶ πολυπόδων.] Ῥινῶν θεραπεία κοινὴ ὀζαινῶν πολύπων. ξηρᾶναι πρῶτον καὶ ῥῶσαι τὴν κεφαλὴν, ἐπιτιθέντας ἢ τὴν δι' ἰτεῶν, ἢ ἀνεμωνίτην, ἢ τὴν διὰ κοχλιῶν. ἡ δὲ σύνθεσίς ἐστιν ἥδε. ♃ σμύρνης γο. α'. λιβάνου γο. α'. κοχλίας ὁλοκλήρους β'. ᾠῶν τὰ λευκὰ β'. ὁλμοκοπήσας μίξας ἅπαντα κατάχριε, ἐντιθεὶς ὀθόνῃ ἐπὶ ἡμέρας θ'.

dum, quoad fedentur dolores. At fedato dolore haec discutientia aderunt. Ex arnogloffo contufo cum fale fac cataplasma. *Vel.* Cocta rumicis radix ex vino admoveatur. *Vel.* Sulphur vivum et cimolia cum aceto fici in muria cocti, fubacti, impofiti. *Vel.* Marrubium cum fale. *Vel.* Sal tritum cum butyro fuccida lana admotum maxime ad incipientes parotidas, potiffimumque in tenera carne donatis. In *parotidibus* vero dolore carentibus et induratis ftercus caprinum cum aceto admotum. Sed certe in quibus celeriter pus movere volumus, parotidas aqua calida fovebimus et farina hordeacea oblinemus.

Cap. IV. [*Ad narium affectiones, primumque ad ozaenam et polypum.*] Narium affectarum curatio ozaenis et polypis communis. Primo exiceandum roborandumque caput eft impofitis emplaftris vel de falicibus, vel de anemonite, vel barbaro, vel de limacibus, cujus haec eft compofitio. Recipe myrrhae unc. j, thuris unc. j, limaces integros ij, ovorum alba ij, omnia contufa in pila mi-

καὶ οὕτως τοῖς τοπικοῖς χρῶ. ἔστι δὲ τάδε. καλαμίνθης χυλῷ ἐγχυμάτιζε. ἢ αὐτὴν ξηράνας τὴν καλαμίνθην ἐμφύσα διὰ καλάμου. ἄλλο. βατραχείῳ χυλῷ μετὰ μέλιτος ἐγχυμάτιζε εἰς τὴν ῥῖνα ὕπτιον κατακλίνας καὶ κέλευε ἀνασπᾷν. ἄλλο. ῥοιᾶς χυλὸν ἐν χαλκῷ ἀγγείῳ ἑψήσας, ἔα παχυνθῆναι, εἶτα ἐγχυμάτιζε. ἄλλο. κηκῖδας καὶ σμύρναν ἴσα κόψας προσφύσα.

[Περὶ πολύπων.] ℞ Χαλκάνθου κεκαυμένου λίτρας δ'. μίλτου γο. α'. λεάνας ἐμφύσα διὰ καλάμου. ἄλλο. βρυωνίας ῥίζης κεκαυμένης ἐμφύσα. ἄλλο. χαλκάνθου καὶ σανδαράχης ἴσα, λεῖα ἐμφύσα. ἄλλο. κέρατος ἐλαφείου κεκαυμένου καὶ σανδαράχης ἐμφύσα. ἄλλο. μόλυβδον κατακαύσας, καὶ οἴνῳ ἀναλαβὼν κατάχριε. ἄλλο. ῥοιᾶς ὀξείας χυλὸν ἐν χαλκῷ ἀγγείῳ βαλὼν, ἑψήσας, ὡς μέλιτος πάχος ἔχῃ, καὶ διάχριε. ἄλλο. ἀρσενικὸν τρίψας μήλῃ προσάπτου. ἄλλο. ἀρσενικὸν καὶ ἄσβεστον ἴσα λειώσας πρόσαπτε.

[Περὶ τῆς ἐκ ῥινῶν αἱμοῤῥαγίας.] Τοὺς θρόμβους

ſceantur, linteo excepta per dies ix, admove. Sicque topicis utitor. Haec autem ſunt. Calaminthes ſuccus naribus infuſus. Vel ipſam arefactam ac tritam calaminthem calamo inſpira. *Aliud.* Ranunculi ſuccum cum melle ſupine jacentis naribus infunde et ut attrahat praecipe. *Aliud.* Mali punici ſuccum aereo vaſe decoquito, quoad craſſeſcat, deinde naribus infundito. *Aliud.* Gallas ac myrrham pari portione conterito ac inſpirato.

[*Ad polypos.*] Recipe chalcanthi uſti lib. iv, minii unc. j, trita calamo inſpira. *Aliud.* Recipe bryoniae radicis uſtae pulverem, inſpira. *Aliud.* Recipe chalcanthi et ſandarachae paria, trita inſpira. *Aliud* Recipe cornucervi uſti et ſandaraches par pondus, inflato. *Aliud.* Plumbum uſtum et vino exceptum illine. *Aliud.* Recipe acidi mali punici ſuccum, in aereo vaſe coquito, ut mellis conſiſtentiam ſortiatur et illinito. *Aliud.* Arſenicum tritum ſtillo applicato. *Aliud.* Arſenicum et calcem pari pondere trita applicato.

[*Ad ſanguinis e naribus profluvia.*] Grumos prius

πρότερον ἐκκαθάρας τοῦ στόματος μηλωτῇ ἔριον ἐχούσῃ βεβρεγμένον ὕδατι, οὕτως λύκιον ἀναλύσας, ὕδατι διάβρεχε, καὶ στρεπτὸν ποιήσας δι᾽ ὀθόνης καὶ βρέξας λυκίῳ διασφήνου. ἄλλο. στρεπτὸν καύσας ἐναπόσβεσον χυλῷ πολυγόνου ἢ πράσου καὶ θὲς εἰς τὸν μυκτῆρα. ἄλλο. ὄξος δριμύτατον ζέσας καὶ ἀποβρέξας σπόγγον, διασφήνου τοὺς μυκτῆρας, ἵνα δὲ εὐχερῶς ἔχῃς ἐξέλκειν τὸν σπόγγον, ὅτε βούλει, λίνῳ ἀπόδησον, ὡς ἀπηρτῆσθαι τοῦ μυκτῆρος. ψῦχε δὲ τὸ μέτωπον σπόγγοις καὶ μετέωρον ἔχειν τὴν κεφαλὴν κέλευε. διαδέσμει δὲ χεῖρας καὶ (476) πόδας καὶ ὦτα ἔμφραττε. ἄλλο. γύψῳ ἢ πηλῷ κεραμικῷ τὸ μέτωπον κατάχριε. ἄλλο. σικύαν σφοδρὰν ἐὰν μὲν ἀπὸ δεξιοῦ μυκτῆρος φέρηται, τῷ ἥπατι πρόσβαλε, ἐὰν δ᾽ ἀπὸ ἀριστεροῦ τῷ σπληνὶ, ἐὰν δ᾽ ἀπὸ ἀμφοτέρων, εἰς ἑκάτερα πρόσβαλε.

[Πρὸς τὰς ἀπὸ μυκτήρων αἱμοῤῥαγίας.] Πύρινα ἄλευρα χυλῷ πράσου ἀναλαβὼν καὶ στρεπτὸν ποιήσας καὶ χρίσας ἐντίθει τῷ αἱμοῤῥαγοῦντι μυκτῆρι. ἄλλο. στρεπτὸν δι᾽ ὀθόνην ποιήσας συναπόβρεχε ὄξει δριμεῖ καὶ λύχνῳ καύσας ἐμ-

oris specillo lanam aqua madentem continente abſterge. Ita lycium aqua diſſolutum perſunde, penecilloque intorque ac impinge. *Aliud.* Linamentum tortile igne accenſum et polygoni aut porri ſucco extinctum naribus inſerito. *Aliud.* Acetum acerrimum coquito et inebriata eo ſpongia in nares impinge: ut vero tempeſtive ſpongiam extrahere queas, quum volueris, eam lineo filo deligato, ita ut naribus id appendatur. Frontem praeterea ſpongiis refrigera et erectum habere caput impera; manus et pedes vinculis conſtringito et aures obturato. *Aliud.* Gypſo aut luto figulino fronti admove. *Aliud.* Cucurbitulam magnam admove, hepati quidem, profluente e dextra nare ſanguine; lieni vero, ſi e ſiniſtra, ſin ex utraque nare effluat, utrique viſceris regioni.

[*Ad ſanguinis e naribus profluvium.*] Ex triticea farina porri ſucco excepta verſatilem turundam forma, narique ſanguinem profundenti inſerito. *Aliud.* Tortile linamentum aceto acri madens ad lucernam urito et nari

βαλε τῷ μυκτῆρι. ἄλλο. ὀνίδος θερμῆς χυλὸν ἴσῳ ὄξει μίξας καὶ ἐπιβαλὼν πύρινα ἄλευρα, ποίει γλοιῶδες καὶ χρίσας στρεπτὸν ἐπιτίθει. χρῶ δὲ καὶ διαδέσμοις κατά τε τῶν ποδῶν καὶ τῶν χειρῶν καὶ ψῦχε τὴν κεφαλήν. καὶ σικύαις χρῶ κατὰ τῶν ὑποχονδρίων· δεξιοῦ μὲν μυκτῆρος αἱμοῤῥαγοῦντος, ἐπὶ τοῦ ἥπατος σφοδρὰν τίθει τὴν σικύαν· ἐπὶ δὲ ἀρι [584] στεροῦ κατὰ τοῦ σπληνός. περὶ δὲ ἀναγωγῆς αἵματος μικρὸν ὕστερον εἴρηται.

[Περὶ τῆς ἐκ τραυμάτων αἱμοῤῥαγίας.] Εἰ δὲ ἐπὶ τραύματος αἱμοῤῥαγία γένηται, λειώσας σμύρναν καὶ λίβανον καὶ ἀναλαβὼν ᾠοῦ τῷ λευκῷ ἐπίβαλε, χρώμενος ἐπεικασμῷ πρὸς τετυπωμένον. ἄλλο. βάτραχον καύσας τῇ σποδιᾷ τὸ τραῦμα κατάπλασσε. χρῶ δὲ καὶ ὀξυκράτῳ, ὡς σπόγγους ἐπιτιθεὶς συνεχῶς περὶ τῆς χρήσεως τοῦ ξηροῦ. ἄλλο. ὀνίδα θερμὴν καταπλάσας ἐπιδέσμει. εἰ δὲ ξηρὰ εἴη, ὄξους πρόσβαλε βραχέως.

Κεφ. ε'. [Πρὸς τὰ τῶν ὀφθαλμῶν πάθη.] Ἅπαντα μὲν τὰ μόρια τοῦ σώματος ἀκριβεστάτων χρήζει διορισμῶν ἐν

infere. *Aliud.* Afinini fimi calentis fuccum mixtum cum aequali aceto et adjecta farina triticea ftrigmenti craffamentum efforma et illitum eo linamentum impone. Utere vero tum pedum tum manuum vinculis et caput refrigera. Ufurpa quoque cucurbitulas hypochondriis affigendas; profundente quidem dextra nare fanguinem, hepatis regioni magnam cucurbitulam admove; profluente vero e finiftra fanguine, fplenis regioni. De fanguinis autem rejectione paulo poft dictum eft.

[*De fanguinis profluvio e vulnere.*] Sed fi e vulnere fanguinis profluvium oriatur, myrrham et thus trita et ovi albo excepta partis percuffae ratione impone. *Aliud.* Uftae ranae cinere vulnus obtura; utere quoque oxycrato, ut eo inebriatos fpongias frequenter ficcitatis ratione fuperponas. *Aliud.* Afininum fimum calidum cataplasmatis modo alliga: quod fi aridus fuerit, aceti pauxillum adjice.

Cap. V. [*Ad oculorum affectiones.*] Omnes fane corporis partes in morborum curationibus accuratiffimis

ταῖς θεραπείαις, εἰ μέλλοιεν ὄντως ἰαθήσεσθαι. ὀφθαλμοὶ δ' ὅσον κυριωτάτην ἔχουσι τὴν χρείαν, καὶ οὐκ ὀλίγον τῶν ἄλλων διαφέρουσιν, ἀκριβεστάτης ἐπισκέψεως δέονται, συχνῶν τῶν περὶ αὐτοὺς παθῶν γιγνομένων, καὶ ἐπὶ ποικίλαις καὶ διαφόροις αἰτίαις συνισταμένων τε καὶ παροξυνομένων. ἀλλ' ὁ μὲν τελειότατος καὶ ἀκριβέστατος περὶ αὐτῶν λόγος ἑτέρας ἐστὶ πραγματείας· ὁ δὲ ἐνεστὼς τῆς προκειμένης πραγματείας στοχαζόμενος διδάσκει τὸ χρήσιμον κατὰ τὸ ἐνδεχόμενον. αἱ τοίνυν περὶ τοὺς ὀφθαλμοὺς διαθέσεις ὁτὲ μὲν μετὰ πυρώσεως συνίστανται, ὁτὲ δὲ μετὰ ψύξεως καὶ ναρκώδους αἰσθήσεως, καὶ ποτὲ μὲν μετὰ φλεγμονῆς, ποτὲ δὲ χωρὶς φλεγμονῆς, καὶ ἔσθ' ὅτε μὲν μετὰ δαψιλοῦς ῥεύματος, ἔσθ' ὅτε δὲ χωρὶς ῥεύματος, καὶ ποτὲ μὲν μετὰ βάρους καὶ ὀδύνης, ποτὲ δὲ καὶ χωρὶς τούτων. τὰς μὲν οὖν μικρὰς καὶ πυρώδεις ταράξεις ἱκανὸν καὶ ὀξύκρατον ἀποκρούσασθαι, ὥσπερ τὰς ἐκ ψύξεως αἱ διὰ σπόγγων ἐξ οἴνου κεκραμένου λευκοῦ πυρίαι· τὰς δὲ ἰσχυρὰς διαθέσεις καὶ σὺν φλεγμονῇ μεγάλῃ καὶ βαρείᾳ, ἐὰν μὲν τὰ κατὰ τὸ μέτωπον ἀγγεῖα πλήρη ᾖ, καὶ διατετα-

egent diſtinctionibus, ſi revera ſanitatem adepturae ſint. Verum oculi quo praeſtantiſſimum habent uſum, neque paululum ab aliis diſcrepant, eo accuratiſſimam conſiderationem efflagitant, quum frequentes ipſis oboriantur affectus, qui ex variis ac diſcrepantibus cauſis conſtituuntur et exacerbantur. Verum perfectiſſima et accuratiſſima de his oratio alterius eſt operis; ſed quae praeſens propoſitum opus reſpicit, utile quantum poteſt edocet. Affectus igitur oculorum interdum ab aeſtu ortum habent, interdum a frigore et ſtupente ſenſu; interdum etiam cum inflammatione, interdum citra inflammationem, interdum quoque ab exuperante humorum defluxu, interdum etiam citra defluxum; nonnunquam cum gravitate et dolore, nonnunquam etiam ſine his. Equidem leves et fervidas oculorum perturbationes abunde poſca reprimit, quemadmodum ex frigore obortos ſpongiis vino albo diluto inebriatis fotus. At vehementes affectus et cum magna gravique inflammatione, ſi frontis vaſa repleta ac diſtenta

μένα, καὶ αὐτόθεν ἐμφαίνει τὸ πλῆθος τοῦ αἵματος, φλεβοτομία μὲν ἐν ἀρχῇ, εἰ μή τι κωλύει· τὰς δ' ἐφ' ἑτέρας γιγνομένας καὶ παροξυνομένας διὰ ἔμφραξιν ἡ διὰ τῆς κάτω γαστρὸς κάθαρσις· χρῆσθαι δὲ δεῖ τοῖς ἐγχύτοις τήξεως χυλῷ μάλα καλῶς κατεσκευασμένῳ. καλῶς δ' ἂν γένοιτο, εἰ πλυθείη ἡ τῆλις ἐπιμελῶς ὕδατι γλυκεῖ, ἑψηθεῖσά τε ἐπ' ὀλίγον, ὡς ἅπαν τὸ ἐν αὐτῇ δριμὺ ἀποθέσθαι, εἶτ' αὖθις ἑτέρῳ ὕδατι ἑψηθεῖσα ἀποχυθέντος τοῦ προτέρου. χρήσιμον δὲ καὶ τοῦ ὠοῦ τὸ λευκὸν καὶ λεπτὸν, συνεχῶς ἐγχεόμενον, καὶ γάλα γυναικεῖον ἐκ τῶν μαζῶν αὐτῶν ἐκθλιβόμενον τοῖς ὀφθαλμοῖς. ἔστω δὲ εὔχυμον τὸ γάλα. παρηγορεῖν δὲ καὶ καταπλάσμασι κούφοις τὰς φλεγμονὰς διά τε ὠοῦ λεπιοῦ καὶ λεκίθου καὶ μελιλώτου καὶ ἄρτου καὶ ῥοδίνου. εἰ δὲ καὶ κολλυρίων εὐπορία ἐπιτηδείων, ἃ διὰ τῆς μακρᾶς πείρας σχεδὸν πᾶσίν ἐστι γνώριμα, ἄλλων ἄλλοις συνειθισμένων χρῆσθαι, καὶ τούτοις μετὰ τοῦ λεπτοτάτου ὠοῦ, κούφως δὲ καὶ ἀθλίπτως φέρειν· καὶ τὰς ἐμφερομένας τοῖς ὀφθαλμοῖς λήμας σπόγγῳ ἁπαλῷ δι' ὕδατος θερμοῦ ἀφαιρεῖν, καὶ λε-

fint, indeque fefe prodat fanguinis plenitudo, curat per initia venae fectio, nifi quid prohibeat: ab alia vero caufa factas atque per obftructionem concitatas ventris per inferiora vacuatio; poftea infufis utendum eft ex foenigraeci fucco pulcherrime praeparato. Quod recte fiet, fi lotum diligenter in aqua dulci foenumgraecum leviter coquatur, ut quicquid acre in fe habet, abjiciat; deinde rurfus alteri aquae incoquatur affufa priore. Utile etiam eft ovi candidum ac tenue frequenter inftillatum et lac muliebre ex mammis ipfis in oculos emulfum. Sit autem lac optimi fucci. Leniendae porro cataplasmatis levibus inflammationes ex ovi tenui luteo, meliloto, pane et rofaceo. Quin utendum etiam collyriis pro facultate idoneis, quae longa experientia prope omnibus innotefcunt, aliis alio uti confuetis, haecque cum tenuiffimo ovo leviter et citra laborem adhibenda. Gramiae porro oculis illatae fpongia molli ex aqua calida abftergendae, tenuiffimoque victu utendum. Quod fi immoderata fuerit ca-

πτοτάτη διαίτη χρῆσθαι. εἰ δ' ἄμετρον εἴη τὸ τῆς κεφαλῆς βάρος, ἀφαιρεῖν τε τὰς κόμας καὶ σικύᾳ χρῆσθαι κατὰ τοῦ ἰνίου μετ' ἐγχαράξεως, συχνὸν τοῦ αἵματος ἀποσχέοντας. ἀτμῶν δὲ πεπληρωκότων τὴν κεφαλὴν καὶ φλέγματος ὄντος τοῦ ἐμφράττοντος τὰς διεξόδους τῶν πόρων, πταρμικοῖς τε τοῖς ἐπιεικεστέροις, καὶ δι' ἀποφλεγματισμῶν κενώσομεν [585] καὶ διαλύσομεν τὴν σφήνωσιν, πταρμικῷ μὲν πεπέρι λείῳ χρώμενοι, κελεύοντες τοῖς μυκτῆρσιν ἀνέλκειν τοὺς πεπονθότας, ἀποφλεγματισμοῖς δὲ τοῖς διὰ νάπυος λειουμένου εὖ μάλα τοῦ νάπυος, καὶ προσλαμβάνοντος ὄξους λευκοῦ συμμέτρου, καὶ μέλιτος καὶ ὕδατος, ὅπως ὑγρὸν γενόμενον διακρατεῖητο καὶ ἀναγαργαρίζοιτο· ῥᾳδίως γὰρ δύνανται ὄντως καὶ αὐτῶν διὰ τῶν μυκτήρων καὶ τοῦ οὐρανίσκου τῆς κενώσεως δαψιλοῦς γενομένης, τὰς περὶ τὴν κεφαλὴν σφηνώσεις διαλυθῆναι. ὅτι δὲ τὸ προηγούμενον καὶ οἷον κεφάλαιον τῆς θεραπείας οὐκ ἐπὶ ὀφθαλμιώντων μόνον, ἀλλὰ καὶ ἐπὶ πάντων σχεδὸν τῶν ἄλλων παθῶν, ἐν τῇ ἀκριβείᾳ μάλιστα τῆς διαίτης κεῖται, οὐδένα οἶμαι τοῦτο ἀγνοεῖν. χρώμεθα δὲ πρὸς τὰς θε-

pitis gravitas et capillitium auferendum eſt et cucurbitula occipitio affigenda cum ſcarificatione, copioſusque ſanguis detrahendus. Quum autem vapores caput repleverint, ac pituita pervios meatus obſtruat, ſternutatoriis mitioribus et apophlegmatismis vacuabimus, ſtipationemque diſſolvemus. Sternutatoriis quidem ex pipere trito utimur, quod naribus aegrotos attrahere imperamus; apophlegmatismis vero ex ſinapi accuratiſſime laevigato additis aceto albo moderato et melle et aqua, ita ut quod liquidum factum eſt retineatur et gargarizetur. Ita enim facile his per nares et palatum facta evacuatione copioſa capitis obſtructiones diſſolvi queunt. Quod autem primarius praecipuusque ſcopus curationis non ſolum ophthalmia laborantium, verum etiam caeterorum prope omnium morborum in accurata victus ratione conſtet, neminem ignorare arbitror. Caeterum ad aeſtivas ophthalmias aridarum roſa-

ρινὰς ὀφθαλμίας καὶ ῥόδων ἀφεψήματι ξηρῶν, τούτῳ συνεχῶς ἀποσπογγίζοντες τὰ βλέφαρα.

[Πρὸς τὰς ἐκ χρόνων ὀφθαλμίας.] Πυρῆνα μήλης καθέντες εἰς σκόροδον, ὡς χρωσθῆναι τῷ χυλῷ ἐγχρίομεν. ἄλλο. πυροὺς ἐπὶ διαπύρων σιδήρων ὀπτήσαντες σὺν οἴνῳ καταχρίομεν τὰ βλέφαρα. ἄλλο. χάλκανθον λειώσαντες ἐν μέλιτι, χρίομεν τὸ μέτωπον καὶ τὰ βλέφαρα.

[Ἀρχιγένους ἐκλογαὶ ἐκ τῶν συνθέτων περὶ τῶν εἰς τοὺς ὀφθαλμοὺς ῥευμάτων.] Ἐπὶ τῶν κατὰ τοὺς ὀφθαλμοὺς ῥευματισμῶν ἐν ἀρχῇ μὲν ἁρμόζει ὀλιγοσιτία καὶ ὑδροποσία καὶ πάντων μᾶλλον συνουσίας ἀποχὴ, καὶ ἡ κοιλία ὑποσυρέσθω, καὶ πολυ ψυχρὸν τὸ ποτὸν, εἶτα καὶ ὀλίγου ὄξους ὕδατι μιγέντος, συνεχῶς τὸ πρόσωπον προσκλυζέσθωσαν. ἔνιοι δὲ χάλκανθον ὕδατι δεύοντες διδόασι προσκλύζεσθαι. περικαμπτέσθωσαν ὀσμὰς δριμείας, κονιορτοὺς, καπνόν τε καὶ τὴν ἀφ' ἡλίου καὶ τὴν ἀπὸ λύχνου αὐγήν. εἰς νύκτα δὲ ἔρια καθαρὰ ἐξ οἴνου, ἢ ῥυπαρὰ ἐξ ὕδατος ψυχροῦ ἐπιτιθέσθωσαν, ἕωθεν δὲ, ὡς εἴρηται, προκλυζέσθωσαν. εἰ δ'

rum decocto utimur, eo fpongiis inebriatis oculorum palpebras crebro foventes.

[*Ad diuturnas lippitudines.*] Mucronem fpecilli allio infertum quoad fucco tingatur, inducimus. *Aliud.* Triticum ignitis ferreis laminis incoctum ex vino palpebras illinimus. *Aliud.* Vitriolo in melle trito et frontem et palpebras inungimus.

[*Archigenis fecreta ex compofitis pro oculorum fluxionibus medicamentis.*] Ad irruentes in oculos fluxiones inprimis conducunt paucitas tum cibi, tum potus, aquae potus ac prae omnibus abfoluta a coitu continentia, ventris inferioris fubductio, frigidae multae potio, deinde frontis frequens irroratio ex aqua aceti pauxillo admixta. Nonnulli chalcanthum aqua perfundentes ad fotum tradunt. Fugiant odores acres, pulverem, fumum et fplendorem tum a fole tum a lampade prodeuntem. Noctu lana munda ex vino, aut fordida ex aqua frigida; mane vero, ut dictum eft, abluantur. At fi fluxio ingravefcat, fuccedatque dolor,

ἐπιτείνοιτο ὁ ῥευματισμὸς καὶ ἀλγηδὼν ἐπιγένηται, φλεβοτομία τε ἁρμόζει, καὶ τελέως ἀσιτία καὶ δίψα, εἰ μὴ ἐκκενοῖτο καὶ ἐπιτείνοιτο· κοιλίας εὔτονος λύσις, ἤτοι διὰ συμφώνου καθαρτικοῦ, ἢ διὰ κλυστήρων εὐτόνων. μετὰ ταῦτα δὲ κατὰ τοῦ μετώπου ἀμπέλου φύλλα χλωρὰ συνεχῶς ἐπιτιθέμενα ὠφελεῖ, ἢ μυρσίνης, ἢ σχίνου, ἢ βάτου χύλισμα, ἢ κράμβης, ἢ ἀμπέλου φύλλα μετὰ λεπτοῦ ἀλφίτου, ἢ σαμψύχου, ἢ ἀειζώου, ἢ ἀνδράχνης, ἢ κυδωνίων. τὰ δ' ἁπαλὰ φύλλα ἕκαστα αὐτῶν μετ' οἴνου, καὶ τοῦ λεπτοῦ τῶν ἀλφίτων ἐπὶ τοῦ μετώπου καταπλασσόμενα. κατ' αὐτῶν δὲ τῶν ὀφθαλμῶν καθαρὸν ἔριον ὠοῦ τῷ λευκῷ διαβρέχων, καὶ ὠοῦ λέκυθον ἑφθὴν μετ' οἴνου, καὶ τοῦ λεπτοῦ τῶν ἀλφίτων ἐπὶ τὸ μέτωπον ἐπιπλαττόμενα, ἢ καὶ ἐπ' αὐτοὺς ἐπιτιθέμενα τοὺς ὀφθαλμοὺς, καὶ ἠρυγγίου ῥίζαν λείαν μεθ' ὕδατος, καὶ κωνείου σπέρμα τὸν αὐτὸν κατασκευαζόμενα τρόπον ὠφελεῖ. καὶ τυρὸς ἁπαλὸς νεαλὴς μετὰ σελίνου φύλλων καταπλασσόμενος, καὶ ἄρτος ἐξ οἴνου, ἢ ῥοδίνου φυραθεὶς ὠφελεῖ θαυμαστῶς. καὶ καθόλου πᾶν τὸ τῶν στυφόντων γένος, καὶ

convenit venae ſectio et ſumma inedia et ſitis, niſi exhauriantur *aegri* et ingraveſcat morbus. Sit alvi vehemens ſolutio, aut idoneo medicamento purgante, aut validioribus clyſteribus. Poſt haec fronti vitis ſolia viridia continue appoſita juvant, aut myrti, aut lentisci, aut ſuccus rubi vel braſſicae, aut vitis folia cum tenui polenta; vel ſampſuchi, vel ſempervivi, vel portulacae, vel cotoneorum. Eorum enim quoque ſolia tenera cum vino et tenui polenta in cataplasmatis forma fronti admoventur. Ipſis autem oculis munda lana ovi alba imbuta, nec non coctum ovi luteum cum vino et tenui polenta, ad ſormam emplaſtri fronti, aut ad formam epithematis ipſis oculis admovetur. Juvat quoque eryngii radicem tritam ex aqua et cicutae ſemen eodem modo comparare. Etiam caſeus mollis recens cum apii ſoliis in cataplasmate poſitus juvat, et panis ex vino vel roſaceo ſubactus mirabiliter confert. In ſumma adſtringentium genus omne et

ἀποκρουομένων ἐν ἀρχαῖς, ὅσα ἐστὶ κώνειόν τε καὶ ψύλλιον, σέλινον, στρύχνον καὶ οἱ ἐπὶ τῶν τελμάτων φακοὶ, ἕρπυλλον, σάμψυχον, φύλλα ἀμπέλου, κόριον, ἀνδράχνη, φακὸς ὁ ἐπὶ τοῦ ὕδατος. τούτων ἕκαστον λεαίνων μετ' οἴνου κατάπλασσε. τὸ δὲ ψύλλιον μεθ' ὕδατος καὶ τὸν ἀπὸ τῶν τελμάτων φακόν.

[*Πρὸς θερμὰ ῥεύματα.*] *Κράμβη* λεῖα μετ' ἀλφίτου λείου σὺν ὕδατι καταπλασθεῖσα· καὶ ὠκίμου φύλλα ὁμοίως, ἢ σαμψύχου πέταλα λεῖα κατάπλασσε. ἵστησι δὲ πολὺ ῥεῦμα, κωδεία καὶ ὑοσκύαμος μετὰ ἀλφίτου λεπτοῦ σὺν οἴνῳ, προπυρία δὲ καὶ [586] οὕτως κατάπλασσε. εἰ δὲ διάτασις εἴη τῶν δύο βλεφάρων, ὀθόνην βουτύρῳ βρέξας ἐπιτίθει τοῖς ὀφθαλμοῖς, ἐφ' ὧν δὲ χύμωσις ἰσχυρὰ γέγονε, καλεῖται δὲ χύμωσις ἡ ἐπὶ τῷ κερατοειδεῖ ἐρυθρὰ καὶ σαρκώδης φλεγμονὴ, σάρκας μυῶν ἐπιμελῶς λεάνας, καὶ προσβαλὼν ὠοῦ λέκυθον, ὠμὴν συλλείου, καὶ ὅταν κερατοειδὲς γένηται, εἰς ὀθόνην ἐμπλάσας ἐπιτίθει, καὶ παραχρῆμα παύει.

repellentium per initia, qualis eſt cicuta, pſyllium, apium, ſolanum, lenticulae paluſtres, ſerpillum, ſampſuchum, folia vitis, coriandrum, portulaca, lens aquis innatans. Horum quodque ex vino tritum in cataplasmatis forma admove, pſyllum ac lenticulas paluſtres ex aqua.

[*Ad calidas fluxiones.*] Braſſica tuſa et farina trita cum aqua cataplasmate imponitur. Eodem modo ocimi feria vel ſampſuchi ſolia trita admove. Sistunt fluxionem papaveris caput et hyoscyamus cum polenta tenui ex vino, fotumque primo, deinde cataplasma admove. Quod ſi duarum palpebrarum diſtenta ſit, linteo butyro madens oculis admove. In quibus ſi gravis ſit chymoſis (vocatur autem chymoſis rubra carnoſaque corneae oculi tunicae inflammatio) ipſi medentur accurate detritae murium carnes cum crudo ovi luteo ſimul ſubactae, quod quum ad cerae conſiſtentiam pervenerit, ex panno lineo in forma cataplasmatis impone, et quamprimum ſedat.

[Περίχρισμα ὀφθαλμῶν.] Ἄρτος καθαρὸς κεκαυμένος, μιγεὶς ἀκακίᾳ καὶ κυτίνῳ σὺν ὕδατι.

[477] [Πρὸς τὰς περιωδυνίας.] Ῥόδα ξηρὰ ἢ χλωρὰ ἐν γλυκεῖ βρέξας ὕδατι λέαινε, μίξας ὠοῦ λευκοῦ λέκιθον καὶ κρόκου τὸ ἀρκοῦν κατάπλασσε· ἢ κρίθινα ἄλευρα ἐν γλυκεῖ ἡψημένα. ἐὰν δὲ μείζων εἴη ἡ ὀδύνη, πρόσμισγε ὑοσκυάμου φύλλα, ἢ πέπονος, ἢ σικύου τὴν σάρκα μετ' ὠοῦ ὀπτοῦ ἢ λεκίθου, καὶ ὀλίγου οἴνου, κατάπλασσε.

[Κατάπλασμα ὀφθαλμῶν.] Καλῶς ποιεῖ πίτυος φλοιὸς καὶ ἄλφιτα σὺν οἴνῳ.

[Πρὸς σφοδρὰς περιωδυνίας.] Κορίου χυλὸν μετὰ γυναικείου γάλακτος εἰς τοὺς κανθοὺς ἔνσταζε, ἢ φύλλα πλατάνου λεῖα μετὰ τῶν λεπτῶν ἀλφίτων, ἄνωθεν ἐπὶ τοὺς ὀφθαλμοὺς ἐμπλαττόμενα.

[Ἐπὶ τῶν ῥευμάτων καταπλάσματα.] Κυπάρισσος χλωρὰ ἢ βράθυ χλωρὸν μετ' οἴνου· ἢ παλιούρου φύλλα, ἢ ἀνδράχνη λεία μετὰ στέατος χηνείου καὶ κρόκου, ἢ ἶρις

[*Linimentum oculorum.*] Panis purus tostus, acaciae et cytino ex aqua mixtus.

[*Ad oculorum dolores.*] Rofas aridas aut virides in aqua dulci maceratas ac laevigatas et cum ovi candidi luteo et croci q. f. commixtas in forma cataplasmatis admove: aut hordeaceam farinam in aqua dulci elixam. Quod fi gravior fuerit dolor, hyoscyami folia, aut carnem vel peponis, vel cucumeris cum ovo cocto vel ovi luteo et pauco vino ut cataplasma admove.

[*Cataplasma oculorum.*] Pulchre facit pini cortex et farina cum vino.

[*Ad vehementes oculorum dolores.*] Coriandri fuccum cum muliebri lacte in angulos inftillato. Aut platani folia trita cum tenui farina in modum emplaftri oculis furfum impofita.

[*Ad fluxiones cataplasmata.*] Cupreffus viridis vel fabina viridis cum vino. Vel paliuri folia, aut portulacae detrita cum pinguedine anferina et croco. Vel iris

ξηρὰ μετὰ μέλιτος, ἢ σελίνου φύλλα μετὰ ἀλφίτων. ἐπὶ δὲ τῶν μεγάλων ῥευμάτων γλήχωνος προσφάτου καρπὸν, καὶ μάλιστα χυλὸν σὺν ὄξει, μαλαγματῶδες ποιήσας ἐπιτίθει κατὰ τοῦ βρέγματος, καὶ ἐπάνω ἔρια, καὶ ἐπιδέσμει ἐλαφρῶς· ἢ ῥόδα καὶ μελίλωτα ἑφθὰ μετὰ ἀμύλου αὐτοὺς τοὺς ὀφθαλμοὺς κατάπλασον, ἢ ἄμυλον σὺν οἴνῳ λευκῷ, ἢ ὠοῦ λευκῷ.

[*Ἀνακολλήματα πρὸς ῥεύματα.*] *Κοχλίαν* μετὰ τοῦ ὀστράκου κόψας, ἀπὸ τοῦ κροτάφου ἐπὶ τὸν κρόταφον κατάχριε.

[*Πρὸς τὰς αἱμάλωπας καὶ ὑποσφάγματα.*] Πρὸς τὰς περὶ τοὺς ὀφθαλμοὺς γινομένας πληγὰς καὶ διὰ τοῦτο συμβαινούσας αἱματώδεις ὑποχύσεις, εὐθέως ἐν ἀρχῇ πρὸς τὰς φλεγμονὰς καὶ τὸ ἄλγημα, ποιεῖ περιστερᾶς ἐνσταζόμενον αἷμα, καὶ μάλιστα τὸ ἐκ τῶν ἁπαλῶν πτερῶν ἐκπιεζόμενον, καὶ τὸ λευκὸν τοῦ ὠοῦ, τὸν αὐτὸν τρόπον εἰς τὸν ὀφθαλμὸν ἐγχεόμενον, ἔτι δὲ ἐρίῳ καθαρῷ προσαναλαμβανόμενον, καὶ ἄνωθεν ἐπιτιθέμενον. εὐθετεῖ δὲ καὶ λέκιθος ὠοῦ κατωπτημένη, καὶ μετὰ οἴνου καταπλασσομένη. ἔτι δὲ ῥόδων τὰ

ſicca cum melle. Vel apii ſolia cum polenta juvant. Ad magnas autem fluxiones pulegii recentis ſemen, ac maxime ſuccum cum aceto ac malagmatis craſſitiem redactum ſyncipiti admove, ac ſuperpone lanam, ſuaviterque illigato. Vel ex roſis et meliloto cum amylo coctis cataplasma ipſis oculis admove. Vel amylum cum vino aut ovi albo.

[*Ad fluxiones oculorum frontalia.*] Limacem cum teſta contuſam a temporibus ad tempora fronti admove.

[*Ad haemalopas et hypoſphagmata.*] Ad illatos oculis ictus, ac proinde oborientes cruentas ſuffuſiones. Quamprimum ab initio ad inflammationes *prohibendas* et dolorem *mitigandum*, facit columbinus ſanguis inſtillatus, potiſſimum ex tenellis albis expreſſus, et ovi album eodem modo in oculum infuſum, deinde lana munda exceptum ac deſuper admotum. Apte quoque admovetur aſſum ovi luteum et cum vino in cataplasma efformatum. Praeterea roſarum ſolia et flores per ſe aut cum vino ſimul ſubacta,

φύλλα καὶ τὸ ἄνθος ἰδίᾳ, καὶ μετ' οἴνου ὁμοῦ τριβόμενα, καὶ μετὰ χνοώδους ἀλφίτου καταπλασσόμενα.

[Πρὸς τὰ γινόμενα περὶ τοὺς ὀφθαλμοὺς οἰδήματα διὰ πληγάς.] Λίαν ἁρμόττει πυρία ἐξ ὀξυκράτου μαλακῷ σπόγγῳ συνεχῶς γινομένη, εἶτ' ὄξει βρεχόμενος καὶ κεκραμένος καινὸς σπόγγος, καὶ ἐπιτιθέμενος.

[Πρὸς τοὺς ὀφθαλμοὺς διὰ τὸν ἥλιον καὶ κονιορτὸν ψωροφθαλμιῶντας.] Ὕδωρ πλεῖον προσκλυζόμενον, θέρους ψυχρὸν, χειμῶνος θερμὸν, καὶ πυρία διὰ σπόγγων ἁρμόζει ἐκ φακῶν ἀφεψήματος. καὶ αὐτοῖς δὲ προσάγειν τοῖς κανθοῖς, ἢ βάτου, ἢ ῥόδων χυλὸν κατ' ἰδίαν ἑκάστου σὺν ὕδατι· ἢ ῥόδα ξη- [587] ρὰ τριβόμενα σὺν οἴνῳ. χριέσθωσαν δὲ καὶ ἐλαίῳ παλαιῷ καθεύδοντες, ἀπεχέσθωσαν δὲ πάντων τῶν δριμέων καὶ ὀξέων.

[Πρὸς τὰς χρονίας περὶ τὰ βλέφαρα διαθέσεις καὶ τετυλωμένας.] Ἀμόργην ἑφθὴν καὶ μετὰ ἐλαίου λειοτριβουμένην ἔγχριε.

[Πρὸς πτίλους καὶ τρίχας μὴ ἔχοντας, ἄκρως ποιεῖ,

et cum tenui polenta mixta, ad cataplasmatis formam admovetur.

[*Ad oculorum tumores ex ictu obortos.*] Admodum conducit fotus ex poſca molli ſpongia frequenter admotus, deinde ſpongia nova aceto aqua temperato inebriata et admota.

[*Ad oculorum pſorophthalmiam pruriginoſam ſcabiem a ſole et pulvere.*] Aqua liberalius affuſa, aeſtate frigida, hieme calida, ac fotus ſpongiis factus ex lentium decocto congruit. Atque ipſis oculorum angulis admove vel rubi vel roſarum ſuccum, quemque ſigillatim ex aqua; aut applicare roſas aridas ex vino ſubaatas. Quin et illinantur dormituri oleo veteri et ab omnibus tum acribus tum acidis abſtineant.

[*Ad inveteratos callentesque palpebrarum affectus.*] Amurcam coctam et cum oleo ſubactam illine.

[*Ad ciliis depilatos pilisque carentes palpebras ſum-*

καὶ τρίχας ἀνάγει.] Μυόχοδα καὶ κόπρους τράγου ἴσα κεκαυμένα καλάμου Ἑλληνικοῦ διπλοῦν σὺν μέλιτι ἐγχριόμενα. τοῦτο καὶ ἀλφοὺς ὠφελεῖ.

[Πρὸς τὰς ἐπιφυομένας ἐν τοῖς βλεφάροις τρίχας.] Προεκτίλας τὰς τρίχας ἐκ ῥιζῶν αἵματι κόρεως κατάχριε, καὶ οὐ μὴ φυήσονται· ἢ κρότωνος ἀπὸ κυνὸς αἵματι ἄκρως ποιεῖ. χρῶ δὲ ἐκ ῥιζῶν τίλλων τρίχας, ἢ χολῇ τραγείᾳ, τίλλων εὐθέως κατάχριε· ἢ αἰγείᾳ χολῇ μετὰ χυλοῦ κράμβης.

[Πρὸς λευκώματα.] Ταχέως ἰᾶται νίτρον μετ' ἐλαίου παλαιοῦ λεανθὲν ἐπιμελῶς καὶ ἐπιχριόμενον· ἢ σαύρας ἀφόδευμα ἔγχριε· ἢ νυκτικόρακος ὠὸν ἔγχριε, καὶ βάψεις αὐτούς.

[Πρὸς ἀμαύρωσιν ὀφθαλμῶν.] Ἀμαύρωσιν πᾶσαν καὶ ἀρχομένην ὑπόχυσιν θεραπεύει γυπὸς χολὴ μετὰ πρασίου χυλοῦ καὶ μέλιτος Ἀττικοῦ· εἰ δὲ μὴ παρείη καὶ τῷ ἁπαλῷ χρῆσθαι μέλιτι. ἔστω δὲ ὅ τε χυλὸς τοῦ πρασίου, καὶ τὸ μέλι ἑκάστου διπλάσιον τῆς χολῆς· ἢ μαράθρου χυλὸν καὶ χολὴν

mopere confert, pilosque producit.] Muscerda et fimum caprinum pari pondere et calami Graeci duplum torrefacta ex melle illinuntur. Id quoque vitiligines curat.

[*Ad noxios pilos palpebris adnascentes.*] Evulsis radicitus pilis, cimicis sanguine locum illine et nunquam renascentur. Etiam pediculi canini sanguis summe juvat. Utere vero evulsis radicitus pilis, felle hyenae, vel felle hirci statim ab evulsione pilorum, illine, vel felle caprino cum brassicae succo *utere.*

[*Ad oculorum albugines.*] Celeriter his medetur nitrum accurate contritum ex oleo veteri et illitum. Vel lacertae fimum illine; vel nycticoracis ovum admove et ipsos colorabis.

[*Ad oculorum obscurationem, amaurosin.*] Omnem amaurosin incipientemque suffusionem curat fel vulturis cum marrubii succo et melle Attico: si non suppetat, tenero melle utere. Esto autem tum succi marrubii, tum mellis dupla ad ipsum fel portio. Aut fel taurinum li-

ταυρείαν ὑγρὰν ἴσα, μετὰ διπλασίονος μέλιτος ἔγχριε· ἢ χολὴ ἀρκεία μετὰ ὕδατος διπλασίου.

[Πρὸς πτερύγια.] Αἰγείρου ὀπῷ μετὰ μέλιτος διπλοῦ ἔγχριε.

[Πρὸς νυκτάλωπας.] Ἧπαρ τράγειον ὀπτήσας, τὸν ἐν τῇ ὀπτήσει ἀποῤῥέοντα τὸν ἰχῶρα συναγαγὼν ἔγχριε, καὶ αὐτὸ τὸ ἧπαρ δίδου ἐσθίειν. ὠφελεῖ καὶ αἷμα περιστερᾶς ἐγχριόμενον, καὶ χολὴ αἰγεία· ἢ ἧπαρ αἰγὸς ἑνέψων κέλευε αὐτοὺς περικαλυψαμένους ἀτενίζειν εἰς τὴν χύτραν, καὶ δέχεσθαι τὴν ἀμίδα τοῖς ὀφθαλμοῖς· ἢ ὀνίδα πρόσφατον χυλώσας ὑπάλειφε.

[Πρὸς τὰς ἐπιγενομένας ἐπὶ τῶν ὀφθαλμῶν κριθάς.] Κηρῷ λευκῷ πυρία· ἢ μυιῶν τὴν κεφαλὴν ἀποβαλὼν, τῷ λοιπῷ σώματι παράτριβε τὴν κριθήν.

[Πρὸς ὑπώπια.] Ὑπώπια παραχρῆμα καταπλασσομένη ἡ ῥάφανος λεία αἴρει· αἴρει δὲ αὐτὴν ὅταν ἄρξηται δάκνειν· ὁ τυρὸς νεαλὴς καταπλασσόμενος· ἢ κηρωτὴ μετὰ

quidum cum fucci foeniculi aequali pondere et mellis duplo; vel fel urfinum cum aquae duplo.

[*Ad pterygia, ungues in oculis.*] Populi nigrae liquorem cum dupla mellis portione mixtum illine.

[*Ad lufcitionem, nyctilopa.*] Jecur hircinum affa, interque affandum defluentem faniofum humorem, collectum oculis infrica ipfumque jecur edendum praebe. Juvat etiam columbae fanguis inftillatus et fel caprae. Aut caprae jecur decoquens praecipe, ut habentes caput pannis circumvolutum teneant intentos in ollam oculos, fufcipiantque vaporem. Vel expreffum ex recenti ftercore afinino fuccum oculis illine.

[*Ad hordea oculis oborientia.*] Cera alba foveto. Aut mufcae reliquum corpus praecifo capite hordeolo infricato.

[*Ad fugillatam.*] Sugillata quamprimum raphanus tritus et impofitus tollit; tollit autem ipfa, quum erodere incipit. Levat etiam impofitus cafeus recens falfus; aut

ἀψινθίου, ἢ χυλῷ ῥαφάνου ἀναλειφθεῖσα· ἄκρως ποιεῖ πρὸς τὰ πρόσφατα καὶ πέλια τῶν ὑπωπίων σπόγγος ἐν ἅλμῃ ἀποβαπτόμενος καὶ συνεχῶς προστιθέμενος. μετὰ τοῦτο δὲ πυρία συνεχὴς διὰ ὕδατος θερμοῦ. ταῦτα πρὸς τὰ πέλια τῶν ὑπωπίων· ἐφ᾽ ὧν δὲ αἱματώδη εἰσὶν, ἢ ὑπόξανθα, ἢ ὕπωχρα, φεύγειν χρὴ τὴν ἅλμην, καταπλάσσειν δὲ βατίνῳ, ἢ ἀψινθίῳ, ἢ ὑσσώπῳ καὶ ὀριγάνῳ, ἢ ῥαφάνου φλοιῷ, ἢ σταφίδι χωρὶς τῶν γιγάρτων· κατ᾽ ἰδίαν ἕκαστον μετὰ μέλιτος, ἢ ὄξους, ἢ ὕδατος ἀνέφθου καὶ λευκὸς βολβὸς μετ᾽ ὠοῦ καὶ μέλιτος, ἢ κυκλάμινος μετὰ σταφίδος. ἐπὶ δὲ τῶν κεχρονισμένων καὶ μεμελανωμένων νᾶπυ μετὰ στέατος προβατείου διπλασίονος· ἢ κυάμινον ἄλευρον μετὰ μέλιτος φυραθὲν, καὶ μασηθὲν, καὶ σὺν σιέλῳ καταχρισθέν· ἢ κύμινον ῥάκει ἐνδή- [588] σας, καὶ εἰς ζεστὸν ἀποβάπτων πυρίαζε. ἢ κρίθινον ἄλευρον μετ᾽ ὀξυμέλιτος ἑψημένον· μαράθρῳ λείῳ μετὰ κηρωτῆς.

[Πρὸς ὑπώπια μετὰ οἰδήματος.] Σπόγγον ὄξει καταβρέξας ἐπιτίθει, καὶ κατάπλασσε ἀλεύρῳ κριθίνῳ μετ᾽ ὀξυ-

ceratum cum abſinthio vel raphani ſucco impoſitum. Summopere confert ad recentia et livida ſugillata ſpongia muriae immerſa aſſidue admota. Praeter haec frequens ſotus ex aqua calida plurimum facit ad livida ſugillata. Quibus cruenta ſunt, aut ſubflava, aut ſubpallida, muria vitanda eſt, imponendumque cataplasma ex rubo, aut abſinthio, aut hyſſopo, aut origano, aut raphani cortice, aut uva paſſa absque acinis: horum enim quodque ſingulatim imponitur; aut ex melle, aut aceto, aut incocta aqua. Nec non bulbus candidus cum ovo ac melle; aut cyclaminum cum uva paſſa. At vetuſtis jam et denigratis ſinapi cum duplo adipis ovini; vel fabacea farina cum melle mixta, aut manſa et cum ſalina inuncta. Aut cuminum veteri linteo illigatum intinge ferventi aquae, oculosque hoc ſove. Aut hordeaceam ſarinam cum oxymelite coctam applicato. Aut tritum ſoeniculi ſemen cum cerato.

[*Ad ſugillationes cum oedemate.*] Spongiam aceto inebriatam impone, et cataplasmate utere ex ſarina hor-

μέλιτος ἡψημένου μέχρι καταστολῆς, καὶ ὕστερον ἐπιτίθει φακὸν ἑφθὸν λεῖον μετὰ μέλιτος.

[Πρὸς ὑπώπια πρόσφατα.] Κώνειον λεῖον μετὰ ὕδατος κατάπλασσε, ἢ βρυωνίας ῥίζαν τρίψας, μετ' οἰνομέλιτος ἐπιτίθει.

(478) Κεφ. στ'. [Περὶ τῶν κατὰ τὸ πρόσωπον παθῶν, καὶ πρῶτον περὶ ἰόνθων.] Ὄγκος μικρὸς καὶ σκληρὸς ἐν τῷ κατὰ τὸ πρόσωπον δέρματι καλούμενος ἴονθος γίνεται. διαφέρει δὲ τῶν συκωδῶν ὄγκων ἐπὶ τοῦ γενείου γιγνομένων τῷ μὴ μόνον παχὺν εἶναι τὸν ἐργαζόμενον χυμὸν, ἀλλὰ καὶ λεπτότητος ἰχωρώδους μετέχειν, δι' ἣν καὶ ταχέως ἑλκοῦται, μὴ θεραπευόμενος ὡς προσήκει.

[Πρὸς ἰόνθους τοὺς ἐν τοῖς προσώποις.] Ὄξους δριμυτάτου μετὰ ἴσου μέλιτος μίξας ἐπιμελῶς ἐπίχριε, τῷ δακτύλῳ διατρίβων. ἄλλο. ἀμύγδαλα πικρὰ ὄξει διαλύσας καὶ τρίψας ἐπιμελῶς ἀνάπλασσε τροχίσκους, καὶ ξήραινε ἐν σκιᾷ. ἐπὶ δὲ τῆς χρήσεως ὄξει διαλύων ἐπίχριε, ὅταν δὲ ξηρανθῇ, σαπῶνι ἀπόσμηχε. ποίει τοῦτο πρὸς τὰς ὀχθώδεις

deacea cocta cum oxymelite, donec tumor reprimatur; poſt haec apponito coctam lentem et cum melle tritam.

[*Ad recentia ſugillata.*] Cicutam ex aqua tritam, aut admodum detritam vitis albae radicem ex mulſo impone.

Cap. VI. [*De faciei affectibus, primumque de varis.*] Tumor in faciei cute parvus durusque, vocatus varus, nascitur. Differt autem a ficoſis tumoribus in mento provenientibus, non ſolum quod ex craſſo humore conſiſtat, verum etiam quod participet tenui quadam ſanie, cujus ratione cito ulceratur, ubi prout deceat, non curatur.

[*Ad varos in facie.*] Acetum acerrimum cum melle aequali menſura mixtum varis accuratius illine, digito infricans. *Aliud.* Ex amygdalis amaris aceto diſſolutis et accurate tritis conformato paſtillos, atque in umbra deſiccato. In uſu, dilutum ex his aliquem aceto varis inducito et ſimul atque aruerit, tunc ſapone abſtergito. Fac

διαθέσεις, καὶ τοὺς ἐπὶ προσώπου κνησμοὺς καὶ τὴν ἀρχὴν ἐλεφαντιάσεως.

[Πρὸς τὰς ἐπὶ γενείου συκώδεις ἐπαναστάσεις.] Ἅλας ὀρυκτοὺς μετ' ὄξους κατάπλασσε, ἢ λεπίδος χαλκοῦ καὶ χαλκάνθου, ἢ κόλλαν τεκτονικὴν μετὰ μίλτεως κατάχριε.

[Πρὸς τοὺς ἐπὶ τοῦ γενείου λειχῆνας.] Πυροὺς πολλοὺς λαβὼν ἐπιτίθει ἐπὶ ἄκμονος, εἶτα πλάτυσμα χαλκοῦ πυρώσας ἐπιτίθει τοῖς πυροῖς, καὶ τὸ ἀνιέμενον ἐξ αὐτῶν ὑγρὸν ἔτι θερμὸν ἐπίχριε.

[Πρὸς χρονίους λειχῆνας.] Καππάρεως φύλλα τρίψας μετ' ὄξους δριμυτάτου μετὰ ἴσου μέλιτος ἐπιτίθει. ἄλλο. λαπάθου φλοιὸν τῆς ῥίζης μετὰ ὄξους λειώσας, κατάπλασσε προεκνιτρώσας. ἄλλο. χαμαιλέοντος ῥίζαν ἐν ὄξει ἑψήσας καὶ τρίψας κατάπλασσε. ἄλλο. λαπάθου ῥίζαν λεάνας καὶ κρίθινα ἄλευρα μετὰ ὄξους δριμυτάτου κατάπλασσε.

[Πρὸς ψωρώδεις λειχῆνας.] Ἀμύγδαλα πικρὰ λειώσας κατάχριε συνεχῶς.

hoc ad tumidos affectus, faciei pruritus et principium elephantiafis.

[*Ad fiscofas in mento excrefcentias.*] Salem foffilem ex aceto, aut fquamam aëris et chalcanthum, aut glutinum fabrile cum rubrica illine.

[*Ad menti impetigines.*] Acceptum magna copia triticum incudi impone; cui deinde applicato candentem laminam aeream, quique effluit humorem etiamnum calentem affectui infrica.

[*Ad diuturnas impetigines.*] Trita capparis folia ex aceto acerrimo cum aequali melle imponito. *Aliud.* Radicis ramicis corticem ex aceto tritum nitro prius perfricans illine. *Aliud.* Chamaeleontis radicem in aceto decoctam ac laevigatam fuperdato. *Aliud.* Detritam ramicis radicem et hordeaceam farinam ex acerrimo aceto admove.

[*Ad fcabras impetigines.*] Tritis amygdalis amaris frequenter ipfas inungito.

Ed. Chart. X. [588. 589.] Ed. Baf. II. (478.)

[Πρὸς λειχῆνα.] Τηλέφιον καὶ σκόροδον καὶ ὄξος δριμὺ λειώσας, προτρίψας ἐρίῳ ἢ ῥάκει, τὸν λειχῆνα περίχριε.

[Πρὸς τὰ ἐπὶ τῶν γενείων ἐξανθήματα.] Σίδηρον πεπυρακτωμένον ἐπίβαλε ξύλῳ καλουμένῳ παλιούρῳ, καὶ τὸ ἐπιγιγνόμενον ὑγρὸν λαβὼν κατάχριε. ἄλλο. μύρτα λειώσας σὺν οἴνῳ κατάχριε.

[589] Κεφ. ζ'. [Πρὸς τὰ ἐν τοῖς ὀδοῦσι πάθη καὶ πρῶτον πρὸς ἀλγήματα.] Ἀλγοῦντες ὀδόντες διακλυζέσθωσαν ὄξει θερμῷ μετὰ κηκίδων, ἢ δαδίοις λιπαροῖς ἀνεζεσμένοις ἐν ὄξει, ἢ ὑοσκυάμου τῷ σπέρματι καὶ τοῖς φλοιοῖς σὺν ὄξει, ἢ κεδρείᾳ, ἢ προπόλει, ἢ στρύχνῳ, ἢ καππάρει, ἢ σκορόδοις, ἢ μυρσίνης κλωνίοις μετ' ὄξους ἀνεζεσμένοις, ἢ οἴνου τρυγὶ θερμῇ, ἢ πολίου φλοιῷ, ἢ καὶ αὐτῇ τῇ βοτάνῃ, ἢ πρασίῳ, ἕκαστον αὐτῶν ὠφελεῖ σὺν ὄξει. ἢ πλατάνου σφαιρία, ἢ ῥόδα ξηρὰ ἕψει ἐν οἴνῳ λευκῷ μέχρι τὸ τρίτον ἀπολειφθῇ, καὶ συνεχῶς δίδου διακλύζεσθαι. ὁμοίως δὲ καὶ εὐπατορίου ῥίζα καθεψηθεῖσα ἐν οἴνῳ, ἢ γλήχων

[*Ad impetiginem.*] Recipe telephium et allium et acetum acre, quibus laevigatis praefrictam cana aut panniculo impetiginem illine.

[*Ad genarum papulas.*] Ferrum candens paliuri ligno vocato imponito, acceptumque qui ex hoc defluit humorem illinito. *Aliud.* Contritas myrti baccas ex vino inungito.

Cap. VII. [*Ad dentium affectiones, primumque ad dolores.*] Collue dentes dolentes calido gallarum ex aceto decocto, aut pinguium facularum, aut alterci tum feminum, tum corticum, aut cedrini liquoris, vel propoleos, vel folani, vel capparis vel allii, vel myrti ramulorum in aceto decoctorum, aut calidae vini faecis, aut polii corticis, aut etiam ipfiusmet herbae, aut marrubii; horum unumquodque cum aceto juvat. Vel platani pilulae et rofae aridae, decoctae in vino albo ad tertias usque, quo dentes frequenter colluantur. Idem efficit tum eupatorii radix cocta in vino,

βοηθεῖ. ἢ κέρας ἐλάφειον ἐν ὀξυγάρῳ ἑψήσας ἐπὶ πολὺ διακλύζου. ἢ σκίλλης τὸ ἐντὸς εἰς λεπτὰ τεμὼν ἐπὶ τὸν ξέστην τοῦ ὄξους βαλὼν εἰς ἄγγος ταρίχευσον ἐν ὀνίδι κατορύξας ἐφ' ἡμέρας λ'. καὶ χρῶ διακλύσματι. ἢ ὀνείῳ γάλακτι διακλλύζου, τοῦτο καὶ τοὺς κινουμένους ὀδόντας στερεοῖ. ἢ τιθυμάλλου ῥίζαν ἐν ὀξυμέλιτι ἑψήσας μέχρι τὸ ἥμισυ λειφθῇ, ἢ ὑοσκυάμου ῥίζαν ἐν ὀξυμέλιτι ἑψήσας διακλύζου. ἢ συκαμίνου γάλα εἰς οἶνον ἐγχέας ἐναπόθλιβέ τε καὶ χλιάνας διακλύζου. ἄλλο. σκορόδου καὶ εὐζώμου σπέρματος, καὶ νίτρου ἀφεψήματι διακλύζου.

[Περὶ πυρίας πρὸς ὀδονταλγίαν.] Πυρίαν δὲ ποιοῦσι πρὸς ὀδονταλγίαν ἔξωθεν μὲν αἱ δι' ἁλῶν πεφρυγμένων, ἢ κέγχρων εἰς μαρσύππιον βεβλημένων, ἢ καὶ διὰ ῥυπαρῶν ῥακίδων εὖ μάλα θερμανθέντων. καὶ αὐτοῦ δὲ τοῦ ἀλγοῦντος ὀδόντος πυρίᾳ οὕτως χρηστέον. ὀριγάνου ξηροῦ κλωνίον εἰς ζεστὸν ἔλαιον βάπτων, τῷ πονοῦντι ὀδόντι ἄνωθεν ἐπέρειδε. ἢ κίκεως καυλὸν ὁμοῦ καὶ κηρὸν ἐπιτίθει τῷ ἀλ-

tum pulegium. Aut decoquito cervinum cornu in oxygaro, ſaepeque os eo abluito. Aut ſcillae interiora in minutas ſecato particulas, additoque aceti ſextario in vas conjicito, ſinitoque haec in ſimo aſinino defoſſa macerari diebus triginta eaque collutione utere; vel aſinino lacte collue, id etiam motos dentes confirmat. Aut tithymalli radicem in oxymelite ad medias usque incoquito; aut etiam hyoscyami radicis in oxymelite decocto dentes collue. Item lacte mori commixto probe cum vino, deinde tepefacto collue dentes. *Aliud.* Decocto quoque allii, ſeminis erucae et nitri collue.

[*De fomentis ad dentium dolores.*] Extrinſecus ad dentium dolorem conveniunt fomenta ex fricto ſale, vel milio in ſacculum conjecto; aut etiam ex ſordidis panniculis admodum calentibus. At vero dolentis dentis fomento ſic utendum eſt. Aridi origani ramulum in fervens oleum demiſſum ſuperne affecto denti applicato. Vel, ricini fruticis coliculum ſimul cum cera imponito dolenti denti. Aut tange hanc frequenter ſpecilli mucrone vehe-

Ed. Chart. X. [589.] Ed. Baf. II. (478.)

γοῦντι ὀδόντι. ἢ πυρῆνι μήλης θερμοτάτῳ προσάπτου συνεχῶς. χρῶ δὲ καθόλου ταῖς πυρίαις ταῖς τε ἔξωθεν καὶ ἔσωθεν, ἢ πρὸ τροφῆς, ἢ πολὺ λίαν ἀποστησάντων ἀπὸ τροφῆς.

[*Ἀποφλεγματισμοὶ ὀδόντων.*] *Ἀποφλεγματισμοὶ* ἄριστοι τοῖς ὀδονταλγοῦσιν, σταφὶς ἀγρία διαμασηθεῖσα ἰδίᾳ καὶ μετὰ γλήχωνος· ἢ κηκίδος τὸ ἔνδοθεν μέλαν δακνέτω τῷ ἀλγοῦντι ὀδόντι, καὶ ἐάτω ἀποῤῥεῖν. ἢ σκορόδων πυρῆνας ε΄. καὶ μυρσίνης μελαίνης φύλλα ὀλίγα ἕψει σὺν ὄξει, σπάθῃ κινῶν δαδίνῃ μέχρι ἡμίσεος, καὶ δίδου διακλύζεσθαι καὶ διακρατεῖν, εἶτα χήναντες ἐάτωσαν ῥεῖν τὸ φλέγμα, καὶ μετὰ τοῦτο ῥοδίνῳ διακλυζέσθωσαν.

[*Ἔγχυτον εἰς τὰς ῥῖνας πρὸς ὀδονταλγίαν.*] *Σεύτλου* ῥίζης τὸν χυλὸν αὐτὸν καθ' ἑαυτὸν ἔγχεε εἰς τὰς ῥῖνας, καὶ λύσεις τοὺς πόνους τῶν ὀδόντων.

[*Πρὸς ὀδόντας μεμελασμένους.*] *Ἅλας* ὀρυκτὸν μέλιτι φυράσας, ὄπτησον ἐπὶ κληματίδων, καὶ τρίψας μῖξον σμύρνης βραχὺ καὶ χρῶ ἀποτρίβων τοὺς ὀδόντας.

mentiſſime calente. Sed utere fomentis id genus omnibus tam iis quae extrinſecus, quam quae intrinſecus adhibentur, aut ante cibum, aut longo poſt aſſumptum cibum tempore.

[*Apophlegmatismi pro dentium dolore.*] Apophlegmatismi optimi dentium doloribus ſunt, herba pedicularis maſticata aut per ſe, aut cum pulegio. Vel quod in galla nigrum interius eſt, affecto dente commordeto, ſinitoque effluere. Aut quinque allii nucleos cum nigrae myrti pauculis foliis in aceto ad dimidias decoquito taedae rude aſſiduo commiſcens, ac eluito eo dentes, oreque contincto; poſt haec hiato, donec pituitae ſatis profluat; demum roſaceo os colluito.

[*Infuſum in nares pro dentium dolore.*] Succum radicis betae in nares infunde et dentium ſolves dolorem.

[*Ad dentes denigratos.*] Praerigatum melle foſſilem ſalem torreto ſuper igne ex ſarmentis vitis, teritoque, deinde adjecta paucula myrrha dentibus infricato.

[*Διάκλυσμα ὀδόντων.*] *Διακλύσματι δὲ χρῶ ἀπὸ τούτων οἴνῳ εὐώδει, ἐν ᾧ ἀφέψηται ἡ ἶρις ξηρά.*

[590] [*Οὔλων διάκλυσμα.*] *Ὄξος, ἐναφηψημένης ὑοσκυάμου ῥίζης, διακλύζου.*

[*Προφυλακτικὸν ὀδονταλγιῶν.*] *Τιθυμάλλου ῥίζας ἑψήσας ἐν οἴνῳ μέχρι ἡμίσεος, δὶς τοῦ μηνὸς διακλύζου, καὶ οὐδέποτε ἀλγήσεις.*

[*Ἄριστα ποιεῖ πρός τε φυλακὴν ἀλγημάτων, καὶ ῥῶσιν τῶν οὔλων καὶ τῶν ὀδόντων, ἔτι τε εὐπρέπειαν καὶ τὰ ὑποτεταγμένα σμήγματα.*] *Ἔρια οἰσυπηρὰ ὀθονίῳ ἐνδήσας, καῦσον, εἶτα ἁλῶν τὸ τρίτον μίξας καὶ λειώσας, εὖ μάλα σμῆχε. ἢ δασύποδος κεφαλὴν κεκαυμένην λειάνας χρῶ. ἄλλο. ἅλας καὶ μέλι λειάνας μέχρι κηρῶδες γενέσθαι καθαρῷ ὀθονίῳ ἐνδήσας καὶ καύσας, εἶτα μίξας ἶριν ὀλίγην, σμῆχε τοὺς ὀδόντας.*

[*Πρὸς στόματος δυσωδίαν.*] *Κριθὰς λεάνας μέλιτι*

[*Collutio dentium.*] Collutione vini odorati, in quo iris cocta fit, utere.

[*Collutio gingivarum.*] Gingivas aceto, in quo coctus fit hyofcyamus, colluito.

[*Dentes a doloribus praefervantia.*] Lavato dentes bis menfibus fingulis vino, in quo ad medias decocta fit tithymalli radix et nunquam dolebunt.

[*Subfcripta dentifricia maxime faciunt ad dentium a dolore praefenvationem et ad confirmandum tam dentes quam gingivas, conciliandumque dentium candorem.*] Lanam fuccidam linteolo alligatam torreto; adjecta deinde tertia falis portione, terito omnia fimul, et perfricato *hoc pulvere* dentes. Vel ufto contritoque leporis capite utitor. *Aliud.* Contritum ex melle falem ad cerae craffitiem linteoque mundo illigatum, urito; quo deinde addita iridos portiuncula, perfricato dentes.

[*Ad oris graveolentiam.*] Hordeum melle et vino

καὶ οἴνῳ δεύσας ἔνδησον χάρτῃ, καὶ καύσας, καὶ λειώσας τρῖβε τὰ οὖλα.

[Πρὸς ὀδόντας σειομένους ἵνα παγῶσι.] Χάλκανθον τρίψας μετὰ ἐλαίου, παράπτου τῶν ῥιζῶν ἔριον ἀποβρέξας. ἢ πτελέας φλοιὸν ἐν οἴνῳ ἑψήσας διακρατείτω· στερεοῖ γὰρ τοὺς ὀδόντας.

[Πρὸς βεβρωμένους ὀδόντας.] Καππάρεως φύλλα ἐν ὄξει δριμεῖ ἕψει εἰς ἥμισυ, καὶ χλιαρῷ διακλύζου· ὁμοίως δὲ ποιεῖ ὁ φλοιός. τὸ δ' αὐτὸ καὶ (479) πρὸς πόνους ποιεῖ.

["Αλλο σπουδαῖον.] Μελάνθιον φρύξας, καὶ τρίψας μετ' ὄξους δριμέος, κατάπλασσε τὸ βρῶμα, καὶ οὐκέτι βρωθήσεται, ἀλλὰ μενεῖ οἷόν ἐστιν.

[Πρὸς βεβρωμένους ὀδόντας.] Θαλάσσιον σκορπίον λευκὸν θὲς ἐπ' ἀνθράκων, χερσαῖον δὲ καὶ πώμαζε χωνείῳ ὀστρακίνῳ, καὶ κέλευε τὸν πάσχοντα δέχεσθαι τὸν ἀτμὸν τοῦ σκορπίου διὰ τῆς ὀπῆς τοῦ χωνείου, καὶ πάντοτε ἄπονος ἔσται.

Κεφ. η'. [Πρὸς πάσας τὰς ἐν τῷ στόματι καὶ τῷ

praemaceratum illigatur chartae, teriturque, quo deinde confricantur gingivae.

[*Ad motos dentes, ut confirmentur.*] Teritur ex oleo vitriolum, quod lana exceptum, dentium applicatur radicibus. Vel ulmi corticem in vino decoctum ore contine; confirmat dentes.

[*Ad erosos dentes.*] Folia capparis in aceto acerrimo ad dimidias coquito, ac tepido eo lavato dentes. Idem et poteſt cortex. Idem vero et ad dolores efficit.

[*Aliud expertum.*] Nigellam praefrictam, deinde tritam ex acri aceto, eroſioni imponito; ſic enim non amplius erodetur, ſed qualis eſt perdurabit.

[*Ad erosos dentes.*] Recipe ſcorpium album, pone ſupra carbones, terreſtre vero operi cruſibulo ſictili, aegrotumque ſcorpii ſumum excipere impera et doloris expers ſemper erit.

Cap. VIII. [*Ad omnes tam oris, quam columellae,*

κίονι καὶ τῷ φάρυγγι φλεγμονὰς καὶ διαθέσεις, κἂν ἕλκος γένηται, καὶ ἐσχάρα καὶ σηπεδών.] Κοινὸν μὲν παράγγελμα, ὡς τὸ ἐκ τῆς κεφαλῆς ἐπιῤῥέον κατ᾽ ἀρχὰς ἀναστέλλειν καὶ ἀποκρούεσθαι προσήκει, τὸ δὲ μετὰ τὴν ἀρχὴν ἄχρι τοῦ τέλους ἐκ μικτοῦ τινος εἶναι, τοῦ τε ἀποκρουομένου καὶ τοῦ διαφοροῦντος. χρὴ δὲ ἀποκρούεσθαι βουλομένους τῷ διὰ μόρων ὀνομαζομένῳ φαρμάκῳ. χρήσῃ δὲ καὶ ὄμφακος χυλῷ, μέλιτι βραχεῖ προσπλέκων, ἢ ῥόδων ἄνθος, ἢ αὐτὰ τὰ ῥόδα ξηρὰ ὕδατι ἀφέψων, ἢ πίτυος φλοιοῦ ἀφεψήματι. μετὰ δὲ τὴν ἀρχὴν, ὅτε κἀκ τῆς κεφαλῆς ἐπιῤῥέοιτο ῥεῦμα, ἄλλης διαφορήσεως χρεία, προσπλέκων ἀφρόνιτρα ἑνὶ τῶν εἰρημένων, ἢ νίτρον, τὸ βερονικάριον λεγόμενον· ἢ ἑψήματι ἐνεψούμενον γλήχωνα, ἢ θύμβραν, ἢ θύμον, ἢ καλαμίνθην. δυνήσεται γάρ τις καὶ ἀθρόως ἐμπίπτοντος τοῦ χυμοῦ γινώσκειν τὰ τοσαῦτα τῶν βοηθημάτων, ἐάν τε κυνηγετῇ κατ᾽ ἀγρὸν, ἐάν τε διαπράττηταί τι τῶν κατ᾽ ἀγρὸν ἔργων, ἐάν τε ἐν ὁδοιπορίαις τότε ἀπορῇ φαρμάκων, ἢ διὰ βάτου

ac faucium inflammationes, caeterosque affectus, ſeu ulcera ſint, ſeu cruſta, ſeu putredo.] Commune equidem praeceptum eſt, reprimendum repellendumque eſſe mox ab initio quod e capite defluit. At ab elapſo jam morbi initio, ad ipſius finem usque utendum mixto quodam reprimente et diſcutiente. Oportet autem eos qui reprimere volunt, uti medicamento de moris appellato. Uteris etiam et uvae immaturae ſucco, admixto pauxillo melle; et florum roſarum, aut ipſarummet roſarum ſiccarum, ſicut et pini corticis ex aqua decocto. At poſt initia, quum adhuc a capite defluxio ruit, alia diſcutiendi ratione eſſet opus. Tum adjice cuivis praedictorum aphronitrum, aut nitrum beronicarium dictum, vel incoque in ſapa pulegium aut ſatureiam aut thymum aut calaminthem. Poterit enim quivis conſertim irruente humore tot copioſa remedia nota habere, ſeu venator erret per agros, ſeu opus ruſticum in agro ſaciat, ſeu etiam viator iter ſuum medicamentorum indigus, aut rubi ſuccum, aut dictorum etiam quemvis ſibi poterit comparare, imo omnia fere

χυλοῦ, ἢ διά τινος τῶν εἰρημένων δύναται [591] πορίσασθαι παραμυθίαν, καὶ καθόλου σχεδὸν τὰ στύφοντα τοῖς στοματικοῖς πάθεσιν ἐπιτήδεια. χρησιμώτατον δὲ φάρμακον ταῖς περὶ στόμα διαθέσεσι καρύων χλωρῶν τοῦ φλοιοῦ χυλὸς ὀλίγῳ μέλιτι συνεψούμενος. χρήσιμον δὲ καὶ τὸ τῶν κυδωνίων ἀφέψημα, εἰ προσβάλῃς βραχύ τι μέλιτος· χρησιμώτατον δὲ καὶ τὸ διὰ τοῦ χλωροῦ τῶν καρύων, καὶ πρὸς τὰς σφοδρὰς φλεγμονὰς τῶν ἀντιάδων καὶ τοὺς πνιγμούς. ἄλλο. ῥοιᾶς γλυκείας σὺν τοῖς λεπύροις κόψας, καὶ ἐκλειώσας διήθησον, καὶ ἓξ μέρεσι τοῦ χυλοῦ πρόσβαλε μέρος ἓν μέλιτος καὶ ἑψήσας ὡς μέλιτος πάχος ἔχειν, χρῶ. ἄλλο. γλεύκους ξέστην ἕψει μέχρις ἂν τὸ τρίτον λειφθῇ, καὶ μίξον ῥοῦς βυρσοδεψικοῦ γο. δ'. καὶ ἀπάρας χρῶ. ἄλλο. κηκίδας λ'. κόψας, καὶ ἐνεψήσας ξέστην α'. μέλιτος, χρῶ.

[Στοματικὴ καλλίστη.] Ἄνθους ῥόδων γο. β'. πιτυΐδων γο. α'. λεάνας σὺν μέλιτι χρῶ.

[Πρὸς παρίσθμια καὶ σταφυλὴν φλεγμαίνουσαν καὶ σηπεδόνας τὰς ἐν στόματι.] Μόρων χυλοῦ ἢ βάτου γο. α'.

aftringentia, oris affectibus idonea. Utiliffimum tamen ipfis oris affectibus medicamentum fuccus eft corticum nucum viridium una cum pauco melle coctus. Utile etiam ad eosdem decoctum cotoneorum, adjecto mellis pauxillo; fed quod ex viridibus nucibus fit medicamentum, multo eft utiliffimum ad vehementes tonfillarum inflammationes et fuffocationes. *Aliud.* Recipe dulcis mali punici tufi cum fuo cortice expreffum colatumque fuccum, cujus fex partibus addito unam mellis, demum coquito ad mellis craffitudinem, ac utitor. *Aliud.* Mufti fextarium decoquito ad tertias, adjectis rhu coriarii unciis quatuor, demum reponito in ufum. *Aliud.* Tufas gallas xxx. decoque in mellis fextario j, quo utere.

[*Optimum ftomaticum.*] Recipe florum rofarum unc. ij, fructus pini unc. j, tere ex melle, ac utere.

[*Ad inflammationes tonfillarum ac columellae et oris putredines.*] Recipe fucci mororum aut rubi unc. j,

ῥόδων ξηρῶν γο. α'. μέλιτι μίξας, καὶ ἐπ' ὀλίγον ἑψήσας, διάχριε. ἄλλο. κυδωνίων στύφων χυλὸν ἐν ἴσῳ μέλιτι ἑψήσας διάχριε. ἄλλο. ῥοιὰς στυφούσας μετὰ τοῦ λέπους κόψας ἕψει ἐν γλυκεῖ, διηθήσας, χρῶ. ἄλλο. εἰς ἕψημα ἐμβαλὼν γλήχωνα ἢ θύμον ἢ ὀρίγανον ἢ ὕσσωπον ἢ καλαμίνθην, καὶ συνεψήσας αὐτάρκως καὶ διηθήσας δίδου διακρατεῖν.

[Πρὸς τὰς ἐν τῷ στόματι σηπεδόνας καὶ ἐσχάρας.] Κυνείαν λευκήν τινα (ἔστω δὲ τοῦτο ἐὰν ὀστᾶ μόνα πρὸ μιᾶς οἱ κύνες φαγόντες φλαχθῶσι) μετὰ μέλιτος διάχριε, ἢ ῥοὸς τοῦ βυρσοδεψικοῦ τὸ ὕδωρ μέχρι γλοιῶδες γίνηται, ἑψήσας μέλιτι. ἢ χελιδόνων κεκαυμένων μετὰ μέλιτος διάχριε.

[Πρὸς κιονίδας φλεγμαινούσας καὶ κεχαλασμένας.] Φοίνικας ἑψήσας ἐν ὕδατι καὶ βραχέος μέλιτος προσβαλὼν, δίδου ἀναγαργαρίζεσθαι καὶ διακρατεῖν. ἢ ῥόδων, ἢ ἑλίκων ἀμπέλου, ἢ βάτου, ἢ κυνοσβάτου, ἢ μήλων στύφων, ἢ οὔων ἀώρων, ἢ ῥοῦ, τοῦ τ' ἐπὶ τὰ ὄψα καὶ τοῦ βυρσοδε-

rofarum aridarum unc. j, cum melle mixta et modice cocta illine. *Aliud.* Cotoneorum acerborum fuccum cum aequali mellis portione coctum illine. *Aliud.* Aftringens malum punicum cum fuo cortice tufum incoquito paffo, quo colato utitor. *Aliud.* Immittito in fapam pulegium aut thymum aut origanum aut hyffopum aut calaminthem, ac fimul coquito fufficienter, deinde colatum da ore tenendum.

[*Ad oris putredines ac cruftas.*] Album canis fimum (fit autem ejus canis fimum, qui folis vefcitur offibus) cum melle illine. Aut aquam rhu futorii cum melle ad fordium craffitudinem decoctum. Aut etiam uftarum hirundinum cinerem ex melle illinito.

[*Ad columellae inflammationem et laxationem.*] Palmularum ex aqua decoctum, adjecto pauxillo melle, gargarizandum, oreque continendum exhibe. *Vel* decoctum rofarum, vel capreolorum vitis, vel rubi, vel rubicanini, vel pomorum acerborum, vel forborum immaturorum, vel

ψικοῦ, ἢ μυρίκης καρποῦ, καθ' ἑαυτό τε ἕκαστον καὶ σὺν ἀλλήλοις ἀφεψηθὲν ἐν ὕδατι ἀνακογχυλιαζέσθω· ἢ ξηρῷ τινὶ τῶν προειρημένων εὖ μάλα λειωθέντι προσάπτεσθαι τοῦ γαργαρεῶνος, ἠρέμα πως ἀνάγονται. ἐμβάλλειν δὲ αὐτὰ κοχλιαρίῳ, καὶ οὕτως προστιθέναι τῇ κιονίδι. καὶ οἱ χυλοὶ δὲ τῶν προειρημένων ἁπάντων τῶν τε φυτῶν καὶ τῶν καρπῶν αὐτῶν ὁμοίως μέλιτι ὀλίγῳ μιγνύμενοι καὶ διαχριόμενοι ὠφελοῦσιν. ἄλλο. ποιοῦσι πρὸς τὰς κιονίδος φλεγμονὰς ἅλες λεῖοι μετὰ μέλιτος διαχριόμενοι. ἄλλο. φοινίκων ὀστᾶ καὶ καρύων ἁπαλῶν χλωρῶν καὶ ξηρῶν, ἑκατέρου ἴσον, καύσας καὶ λειοτριβήσας, χρῶ ἁπτόμενος. ἄλλο. ῥόδα ξηρὰ πάνυ λειώσας σὺν μέλιτι διάχριε.

[Πρὸς ἄφθας.] Ἀνδράχνην εἰς μέλι βάπτων μασάσθω, ἢ ἐλαίας φύλλοις ἐν οἴνῳ ἡψημένοις διακλυζέσθω.

[Πρὸς ἄφθας μελαίνας καὶ νεμομένας.] Ἀποσμήξας ὀροβίνοις ἀλεύροις καὶ κηκῖδος διάχριε μετὰ μέλιτος, ἢ λυκίου ἀφεψήματι ἀναγαργαριζέσθω, ἢ τρυγὶ οἴνου μετὰ

rhoi quo in cibis utitur et rhoi coriarii, vel fructus myricae; horum enim quodque ſigillatim, aut cuivis ex praedictis adjunctum et ex aqua decoctum gargarizatur. Aut ex his ſiccatum quoddam in pulverem conteritur et columellae apponitur, quae ſenſim ac leniter ſurſum ducitur: ſolet autem is cochleario injectus ita columellae apponi. Quin etiam cujusvis praedictorum, tam plantarum, quam fructuum succus, cum pauculo melle uvae illitus juvat. *Aliud.* Ad vulvae inflammationem conferunt triti et ex melle inuncti. *Aliud.* Palmularum oſſa ac nuces tenerae, virides, aridaeque pari portione utuntur, inque pulverem comminuuntur, quo columella tangitur. *Aliud.* Roſas ſiccas in tenuiſſimum pollinem laevigantes ex melle inducito.

[*Ad aphthas.*] Portulacam melle madentem maſticato. *Aut* foliorum olivae ex vino decoctum gargarizato.

[*Ad aphthas nigras depaſcentes.*] Deterſas prius ervi farina ac gallarum ex melle illinito. Aut lycii deco-

μέλιτος διαχριέσθω. ἢ [592] μυρίκης καρπὸν λειώσας μετὰ μέλιτος διάχριε.

[Πρὸς νεμομένας ἄφθας.] Κηκίδων ἀφέψημα εἰς ἴσον μέλιτι μίξας καὶ ἀναζέσας χρῶ.

[Πρὸς λευκὰς ἄφθας.] Χαλκῖτιν ἐλαίῳ ζέσας διάχριε πτερῷ, καὶ παραχρῆμα αἴρει. ἐπὰν δὲ καθαρὰ γένηται, μυρίκης καρπὸν λεάνας καὶ διεὶς μελικράτῳ ἢ οἴνῳ διάχριε πτερῷ, καὶ παραχρῆμα αἴρει.

[Πρὸς μελαίνας ἄφθας.] Σταφίδι ἐκγεγιγαρτισμένῃ καὶ ἀνίσῳ λείοις κατάχριε μετὰ μέλιτος. ἢ φύλλα κοκκυμηλέας κόψας καὶ γάλακτι μίξας ὀνείῳ, διάκλυζε. ποιεῖ καὶ πρασίου χυλὸς ἢ φακοῦ ἀφέψημα, ἢ βάτου, ἢ κέρας ἐλάφειον λεάνας παράτριβε.

[Πρὸς ἄφθας βρεφῶν.] Φακὴν μετὰ βραχέος ἄρτου καὶ κυδωνίων ὀπῷ μίξας, δίδου, καὶ ῥόδων ἄνθος, καὶ αὐτὰ τὰ ῥόδα ξηρὰ, καὶ διακλύσματι διὰ τῶν μετρίως στυφόντων. ἔλαιον δὲ ἐναντιώτατόν ἐστι τῇ διαθέσει τῆς ἄφθης,

ctum gargarizato. Aut faece dulcis vini ex melle perfricato. Aut tamaricis fructum cum melle tritum infricato.

[*Ad depafcentes aphthas.*] Gallarum decocto cum mellis aequali menfura mixto fervefactoque utitor.

[*Ad aphthas albas.*] Pluma oleum in quo chalcitin praecoxeris illine et confeftim curabit. Aut deterfo nunc mundatoque loco affecto, tritum tamaricis fructum ex melicrato aut vino pluma fimiliter inducito et cito fanabit.

[*Ad aphthas nigras.*] Uvam paffam fine acinis et anifum tere, locoque affecto ex melle infrica. Aut pruni folia concifa afinino lacte misceto, osque ex eo colluito. Idem poffunt marrubii fuccus et lentis ac rubi decoctum; nec non tritum cornu cervinum, infricatum.

[*Ad aphthas infantium.*] Lentem cum pauco pane et cotoneorum fucco mixtam exhibe et rofarum florem; quin ipfas etiam rofas aridas; utitor autem oris collutione ex rebus mediocriter adftringentibus. Sed oleum aphthis ipfis adverfiffimum eft et vehementer acria; illud quidem,

καὶ τὰ πάνυ δριμέα· τὸ μὲν γὰρ ὑγραίνει τε καὶ ῥυπαίνει, τῇ τήξει δὲ τὰ δριμέα βλάπτει.

Κεφ. θ'. [Πρὸς τὰ πάθη ὀργάνων τῶν τῇ φωνῇ καὶ ἀναπνοῇ ὑπηρετεόντων καὶ πρώτως πρὸς τραχύτητας τῆς ἀρτηρίας.] Γλυκυῤῥίζης γο. γ'. λειώσας πάνυ, καὶ ἀποβρέξας κόμμεως τραγακάνθης γο. α'. γλυκεῖ ἀναλάμβανε, καὶ ποιήσας κυαμιαῖα, δὸς ὑπὸ τὴν γλῶσσαν καθεύδοντι.

[Πρὸς ἀποκεκομμένην φωνήν.] Σῦκα καὶ ἠρύγγια ἑψήσας καλῶς, τῷ ἀφεψήματι μίσγε κόμμεως βραχὺ, ὥστε γενέσθαι μέλιτος σκληρότερον, καὶ δίδου εἰς νύκτα. ἄλλο. κράμβης χυλὸν μετὰ μέλιτος ἑψήσας δίδου ἐκλείχειν, ποιεῖ καὶ πρὸς βῆχα. ἄλλο. (480) λινοσπέρμου κεκαυμένου καὶ σεσησμένου, σταφίδων λιπαρῶν χωρὶς τῶν γιγάρτων, στροβίλων πεφρυγμένων, καρύων Ποντικῶν κεκαθαρμένων ἴσα λεάνας, καὶ μέλιτι ἀπέπτῳ ἀναλαβὼν, δίδου κοχλιάριον ἕν.

[Βηχικὸν ἐκλεικτόν.] Πυρήνων, ἤτοι στροβίλων γο.

quod humectet fordidetque, acria vero, quod morfu laedant.

Cap. IX. [*Ad inftrumentorum voci refpirationique defervientium affectus, et primo ad vocalis arteriae afperitatem.*] Recipe dulcis radicis unc. iij, minutim eas admodum contere, deinde macerata gummi tragacanthae uncia una excipe paffo et forma ad fabae magnitudinem pilulas; unamque fub lingua dormituro continendam exhibe.

[*Ad intercifam vocem.*] Ficus et eryngium probe coque, huicque decocto adde gummi pauxillum, ita ut quam mellis craffior fit ipforum confiftentia, et fub nocte exhibeto. *Aliud.* Braffícae fuccum cum melle decoctum lambat; conducit hoc idem ad tuffim. *Aliud.* Lini femen toftum ac per cribrum excretum, uvas paffas pingues fine acinis, pineae nucis nucleos frixos, nuces Ponticas praepurgatas pari portione trita excipe melle crudo; da cochlearium unum.

[*Eclegma tuffículare.*] Recipe nucleorum pineorum

ιβ'. φοινίκων σάρκας β'. εὖ μάλα λείωσας ἀναλάμβανε μέλιτι ἀπέπτῳ.

[Πρὸς τὰς ξηρὰς βῆχας.] Ἶριν ὕδατι ἀφέψας πρόσβαλε μέλιτος βραχὺ καὶ δίδου καταῤῥοφεῖν συνεχῶς.

[Πρὸς αἵματος ἀναγωγὴν καὶ αἱμοπτοϊκούς.] Ῥόδων ξηρῶν γο. η'. κόμμεως τραγακάνθης ἑξάγια γ'. λείου μετὰ ὕδατος καὶ τροχίσκους ποίει ἀνὰ γο. α'. καὶ δίδου ὕδατι. ἄλλο. σικύων ἡμέρων κοιλίαν καὶ ὕδατος ἐπιβαλὼν ξέστην, ἕψει ἕως ἀποτριτωθῇ, καὶ καταπλάσας δίδου καταῤῥοφεῖν. ἄλλο. μίλτου Σινωπικῆς γο. β'. γῆς Σαμίας γο. ιβ'. ἀμύλου γο. γ'. ἀναλάμβανε πολυγόνου χυλῷ καὶ δίδου τριώβολον. ἄλλο. λινοσπέρμου πεφρυγμένου γο. η'. [593] κόμμεως τραγακάνθης γο. ιβ'. ὁμοίως χρῶ. ἄλλο. πολυγόνου ῥίζας ἑψήσας ὕδατι ἀποτριτωθῆναι ποίησον καὶ βραχὺ λείου κόμμεως ἐπιβάλλων, δίδου καταῤῥοφεῖν.

[Πρὸς φθισικοὺς καὶ τὰ περὶ θώρακος πάθη.] Ἴρεως ἀφέψημα μετὰ μέλιτος πότισον. ἢ ὑσσώπου ἀφέψημα μετὰ

unc. ij, carnem duorum dactylorum, admodum terito, melleque crudo excipito.

[*Ad tuffim ficcam.*] Iridis ex aqua decoctum, cui mellis pauxillum adjectum fit, da frequenter forbendum.

[*Ad fanguinis rejectionem.*] Recipe rofarum aridarum unc. viij, gummi tragacanthae hexagia iij, trita ex aqua in paftillos drachmae j, pondere forma; propina ex aqua. *Aliud.* In cucumeris domeftici ventrem infundito aquae fextarium, coquitoque ad tertias, et expreffum cremorem in forbitione dato. *Aliud.* Recipe rubricae Sinopicae unc. ij, terrae Samiae unc. xij, amyli unc. iij, polygoni fucco excipe; dato trium obolorum quantitatem. *Aliud.* Recipe fricti feminis lini unc. viij, gummi tragacanthae unc. xij, fimiliter utere. *Aliud.* Polygoni radices aqua incoquito ad tertias, additoque trito pauco gummi, offerto in forbitionem.

[*Ad tabidos et thoracis affectus.*] Ireos decoctum cum melle potandum dato. Vel forbendum hyffopi decoctum cum melle dato. Vel coctum marrubii herbae

μέλιτος δίδου καταῤῥοφεῖν. ἢ πρασίου βοτάνης χυλὸν σὺν μέλιτι ἑψήσας. ἢ ὀρόβους κιῤῥοὺς φρύξας καὶ λειοτριβήσας εἰκοσαπλασίῳ μέλιτι, δίδου ἔκλειγμα. ἢ ἀμύγδαλα πικρὰ λειώσας σὺν μέλιτι δίδου. ἄλλο. σελίνου σπέρματος γο. στ'. πεπέρεως μέλανος γο. α'. μέλιτος λίτραν α'. λειώσας καὶ ἠρέμα ἑψήσας, δίδου κοχλιάριον. ἄλλο. βούτυρον μέλιτι μίξας καὶ ἠρέμα ἑψήσας δίδου. ἄλλο. σελίνου γο. α'. πεπέρεως κοινὸν, μέλιτος λίτραν α'. λειώσας καὶ ἠρέμα συνεψήσας δίδου. ἄλλο. σκίλλης ὠμῆς τὸν χυλὸν ἔκθλιβε καὶ μίσγε μέλιτος ἴσῳ, καὶ θὲς ἐπ' ἀνθράκων ἕψε καὶ δίδου μύστρον πρὸ τροφῆς καὶ μετὰ τροφήν. ἄλλο. ἀβροτόνου, σταφίδων ἐκγεγιγαρτισμένων λιπαρῶν, πηγάνου ἀκρεμόνων ἑψήσας ἐν ὕδατι καὶ διηθήσας, πρόσβαλλε μέλιτος καὶ πάλιν ἑψήσας δίδου.

[Βοήθημα πρὸς δύσπνοιαν.] Ἀρσενικὸν κάπνισον εἰς βόλβιτα βοϊκὰ, μὴ ἀπὸ τοίχου ξηρανθέντα, καὶ κάπνιζε τὸν κάμνοντα διὰ χωνείου. χανέτω δὲ τὸ στόμα ὅσον δύναται, καὶ μετὰ τοῦτο δίδου αὐτῷ ἄκρατον Αἰγύπτιον. τέταρ-

ſuccum cum melle. Vel ervum rufum frixum ac tritum cum viginti partibus mellis da in eclegmate. Vel amygdalas amaras laevigatas cum melle exhibeto. *Aliud.* Recipe ſeminum apii drach. vj, piperis nigri unc. j, mellis lib. j, trita et ſenſim da cochlearii menſura. *Aliud.* Mixtum cum melle, lentoque igne decoctum, butyrum offerto. *Aliud.* Apii et piperis cujusque uncia una trita, cum mellis libra una, ſenſim decoque et propina. *Aliud.* Scillae crudae expreſſum ſuccum cum mellis aequa portione carbonibus ſuperpoſitum coquito, ac dato myſtrum ante cibum et poſt cibum. *Aliud.* Abrotonum, pingues paſſulas ſine acinis, rutae germina, in aqua decoquito percolatoque, decocto huic mel adjice, rurſusque decoque ac utere.

[*Ad ſpirandi difficultatem remedium.*] Arſenicum ſuffito ad ſtercora bubula non a muro exiccata, et aegrotum ſuffito per infundibulum; hiſcat os quantum poſſit et poſtea da ipſi merum Aegyptium. Quater id effice per

τον τοῦτο ποίει ἐπὶ ἡμέρας γ'. ἐὰν δὲ νοσερὸς εἴη ὁ κάμνων, τοῦτο ποίει· τὸ ἀρσενικὸν κόψας καὶ τρίψας σύμμισγε τῷ ἀκράτῳ καὶ δίδου αὐτῷ ἐπὶ ἡμέρας γ'. νήστει πιεῖν, καὶ ὅτε εὑρήσῃς αὐτὸν ἐλαφρότερον, κάπνισον ὡς προείρηται.

Κεφ. ι'. [Περὶ τῶν κατὰ τὸ στόμα τῆς κοιλίας παθῶν καὶ τῶν αὐτοῖς εὐπορίστων.] Αἱ τοῦ στόματος τῆς κοιλίας φλεγμοναὶ καὶ τοῦ ἥπατος δέονται τῆς τῶν στυφόντων παραπλοκῆς. εἰ μὲν γὰρ ὑπὸ τῆς χαλαστικῆς ἀγωγῆς μόνης θεραπεύονται, κίνδυνον ἐπάγουσι περὶ τῆς ζωῆς, καὶ τοῦτο πάντων μὲν τῶν ἐμπειρικῶν ὑπὸ τῆς πείρας δεδιδαγμένων καὶ ἐπὶ τῶν ἔργων τῆς τέχνης φυλαττόντων. οὐκ ὀλίγοι τῶν νῦν μεθοδικῶν μυρίοις μὲν στομαχικῆς συγκοπῆς αἴτιοι γεγόνασιν, οὐκ ὀλίγους δὲ καὐτῶν ἡπατικῶν ἀναιροῦσι, μόνῃ τῇ ἀγωγῇ τῇ χαλαστικῇ χρώμενοι, ὡς λυθῆναι πολλοῖς τὸ ἧπαρ. εἰ τοίνυν εἴτε ἔλαιον εἴη τὸ ἐπαντλούμενον τοῖς πεπονθόσι τόποις, εἴτε κατάπλασμα, παραπλέκειν τι τῶν στυφόντων, οἷον ἀψίνθιον ἢ νάρδινον μύρον

dies iv. Quod ſi valetudinarius fuerit aeger, id effice. Arſenicum fractum ac tritum commiſce mero, daque ipſi per dies iv. jejuno exhibendum; quumque inveneris ipſum facilius ferentem, ſuffito ut praedictum eſt.

Cap. X. [*De ſtomachi et ventriculi affectibus, eorumque remediis.*] Inflammationes oris ventriculi et hepatis aſtringentium medicamentorum indigent admixtione. Nam ſi qui ſolis laxantibus admotis curationem ſuſcipiant, vitae adducent diſcrimen, idque omnibus empiricis experientia edoctis et in artis operibus obſervantibus. Non pauci hodiernorum methodicorum innumeris ſyncopes ſtomachicae cauſam attulerunt, imo nec paucos etiam hepaticos e vita ſuſtulerunt, ſolis uſi laxantibus, quibus jecur plerisque diſſolvitur. Quare aſtringentium aliquid his ſemper adjiciatur, ſeu oleo affectum locum foveas, ſeu admoto cataplasmate cures; quale abſinthium vel unguentum nardinum vel aloe vel cotoneorum tam deco-

ἢ ἀλόην ἢ μήλινον ἔλαιον ἢ κυδώνιον ἀνέψοντες. καὶ κηρωταῖς δὲ χρηστέον διὰ τῆς ἀλόης καὶ μαστίχης καὶ κηροῦ καὶ νάρδου. σκευάσειας δὲ τὴν κηρωτὴν, βαλὼν κηροῦ γο. α'. μαστίχης γο. δ'. ἀλόης γο. β'. καὶ νάρδου τὸ ἀρκοῦν. εἰ δὲ πλείων εἴη ἡ ἀτονία, ὡς μηδὲ τὰς τροφὰς κατέχειν, μιγνύτωσαν τοῦ ὀμφάκου γο. β'. παρόντος δὲ καὶ ἀψινθίου χυλοῦ, προσπλέκειν καὶ αὐτοῦ γο. α'. ἢ οἰνάνθην, ἢ ῥοῦ χυλόν.

[*Περὶ τῶν θερμῶν τοῦ στομάχου δυσκρασιῶν.*] *Ἐπὶ* δὲ τῶν θερμῶν τοῦ στομάχου δυσκρασιῶν καὶ διὰ στόματος δοτέον τὸ φάρμακον τοῦτο. μαστίχης γο. β'. ἡδυόσμου γο. α'. ἀναλάμβανε χυλῷ ἀρνογλώσ- [594] σου, καὶ δίδου κυάμου μέγεθος μετὰ ὕδατος. ἐφ' ὧν δὲ καταψύχεται ὁ στόμαχος, τῇ προειρημένῃ σκευασίᾳ προσπλέκειν δεῖ καστορίου γο. α'. καὶ διδόναι ὁμοίως. ἐπιγνωσθήσεται δὲ ἡ θερμὴ δυσκρασία, ἐκ τοῦ ποτὲ μὲν καὶ χολῶδές τι ἀνάγεσθαι αὐτοὺς, καθόλου δὲ χολώδους δήξεως αἴσθησιν ἔχειν τοῦ στόματος τῆς γαστρὸς, καὶ ἁπτομένοις εἶναι θερμόν.

ctum quam oleum; atque cerato ex aloe, mastiche, cera et nardo utendum: ceratum autem ita conficies. Recipe cerae unc. j, mastiches unc. iv, aloes unc. ij, nardi quantum satis. Quod si vehemens adeo fuerit ventriculi imbecillitas, ut ne alimentum contineat, adjiciantur his succi uvae immaturae unciae ij, sed si succi absinthii fuerit facultas, addatur et hujus uncia una, aut oenanthe, aut succus rhu.

[*Pro calida ventriculi intemperie.*] In calida ventriculi intemperie medicamentum hoc per os exhibendum. Recipe mastiches unc. ij, mentae unc. j, excipe succo plantaginis et exhibe fabae magnitudinem ex aqua. Si contra ventriculus frigida afficiatur intemperie, dictae confectioni adjiciendum castorei unc. j, exhibetoque similiter. Cognoscetur autem calida *ventriculi* intemperies tum ex bilioso vomitu, tum ex sensu morsus biliosi in ore ventriculi percepti, tum quod tangentibus calidum appareat.

[Περὶ τῶν κατεψυγμένων στομάχων.] Ἐπὶ δὲ τῶν κατεψυγμένων στομάχων, καὶ ἐπὶ τῶν διὰ πάχους τοῦ φλέγματος θερμαίνεσθαί τε καὶ τέμνεσθαι δεομένων, χρήσιμόν ἐστι μαράθρου ῥίζης φλοιοῦ γο. στ'. ὄξους λίτραν α'. μέλιτος λίτραν α'. αἱ ῥίζαι σὺν τῷ ὄξει ἕψονται, εἶθ' ὅταν ἑφθαὶ γένωνται, ἐκθλιβόμεναι ῥίπτονται, καὶ ἐπιχεομένου τοῦ μέλιτος αὖθις ἕψεται τὸ φάρμακον μέχρι συστάσεως, καὶ δίδοται κοχλιάρια γ'. σὺν ὕδατι.

[Περὶ τῶν ἀποξυνόντων τὴν τροφήν.] Ἐπὶ δὲ τῶν ἀποξυνόντων τὴν τροφὴν χρήσιμον τόδε τὸ φάρμακον. πεπέρεως γο. α'. ἀνήθου σπέρματος γο. α'. κυμίνου γο. δ'. εὖ μάλα λειώσας, δίδου εἰς κοίτην κοχλιάριον ὕδατι ἐν οἴνῳ κεκραμένῳ.

[Πρὸς ἀνατροπὰς στομάχων.] Πρὸς δὲ τὰς ἀνατροπὰς καὶ ναυτίας τοῦ στομάχου, ῥοιᾶς ὀξείας πυρήνων τεθλασμένων τοῦ χυλοῦ μέρη γ'. ἡδυόσμου χυλοῦ μέρος α'. μέλιτος Ἀττικοῦ μέρος ἕν· βαλὼν εἰς κεράμειον ἀγγεῖον ἕψει,

[*Ad ventriculum refrigeratum.*] Ad ventriculum refrigeratum, quique ob pituitae in ipfo haerentis craffitudinem opus habet et calefacientibus et incidentibus aptum eft medicamentum, quod conftat corticis radicis foeniculi unciis vj, aceti libra j, mellis libra una. Decoquuntur primum radices cum aceto, ac coctae tunc exprimuntur abjiciunturque; demum affufo melle incoquitur rurfus medicamentum ad confiftentiam; propinantur cochlearia tria ex aqua.

[*Ad eos quibus in ventriculo cibus acefcit.*] Quibus affumptus cibus acefcit, medicamentum hoc accommodatum eft. Recipe piperis unc. j, feminum anethi unc. j, cumini unc. iv, omnibus diligenter tritis propinatur dormituris cochlearium ex aqua vino mixta.

[*Ad ventriculi fubverfiones.*] Ad fubverfiones et naufeas ventriculi. Recipe fucci mali punici acidi cum fuis acinis expreffi partes iij, fucci mentae partem j, mellis Attici partem j, decoque haec conjecta in vas fictile, affidue mifcendo; quumque craffefcunt, fublata reponuntur

κινῶν συνεχῶς. καὶ ὅταν συστραφῆ, ἄρας ἀπόθου. ἐν δὲ τῇ χρήσει δίδου πρὸ τροφῆς μύστρον α'. ἤτοι γο. β'.

[Πρὸς δυσεντερικοὺς καὶ τὴν τροφὴν ἐμοῦντας.] Κυδωνίας μηλέας τῆς ῥίζης λίτραν α'. οἴνου μυρτίτου ξ. γ'. ἕψει μέχρις ἂν ἀποτριτωθῇ, ἔπειτα ἐκθλίψας τὸ ὑγρὸν, ἐπίβαλε μέλιτος ἡμίλιτρον, καὶ πάλιν ἕψει κινῶν συνεχῶς, καὶ ἀνελόμενος, δίδου πρὸ τροφῆς μύστρον.

[Πρὸς στομάχου ἀνατροπὴν, καὶ κοιλιακοὺς, καὶ δυσεντερικούς.] Μῆλα κυδώνια ἀριθμῷ δ'. ῥοὰς ὁλοκλήρους ι'. οὖα ἀριθμῷ η'. ὕδατος Ἰταλικοῦ ξ γ'. καὶ ἕψει φιλοπόνως, καὶ ὅταν διαλυθῇ, ἔκθλιβε τὸ ὑγρόν· καὶ πᾶν τὸ ἀχυρῶδες τῶν ὀπωρῶν ἐκβαλὼν, πάλιν ἕψει, καὶ ὅταν τὸ τρίτον τοῦ ὑγροῦ ἀπολειφθῇ, βάλε μέλιτος καλοῦ λίτρας δ'. καὶ ἕψει ἐπ' ἀνθράκων, κινῶν συνεχῶς, καὶ ὅταν συστραφῇ, ἀπόθου, καὶ χρῶ ὁμοίως.

[Πρὸς χολέραν.] Εἰ χωρὶς πυρετοῦ γένοιτο καὶ τῆς ἄλλης καθάρσεως, δίδου ψωμοὺς ἐν οἴνῳ κεκραμένῳ, καὶ

in ufum. Datur poftulante neceffitate ante cibum myftrum j, aut unc. ij.

[*Ad dyfentericos et cibum vomitu rejicientes.*] Recipe radicis arboris cotoneae lib. j, decoque in vini myrtei fextariis iij, ad tertias usque; expreffo deinde cremori adde mellis libram dimidiam, coquitoque rurfus affidue mifcendo; tandem reponito in ufum: datur ante cibum myftrum.

[*Ad ventriculi fubverfionem, coeliacos et dyfentericos.*] Recipe mala cotonea numero iv, integra mala punica x, forba numero viij, in aquae Italicis fextariis tribus accurate decoquito; quumque omnia diffoluta jam fuerint, liquorem exprimito; demum ejectis craffis fructuum partibus, cremorem eum iterum coque ad tertias ufque; poftremo additis generofi mellis libris quatuor, rurfumque coquito impofitum carbonibus, continuo miscendo, quumque coctus fuerit, reconde, ac fimiliter utere.

[*Ad choleram.*] Si fine febre et intempeftiva purgatione eveniat, da bucellam panis ex vino diluto, daque

ψυχρῷ πότιζε, καὶ σικύας τίθει σφοδρὰς κατὰ τοῦ μέσου. εὐέκτου δὲ ὄντος τοῦ πάσχοντος, καὶ εἰς ψυχρὰν δεξαμένην ἐπὶ πλεῖστον ἐγκάθιζε. δίδου δὲ καὶ τροφὰς στυφούσας, καὶ τῶν ὀπωρῶν, μῆλον κυδώνιον, καὶ ῥοὰς στυφούσας.

[*Πρὸς ἐκκαιομένους ἄδιψον καταπότιον.*] Σικύου ἡμέρου σπέρματος γο. η'. ἀνδράχνης σπέρματος γο. η'. τραγακάνθης γο. δ'. διάλυε τὴν τραγάκανθαν ᾠῶν ὠμῶν προσφάτων τῷ λευκῷ, καὶ ὅταν διαλυθῇ, τρίψας ἐπιμελῶς, ἐπίβαλε τοῖς λοιποῖς, καὶ μίξας ἀνάπλαττε καταπότια, καὶ ξήραινε ἐν σκιᾷ, καὶ δίδου ἓν ὑπὸ τὴν γλῶτταν κατέχειν, καὶ τὸ διαλυόμενον ὑγρὸν καταπινέτω.

[595] (481) [*Πρὸς ἀνατροπὴν στομάχου, ἢ καυσώδεις ἀναθυμιάσεις.*] Ἀνίσου γο. β'. σελίνου γο. β'. κυμίνου γο. α'. λειώσας ἐπιμελῶς δίδου ὅτε μὲν νήστει κοχλιάριον α'. ἐν ὕδατι, ὅτε δὲ πρὸς τὴν κοίτην, ἐν οἴνῳ. ἄλλο. ἀψινθίου ἀπόβρεγμα τριῶν ἐφεξῆς ἡμερῶν πότιζε.

[*Πρὸς καταψύξεις καὶ λυγμοὺς τοῦ στομάχου.*] Πε-

potu frigidam et cucurbitulas magnas medio affige ventri. Quod fi aegrotus bono fit habitu, eum in frigidum lavacrum inducito, in quo diutius permaneat, da quoque cibum aftringentem, ut ex autumnalibus fructibus mala tam cotonea, quam punica.

[*Immodicam ex nimio ardore fitim extinguentia catapotia.*] Recipe feminum cucumeris domeftici unc. viij, feminum portulacae unc. viij, tragacanthae unc. iv, diffolve tragacantham recentium crudorum ovorum albis, diffolutamque affundito caeteris probe tritis; formatoque ex omnibus mixtis catapotia, in umbra deficca; tenendum ex ipfis unum fub lingua dato, folutusque faliva humor paulatim deglutiatur.

[*Ad ventriculi fubverfionem, vel fervidos halitus.*] Recipe anifi unc ij, apii unc. ij, cumini unc j, propinato ex his bene laevigatis, jejuno quidem cochlearium ex aqua, fub fomnum autem aliquando ex vino. *Aliud.* Bibatur tribus continuis diebus abfinthii dilutum.

[*Ad ventriculi refrigerationem et fingultum.*] Recipe

πέρεως γο. β΄. καστορίου γο. α΄. δίδου κοχλιάριον σύμμετρον νήστει ἐν ὕδατι. εἰ δὲ ἀπὸ θερμῶν χυμῶν τῶν κατὰ τὴν πέψιν διεφθορότων ὁ λυγμὸς γίνεται, ὃ καὶ διὰ καύσεως καὶ δηγμοῦ τοῦ στομάχου αἰσθάνοιτο, ὕδωρ χλιαρὸν πίνοντας κέλευε πολυεμεῖν, καὶ αὐτίκα παύσεται ὁ λυγμός. καὶ πταρμὸς ἐπιτηδευθεὶς παύει λυγμὸν καὶ ὄξος καταῤῥοφούμενον.

[Πρὸς καυσούμενον στόμαχον.] Τοῖς δ᾽ ἐγκαυσουμένοις τὸν στόμαχον μετ᾽ ἐκλύσεως ἢ λειποθυμίας, εἰ μὴ πυρέττοιεν, κυάθους γ΄. ἢ δ΄. δίδου ψυχροῦ ὕδατος καταπίνειν ἐκ διαλειμμάτων, καὶ εἰ μὲν παρηγοροῖτο τοῦτο, αὐτὸς ἀνακτησάμενος τροφὴν δίδοσο. εἰ δὲ ἐπιμένοι, διακρατουμένων τε καὶ ἡνωμένων τῶν ἄκρων, καὶ ἀπόβρεγμα συνεχῶς καταῤῥοφεῖν δίδου, ἢ μήλων κυδωνίων, ἢ ἀπίων, ἢ μεσπίλων, ἢ ἀρκευθίδων, ἢ ἑλίκων ἀμπέλου, ἢ ῥόδων, ἢ ῥοᾶς χυλοῦ, ἢ ὄμφακος χυλοῦ, ἢ κλώνιον ἡδυόσμου λεάνας, δὸς πιεῖν, ἢ οἰνάνθην, καὶ ἔα ἠρεμεῖν.

[Πρὸς σιελίζοντας ἐκ στομάχου.] Τοῖς δὲ σιελίζουσιν

piperis unc. iij, caſtorei unc. j, mediocris cochlearii quantitas, ex aqua jejuno datur. At ſi ex calidis ſuccis in ipſa ventriculi concoctione corruptis ſingultus ortum habeat, quod ex ventriculi ardore mordicationeque cognoſces, aqua tepida epota, jube affatim vomant, et ceſſabit confeſtim ſingultus. Porro ſternutamentum in tempore factum ſedat ſingultum et acetum in ſorbitione acceptum.

[*Ad aeſtuantem ventriculum.*] Quibus ventriculus aeſtuat cum exolutione aut animi deſectu, niſi febricitent, dato in potu frigidae cyathos iij, aut iv, idque per intervalla. Quod ſi malum miteſcat, ipſos reficiendo cibum exhibeto; ſin vero perduret, adſtrictis conjunctisque extremis, ei praebeto ſorbendum aſſidue dilutum vel malorum cotoneorum, pyrorumve, aut meſpilorum, aut baccarum juniperi, aut pampinorum vitis, aut roſarum, vel ſucci mali punici, vel uvae acerbae: vel dato, quem bibat, tritum menthae ramulum, aut oenanthem, et ſinito quieſcere.

[*Ad exuberantem e ventriculo ſalivam.*] Diſſluen-

ὄρυζαν ξηρὰν δίδου μασᾶσθαι. ἐπιτίθει δὲ καὶ ἔξω ἐπὶ τὸν στόμαχον ἀμπέλου φύλλα χλωρὰ λεῖα, ἢ μῆλα κυδώνια, ἢ χλωρὰν ἀνδράχνην, ἢ κολοκύνθης ξύσμα.

[Πρὸς πόνον στομάχου.] Τὰ δὲ ἀλγήματα τοῦ στομάχου πραΰνει καὶ μαλάσσει, ἐφ᾽ ὧν δυσφορία τις ἢ ἀπορία τρέπεται, γάλα βόειον ἢ ὄνειον, κοχλάκων ἐναφηψημένων πινόμενον· ἢ ἀπόζεμα ῥόδων, ἢ ᾠοῦ λέκυθον ὀπτὴν μετὰ ἀλφίτου πότιζε.

[Πρὸς στόμαχον ἐμοῦντα χολὴν μέλαιναν.] Ἐπὶ δὲ τῶν χολὴν μέλαιναν γεννώντων καὶ ἐμούντων, καὶ φυσωμένων τὸν στόμαχον, καὶ μάλιστα ἐν ταῖς ἐκμασήσεσι, σπόγγους ὄξει δριμυτάτῳ θερμῷ βεβρεγμένους στομάχῳ ἐπιτίθει, ἢ κισσοῦ φύλλοις ἑφθοῖς ἐν οἴνῳ κατάπλασσε, καὶ τροφὴν εὔχυμον δίδου. ἔστι δὲ εὔχυμος τροφὴ διά τε τῶν ᾠῶν, καὶ ἄλικος, καὶ ζωμῶν, οἷς ἐνήψηται ἢ ὀρνίθια, ἢ ὄνυχες χοίρων, ἢ φασιανοῦ κρέας, ἢ νεαροῦ πέρδικος, καὶ πάντων τῶν τούτοις ὁμοίων.

tes faliva mafticent ficcam oryzam. Extrinfecus etiam impone ventriculo contrita vitis viridia folia, aut mala cotonea, aut viridem portulacam, aut etiam cucurbitae ramentum.

[*Ad dolorem ventriculi.*] Ventriculi ex jactatione aut anxietate dolores fedat, ac mitigat potum lac bubulum, aut afininum, cui incocti fint lapilli; aut rofarum decoctum, aut affum ovi luteum cum polenta potato.

[*Ad ftomachum bilem nigram evomentem.*] Ad nigram bilem procreantes et vomentes, ventriculique flatibus diftentos et potiffimum inter manducandum, fpongias aceto acerrimo calido inebriatas ventriculo admove. Aut hederae folia vino decocta in cataplasma admove. Da quoque cibum boni fucci. Eft autem boni fucci cibus, tum qui ex ovis et alica, tum qui ex jusculis fit, quibus aut aviculae, aut extremae porci partes, aut phafiani, aut juvenis perdicis, omniumque his fimilium carnes incoctae fuerint.

[Πρὸς πνευμάτωσιν στομάχου.] Τοὺς δὲ πνευματουμένους καὶ διατεινομένους τὸν στόμαχον πολίου δεσμίδιον κατέχων καὶ καθέψων πότιζε. ἢ καλαμίνθης ἀφέψημα μίξας ὀλίγον μέλιτος καὶ πεπέρεως γο. α΄. χρῶ.

[Ἀνώδυνον στομαχικοῖς.] Κύμινον πεφρυγμένον καὶ σέλινον ὀλίγον ποτιζόμενον ἐν ὕδατι, ἢ ἀβροτόνου καὶ θύμου ἀνὰ δύο ὀβολοὺς δὸς πιεῖν.

[Πρὸς τοὺς βουλιμιῶντας ἐν ταῖς ὁδοῖς.] Τοὺς δὲ βουλιμιῶντας ἐν ταῖς ὁδοῖς, ἢ ἄλλως πως, ἀνακτησόμεθα ὄξει ὀσφραίνοντες, ἢ γλήχωνι, ἢ γῆν ὄξει βρέξαντες, ἢ μήλοις, ἢ ἀπίοις, ἢ ἄλλοις καρποῖς [596] ὁμοίοις τοῖς παροῦσιν, ἢ ἄρτον μετὰ οἴνου προσφέρεσθαι ἀναγκάζοντες.

[Πρὸς τοὺς λύζοντας.] Ἐπὶ δὲ τοῖς λύζουσι πήγανον μετὰ οἴνου δίδου καταῤῥοφεῖν, ἢ νίτρον ἐν μελικράτῳ, ἢ σέλινον, ἢ καστόριον, ἢ ἀβρότονον, ἢ ἀριστολοχίαν, ἢ κύμινον, ἢ ἄνισον, ἢ καλαμίνθην.

Κεφ. ια΄. [Πρὸς τὰ ἥπατος πάθη, καὶ πρῶτον πρὸς ἔμφραξιν ἥπατος.] Ἀμυγδάλων πικρῶν γο. γ΄. κυμίνου γο.

[*Ad ventriculi inflationem.*] Inflato diftentoque ventriculo laborantes juvat polii fasciculus foris impofitus, nec non potum ejusdem decoctum; aut calaminthae decoctum admixto mellis pauco et piperis drach. j, ufurpatur.

[*Doloris ftomachi mitigatorium.*] Cuminum affum et apii pauxillum potui ex aqua datur; aut abrotoni ac thymi, utriusque obolos duos potui dato.

[*Ad vehementer efurientes in itineribus.*] Bulimo laborantes feu in itinere, feu modo alio eos reficimus porrigentes olfaciendum acetum, aut pulegium, aut terram aceto madentem, aut poma, aut pyra, aut his fimiles fructus alios obvios; aut etiam panem ex vino eos affumere cogentes.

[*Ad fingultientes.*] Singultientibus da rutam cum vino in forbitionem, aut nitrum ex melicrato, vel apium, vel caftoreum, vel abrotonum, vel ariftolochiam, vel cuminum, vel anifum, vel calaminthem.

Cap. XI. [*Ad hepatis affectus et primo ad obftru-*

α΄. σελίνου σπέρματος γο. α΄. δίδου πιεῖν κοχλιάριον ἐν οἴνῳ. ἄλλο. πάνακος ῥίζης γο. γ΄. ἐρυθροδάνου < α΄. σελίνου < α΄. πεπέρεως < β΄. ἀριστολοχίας < α΄. γεντιανῆς ῥίζης ἐπιμελῶς λειωθείσης, κοχλιάριον α΄. ἐν οἴνῳ δίδου. ἄλλο. ἀρκευθίδων γο. γ΄. κράμβης σπέρματος γο. α΄. εὐζώμου σπέρματος γο. β΄. μέλιτι ἀπέπτῳ ἀναλαβὼν, δίδου κοχλιάριον ἕν. ἄλλο. κιχωρίου χυλίσματος κύαθον δίδου μετὰ ὕδατος θερμοῦ κυάθων β΄. ἐπιβάλλων μέλιτος κοχλιάρια β΄. μετὰ ὕδατος θερμοῦ. ἄλλο. ἀνήθου χυλοῦ κύαθον μετὰ μελικράτου θερμοῦ κυάθων γ΄. καὶ ξηρὰ δὲ γενόμενα τὰ προειρημένα, καὶ κοπτόμενα καὶ ἐπιπασσόμενα, ἀφεψήσας ἕκαστον αὐτῶν πινέτω. ἄλλο. χαμαιπίτυος ἀφέψημα μετὰ βραχέος μέλιτος δίδου πιεῖν. ἄλλο. χαμαιπίτυος ἀφεψήματος γο. η΄. κιχωρίου ῥίζης γο. δ΄. κόπτε καὶ ἀναλάμβανε μέλιτι ἑφθῷ, καὶ δίδου καρύου Ποντικοῦ μέγεθος μεθ᾽ ὕδατος θερμοῦ.

[*Τροχίσκος ἡπατικός.*] Ἀνίσου, σελίνου σπέρματος, ἄρου, ἀμυγδάλων πικρῶν κεκαθαρμένων, ἀψινθίου ἀνὰ γο. α΄.

ctionem.] Recipe amygdalarum amararum unc. iij, cumini unc. j, ſeminum apii unc. j, da cochlearium ex vino. *Aliud.* Recipe radicis panacis unc. iij, rubiae drach. j, apii drach. j, piperis drach. ij, ariſtolochiae drach. j, radicis gentianae diligenter tritae cochlearium j, dato ex vino. *Aliud.* Recipe baccarum juniperi unc. iij, ſeminum braſſicae unc. j, ſeminum erucae unc. ij, excipe melle crudo, daque cochlearium unum. *Aliud.* Succi cichorii cyathum da cum aquae calidae cyathis ij, et mellis cochleariis duobus cum aqua calida exhibeto. *Aliud.* Succi anethi cyathus cum tribus cyathis aquae mulſae calidae. Dictorum autem ipſorum quodque ſeorſum aridum, tuſum, aut cibo inſpergitur, aut coctum bibitur. *Aliud.* Chamaepityos decoctum cum pauxillo melle bibendum exhibe. *Aliud.* Chamaepityos decocti unc. viij, radicis cichorii unc. iv, contunde et excipe melle cocto, da avellanae magnitudinem ex aqua calida.

[*Trochiscus hepaticus.*] Recipe aniſi, ſeminum apii, ari, amygdalarum amararum mundatarum, abſinthii, cu-

ὕδατι ἀναπλάττων τροχίσκους ἔχοντας ἀνὰ < α'. ἀπυρέτοις μετὰ οἴνου κεκραμένου δίδου, πυρέσσουσι μετὰ ὑδρομέλιτος. ἄλλο. ἠριγέροντος ἀφέψημα δίδου πιεῖν. ἄλλο. ἀριστολοχίας ἡμίδραχμον λειώσας, πότιζε πυρέσσοντας ὕδατι, ἀπυρέτους μετ' οἴνου. ἄλλο. τρίφυλλον βοτάνην ἀποτριτώσας δίδου πιεῖν.

[Πρὸς ἰκτεριῶντας.] Λοῦε αὐτοὺς ἐν λουτροῖς ὑδάτων ποτίμων, καὶ τρῖβε αὐτῶν ὅλον τὸ σῶμα ἐλαίῳ ἀνηθίνῳ. εἰ δὲ μὴ πυρέττοιεν, εἰς κολοκυνθίδος κέλυφος ἐμβαλὼν οἶνον καὶ θερμάνας δίδου πιεῖν. ἄλλο. στρουθίον λειώσας δίδου κοχλιάριον α'. ὕδατι ἢ οἰνομέλιτι ἀπυρέτοις. ἄλλο. κιχωρίου κυάθους γ'. δίδου πυρέττουσι μὲν καθ' ἑαυτὸ, ἀπυρέτοις δὲ μετὰ οἰνομέλιτος κεκραμένου. ἄλλο. ἐρεβίνθους τοὺς καλουμένους κριοὺς, καὶ μάραθρον ἑψήσας, δίδου τὸν χυλὸν, ἀπυρέτοις μετ' οἴνου κεκραμένου. ἄλλο. καρδάμου χλωροῦ τὰ ἁπαλώτατα φύλλα, λιβανωτίδος χλωρᾶς τὰ ἁπαλώτατα φύλλα τρίψας, καὶ τούτων τὸ ὑγρὸν ἐκθλίψας, χρῶ μετ' οἰνομέλιτος ἐπὶ τῶν ἀπυρέτων. ἄλλο. ἐλατήριον μετὰ γά-

jusque unc. j, forma ex aqua trochiscos drach. j, continentes, exhibe non febricitantibus ex vino diluto, febricitantibus ex mulſo. *Aliud.* Senecionis da bibendum decoctum. *Aliud.* Ariſtolochiae drachmam dimidiam tritam da potui, febrientibus ex aqua, ex vino non febrientibus. *Aliud.* Trifolii herbae ad tertias decoctum dato potui.

[*Ad aurigine laborantes.*] Affectos aurigine lavato in balneo aquae poculentae, totumque eorum corpus oleo confricato anethino. Quod ſi febre vacet, in colocynthidos corio calefactum vinum propinato. *Aliud.* Lanariae tritae cochlearium ex aqua dato; aut ex mulſo liberis a febre. *Aliud.* Cichorii ſucci cyathos tres propinato, febrientibus quidem per ſe, non febrientibus vero ex mulſo mixto. *Aliud.* Ciceris dicti arietini et foeniculi coctorum cremorem exhibeto; febre carentibus cum vino mixto. *Aliud.* Tenerrima folia tam naſturtii viridis, quam roris marini etiam viridis terito; expreſſoque ex his ſucco utitor ex mulſo, ſi febre careant. *Aliud.* Elaterium tritum

λακτος γυναικείου τρίψας, ἐγχυμάτιζε εἰς τοὺς μυκτῆρας, κελεύων ἀνασπᾷν. ἄλλο. κυκλαμίνου χυλὸν ὕδατι διαλύσας, χρῶ καθὰ προείρηται. ἄλλο. τὸν πυῤῥὸν καρπὸν τῆς κυνοσβάτου ἐσθίειν δίδου. ἄλλο. χελιδονίας βοτάνης χυλὸν μετὰ οἴνου καὶ ὑδρομέλιτος δίδου τοῖς ἀπυρέτοις. ἄλλο. ὑπερικοῦ < α'. πότιζε μετὰ ὑδρομέλιτος καὶ ἀσίτοις δίδου ἐσθίειν ἀμύγδαλα πικρά.

[597] Κεφ. ιβ'. [Πρὸς σπληνικούς.] Χαμαίδρυος ἀφεψήματι πότιζε, ἢ χαμαιπίτυος, ἢ πολίου, ἢ ἐρυθροδάνου, ἢ καθ' ἑαυτά, ἢ ὀξυμέλιτος τοὺς ἀπυρέτους. ἄλλο. κισσοῦ λευκοῦ τῶν κορύμβων δίδου κόκκους γ'. καταπιεῖν, καὶ ὀξύμελι ἐπιπίνειν. ἄλλο. καππάρεως ῥίζαν ἑψήσας, πότιζε μετ' ὀξυμέλιτος τοὺς ἀπυρέτους. ἄλλο. μυρίκης καρποῦ κόψας καὶ σήσας, (482) δίδου κοχλιάρια β'. μετ' ὀξυμέλιτος. ἄλλο. σίδηρον πυρακτώσας ἐναπόσβεσον ὕδατι, καὶ δίδου πιεῖν ἀπυρέτοις ἐν οἴνῳ.

['Επίθεμα σπληνικόν.] Τήλεως γο. δ'. κριθῶν ἀλεύρων γο. γ'. καρδάμου σπέρματος γο. γ'. πυρέθρου γο. β'.

cum lacte muliebri maceratum naribus infundito et jubeto furfum attrahi. *Aliud.* Cyclamini fucco aqua diluto, ut dictum eft, utitor. *Aliud.* Edendum rubicanini rufum fructum dato. *Aliud.* Chelidonii herbae fuccum cum vino et aqua mulfa porrigito non febricitantibus. *Aliud.* Hyperici drach. j, propinato ex aqua mulfa, et jejunis dato in cibum amygdalas amaras.

Cap. XII. [*Ad lienofos.*] Da his potui decoctum chamaedryos, vel chamaepityos, vel polii, vel rubiae, aut per fe, aut cum oxymelite non febricitantibus. *Aliud.* Albae hederae corymbos numero tres dato devorandos et fuperbibendum acetum mulfum. *Aliud.* Radicis capparis ex oxymelite decoctum non febricitantibus dato. *Aliud.* Tamaricis fructum tritum et cribratum, duo cochlearia dato ex oxymelite. *Aliud.* Ferrum ignitum aqua reftinguito, quam potui dato non febricitantibus cum vino.

[*Epithema fplenicum.*] Recipe foenigraeci unc. iv, hordeaceae farinae unc. iij, feminum nafturtii unc. iij,

λιβάνου γο. S''. σινάπεως γο. S''. σύκων λιπαρῶν λίτραν α'. περιστερεῶνος βοτάνης γο. α'. ἀποβρέξας τὰ σῦκα ὄξει δριμεῖ, καὶ εὐτόνως κόψας ἐν ὅλμῳ, ἐπίβαλε τὰ λοιπὰ καὶ ἐνώσας χρῶ. ἄλλο. μώλυος βοτάνης χλωρᾶς ἔτι μετὰ τοῦ σπέρματος ἐμβαλὼν ἐν χύτρᾳ, καὶ διαμάξας ἐπιμελῶς ἐπίπλασσε καὶ ἕψει μαλακῷ πυρὶ ἐπὶ πλεῖστον, καὶ ὅταν καθεψηθῇ, ὁλμοκοπήσας ἐπιτίθει, μὴ λύων μέχρι τῆς τρίτης.

[Πρὸς σπλῆνα.] Σκορόδου ὄνυχας ζ'. λεπτὰ λεπίσας εἰς ἄκρατον ἐξαιθρίασον, καὶ πρωῒ νῆστις λάμβανε α'. συνθλάσας αὐτὸν, καὶ κατάπιε ἐφ' ἑκάστου ὄνυχος βρόχθον α', πεπείραται, συνεχῶς ποίει. εἰ δέ γε θέλεις καὶ κατάπλασμα πεπειραμένον, ἔμβαλε ῥίζας καππάρεως ἐν ὄξει καὶ ἰσχάδας καὶ ζέσον, μετὰ δὲ ταῦτα κρίθινον ἄλευρον καὶ μέλι προσβαλὼν τῷ ὄξει, καὶ τὰς ἰσχάδας λελειωμένας εὖ μάλα ἑψήσας οὕτως κατάπλασσε.

Κεφ. ιγ'. [Πρὸς ἄλλα τοῦ ἐπιγαστρίου πάθη, καὶ

pyrethri unc. ij, thuris unc. S, ſinapi unc. S, caricarum pinguium lib. j, verbenacae herbae unc. j, caricas acerrimo aceto maceratas contundito fortiter in pila; adjiciens caetera unito ac utitor. *Aliud.* Moly herbam etiamnum virentem cum ſuo ſemine in ollam conjicito, in qua diligenter obturata coquito plurimum lento igni; coctamque nunc et in pila tritam imponito lieni, ante tres dies non ſoluturus.

[*Ad ſplenem.*] Recipe allii ſegmenta vij, tenuibus purgatis pelliculis in merum projecta in ſole, maneque jejunus unum ſume, contunde ipſum et in cujusque ſegmenti poculo uno aſſume, expertum eſt, continuo eſſice. Si velis etiam cataplasma expertum, injice radices capparis in acetum et raphanos ſilveſtres et elixa, poſtea vero hordeaceam farinam et mel adjice aceto et raphanos ſilveſtres laevigatos et probe admodum elixos forma cataplasmatis admove.

Cap. XIII. [*Ad alios abdominis affectus, ac pri-*

πρῶτον πρὸς ὑδρωπικούς.] Τήλεως γο. α'. κριθῶν ἀλεύρων γο. γ'. κόπρου περιστερᾶς γο. δ'. ῥητίνης φρυκτῆς λίτραν α'. πίσσης λίτραν α'. κηροῦ λίτραν α'. ἀξουγγίου παλαιοῦ λίτρας β'. τὰ τηκτὰ τήξας κατάχεε, τῶν ἄλλων προλελειωμένων ἐν ὄξει, καὶ χρῶ. ἄλλο. βολβίτου αἰγείου ξηροῦ λίτρας β'. ἕψει ἐν ὀξυκράτῳ καὶ κατάπλασσε.

[Πρὸς κωλικούς.] Ἄνηθον καὶ κύμινον ἐνεψήσας εἰς ἐλαίου γο. γ'. δίδου ἅμα καὶ διάκλυζε. ἄλλο. πήγανον ὁμοίως ἐνεψήσας ἴσῳ ἐλαίῳ, καὶ ἐμβαλὼν ῥητίνης τερμινθίνης ὅσον κοχλιάριον χρῶ.

[Πρὸς τοὺς ὄντας κατεψυγμένους.] Ἀνηθίνῳ ἐμβαλὼν κοχλιάριον καστορίου λελειωμένου χρῶ.

[Πρὸς τὰς φλεγμονάς.] Ἀνηθίνῳ ἀναμίξας κοχλιάρια β'. ἀνάλου τυροῦ χρῶ. ὁμοίως καὶ στέαρ χήνειον, ἢ μυελὸν ἐλάφου.

[Πρὸς δυσεντερικούς.] Ἐπὶ δὲ δυσεντερικοῖς εἰδέναι αναγκαῖον ὅτι ἐξαίρε- [598] τον δυσεντερίας ἐστὶ φάρμακον, ὀλιγοσιτία. χρὴ δὲ καὶ τὰ προσφερόμενα ὡς ἐνὶ

mum ad hydropicos.] Recipe foenigraeci unc. j, hordeaceae farinae unc. iij, ſtercoris columbini unc. iv, frixae reſinae lib. j, picis lib. j, cerae lib. j, axungiae veteris lib. ij, liquato liquanda, demum addito caetera ex aceto trita, ac utitor. *Aliud.* Recipe fimi caprilli ſicci lib. ij, coque in oxycrato et cataplasma impone.

[*Ad colicos.*] Anethum et cuminum in olei unc. iij, coquito et ſimul exhibeto et injicito. *Aliud.* Rutam coctam ſimiliter in pari olei menſura, adjecto reſinae terebinthinae cochleario, praebeto.

[*Ad refrigeratos.*] Anethino cui additum ſit triti caſtorei cochlearium, utere.

[*Ad inflammationes.*] Anethino utitor, cui admixta ſint caſei non ſaliti duo cochlearia. Additur ſimiliter vel pinguedo anſerina, vel cervi medulla.

[*Ad dyſentericos.*] In dyſentericis curandis ſcire neceſſarium eſt eximium dyſenteriae remedium cibi eſſe paucitatem. Oportet autem et quae exhibentur, ea quan-

μάλιστα κοῦφα καὶ ἀβαρῆ τυγχάνειν, καὶ πρὸς τὰς πέψεις εὐκόλως ἔχοντα. ποτίζειν δὲ καὶ ἐνιέναι τούτοις ῥοᾶς ὁλοκλήρους καὶ κυδώνια ἀφεψήσαντας ἐνιέναι τῷ ἀφεψήματι, καὶ καταῤῥοφεῖν διδόναι. ἄλλο. ἀρνόγλωσσον βοτάνην ὀρύζῃ συνεψήσαντας ἐπιμελῶς ἐσθίειν διδόναι, καὶ τῷ χυλῷ δὲ τῷ αὐτῷ προσπλέξαντας στέαρ τράγειον διδόναι. ἄλλο. μυρσίνας ἑψήσαντας οἴνῳ, εἰ ἀπύρετοί εἰσιν, ἐνιέναι· εἰ δὲ πυρέττοιεν, ὕδατι. ἄλλο. κοχλιῶν ὁλοκλήρων κεκαυμένων γο. α΄. κέρατος ἐλαφείου κεκαυμένου γο. β΄. ἀναλάμβανε χυλῷ ἀρνογλώσσου, καὶ δίδου κυάμου μέγεθος, ἀπυρέτοις οἴνῳ, πυρέσσουσιν ὕδατι.

[Πρὸς κοιλιακοὺς καὶ δυσεντερικούς.] Μύρτων ξηρῶν κεκομμένων γο. α΄. ῥόδων ξηρῶν γο. α΄. ἀρκευθίδων τὸν ἀριθμὸν ι΄. ἀπίων ξηρῶν κεκομμένων κγ΄. κερατίων κεκομμένων γο. α΄. πίτυος φλοιοῦ γο. δ΄. δίδου ξηρὸν ἐν οἴνῳ κοχλιάριον. τὸ δὲ ἁδρομερὲς φοίνιξι λιπαροῖς ἀναλαβὼν ἐπιτί-

tum licet levia, minime gravia et concoctu facilia esse. Porro decoctum malorum punicorum integrorum et cotoneorum his tum ad sorbendum propinatur, tum per clysterem injicitur. *Aliud.* Plantaginem herbam cum oryza exacte decoctam da in cibo; quin hujus ipsius succum adjecta pinguedine hircina commode subministrabis. *Aliud.* Myrti baccas vino incoquito, si febre careant; si vero febricitent, aquae; ac immittito. *Aliud.* Recipe cochlearum integrarum ustarum unc. j, cornu cervi usti unc. ij, excipe succo plantaginis, exhibetoque fabae magnitudinem, febrem carentibus cum vino, cum aqua febricitantibus.

[*Ad coeliacos et dysentericos.*] Recipe baccarum myrti siccarum contusarum unc. j, rosarum aridarum unc. j, baccas juniperi decem, pyra arida tusa xxiij, silicarum contusarum unc. j, corticis pini unc. iv, propinato excreti ex his pulvisculi aridi cochlearium ex vino. Porro quod crassiorum est partium, pinguibus palmulis coactum ventri imponito. *Aliud.* Potum leporis, tum hinnuli, tum

θει τῇ γαστρί. ἄλλο. πιτύαν λαγωοῦ ἢ νεβροῦ ἢ αἰγάγρου οἴνῳ πότιζε, καὶ ἐνιέμενον δὲ μετὰ χυλοῦ ὀρύζης βοηθεῖ.

[Πρὸς τὰς κεχρονισμένας δυσεντερίας.] Χάρτου κεκαυμένου γο. α'. ἀσβέστου γο. α'. ὄμφακι σταφυλῆς ἀναλαβὼν, ποίει τροχίσκους ἔχοντας < γ'. καὶ β'. καὶ α'. ὡς ἐπὶ πάσης ἡλικίας ἔχειν τὸ μέτρον. ἐπὶ δὲ τῆς χρείας οἴνῳ αὐστηρῷ λύσας, καὶ μίξας ὀρύζης χυλὸν, ἐνίεσθαι κέλευε. ἄλλο. ᾠοῦ χηνείου ἑψηθέντος τὸ λέπυρον λειώσας ἐπιμελῶς, πότιζε ἡμίδραχμον οἴνῳ.

Κεφ. ιδ'. [Περὶ των τῆς ἕδρας παθῶν, καὶ τῶν ἑδρικῶν φαρμάκων.] Περὶ τὴν ἕδραν γίνεται διάφορα πάθη, ῥαγάδες τε καὶ κονδυλώματα, καὶ ἄλλαι φλεγμοναί. ἁρμόζει δ' ἐπ' αὐτῶν τὰ ἁπαλὰ τῶν φαρμάκων καὶ ἄδηκτα διαχριόμενα.

[Ἑδρικὸν πρὸς τὰς πυρώδεις ὀδύνας.] Ὠοῦ τὸν λέκυθον λειώσας οἴνῳ λευκῷ καὶ ῥοδίνῃ κηρωτῇ ἀναλαβὼν, διάχριε, καὶ ἐμπλάστρῳ χρῶ. ἁρμόζει δ' ἐπ' αὐτῶν τὰ ἁπαλὰ

etiam capreae coagulum ex vino, nec non immiſſum cum oryzae cremore juvat.

[*Ad diuturnam dyſenteriam.*] Recipe chartae uſtae unc. j, calcis vivae unc. j, uvae immaturae ſucco excipiens in paſtillos formato, continentes alios drach. iij, alios drach. ij, alios drach. j, ut cuique aetati apta ſit ad manum quantitas. At in uſu unum vino auſtero diſſolve, et adjecto oryzae cremore per clyſterem injice. *Aliud.* Cocti anſerini ovi putamen minutiſſime tritum dimidiae drachmae quantitate ex vino propinato.

Cap. XIV. [*De ſedis affectibus ac propriis ſedi medicamentis.*] Sedi diverſi oboriuntur affectus, rhagades, condylomata, aliaeque inflammationes. His autem conveniunt quae tenera, mollia, omnisque morſus expertia medicamenta illinuntur.

[*Ad ſedis ex ardore dolores topicum.*] Ovi luteum ex vino albo tritum et roſaceo cerato exceptum illine, emplaſtrique modo utere. Conveniunt autem his quae

τῶν φαρμάκων καὶ ἄδηκτα διαχριόμενα. ἄλλο. στέαρ χήνειον νεαρὸν διάχριε καὶ ἐμπλάστρῳ χρῶ. ἁρμόζει δ' ἐπ' αὐτῶν καὶ κατάπλασμα ἄρτου καθαροῦ λυομένου καὶ ἑψουμένου ὕδατι καὶ ῥοδίνῳ· κάλλιον δὲ γίνεται, εἰ προσβάλλῃς καὶ λεκύθους ᾠῶν ὠπτημένους. ἄλλο. τῆλιν ἑψήσας καὶ λειώσας κατάπλασσε, προσβάλλων καὶ βούτυρον. ἄλλο. στέατι χηνείῳ διάχριε. ἄλλο. ῥόδων γο. γ'. ᾠῶν ὀπτῶν λεκύθους β'. οἴνω λευκῷ λείωσας καὶ ῥοδίνῃ κηρωτῇ ἀναλαβὼν διάχριε.

[Πρὸς τοὺς ἐν δακτυλίῳ κνησμούς.] Γῆν τὴν καλουμένην κιμωλίαν οἴνῳ λειώσας, ἀναλάμβανε κηρωτῇ μυρσίνῃ καὶ χρῶ.

[Πρὸς τοὺς προσπίπτοντας ἀρχούς.] Σκωρίας μολύβδου γο. α'. ῥόδων ξηρῶν γο. δ'. εὖ μάλα λειώσας ξη [599] ρα προσάπτου, προαπονίπτων οἴνῳ μυρσίνῳ. ἄλλο. κυκλαμίνου χυλοῦ καὶ μέλιτος ἴσον ἕψει ἐν ἀγγείῳ χαλκῷ, ὥστε κηρωτῆς ἔχειν πάχος, καὶ κατάχριε.

Κεφ. ιε'. [Περὶ τῶν ἐν νεφροῖς τε καὶ κύστει πα-

mollia et morſu carentia medicamenta illinuntur. *Aliud.* Recentem anſeris adipem inungito et ut emplaſtro utitor: utile his etiam cataplasma ex pane puro ſoluto coctoque in aqua et roſaceo; quod fuerit efficacius, additis ovorum luteis aliquot coctis. *Aliud.* Foenumgraecum elixum tritumque adjecto butyro ut cataplasma applicato. *Aliud.* Anſerinum adipem inungito. *Aliud.* Recipe roſarum unc. iij, coctorum ovorum lutea duo, trita ex vino albo, roſaceoque cerato excepta, illine.

[*Ad ani pruritus.*] Recipe terram vocatam cimoliam, tritam cum vino, qua cerato myrteo excepta utere.

[*Ad procidentem anum.*] Recipe recrementi plumbi unc. j, roſarum ſiccarum unc. iv, accurate admodum trita, ſicca ano appone, eloto prius vino myrteo. *Aliud.* Cyclamini ſuccum et mel aequa portione decoque in vaſe aereo, donec cerati habeat craſſitudinem, et inunge.

Cap. XV. [*De renum et veſicae affectibus.*] [*Potio

θῶν.] [Πρὸς τὰς φλεγμονώδεις διαθέσεις καὶ ἑλκώσεις τῶν νεφρῶν καὶ τῆς κύστεως πότιμα.] Λινοσπέρμου γο. β΄. ἀμύλου γο. α΄. δίδου ἐν ὕδατι κοχλιάριον.

[Πρὸς ἡλκωμένην κύστιν καὶ δυσουρίαν.] Στροβίλους, ἀμύγδαλα ἀνὰ κ΄. φοινίκια ιε΄. τραγακάνθης γο. δ΄. δίδου μεθ' ὕδατος.

[Πρὸς ἔμφραξιν νεφρῶν.] Σελίνου ἀφέψημα πότιζε ἀπυρέτους κονδίτῳ, πυρέσσοντας ὕδατι. ἄλλο. ἐρεβίνθων τῶν καλουμένων κριῶν ἀφέψημα μετὰ κονδίτου προπότιζε.

[Πρὸς λιθιῶντας.] Λινόσπερμον λειώσας ἐπιμελῶς, πότιζε μετὰ κονδίτου. ἄλλο. σικύου ἡμέρου σπέρματος πεφρυγμένου γο. στ΄. μαλάχης καρποῦ γο. ε΄. στροβίλων πεφρυγμένων γο. στ΄. σελίνου σπέρματος γο. η΄. ἀμυγδάλων πικρῶν κεκαθαρμένων γο. θ΄. ἀναλάμβανε γλυκεῖ καὶ δίδου κοχλιάριον καθὰ προείρηται.

Κεφ. ιστ΄. [Πρὸς ἰσχιάδας καὶ ποδάγραν καὶ ἀρθρῖτιν.] Ὁμογενῆ εἰσὶ ταῦτα ἀλλήλοις τὰ νοσήματα, διὸ

ad renum et veſicae affectus inflammatiorios et exulcerationes.] Recipe ſeminum lini unc. ij, amyli unc. j, propinato ex aqua cochlearium.

[*Ad veſicam ulceratam et urinae difficultatem.*] Recipe pineos nucleos et amygdala ana xx, palmulas xv, tragacanthae unc. iv, dato cum aqua.

[*Ad renum obſtructionem.*] Apii decoctum dato in potu febre carentibus ex condito; febrientibus ex aqua. *Aliud.* Decoctum cicerum arietinorum appellatorum cum condito detur in potu.

[*Ad calculoſos.*] Lini ſemen exacte tritum da bibendum cum condito. *Aliud.* Recipe ſeminum cucumeris domeſtici frixi unc. vj, ſeminum malvae unc. v, nucleorum pineorum frixorum unc. vj, ſeminum apii unc. viij, amygdalorum amarorum mundatorum unc. ix, paſſo excipe, da cochlearium, ut ante dictum eſt.

Cap. XVI. [*Ad ischiades, podagram et arthritidem.*] Hi morbi ejusdem inter ſe ſunt generis, proinde

καὶ τῆς αὐτῆς σχεδὸν θεραπείας χρήζει, διαφορὰ δὲ τῶν ποιούντων αὐτὰ ῥευμάτων. τὰ μὲν γὰρ αὐτῶν εἰσὶ θερμὰ, τὰ δὲ ψυχρά. διάγνωσις δ' αὐτῶν ἐπὶ μὲν τοῖς θερμοτέροις, ἔρευθος καὶ πύρωσις, κἂν ᾖ φλεγμονή τε καὶ ἀλγήματα σφοδρά. ἐπὶ δὲ τῶν ψυχροτέρων οἴδημα λευκὸν ἔνσομφον. ἑκατέρων (483) δὲ ἴασις αὕτη ἐστί. ἐπὶ μὲν τῶν θερμῶν τὰ ψύχοντα, ἐπὶ δὲ τῶν ψυχρῶν τὰ θερμαίνοντα καὶ διαφοροῦντα. εἰ μὲν οὖν πολὺς εἴη ὁ ἐνοχλῶν χυμὸς, καθάρσει πρῶτον χρηστέον τοῦ λυποῦντος χυμοῦ. εἰ δὲ πληθωρικὸν εἴη τὸ σῶμα, πρώτης ἁπάντων παραλαμβανομένης φλεβοτομίας, ἀποκρουομένων τὰ ῥεύματα ὀξυκράτῳ, καὶ τοῖς ψυχροτέροις φαρμάκοις χρωμένων. (εἴρηται δὲ ἡμῖν περὶ τούτων ἐπὶ πλεῖστον ἐν τοῖς ἐμοῦ πρὸς Γλαύκωνα θεραπευτικοῖς γεγραμμένοις δυσὶ βιβλίοις, καὶ ἐν ἄλλοις πλείοσι, διὸ βραδύνειν οὐ χρὴ ὡς ἐν εὐποριστοις περὶ τούτων λέγοντα.) ἐπὶ δὲ τῆς κατ' ἰσχίον διαρθράσεως φυλαττομένων τοῦτο δρᾷν. ἐν βάθει γὰρ οὔσης αὐτῆς, συνελαύνεται τὸ ἐκ τῶν περιεχομένων ἀγγείων τε καὶ μυῶν αἷμα πρὸς

eandem fere poſtulant curationem. Hi differunt efficientibus ipſos fluxionibus, quarum hae calidae ſunt, illae frigidae. Dignoscuntur autem, quod calidiorem fluxionem comitentur rubedo, incendium et, ſi fuerit inflammatio, vehementes dolores. Frigidiorem vero tumor albus, laxus, mollis. Porro utriusque curatio haec eſt, ut calidae refrigerantia, frigidae calefacientia discutientiaque applicentur. Itaque ſi copioſus vexans humor fuerit, purgatione primum utendum eſt vexantis humoris. Quod ſi corpus plethoricum fuerit, omnium primam venae ſectionem praeſcribimus, ac repellimus fluxiones oxycrato, etiam frigidioribus medicamentis utentes. (De his autem nobis abunde ſcriptum eſt tum in meis ad Glauconem curationum libris duobus, tum in caeteris pluribus; proinde mihi in parabilibus haud immorandum eſt de his differenti.) Caeterum in iſchii dearticulatione *affecta ſeu iſchiade* id moliri cavemus. Quum enim haec in alto ſit, ad eam a circumſtantibus vaſis musculisve ſanguis compellitur ve-

ἐκείνην καὶ ἄγαν λυπεῖ. παρηγορικῶν γοῦν δέονται φαρμάκων· ἐπὶ γὰρ τῆς κατ᾽ ἰσχίον ὀδύνης οὔτε ψυχρῶν σφοδρῶς οὔτε θερμαινόντων ἰσχυρῶς χρεία. παροξύνεται γὰρ ὑπ᾽ αὐτῶν τὰ ῥεύματα, τῆς μὲν πολλῆς θερμασίας ἑλκούσης αὐτὰ μᾶλλόν τε κωλυούσης διαφορεῖσθαι, τῆς δὲ ψύξεως πήξει τι ὅμοιον ἐργαζομένης καὶ δυσδιαφόρητα ποιούσης τὰ ῥεύ- [600] ματα, ὠφελοῦσι δ᾽ ἔμετοι μᾶλλον τοὺς ἰσχιαδικοὺς τῶν διὰ τῆς ἄνω γαστρὸς κενώσεων ἀντισπῶντες τὴν κάτω ῥοπὴν τῶν χυμῶν. χρηστέον δ᾽ αὐτοῖς ἐν ἀρχῇ μετὰ τὴν τροφὴν, ὕστερον δὲ καὶ διὰ ἐμετικῶν βολβῶν τε καὶ ῥαφανίδων. δεῖ δὲ τοὺς μὲν βολβοὺς ἐν ὕδατι ἕψοντας μετ᾽ ὀξυμέλιτος προσφέρειν, τὰς δὲ ῥαφανῖδας εἰς λεπτὰ κόψαντας καὶ ἐναποβαλόντας ὀξυμέλιτι ἐσθίειν, καὶ ὥραν πολλὴν διαλιπόντας ἐπὶ τοὺς ἐμέτους ἄγειν, κἄπειτα ἑξῆς μακρὸν διαλιπόντας χρόνον λούειν· εἶτ᾽ αὖθις διαλιπόντας ὡς ἅπασαν καταστῆναι τὴν ταραχὴν λεπτῶς διαιτᾷν.

[Πρὸς παροξυσμοὺς ποδαγρικούς.] Κράμβης φύλλα

hementerque cruciat. Mitigantibus itaque medicamentis utendum eſt. Nam in iſchii dolore neque magnopere refrigerantium neque vehementer calefacientium uſus eſt. Ab his enim fluxiones exacerbantur, quam ipſas quidem multus calor attrahat, magisque discuti prohibeat; frigus vero concretioni quiddam ſimile moliatur, fluxionesque discuſſu difficiles efficiat. Sed iſchiadicos juvant magis vomitus, qui vacuationibus ad ſuperiorem ventrem humorum deorſum irruentium impetum revellunt. Hi vomitus per initia provocandi ſunt ab accepto cibo *ſpontanei*, imo etiam poſtea bulbis vomitoriis et raphanis. Exhibentur autem in aqua cocti bulbi cum oxymelite: radicula vero ni tenues partes conciſa et oxymelite immerſa editur. Atque his uſi quum diuturnam horam intermiſerint, ad vomitum ducendi ſunt, poſteaque deinceps longo interjecto tempore lavandi; rurſusque demum ipſi quiescentes quoad omnis turbatio deſierit, tenui victu reficiendi ſunt.

[*Ad podagricas acceſſiones.*] Braſſicae foliis decoctis

καθεψήσας καὶ λειώσας πρόσβαλε τρύγα ὄξους καὶ ὠῶν ἀνέφθων λεκύθους β'. καὶ βραχὺ ῥόδινον καὶ μίξας ἐπιμελῶς καὶ χλιάνας κατάπλασσε ἀμείβων συνεχῶς. ἄλλο. τῷ καταπλάσματι τῷ συνήθως διὰ τῶν σύκων ἡψημένῳ πρόσβαλε ὑοσκυάμου φύλλα καὶ συνεψήσας κατάπλασσε.

[Πρὸς πυρώδεις φλεγμονάς.] Φακὸν τὸν ἐπὶ τῶν τελμάτων ὄξει καὶ ῥοδίνῳ κατάπλασσε. ἄλλο. πτελέας φύλλα χυλίσας καὶ ἑψήσας κηρωτῇ κατάχριε.

[Πρὸς τὰς ὑπερβαλλούσας πυρώσεις.] Θριδακίνης φύλλα ἐπιμελῶς τρίψας σὺν ἄρτῳ κατάπλασσε συνεχῶς ἀμείβων. ἄλλο. κορίανδρον τὸ χλωρὸν λειώσας σὺν ἀλφίτῳ κατάπλασσε.

[Πρὸς τὰς χαύνας φυσιώσεις.] Ἅλαιον ἐπιμελῶς λειώσας κατάπλασσε, ἐπιτιθεὶς οἰσυπηρὸν ἔριον.

[Πρὸς ἰσχιαδικούς.] (484) Σκορόδων ὄνυχας τρεῖς καθαρίσας ὑγιεῖς κατάπιε μετὰ τὸ δειπνῆσαι πίνων συγκεραστικόν· τοῦτο συνεχῶς ποιεῖν πεπείραται. ἄλλο. χελιδόνιον ἄγρευσον, καὶ ἐὰν ᾖ ὁ δεξιὸς ποὺς ὃν πάσχεις, τῇ δεξιᾷ

ac contritis addito aceti faecem, lutea duorum ovorum crudorum ac rofacei parum; quae accurate mixta in modum cataplasmatis tepida imponito frequenter renovans. *Aliud.* Cataplasmati vulgari et ufitato ex caricis elixo adjecta hyoscyami folia incoque et admove.

[*Ad fervidas inflammationes.*] Lenticulam paluftrem ex aceto et rofaceo imponito. *Aliud.* Ulmi foliis expresfum fuccum et coctum cum cerato illine.

[*Ad exuperantes ardores.*] Lactucae folia exacte cum pane trita applica frequenter iterando. *Aliud.* Coriandrum viride tritum cum polenta admove.

[*Ad laxas inflationes.*] Salem ex oleo diligenter tritum fuccidaque lana exceptum ut cataplasma admove.

[*Ad ifchiadicos.*] Alliorum aglitas tres purgatas integras deglutiendas exhibe poft coenam, contemperatum bibens; id crebro effice, expertum eft. *Aliud.* Hirundinem cape, atque fi fit pes dexter quo laboras, dextra

χειρὶ τὰ πτερὰ πατήσας τῷ πάσχοντι καὶ κνήσας ἕλκε τὸ αἷμα ἀπὸ ἄνωθεν τῆς κοτύλης ἕως τοῦ ἀστραγάλου σύρων τὸ αἷμα ὅλῳ τῷ χελιδονίῳ, καὶ λεπίσας καὶ ὀπτήσας φάγε μηδὲν βαλὼν ἔξω καὶ φαγὼν παραυτίκα ἄλειψον ἐλαίῳ ἕως ἐπὶ τὸν ἀστράγαλον ἐπὶ τρεῖς ἡμέρας, καὶ θαυμάσεις. πεπείραται δὲ πάνυ καὶ τοῦτο. ἄλλο. κορώνην ἀγρεύσας σπούδασον ἀσινῆ διαφυλάξαι, καὶ ἐὰν μὲν τὰ δεξιὰ μέρη τὰ πάσχοντα ᾖ, τὸν μικρὸν δάκτυλον τὸν ὄπισθεν τῆς κορώνης τοῦ δεξιοῦ ποδὸς κόψας περιτίθει. μύρῳ δὲ χρίσας τὰς πτέρυγας τῆς κορώνης ἔα ἵπτασθαι. ἐὰν δὲ ἀριστερὰ μέρη πάσχῃ, τοῦ ἀριστεροῦ ποδὸς τὸν προδεδηλωμένον κόψας περιτίθει. ποίει δὲ τἄλλα ὡσαύτως, πεπείραται δὲ τοῦτο συνεχῶς.

Κεφ. ιζ'. [Περὶ θανασίμων φαρμάκων.] (483) Περὶ τῶν θανασίμων φαρμάκων οὔτε ἀδιορίστως ἐνθάδε γράφειν ἀσφαλὲς καὶ ἕκαστον αὐτῶν ἐκτιθέμενον κατὰ τῶν ἑπομένων συμπτωμάτων ἐπάγειν οὕτως τὰς θεραπείας χαλεπόν. παρέχοι γὰρ ἂν ἡ τοιαύτη πραγματεία ἀφορμὴν κακίας τοῖς κακουργεῖν

manu alas contere aegrotanti, incide, trahe ſanguinem a ſuperiore acetabuli parte adusque talum trahens ſanguinem ex tota hirundine et extracta pelle et aſſa comede nihil foras projiciens et confeſtim comedens inunge oleo usque ad talum per tres dies et miraberis. Expertum eſt admodum. *Aliud.* Cornicem capies, ſtude illaeſam conſervare, et ſi dextrae partes affectae ſint, parvum digitum poſteriorem cornicis dextri pedis conciſum circumpone, unguento vero illitas alas cornicis ſinito volare. Si vero ſiniſtrae partes aegrotent, ſiniſtri pedis prius declaratum digitum conciſum admove. Effice et alia eodem modo, id ſaepe exploratum eſt.

Cap. XVII. [*De mortiferis medicamentis.*] De letalibus medicamentis neque indiſtincte hic ſcribere tutum eſt, neque parvi laboris de omnibus ſingulatim deque comitantium haec ſymptomatum curatione differere. Ejusmodi autem tractatio iis malitiae occaſionem praeberet

βουλομένοις. ἃ δὲ κοινῶς βοηθεῖν πεπίστευται τοῖς εἰληφόσι τὰ δηλητήρια, ταῦτα γράφω. παραυτίκα μὲν πεπωκότας ἐμεῖν κέλευε, ποτίζων πλεῖστον ὑδρέλαιον συνεχῶς καὶ παντοδα [601] πὰ σιτία δίδου, εἰς καιρὸν αὖθις δ' ἐμεῖν κέλευε· ἢ γὰρ συνεξεργασθήσεται τὸ φάρμακον, ἢ ἐπικραθὲν ἀμβλυωτέραν ἕξει τὴν δύναμιν. εἰ δὲ διακαίοιντο τὴν γαστέρα μετὰ τὸν ἔμετον, ὑδροροδίνῳ ποτίσας αὖθις ἐμεῖν κέλευε. δίδου δὲ, εἰ χρὴ, καὶ τῆς θηριακῆς μετὰ οἴνου ἢ ἀρκευθίδας θ'. καὶ πηγάνου κ'. φύλλα λειώσας ποτίζειν, ἢ χαμαιπίτυος βοτάνης. καὶ ὕπνου παντελῶς εἶργε καὶ ψηλαφίᾳ τῶν ἄκρων χρῶ. εἰ δὲ καὶ ὑποβιασθῆναι τὸ κακὸν ἔμφασιν ἔχοι, δακνομένης καὶ ἐρεθιζομένης τῆς κάτω γαστρὸς, κλυσμοῖς δριμέσι χρηστέον, μέλι δαψιλὲς καὶ ἀφρόνιτρον ἢ ἕτερόν τι τῶν συνταραττόντων συμπλέκοντας. τοὺς δ' ἀπὸ μυκήτων πνιγμοὺς κουφίζει ὀξύμελι μετὰ νάρδου πινόμενον καὶ ὀρνίθων τῶν κατοικιδίων ἄφοδος μετ' ὀξυμέλι-

quibus maleficiendi eſt animus. At ea ſcribo quae vulgo creduntur iis opitulari qui letalia medicamenta devoraverint. Quamprimum jube eos vomere, epoto prius hydrelaeo et plurimo et frequenter, et varia cibaria exhibe, a quibus tempeſtive rurſum vomant jubeto: ſic enim aut ſimul rejicietur mortiferum medicamentum, aut evictum obtuſiorem habebit facultatem. Quod ſi ventriculus a vomitu aduratur, aquam roſaceo oleo mixtam potui offerto et eos vomere rurſus jubeto. Da vero ſi ſit opus et theriacen bibendam ex vino, aut juniperi baccas novem et rutae trita viginti ſolia aut herbae chamaepityos. A ſomno prorſus arce extremarumque partium utitor frictione. Quod ſi malum videatur tibi altius in ventrem nunc deſcendiſſe, quod ex ventris inferioris irritatione cognoſces, utendum acribus clyſteribus, cujus generis ſunt qui ex melle copioſiori et aphronitro conſtant aut alio quovis, cui irritandi ventris ſit facultas. At ſtrangulationi a devoratis ſungis medetur nardus ex oxymelite pota. Idem poteſt gallinarum domeſticarum ſimum ex oxymelite. Cae-

τος. ἐπὶ δὲ τυρωθέντος γάλακτος καὶ διὰ τοῦτο πνιγμὸν ἐπάγοντος πιτύαν ἐν οἴνῳ διεὶς πότιζε.

(484) Ὁ μὲν οὖν τέταρτός μοι λόγος, ὦ Γλαύκων, ἐνθάδε πέρας ἐχέτω· εἰ δέ σοι χρεία γένηται καὶ τοῦ πρὸς Σαλομῶντα τὸν ἀρχίητρον γεγραμμένου ἡμῖν συντάγματος, δηλώσας ἑτοίμως λήψῃ, θαυμάσεις δὲ πάνυ δεξάμενος.

terum ſuffocationi ex concreto in ventriculo lacte auxiliatur potum cum vino coagulum.

Quartus itaque mihi liber, o Glauco, hic finem habeto. Quod ſi *pluribus* tibi opus ſit, ea in eo quod ad Salomonem medicorum principem ſcriptum eſt opere declaravi facile, uſurpabis et admodum probata admiraberis.

ΓΑΛΗΝΟΥ ΠΕΡΙ ΕΥΠΟΡΙΣΤΩΝ ΒΙΒΛΙΟΝ ΔΕΥΤΕΡΟΝ.

Ed. Chart. X. [602.]

[602] *Προοίμιον.* Ἐπειδὴ μὲν ἠξίωσας ὡς περὶ εὐπορίστων σοι γράφειν, ὦ Σόλων τιμιώτατε, χαρίζεσθαί σοι νενόμικα τά μοι διὰ τῆς πείρας ἐγνωσμένα γράφειν τε καὶ σοι ἐπιστέλλειν, ἀπὸ τῶν τριχῶν πρὸς τὰς πόδας προβαίνων, ὅπως ἄνθρωπος ῥᾳδίως αὐτὰ προσλαμβάνειν δύνηται. ἀρχόμεθα μὲν οὖν πρῶτον ἀπὸ τῶν τριχῶν.

Κεφ. α΄. [Περὶ εὐπορίστων τῶν ταῖς ἔξωθεν τῆς κεφαλῆς διαθέσεσι θεραπευομέναις προσηκόντων.] [Περὶ βαμμάτων τῶν τριχῶν.] Καταχρίσεις τῶν τριχῶν, ὡς

GALENI DE REMEDIIS PARABILIBUS LIBER SECUNDUS.

Prooemium. Quia petiisti ut de facile parabilibus remediis ad te scriberem, Solon carissime, gratum tibi esse putavi quae mihi per experientiam cognita sunt scribere et ad te mittere, a capillis usque ad pedes procedens, ut homo facile possit ipsa adipisci. Incipiamus igitur primo a capillis.

Cap. I. [*Parabilia externis capitis affectibus curandis idonea.*] [*De tincturis capillorum.*] Unctiones ca-

αἱ πολιαὶ μελάνοχροι γένηται. σκορίαν σιδηροῦ καὶ μόλυβδον ἐν ὄξει ἑψήσας μέχρι τὸ τρίτον λειφθῇ ἐπιχρίου, ἐλαίου ἀπεχόμενος τῶν τριχῶν ἅπτεσθαι. ἄλλο. καππάρεως ῥίζα λεία σὺν γάλακτι ὀνείῳ μέχρι τὸ τρίτον λειφθῇ ἑψήσας καὶ χρῶ. τοῦτο φύλαττε, τελέως γὰρ τὰς τῆς κεφαλῆς τρίχας μελαίνει. ἄλλο. χολὴν τῆς χελώνης θαλασσίας διαλύσας σὺν ἐλαίῳ καὶ τὰς τρίχας κατάχριε. ἄλλο. ἀπὸ καρύας τὰ ὡσανεὶ βοτρύδια ἐλαίῳ ἑψήσας ὑγρὰν ἄσφαλτον μίξον καὶ κατάχριε. ἄλλο. μόλυβδον σὺν ἐλαίῳ ἐν τῷ ἀγγείῳ ἀπολαβὼν αὐτῷ τὰς τρίχας κατάχριε. ἄλλο. χερσαῖον ἐχῖνον κατακαύσας καὶ σὺν ἐλαίῳ διαλύσας τὰς τρίχας κατάχριε καὶ ἔα διὰ τῆς ὅλης νυκτός. ἄλλο. προφυλακτικὸν ὥστε μὴ γενέσθαι πολιάς. κολοκυνθίδα ἀγρίαν τρυπήσας κάθαρον τὰ ἔσω εὖ μάλα. εἶτα πλήρωσον αὐτὴν ἐλαίου δαφνίνου καὶ πρόβαλλε [603] ὑοσκυάμου λευκοῦ σπέρματος μὴ τρίψας· καὶ ἄφες αὐτὸ μίαν ἡμέραν, καὶ ἄλειφε χρησίμως ἅπαξ τοῦ ἐνιαυτοῦ. πρὸς τὸ λευκὰς ποιῆσαι τρίχας. χελιδόνος κόπρον τρίψας σὺν χολῇ ταυρείᾳ μίσγε, καὶ γίνονται

pillorum, ut etiam cani fiant nigri. Scoriam ferri et plumbum coque in aceto usque ad tertiam partem et illine, et oleo tangi capillos prohibe. *Aliud.* Radices capparis tere et coque in lacte asinae usque ad tertiam partem et utere; hoc serva, quia prorsus denigrat pilos capitis. *Aliud.* Testudinis marinae fel dissolve cum oleo et unge capillos. *Aliud.* Racemulos in nucibus pendentes in oleo coque, bitumen liquidum adde et unge. *Aliud.* Plumbum cum oleo repone in vase plumbeo et eo unge capillos. *Aliud.* Echinum terrestrem combure et cum oleo dissolvens unge capillos et dimitte per totam noctem. *Aliud* quod ne cani fiant prohibet. Recipe colocynthidem et perfora eam et purga ipsam bene ab iis quae sunt intus; deinde imple oleo laurino et adde semen hyoscyami non contritum, dimitte unum diem et unge semel in anno. *Ad dealbandos capillos.* Stercus hirundinis terens cum felle tauri unge et albi fient. *Aliud.* Verbasci albi

Ed. Chart. X. [603.]
λευκαί. ἄλλο. φλόμου λευκῆς τὸ ἄνθος καύσας ὄξει σβέσον καὶ συμμίξας καὶ σμήγματι χρῶ. πρὸς τὸ πυῤῥὰς ποιῆσαι τρίχας. τὴν στυπτηρίαν ἐν ὕδατι ἑψήσας καὶ διάβρεχε δυοῖν ἡμερῶν τὰς τρίχας, καὶ μετὰ τοῦτο διάκλυζε σὺν ὕδατι, ἐν ᾧ τρυγίας κεκαυμένος διαλελυμένος ᾖ. ἄλλο. ἑψήματι τῶν θερμῶν πικρῶν τὰς τρίχας διάβρεχε, ἢ αὐτοὺς θερμοὺς πικροὺς τρίψας καὶ διαμίξας σὺν ὕδατι κατάχριε. ἄλλο. τρυγίαν οἴνου παλαιοῦ κεκαυμένην καὶ σὺν ἐλαίῳ βαλανίνῳ λειουμένην συμμίξας πρὸς τῆς κηρωτῆς πάχος καὶ τρίχας σύγχριε, ὅταν μέλλῃς καθεύδειν. ἄλλο. κύπρου φύλλα λεῖα τῷ στρουθίου χυλῷ ἐπίβρεχε καὶ χρῶ τούτῳ ἀποβρέγματι. ἄλλο. ἐρυθρόδανον, στοιχάδα κιτριοειδῆ, πολύτριχον, ἀψίνθιον καὶ θερμοὺς ἐς τὸ ὕδωρ κατάβαλλε, ἀναθήσας ἐν τῷ ἀγγείῳ ὑαλίνῳ, καὶ ἄφησον ἡμερῶν ἐννέα, ἀνακινέων δὶς ἐν ἡμέρᾳ· τῷ δὲ χρήσεως χρόνῳ ἀπολαβὼν τὸ προειρημένου ὕδατος ἱκανὸν, ἐπιβάλλων εἰς τὸ τοῦτο σπογγίαν καὶ τὴν ἀφήσας τὸ ὕδωρ ἐναποληψομένην· καὶ ὅταν ἐξηρανθεῖσαι τρίχες ὦσιν αἱ τούτῳ ὕδατι προκαταβραχεῖσαι, αὐτὰς μετὰ τοῦ θερμοῦ ὕδατος καὶ σάπωνος ἔκκλυζε.

combure florem et extingue aceto et misce et mixtura utere. *Ut flavi fiant capilli.* Alumen coque in aqua et madefacito capillos duobus diebus, et post hoc lava cum aqua, in qua est dissoluta faex vini usta. *Aliud.* Decocto lupinorum amarorum madefacito capillos; vel ipsos lupinos amaros crudos terens et permiscens cum aqua illine. *Aliud.* Faecem vini veteris ustam ac tritam permisce cum oleo balanino ad cerati crassitudinem et unge caput. quando vadis dormitum. *Aliud.* Folia ligustri trita infunde in succo lanariae et utere hoc diluto. *Aliud.* Rubiam, stoechadem citrinum, polytrichum, absinthium et lupinos conjice in aquam, reponens in vase vitreo, et dimitte per novem dies, movens bis in die; tempore vero usus accipiens dictae aquae quod sufficit, mitte in eam spongiam et dimitte, ut imbibat aquam: et quando fuerint desiccati capilli ea aqua prius irrigati, ablue cum aqua calida et sapone.

Ed. Chart. X. [603.]

[β'. Περὶ ῥεουσῶν τριχῶν.] Πρὸς ῥύσιν τριχῶν τὴν πτελέας ῥίζαν τε καὶ φύλλων δράγμα α'. ἐναποβρέξας τοῖς ὕδατος κυάθοις δ'. κατάχριε καὶ μετὰ τοῦτο τῷ ἐλαίῳ σύγχριε. ἄλλο. ἀκτὴν καύσας καὶ μετὰ κηρωτῆς ὑγροτάτης μίξας χρῖε. ἄλλο. ἀλόην μίξας σὺν οἴνῳ αὐστηρῷ μέλανι ἐπίχριε. ἄλλο. σμύρναν καὶ λάδανον σὺν οἴνῳ ἢ ἐλαίῳ μυρσίνῳ κατάχριε. ἄλλο. λαβὼν μελίσσας τὰς πλείστας καὶ συγκαύσας καὶ μίξας ἐλαίῳ καὶ τὰς τρίχας κατάχριε, φυλάττων ἵνα μὴ τὰ πέριξ καταχρίῃς. ἄλλο. μελάνθιον καύσας καὶ μετὰ ὕδατος τρίψας καὶ μίξας κατάπλαττε· μάλιστα δὲ τοῦτο τοῖς ὀφρύσιν συμφέρει.

[γ'. Πρὸς τὰς ἐκ νόσου ἀποῤῥεούσας τοῖς ἀναλαμβανομένοις τρίχας.] Λάδανον σὺν οἴνῳ καὶ ἐλαίῳ ῥοδίνῳ ἑψήσας πρὸς τῆς κηρωτῆς πάχος καὶ κατάχριε. ἄλλο. ῥίζαν τῆς μορέας φλοισθεῖσαν σύγκαιε καὶ ἕψε, ὡς εἴρηται. ἄλλο. τὸ ψυλλίου σπέρμα τρίψας τίθετι ἐν τῇ κονίᾳ καὶ τὴν κεφαλὴν σύγκλυζε. ἄλλο. ᾧ ἐν τῷ ἀπὸ τοῦ πυρὸς περικεκαυμένῳ τόπῳ αἱ γίγνωνται τρίχες. φύλλα τῆς συκέας τρι-

[2. *De capillorum defluvio.*] Ad casum capillorum ulmi radicem et foliorum manipulum j, macera in iv cyathis aquae et unge et post hoc unge cum oleo. *Aliud.* Sambucum combure ac misce cum cerato liquidissimo et unge. *Aliud.* Aloën permisceto cum vino nigro austero et ungito. *Aliud.* Myrrham et ladanum illine cum vino aut oleo myrtino. *Aliud.* Accipe apes multas et combure et misce cum oleo et unge, cavens ne ungas ea quae sunt circa. *Aliud.* Recipe nigellam, combure et tritam miscens cum aqua illine; maxime autem confert superciliis.

[3. *De capillis, qui cadunt iis qui reficiuntur ex morbo.*] Ladanum cum vino et oleo rosaceo coquito ad crassitudinem cerati et ungito. *Aliud.* Radicem mori decortica et combure et coque, ut dictum est. *Aliud.* Pulicariae semen terens, pone in lixivio et lava caput; deinde coque lentiscum et collue caput. *Aliud*, quo in loco

βέσθωσαν καὶ εἰς ἄλευρον στρεφέσθωσαν καὶ τόπῳ ἐπιτιθέσθωσαν.

[δ'. Ψίλωθρα.] Ἐγκέφαλον νυκτερίδος τρίψας μετὰ γάλακτος γυναικείου καὶ ἐπίχριε. ἄλλο. χολὴν θύννου κισσοῦ τοῦ δακρύου ἢ κόμμεως καὶ κατάχριε. ἄλλο. λαβὼν τὸ αἷμα λαγωοῦ θαλαττίου νεογενὲς ἐπιτίθετι. ἄλλο. αἷμα τοῦ ἐλάφου συμμίξας ὄξει καὶ ἐπίχριε. ἄλλο. τὸ κνήδης ἀγριοστέρας σπέρμα λαβὼν, σὺν ἐλαίῳ τρίψας καὶ αὐτῷ τὸν τόπον τρῖβε. ἄλλο. νυκτερίδας πλείστας ζωὰς τίθετι ἐν ἀσφάλτῳ καὶ ἔασας ὡς σήπωνται καὶ τόπον ὀντιναοῦ κατάχριε.

[ε'. Πρὸς ἀλωπεκίας.] Μύα καύσας καὶ λεῖον ἀρκτείῳ στέατι μίξας κατάχριε, προανατρίβων κρομμύῳ λευκῷ τὸν τόπον. ἄλλο. κανθαρίδας κατακαύσας καὶ τρίψας, κόνιτρον τῷ μέλιτι ἀναλαβὼν, κατάχριε. ἄλλο. τοῖς φύλλοις συκίνοις τρῖψον ἀκριβῶς, [604] ἔπειτα χρῖε σὺν τῷ ἀρκτείῳ στέατι. ἄλλο. ἀφρὸν θαλάσσης συγκαύσας καὶ τρίψας καὶ συμμίξας ἐλαίῳ κατάχριε. ἄλλο. βατράχιον τὸ μακροσκελὲς

combuſto ab igne oriantur capilli. Folia ficus terantur et in farinam vertantur et apponantur loco.

[4. *Pſilothra.*] Cerebrum veſpertilionis terito cum lacte mulieris et illine. *Aliud.* Fel thunni miſce cum lacrima vel gummi hederae et illine. *Aliud.* Accipe ſanguinem recentem leporis et adhibe. *Aliud.* Sanguinem cervi permisce cum aceto et obline. *Aliud.* Semen urticae ſilveſtris accipe, tere cum oleo et frica ipſo locum. *Aliud.* Veſpertiliones plures vivos pone in bitumine et dimitte ut putrefiant et unge quemvis locum.

[5. *Ad alopecia.*] Murem combure et tere et pulverem permiſce cum adipe urſino et unge, prius fricans locum cepa alba. *Aliud.* Cantharidas combure et tere et pulverem permiſce cum melle et ungito. *Aliud.* Foliis ficulneis frica diligenter, deinde unge cum adipe urſino. *Aliud.* Spumam maris combure et terens permisce cum oleo et unge. *Aliud.* Ranam habentem longa crura com-

Ed. Chart. X. [604.]
κατακαύσας καὶ λεῖον μετὰ πίσσης ὑγρᾶς καὶ προανατρίβων τὸν τόπον αὐτὸν κατάχριε. ἄλλο. ἵππου ποταμίου τὸ δέρμα συγκαύσας κατάχριε τὸν τόπον. ἄλλο. τῷ αἵματι χελώνης θαλασσίας τὸν τόπον κατάχριε. ἄλλο. λαβὼν μυόχοδον καὶ τρίψας καὶ συμμίξας τῷ ὄξει πρὸς τῷ μέλιτος πάχος καὶ προανατρίβων τὸν τόπον κατάχριε. ἄλλο. ἀσφόδελον τρίψας καὶ μίξας τῷ ὄξει ἢ τῷ οἴνῳ, καὶ προξυρεύσας, τόπον τρῖβε τοῖς συκέας φύλλοις ἢ τῷ πανίῳ ὑφάσματι τραχεῖ καὶ κατάχριε. ἄλλο. ῥίζαν καλάμου καύσας καὶ μίξας τῷ ἀρκτείῳ στέατι καὶ κατάχριε. ἄλλο. τιθύμαλλον τρίψας κατάχριε τὸν τόπον.

[στ'. Περὶ πιτυριάσεως.] Κιμωλίαν προβρέξας ὕδατι, μῖξον χυλὸν τεύτλου καὶ κατάχριε καὶ ἔα ἕως ἂν ἀποξηρανθῇ εἶτα ἀποπλύνας λεῖον λιβανωτὸν σὺν οἴνῳ καὶ ἐλαίῳ κατάχριε καὶ ἔα ἕως ἂν ἀποξηρανθῇ· τῇ ὑστεραίᾳ ἡμέρᾳ σταφίδα ἀγρίαν βοτάνην σὺν ἐλαίῳ κατάχριε. ἄλλο. λαβὼν νίτρου καὶ τρυγὸς οἴνου καὶ μυροβαλάνων, ἀνὰ λίτραν α'. βοτάνης σταφίδος ἀγρίας λίτραν α'. καὶ S''. μίξας ἐλαίῳ

bure et terens misce cum pice liquida et unge locum praefricando ipsum. *Aliud.* Equi fluvialis pellem combure et unge locum. *Aliud.* Sanguine testudinis marinae unge locum. *Aliud.* Accipe muscerdam et tere et permisce cum aceto ad mellis crassitudinem et unge praefricato loco. *Aliud.* Asphodelum tere et permisce cum aceto vel vino, et praeradens locum frica foliis ficus vel panno aspero, et illine. *Aliud.* Radicem cannae urito et permisceto cum adipe ursi et ungito. *Aliud.* Tithymallum tere et unge locum.

[6. *De porrigine.*] Cimoliae aqua prius maceratae misce succum betae et illine et sinito dum inaruerint; deinde lava; post thus masculum tere, permisce cum vino et oleo atque unge, ac sinito quousque desiccetur; sequenti vero die herbam pedicularem ex oleo illinito. *Aliud.* Accipe nitri, faecis vini, mirobolanorum, singulorum libram, herbae pedicularis sesquilibram, permisce

παλαιῷ κατάχριε. ἄλλο. πρὸς δὲ τὰς ὑγροτέρας πιτυριάσεις ἅλμῃ ἀπόκλυζε, ἢ θερμῶν ἀποβρέγματι· πεπείραται γάρ. ἄλλο. τῷ τῆς ἀνδράχνης χυλῷ τὴν κεφαλὴν ἀπόκλυζε. ἄλλο. κατάχριε τὴν κεφαλὴν χυλῷ τεύτλου ἑψηθέντι, ἢ ὠμῷ τῷ μέλιτι μεμιγμένῳ. ἄλλο. κιμωλίαν μίξας τῷ τήλεως ἑψήματι κατάπλασσε. ἄλλο. σικύου ἀγρίου ῥίζαν ἑψήσας τῷ ἀφεψήματι χρῶ. ἄλλο. σκίλλαν ὀπτήσας καὶ ὅταν μαλακὴ γένηται, ἐκπιάσας τὸν χυλὸν, καὶ μίξας ἐλαίῳ, κατάχριε.

[ζ'. Πρὸς ψυδράκια καὶ ἐξανθήματα γιγνόμενα ἐν τῇ κεφαλῇ.] Ψυδράκιά εἰσι μικραὶ τῆς κεφαλῆς ὑπεροχαὶ φλυκτίσιν ὅμοιαι, ὑπερκείμεναι τῆς ἐπιφανείας. τὰ δὲ ἐξανθήματα κατὰ τὴν ἐπιφάνειαν ἐπιπόλαιαι ἑλκώσεις ὑπέρυθροι καὶ τραχεῖαι. ἀμφότερα δὲ θεραπεύονται δυνάμεσι ταῖς ὑποτεταγμέναις. πρῶτον λαβὼν τὸ λείωμα καὶ προσβαλὼν ἐν τῷ οἴνῳ καὶ ᾧ κηρωτὴν προστιθέντι. ἄλλο. ποίει κηρωτὴν ἐκ κύπου καὶ τοῦ ψιμυθίου καὶ κατάχριε. ἄλλο. προσλαμβάνων ἀμύλου, ψιμυθίου, στυπτηρίας, πηγάνου

cum oleo antiquo et unge. *Aliud.* Humidas autem porrigines aqua ſalſa vel decocto lupinorum ablue; eſt enim uſu probatum. *Aliud.* Lava caput ſucco portulacae. *Aliud.* Unge caput ſucco betae cocto vel crudo permixto cum melle. *Aliud.* Cimoliam permiſce cum decocto foenigraeci et impone. *Aliud.* Radicem cucumeris ſilveſtris coque et ejus decocto lavato. *Aliud.* Scillam coque, ubi fuerit mollis, exprime ſuccum et ei parum olei admisce et unge.

[7. *De pſydraciis et exanthematibus capitis.*] Pſydracia ſunt parva tubercula facta in capite, ſimilia veſicis eminentibus in ſuperficie. Exanthemata vero ſunt ulcerationes factae in ſumma cutis ſubrubicundae et asperae. Curantur autem utraque remediis ordine ſubſequenti poſitis. Primum accipe lomentum et funde in vinum et appone ut ceratum. *Aliud.* Fac ceratum ex liguſtro et ceruſſa et illine. *Aliud.* Accipe amyli, ceruſſae, aluminis, foliorum viridium rutae, ſingulorum drachmas quatuor,

Ed. Chart. X. [604.]

φύλλων χλωρῶν ἀνὰ < δ'. σὺν ὄξει μίξας καὶ ἐλαίῳ μυρσίνῳ κατάχριε. ἄλλο. προσλάμβανε λιθαργύρου, ψιμυθίου ἀνὰ < αβ'. θείου ἀπύρου < η'. ἐλαίῳ μυρσίνῳ ἀναλάμβανε καὶ κατάχριε.

[η'. Περὶ ἀχώρων καὶ κηρίων.] Ἀχὼρ πάθος ἐστὶν ἐν τῇ κεφαλῇ γινόμενον, τὸ λεπτοῖς πάνυ τρήμασι τὸ δέρμα κατατῆρον, δι' ὧν ἰχὼρ ἀποδίδοται γλίσχρος. ὅμοιον δὲ αὐτῷ πάθος κηρίον, ἀλλὰ τὰς κατατρήσεις ἔχει μείζονας ὑγρότητος μελιτώδους περιεκτικάς. οὕτω δὲ θεραπεύονται. ξυρήσας τὰς τρίχας πυρία δὶς ἢ καὶ τρὶς ἢ καὶ πλεονάκις ὕδατι θερμῷ ἐναφηψημένης μυρσίνης ἢ βάτου ἢ φακοῦ ἢ πικρῶν θερμῶν ἢ ἀσπαράγου ῥίζης· ὅταν δὲ πλείονες ἰχῶρες ῥέωσι, κατάπλασσε φύλλοις ἰτέας μεθ' ὕδατος, ἢ φακῷ ἐν ὕδατι ἑψηθέντι. συμφέρει δὲ τὴν κεφαλὴν τῷ θείῳ τε καὶ περδικιάδος καὶ σάπωνι προχρίειν. λαβὼν λιθαργύρου < ιστ'. πηγάνου φύλλων < η'. σταφίδος ἀγρίας < δ'. χαλκάνθου < β'. ὄξει καὶ μυρσίνῳ ἐλαίῳ ἀναλάμβανε.

permisce cum aceto et oleo myrtino et unge. *Aliud.* Accipe ſpumae argenti, ceruſſae, ſingulorum ſesquiunciam, ſulfuris ignem non experti drachmas octo, dilue oleo myrtino et unge.

[8. *De achoribus et favis.*] Achor eſt affectio oriens in capite, perforans cutim tenuibus foraminibus, per quae exit ſanies parum viscoſa. Affectio ſimilis eſt favus, ſed facit foramina majora continentia humiditatem melli ſimilem. Curantur autem ſic. Abraſum caput ſove bis aut ter aut ſaepius aqua calida decocti myrti aut rubi aut lentis aut lupinorum amarorum aut radicis asparagi; quum autem effluet multa ſanies capiti, folia ſalicis aut lentem coctam in aqua imponito: confert etiam ante caput ſulfure et parietaria et ſapone oblinere. *Aliud.* Accipe lithargyri drach. xvj, foliorum rutae drach. viij, herbae pedicularis drach. iv, attramenti ſutorii drach. ij, aceto et oleo myrtino excipito.

Κεφ. β'. [*Περὶ τῶν τῆς κεφαλῆς παθῶν.*] [605] [*α'. Περὶ τρυμοῦ τῆς κεφαλῆς.*] *Στοιχάδα δίδου πίνειν σὺν ὕδατι. ἄλλο. ἀρτεμισίας λεπτοφύλλου χυλὸν μίξας ἐλαίῳ ῥοδίνῳ καὶ τὰ τῶν νεύρων ῥίζια κατάχριε. ἄλλο. ἀκάνθας λευκῆς σπέρμα δίδου πίνειν. ἄλλο. καστόριον ὕδατι διακλύσας δίδου πίνειν.*

[*β'. Περὶ κεφαλαλγίας.*] *Κέρας ἐλάφου καύσας καὶ τρίψας καὶ μίξας ἐλαίῳ ῥοδίνῳ κατάχριε τὸ μέτωπον καὶ κροτάφους. ἄλλο. ἐγκέφαλον γύπειον τρίψας τὴν κεφαλὴν κατάχριε καὶ κροτάφους. ἄλλο. ψύλλιον κατάχεε ἐλαίῳ ῥοδίνῳ μίξας καὶ χρῶ. τοῦτο δὲ συμφέρει καὶ πρὸς τὴν ἡμικρανίαν. ἄλλο. στύρακα τὴν ὑγρὰν μίξας ἐλαίῳ παράπλεκε. ἄλλο. ὀνίσκους τοὺς ὑπὸ ὑδρίαις διαγομένους ἐν ἐλαίῳ ἑψήσας τὴν κεφαλὴν κατάχριε. ἄλλο. κυτίνους ἢ τὰ βαλάντια ἐν οἴνῳ ἑψήσας ἢ ὕδατι θαλασσίῳ μέχρι τῆς τρίτου τοῦ μέρους καταναλώσεως, καὶ τρίψας καὶ μετὰ κηρωτῆς μίξας κατάχριε. ἄλλο. τῷ γλήχωνι καὶ μαράθρου ῥίζῃ σὺν ἀλεύρῳ*

Cap. II. [*De internis capitis affectibus.*] [1. *De tremore capitis.*] Stoechadem da bibendam ex aqua. *Aliud.* Artemiſiae ſuccum parva habentis folia permisce cum oleo roſaceo et unge nervorum origines. *Aliud.* Spinae albae ſemen bibendum exhibe. *Aliud.* Caſtoreum aqua dilue et bibendum praebe.

[2. *De dolore capitis.*] Cornu cervi combure et tere et permisce cum oleo roſaceo et unge frontem ac tempora. *Aliud.* Cerebrum vulturis terens illine caput et tempora. *Aliud.* Pſyllium ſuffundens oleo roſaceo permisce et utere; hoc autem confert et ad hemicraniam. *Aliud.* Styracem liquidam permisce cum oleo et applica. *Aliud.* Aſellos ſub hydriis degentes coque in oleo et unge caput. *Aliud.* Flores mali punici vel ipſa balauſtia coque in vino aut aqua marina usque ad conſumptionem tertiae partis et tere et cum cerato permiscens admove. *Aliud.* Pulegio et foeniculi radice cum farina hordei line

Ed. Chart. X. [605.]
κριθίνῳ τοὺς κροτάφους κατάχριε. ἄλλο. ἡδύοσμον ἢ σίνηπι σὺν ὄξει μίξας κατάχριε κροτάφους δὶς ἐν ἡμέρᾳ.

[γ΄. Πρὸς τῆς κεφαλῆς τε καὶ τῶν κροτάφων ἀλγήματα.] Προςλάμβανε ὀπίου τὸ κυάμου μέγεθος καὶ γλήχωνος καὶ σχίνου μερίδας ἕξ, καὶ ἀναλαβὼν ὄξει καὶ ἐλαίῳ ῥοδίνῳ κατάχριε. ἄλλο. ὀξυλάπαθον καὶ τὴν κικίδα τρίψας τὸ μέτωπον καὶ κροτάφους κατάχριε. ἄλλο. καστόριον διαλύσας ἐλαίῳ ῥοδίνῳ καὶ ὄξει κατάχριε μέτωπον καὶ κροτάφους. ἄλλο. ἶριδα ξηρὰν καὶ καρδάμωμον ἔλαττον ὄξει ἀναλύσας χρῖε τρίχας ὡς γυναῖκες ποιοῦσιν αὐτὰς καταχρίουσαι. ἄλλο. χυλὸν πευκεδάνου ἐλαίῳ ἰρίνῳ διαλύσας ἐπιτίθετι. ἄλλο. νεοττείαν χελιδόνων μὴ συγχωρέῃς εἰς γῆν πίπτειν καὶ πηλὸν τὸν τῷ κόπρῳ μεμιγμένον λαβὼν καὶ τῷ ὄξει ἐν ἀγγείῳ ξυλίνῳ συμβρέξας καὶ ὑπάξας τὸ μέτωπον κατάχριε. ἄλλο. τὸ κόμμι κισσοῦ τῷ ὄξεῖ τε καὶ ἐλαίῳ ῥοδίνῳ διαλύσας τοὺς κροτάφους κατάχριε. ἄλλο. βοήθημα σπυράθους, τουτέστιν ἀφοδεύματα αἰγὸς σὺν ὄξει καὶ ἐλαίῳ ῥοδίνῳ λειοτριβήσας κατάχριε τὸ μέτωπον καὶ κατάδησον φασκίᾳ·

tempora. *Aliud.* Mentem aut ſinapi cum aceto permisce et madefac tempora bis in die.

[3. *Ad dolorem capitis et temporum.*] Accipe opii magnitudinem fabae et pulegii partes ſex et lentisci et excipe aceto, ac oleo roſaceo et ungito. *Aliud.* Rumicem acidum et gallam tere et unge tempora et frontem. *Aliud.* Caſtoreum diſſolve cum oleo roſaceo et aceto; unge frontem et tempora. *Aliud.* Iridem ſiccam et cardamomum minus aceto reſolve et line capillos, ſicut faciunt mulieres quum inungunt eos. *Aliud.* Succum peucedani oleo irino diluens imponito. *Aliud.* Hirundinum nidum ne permittas in terram cadere, et lutum, quod eſt ſtercori mixtum capito, et aceto in vaſe ligneo ſubigito et illine frontem. *Aliud.* Gummi hederae aceto et oleo roſaceo diluens ungue tempora. *Aliud remedium.* Pilulas, hoc eſt caprinum ſtercus, ex aceto et oleo roſaceo terito, fronti illinito et ſascia deligato; id facito mane ac vesperi et caput dolentem ſanitati reſtitues. *Aliud.* Euphor-

ποίει δὲ πρωῒ καὶ δείλης καὶ ἰάσῃ τὸν κεφαλαλγοῦντα. ἄλλο. εὐφόρβιον καὶ μέλαν γραφικὸν λειώσας μετ' ὄξους κατάχριε τὸ μέτωπον. ἄλλο. παῖς ἄφθορος οὐρησάτω ἐπὶ τὴν οὐδὸν τῆς θύρας τοῦ πάσχοντος. σὺ δ' ἐπιβάλλων ὄξος τρῖβε ἀμφότερα εἰς ἓν ἐπὶ τὴν οὐδὸν, ὡς γλοιοῦ γίνεσθαι πάχος, καὶ κατάχριε τὸ μέτωπον αὐθωρόν. ἄλλο. ἐάν τις τίκτουσα κεφαλὴν πονῇ, σποδὸν ὄξει φυράσας κατάχριε. ἄλλο. δάκρυον κισσοῦ, μετ' ὄξους καὶ ῥοδίνου λειώσας, κατάχριε τὸ μέτωπον καὶ κροτάφους. ἐπίθεμα πρὸς ταυτά. κάρδαμον φυράσας ὄξει καὶ ῥοδίνῳ καὶ ποιήσας κηρωτῆς τὸ πάχος ἐπιτίθει ἀπὸ κροτάφου ἐπὶ κρόταφον. παραχρῆμα τὴν ὀδύνην παύει.

[δ'. Πρὸς ἑτεροκράνιον.] Ἀκακίαν λαβὼν κηρωτῇ ῥοδίνῃ χρῶ. ἄλλο. κιχώριον ἐπιτιθέμενον καὶ πόνους κεφαλῆς καὶ τὰς ἐγκαύσεις τὰς γινομένας ἀφ' ἡλίου παύει.

[606] [ε'. Πρὸς ἐπιληπτικοὺς πότημα.] Ἰκτῖνον καύσας ζῶντα ἐν χύτρᾳ, δίδου πίνειν τὴν τέφραν καὶ ὑγιάσεις. ἄλλο. ἧπαρ αὐτοῦ καύσας καὶ τρίψας δίδου δι'

bio et atramento fcriptorio una cum aceto detritis frontem illine. *Aliud.* Puer impubes in limine aegroti januae mingat; tu vero acetum infundito, atque utrumque in unum fuper limen commisceto, donec fordium acquirat craffitudinem, ac eadem illa hora fronti imponito. *Aliud.* Si qua ex partu capitis dolore tentetur, cinerem cum aceto admiscens fronti fuperdato. *Aliud.* Hederae lacrima cum aceto et rofaceo mixta tempora et frontem obline. Epithema ad idem. Nafturtium cum aceto et rofaceo misceto ad cerati craffitudinem imponitoque ita, ut a tempore ad tempus pertineat; illico dolorem auferes.

[4. *Ad eos qui ex altera capitis parte dolent.*] Acaciam rofaceo cerato excipiens utere. *Aliud.* Cichorium impofitum et capitis dolores et exuftiones a fole factas tollit.

[5. *Ad comitialem morbum.*] Milvum in olla cremato viventem cineremque propinato et fanabis. *Aliud.* Ejusdem jecur uftum et tritum ex aqua potui dato. *Aliud.*

Ed. Chart. X. [606.]
ὕδατος. ἄλλο. κόπρον ὀνείαν φρύξον καὶ λάμβανε ἀπ' αὐτῆς ὅσον κοχλιάρια β'. καὶ πότιζε καθ' ἡμέραν, καὶ ἀπαλλαγήσεται τοῦ πάθους· τοῦτο τῶν λίαν πεπειραμένων ἐστίν. ἄλλο. οὖρον κάπρου ἐν κάπνῳ ξηρὸν ποίει, ποτιζόμενον δι' ὀξυμέλιτος· ἔστω δὲ τοῦ οὔρου τὸ μέγεθος κυάμου Αἰγυπτίου, μάλιστα δὲ συάργου. ἄλλο. κόπρος τράγειος ποιεῖ διδομένη ἕως πεντεκαίδεκα σπυράθων. ἄλλο. μαλάχης ἀγρίας χυλὸν δίδου ἐπὶ ἡμέρας λ'. πίνειν νηστικῷ, καὶ ἰάσῃ. ἄλλο. γαλῆς αἷμα κατάξηρον δίδου δι' ὕδατος. τοῦτο δὲ ποίει, ὅταν ᾖ παραυτικα πεσούμενος ὁ κάμνων. ἄλλο. ὀλίγον ἐλαίου τῇ λάγωῃ πητύᾳ κατάχεε καὶ καταπότια ποίεε, ἐξ ὧν [ὅθ' ἓν, ὁτὲ δύο δίδου. ἄλλο. γαλῆς αἷμα περίχριε καὶ τὴν γαλῆν δίδου φαγεῖν, ἀποκόπτων αὐτῆς τοὺς πόδας καὶ τὴν κεφαλήν· ποιεῖ ὁμοίως καὶ πρὸς χοιράδας διδομένη γαλῆ. ἄλλο. μῦν ἀνατεμὼν ἐν ληγοσεληνίῳ δέξαι αὐτοῦ τὸ ἧπαρ καὶ ὀπτήσας δὸς φαγεῖν τῷ πάσχοντι. ὠφελεῖ καὶ τὸ ὀξύμελι σκιλλιτικὸν καὶ τὸ Ἰουλιανοῦ καὶ ἡ θηριακή.

Asini stercus frictum cochleariorum duorum pondere quotidie exhibeto, atque aegrotus morbo liberabitur; id remedium longa experientia comprobatum est. *Aliud.* Urina verris in fumo arefacta ex oxymelite pota bene facit; esto autem urinae portio ad Aegyptiae fabae magnitudinem, sed optima est apri. *Aliud.* Hircinum stercus ad morbum comitialem proficit, si ex eo quindecim globuli ad summum exhibeantur. *Aliud.* Agrestis malvae succum aegrotus per triginta dies jejunus bibat et curabitur. *Aliud.* Mustellae jecur aridum ex aqua propinato; id facias autem, quum aegrotus mox est casurus. *Aliud.* Parum olei leporis coagulo infundito et pilulas facito; ex quibus modo unam, modo duas praebeto. *Aliud.* Mustellae sanguine oblinito ac mustellam pedibus capiteque abjectis edendam apponito. Pariter et strumis exhibita mustella prodest. *Aliud.* Murem dissecans per lunae silentium jecur ipsius extrahito et assum aegro, ut comedat, exhibeto. Juvat etiam oxymel scilliticum et Juliani et theriaca.

[στ'. Ἄλλο ὀσφραντικὸν πρὸς ἐπιληπτικούς.] Τιθύμαλλον τρίψας μετὰ ὄξους καὶ ἀλφίτων, μαζία ποιήσας δίδου ὀσφραίνεσθαι τῷ ἐπιληπτικῷ καὶ οὐ πεσεῖται. καὶ συμφέρει τοῦ πευκεδάνου τε καὶ πίσσης ὀσφρᾶσθαι.

[ζ'. Ἐπιθυμίαμα τῷ γνῶναι εἰ ἔστιν ἐπιληπτικός.] Λίθον ἐπιθυμίασον τὸν γαγάτην, αὐτῷ συμπεριβαλὼν, ὡς μὴ διασκίδνασθαι τὴν οσμὴν καὶ καταπεσεῖται εἴπερ ἑάλῳ τῷ πάθει.

[η'. Πότημα πρὸς τὸ γνῶναι εἰ ἀθεράπευτοί εἰσιν οἱ ἐπιληπτικοί.] Ἀκακίας δραχμὴν ὕδατι διεὶς πότιζε· ἐὰν ἐμέσῃ, ἀνίατόν ἐστιν· ἐὰν δὲ πυρέξῃ, πότερον συμφέρει αὐτῷ.

[θ'. Ἀστροπλήκτων θεραπεία.] Ὄνου οὖρον κατάχεε αὐτοῖς καὶ θεραπεύονται.

[ι'. Ἐὰν πεπτωκότα ἐπιληπτικὸν θέλῃς ἐγεῖραι παραχρῆμα.] Θύμον ἢ γλήχωνα τρίψας προσένεγκε αὐτοῦ τοῖς μυκτῆρσι.

[ια'. Καθαρτικὸν διὰ μυκτήρων.] Ἀναγαλλίδος τῆς

[6. *Aliud odorabile ad comitialem affectum.*] Tithymallum cum aceto et polenta terens placentulas conficito olfaciendasque laboranti offerto et non cadet. Confert etiam odorari peucedanum et picem.

[7. *Suffimentum comitialem morbum detegens.*] Lapidem gagatem suffito, ipsum circumvelans, ne odor dissipetur, cadetque si re vera comitiali morbo affectus est.

[8. *Potiones, per quas dignoscitur, utrum comitialis morbus sanabilis sit.*] Acaciae drachmam aqua diluens bibendam dato; si vomuerit, insanabile malum est, sin autem febricitaverit, potio ipsi prodest.

[9. *A sidere percussorum curatio.*] Asini lotio ipsos consperge et sanescent.

[10. *Si comitiali morbo humi prostratum confestim excitare vis.*] Thymum aut pulegium conterens ejus naribus admoveto.

[11. *Materiam per nares detrahentia.*] Anagallidis

τὸ κυανοῦν ἄνθος ἐχούσης τὸν χυλὸν εἰς τοὺς μυκτῆρας ἐνθεὶς κέλευε ὕπτιον ἀνανεύσαντα. τοῦτο δὲ βοηθεῖ πᾶσι τοῖς περὶ κεφαλὴν ὀχλουμένοις. ἄλλο. χυλὸν τοῦ κισσοῦ λευκοῦ ἔγχει εἰς μυκτῆρας. ἄλλο. μελάνθιον χυλίσας μετὰ ὑδρομέλιτος καὶ ἶριν, οὕτως χρῶ, ἔλαιον παλαιὸν μίξας. ἄλλο. σεύτλου ῥίζαν χυλίσας ἔγχει εἰς μυκτῆρας καὶ καθαίρει.

Κεφ. γ'. [Πρὸς τὰ ὤτων πάθη] [α'. Πρὸς τὰς διαθέσεις τὰς ἐν τοῖς ἀκουστικοῖς πόροις.] Ἐγκλύσας οἴνῳ κεκραμένῳ ἢ ὑδρομέλιτι τὸ οὖς ἔνσταζε λύκιον, λεάνας ἐν λεπυρίαις.

[607] [β'. Πρὸς φλεγμονὰς καὶ πόνους.] Σκορόδου τὸ ἐντὸς ἀμυγδαλοειδὲς θλάσας μετὰ ἐλαίου εἰς ξύστραν θερμάνας, ἔγχει τὸ ἔλαιον εἰς οὖς καὶ ἄπονος ἔσται.

[γ'. Πρὸς περιωδυνίαν.] Ἧπαρ χήνειον τεταριχευμένον τήξας μετὰ νάρδου καὶ ἀπομάξας εἰς τὸ οὖς ἐντίθει.

[δ'. Πρὸς ὦτα πυοῤῥοοῦντα.] Στυπτηρίαν ὑγρὰν ἀνεὶς ὕδατι ἔμβαλον εἰς ὑέλινον ἀγγεῖον καὶ λειάνας ἔνσταζε.

caeruleum habentis florem ſuccum naribus inſtillato, jubetoque ſupinum aegrotum ſpiritum adducere; hoc enim omnibus ex capite laborantibus opitulantur. *Aliud.* Succum hederae albae naribus inſtillato. *Aliud.* Nigellae expreſſum ſuccum cum mulſa inſtilla. Ad eundem modum et iride veteri oleo admixto utitor. *Aliud.* Betae radicis ſuccum in nares inſunde et caput purgat.

Cap. III. [*Ad aurium affectiones.*] [1. *Ad eas quae in auditoriis meatibus fiunt.*] Vino diluto aut mulſa aurem ſubluito, ac lycium in ovi putamine macerans inſundito.

[2. *Ad inflammationes et dolores.*] Allii capitula contuſa cum oleo in olla caleſacito, oleumque in aurem inſundito et dolor ſedabitur.

[3. *Ad magnum dolorem.*] Anſerinum jecur ſalſum cum nardo eliquato et repurgans in aurem indito.

[4. *Ad aures ſanie manantes.*] Liquidum alumen aqua diluens in vitreum vas conde et maceratum inſtilla.

Ed. Chart. X. [607.]

[ε'. Πρὸς τὰ πυοῤῥοοῦντα καὶ περιωδυνῶντα.] Πράσου χυλὸν μέλιτι διεὶς χρῶ. ἄλλο. ὄπιον ἀνιεὶς γλυκεῖ εἰς τὸ οὖς ἔνσταζε χλιαίνων. ἄλλο. κεδρίαν ἐν ὀλίγῳ νάρδῳ ἔνσταζε. ἄλλο. μέλι καὶ ἔλαιον ἐν κενώμασι προχλιάνας ἔνσταζε.

[στ'. Πρὸς τερηδόνας καὶ πυοῤῥοοῦντας.] Στυπτηρίαν σχιστὴν μετ' ὄξους καὶ γλυκέος ἑψήσας ἔνσταζε ποιῶν μέλιτος πάχος, ἐνεργὲς ἐπὶ προσφάτου καὶ ἐπὶ χρονίου.

[ζ'. Πρὸς ἤχους καὶ περιωδυνίας.] Κεδρίαν μέλιτι μίξας ἔνσταζε. ἄλλο. ἀλόην ἡπατικὴν μετὰ οἰνομέλιτος, ποιῶν γλοιοῦ πάχος, ἔνσταζε. ἄλλο. ἀλώπεκος στέαρ ἀνειμένον ἔνσταζε. ἄλλο. νάρδον χλιαρὰν ἔνσταζε. ἄλλο. κασίαν μετὰ ῥοδίνου ἔνσταζε. ἄλλο. σίλφας τὰς κατοικιδίους μετὰ ῥοδίνου θερμαίνων ἔνσταζε.

[η'. Πρὸς τὰς κατὰ μικρὸν περιωδυνίας.] Ἔρια οἰσυπηρὰ περιζέσας ὄξει ἐγχυμάτιζε καὶ ἐξ αὐτοῦ τοῦ ἐρίου ἐντίθει εἰς τὸ οὖς. ἄλλο. ῥοιᾶς ἀώρου τῷ χυλῷ μετὰ μέλιτος χρῶ, ἢ σχίνου τῷ χυλῷ ἢ περδικίου βοτάνης ἢ κύ-

[5. *Ad aures purulentas et graviter dolentes.*] Porri ſucco melle diluto utere. *Aliud.* Opium dulci vino eliquans ac tepeſaciens, in aurem injice. *Aliud.* Cedri lacrimam ex pauca nardo immittito. *Aliud.* Mel et oleum una in vasculo prius tepefacta inſtillato.

[6. *Ad teredines et ſaniem.*] Alumen ſciſſile cum aceto et dulci vino elixum ad mellis craſſitudinem infuſum tam in recentibus quam antiquis vitiis efficax eſt.

[7. *Ad ſonitus aurium intra ſeipſas et acres dolores.*] Cedri lacrimam cum melle mixtam inſtilla. *Aliud.* Aloen jecorariam cum mulſo ad ſordium craſſitudinem temperatam infunde. *Aliud.* Vulpis adipem eliquatam infunde. *Aliud.* Nardum tepefactum infundito. *Aliud.* Caſſiam ex roſaceo injicito. *Aliud.* Blattas domeſticas oleo roſaceo inſerveſactas inſtilla.

[8. *Ad dolores paulatim ingruentes.*] Lanam ſuccidam in aceto fervefactam exprimito et humorem ex ipſa lana in aurem impone, ſuperpoſita lana. *Aliud.* Mali punici immaturi ſucco cum melle utere, aut ſucco lentisci

πρου ἢ βάτου. τούτων τὸν χυλὸν κατ' ἰδίαν ἑκάστου ἢ καὶ μετὰ μέλιτος μίσγων καὶ ἑψῶν χρῶ. ἢ ἀρνογλώσσου ἢ θριδακίνης ἢ πολυγόνου χυλοῦ ὁμοίως χρῶ.

[θ'. Πρὸς πόνους χωρὶς ἑλκώσεως.] Θεῖον ἄπυρον ἐμφύσα διὰ συριγγίου. ἄλλο. ὄπιον ἀνιεὶς γυναικείῳ γάλακτι ἔνσταζε.

[ι'. Πρὸς δυσηκοοῦντας.] Ἀψίνθιον ἀφέψων διὰ ὕδατος κλύζε τὸ οὖς τῷ ἀφεψήματι.

[ια'. Πρὸς τοὺς ἐκ γενετῆς κωφούς.] Αἰγὸς νεωστὶ ἐσφαγμένης τὸ κέρας πλῆσον οὔρου αἰγὸς καὶ κρέμασον εἰς καπνὸν ἐπὶ ἡμέρας θ'. καὶ χρῶ.

[ιβ'. Πρὸς τοὺς ἐκ βάθους ἤχους.] Ὄξος καὶ ῥόδινον, πήγανον, κύμινον λεάνας μετὰ μέλιτος χρῶ.

[ιγ'. Πρὸς βόμβους καὶ ἤχους ἐξαπίνης γινομένους.] Ὄξος δριμὺ χλιαίνων ἔνσταζε. ἄλλο. βρυωνίας, μέλιτος καὶ ἐλλεβόρου λευκοῦ καὶ ῥοδίνου λεάνας ἔνσταζε.

aut herbae parietariae aut liguſtri aut rubi; horum cujusque ſuccum aut per ſe aut melli admiſcens et elixans utere; aut plantaginis aut lactucae aut ſanguinalis ſucco ſimiliter utere.

[9. *Ad dolores absque ulcere.*] Sulfur ignem non expertum per calamum naribus inſuſſletur. *Aliud.* Opium muliebri lacte temperatum inſtilla.

[10. *Ad gravem auditum.*] Abſinthium in aqua decoquens aurem decocto eluito.

[11. *Ad ſurditatem naturalem.*] Caprae nuper jugulatae cornu caprino lotio impleto et fumum per dies ix, ſuſpendito et utere.

[12. *Ad ſonitus ex profundo.*] Acetum et oleum roſaceum, rutam et cuminum cum melle macerans utitor.

[13. *Ad tinnitus ſonosque repente exortos.*] Acetum acre tepefactum in aurem demitte. *Aliud.* Vitis albae, mellis, veratri albi et roſacei olei portionem, in unum permiscens, in aurem dato.

Ed. Chart. X. [607. 608.]

[ιδ΄. Πρὸς ἀλγοῦντα καὶ πυοῤῥοοῦντα.] Ὄξος καὶ μέλι καὶ ῥόδινον μίξας χλιάνας χρῶ.

[ιε΄. Πρὸς περιωδυνίας.] Εὐθύπαστον ἐλαίῳ στέαρ ἔνσταζε, καὶ σπόγγῳ τόπον ἔπεχε· ποιεῖ καὶ πρὸς τὰ νευρώδη μισγόμενον καὶ μετὰ ἀλωπεκίου στέατος καὶ ὕου, ἴσα ἴσοις.

[ιστ΄. Πρὸς ἀλγηδόνας καὶ φλεγμονάς.] Ἀσφοδέλου ῥίζαν καθάρας βάλλε εἰς ἔλαιον ἐν ἀγγείῳ ὑελίνῳ καὶ ἡλίαζε ταῖς ὑπὸ κυνὸς καύμασιν [608] ἡμέραις μ΄. καὶ χρῶ.

[ιζ΄. Πρὸς τὰ ἡλκωμένα καὶ πυοῤῥοοῦντα.] Σαύρας τὰς μικρὰς λαβὼν τῆξον ἐλαίῳ καθαρῷ, καὶ οὕτως ἐγχυμάτιζε καὶ ἐὰν σκώληκας ἔχῃ, ἰᾶται.

[ιη΄. Πρὸς τὰ ἐν ὠσὶ σκωλήκια παρεισδυόμενα εἰς τὰς ἀκοάς.] Κρόμμυα καὶ ὕσσωπον τρίψας οὔρῳ παλαιῷ ἐγχυμάτιζε. ἄλλο. κολοκυνθίδος τοῦ σπέρματος τῆς ἐντεριώνης, στυπτηρίας Αἰγυπτίας ἴσα, μετὰ κεδρίνου ἐλαίου λειώσας ἐγχυμάτιζε.

[14. *Ad aurem dolentem et ſanie manentem.*] Acetum, mel roſeumque permisce et tepeſactis utere.

[15. *Ad acerbos dolores.*] Subactam oleo adipem infundito et ſpongia locum occludito; facit et ad nervorum morbos cum vulpino adipe atque ſuillo aequa portione permixta.

[16. *Ad dolores aurium ac phlegmonas.*] Haſtulae regiae radicem mundato et in oleum vaſe vitreo contentum demittito et per continuos quadraginta dies ſub canis aeſtu inſolato, deinde utitor.

[17. *Ad ulceratas aures et purulentas.*] Lacertas puſillas venatus mundo oleo eliquato, atque ita in aurem demittito et vermes, ſi in aure ſuerint, ſanabis.

[18. *Ad aurium vermiculos et ad ea quae in aurem ſubierunt.*] Caepas et hyſſopum in lotio vetere conterens inſtillato. *Aliud.* Partis interioris colocynthidis ſeminum, aluminis Aegyptii, pares portiones in cedrino oleo macerans infundito.

Ed. Chart. X. [608.]

[ιθ'. Πρὸς τὸ ῥύπον ἐξελεῖν.] Κροκίδα βρέξας μυροβαλάνῳ ἔνθες καὶ εὑρήσεις τὴν κροκίδα πλήρη τοῦ ῥύπου. ἄλλο. νίτρον λεπτὸν ἔμβαλλε εἰς τὸ οὖς καὶ ἐπίσταξον ὄξος καὶ πρόσθες ἔριον, ἔασον ἐννυκτερεῦσαι· τῇ δὲ ἐπιούσῃ κλύσον ὑδρελαίῳ θερμῷ.

[κ'. Πρὸς ὠταλγίαν.] Ἁλὸς ἄνθος μετὰ ῥοδίνου καὶ ὄξους ἔνσταζε.

[κα'. Πρὸς τὰ πυοῤῥοοῦντα καὶ περιωδυνῶντα.] Νίτρον μετὰ ῥοδίνου διεὶς ἐγχυμάτιζε τὸ οὖς. ἄλλο. ἐλλέβορον λευκὸν μετὰ οἴνου ἢ ὄξους ἔνσταζε σὺν στυπτηρίᾳ· καὶ χυλὸν καλαμίνθης ῥίζης συλλειοτριβήσας μετ' ὄξους ἐγχυμάτιζε.

[κβ'. Πρὸς τὰ χρόνια.] Λύκιον καὶ μέλι ἴσα μίξας χρῶ.

[κγ'. Πρὸς φλεγμαίνοντα.] Σκωδειῶν κελύφη κόψας εἰς ὠμὴν λύσιν ἕως τρίτου μέρους, καὶ ἑψήσας ἐν γλυκεῖ κεκραμένῳ κατάπλασσε.

[19. *Ad ſordes aurium educendas.*] Lanam unguentaria glande madidam in aurem demitte et lanam ſordium plenam invenies. *Aliud.* Nitrum tenue in aurem conjicito acetumque inſtillato; ſuper lana mollis addenda eſt et per noctem relinquenda; ſequenti vero die calida aqua et oleo aurem eluito.

[20. *Ad aurem dolentem.*] Salis flos cum roſaceo et aceto infundendus eſt.

[21. *Ad ſaniem aurium et magnum dolorem.*] Nitrum roſaceo dilutum in aurem demitte. *Aliud.* Album veratrum ex vino aut aceto cum alumine infunde; radicis praeterea calaminthae ſuccus aceto maceratus inſtilletur.

[22. *Ad diuturna vitia.*] Lycii et mellis aequas portiones commiscens utere.

[23. *Ad inflammatas aures.*] Capitulorum papaveris cortices contere et tertiam partem cum hordeacea farina permisce et in dulci diluto incoque, cataplasmaque conſice.

Ed. Chart. X. [608.]

[κδ'. Πρὸς τὰ πυοῤῥοοῦντα καὶ περιωδυνῶντα.] Μυελὸν μόσχειον χυλίσας ἔνσταζε. ἄλλο. σκωρίαν σιδήρου τρίψας ἐν τῷ ὄξει δριμυτάτῳ ἔνσταζε.

[κε'. Πρὸς χοιράδας καὶ παρωτίδας.] Χοιράδας κοινῇ μὲν θεραπείᾳ τὰ τῶν σκιῤῥῶν διαφορητικὰ διαφορέουσι· ἰδίᾳ δὲ οὕτως. ἄλευρον θερμῶν πικρῶν ἑψήσας ἐν τῷ ὀξυμέλιτι κατάπλασσε. ἄλλο. βοείαν κόπρον ἢ αἰγείαν ἐν ὄξει ἑφθὴν ἐπιτίθετι. ἄλλο. ἄσβεστον μέλιτι ἢ ἐλαίῳ ἢ στέατι χοιρείῳ ἀναληφθεῖσαν ἐπιτίθετι. ἄλλο. ἄλευρον ἴριδος καὶ κόπρον περιστερᾶς ἑψήσας οἴνῳ κατάπλασσε. ἄλλο. λαβὼν στέατος παλαιοῦ καὶ σπέρματος ὑοσκυάμου καὶ πίσσης καὶ ἐλαίου παλαιοῦ καὶ κόπρου ἀλεκτορίδος μελίνης τὰ ἴσα συμμίξας κατάπλασσε.

Κεφ. δ'. [Εὐπόριστα φάρμακα πρὸς τὰ τῶν ὀφθαλμῶν πάθη.] [α'. Πρὸς ὀφθαλμίαν ἀρχομένην.] Χυλὸν ἡδυόσμου ἔνσταζε, διαλύει γάρ· ἔστι δὲ βέλτιον τὸ περιστερᾶς αἷμα. ἄλλο. μαράθρου χυλὸν ἐκπιέσας καὶ χρῶ· παλαιὸς μέν ἐστιν ἀμείνων. αὐτὸν δὲ τῷ ὕδατι μίξας χρῶ.

[24. *Ad aures ſanie manantes et dolentes.*] Medullam vituli liquefaciens inſtilla. *Aliud.* Scoriam ſerri terens in aceto acerrimo inſtilla.

[25. *Ad ſtrumas et parotidas.*] Scrophulas communi quidem curatione discutiunt ea, quae ſcirrhos, propria vero ita. Farinam lupinorum amarorum coque in oxymelite et illine. *Aliud.* Stercus bovis aut caprae coque in aceto et appone. *Aliud.* Calcem melli aut oleo aut adipi porci permiſce et appone. *Aliud.* Farinam iridis et ſtercus columbi coque in vino et adhibe. *Aliud.* Accipe axungiae veteris, ſeminis hyoscyami, picis, olei antiqui ſtercoris citrini gallinae ſingulorum pares portiones, commisce et admove.

Cap. IV. [*Parabilia medicamenta ad oculorum morbos.*] [1. *Ad ophthalmiam incipientem.*] Succum menthae infunde, reſolvit enim; ſed melior eſt ſanguis columbi. *Aliud.* Foeniculi ſuccum exprime et utere; antiquus autem eſt melior; permisce autem eum aquae et

ἄλλο. ἐκ τοῦ πηγάνου προσφάτου χυλὸν ἐκπιέσας τίθετι ἐν τῇ πυξίδι τοῦ χαλκοῦ ἐρύθρου καὶ χρῶ. ἄλλο. ἐκ κυδωνίων ἑψηθέντων καὶ ἀλφίτου καὶ οἴνου λευκοῦ κατάπλασμα ποίει. ἄλλο. φύλλα μήκωνος καὶ σιδία σὺν παιπάλῃ κριθίνῃ ἐπιτίθετι. ἄλλο. ῥόδα ἑψήσας καὶ τρίψας κατάπλασσε. ἄλλο. ἀφέψημα μελιλώτου ἔνσταζε. ἄλλο. ἐκ [609] φύλλων κοκτόνου τετριμένων ποίει κατάπλασμα σὺν οἴνῳ καὶ ἀλεύρῳ.

[β΄. Πρὸς ὄνυχα.] Ὄνυξ μὲν λέγεται ἡ ὀφθαλμοῦ νόσος, ὅταν κερατοειδὴς ποτὲ μὲν διὰ βάθος, ποτὲ δὲ ἐπιπολῆς, ὄνυχι προσεοικότος τοῦ πύου κατὰ τὸ σχῆμα, διὸ καὶ τὸ πάθος ὄνυχα προσαγορεύουσι. πρὸς τοὺς μὲν οὖν μετρίους ὄνυχας συντέλει μελίκρατον καὶ τῆς τήλεως ὁ χυλὸς καὶ κολλούριον τὸ διὰ λιβάνου γινόμενον· πρὸς τοὺς δὲ μείζονας λαβὼν ἀλόης, σμύρνης, κρόκου ἀνὰ μέρος α΄. οἴνου μέρει γ΄. μέλιτος μέρει στ΄. λειοῦται ὁ κρόκος σὺν ὀλίγῳ οἴνῳ, εἶτα ἀλόη καὶ σμύρνα καὶ ἐπειδὰν παχυνθῇ ἐπίβαλλε τὸ μέλι καὶ ἑνώσας ἀπόθου ἐν ὑέλῳ ἀγγείῳ, χρῶ

utere. *Aliud.* Ex ruta recente ſuccum exprime et pone in pyxide aeris rubri et utere. *Aliud.* Ex cotoneis coctis et farina hordei et vino albo cataplasma facito. *Aliud.* Folia papaveris et cortices granatorum cum polline hordei ſuperdato. *Aliud.* Roſas coctas et tritas impone. *Aliud.* Decoctum meliloti infunde. *Aliud.* Ex foliis coctani tritis ſac cataplasma cum vino et polenta.

[2. *Ad ungulam.*] Dicitur ungula morbus oculi, quando cornea aliquando quidem ſuperficie tenus, aliquando vero in profundo pus continet, et aſſimilatur parvae ungulae, quare morbus ille vocatur ungula. Ad mediocres ergo ungulas confert mulſa et ſuccus foenigraeci et collyrium quod ſit ex thure. Ad majores autem accipe aloes, myrrhae, croci, ſingulorum partem j, vini partes iij, mellis partes vj, diſſolvas crocum cum modico vini, deinde aloen et myrrham, deinde et ubi craſſa ſuerint, adjicito mel et

δὲ δὶς τῆς ἡμέρας· ὀφθαλμὸν γὰρ ἅμα καθαίρει, σαρκὶ ἀπουλοῖ.

[γ'. Πρὸς ὑπώπια.] Σίνηπι λεῖαν κηρωτῇ ἀναλαβὼν ἐπιτίθετι. ἄλλο. ὄστρακα τῆς σηπίας λεάνας καὶ ὄξει μίξας νυκτὸς κατάχριε· ἀφαιρεῖ γὰρ αὐτά. ἄλλο. ῥίζαν σίκυος ἀγρίου μέλιτι συμμίξας ἐπιτίθετι.

[δ'. Πρὸς τῶν ὀφθαλμῶν πελιώματα.] Ὕσσωπον τρίψας, εἰς ῥάκος ἐνδήσας καὶ εἰς ζέον ὕδωρ ἀποβάπτων ἡσυχῇ ἀποπυρία καὶ πελιώματα θίγε. ἄλλο. ἄλευρον ἴριδος μίξας τῷ μέλιτι καὶ κατάπλασσε. ἄλλο. κύμινον τετριμμένον συμμίξας γάλακτι γυναικείῳ ἐπιτίθετι· ἢ ὀρίγανον ἐπιτίθετι ὁμοίως. ἄλλο. εὐζώμου σπέρμα τρίψας σὺν χολῇ βοείᾳ ἐπιτίθετι.

[ε'. Πρὸς τὰ πτερύγια.] Τὸ πτερύγιον νευρώδης ἐστὶ τοῦ ἐπιπεφυκότος ὑμένος ὑπεροχή· ἐκφυομένη μὲν ἀπὸ τοῦ κανθοῦ, προϊοῦσα δὲ μέχρι τῆς στεφάνης. ὅταν δὲ ὑπεραυξηθῇ, καὶ τὴν κόρην καλύπτει. τὰ μὲν οὖν μεγάλα καὶ χρόνια τῶν πτερυγίων διὰ μόνης χειρουργίας ἐκτέμνε-

uniens in vafe vitreo reconde et utere bis in die: expurgat enim oculum fimul, carnem gignit et folidat.

[3. *Ad fugillata.*] Sinapin tere et appone cum cerato. *Aliud.* Offa fepiae tere fubtiliffime et permiscens aceto illine noctu; tollit enim ea. *Aliud.* Radicem cucumeris agreftis melli commisce et impone.

[4. *De livoribus oculorum.*] Hyffopum tritam liga in panno et infunde in aqua calida et tange livores, fomentum faciens. *Aliud.* Farinam iridis melle admifce et adhibe. *Aliud.* Cuminum tritum admifce lacti mulieris et appone; vel origanum appone fimiliter. *Aliud.* Erucae femen terens cum felle bubulo imponito.

[5. *De pterygiis.*] Pterygium dicitur nervofa fupernatae oculo membranae eminentia, incipiens ab angulis et procedens ufque ad coronam; quando vero amplius augetur, cooperit et pupillam. Magna igitur et diuturna pterygia per chirurgiam inciduntur; recentia vero et mode-

Ed. Chart. X. [609.]
ται· τὰ δὲ νεώτερα καὶ σύμμετρα τῷ μεγέθει τὰ σμηκτικὰ δαπανᾷ, ὡς χαλκὸς κεκαυμένος ἢ χάλκανθος ἅμα χορείᾳ χολῇ. ἄλλο δραστικώτερον. χαλκάνθου μέρος α'. κόμμεως Ἀραβικοῦ μέρος S''. οἴνῳ ἐκλείων κατάχριε. τινὲς δὲ χολὴν αἰγὸς μέλιτι μίξαντες ἐγχρίουσιν. ἄλλο. λύκιον καὶ κύπρον καὶ σὺν ὕδατι ποίει τὸ κολλύριον καὶ ἐπίχριε.

[στ'. Πρὸς τὰς ἐν ὀφθαλμοῖς οὐλὰς καὶ λευκώματα.] Τὰς ἐπιπολῆς μὲν γινομένας ἐν τοῖς ὀφθαλμοῖς τὰ νεφέλια καλοῦσι, τὰς δὲ διὰ βάθους, λευκώματα. τούτων δὲ τὰ ῥυπτικά τε καὶ σμηκτικὰ λεγόμενά εἰσιν ἰάματα. τὰ μὲν οὖν νεφέλια τῆς ἀνεμώνης ὁ χυλὸς ἀποσμήχει καὶ τοῦ μικροῦ κενταυρίου ὁ χυλὸς μετὰ μέλιτος. ἄλλο. ἀναγαλλίδος τῆς τὸ κυανοῦν ἄνθος ἐχούσης χυλὸν σὺν μέλιτι ἔγχριε· τὰ δὲ χρονιώτερα ἡ κεδρία λεπτύνει καὶ ὁ χαλκὸς μόνος ὕδατι λειούμενος ὡς κολλύριον. τὰ δὲ λευκώματα νίτρον μετὰ ἐλαίου παλαιοῦ λειωθὲν ἐπιμελῶς καὶ ἐγχρειόμενον καλῶς ἀποσμήχει. ἄλλο. ἐπιλαβὼν δρακουντίου χυλὸν καὶ μίξας μέλιτι ἀπέπτῳ ἐπίχριε. ἄλλο. χολῇ τραγείῳ κατάψηχε τὸν

ratae magnitudinis detergentia consumunt, ut aes combustum vel atramentum sutorium cum felle porcino. *Aliud bonum.* Recipe atramenti sutorii partem j, gummi arabici partem mediam, dilue vino et unge. Quidam autem hepar caprae melli miscentes inungunt. *Aliud.* Accipe lycium et ligustrum et cum aqua fac collyrium et illine.

[6. *De cicatricibus oculorum et albuginibus.*] Cicatrices, quae fiunt in oculis superficie tenus, nebulas nominant; qua vero profundum petunt, albugines. Harum autem medelae detergentia et expurgantia dicta sunt medicamenta. Nebulas ergo succus anemones expurgat et succus centaurii minoris cum melle. *Aliud.* Recipe anagallidis caeruleum florem habentis, succum cum melle admove. Diuturnas vero extenuat cedria et aes ustum solum dissolutum aqua in modum collyrii. Albugines autem expurgat nitrum dissolutum diligenter oleo et illitum. *Aliud.* Accipe succum dracunculi et misce cum melle crudo et unge. *Aliud.* Felle hirci confrica oculum. *Aliud.* Os

Ed. Chart. XIII. [609. 610.]
ὀφθαλμόν. ἄλλο. τῆς σηπίας τὸ ὄστρακον καυθὲν μετὰ μέλιτος καὶ λειωθὲν ἐπιτίθετι. ἄλλο. ἐκ κόπρου τῆς σαύρας ποιήσας κολλύριον σὺν ὕδατι προστίθετι. ἄλλο. χολῇ κυνὸς θαλασσίας κατάχριε, ἢ ῥαφάνου χυλῷ ἢ χολῇ τοῦ ἀλέκτορος. ἄλλο. λαβὼν χυλὸν τῆς ῥοίας καὶ ἐν τῷ κεραμίῳ τήσας καὶ τῷ ῥακέει κατακαλύψας ἡλίαζε ἕως ἔχῃ τὸ μέλιτος πάχος, καὶ τούτῳ ἴσον τοῦ μέλιτος καὶ τήρει. πεπαλαιωμένον γάρ ἐστι δραστικώτερον· καὶ ὅταν καθευ- [610] σόμενος ᾖ ὁ κάμνων, ὀφθαλμοὺς κατάχριε. ἄλλο. χολὴν λέοντος μετὰ μέλιτος ἐντίθετι. ἐὰν δὲ παιδίῳ σμικρῷ λεύκωμα γένηται, εἰς τὸν ὀφθαλμὸν ἡ μήτηρ τοῦ παιδίου ἀμμωνιακὸν μασησαμένη, ἐμφυσάτω εἰς τὸν τοῦ παιδίου ὀφθαλμόν· ὁμοίως χριέτω ὀφθαλμὸν καταμηνίῳ τῆς τινὸς ἐκ τῇ ἰδίᾳ συγγενείᾳ· καὶ ὁμοίως τούτου μήτηρ ἐντεμνέτω μικρὸν δάκτυλον ὄν, καὶ τῷ αἵματι ῥευθέντι τὸν ὀφθαλμὸν καταβρεχέτω.

[ζ'. *Πρὸς τὰ νεφέλια καὶ ἀχλύας τῶν ὀφθαλμῶν.*] Ὀφθαλμοὺς χυλῷ φύλλων τοῦ δρακοντίου κατάχριε. ἄλλο. χυλὸν τοῦ κέστρου σὺν μεμιγμένῳ οἴνῳ ἔνσταζε.

ſepiae combure et diſſolve cum melle et impone. *Aliud.* Ex ſtercore lacertae faciens collyrium cum aqua indito. *Aliud.* Felle canis marini unge, vel raphani ſucco, vel felle galli. *Aliud.* Sumito ſuccum malorum granatorum et pone in vaſe terreo et contege panno et expone ſoli, donec habeat mellis craſſitudinem, et ei miſce mellis tantundem et ſerva, quia inveteratum valet magis et quum it dormitum patiens, unge oculos. *Aliud.* Fel leonis cum melle indito. Si vero puer parvus habet albuginem, mater infantis mandat ammoniacum et inſufflet in oculum; ſimiliter ungat oculum menſtruo alicujus de cognatione ſua et ſimiliter mater ejus incidat parvum digitum ſuum et ſanguine qui effluxerit perſundat oculum.

[7. *Ad caliginem et nebulas oculorum.*] Illine oculos ſucco foliorum dracunculi. *Aliud.* Succum betonicae mixto vino calido inſtilla.

Ed. Chart. X. [610.]

[η'. Περὶ κριθῆς.] Τῷ ὕδατι ἀφεψήματος τῆς κριθῆς πυρία τοὺς ὀφθαλμοὺς, ἢ τῷ κήρῳ λευκῷ. ἄλλο. μυίας τὴν κεφαλὴν ἀπολαβὼν τῷ λοιπῷ σώματι παράτριβε τὴν κριθήν.

[θ'. Πρὸς μαδάρωσιν.] Μαδάρωσις καὶ μίλφωσις τοῦ βλεφάρου τριχῶν ἀπόπτωσις. θεραπεύονται δὲ τούτοις. προσλάμβανε πυρήνων τῶν φοινίκων κεκαυμένων < γ'. στάχυος < β'. τρίψας χρῶ. ἄλλο. στίμμεως κεκαυμένης πεπέρεως ἀνὰ < α'. ναρδοστάχυος < γ'.

[ι'. Ἄλλο ποιέον πρὸς ἀπόπτωσιν τριχῶν τῶν βλεφάρων.] Λεπτοκάρυα συγκαύσας καὶ μίξας στέατι ἀρκτείῳ ἢ αἰγὸς κατάχριε.

[ια'. Ἄλλο καὶ τὸ συμφέρον πρὸς ἀλωπεκίαν τοῦ πώγωνος.] Ὑοσκυάμου < β'. μυοκόου < α'. πολυτρίχου < β'. ἐλαίου ἰρίνου κυάθους δ'. τρίψας καὶ διαμίξας ἐλαίῳ καὶ προπυριάσας ἐπίχριε. ἄλλο. ὄφεος γῆρας συγκαύσας ἐπίπασσε· γένεσιν γὰρ τῶν τριχῶν ποιεῖ. ἢ μελανθίου τρίψας καὶ ποίει ὁμοίως.

[8. *De hordeolo.*] Aqua decoctionis hordei fove oculos, vel cera alba. *Aliud.* Accipe muſcas et abſcinde capita earum, poſtea reliquo corpore frica hordeolum.

[9. *De madaroſi.*] Madaroſis et milphoſis eſt caſus pilorum palpebrarum. Curantur autem his. Accipe nucleorum palmularum uſtorum drach. iij, ſpicae drach. ij, tere et utere. *Aliud.* Stibii aſſi, piperis ana drach. j, ſpicae drach. iij.

[10. *Aliud faciens ad caſum pilorum ſuperciliorum.*] Avellanas combure et permiſce cum adipe urſi aut caprae et unge.

[11. *Aliud quod etiam confert ad alopeciam barbae.*] Alterci drach. ij, muſcerdae drach. j, polytrichi drach. ij, olei irini cyathos quatuor tere et permiſce oleo et praefovens ungito. *Aliud.* Vernationem anguis combure et inſperge; facit enim nasci pilos. *Vel* nigellam tere et fac ſimiliter.

Ed. Chart. X. [610.]

[ιβ'. Πρὸς τὴν τῶν ὀφρύων τριχίασιν.] Ὀρίγανον συγκαύσας καὶ τρίψας προεκτίλας τρίχας ἐπιτίθετι. ἄλλο. σαῦραν χλωρὰν ἐν ἐλαίῳ ἑψήσας καὶ τρίχας προεκτίλας τόπον κατάχριε. ἄλλο. χαμαιλέοντος λευκοῦ ἢ τῆς χαμελαίας ῥίζαν διαμίξας τῷ αἵματι τοῦ βατραχίου τόπον κατάχριε.

[ιγ'. Πρὸς γλαυκοφθάλμους ὥστε μέλανας ἔχειν τὰς κόρας.] Τὰς γλαυκοφθάλμους γυναῖκας ποιεῖ ὑοσκυάμου τὸ κυανοῦν ἄνθος ξηραινόμενον ἐν σκιᾷ, ἐπὶ δὲ τῆς χρήσεως οἴνῳ αὐστηρῷ μεμιγμένον καὶ καταχρισθέν.

[ιδ'. Πρὸς ὑποχύματα.] Θηριακὴν τὴν ἐξ ἐχέων παρασκευαζομένην τῷ μέλιτι διαμίξας ἄνευ καπνοῦ ἐπιτίθετι. συμφέρουσι καὶ οἱ ἀποφλεγματισμοὶ καὶ κάθαρσις σὺν ἱερᾷ καὶ πυρία σὺν ἀφεψήματι τοῦ μαράθρου καὶ σαγαπηνοῦ καὶ ἐλλέβορος λευκὸς σὺν μέλιτι παρατεθειμένος, ἢ τὸ μέλι σὺν χυλῷ τοῦ μαράθρου.

[ιε'. Πρὸς τοὺς αἰγίλωπας.] Ὁ μὲν αἰγίλωψ ἀπόστημά ἐστι σμικρὸν μεταξὺ τοῦ μεγάλου κανθοῦ καὶ τῆς ῥινὸς, καὶ εἰ ἀμεληθείη συριγγούμενον ἕως ὀστέου, πρινὴ δὲ

[12. *Ad ſupercilia piloſa.*] Origanum combure, tere et applica; prius tamen evelle pilos. *Aliud.* Lacertam viridem coque in oleo et poſtquam evulſeris pilos, unge locum. *Aliud.* Chamaeleontis ſeu chamelaeae radicem permiſce cum ſanguine ranae et unge locum.

[13. *Ad habentes oculos glaucos, ut nigros habeant pupillas.*] Glaucos mulierum oculos nigros reddit hyoscyami flos caeruleus ſiccatus in umbra et tempore uſus permixtus vino auſtero et illitus.

[14. *Ad ſuffuſiones.*] Theriacam, quae fit ex viperis, permiſce melle ſine fumo et impone. Conſerunt etiam caput purgantia et purgatio cum hiera et fomentum cum decocto foeniculi et ſagapenum et helleborus albus cum melle appoſitus, vel mel cum ſucco foeniculi.

[15. *Ad aegilopes.*] Aegilops eſt abſceſſus parvus inter magnum oculi angulum et nares; qui ſi negligatur, ſiſtulatur usque ad os et dicitur anchilops, antequam ſiſtu-

Ed. Chart. X. [610. 611.]
εἰς ἕλκος ἐκραγῇ τὸ ἀπόστημα, ἀνχίλωψ καλῶ. ποιεῖ καὶ γλαύκιον καὶ κρόκος ἅμα χυλῷ περδικιάδος ἐπιτιθέμενα· συνεχῶς δὲ ἀλλάσσειν χρή. ἄλλο. κοχλίους μετὰ τῶν ὀστράκων λειώσας ἐπίθες· ἔνιοι δὲ μιγνῦσι καὶ ἀλόην ἢ σμύρνην. ἄλλο. χολὴν χοιρίαν ξηράνας ἐπίθες. ἄλλο. ἐκ περδικιάδος τὸ κατάπλασμα ποίει. ἄλλο. ἐξ αἰγίλωπος βοτανίου κατάπλασμα ἐπίθες. ἄλλο. ἀνδράχνην ἀγρίαν καὶ λίβανον ἐπίθες. ταῦτα δὲ προμασσάου προμασσήσῃ νῆστις. ἄλλο. κράνιον ἀνθρώπινον τρίψας ἐπιτίθετι.

[611] [ιϛ'. Πρὸς νυκτάλωπας.] Ἧπαρ τράγου καῦσον καὶ τῷ ἀποῤῥέοντι ἰχῶρι ὀφθαλμὸν ἔγχριε. ὠφελεῖ γὰρ ὁ δωδεκάκις καταχρισθείς.

[ιζ'. Πρὸς τοὺς ἐν βλεφάροις φθεῖρας.] Θαλάσσῃ τῷ ὕδατι χλιαρῷ πυρία.

Κεφ. ε'. [Πρὸς τὰ μυκτήρων πάθη εὐπόριστα.] [α'. Πρὸς πολύποδας καὶ ὀζαίνας.] Χάλκανθον τρίψας σὺν ὄξει ἐπίθες· ἢ χάλκανθον ἀναλαμβανομένην μέλιτι ἑφθῷ ἐπίθες. ἄλλο. σιδίων < ιστ'. χολῆς ταύρου, ἀμώμου,

latur. Huic confert glaucium et crocum ſimul cum ſucco perdicii appoſitum; oportet autem frequenter ea permutare. *Aliud.* Conchulas cum teſtis ſuis tere et appone. Aliqui vero miſcent et aloen vel myrrham. *Aliud.* Fel porcinum ſicca et appone. *Aliud.* Ex perdicio cataplasma facito. *Aliud.* Ex aegilope herba cataplasma impone. *Aliud.* Portulacam ſilveſtrem et thus maſculum appone; prius tamen ea manducabis jejunus. *Aliud.* Calvariam hominis tere et appone.

[16. *Ad nyctilopas.*] Hepar hirci aſſa et unge liquore, qui defluit oculum: juvat enim duodecies illitus.

[17. *Ad pediculos palpebrarum.*] Aqua marina tepida fove.

Cap. V. [*Ad affectus narium parabilia.*] [1. *Ad polypos et ozaenas.*] Vitriolum terens ex aceto illine, aut vitriolum melle cocto exceptum illine. *Aliud.* Recipe corticum granatorum drach. xvj, fellis tauri, amomi,

Ed. Chart. X. [611.]

σμύρνης, καλαμίνθης, πρασίου, ἀνὰ < η'. κρόκου < β'. ἐλλεβόρου λευκοῦ < β'. χρῶ ξηρῷ.

[β'. Πρὸς δυσωδίαν μυκτήρων.] Ἀμώμου, σμύρνης, κασίας, ῥόδων ξηρῶν ἑκάστου τὸ ἴσον μέρος κόψας καὶ μετὰ νάρδου μύρου ἀνέσας κατάχριε· συμφέρει δὲ καὶ κατάχρισις σὺν ἡδυχρόῳ μαλάγματι.

[γ'. Πρὸς τὰ ἐν μυκτῆρσιν ἕλκη.] Λιθαργύρου < δ'. πηγάνου νεαροῦ < δ'. στυπτηρίας σχιστῆς < β'. ἐλαίῳ μυρσυνίνῳ καὶ ὄξει διάκλυζε. ἄλλο. ψιμυθίου < α'. λιθαργύρου < γ'. σκωρίας μολίβδου ἢ μολίβδου κεκαυμένου < γ'. πάντα δὲ πεπλυμένα καὶ ἀναλαμβανέσθω ἐλαίῳ μυρσυνίνῳ.

[δ'. Πρὸς τὸ ἐφέλκειν αἷμα ἀπὸ μυκτήρων.] Ἀγρώστεως ἄνθος ἐντίθετι. ἄλλο. ἐρυθρόδανον τρίψας σὺν ἐλαίῳ ἀναλαβὼν τὰς μυκτῆρας κατάχριε.

[ε'. Πρὸς τὰς ἐκ ῥινῶν αἱμοῤῥαγίας.] Κέλυφος ὠοῦ συγκαύσας καὶ λαβὼν μέρος α'. καὶ κηκίδος μέρος ἥμισυ καὶ ἐμφύσα. ἄλλο. λύκιον ἐπίθες. ἄλλο. ὀνείαν κόπρον καύσας ἐμφύσα τὴν σποδόν· ἢ χυλὸν ἐκπιέσας ἔνσταζε.

myrrhae, calaminthae, marrubii, ana drach. viij, croci drach. ij, ellebori albi drach. ij, utere ſicco.

[2. *Ad foetorem narium.*] Recipe amomi, myrrhae, caſiae, roſarum ſiccarum pares portiones cum oleo nardino et unge; conſert autem et unctio cum hedychroe magmate.

[3. *Ad ulcera narium.*] Recipe lithargyri drach. iv, rutae recentis, aluminis ſciſſi drach. ij, dilue oleo myrtino et aceto. *Aliud.* Recipe ceruſſae drach. j, lithargyri drach. iij, ſcoriae plumbi vel plumbi combuſti drach. iij, omnia laventur et excipiantur oleo myrtino.

[4. *Ad extrahendum ſanguinem e naribus.*] Florem graminis impone. *Aliud.* Rubiam cum oleo accipe et unge nares.

[5. *Ad fluxum ſanguinis e naribus.*] Corticem ovi combure et accipe partem unam et gallae partem mediam et inſuſſla. *Aliud.* Lycium impone. *Aliud.* Aſini ſtercus comburens inſuſſla cinerem ejus; aut exprimens inſtilla

Ed. Chart. X. [611.]
ἄλλο. λίθον μυλίτην πυρώσας σβέννυε ἐν ὄξει δριμυτάτῳ καὶ πρόσαγε ταῖς ῥισὶ τὴν ἀτμίδα, καὶ στήσεται. ἄλλο. λίβανον καὶ τὴν ἀλόην ὠοῦ τῷ λευκῷ ἀναλαβὼν καὶ ποίει τὸν μοτὸν καὶ ἐπιτίθετι, προστίσας τὰς τοῦ λαγόου τρίχας. ἄλλο. σικύαν εὐμεγέθη πρόσβαλλε τῷ ὑποχονδρίῳ κατ' ἴξιν τῆς ῥινὸς πασχούσης· χρηστέον δὲ τοῖς στύφουσί τε καὶ τοῖς τὴν αἱμοῤῥαγίας ὁρμὴν κωλύουσι.

[στ'. Πρὸς μυκτῆρας ἡλκωμένους καὶ πολύποδας καὶ ὀζαίνας.] Ἀφρονίτρῳ παράπτου διαστέλλων τοὺς μυκτῆρας· καὶ πρὸς εὐωδίαν λευκοίου ἄνθους μήπω ἐκπεπτωκότος τοῦ βλαστοῦ ἐπιμύων, τρίβων τε μεθ' ὕδατος, πάχος ποιῶν μέλιτος ἀφάπτου τῶν ἡλκωμένων. ἄλλο. ἰὸν ἑφθὸν μετὰ μέλιτος παράπτου.

[ζ'. Πρὸς τὰς ἐνδοτέρω φλεγμονάς.] Στέαρ χήνειον χυλῷ πράσου καὶ στρύχνου διεὶς ἴσον διάχριε τῆς ἡμέρας.

[η'. Πρὸς τὰ ἐν μυκτῆρσι ἕλκη σκληρώδη.] Μόλιβδον λεάνας ἐπίχεε οἶνον ἀπαράχυτον καὶ μυρσινελαίου τὸ

ſuccum. *Aliud.* Lapidem molarem candentem extingue in aceto et olfaciendum naribus admove vaporem, et ſiſtetur. *Aliud.* Thus masculum et aloen albo ovi excipe et fac linamentum et impone addens pilos leporis. *Aliud.* Cucurbitulam magnam affigito hypochondrio e regione naris patientis. Oportet autem et iis quae adſtringunt et prohibere poſſunt impetum ſanguinis uti.

[6. *Ad nares ulceratas et polypos et ozaenas.*] Spuma nitri attinge nares apertas. Et ad probum ſpiritus odorem conciliandum albae violae florem nondum ex coliculo delapſum lege tereque ex aqua, donec mellis craſſitudo fiat; tange ulceratas nares. *Aliud.* Aerugine ex melle decocta locum attinge.

[7. *Ad interiores phlegmonas.*] Adipe anſerino cum porri ſolanique ſucco aequis portionibus diluto interdiu obline.

[8. *Ad narium ulcera cum duritie.*] Plumbum tritum vino puro macera myrteique olei quod ſatis

Ed. Chart. X. [611. 612.]
ἀρκοῦν, ἵνα ἔχῃ μέλιτος πάχος. ἄλλο. λεπίδα ἑψήσας μετὰ μέλιτος χρῶ.

[θ'. Αἷμα ἀπὸ μυκτήρων ἀποσπᾶσαι.] Ἡδύοσμον ἀναλαβὼν μέλιτι καὶ κολλύρια ποιήσας θὲς εἰς τοὺς μυκτῆρας.

[612] [ι'. Πρὸς τοὺς ἀπὸ μυκτήρων αἱμοῤῥαγοῦντας.] Πήγανον τρίψας ἀναλάμβανε ἐλαίῳ καὶ εἰς τοὺς μυκτῆρας ἐπιτίθει. ἄλλο. κόμμι καὶ λιβανωτὸν λεάνας καὶ δεύσας ἐν ὄξει τίθει. ἄλλο. σποδὸν κυπρίαν μετὰ πράσου χυλοῦ δεύσας χρῶ. ἄλλο. σπόγγον κεκαυμένον μετὰ πίσσης ξηρᾷ χρῶ. ἄλλο. ὀξυσχοίνου ἄνθος ἐντίθει τοῖς μυκτῆρσιν.

[ια'. Πρὸς τὰς ἀκαταχέτους αἱμοῤῥαγίας καὶ μάλιστα ὅταν χρονίως πυρέξαντες αἱμοῤῥαγῶσιν.] Πυρίον ἐντίθει ὁτὲ μὲν ξηρὸν, ὁτὲ δὲ κολλύριον ποιῶν ἰσομέγεθος τοῖς μυκτῆρσι καὶ οὕτως ἐπιτίθει· κατάπλασσε τούτοις καὶ τοὺς μυκτῆρας καὶ τὰς παρειὰς καὶ τὸ μέτωπον. ἄλλο. διφρυγὲς καύσας καὶ λειοτριβήσας μετὰ ὄξους κατάπλασσε. ἄλλο. ἔριον βρέξας εἰς τὸ λευκὸν τοῦ ὠοῦ ἐντίθει. ἄλλο. πολυ-

eſt adde ad mellis ſpiſſitudinem. *Aliud.* Aeris ſquama ex melle decocta utere.

[9. *Sanguinem per nares evocantia.*] Mentam excipiens melle et collyrium faciens in nares mitte.

[10. *Ad profluvium ſanguinis e naribus.*] Rutam tritam oleo excipito et intra nares conjicito. *Aliud.* Gummi ac thus contrita et aceto liquata in nares da. *Aliud.* Cinerula Cypria cum ſucco porri temperata utere. *Aliud.* Spongiam uſtam pici admixtam et areſactam linamento inſperſam in nares pellito. *Aliud.* Acuti junci florem naribus imponito.

[11. *Ad ſanguinis eruptiones, quae ſupprimi nequeunt, praeſertim cum diutius febricitantibus ſanguis effunditur.*] Pyrion imponito nonnunquam aridum, nonnunquam linamentum illitum et craſſitudinem cavis naſi reſpondentem faciens ita immittito, iisdem et nares et tempora et frontem illinito. *Aliud.* Diphryges uſtum et ex aceto tritum ſuperimpone. *Aliud.* Lanam ovi albo

Ed. Chart. X. [612.]

γόνου χυλῷ βρέχων ἔριον ἐπιτίθει· ἢ στρύχνου χυλῷ. ἄλλο. πήγανον τρίψας λεῖον μετ᾽ ὄξους κατάπλασσε καὶ ἐπιθυμία· δεῖ δὲ χρῆσθαι τοῖς δυναμένοις ἐπιστύφειν καὶ ἐπουλεῖν τὴν φορὰν τοῦ αἵματος, τοιούτοις οὖσιν, οἷον κώνιον ὑποθυμία τοῖς μυκτῆρσι καὶ τὴν ἀποφορὰν ἕλκε· προσπιέζειν δὲ καὶ τοῖς δακτύλοις τοὺς μυκτῆρας. μύε δὲ τὰς ἀκοὰς κηρωτῇ ἢ ἄλλῳ τινὶ ἐπιμελῶς. ἢ καὶ τὴν ἀκροποσθίαν ἐπιδεσμεῖν παπυρίῳ, ἐπὶ δὲ γυναικῶν θηλὴν τοῦ μαζοῦ ὁμοίως. χρῆσθαι δὲ καὶ τοῖς ψύχειν δυναμένοις κατὰ τοῦ μετώπου καὶ τῆς κεφαλῆς. εὔθετον δὲ σικύαν τῇ κεφαλῇ προσάγειν ἢ καὶ τὴν ἐν μετώπῳ φλέβα λύειν. ποιοῦσι δὲ καὶ οἱ πταρμοὶ πολλάκις στῆναι· ἢ βούγλωσσον τὴν βοτάνην ὁμοίως ἢ ὀνίδα δεύσας ἐν ὄξει προστίθει τοῖς μυκτῆρσιν.

[ιβ'. Πρὸς τοὺς ῥέγχοντας.] Ἄνηθον ὑποτίθει ὑπὸ τὴν κεφαλὴν μὴ γινώσκοντος, ποιεῖ δὲ τοῦτο καὶ πρὸς τοὺς ἐκ σκιμπόδων ἐξαλλομένους.

[ιγ'. Πρὸς στίγμα καὶ αἶραν χωρὶς οὐλῆς καὶ ἕλκους.]

madentem admove. *Aliud.* Lanam ſanguinalis aut ſolani ſucco imbutam in nares dato. *Aliud.* Rutam ex aceto tritam impone et ſuffito. Utendum praeterea eſt reprimere cohibereque ſanguinis impetum valentibus, ut cicutam naribus ſuffito, odoremque aeger attrahito; nares etiam digitis comprimito; aut cerato, aut alio quopiam diligenter occludito; quin etiam penis extremum papyro deligato. in mulieribus vero mammarum papillas ſimiliter. Item refrigerare potentibus frontem caputque oblinito et conſpergito. Praeſentiſſimum remedium eſt capiti cucurbitulam affigere; vel etiam frontis venam ſolvere. Sternutamenta quoque plerunque ſanguinem revocant. Aut herbam bugloſſon aut aſini ſimum ex aceto in nares conjice.

[12. *Ad ſtertentes.*] Anethum capiti clam ſubjicito; id et proſilientibus ex lectulo remedio eſt.

[13. *Ad puncta et aeram vocatam absque cicatrice*

Ed. Chart. X. [612.]

Ἀποσμήξας τὸν τόπον νίτρῳ ῥητίνη τερεβινθίνη κατάπλασσε καὶ ἔασον ἡμέρας ε΄. καὶ οὕτως λύσας κατακέντησον τὰ στίγματα γραφείῳ, ἔπειτα λιβάνῳ χρῶ μετὰ νίτρου καὶ μετὰ μέλιτος ἴσον ἑκάστου κατάπλασσε, ὡς πάχος κηρωτῆς ὑγρᾶς, λῦε δὲ καὶ κατάντλει. ἄλλο. ἐλλέβορον λεῖον μετ᾽ ἄρτου κατάπλασσε ἢ ὀξύγαλα καθ᾽ ἑαυτὸ κατάπλασσε. ἄλλο. συκῆς φλοιὸν λεῖον κατάπλασσε. ἄλλο. σταφίδα ἀγρίαν κατάπλασσε.

Κεφ. στ΄. [α΄. Πρὸς ἀλφοὺς καὶ ἔφηλιν καὶ φακοὺς καὶ τὰ τοιαῦτα προσώπου πάθη.] Σικύου ἀγρίου ῥίζης χυλοῦ κεκομμένου καὶ σεσησμένου σμῆχε τὸ πρόσωπον. ἄλλο. ἀλκυόνιον μετὰ οἴνου τρίψας κατάπλασσε. ἄλλο. ἀγρίαν ἄμπελον κόψας μετὰ οἴνου Αἰγυπτίου κατάχριε λειοτριβήσας. ἄλλο. εὐζώμου ἀγρίου ῥίζαν τρίψας καὶ ἀναλαβὼν χολῇ προβατείᾳ κατάχριε τὸ πρόσωπον νίτρῳ. ἄλλο. ἐλατήριον λειοτριβήσας μετὰ ὄξους καὶ ποιήσας μέλιτος πάχος, κατάχριε, μετὰ κηρωτῆς μίξας. ἄλλο. κιννάβαρι μετὰ μέλιτος χρῖε τὸ πρόσωπον. ἄλλο. κάγχρυος σπέρμα λειώσας

et ulcere.] Nitro locum detergens refinam terebinthinam fuperdato et per dies quinque dimittito; mox locum folvens puncta fcriptorio fpecillo perforato: deinde thus nitrum ac mel pari modo mixta, ut cerati craffitudo fit, imponito; poft folve et ablue. *Aliud.* Ex trito veratro cum pane aut ex acido lacte per fe cataplasma facito. *Aliud.* Fici trito cortice illine. *Aliud.* Uvam taminiam in cataplasmatis modum imponito.

Cap. VI. [1. *Ad vitiligines, ephelidas, lenticulas et alias id genus faciei affectiones.*] Cucumeris filvatici radicis tritae et cribratae fucco faciem deterge. *Aliud.* Alcyonio ex vino trito faciem obline. *Aliud.* Vitem filveftrem contufam et vino Aegyptio maceratam et in farinam redactam fuperdato. *Aliud.* Erucae agreftis radice trita et ovis felle excepta utitor, facie prius nitro perfricata. *Aliud.* Elaterium ex aceto terens et ad mellis craffitudinem redigens ceratoque admifcens inunge. *Aliud.* Cinnabari ex melle faciem illine. *Aliud.* Canchrys femine

Ed. Chart. X. [612. 613.]
αὐτοὺς τοὺς φακοὺς κατάχριε καὶ ὅταν ξηρανθῇ, ἔκκλυζε. ἄλλο. σικύου ἀγρίου τὴν ῥίζαν καὶ συκῆς τοὺς ἀκρέμονας ἕψει ἐν ὄξει καὶ λείοις κατάπλασσε. ἄλλο. κοτυληδόνος ῥίζας λειώσας μετὰ [613] μέλιτος κατάχριε τὸ πρόσωπον. ἄλλο. ἐρυθρόδανον ποιεῖ πρὸς ἔφηλιν καὶ ἀλφοὺς ἤγουν κόψας μετὰ ἐλαίου κατάχριε. ἄλλο. ζόγχον πικρὸν λειώσας μετὰ μέλιτος κατάχριε. ἄλλο. ἀνήθου σπέρμα τρίψας μετὰ οἴνου παλαιοῦ καὶ ποιῶν μέλιτος πάχος ἐπίχριε τὸ πρόσωπον καὶ ἐννυκτέρευε· πρωῒ δι' ἑτέρων μεμασημένου δὲ αὐτοῦ πρὸς ἔφηλιν καὶ φακούς. ἄλλο. τῷ λευκῷ ἴῳ μετὰ ὕδατος κατάχριε. ἄλλο. ἀφρόνιτρον λειώσας μετὰ κηρωτῆς ἐσκευασμένης διὰ κηροῦ Τυῤῥηνικοῦ κατάχριε τὸ πρόσωπον.

[β'. *Πρὸς ἀλφοὺς καὶ χρῶμα λευκόν.*] Ἀλκυόνιον καύσας μῖξον μέλιτι καὶ κατάχριε καὶ ἀλεύρῳ μίξας ὀροβίνῳ καὶ σιτίνῳ σμηχέσθω θερμῷ ὡς τὰ μάλιστα. ἄλλο. ἀμύγδαλα πικρὰ λελεπισμένα ὄξει δριμεῖ ἀναλαβὼν κατά-

trito ipſas lenticulas inunge et arefactum ablue. *Aliud.* Silvatici cucumeris radicem ficique ſummos ramulos in aceto decoctos tritosque imponito. *Aliud.* Veneris umbilici radicibus ex melle contritis faciem illine. *Aliud.* Rubia ad maculas a ſole contractas et vitiligines beneſacit, ſi ea trita ex oleo facies inungatur. *Aliud.* Zonchum amarum terens ex melle faciei imponito. *Aliud.* Anethi ſemen ex vino vetere tritum et ad mellis ſpiſſitudinem redactum faciei obducito, atque ita per integram noctem remaneto; ſequenti mane illud removeto recensque aliud reponito. Eodem quoque ſemme commanducato ephelidas et lenticulas utiliter illinito. *Aliud.* Alba viola ex aqua ad eadem proficit. *Aliud.* Aphronitrum tritum cum cerato ex Tyrrhenica cera confecto faciei ſuperdato.

[2. *Ad vitiligines et album colorem.*] Alcyonium uſtum mellique admixtum illitum prodeſt; eodem quoque cum ervi farina et tritici mixto quam maxime calido faciem detergito. *Aliud.* Amara amygdala cortice ſpoliata aceto acri excipito et cataplasma facito. *Aliud.* Ocimi

πλασσε. ἄλλο. ὠκίμου σπέρμα τρίψας μετ' ὀρνιθείου στέατος ἢ χηνείου κατάχριε. ἄλλο. τῆλιν μετ' ὄξους λείαν κατάχριε, ἀφίστησι λεπίδας.

[γ'. Πρὸς ἔφηλιν καὶ φακούς.] Σμύρναν καὶ κρόκον μεθ' ὕδατος λεάνας κατάχριε. ἄλλο. πορφύρας ἢ κήρυκας λαβὼν εἰς πολταρίδιον δὸς εἰς κάμινον ὀπτηθῆναι καὶ λειάνας μετὰ μέλιτος χρῶ.

[δ'. Ποιοῦν λευκὸν καὶ τεταμένον τὸ πρόσωπον.] Σικύου ἀγρίου τὰς ῥίζας τεμὼν ψῦξον καὶ ἑψήσας δι' ὕδατος τρῖψον λεῖον κατάπλασσε.

[ε'. Στίλβον ποιοῦν τὸ πρόσωπον.] Ὀρόβους οἴνῳ εὐώδει λειώσας κατάπλασσε. ἄλλο. σεμιδάλεως χυλὸν καταστήσας ἀπόχεε τὸ ὑγρὸν καὶ τῇ ὑποστάθμῃ πρόσμιξον ὠοῦ τὸ λευκὸν, ποιῶν μέλιτος πάχος, καὶ τούτῳ χρίων τὸ πρόσωπον ἐλαίῳ διάτριβε. ἀπὸ δὲ τοῦ ἡλίου γενόμενος ψυχρῷ πρόσκλυζε πολλῷ, ὥστε εὔχρουν ποιεῖν εἰς μίαν ἡμέραν. φῦκος ἑψήσας ἔμβαλλε στυπτηρίαν ὀλίγην, εἶτα κονίαν προσμίξας, τρίψας χρῶ, πολλῷ χριόμενος ἐλαίῳ, ὥστε εὔχρουν τὸ πρόσωπον καὶ τὸ χρῶμα ποιῆ-

semen cum gallinaceo aut anserino adipe tritum benefacit. *Aliud.* Foenum graecum ex aceto tritum squamulas, si illinatur, detrahit.

[3. *Ad ephelidas et lentigines.*] Myrrha et crocum si aqua macerentur, illita juvant. *Aliud.* Purpuras aut buccina expiscatus in ollulam conjice et in furnum assandas mitte, deinde ex melle tritis utere.

[4. *Ad faciem albam et extenta cute reddendam.*] Cucumeris silvestris radices in frusta divide et refrigera; deinde aqua elixatis ac tritis in cataplasma utere.

[5. *Aliud faciem splendidam reddens.*] Ex ervo bene olente vino macerato ac trito cataplasma facito. *Aliud.* Siliginis succum exprimens humidiorem partem abjice; parti illi autem, quae subsedit, ovi album commisceto ad mellis spissitudinem; atque hoc faciem perunctam oleo deterge. A sole autem maculatam faciem frigida multa lavato et per unum diem facies coloratior redditur. Fucum elixans parum aluminis injice; deinde lixivium ad-

σαι ἡδὺ ὄζον. πελεκήματι κυπαρίσσου καὶ πρίνου ἐν τῷ αὐτῷ ζέσας ἄλειφε ὅλον τὸ σῶμα. ἄλλο. λιβανωτὸν καὶ παιδέρωτα ἴσα μίξας μετὰ μέλιτος τρίψας χρῖε τὸ πρόσωπον καὶ ἔα δι' ὅλης ἡμέρας, εἶτα ἀπόκλυζε. ἄλλο. λίνου μίξας τρύγα σύγχριε εἰς τὸν ἥλιον, μέλλων πορεύεσθαι προεκνιτρώσας τὸ σῶμα.

[στ'. *Πρὸς τὸ μὴ ὑπὸ ἡλίου ὑποκαίεσθαι, ἀλλὰ καὶ τὴν ἐκκαυθεῖσαν ὄψιν ἰάσασθαι.*] Βολβὸν λευκὸν λεῖον μετὰ μέλιτος κατάχριε. ἐὰν οἰδῇ τὸ πρόσωπον χωρὶς φλεγμονῆς, γῆν μέλαιναν τρίψας δι' ὕδατος κατάχριε. ἄλλο. ἀλκυόνιον μετὰ νάρδου Κελτικῆς λείοις ἅμα.

[ζ'. *Πρὸς φύγεθλον καὶ φακούς.*] Δρακοντίου ῥίζαν σὺν μέλιτι κατάπλασσε. ἢ μελάνθιον σὺν ὄξει· ἢ πενταφύλλου σπέρμα.

[η'. *Πρὸς ποιεῖν τὸ πρόσωπον ἐρυθραῖον.*] Ἐρυθρόδανον τρίψας καὶ διαμίξας ἐλαίῳ κατάχριε. ἄλλο. βολβὸν πικρὸν τρίψας καὶ μίξας ἐλαίῳ κατάχριε. ἄλλο. λαβὼν

miſcens ac terens utere multo inungens oleo: ſic enim facies grati coloris bonique odoris os ſpirans efficitur. Cupreſſi atque ilicis ramenta una fervefaciens decocto corpus totum madefacito. *Aliud.* Thuris et paederotis aequas portiones misce et ex melle tere; ita faciem inunge, atque integrum diem ſic dimitte, deinde ablue. *Aliud.* Lini faecem melli admiscens ſub ſole iter facturus corpus inungito, eo tamen prius nitro perſricto.

[6. *Ad impediendum ſolis exuſtionem et exuſtam faciem ſanandam.*] Bulbo candido trito ex melle inungito. Quod ſi facies citra phlegmonem tumefacta fuerit, nigram terram ex aqua conterens ſuperdato. *Aliud.* Alcyonio et nardo Celtica ſimul tritis utere.

[7. *Ad panum et lentigines.*] Dracunculi radicem cum melle in cataplaſma redige: vel nigellam cum aceto, vel pentaphylli ſemen.

[8. *Ad faciendam faciem rubicundam.*] Rubiam tere et permiſce cum oleo et unge. *Aliud.* Bulbum amarum terens permiſce cum melle et unge. *Aliud.* Accipe cice-

κρόκου, ἐρεβίνθου, λιβάνου, σμύρνης, ἐρυθροδάνου ῥίζης ἀνὰ < β'. ἀναλάμβανε στέατι μοσχίῳ καὶ μαστιχίνῳ ἐλαίῳ, εἶτα ἐπίχριε· καὶ διαστήσας περίματτε σπόγγῳ θερμῷ.

[614] Κεφ. ζ'. [Πρὸς τὰ κατὰ στόμα πάθη καὶ πρῶτον πρὸς τὰ χείλη κατεῤῥωγότα.] Κηκίδα ὀμφακίνην λείαν ἀναλάμβανε καὶ ῥητίνην τερεβινθίνην σὺν ὑσσώπῳ καὶ μέλιτι καὶ ἐπίχριε.

[β'. Πρὸς τὰς βαθυτέρας ἐπιῤῥήξεις.] Ἐνάλειφε αἰγείῳ τεθεραπευμένῳ λίπει. ἄλλο. στέαρ χήνειον, μετὰ μέλιτος τερεβινθίνης ἴσα, ῥόδων ἄνθους, ὑσσώπου ξηροῦ, μαστίχης γένηται ἔγχρισις.

[γ'. Πρὸς . εὐωδεῖν τὸ στόμα.] Ἶριν ἀποβρέξας οἴνῳ παλαιῷ εὐώδει διακλύζου συνεχῶς, κατέχων ὀλίγον ἐν τῷ στόματι χρόνον. ἄλλο. ἕρπυλλον ἀποβρέχων οἴνῳ διακλύζου ἐπ' ὀλίγον.

[δ'. Πρὸς δυσφόρους ὀσμὰς χωρὶς ἑλκῶν γινομένας.] Τινὲς ἀκράτῳ διακλύζονται μετὰ σμύρνης· καὶ τοῦ σχοίνου δὲ ἄνθος λεάναντες παρατρίβουσι τὰ αὐτὰ καὶ κιμωλίαν

ris, rubiae, thuris, myrrhae ana drach. ij, excipe adipe vituli et oleo maſtichino et unge: et poſt ſpatium abſterge ſpongia calida.

Cap. VII. [*Ad oris vitia et primo ad labiorum rimas.*] Immaturam gallam tritam accipito et reſinam terebinthinam cum hyſſopo et melle atque his perunge.

[2. *Ad altiores ſciſſuras.*] Caprino adipe mundato illine. *Aliud.* Adeps anſeris et mel et terebinthina aequis portionibus, addito flore roſarum, hyſſopo arido et maſtiche fiat inunctio.

[3. *Ad ſuavitatem odoris ori conciliandam.*] Vino vetere bene olente, in quo iris maduerit, os collue adſidueque in ore brevi tempore contine. *Aliud.* Vino paulisper os ſublue, in quo ſerpillum maduerit.

[4. *Ad oris tetros absque ulcere odores.*] Nonnulli meraco vino, cui myrrha admixta ſit, os eluunt, atque odoratum juncum terentes partes oris internas perſricant

Ed. Chart. X. [614.]

ποιήσαντες μεθ᾽ ἁλὸς παρατρίβουσιν, ὁμοίως καὶ μαρμάρῳ ὀπτῷ μετ᾽ ἀνίσου. ὁμοίως δὲ καὶ κριθὰς μετὰ ἁλὸς καὶ μέλιτος. τινὲς δὲ καὶ ὀθόνιον καίουσι καὶ οἴνῳ ἐμβάλλουσι καὶ οὕτω λείῳ χρῶνται καὶ κισσήρει καὶ νάρδῳ καὶ σμύρνῃ μετὰ μέλιτος. καὶ σεμίδαλιν καὶ ἶριν μέλιτι μίξαντες καίουσι καὶ τούτῳ χρῶνται. καὶ τῶν ὀστρέων τῇ πορφύρᾳ καὶ κήρυκι καὶ σμύρνῃ καὶ ὅταν πρὸς κοίτην ἀπέρχωνται, ὄξει δριμεῖ διακλύζονται. διαμασῶνται δέ τινες καὶ τὰ τῆς πίτυος φύλλα, ὅταν ἐκπορεύωνται, καὶ ὕδατι διακλύζονται. τινὲς δὲ καὶ ἄνισον διαμασῶνται ἢ γλυκύῤῥιζον ἢ ἶριν ἤ τι τοιοῦτον ἐκπορευόμενοι.

[έ. *Πρὸς τὰ ἐν τῷ στόματι ἕλκη καὶ σηπεδόνας.*] Μελαντηρία κεκομμένη ὠφελεῖ. ποιεῖ δὲ πρὸς ταῦτα καὶ τὸ ὀμφάκινον κατ᾽ ἰδίαν καὶ μετὰ μέλιτος πινόμενον. ποιεῖ δὲ καὶ ἡ γλαύκουρις. θλασθεῖσα μετὰ μέλιτος καὶ ὕδατος ἴσου διδομένου τοῦ χυλοῦ ἀναγαργαριζέσθω.

[στ΄. *Πρὸς αἱμοῤῥαγίαν ἐκ τοῦ στόματος.*] Συγκλύζηται τὸ στόμα ἀφεψήματι τῶν ῥόδων ἐν ὀξυκράτῳ, ὅταν

et cimoliam cum ſale tritam affricant; perinde et marmore uſto cum aniſo utuntur: ita et hordeo cum ſale et melle. Quidam et linteolum cremant et vino injiciunt, atque ita trito utuntur et pumice et nardo et myrrha ex melle. Siliginem quidam et irin cum melle miſcentes comburunt atque ita utuntur, et ex oſtreis purpura et buccino cum myrrha quum cubitum eunt aceto acerrimo colluunt. Commanducant autem nonnulli domum egreſſuri piceae folia et aqua os ſubluunt. Quidam praeterea et aniſum aut dulcem radicem aut irin idque genus alia aliqui iter facturi commanducant.

[5. *Ad oris ulcera et putredines.*] Melanteria contuſa prodeſt. Ad eadem benefacit oleum immaturum per ſe aut cum melle propinatum. Prodeſt etiam glaucuris vocata contuſa, ejus ſuccum ex melle et aqua paribus portionibus ad gargarizandum exhibeto.

[6. *Ad fluxum ſanguinis ab ore.*] Colluatur os ex decoctione roſarum in poſca, poſtquam erit frigida et de-

Ed. Chart. X. [614. 615.]

καταψυχθῇ καὶ καταπίνηται. ἄλλο. γαργαριζέτω ὁ πάσχων καὶ συγκλυζέτω τὸ στόμα ἑψήματι τῶν ῥόδων ψυχρῷ, ἢ ἑλίκων ἀμπέλου ἢ σχίνου φύλλων ἢ βάτου ἢ μήλων κυδωνίων ἢ ῥόδων ἢ γιγάρτων ἢ ῥοιᾶς. ἄλλο. σπέρμα ῥόδου σὺν μαστίχῃ δίδου σὺν οἴνῳ στυπτικῷ πίνειν ἢ σὺν οἴνῳ ἑψήματος τῆς βάτου ἢ ῥόδων.

[ζ'. Πρὸς τὰ τοῦ στόματος ἕλκη.] Κηκίδα ἐν τῷ οἴνῳ ἑψήσας σύγκλυζε τὸ στόμα, ἔπειτα προστίθει κηκίδα τετριμμένην τὴν σὺν μέλιτι διαμεμιγμένην ἢ τὸ ῥόδων ἄνθος· σύγκλυζε καὶ στόμα ἑψήματι τῶν τῆς ἐλαίας φύλλων.

Κεφ. η'. [α'. Πρὸς τὸ λευκαίνειν ὀδόντας καὶ τὰ πάθη αὐτῶν.] Χρῶνται δὲ καὶ ὀδοντοτρίμμασι τοιούτοις τισὶ, ποιοῦσιν ἅμα πρὸς τὰ οὖλα καὶ ὀδόντας λευκαίνουσι καὶ στεροῦσι, [615] γῆν ἐρετριάδα καύσαντες καὶ λειώσαντες χρῶνται· λευκαίνει τοῦτο τοὺς ὀδόντας σφόδρα καλῶς. ὀροβίνῳ βρέχων ἐν οὔρῳ λεῖον κατάχριε. ἄλλο. δασύποδος κεφαλὴν καύσας μίξον τῷ μαράθρῳ ὡς λευκοτάτῳ καὶ σηπίας ὀστράκοις λείοις χρῶ. ἄλλο. ἐλάφειον ὀστοῦν καύσας

glutiatur. *Aliud.* Gargarizet patiens et colluat decoctione rosarum frigida aut extremitatum vitis aut foliorum lentisci aut rubi aut cydoniorum aut vinaciorum aut mali punici. *Aliud.* Semen rosae cum mastiche da ex vino astringente bibendum vel ex vino decoctionis rubi, aut rosarum.

[7. *Ad oris ulcera.*] Gallam in vino coquens collue os, deinde appone gallam tritam permixtam cum melle aut florem rosarum; collue etiam os decoctione foliorum oleae.

Cap. VIII. [1. *Ad dealbandos dentes aliaque eorum vitia sananda.*] Utuntur autem et hujusmodi quibusdam dentifriciis, quae una et gingivis prosunt et dentes candidos firmioresque reddunt. Terram eretriada vocatam ustam tritamque adhibent; hoc valde bene splendidos dentes reddit. Farina ervi lotio subactam illine. *Aliud.* Cuniculi caput ustum cum foeniculo quam albissimo sepiae tritis ossibus admiscens utere. *Aliud.* Cornu cer-

καὶ λειώσας χρῶ. τοῦτο καὶ τοὺς πόνους τῶν ὀδόντων ἰᾶται καὶ μετὰ ῥοδίνου χριόμενον κεφαλαλγίας παύει. ἄλλο. γλήχωνα καὶ ἁλὸς πεφρυγμένον μίξας εἰς τὰ αὐτὰ λείοις χρῶ. ἄλλο. ἀστράγαλον προβάτειον καύσας ὁμοίως χρῶ. ἄλλο. κριθὰς ὀπτήσας μεθ' ἁλὸς λείοις χρῶ.

[β'. *Διάκλυσμα πρὸς ἕλκη καὶ ὀδόντας σειομένους καὶ ἀστατοῦντας.*] Ἀλυκακάβου ῥίζαν καθεψήσας μετὰ σιδίων λιπαρῶν κατάχριε. ἄλλο. λευκῆς ῥίζαν καὶ περιστερεῶνος βοτάνης τὴν ῥίζαν ἢ ἠρυγγίου ῥίζαν ἢ αὐτὸ τὸ ἠρύγγιον ἢ πολίου ῥίζαν λειώσας κατάχριε.

[γ'. *Πρὸς κινουμένους ὀδόντας.*] Ὄνου χηλήνιον καύσας τρῖψον ὄξει ἀναλάμβανε καὶ ποιῶν κυκλίσκια ἀπόθου καὶ χρῶ, ἀνιοὶν ὄξει, ἕνα κυκλίσκον δίδου διακλύζεσθαι, παύει παραχρῆμα τοὺς πόνους καὶ ἵστησιν. ἄλλο. χαμαιλέων μέλας διακλυζόμενος παύει ὀδονταλγίας. τοῦτο καὶ μῦς κτείνει. ἄλλο. σεύτλου διακλυζόμενος χυλὸς ὀδονταλγίας παύει παραχρῆμα. ἄλλο. ὑοσκυάμου ῥίζαν διάκλυζε θερμοτέρως καὶ ἄπονος ἔσται. ἄλλο. πήγανον καὶ ὕσσωπον καὶ

vino usto tritoque utitor; hoc et dentium dolores tollit et ex rosaceo impositum capitis dolores sedat. *Aliud.* Pulegio et sale fricto mixtis ad eadem tritis utere. *Aliud.* Ovillo talo usto ad similia utitor. *Aliud.* Hordeo tosto et sale mixtis tritisque utere.

[2. *Lavatio ad ulcera et dentes titubantes infirmosque.*] Alycacabi radicem una cum malicorio crassiore elixam imponito. *Aliud.* Recipe albae populi aut verbenacae radicem aut eryngii radicem vel ipsum eryngium aut polii radicem terens apponito.

[3. *Ad concussos dentes et dolentes.*] Asini ungulam ustam tritamque aceto excipe et orbiculos faciens repone; ad usum aceto orbiculum unum liquato datoque ore continendum, illico enim dolorem sedat tollitque. *Aliud.* Nigri chamaeleonis decocto si foveas, dolorem dentium curabis; id et mures necat. *Aliud.* Betae succo si fiat collutio, confestim dolor dentium finitur. *Aliud.* Alterci radicis calidiore decocto si foveas, dolor quiescit. *Aliud.*

σμύρναν μετ᾿ οἴνου λεάνας διακρατείτω. ἄλλο. φλόμου ῥίζαν ἑψήσας μετ᾿ ὄξους ἢ οἴνου ἢ ὀξυκράτου δίδου διακλύζεσθαι. ἄλλο. νίτρον σὺν ἐλαίῳ δίδου διακλύζεσθαι, καὶ ἄπονον ποιεῖ. ἄλλο. σφαιρία κυπαρίσσου ἑψηθέντα διὰ οἴνου καὶ ῥόδου διακλυζέσθω. ἐὰν δὲ ὅλοι πονῶσιν οἱ ὀδόντες, κεδρίαν διακλύζων, ἄπονον ποιεῖς παραχρῆμα. ἄλλο. μύλη ἐὰν ἀλγοῦσα εἴη, μονοκλώνου μαλάχης ῥίζαν ἐφάπτου καὶ ἄπονος ἔσται. δίδου διαμασήσασθαι τοῖς ἀλγοῦσι τοὺς ὀδόντας, περδικίου τῆς βοτάνης ῥίζαν, εἰσερχομένοις εἰς τὸ βαλανεῖον, καὶ διακρατείτω τὴν μύλην μέχρις ἂν ἐξέλθῃ, καὶ ἄπονος ἔσται. ἄλλο. πυρέθρου ῥίζα διαμασηθεῖσα αὐθήμερον τὸν πόνον παύει. ἄλλο. βοτάνης ποντίτιδος ῥίζα διαμασηθεῖσα παύει τὸν πόνον.

[δ'. Ὑποθυμίαμα τοῖς ἀλγοῦσιν ὀδοῦσιν.] Ἀλκυόνιον ὑποθυμία καὶ εὐθέως ἄπονος ἔσται. ἄλλο. ὑοσκυάμου σπέρμα ὑποθυμιασθὲν ἄπονον ποιεῖ.

[ε'. Πρὸς εὐωδίαν ὀδόντων.] Κιμωλίαν μεθ᾿ ἁλὸς

Rutam, hyſſopum et myrrham ex vino tritas ore contineto. *Aliud.* Si ex aceto, poſca aut vio, ubi verbaſci radix incocta ſit, os colluatur, bene facit. *Aliud.* Ex nitro cum oleo facta collutio dolorem pellit. *Aliud.* Cupreſſi baccis ex vino et roſa elixis os ſove. Quodſi dentes omnes doluerint, cedri liquore os ſi collues, protinus dolori ſuccurres. *Aliud.* Dens molaris ſi doleat, malvae unicum habentis cauliculum radice ſi tangas, dolor abibit. Dentes dolentibus herbae muralis radicem quum balneas ingrediuntur commanducandam praebeto, quam ſub molari dente quoad ex balneis egrediantur retineto et dolor evaneſcet. *Aliud.* Pyrethri radicala commanducata eodem die fugat dolorem. *Aliud.* Herbae pontidis vocatae radix manducata dolorem finit.

[4. *Suffimentum dentes dolentibus.*] Alcyonii ſuffitu quam primum dolor tollitur. *Aliud.* Alterci ſemen ſuffitum dolori medetur.

[5. *Ut dentes bene oleant.*] Cimoliam cum ſale terito

Ed. Chart. X. [615. 616.]
διάτριβε, χρίσας τοὺς ὀδόντας. ἄλλο. ὀδόντα κυνὸς λαβὼν ἐπὶ πῦρ ἐπίθες καὶ ὑποθυμία· ἅμα γὰρ τῷ καίεσθαι στερεοῦται.

[στ'. Πρὸς βεβρωμένους ὀδόντας.] Πρὸς τοὺς δὲ βεβρωμένους ὀδόντας ἔμβαλε πέπερι λευκὸν λείῳ ἀνειμένον χαλκάνθῳ ἢ κηκίδα. ἢ μετὰ μέλιτος σχιστὴν ἐντίθει εἰς τὸ βρῶμα καὶ ἄπονον ποιήσει. ἄλλο. τὸν τοῦ λίμακος λίθον θραύσας εἰς σησαμοειδῆ μεγέθη καὶ ἐπίθες εἰς τὸ βρῶμα τοῦ ὀδόντος καὶ παραχρῆμα ἄπονον ποιεῖ, ἐπιπωμάτιζε δὲ κηρῷ. ἄλλο. ἧπαρ ταύρου ἡσύχως πεφρυγμένον καὶ ἐντιθέμενον εἰς τὸν ὀδόντα ἅμα τῇ θίξει ἄπονον ποιεῖ. ἄλλο. ὄνυξ χελώνης ἐντιθέμενος τῇ βεβρωμένῃ μύλῃ ποιεῖ καλῶς. ἄλλο. χολὴ ἄρκτου ἐντεθεῖσα αὐτίκα ἀπόνους ποιεῖ, θεραπεύει [616] δὲ καὶ πάντα τρόπον ἐπιχριομένη.

[ζ'. Πρὸς κινουμένους ὀδόντας.] Τὸ τῆς χελώνης αἷμα διακρατούμενον ἐν τῷ στόματι στερεοῖ. ἄλλο. ἀλκυόνιον Ἰνδικὸν ἐν οἴνῳ τριπτὸν διακλυζέσθω καὶ ἵστησι τὴν κίνησιν.

dentesque fricato. *Aliud.* Dentem canis accipito et in ignem conjice fuffitumque facito; dum enim crematur, fimul dentes confirmat.

[6. *Ad exefos dentes.*] Ad exefos autem dentes vitriolo trito permixtum piper accipito aut gallam. Aut ex melle fiffum alumen in cavum dentis inferito et dolorem levabis. *Aliud.* Limacis lapidem in fruftula fefami magnitudinem aequantia confringe et in dentis foramen immitte, illico dolorem fedat, fed ex cera operculum facito. *Aliud.* Taurinum jecur lento igne frictum dentique impofitum, fimulatque tetigit, dolorem discutit. *Aliud.* Teftudinis unguis in maxillaris dentis exefi foramen conjectus multum proficit. *Aliud.* Fel urfi impofitum illico dolorem levat; curat autem etiam quoquo modo illinatur.

[7. *Ad dentes motos et labantes.*] Teftudinis fanguis diu ore contentus dentes roborat. *Aliud.* Alcyonio Indico ex vino trito fi os colluatur, motus fiftitur.

Ed. Chart. X. [616.]

[η'. Πρὸς τοὺς ἐκ πληγῆς κινουμένους ὀδόντας.] Κοράλλιον ἐπιτίθει καὶ κράτει ἐπὶ ἱκανὸν χρόνον.

[θ'. Πρὸς αἱμωδίαν.] Ἄῤῥωστος διαμασαέσθω] τὴν ἀνδράχνην· ἢ ἐλαίῳ ὠμοτρίβει παρατριβέσθω ἢ ἀμόργῃ ἐν χαλκῷ ἑψηθείσῃ μέχρι μελιτώδους στάσεως· ἡ γὰρ παλαιωθεῖσα διαχριομένη πάνυ ποιεῖ.

[ι'. Χωρὶς σιδήρου ἀπόνως ἆραι ὀδόντας.] Περιπλάσας ζύμην ἔασον αὐτὸν ὀλίγον· εἶτα περίχυσον αὐτὸν σαύρας αἵματι, καὶ ἐκπεσεῖται.

[ια'. Ὥστε αὐτόματον ἐκπεσεῖν.] Πύρεθρον ἐν ὄξει φυράσας καὶ ταριχεύσας ἐπὶ ἡμέρας λ'. ἐν τούτῳ περίπλασσε τὸν ὀδόντα καθάρας. ἄλλο. ἀρτεμισίαν τὴν βοτάνην ἐν ὄξει τρίψας περίπλασσε. ἄλλο. περιχαράξας τὸν ὀδόντα κάμπαις ταῖς εὑρισκομέναις ἐπὶ ταῖς ἀκρέμοσι τῶν βοτανῶν καὶ κραμβῶν κατάχριε, φυλασσόμενος τοὺς ἄλλους ὀδόντας· εἰ δὲ τοὺς κάτω ἆραι θέλεις, ταῖς εὑρισκομέναις ὑποκάτω χρῶ. ἄλλο. σανδαράχην ἐν ὄξει τρίψας χρησίμως ἔασον ξηραν-

[8. *Ad dentes ex ictu concuſſos.*] Corallium imponito et ſatis diu contineto.

[9. *Ad dentium ſtuporem.*] Aegrotus portulacam mandito. Aut oleo omphacino perungito aut amurca olei in vaſe aeneo ad mellis conſiſtentiam cocta; haec enim vetuſta inuncta valde prodeſt.

[10. *Ad dentes eximendos ſine ferramento et absque dolore.*] Fermentum denti circumdato et paulisper relinquito; mox dentem lacertae ſanguine circumfundito et excidet.

[11. *Ut ſponte dens excidat.*] Pyrethrum aceto mollitum ſaleque per triginta dies maceratum denti prius mundo facto circumponito. *Aliud.* Artemiſiam herbam ex aceto tritam obline. *Aliud.* Dentem circumſuffodiens vermiculis, quas campas vocant, in ſummis braſſicarum aliarumque herbarum foliis repertis illine, ab aliis dentibus cavens. Quod ſi inferiores dentes eximere voles, illis vermiculis utere, qui in inferiore parte illarum herbarum

Ed. Chart. X. [616.]
θῆναι καὶ χρῶ ξηρῷ αἱμάξας τὴν μύλην, ἐάσας γὰρ βραχὺ ἑλκύσεις τοῖς δακτύλοις αὐτὴν, ἢ κολοκυνθίδος ἀγρίας ἐντίθει ῥίζαν τῷ ὀδόντι. ἄλλο. μοίδου ὀμφακίτου ῥίζαν ξηράνας ἐν σκιᾷ καὶ κόψας καὶ σήσας περίπασσε τὰς ῥίζας καὶ μετ᾽ ὀλίγον ἐπιλαμβάνου τοῖς δακτύλοις καὶ ἀκολουθεῖ, ἢ τῷ τῆς Αἰθιοπικῆς ἐλαίας δακρύῳ παράπτου τοῦ πεπονθότος ὀδόντος. ἄλλο. σαῦραν ἀγρίαν ξηράνας καὶ ἀνασχίσας καὶ κόψας ἀπόθου. ὅταν περικαθάρῃς τὸν ὀδόντα, ἐντίθει καὶ μετ᾽ ὀλίγον ἕλκε καὶ ἀκολουθήσει. ἄλλο κόκκους κνίδης μίξας μετὰ χαλβάνης περίπλασσε τῷ πάσχοντι, καὶ παραχρῆμα πεσεῖται.

[ιβ΄. Ἀπόνως ἆραι ὀδόντας.] Ἡ τῆς ξανθοῦ βοτάνης ῥίζα θερμαινομένη καὶ πρὸς τῷ ὀδόντι εὐθέως θεῖσα αἴρει τοῖς δακτύλοις.

[ιγ΄. Ὥστε τοῖς δακτύλοις αἴρειν.] Κολοκυνθίδας ἀγρίας κόψον καὶ ὄξει ἀπόβρεξον, ὥστε πάχος σχεῖν μέλιτος, καὶ ἀπόβαπτε εἰς τὸ φάρμακον τὸ περιχαρακτήριον περιχάρασσε·

reperiuntur. *Aliud.* Sandaracham ex aceto tritam ſiccari permitte et ſicca utiliter utitor, prius ſanguinem circum dentem eliciens; ſic enim pauliſper dimittens digitis ipſum eximes. Aut agreſtis cucurbitulae radicem in foramen dentis conjice. *Aliud.* Moedi immaturi radicem in umbra areſactam, tritam et cretam radicibus dentis circumda et paulo poſt digitis apprehende, ſequetur enim; aut Aethiopicae oleae lacrima affectum dentem tangito. *Aliud.* Lacertam agreſtem areſactam, diſſectam contritamque repone; quum dentem circum purgaveris, imponito et paulo poſt attrahito et ſequetur. *Aliud.* Urticae ſemina cum galbano mixta affecto denti circumline et protinus excidet.

[12. *Ad eximendos ſine dolore dentes.*] Herbae lappae radix caleſacta et denti appoſita facit, ut ſtatim digitis tollatur.

[13. *Ut dentes digitis evellantur.*] Silveſtres cucurbitulas contunde et aceto macera ad mellis ſpiſſitudinem, deinde ferramentum ad ſcalpendos dentes in medicamen-

Ed. Chart. X. [616. 617.]
καὶ κέλευε συμμῦσαι τὸ στόμα ἐπ' ὀλίγον. εἶτα ἐπιλαμβανόμενος τοῖς δακτύλοις ἕλκε τὸν ὀδόντα, ἀπόνως ἀκολουθεῖ. ἄλλο. ἄλευρον μετὰ ὀποῦ τιθυμάλλου ἐπιθὲς καὶ ἐπάνω κισσοῦ φύλλον, καὶ ἔασον ὥραν· αὐτομάτως γὰρ θρυβήσεται.

[ιδ'. Πρὸς τὸ λευκαίνειν ὀδόντας.] Τὸ νίτρον, σηπίας ὄστρακον καὶ φοινίκων ὀστοῦν τρίψας χρῶ. ἄλλο καλόν. κοράλλιον ἐρυθρὸν, κίσσηριν, φοινίκων ὀστᾶ, σηπίας ὄστρακα καὶ τοὺς ἅλας κεκαυμένους τρίψας χρῶ.

[ιε'. Πρὸς ὀδονταλγίαν.] Σκινελαίῳ μὴ παλαιῷ ὀδόντας σύγκλυζε. ἄλλο. συγκλυζέσθω τὸ στόμα σὺν τοῖς πηγάνου φύλλοις ἐν ὀξυμέλιτι ὠπτημένοις, ἢ συγκλυζέσθω σὺν ὄξει σκιλλιτικῷ· ἢ ἑψέσθω ἐν ὄξει πύρεθρον καὶ ὕσσωπον. χρὴ δὲ καὶ τὸ ὑγρὸν καὶ τὸν χυμὸν κενοῦν.

[617] Κεφ. θ'. [Πρὸς τὰ τῶν οὔλων πάθη.] [α'. Πρὸς διαβεβρωμένα οὔλη.] Ῥόδων ἄνθους < η'. κηκίδων < δ'. σμύρνης < β'. καὶ μίξας πρόσθες. ἄλλο. γάλακτι ὀνίῳ τὰ οὔλη διάκλυζε. ἄλλο. ἐλαίας φύλλων ἀφε-

tum demitte, eoque dentem circum ſcarifica atque os paulisper clauſum haberi praecipe; deinde apprehende digitis dentem et attrahe; absque dolore ſequitur. *Aliud.* Farinam ex lacte tithymalli admove et hederacea folia ſuperimpone, per horamque dimitte; frangetur enim ſine dolore.

[14. *Ad dealbationem dentium.*] Nitrum, os ſepiae et os palmularum terens utere. *Aliud bonum.* Corallium rubrum, pumicem, oſſa palmularum, oſſa ſepiae et ſalem aſſum terens utere.

[15. *Ad dolorem dentium.*] Oleo lentisci non antiquo colluantur dentes. *Aliud.* Colluatur os cum foliis rutae coctis ex oxymelite; vel colluatur cum aceto ſcillitico; vel coquatur in aceto pyrethrum et hyſſopum: oportet autem humiditatem et humorem evacuare.

Cap. IX. [*Ad gingivarum affectus.*] [1. *Ad gingivas corroſas.*] Recipe florum roſarum drach. viij, gallarum drach. iv, myrrhae drach. ij, commiſce et appone. *Aliud.* Lacte aſinae gingivas collue. *Aliud.* Foliorum oleae

Ed. Chart. X. [617.]
ψήματι στόμα διάκλυζε. ἄλλο. ὄξει σκιλλιτικῷ οὖλη ἔκκλυζε. ἄλλο. ἰὸν σιδήρου καὶ βαλαύστια ξηρὰ προσθές.

[β'. Πρὸς τὰ οὖλη οἰδοῦντα καὶ ἐκσαρκοῦντα.] Ὠφελεῖ ἀνδράχνης χυλὸς διαβρατούμενος ἢ ἅλμη κολυμβάδων ἐλαιῶν, ἢ ἔλαιον θερμὸν ὠμοτριβὲς, ἢ σχίνινον, ἢ ἀμόργη. ξηρὰ δὲ προσαπτόμενα συμφέρουσι, ἰὸς σιδήρου ἢ χαλκοῦ, ἀριστολοχίας ῥίζα, ἀρνογλώσσου σπέρμα, διφρυγὲς, χάλκανθος ὀπτὴ, κύτινοι.

[γ'. Πρὸς παρουλίδας.] Ἀφεψήματι φύλλων ἐλαίας διάκλυζε καὶ προσθὲς κηκίδα. ἄλλο. ἕψε ἐν ἑψήματι φύλλα ἐλαίας καὶ κηκίδα.

[δ'. Πρὸς οὖλα ἀπομελανθέντα καὶ σαπρά.] Ποιεῖ τρίψις ἐξ οἴνου τρυγὸς κεκαυμένης· ῥύπτει γὰρ, καθαρίζει καὶ ἀπολευκαίνει.

[ε'. Πρὸς αἱμασσόμενα οὖλα.] Ποιεῖ ἡ τοῦ αἵματος ἀφαίρεσις ἐκ τῆς κεφαλικῆς καὶ ὁ τῶν οὔλων σχασμός· ποιεῖ καὶ ὑοσκυάμου φύλλων χυλὸς ἢ τὸ αὐτοῦ ἀφέψημα σὺν

decocto os collue. *Aliud.* Aceto ſcillitico gingivas ablue. *Aliud.* Rubiginem ferri et balauſtia ſicca appone.

[2. *Ad gingivas tumidas et carnis incrementum.*] Confert ſuccus portulacae ore detentus vel aqua ſalita olivarum colymbadum vel oleum ex immaturis olivis expreſſum calidum vel lentiscinum vel de cotoneis aut amurca. Sicca vero, quae proſunt, ſunt rubigo ferri, aut aeris, radix ariſtolochiae, ſemen plantaginis, atramentum ſutorium aſſatum et balauſtia.

[3. *Ad inflammationem gingivarum.*] Collue decocto ſoliorum oleae et appone gallam. *Aliud.* Coque in ſapa folia oleae et gallam.

[4. *Ad gingivas denigratas et putridas.*] Confert fricatio ex faece vini uſta; abſtergit enim, mundat dealbatque.

[5. *Ad gingivas cruentas.*] Confert miſſio ſanguinis e cephalia et ſcarificatio gingivarum; confert etiam ſuccus hyoscyami vel ejus decoctum ex ſapa aut cum palma-

ἑψήματι ἢ στάγματι θερμὸν διακρατούμενον ἐν τῷ στόματι. ἄλλο. σχίνου ἀκρεμόνας καὶ τὰ βαλαύστια ἑψήσας ἐν ὀξυκράτῳ σύγκλυζε. ἄλλο. ῥίζαν βάτου ἑψήσας ἐν οἴνῳ τὸ στόμα σύγκλυζε· ἢ ῥοῦν καὶ κηκίδα ἐν οἴνῳ ἑψήσας ὁμοίως χρῶ.

Κεφ. ι'. [Πρὸς κιονίδας.] Κηκίδα λείαν καθ' αὑτὴν προσάπτου, βρέχων τὸν δάκτυλον εἰς ἔλαιον ἢ εἰς κοχλιάριον βαλὼν παράπτου. ἄλλο. ἀκάνθης Αἰγυπτίας τὸ σπέρμα λειώσας ξηρῷ παράπτου. ἄλλο. ἰσχάδας νήστει μετὰ φύλλων ἐλαΐνων δὸς φαγεῖν. ἄλλο. ὀπὸν Κυρηναϊκὸν μεθ' ἁλὸς λεάνας ξηρῷ προσάπτου, πρότερον ἀναγαργαρίσας ὕδατι θερμῷ· ἢ σχιστὴν καύσας ἐπιμελῶς παράπτου· ἢ ἀσκαλαβώτην ἐπ' ἀμπελίνοις ξύλοις παράπτου, ποιεῖ καλῶς. ἄλλο. βάτου τοὺς καυλοὺς μετὰ μέλιτος καὶ πίσσης ὑγρᾶς λειώσας κατάπλασσε. ἄλλο. λίθου ἀγηράτου ἄνθος μίξας δίδου ἀναγαργαρίζειν ἢ κράμβης χυλῷ μίξας στυπτηρίαν σχιστὴν ἀναγαργαριζέτω, ὠφελεῖ καλῶς.

[Καυστικὸν κιονίδος.] Μίσυ καὶ ἄσβεστον ἀναλαβὼν

rum ſtillamento calidum ore retentum. *Aliud.* Camulos lentisci et balauſtia coque in posca et collue. *Aliud.* Radicem rubi coque in vino et os collue; vel rhun et gallam coque in vino et utere ſimiliter.

Cap. X. [*Ad columellae morbos.*] Gallam tritam per ſe admoveto, digito oleo intincto aut in cochlearium injiciens applica. *Aliud.* Spinae Aegyptiae ſemen tritum atque aridum appone. *Aliud.* Caricas cum oleae foliis eſui dato. *Aliud.* Succum Cyrenaïcum cum ſale arefactum apponito, prius gargarizatione ex aqua calida facta. Aut fiſſum alumen uſtum diligenter admotum juvat. Aut ſtellionem viteis lignis crematum imponito, et bene facit. *Aliud.* Rubi cauliculos ex melle et pice liquida maceratos admove. *Aliud.* Lapidis agerati florem admixtum gargarizandum da. Aut braſſicae ſucco admixtum alumen fiſſum et gargarizatum recte prodeſt.

[*Uſtorium columellae apponendum.*] Miſy et calcem

ἴσα ῥητίνῃ τερεβινθίνῃ ὑποτίθει καὶ ἔα ὑποκρατεῖν· αἴρει ἐντὸς ὡρῶν τριῶν. ποιεῖ δὲ καὶ πρὸς σταφυλὰς καλῶς τὸ ἀπόῤῥυμμα τῆς πίσσης, τὸ φερόμενον ἀπὸ Κιλικίας λαμβανόμενον εἰς κοχλιάριον καὶ ὑποτιθέμενον. καὶ ὀμφάκιον μετὰ μέλιτος ἢ γλυκέος λίαν. λέγεται δὲ ἀπαθῆ φυλάσσειν τὴν κιονίδα, ἐάν τις ῥᾶγας σταφυλῆς καταπίνῃ νῆστις ἑκάστου ἔτους, καὶ οὐδέποτε ἕξει [618] τὸ πάθος. καὶ τοῖς ἐπὶ τῶν παρισθμίων τεχθησομένοις ἀναγαργαρίσμασι χρηστέον, ἐπὶ σταφυλῆς πασχούσης. πρῶτον καὶ ἐν ἀρχῇ κέλευε ὕδωρ θερμὸν διακρατεῖν καὶ ἀναγαργαρίζεσθαι ψυχρῷ, ἢ ὀξυκράτῳ ἢ ῥοιᾶς γλυκείας χυλῷ καθηψημένῳ, μέχρις ἂν σχῇ πάχος μέλιτος, ἀνεθέντι μετ' ὀξυμέλιτος ἢ ὀξυκράτου ἢ δρακοντίου χυλῷ, καὶ ποιήσουσι καλῶς.

[*Πρὸς σταφυλὴν τῇ φλεγμονῇ ἐπιληφθεῖσαν.*] Σκευαζέσθω γαργάρισμα σὺν χυλῷ τῆς ῥοιᾶς μετὰ μελικράτου, ἢ σὺν ὕδατι τῶν ἀφεψήματος ῥόδων, ἢ σὺν τῷ διάμβαρ ἐξ ὕδατος θερμοῦ. ποιεῖ καὶ ὁ τῆς γλυκυῤῥίζης χυλὸς σὺν

vivam aequis portionibus refina terebinthina excipe et fubde retinendamque permitte: intra horas tres aufert. Item proficit ad uvae affectum picis recrementum, quod ex Cilicia advehitur, cochleario exceptum et fubditum. Et uvae acerbae fuccus ex melle aut praedulci vino. Dicitur autem incolumem fervare columellam, fi quis uvae acinos quotannis jejunus devoret; et nunquam ejus partis affectu vexabitur. Iisdem praeterea gargarismatis in vulvae vitiis utendum eft, quae ad tonfillas affectas defcribentur. Primum atque inter initia jube aqua calida os fovere; deinde frigida gargarizare aut posca aut mali punici dulcis fucco ad mellis craffitudinem decocto et oxymelite eliquato; aut posca aut dracunculi fucco gargarizet et optime proficient.

[*Ad vulvam phlegmonem patientem.*] Fiat gargarizatio cum fucco mali punici ex mulfa vel cum aqua decoctionis rofarum, vel cum diambron ex aqua calida. Confert etiam glycyrrhizae fuccus cum melle appofitus et

Ed. Chart. X. [618.]
μέλιτι παρατεθειμένος καὶ γῆ σφραγὶς, τῆς τε Αἰγυπτίας ἀκάνθου ὁ καρπός. ἀδηκτότερά ἐστι κόμμι Ἀραβικὸν, τραγάκανθα, σαρκόκολλα προστεθειμένα. ἄλλο. τὸν τῆς Αἰγυπτίας ἀκάνθου καρπὸν καὶ ὀπὸν προσθές· ἢ βάτου ἀκρέμονας τρίψας σὺν μέλιτι κατάπλασσε.

Κεφ. ια'. [Πρὸς φλεγμονὰς παρισθμίων καὶ συνάγχας.] Ποιεῖ δὲ τοῦτο καλῶς ἐπὶ παρισθμίων. οἱ τὰ μύρτα κατασκευάζοντες εἰώθασιν ἐν μέλιτι χρίειν καὶ ἀψινθίῳ· τοῦτο οὖν διαχριόμενον ἢ μετά τινος ἀναγαργαριζόμενον θαυμαστῶς ποιεῖ. ἐὰν ἐπιμένῃ τι τῆς φλεγμονῆς μετὰ τοῦ τετραχύνθαι τὰ παρίσθμια, χρηστέον γάλακτι πάντῃ θερμῷ καθ' ἑαυτὸ καὶ μετά τινος τῶν εἰρημένων. ἢ πιτύροις ἀφηψημένοις δι' ὕδατος ἢ ὑδρομέλιτος ἢ πιτύρων ἀποβρέγματι ἢ τράγου ῥᾶγας, ὀρύζης βρέξας ἐν ὕδατι θερμῷ ἄλευρον, δὶς ἢ τρὶς χρῶ τῷ χυλῷ. ἢ ζωμῷ ὀρνιθείῳ ἢ ἐριφείῳ ἢ πτισάνην ἕψει μετὰ σταφίδος καὶ τῷ χυλῷ, ἢ μαλάχης ἀφεψήματι καθ' αὐτό. ἢ καὶ μετὰ μέλιτος ἕψει τὴν μαλάχην ἢ καὶ μετὰ θερμῶν καὶ μετὰ γλυκέος χρῶ.

terra ſigillata et fructus ſpinae Aegyptiacae. Mitiora autem ſunt haec, gummi Arabicum, tragacanthum, ſarcocolla appoſita. *Aliud.* Fructum ſpinae Aegyptiae et ſuccum appone; vel cauliculos rubi terens illine cum melle.

Cap. XI. [*Ad inflammationes tonſillarum et anginas.*] Id vero benefacit in tonſillarum inflammationibus. Myrteas baccas praeparantes melle et abſinthium et dracunculum inungere conſueverunt; hoc autem medicamentum illitum aut cum aliquo gargarizatum mirum in modum prodeſt. Quod ſi aliquae phlegmonis reliquiae ſuperſint tonſillaeque exasperatae ſint, lacte plane calido per ſe aut cum ſuprapoſitorum aliquo utendum eſt. Aut ſurfuribus aqua elixis aut mulſa aut ſurfurum diluto. Aut tragi acinos aut orizae aqua calida farinam ſubigens bis aut ter ſucco utere. Aut gallinae hoedive jusculo; aut hordeum cortice liberatum una cum paſſulis decoque; aut malvae ſucco vel decocto per ſe utere: aut una cum melle malvam elixa aut cum lupinis et paſſo et utitor.

Ed. Chart. X. [618.]

[Πρὸς παρίσθμια καὶ συναγχικούς.] Γλυκυῤῥίζης χυλὸν ἀνεὶς χρῶ· ἐὰν δὲ ἐσχάραι γένωνται, πρὸς τὸ ταύτας σχολάσαι, ὑδρομέλιτι ἀναγαργαρίζεσθαι δεῖ. ἢ φακῆς ἀφεψήματι καθ' αὑτὸ καὶ μετὰ ὑσσώπου ἢ ἴρεως ἢ κολυμβάδων ἐλαιῶν ὕδατι ἀναγαργαριζέσθω, ἢ κρόκου βραχὺ καὶ σμύρνης μετὰ βραχέος γλυκέος ἀναζεσθέντα. ἢ σῦκα παρεψήσας, παρέμπλασον αὐτοῖς ὠμήλυσιν καὶ χυλώσας διήθησον καὶ τῷ χυλῷ χρῶ. ἢ τῷ τῶν σύκων ἀφεψήματι μίξας νᾶπυ ὀλίγον, δίδου ἀναγαργαρίζεσθαι· φλέγμα γὰρ ἄγει καὶ λύει τὴν φλεγμονήν.

[Πρὸς δὲ τὰς ἀποστάσεις τὰς ἐν παρισθμίοις.] Συμφέρει τι τῶν εἰρημένων· ἀφρονίτρῳ λείῳ παράπτου, ἐνίοτε δὲ καὶ ἄνθος νίτρου μίσγε. ἀποχύει γὰρ τὰς ἐσχάρας καὶ τήκει τὰς ἀποστάσεις ἐν διακλύσματι διδόμενον. καὶ στακτῇ κονίᾳ πρασίου χυλὸς διηθείς· ἢ αὐτὸ τὸ πράσιον τὴν βοτάνην ἐν ὑδρομέλιτι ἑψηθεῖσαν· ἢ πηγάνου ἀφέψημα μετὰ πρασίου ἢ καθ' ἑαυτὸ ἢ ἐν ὑδρομέλιτι καθεψηθὲν ποιεῖ. καὶ ὁ χυλὸς ἀναγαργαριζόμενος καὶ ὀρόβων ἀφεψήματι ἀνα-

[*Ad tonfillarum tumores et anginas.*] Dulcis radicis fuccum eliquans utere. Quod fi cruftae factae fint, ad has removendas mulfa gargarizandum eft; aut lentis decocto per fe aut hyffopo aut iride. Vel etiam olivarum falfarum aqua gargarizetur. Aut croci parum et myrrhae cum modico paffi infervescant. Aut ficis elixis hordei farinam permisce fuccumque exprimens percola et fucco utere. Aut ficorum decocto finapis modicum adjiciens gargarizandum propina; pituitam namque detrahit et phlegmonem folvit.

[*Ad abfceffus in tonfillis.*] Aliquod ex iis quae fupra comprehenfa funt proficit. Item aphronitro contrito locum tange; interdum autem et florem nitri adjunge; feparat enim cruftas et abfceffus attenuat, fi per collutionem detur. Ex lixivio percolato marrubii fuccus dilutus utiliter exhibetur; aut ipfum marrubium in mulfa coctum; aut rutae decoctum cum marrubio aut per fe aut in mulfa elixum fubfidio eft. Item et fuccus gargarizatur et ervi

γαργάριζε ἢ μίσυ μίσγων μετὰ κηκίδος ὀμφακίνης καὶ μυρσίνης ἐξ ἴσου λειοτριβήσας μετὰ στυπτηρίας ὑγρᾶς καὶ μέλιτος ἴσον μίσγων διάχριε. τοῦτο οὐ μόνον ἐσχάρας ἐκβάλλει, ἀλλὰ καὶ τὰς ἀντιάδας τήκει θαυμαστῶς. ἢ δέλφακος αἵματι χρίσας τὰς χεῖρας καθάψου τοῦ τραχήλου τρίς. [619] ἄλλο. κοχλίας γυμνοὺς βάλε εἰς πολτάριον καὶ καῦσον καὶ λειώσας τὴν τέφραν ἀναλάμβανε μέλιτι λείῳ, διάχριε· ἀπαράβατόν ἐστιν.

Κεφ. ιβ'. [Πρὸς τὰ τοῦ βρόγχου καὶ φάρυγγος πάθη.] [α'. Πρὸς παρεκκοπὰς καὶ ἐλαττώσεις τῆς φωνῆς.] Βολβοὺς δύο μετὰ μέλιτος δίδου φαγεῖν ὠμούς. ὠφελεῖ δὲ καὶ τὸ σῦκον ἑψόμενον καὶ ἀναγαργαιζόμενον μετὰ λιβάνου καὶ σμύρνης. ποιεῖ δὲ καὶ τὸ θεῖον ἄπυρον μετὰ ᾠῶν λαμβανόμενον κοχλιάρια β'. ἢ γ'. ἄλλο. λαβὼν ἀμύγδαλα πικρὰ κ'. σπέρματος λίνου κεκαυμένου < δ'. τραγακάνθης τῆς ἐν ὕδατι βεβρεγμένης < β'. στροβίλους λ'. τῷ μέλιτι ἀναλαβὼν χρῶ. ἄλλο. τοῦ γλήχωνος < δ'. σπέρματος λίνου,

decoctum fimiliter prodeft, aut mify cum galla immatura mixtum. Aut myrtum liquido alumini ac melli paribus portionibus tritam mifcens illine; hoc remedium non cruftas folum abjicit, verum etiam antiadas glandulas mirifice diffipat. Aut porcelli cruore manus imbuens ter laborantis collum attinge. *Aliud.* Cochleas tefta nudatas in ollam injice, deinde torreas et in cinerem redigens puro melle ac leni excipe atque perunge; vis ejus incredibilis eft.

Cap. XII. [*Ad gutturis et faucium affectus.*] [1. *Ad interruptam fubmiffamque vocem*] Bulbos duos crudos ex melle efui dato. Auxiliatur et fici decoctum cum thure et myrrha gargarizatum. Ad idem facit et fulfur ignem non expertum in ovis devoratum ad cochlearia duo aut tria. *Aliud.* Accipe amygdalas amaras xx, feminis lini affi drach. iv, tragacanthae aqua maceratae drach. ij, nucleos pini triginta; melle excipe et utere. *Aliud.* Pu-

Ed. Chart. X. [619.]
πεπέρεως, καλαμίνθης ἀνὰ < β'. πετροσελίνου < α'. μέλιτος λίτρ. α'.

[β'. Πρὸς τοὺς ἤδη πνιγομένους.] Ἀνθρωπείαν κόπρον εἰς ῥάκος ἐνδήσας καὶ καύσας δίδου πιεῖν· τοῦτο τοῖς ἤδη πνιγομένοις βοηθεῖ. ἄλλο. ποιεῖ δὲ καὶ κόπρος αἰγεία σὺν μέλιτι καὶ πίσσῃ ὑγρᾷ διαχριομένη ἐπὶ τῆς συναγχικῆς ἄκρως. ἢ πηγάνου χυλῷ καὶ γάλακτι κλύζε διὰ κλυστῆρος τὸν φάρυγγα τοῦ συναγχικοῦ· κατασπᾷ γὰρ δάκρυον πολὺ καὶ κουφίζει. ἄλλο. οὖρον συνεχῶς ἀναγαργαριζόμενον ὑγιάζει· δεῖ δὲ συναναγαργαρίζεσθαι καὶ χυλὸν κράμβης.

[γ'. Πρὸς τὰς τῶν παίδων ἐσχάρας.] Τὰς ἐν τῷ φάρυγγι γιγνομένας διάχριε· εἶτα δίδου ἀριστολοχίαν ἐν οἴνῳ ἑψήσας ἀναγαργαρίζεσθαι. τάχιστα θεραπεύει.

[δ'. Πρὸς ὀστᾶ ἀκαφθέντα καὶ πάντα ἐκ τοῦ βρόγχου ἐκβαλεῖν.] Ὕδατος καὶ ἐλαίου τὸ ἴσον εἰς τὸ στόμα ἐγχέας κατεχέτω ἕως ἐκβάλῃ τὸ καταποθέν. ἐάν τις ἐσθίων καὶ καταπίνει καὶ πνίγεται, ἐκ τοῦ αὐτοῦ οὗ τρώγει εἰς ἑκάτερον

legii drach. iv, ſeminis lini, piperis, calaminthi ana drach. ij, petroſelini drachmam j, mellis libram j.

[2. *Ad eos qui prope ſuffocantur.*] Humanum ſtercus in panniculo deligatum et crematum potui dato; hoc his qui jam ſtrangulantur opem fert. *Aliud.* Et caprinum ſtercus cum melle et liquida pice illitum angina laborantibus ſumme prodeſt. Aut rutae ſucco et lacte per clyſterem transmiſſo laborantis fauces collue; multam enim lacrimam detrahit et malum levat. *Aliud.* Urina aſſidue gargarizata ſanitatem reſtituit; una vero et ſuccum braſſicae gargarizare oportet.

[3. *Ad puerorum cruſtas in faucibus.*] Cruſtas in faucibus factas prius inungito; deinde vinum, in quo ariſtolochia decocta fuerit, gargarizetur; citiſſime curabitur.

[4. *Ad oſſa devorata aliaque omnia ex gutture excutienda.*] Aquae et olei parem modum in os fundens contineto, quo ad rem devoratam ejiciat. Si quis comedens aliquid devoraverit et ſuffocetur, ex eadem re, quam

Ed. Chart. X. [619. 620.]

ὠτίων ἐπάνω ἐπιτιθέτω καὶ ἐπὶ τὴν κεφαλήν· ὑποβιβάζεται γὰρ τὸ καταποθὲν καὶ πνῖγον.

[ε'. Πρὸς βδέλλας ἐκ βρόγχου ἐκβαλεῖν.] Ἀναγαργαριζέσθω θαλασσίαν ἅλμην. ἄλλο. ἐλαίου ἢ ὀποῦ Κυρηναϊκοῦ τὸ μέγεθος ὀρόβου τρίψας μετὰ ἀκράτου δίδου πιεῖν θερμόν. ἢ χυλὸν ἀναγαλλίδος πότιζε ἢ ὄξος μετὰ θύμου δριμύ· μετὰ δὲ ταῦτα ἀναγαργαριζέσθω θερμῷ ὕδατι.

Κεφ. ιγ'. [Πρὸς τὰ τοῦ θώρακός τε καὶ πνευμόνων πάθη καὶ πρῶτον πρὸς κατάῤῥους.] Τυρὸς παλαιὸς λαμβανόμενος ὠφελεῖ, ἀναξηραίνει γὰρ αὐτούς. ἐν ἐλαίῳ παλαιῷ διάχριε τοὺς μυκτῆρας συνεχῶς, ἢ θείῳ καὶ σμύρνῃ τετριμμένῃ μετ' οἴνου καὶ μέλιτος καὶ ἐλαίου.

[Πρὸς βῆχας.] Σῦκα βαπτόμενα εἰς ἄκρατον καὶ λαμβανόμενα ὠφελεῖ. ἄλλο. ῥητίνην τερεβινθίνην σὺν μέλιτι ἑψῶν δίδου ἐκλείχειν· καὶ οἶνον κεκραμένον γλυκεῖ δίδου ἐπιῤῥοφεῖν.

[620] [Ἄλλο παιδίοις μᾶλλον ἁρμόζον.] Πητυὰν καθαρὰν ἀναλάμβανε μέλιτι ἑψηθέντι καὶ δίδου. ἄλλο. λυ-

comedebat particulam utrique auri ſuperimponat ac ſuper caput; res enim devorata ſtrangulansque deſcendet.

[5. *Ad hirudines ex gutture ejiciendas.*] Marina aqua gargarizetur. *Aliud.* Oleum aut ſuccus Cyrenaïcus ad magnitudinem ervi ex vino puro calidus potui detur. Aut ſuccum anagallidis aut acetum acre cum thymo propina; poſtea calenti aqua gargarizetur.

Cap. XIII. [*Ad thoracis ac pulmonum affectus, primumque ad deſluxiones.*] Caſeus antiquus in cibum ſumptus juvat; ipſas enim reſiccat. Oleo veteri nares aſſidue perunge; aut ſulſure et myrrha contrita cum vino et melle et oleo.

[*Ad tuſſes.*] Fici puro vino madeſacti et in cibum ſumpti bene faciunt. *Aliud.* Reſina terebinthina in melle cocta linctui detur; poſtea vinum dilutum dulci ſorbendum exhibeatur.

[*Aliud pueris magis commodum*] Coagulum purum cocto melle comprehende et exhibe. *Aliud.* Canem licur-

Ed. Chart. X. [620.]

κοῦργον τὸν λεγόμενον κυνὰ ψιλὸν δίδου φαγεῖν. ἄλλο. σκόροδα ἑφθὰ μετὰ μέλιτος ὠφελεῖ. ἄλλο. σκίλλαν λαβὼν περιόρυξον αὐτῆς τὴν κεφαλὴν καὶ βαλὼν ἐκεῖ ὠὸν, περιπήλωσον τὸν τόπον καὶ ὀπτήσας δὸς φαγεῖν.

[Πρὸς τοὺς διηνεκῶς πυρέσσοντας.] Ὑσσώπου δεσμίδιον μετὰ ὕδατος εἰς τρίτον ἑκζέσας δὸς πιεῖν νήστει ἐπὶ ἡμέρας λ'. εἰς θερμὸν, παιδίοις δὲ καὶ μετὰ ἰσχάδων. ἄλλο. πτερίνην κόψας καὶ σήσας ἐπίπασον ὡς ἄλφιτα εἰς τὸν τόπον. ποιεῖ δὲ τοῦτο καὶ πρὸς αἱμοπτοϊκοὺς καλῶς. ἄλλο. σίνηπι κόψας καὶ λειοτριβήσας δίδου κοχλιάριον α'. μετὰ οἴνου κυάθων β'. πίνειν ἑξῆς ἐπὶ ἡμέρας γ'.

[Πρὸς τὰς νυκτερινὰς βῆχας.] Ἡδύοσμον τρίψας βάλε εἰς ὄξος καὶ δίδου ῥοφεῖν.

[Ὑποκαπνισμὸς πρὸς τὴν βῆχα.] Στύρακος, μαστίχης, πεπέρεως, πετροσελίνου ἀνὰ < α'. σανδαράχης < στ'. ἀκρόδρυον τῆς δάφνης α'. τοῖς ἄνθραξιν ἐναπτομένοις ἐπιθὲς καὶ καλάμῳ τὸν καπνὸν ἐν τῷ στόματι δέχηται ὁ πάσχων.

gum vocatum excoriatum epulandum appone. *Aliud.* Allium ex melle decoctum succurrit tussientibus. *Aliud.* Scillam accipito et ejus summum exacuato; in cavo conjice ovum locumque creta obtege et tostum edendum exhibe.

[*Ad tussientes assidue.*] Hyssopi fasciculum in aqua ad tertias decoquens jejuno per triginta dies calidam potui dato; pueris vero etiam cum caricis. *Aliud.* Pernam contundens et instar farinae in potione spargens juvat. Hoc idem et sanguinis ex ore ejectioni succurrit egregie. *Aliud.* Sinapi tusum tritumque cochlearii mensura cum vini cyathis duobus deinceps per dies tres bibendum dato.

[*Ad nocturnas tusses.*] Mentham tritam in acetum conjice et sorbendum praebe.

[*Suffitus ad tussim.*] Styracis, mastiches, piperis, petroselini, ana drach. j, sandarachae drach. vj, baccam lauri unam impone carbonibus accensis et per calamum aeger fumum excipiat.

[Πρὸς ἀσθματικούς.] Σκίλλαν ἑψήσας ἐν οἴνῳ ἢ μελικράτῳ πίνειν δίδου. ποιεῖ καὶ πνεύμων ἀλώπεκος ξηρὸς καταξυόμενος εἰς οἶνον μέλανα καὶ πινόμενος. ἄλλο. κάρδαμον λευκὸν κόψας καὶ μίξας μέλιτι δὸς ἐκλείχειν.

[Πρὸς δυσπνοοῦντας.] Λαβὼν προβάτων τὰς κατὰ τὸν δακτύλιον τρίχας καὶ καύσας καὶ τρίψας ἐν γλυκεῖ δὸς πιεῖν. ἄλλο. θεῖον ἄπυρον δὸς πιεῖν μετὰ οἴνου κοχλιάρια δ'.

[Πρὸς ὀρθοπνοϊκούς.] Στρούθιον ἐν ὕδατι θερμῷ δὸς πιεῖν. ἄλλο. ἀείζωον μετὰ μέλιτος δίδου λεῖον ἐκλείχειν ἢ βολβὸν ἢ ἀβρότονον, ὡς χόνδρον δίδου μεθ' ὑδρομέλιτος ἢ ὑσσώπου ἑφθῶν δίδου σὺν ὑδρομέλιτι, ἢ στοιχάδα τὴν βοτάνην, ἢ καστόριον μετὰ γλυκέος πινόμενον, ἢ σκίλλης τὸ ἐντὸς μετὰ ὀξυμέλιτος.

[Πρὸς αἱμοπτοϊκούς.] Συμφύτου ῥίζαν δὸς φαγεῖν ὅσον δύναται καὶ τῇ αὐτῇ ἡμέρᾳ ὄξος μὴ ἀπτέσθω. ἄλλο. Σαμίας γῆς ἀστέρα δίδου, ὁτὲ μὲν μετὰ πολυγόνου χυλοῦ, ὁτὲ δὲ καθ' ἑαυτό. ἔλεγε δὲ Ἱππίων ὁ Κενταύριος πρὸς

[*Ad aſthmaticos i. e. ſuſpirioſos.*] Vinum aut mulſam, ubi ſcilla decocta fuerit, propinato. Facit et pulmo vulpis ſiccatus et inciſus ex vino nigro potui datus. *Aliud.* Naſturtium album tuſum et melli mixtum lingendum exhibeto.

[*Ad ſpiritus difficultatem.*] Ovium pilos qui circum anum ſunt accipe, hosque uſtos ac tritos in paſſo propinato. *Aliud.* Sulfur ignem non expertum ex vini cyathis quatuor potui dato.

[*Ad recta cervice ſpirantes.*] Struthium ex aqua calida propinato. *Aliud.* Sedum ex melle tritum linctui dato; aut bulbum aut abrotonum aut halicam ex mulſa aut hyſſopum in mulſa coctum aut herbam ſtoechada aut caſtoreum ex dulci vino aut ſcillae intranea ex aceto mulſo.

[*Ad ſanguinem ſpuentes.*] Symphyti radici quanta poteſt vescatur, eodemque die acetum ne guſtato. *Aliud.* Terram Samiam dato interdum cum ſucco ſanguinalis, interdum per ſe. Dicebat autem Hippio Centaurius: ad

αἱμοπτοϊκούς· καλῶς ποιεῖ κνίδης χυλὸς διδόμενος σὺν οἴνῳ κυάθων γ'. ποιεῖ δ' ἐπὶ τούτῳ καὶ ὄξος ῥοφόμενον καὶ μάλιστα ὁ σκιλλίτης. ἔτι δὲ χυλὸς ἡδυόσμου καὶ τραγακάνθης ὑπὸ τὴν γλῶσσαν κατεχόμενος.

[Πρὸς τοὺς ἔκ τινος βίας εἰς τὰ ἔνδον αἱμοῤῥαγοῦντας.] Λαβὼν ἀμπελίνην σποδὸν ὄξει κατάσβεσον καὶ ἐπιχέας πλεῖον ὄξος δεῦσον καὶ διήθησον διὰ ῥάκους, καὶ μίξας ὕδατι ὀλίγῳ δὸς πιεῖν ὅσον κοχλιάρια στ'. τοῦτο καὶ στύφει τὸν αἱμοῤῥαγήσαντα τόπον καὶ τὸ πηχθὲν αἷμα καὶ βρωθὲν ἐκκρίνει καὶ ἵστησι τὴν αἱμοῤῥαγίαν. ἴσχαιμον γάρ ἐστι τῶν ἐντὸς αἱμοῤῥαγιῶν.

[Πρὸς πᾶσαν αἱμοῤῥαγίαν.] Συμφύτῳ μετ' ὄξους κατάπλασσε τὸ πρόσωπον, ἐὰν μὲν ἀπὸ μυκτῆρος ᾖ· ἐὰν δὲ ἀπὸ θώρακος τὸ στέρνον· ἐὰν δὲ ἀπὸ κύστεως ἢ μήτρας ἢ νεφρῶν καὶ τὰ ἰσχία κατάπλασσε.

[621] [Πρὸς ἀναφορικοὺς καὶ φθισικούς.] Κόμμεως τὸ μέλαν καθεψήσας διὰ γλυκέος δίδου ὑπὸ γλῶσσαν

ſanguinem ſpuentes magnifice proficit urticae ſuccus ex vini cyathis tribus epotus. Juvat praeterea acetum abſorptum praecipue ſcillinum, item et menthae ſuccus et tragacanthae ſub lingua contentus.

[*Ad eos quibus ex aliqua vi interior ſanguis erupit.*] Accipe vitis cinerem aceto exſtinctum plusque aceti ſuperfundens madefacito et per panniculum excola; id modica aqua temperatum propina cochleariorum ſex menſura; hoc et locum ſanguinem fundentem aſtringit et concretum ſanguinem devoratum excernit et cruoris profluvium compescit; nam ſanguinis in interioribus locis exitum coërcet.

[*Ad omne ſanguinis profluvium.*] Symphyton ex aceto faciei ſuperdato, ſi ex naribus ſanguis decurrat; ſi ex thorace feratur, oſſi pectoris; ſi ex veſica aut utero aut renibus, coxendicibus imponito.

[*Ad ſanguineum ſputum et tabem vel phthiſim.*] Gummi partem nigram paſſo elixam exhibe ſub lingua

κατέχειν καὶ καταπίνειν· ποιεῖ γὰρ πρὸς ἀναφορικοὺς κόμμεως τὸ μέλαν καὶ πρὸς βῆχα καλῶς.

[Φθίσιν μὴ τελείαν παῦσαι.] Πνεύμονα ἐλάφου καλάμῳ ἐξελὼν καὶ ξηράνας λειοτρίβησον καὶ δίδου κοχλιάρια γ'. μετὰ μέλιτος κυάθων γ'. εἶτα διαστήσας ὀλίγας ἡμέρας δὸς πάλιν πιεῖν.

[Ἐπὶ τῶν φθισικῶν καὶ τῶν ἀγόντων αἱμόπυα.] Χρώμεθα τῷ ταρίχῳ μετ' ἄρτου διδόντες ἐσθίειν, οὕτως βρέχοντες αὐτὸ εἰς ὕδωρ τρὶς ἢ τετράκις, ἕως οὗ πλυνόμενον τὸ ὕδωρ μὴ ἐνδιδοῖ ἅλμην εἰς αὐτὸ, ἐνδεσμεύοντες αὐτὸν εἰς χάρτην ὀπτῶμεν καὶ δίδομεν χωρὶς οἰνομέλιτος ὀλίγον ἐπιχέοντες. Ἡρόφιλος δὲ ἐπ' αὐτῷ χωρὶς τινὸς δίδωσι ταρίχους σὺν ἄρτῳ καὶ ἐπιπίνειν ὕδωρ κελεύει, λέγων ὅτι ἐπείπερ ἅλες ἐπὶ ταρίχῳ συστρέφουσι τὴν κοιλίαν, οἶνος δὲ δοθεὶς λύει. χρώμεθα δὲ καὶ σκίλλῃ ὀπτῇ καὶ μετὰ ταρίχου ἐν αὐτῇ καὶ ἀνακαθαίρονται ἰσχυρῶς. καὶ πράσοις δὲ μετὰ ἄρτου. εἶτα ὅταν δόξωσιν ἀνακεκάρθαι ἐπιμελῶς καὶ εἰ ἀσθενέστεροι ὦσιν, ἀνατρέφομεν αὐτοὺς κρέασι καὶ τοῖς

continendam ac devorandam; ad ſputum enim ſanguinis et tuſſim gummi nigra pars vehementer facit.

[*Ad phthiſim non perfectam ſanandam.*] Pulmo cervi calamo extractus et arefactus conteratur; ipſius cochlearia tria ex mellis cyathis tribus exhibeantur; deinde paucis diebus interpoſitis iterum propinetur.

[*Ad phthiſicos et purulenta ſanguineaque ſputa rejicientes.*] Utimur ſalſamento cum pane eſui dantes, ipſum ita colluentes aqua ter et quater, donec aqua ſalſa non reddatur; ipſum deinde charta involventes cremamus, damusque ſine oleo exiguum mulſi infundentes. Herophilus autem ſalſamentum cum pane exhibet; poſtea vero aquam potare jubet, dicens, quum ſal in ſalſamento alvum perturbat, vinum quidem datum ſolvit. Utimur et ſcilla toſta cum ſalſamento in ipſa et vehementer purgantur; item et porro cum pane. Poſtea quum diligenter purgati eſſe videbuntur, ſi infirmiores fuerint, ipſos carnibus et aliis id genus reficimus. Eadem ratione utimur

ὁμοίοις, τῇ αὐτῇ δ' ἀγωγῇ χρώμεθα καὶ ἐπὶ τῶν συῤῥαγέντων ἀποστημάτων ἐν τοῖς πρὸς κάθαρσιν. καὶ ἰχθὺς δὲ ἡ βοτάνη μετὰ ἀξουγγίου ἀνάλου διδομένη τρώγειν τοὺς ἀναφορικοὺς καὶ βήσσοντας ποιεῖ καλῶς.

[*Πρὸς τὴν αἵματος πτύσιν ἢ ἀναγωγήν.*] *Ποιεῖ* καὶ γῆ σφραγὶς καὶ οἱ τροχίσκοι ἐκ τοῦ ἠλέκτρου καὶ τροχίσκοι ἐκ κοραλλίου καὶ ἡ θηριακὴ ἐν κλίνῃ διδομένη.

Κεφ. ιδ'. [α'. Πρὸς πλευριτικούς.] Φλοιοῦ ῥίζης δίδου πίνειν. κυμίνου ἐπὶ τὰ ὄψα ἐπίπασον ὕδατι καὶ δὸς πιεῖν. ἄλλο. πηγάνου κλωνία ε'. δίδου λειάνας καθ' ἡμέραν. ἢ στοιχάδος βοτάνης τρισὶ δακτύλοις δίδου. τριφύλλου σπέρμα πότιζε. πάνακος ῥίζαν πότιζε. χαμαιπίτυν ὁμοίως.

[β'. Πρὸς πλευρίτιδα.] Εἰ μὲν οὖν ἄχρι κλειδὸς ἡ ὀδύνη διατείνῃ, φλεβοτομητέον αὐτούς. εἰ δὲ εἰς ὑποχόνδριον κάτω, καθαρτέον καὶ κλυσμοῖς δριμέσι χρηστέον. καὶ εἰ μὲν μέτριον ᾖ τὸ ἄλγημα, μετὰ τὸ κλύσμα δοτέον αὐτοῖς μελίκρατον καὶ τὸν πτισάνης ἢ τοῦ χόνδρου χυλόν· παρα-

in iis, quae ad purgationem attinent, ubi abſceſſus eruperint. Herba quoque piſcis vocata cum axungia non ſalita eſui data ſanguinem rejicientes ac tuſſientes mirifice adjuvat.

[*Ad ſputum ſanguinis.*] Juvat etiam terra ſigillata et trochisci ex electro et trochisci ex corallo et theriaca data in lecto.

Cap. XIV. [1. *Ad pleuriticos.*] Radicis corticem in potum exhibe. Cuminum, in obſoniis utimur, in aquam injice et bibendum praebe. *Aliud.* Rutae coliculos quinque contritos quotidie dato; aut herbae ſtoechadis quantum tribus digitis capi poteſt. Item trifolii ſemen aut panacis radicem aut ajugam ſimiliter potui dato.

[2. *Ad pleuritidem.*] Si quidem usque ad claviculam pervenerit dolor ipſis mittendus, ſanguis eſt; ſi vero ad hypochondrium deſcendat, corpus eſt purgandum et utendum clyſteribus valentibus. Si dolor fuerit moderatus, poſt clyſteres danda eſt aqua mulſa et ptiſanae cre-

κμάσαντος δὲ τοῦ πάθους, ἐμβλητέον τοῖς χυλοῖς καλαμίνθην ἢ πράσιον. ποιεῖ καὶ τῆς κνίδης σπέρμα σὺν μέλιτι. πρὸς τὰ δὲ σφοδρὰ τῶν ἀλγημάτων μετὰ τὴν κένωσιν παρηγορητέον, ὡς ταῖς διὰ κέγχρον καὶ πιτύρων ἐν μαρσίππῳ πυρίαις ἢ διὰ θερμοῦ ὕδατος ἢ ἐλαίου ἐν κύστῃ ἢ διὰ ἐρίου οἰσυπηροῦ σὺν ἐλαίῳ καὶ οἴνῳ τεθαλασμένῳ ἐπιτιθεμέναις. περὶ δὲ τὴν τετάρτην ἡμέραν θρέψον τοῖς ῥοφήμασι σὺν ὀλίγῳ μέλιτι. μετὰ δὲ τὴν ἑβδόμην καὶ τῇ πηγανερᾷ ἐμπλάστρῳ κατὰ τῶν ὀδυνωμένων χρησώμεθα τόπων. καὶ βολβοὶ δὲ σὺν ὀξυγγίᾳ τεθέντες πολλάκις ἤρκεσαν. δοτέον ἔκλεγμα διὰ στροβιλίων καὶ ἀμυγδάλων πικρῶν καὶ λινοσπέρμου καὶ ἀμύλου.

[γ'. Τὸ χρίσμα καλόν.] Λαβὼν βδέλλιον, κόστον, κράμβης καυλοὺς καυθέντας τῇ τέφρᾳ καὶ στέατι μιγισμένα. διαφορητικὸν καὶ ἰσχυρῶς ἐστὶ τὸ φάρμακον.

[622] Κεφ. ιε'. [Πρὸς τὰ μαστῶν πάθη.] [α'. Πρὸς τοὺς μαστοὺς κεκλιμένους ὀρθῶσαι.] Λαβὼν γῆν γραφικὴν, μετὰ μέλιτος ἑψήσας εἰς ῥάκος ἐπιτίθει ἀπὸ

mor aut chondri; in proceſſu vero morbi permiſcendum ſorbitioni calamentum, vel marrubium; confert etiam ſemen urticae cum melle. Ad fortiores autem dolores poſt vacuationem lenientibus utendum eſt, ſacculis e milio et furſure vel fomentis ex aqua calida aut oleo in veſica poſito vel lana ſuccida perfuſa oleo et vino habente ſal. Circa vero quartum diem ſorbitionibus cum pauco melle nutrito. Poſt ſeptimum vero diem et emplaſtro dicto rutaceo ad locos dolentes utemur. Multoties autem bulbi cum axungia ſuffecerunt. Dandum eſt et eclegma, quod fit ex nucleis pineis et amygdalis amaris et ſemine lini et amylo.

[3. *Unguentum bonum.*] Accipe bdellium, coſtum, cauliculos braſſicae uſtos et redactos in cinerem, permiſce cum adipe; hoc enim medicamentum praeclare discutit.

Cap. XV. [*Ad mammarum affectus.*] [1. *Ad extollendas diſtendendasque mammas pendulas ac flaccidas.*] Recipe terram pictorum et cum melle elixam panniculo illitam imponito a ſummo mane usque ad veſpe-

Ed. Chart. X. [622.]

ὄρθρου ἕως ἑσπέρας. εἶτα σπόγγον ἐκ χύτρας ἐπιτίθει, ἕως ἀποσπάσῃς τὸ κατάπλασμα. ποιεῖ δὲ τοῦτο καὶ ὀρθοὺς καὶ τεταμένους. κατάπλασσε δὲ ἐπὶ πάχος, ἐὰν θέλῃς ἐνεργότερον αὐτὸ ποιῆσαι κηκῖδος ὀμφακίτιδος γο. ι'.

[β'. *Μαστοὺς μένειν ἁπαλοὺς ἐπὶ πολλὰ ἔτη.*] Κωνείῳ κατάπλασσε καρυϊστίῳ.

[γ'. *Μαστοὺς μείζονας μὴ γίνεσθαι.*] Χοῖρον ἐκτεμὼν τῷ αἵματι κατάχριε τοὺς μαστοὺς καὶ οὐκ αὔξονται.

[δ'. *Πρὸς τὸ ξηραίνειν τὸ γάλα.*] Κρητάριον λειωθὲν ὄξει καὶ καταχρισθὲν καὶ ἐπιτιθέμενα τὸ γάλα ἵστησι.

[ε'. *Πρὸς φλεγμονὴν ἢ ἀπόστημα τῶν μαστῶν.*] Κιμωλίαν, λίβανον καὶ ἔλαιον ῥόδινον διαμίξας ἐπιτίθει. ἄλλο. κατ' ἀρχὰς μὲν σπόγγον ἁπαλὸν ὀξυκράτῳ χλιαρῷ βρέξας καὶ ἐκπιάσας ἐπιτίθει καὶ ἐπιδέσμει. ἄλλο. φοίνικας καὶ ἄρτου ψίχιον συντρίψας ὀξυκράτῳ καὶ χλιαρὸν ἐπιτίθει. ἄλλο. κορίαννον, στυπτηρίαν καὶ ψύλλιον μετὰ κηρωτῆς ἐπιτίθει. ἄλλο. ἄρτον μετὰ περδικιάδος χλωρᾶς ἅμα κηρωτῇ ἐπιτίθετι τὴν ἡμέραν. ἄλλο. ἄρτον σὺν μελικράτῳ ἢ μέλιτι ἢ οἴνῳ

ram; deinde ſpongiam ex olla ſuperpone, quoad cataplasma abduxeris; hoc autem et erectas et turgidas mammas facit; craſſius autem cataplasma imponas, ſi vis ipſum efficacius reddere, gallae acerbae uncia una misceatur.

[2. *Ut mammae plures annos molles ſint.*] Ex cicuta cariſtia cataplasma facito.

[3. *Ut mammae majores non ſiant.*] Porcellum diſſecans cruore mammas obline; amplius non augeſcent.

[4. *Ad lac ſiccandum.*] Cretarium aceto maceratum, illitum et impoſitum lac areſacit.

[5. *Ad phlegmonem ſeu abſceſſum mammarum.*] Cimoliam, thus et oleum roſatum permiſce et appone. *Aliud.* Principio inſunde ſpongiam mollem in poſca tepida et exprime et appone et ſuperliga. *Aliud.* Palmulas et micam panis tere, permisce cum posca et appone tepidum. *Aliud.* Coriandrum, alumen et pſyllium cum cerato appone. *Aliud.* Panem et herbam muralem viridem cum cerato imponito per diem. *Aliud.* Panem cum aqua mulſa

κατάπλασσε. εἰ δὲ μὴ φέροιεν τὸ βάρος καταβροχῇ διὰ γλυκέος ἐλαίου χρηστέον θερμοῦ δι' ἐρίων τρυφερῶν. πυριατέον δὲ αὐτοὺς ἀτμῷ θερμοῦ ὕδατος ἢ ἀφεψήματι τήλεως ἢ ἀλθαίας ἢ σελινοσπέρμου.

[στ'. *Πρὸς ἐφέλκειν τὸ γάλα.*] Ῥάφανον σὺν πιτύροις ἐν οἴνῳ ἑψήσας καὶ ἠθήσας δίδου πίνειν. ἄλλο. σήσαμον σὺν οἴνῳ γλυκεῖ δίδου πίνειν. ἄλλο. ἄνητον ἢ αὐτοῦ σπέρμα ἑψήσας σὺν σαρξὶ ἢ τοῖς τὴν γάλακτος εὐπορίαν ποιέουσιν. ἄλλο. πίτυρα σὺν ῥίζαις τοῦ μαράθρου ἑψήσας ἐν ὕδατι δίδου πίνειν. ἄλλο. μελανθίνου < α'. τίθετι ἐν μελικράτῳ καὶ δίδου. ἄλλο. πράσον ἑψήσας ἐν ὕδατι καὶ δίδου πίνειν αὐτοῦ ἀφέψημα. ἢ πράσον τρίψας καὶ ἠθήσας δίδωτι τὸ ὕδωρ πίνειν. ἄλλο. χυλὸν μαράθρου δίδου πίνειν. ἄλλο. ῥίζαν μαράθρου καὶ ῥηθὴν κεκαυμένην ἑψήσας ἐν ὕδατι καὶ τὸ βούτυρον διαμίξας δίδου πίνειν. ἄλλο. ἀφέψημα ἱππομαράθρου δίδου πίνειν. ἢ δίδου καὶ κατεσθίειν αὐτὸν ἱππομάραθρον. ἄλλο. καρδάμωμον σὺν οἴνῳ δίδου πίνειν. ἄλλο. σπέρμα τοῦ ἄγνου δίδου σὺν οἴνῳ

vel melle et vino admoveto; ſi vero non tolerant gravitatem mammae, perſunde oleo calido et lana ſuccida molli, fovendum vero ipſas decoctione foenigraeci vel althaeae vel ſeminis lini.

[6. *Ad attrahendum lac.*] Raphanum cum furfuribus in vino coque, cola et propina. *Aliud.* Seſamum ex vino dulci da potui. *Aliud.* Anethum vel ſemen ejus coque cum carnibus vel cum ſacientibus lactis copiam. *Aliud.* Furfures cum radicibus foeniculi coque in aqua et da potui. *Aliud.* Nigellae drach. j, pone in mulſa et propina. *Aliud.* Porrum coque in aqua et da bibendum ejus decoctum. Vel porrum tere et cola et da aquam potui. *Aliud.* Succum foeniculi da bibendum. *Aliud.* Radicem foeniculi et hordeum aſſum coque in aqua et permiſce butyrum et da bibendum. *Aliud.* Decoctum erratici foeniculi da bibendum: da etiam eſui ipſum foeniculum. *Aliud.* Cardamomum cum vino da potui. *Aliud.* Semen viticis da cum vino bibendum. *Aliud.* Succum

πίνειν. ἄλλο. χυλὸν τεύτλου δίδου πινόμενον. δεῖ δὲ τοῖς δριμέσι καὶ ἁλμυροῖς καὶ ὀξέσι καὶ λαχάνοις ἀπέπτοις ἀπέχεσθαι.

[ζ'. Πρὸς κωλύειν τὸ γάλα.] Μαστοὺς τῷ ὕδατι θαλασσίῳ πυριάσας καὶ αὐτοῖς τὰ στυπτικά τε καὶ ξηραντικὰ πρόσθες.

[η'. Διαφυλακτικὰ μαστῶν, οἷς αὐταὶ διὰ πολλοῦ τεταμέναι καταμένουσι.] Κιόνιον λεάνας μαστῷ ἐπιτίθει ἐπὶ ἡμέρας θ'. καὶ τὸ σπόγγον ἔξωθεν τῷ ὀξυκράτῳ βρεχόμενον. ἄλλο. κύμινον σὺν ὕδατι τρίψας κατάπλαττε τοὺς τιτθοὺς, εἶτα ἔξωθεν ἐπιθεὶς σπόγγον ἀπὸ ὀξυκράτου σφίγγε τὸ στῆθος δεσμίδι· μετὰ δὲ τρεῖς ἡμέρας τὸ κύμινον ἄρας κατάπλαττε τοὺς τιτθοὺς κρίνου βολβῶν μετὰ μέλιτος· καὶ δήσας πάλιν ἔα τρεῖς ἡμέρας. καὶ τοῦτο ποίει τρεῖς τοῦ μηνός.

[623] Κεφ. ιστ'. [Πρὸς δυσώδεις ἱδρῶτας καὶ μασχάλας.] Ἀσάρῳ χρῖε τὰς μασχάλας ἀπὸ βαλανείου καὶ πρωῒ καθ' ἡμέραν. ἢ στυπτηρίαν ὑγρὰν κατάχριε καθ' ἡμέραν. ἢ ὠκίμου σπέρμα δι' οἴνου καὶ μέλιτος κατάχριε· τοῦτο αἴρει τὰς δυσωδίας τῶν μασχαλῶν. ἢ κονίαν πρόσπλασσε λεπτήν. ἄλλο. μολύβδαινον καύσας καὶ οἴνῳ εὐώδει κατα-

betae da bibendum. Oportet autem abſtinere ab acribus et ſalſis et acidis et oleribus crudis.

[7. *Ad prohibendum lac.*] Fove mammas ex aqua marina et eis admove aſtringentia et ſiccantia.

[8. *Mammas conſervantia, quibus hae remanent tenſae diu.*] Cicutam mammae imponito per dies novem ſpongiamque posca madentem ſuperdato. *Aliud.* Cuminum terens impone cum aqua, deinde ſpongiam perſuſam posca ſuperappone et liga; poſt tres autem dies aufer cuminum et tege mammillas cum radice lilii et melle et dimitte tribus diebus et hoc fac ter in menſe.

Cap. XVI. [*Ad foetidos ſudores et axillarum tetros odores.*] Aſaro axillas ſubline a balneo et ſummo mane quotidie. Aut alumine liquido perunge quotidie. Aut ocimi ſemine ex vino et melle illinito; hoc odores foedos axillarum discutit. Aut pulverem tenuem admove. *Aliud.* Plumbaginem uſtam et vino odoro extinctam cum

σβέσας τρῖβε μετ' οἴνου ὀλίγον σμύρνης ἐπιβάλλων ἄχρι γλοιοῦ πάχους καὶ χρῶ.

Κεφ. ιζ'. [α'. Πρὸς στομαχικούς.] Κεδρίας κοχλιάρια δύο, ἐλαίου ὠμοτριβοῦς κύαθον ἴσα μίξας δὸς ῥοφῆσαι. τοῦτο πάντα πόνον παντελῶς ἀποθεραπεύει. ἔστι δὲ τοῦ Σεραπίωνος ἀπαράβατον. ἄλλο. ἄνισον εἰς ὀθόνιον ἐνδήσας κάθυγρον καὶ ἀποβρέξας εἰς ὕδωρ θερμὸν δίδου καταῤῥοφεῖν.

[β'. Πρὸς ἀτόνους καὶ ναυτιῶντας.] Ἡδυόσμου κλῶνας β'. ἢ γ'. ῥοᾶς γλυκείας χυλῷ καὶ ὄξει ἀναζέσας δὸς καταῤῥοφεῖν. ἄλλο. ἀκτέος τὰ ἁπαλὰ φύλλα καθαρίως διὰ ὕδατος δίδου πιεῖν, ἀπαράβατόν ἐστι.

[γ'. Πρὸς δηγμοὺς ἄνευ τοῦ ἀναχεῖσθαί τι χολῶδες.] Τραγορίγανον λεάνας ἐν ὕδατι. ἴσα δίδου καταῤῥοφεῖν γαλακτῶδες ποιῶν τὸ κρᾶμα.

[δ'. Πρὸς τὰς τοῦ στομάχου ἀτονίας.] Σίνηπι πεφρυγμένον λεῖον μετὰ ὕδατος δίδου πίνειν.

[ε'. Ἐπίθεμα πρὸς στομαχικοὺς καὶ ὑποχονδριακούς.]

extinctam cum vino terito, modica myrrha adjecta, donec ſtrigmentitia fiat craſſitudo, et utitor.

Cap. XVII. [1. *Ad vitio ſtomachi laborantes.*] Cedri liquoris cochlearia duo, olei immaturi cyathum in unum miſcens ſorbendum dato; id omnem dolorem funditus tollit: eſt autem id Serapionis exploratiſſimum. *Aliud.* Aniſum in panniculo ſucci plenum deligato et in aquam calidam conjicito et ſorbere jubeto.

[2. *Ad imbecillos et nauſeantes.*] Menthae coliculos duos aut tres mali punici dulcis ſucco, atque aceto inferveſaciens ſorptui dato. *Aliud.* Sambuci tenera folia ex munda aqua bibantur, probatiſſimum eſt.

[3. *Ad morſus ventriculi ſine bilis vomitu.*] Tragoriganum in aqua pari pondere macerans ſorbendum exhibeto, lactis faciens temperaturam.

[4. *Ad ſtomachi imbecillitates.*] Sinapi frictum ex aqua tritum potui dato.

[5. *Epithema ad ſtomachi hypochondriorumque vitio*

Ed. Chart. X. [623.]
Τρύγα ξηρὰν ἀναλάμβανε κηρωτῇ ἢ μυρσίνῃ ἢ ῥοδίνῃ, καὶ χρῶ.

[στ΄. Πρὸς λυγμόν.] Ἐὰν ἅπαξ ἐπαίσθῃ τοῦ λυγμοῦ, τὸν δάκτυλόν σου τῆς ἀριστερᾶς χειρὸς τὸν ἀσπαστικὸν τρὶς κράτησον, ἢ ὄξος ἐπιῤῥοφησάτω, ὥστε καὶ κύμινον καὶ χόνδρον· ἢ ἐμεσάτω καὶ παύσεται· ἢ πνεύματος κατοχὴν ποιείτω· ἢ πταρμοῖς χρήσθω· ἢ πήγανον μετὰ οἴνου πινέτω· ψωμὸν ἐν ὄξει δεύσας καταπινέτω· ἢ ὀστάριον χοίρειον τῇ χειρὶ ἀνατριβέτω. παύει δὲ τοὺς λυγμοὺς καὶ ἔκπληξις.

[ζ΄. Πρὸς τὴν τοῦ στομάχου ὀδύνην.] Καστόριον δίδου πίνειν δι᾽ ὀξυκράτου· καὶ εἰ μὲν φύσημα τὸ αἴτιον ᾖ, ἑψήσας ἐν ἐλαίῳ κύμινον, δαύκου σπέρμα καὶ πετροσέλινον κατάχριε· εἰ δὲ τὸ ψῦχος, ἕψε τὰς ἐν ἐλαίῳ δαφνίδας καὶ πήγανον καὶ μελάνθιον καὶ μαράθρου σπέρμα. ἐπὶ δὲ τῆς μέσης ὀδύνης ποίει τὰ πυρία διὰ κέγχρων. ὠφελεῖ σικύα εὐμεγέθης περιλαμβάνουσα τὸν ὀμφαλόν.

[η΄. Πρὸς ἀτονίαν στομάχου.] Ὠφελεῖ ἔλαιον μήλινον ἢ διὰ χυλοῦ τῶν ῥόδων. ἄλλο. τὸ σινήπεως σπέρμα κεκαυ-

laborantes.] Faecem aridam cerato myrteo aut rosaceo excipe et utere.

[6. *Ad singultum.*] Quum semel singultum sensit, digitum tuum sinistrae manus salutatorium ter ore contineto; aut acetum ei sorbendum dato aut cuminum et alicam; aut vomat; et singultus sedabitur; aut spiritum contineat; aut sternutatione utatur, aut rutam ex vino bibat; aut micam panis aceto madentem bibito; aut porcelli ossiculum manu atterito. Singultus quoque terror incussus finit.

[7. *Ad dolorem stomachi.*] Castoreum da bibendum cum posca et si est status causa, coque in oleo cuminum et semen dauci et petroselinum et unge, et si est frigus, coque in oleo baccas lauri et rutam et nigellam et semen foeniculi. In moderatis autem doloribus fac fomentum cum milio. Confert etiam cucurbitula magna umbilico imposita.

[8. *Ad debilitatem stomachi.*] Confert oleum de succo cotoneorum. *Aliud.* Semen sinapis ustulatum tere

Ed. Chart. XIII. [623. 624.]

μένον τρίψας καὶ σὺν ὕδατι δίδου πίνειν. ἄλλο. λαβὼν μαστίχης, ἀλόης, στύρακος ἀνὰ μέρη β'. ἀψινθίου, οἰνάνθης ἀνὰ μέρη γ'. μηλίνου μέρη δ'. οἴνου τὸ ἀρκοῦν, ῥόδων μέρη β'. ταῦτα λειούμενα ἀναλαμβάνεται πορφύρᾳ ἢ ἐρίῳ καὶ ἐπιτίθεται τῷ στομάχῳ. τινὲς καὶ κῦφι καλούμενον, τινὲς δὲ καὶ κηρὸν προσπλέξαντες κηρωτὴν ποιοῦσιν. ἄλλο. ἡδυόσμου κλῶνας β'. ἢ γ'. ἐν τῷ ῥοιᾶς γλυκείας χυλῷ καὶ τῷ ὄξει δίδου πίνειν.

[624] Κεφ. ιη'. [α'. Πρὸς χολέραν καὶ ἔμετον καὶ εἰλεὸν καὶ κόπρον ἐμοῦντας.] Ὀλβίνος οἶνος ἐπὶ τῶν χολερικῶν εὔθετός ἐστι· καὶ γὰρ εὐστόμαχος καὶ πρὸς κοιλίαν ποιῶν.

[β'. Ἔμετον παῦσαι.] Πολυγόνου χυλῷ χρῖε τὰ ἐσθιόμενα. ἄλλο. ἀψίνθιον ἑψήσας ἐν ὕδατι, εἰς τρίτον μέρος καθεψηθέντος πιεῖν, πρὸς τὴν ἕξιν ἀποβλέπων. ἢ κενταυρίου ἢ θύμου ἢ μυρτίδας μελαίνας.

[γ'. Ὥστε ἐμέσαι ἀλύπως.] Σαμψύχου φύλλα δὸς φαγεῖν. ἄλλο. στακτῇ κονίᾳ χρῖε τὸ ἔσχατον ποτήριον.

et ex aqua propina. *Aliud.* Recipe maſtiches, aloes, ſtyracis ana partes ij, abſinthii, oenanthes ana partes tres, olei melini partes quatuor, vini quod ſufficit, roſarum partes duas; haec trita et mixta aſſume ex purpura aut lana et appone ſtomacho. Quidam addunt cyphi vocatum; quidam apponunt ceram et ceratum faciunt. *Aliud.* Menthae ramos duos vel tres coque in ſucco punici dulcis et aceto ac potui dato.

Cap. XVIII. [*Ad choleram et vomitum et volvulum et vomitum ſtercoris.*] Vinum olbinum in cholera ex uſu eſt; ſtomacho enim commodat et ad ventrem bene facit.

[2. *Ad vomitum ſedandum.*] Sanguinalis ſucco cibos inficito. *Aliud.* Abſinthium in aqua ad tertias decoctum potui dato, habitum aegroti conſiderans. Centaurium praeterea aut thymum aut nigras myrti baccas ſimiliter exhibeto.

[3. *Ut facilis ſit vomitus.*] Sampſuci folia eſui dato. *Aliud.* Lixivio percolato oras poculi oblinito.

Ed. Chart. X. [624.]

[δ'. *Πρὸς εἰλεὸν θαυμαστὸν καὶ κόπρον ἐμοῦσι.*] Ποίησον οὕτω. ἑψήσας ἔλαιον ἐξ ἀνήθου δὸς πιεῖν· ἕως δὲ τοῦτο ἑψηθῇ, αὐτὸν εἰς θερμὸν καχλάζον ἔμβαλε καὶ μετὰ τὸ πιεῖν τὸ ἔλαιον θερμοὺς τοὺς ψωμοὺς δὸς φαγεῖν. σωθήσεται καὶ ἐὰν ἤδη πνίγεται. τούτῳ ἔσωσα ἡγεμόνα κατὰ τὴν ἡμετέραν Ἀσίαν.

[ε'. *Πρὸς τοὺς πυκνὰ ἐμοῦντας.*] Ῥοῦν καὶ κύμινον τρίψας ἐν τῷ αὐτῷ δὸς πίνειν ὀξυμέλιτι κυάθων στ'. οὐγγίαν α'.

[στ'. *Πρὸς χολερικοὺς λίαν καλόν.*] Ἡδύοσμον ἐν οἴνῳ δὸς πιεῖν, ἐὰν ἀπύρετος ᾖ. καὶ βοτάνην πενταδάκτυλον ξηράνας δὸς πιεῖν. λειάνας ἐν οἴνῳ διὰ κυάθων ζ'. ἢ διὰ ὕδατος θερμοῦ κυάθων β'. εὐθέως ἄπονος ἔσται. ἄλλο. κοχλίαν τρίψας σὺν τῷ κελύφει δίδου πιεῖν.

[ζ'. *Πρὸς τὴν τῶν ἐμέτων ἐποχήν.*] Ἀμπέλων φύλλα καὶ ἕλικας χυλίσας μετὰ ἀλφίτων δίδου πιεῖν νήστει ἐν ὕδατι κοχλιάριον ἕν. ἄλλο. πάνακος ὀβολὸν ἐν οἴνῳ καὶ ἐλαίῳ θερμῷ πότιζε.

[4. *Ad volvulum mirum auxilium et ad ſtercus vomentes.*] Ita facito. Oleum, in quo anethum decoctum ſit, propinato; quoad autem elixetur, aegrotum in calidam aquam demitte et ab olei potu calidas micas eſui concedito; ſervabitur enim etiamſi jam ſtranguletur. Hoc ego principem in noſtra Aſia ſervavi.

[5. *Ad eos qui crebro vomunt.*] Rhun et cuminum in unum contundens da ex aceti mulſi cyathis ſex unciam j, in potum.

[6. *Ad cholera vexatos valde efficax.*] Mentha ex vino ſumpta, ſi febris abſit, herba quinquefolia arida trita ex vini cyathis ſeptem aut ex aquae calentis cyathis duobus pota ſtatim dolorem levat. *Aliud.* Cochlea cum teſta contuſa potui danda eſt.

[7. *Ad ſupprimendum vomitum.*] Foliorum et capreolorum vitis ſuccus cum polenta jejuno in potum detur ex aqua cochlearii menſura. *Aliud.* Panacis obolum ex vino et oleo calido propinato.

Κεφ. ιθ'. [*Πρὸς ἡπατικούς.*] *Πετροσελίνου σπέρματος κοχλιάριον α'. ἡδύοσμον πασσόμενον καὶ πινόμενον ὠφελεῖ. ἄλλο. ἡ καλουμένη ἄκαπνος βοτάνη κλυθεῖσα καὶ εἰς τροχίσκους ἀναπλασθεῖσα καὶ ξηρανθεῖσα ἀπονίαν παρέχει· τρίτον δὲ ποθεῖσα μεθ' ὕδατος ἀπαλλάσσει. ἄλλο. λύκου ἧπαρ διδόμενον ὠφελεῖ ὁλκῇ δηναρίου διὰ γλυκέος ξέστου. ἄλλο. πεπέρεως λευκοῦ κόκκους θ'. καὶ σμύρνης μέγεθος καρύου Ποντικοῦ, τρίψας πάντα ὁμοῦ, αἰθρίου ὄντος παρὰ μίαν ποιήσεις ἡμέραν ἢ τρεῖς. ἄλλο. ἧπαρ ἵππου ἀπόθου ἐν κεδρίνῳ γλωσσοκόμῳ. καὶ ἀπὸ τούτου δίδου μετὰ οἴνου Χίου καὶ ὕδατος. οἷς τὸ ἧπαρ ἥλκωται καὶ νομὴν ἴσχει. ἄλλο. μαλάχης χύλισμα πινόμενον μετὰ μέλιτος ἡπατικοὺς ἰᾶται. ἄλλο. ἀσφοδέλου ῥίζα πινομένη ἰᾶται πόνους ἥπατος. ἄλλο. λευκόϊον πινόμενον ἐπὶ ἡπατικῶν ἔξεστιν εὐθὺς ἀπόνους ποιεῖν.*

[*'Επίθεμα πρὸς ἡπατικούς.*] *Σίλφιον κόψας ἀναλάμβανε ἀξουγγίῳ παλαιῷ καὶ ἐμπλάσας εἰς ὀθόνην ἐπιτίθει. ἄλλο. σῦκον ἐν μελικράτῳ ἑψήσας καὶ λειάνας μίσγε. ἀψίν-*

Cap. XIX. [*Ad hepaticos.*] Petroſelini ſeminis cochleario mentha inſperſa et epota proficit. *Aliud.* Herba fumaria vocata in ſuccum ſoluta et in paſtillos redacta aridaque indolentiam praebet; ter autem ex aqua pota liberat. *Aliud.* Lupi jecur denarii pondere ex paſſi ſextario exhibitum bene facit. *Aliud.* Piperis albi grana novem et myrrhae quod avellanae magnitudinem aequat, omnia una contuſa ſereno caelo alternis exhibeto ter aut quater. *Aliud.* Equi jecur penu cedrino reponito; deinde Chio vino et aqua dilutum exhibeto; quibus enim jecur ulceratum eſt, ne amplius exedatur, efficitur. *Aliud.* Malvae ſuccus ex melle potus hepaticis medetur. *Aliud.* Haſtulae regiae radix pota jecinoris dolores levat. *Aliud.* Alba viola pota confeſtim hepaticos dolore liberat.

[*Epithema hepaticis commodum.*] Laſerpitium contuſum veteri axungia comprehende et linteolo illitum ſuperimpone. *Aliud.* Fico in mulſa decocto et trito abſin-

θιον λεῖον εἰς πλεῖστον καὶ χρῶ. [625] ἄλλο. κράμβη ὠμὴ καταπλασσομένη ὠφελεῖ ἡπατικοὺς ἐν τάχει.

Κεφ. κ'. [Πρὸς ἰκτερικοὺς καὶ νεφριτικοὺς καὶ λιθάρια μικρὰ ἐξουροῦντας.] Ἀκάνθου ῥίζας ὃ καλεῖται Ῥωμαϊστὶ τρικαρδουμαίας χλωρὰς γ'. ἐὰν δὲ μὴ, ξηρὰς δ'. μεθ' ὕδατος ἕψει ἕως ἥμισυ λειφθῇ καὶ τὴν ῥίζαν ἐκθλίψας δίδου τὸ ὕδωρ πιεῖν.

[Πρὸς ἴκτερον καλὸν λίαν καὶ ἐπὶ πολλῶν πεπειραμένον.] Ῥαφάνους χλωροὺς σὺν τοῖς φύλλοις λειώσας, τοῦ χυλοῦ μετὰ οἴνου κυάθου α'. ἢ δύο, πότιζε δὲ πρὸ τοῦ βαλανείου, ἐὰν νῆστις ᾖ. καὶ εἰς τὸ θερμὸν ἐμβαίνειν ποίει. ὄψει γὰρ τὸν ἴκτερον εἰς τὸ ὕδωρ ἐπιπλέοντα. ἐὰν δὲ πλείονα νόσον ἔχῃ, τοῦ χυλοῦ δίδου πιεῖν ἢ ἀγχούσης τῆς ῥίζης ξηρᾶς κοχλιάρια β'. λαβὼν μεθ' ὕδατος κυάθων γ'. δίδου πίνειν· ἢ θείου ἀπύρου κοχλιάρια δ'. δίδου ἐν οἴνῳ ἢ βράθυος γο. α'. μετὰ οἰνομέλιτος δίδου πίνειν. ἐγὼ μέντοι καὶ τοιούτῳ χρῶμαι ἐναργῶς ποιοῦντι. ἀφρονί-

thium contufum quamplurimum admifceto et utitor. *Aliud.* Braffica cruda fuperdata hepaticis celeriter opitulatur.

Cap. XX. [*Ad arquatos.*] Radices acanthi, quod Romani tricardumaeam vocant, virides tres aut aridas quatuor in aqua decoquito, donec dimidium relictum fit et expreffis radicibus aquam potui dato.

[*Ad auriginem valde efficax medicamentum et longa experientia comprobatum.*] Raphanos virides cum foliis contunde et unius duorumve fuccum ex vini cyatho uno exhibeto, ante balneum vero, fi jejunus fuerit, propinato et in calidum folium defcendere jubeto, videbis enim auriginem aquae fupernatantem. Quod fi contumacior morbus fuerit, fuccum propina. Aut anchufae radicis aridae cochlearia duo accipiens ex aquae cyathis tribus potandam dato. Aut fulfuris ignem non experti cochlearia quatuor ex vino. Aut herbae fabinae unciam ex mulfo. Ego fane et hoc utor vehementer faciente. Recipe aphronitri uncias ij, in vini Aminaei cyathis duo-

τρου γο. β'. βρέχων ἐν οἴνῳ Ἀμιναίῳ κυάθων β'. καὶ ἐξαιθριάσας τὴν νύκτα ὅλην δίδωμι νήστει πιεῖν· ποιῶ δὲ τοῦτο τριῶν ἡμερῶν ἢ δ'. ἐφεξῆς καὶ ἰῶμαι. ἄλλο. βοτάνην ὑπερικὸν καὶ ἀδίαντον ἐν ὕδατι ἑψήσας δὸς πιεῖν. ἄλλο. μυρίκην μετ' ὄξους τρίψας δὸς πιεῖν, ἰᾶται ἰκτερικούς. ἀπάγων εἰς βαλανεῖον τὸν ἰκτερικὸν καὶ ἐμβιβάσας εἰς τὴν ἐμβατὴν δίδου σχοίνου ἄνθος γο. ιβ'. μετ' οἰνομέλιτος κυάθων γ'. πιεῖν, βάψει τὴν μακρὰν καὶ ἀπαλλαγήσεται. ἄλλο. βοτάνῃ ῥυβίᾳ χρώμενος τῇ καθημερινῇ διαίτῃ χωρὶς χοιρείου κρέως, κόψας ταύτην καὶ σήσας, δίδου ἐπὶ ἡμέρας στ'. τῇ α'. κοχλιάριον μετὰ κοχλιαρίων δ'. οἴνου. εἶτα προσαφαιρῶν τοῦ οἴνου δὸς κοχλιάρια θ'. εἶτα η'. εἶτα ζ'. εἶτα στ'. εἶτα ε'. εἶτα δ'. εἶτα γ'. ἐὰν δὲ τῇ λ'. εἴη κατάλειμμα, δίδου τὰ αὐτὰ ὁμοίως ποιῶν. ἄλλο. ἀνθεμὶς σὺν ὕδατι πινομένη ἴκτερον ἀποκαταστήσει καὶ ἡπατικοῖς ἄκρως ποιεῖ. ἄλλο. στρούθιον μετὰ μέλιτος καὶ γάλακτος ἰᾶται πινόμενον. ἄλλο. ὀνίσκοι οἱ ὑπὸ τῆς ὑδρίας γεννώμενοι, λεῖοι δι' οἰνομέλιτος πινόμενοι ἰῶνται ἴκτερον. ἄλλο. ἕρπυλλον ἑφθὸν σὺν ὕδατι

bus macerans ſub dioque noctem integram exponens do jejuno potandum; idque facio per tres aut quatuor continuos dies et ſanitatem reſtituo. *Aliud.* Herbam hypericon et adianton aquae incoctam potandam offeras. *Aliud.* Myricam ex aceto tritam potui da, arquatos curat. Icterum in balneum abducens et in ſolium deſcendere jubens junci odorati uncias duas ex vini mulſi cyathis tribus potui exhibe; diſcutiet longam auriginem et liberabit. *Aliud.* Herba rubia utere in quotidiano victu absque carne ſuilla; ipſam contundens et cribrans da usque in ſextum diem cochlearium unum ex vini iv, cochleariis; deinde ſemper ſubtrahens dato vini cochlearia novem, deinde octo, deinde ſeptem, poſtea ſex, poſtea quinque, deinde quatuor, deinde tria: quod ſi trigeſimo die fuerint aliquae morbi reliquiae, eandem exhibeto ſimilem ordinem ſervans. *Aliud.* Chamaemelum ex aqua potum icterum pellit et jecinoroſis vehementer auxiliatur. *Aliud.* Radicula ex melle et lacte pota medetur. *Aliud.* Aſelli ſub

Ed. Chart. X. [625. 626.]

πινόμενον ἀποκαταστήσει ἰκτερικούς. ἄλλο. θεῖον ἄπυρον δι' οἴνου πινόμενον θεραπεύει ἴκτερον, ὅσον κοχλιάριον α'. καὶ β'. λαμβανόμενον τοῦ σιδήρου ἰὸς καταστήσει ἐν τάχει. ἄλλο. αἰγὸς βοσκάδος ἄφοδον ξηράνας, κόψας σῆσον, δὸς νήστει λουσαμένῳ, οἴνῳ εὐώδει κυάθους δ'. κοχλιάριον μὴ δειπνήσαντος· πυρέσσουσι δὲ δι' ὕδατος τὸ αὐτὸ πλῆθος. ἄλλο. χολῆς ἀρκείας ὅσον κύαμον Ἑλληνικὸν δίδου, εἶτα ὕδωρ ἐπιπινέτω. ἄλλο. βράθυος κύαθον α'. μετ' οἰνομέλιτος πινόμενον ἰᾶται ἴκτερον. ἄλλο. λίβανον ἀφέψων τῷ ὕδατι πότιζε. ἄλλο. γῆς ἔντερον λειοτριβήσας δίδου πιεῖν. ἄλλο. ἀριστολοχίας δι' ὑδρομέλιτος πότιζε. ἄλλο. κιχωρίου χυλοῦ κυάθους δ'. δὸς πιεῖν καὶ ἰαθήσεται. ἄλλο. εἰς τὸν μέσον οἶκον τοῦ βαλανείου ἱδρώσειν ἐμβίβασον καὶ ἐξελθὼν ἀπο- [626] θήσει. ἄλλο. κυνείας λευκῆς τῆς καλουμένης γενούβεως κοχλιάριον α'. μετ' οἴνου καλοῦ κυάθων γ'. δίδου πιεῖν ἐπὶ ἡμέρας ι'. ποιεῖ δὲ καὶ πρὸς κωλικοὺς καὶ πνευματώσεις ὁμοίως.

aquariis vaſis reperti, triti, ex mulſo poti regio morbo liberant. *Aliud.* Serpillum aquae incoctum et potui datum auriginem ſubmovet. *Aliud.* Sulſur ignem non expertum menſura unius cochlearii aut duorum ex vino potum arquatum curat. *Aliud.* Ferri aerugo cito liberat. *Aliud.* Capreae ſtercus aridum tritum cribratum cochlearii menſura ex vini odorati cyathis quatuor jejuno et loto exhibe; febricitantibus autem ex aqua eandem portionem. *Aliud.* Urſini fellis quantum Graecam fabam aequat, exhibeto, deinde aquam ſuperbibito *Aliud* Sabinae cyathus ex mulſo potus hoc morbo liberat *Aliud* Thus aquae incoctum propinato. *Aliud.* Terreſtrem lumbricum tritum potui dato *Aliud.* Ariſtolochiam ea aqua mulſa exhibeto. *Aliud.* Cichorii ſucci cyathos quatuor ſi biberit, ſanabitur. *Aliud.* In medium balnei conclave deſcendere jubeto, ut ſudet, et egreſſus ſanus erit. *Aliud.* Stercoris canini albi, quod genubeos vocant, cochlearium ex vini optimi cyathis tribus per dies decem propinato Hoc idem ad colicos dolores et inflationes pariter proficit.

Ed. Chart. X. [626.]

[*Ἔῤῥινον πρὸς ἰκτερικούς.*] *Ἐλατήριον ὅσον κύαμον Ἑλληνικὸν διεὶς γάλακτι γυναικείῳ εἰς τοὺς μυκτῆρας ἔγχει. ἄλλο. μελάνθιον ἑψήσας ἐγχυμάτιζε τοὺς μυκτῆρας ἐν βαλανείῳ, ἐκχεῖ τὸν ἴκτερον.*

Κεφ. κα'. [*Πρὸς σπληνικούς.*] *Λαπάθου ἀγρίου ῥίζαν κόψας ἐν ὅλμῳ καὶ τρίψας τὸν χυλὸν δίδου πιεῖν ἐπὶ ἡμέρας γ'. ἀνὰ κύαθον α'. ἄλλο. πάνακος ῥίζαν κόψας δὸς νήστει ἐν ὕδατι θερμῷ κυάθων γ'. κοχλιάριον α'.*

[*Πρὸς σπληνικοὺς, κᾂν ὦσιν ἐσκιῤῥωμένοι.*] *Λαβὼν καππάρεως ῥίζης τοῦ φλοιοῦ γο. β'. ὄξους κοτύλης τὸ ἥμισυ, ὕδατος κοτύλην α'. ἕψει ἕως εἰς τρίτον κατέλθῃ μέρος καὶ δίδου εὐπέπτῳ ὄντι κύαθον α'. ἢ β'. καὶ τοῦτο ποίει ἐκ διαστημάτων. ἄλλο. κισσοῦ φύλλα ἑψήσας ἐν ὄξει καὶ κόψας, ἔκθλιψον τὸ ὑγρὸν, κᾂν ἰσχυρὸς ᾖ, ἄκρατον αὐτῷ δίδου πιεῖν. τοῖς δὲ τῶν τρυφερωτέρων ὕδωρ ἐπιμίσγων τῷ χυλῷ. δεῖ μὲν πρὸ τοῦ πίνειν αὐτοὺς ἀναγκάζειν συχνῶς περιπατεῖν. ἄλλο. κενταυρίου λεπτοῦ γεγηρακότος, κοπτο-*

[*Medicamentum ad morbum regium, quod in nares fundi debet.*] Elaterii quantum fabae Graecae amplitudinem aequat muliebri lacte liquatum in nares fundatur. *Aliud.* Nigella aquae incocta in nares conjecta in balneo auriginem detrahit.

Cap. XXI. [*Ad lienofos.*] Rumicis agreftis radix tundatur in pila et tritae fuccus exprimatur et per tres dies finguli cyathi bibantur. *Aliud.* Panacis radix contufa cochlearii menfura jejuno ex aqua calidae cyathis tribus exhibeatur.

[*Ad lienofos cum praeduro tumore.*] Capparis radicis corticis unc. ij, accipe, aceti fextarium femis, aquae fextarium j, decoque ad tertias; propina a cibi perfecta concoctione cyathum unum duosve et hoc per intervalla facito. *Aliud.* Hederae foliorum aceto incootorum et contuforum fuccus expreffus robuftis purus potui detur; fed delicatioribus aqua dilutus; antequam bibant autem, ipfos concitatius ambulare cogito. *Aliud.* Centauri tenuioris, quod jam confenuerit, in pila contufi cochlearium febre

Ed. Chart. X. [626.]

μένου ἐν ὄλμῳ δίδου κοχλιαρίου τὸ πλῆθος ἀπυρέτοις. ἄλλο. λαγωοῦ σπλὴν πρόσφατος καταπινόμενος, ὥστε τοῖς ὀδοῦσι μὴ ἅπτεσθαι, ὑγιάζει τοὺς σπληνικούς. ἀγνοείτω δὲ ὁ πάσχων ὅ τι κατέπιεν ἐνδεδεμένος τοὺς ὀφθαλμοὺς, ποιεῖ δὲ καὶ ὁ τῶν μήπω βλεπόντων κυνιδίων σπλὴν ὡσαύτως καταπινόμενος. ἄλλο. κυνηγετικοῦ κυνὸς σκυλάκιον λεῖον ξηρὸν δίδου νήστει προσβαλὼν νάρδου ὀλίγης. ἔλεγε δὲ Μάρκελλος ποιεῖν καλῶς πρὸς σπληνικοὺς καρδαμώμου κοχλιάριον α'. ἢ β'. μετὰ ὄξους σκιλλητικοῦ κυάθου α'. ἢ β'. διδόμενον πιεῖν ἐπὶ ἡμέρας β'. νήστει δίδου. ἄλλο. κισσοῦ ῥίζας ἁπαλὰς ἑψήσας δι' οἴνου πότιζε. ἢ ὠμὰς κόψας πότιζε δι' οἴνου. ἄλλο. ὀνίδας ξηρὰς διάλυσον ὄξει καὶ διηθήσας δι' ὀθόνης δίδου πιεῖν. ἄλλο. ῥαφάνου χυλὸν λειοτριβήσας δι' ὀξυμέλιτος δὸς ἐπὶ ἡμέρας γ'. τῆς ἡμέρας ἀνὰ κυάθους β'. πιεῖν. τήκει τὸν σπλῆνα. ἄλλο. σκωρίαν σιδήρου δίδου πιεῖν, ὅσον κοχλιάριον μετὰ ὀξυκράτου. ἄλλο. ἶριν μακρὰν ἑψήσας διὰ ὄξους δίδου πιεῖν τὸ ὄξους ἀπόζεμα. ἄλλο. ἑλκοροδάνου καρδίαν δίδου πιεῖν καὶ ἐσθίειν.

carentibus dato. *Aliud.* Leporinus lien recens ita devoratus, ut ne dentibus attingatur, lienofos fanat; ignoret autem laborans quid devoraverit, oculis fascia velatis. Idem facit et catellorum nondum vifum adeptorum lien fimiliter in ventriculum transmiffus. *Aliud.* Venatorii canis catulum aridum tritum modico nardo adjecto, jejuno exhibe. Dicebat autem Marcellus id quoque ad lienofos vehementer facere, fi cardamomi cochlearium unum aut duo ex aceti fcillini cyatho uno duobusve jejuno dentur; idque per ij, dies continuos facito. *Aliud.* Radices hederae molles elixae ex vino bibantur: aut crudae contufae ex vino itidem. *Aliud.* Afini ftercus aridum aceto diffolve et per linteolum excolatum potui dato. *Aliud.* Raphani fuccus ex oxymelite maceratus per tres dies accipiatur, fingulis diebus cyathi bini; lienem attenuat. *Aliud.* Ferri recrementi cochlearium ex posca potui dato. *Aliud.* Irin longam aceto incoque et acetum propinato. *Aliud.* Elcorodani cor potui efuique exhibeto. *Aliud.* Muxin ex aqua

Ed. Chart. X. [626. 627.]

ἄλλο. μοῦξιν καθεψήσας δι᾽ ὕδατος, ἐὰν ᾖ ξηρὸς, δὸς πιεῖν τὸν χυλόν· μοῦξιν δὲ λέγεται Καππαδοκιστί. ἄλλο. στοιχάδος κοχλιάριον μετὰ οἴνου σχοινίνου κύαθον α΄. λειοτριβήσας δὸς πιεῖν. ἄλλο. ἀμμωνιακοῦ θυμιάματος λειοτριβήσας μετ᾽ ὄξους δίδου πιεῖν κύαθον νήστει. ἄλλο. μυὸς σπλῆνα καὶ πεπέρεως κόκκους ζ΄. εἰς σῦκον ὀπτήσας δὸς λεληθότως φαγεῖν.

[Ἐπίθεμα πρὸς σπληνικούς.] Λίθον ἄσιον ἐμβαλὼν εἰς κύστιν βοείαν καὶ ὄξος δριμὺ ἀποδήσας ἐπιτίθει κατὰ τοῦ σπληνὸς καὶ καταδιέλης. ἄλλο. μυροβάλανον μετ᾽ ὄξους λειοτριβήσας καὶ ποιήσας κηρωτῆς πάχος ἐπιτίθει. ἄλλο. ἀλώπεκος σπλὴν ἐπι- [627] δεσμούμενος ἰᾶται σπληνικούς. ἄλλο. ἐρίφου σπλὴν ἐπιτιθέμενος τήκει σπλῆνα. ἄλλο. ἀγρία κράμβη καταπλασσομένη ἰᾶται σπληνικούς. ἄλλο. Περσικῆς φύλλα καταπλασσόμενα ποιεῖ καλῶς. ἄλλο. μυρίκης καρπὸν ἐν ὄξει καθεψήσας, λεῖον ἑλκύσας ἐπιτίθει. ἄλλο. ἀμμωνιακὸν θυμίασμα λειοτριβήσας μετ᾽ ὄξους ἔνελκε καὶ ἐπιτίθει. ἄλλο. κροκόμαγμα ἐν ὄξει λειοτριβήσας καὶ ποιήσας κηρω-

elixum ſi aridum ſit, ſuccum propinato; muxin vero dicitur lingua Cappadocica. *Aliud.* Stoechadis triti cochlearium ex vini lentiſcini cyatho bibatur. *Aliud.* Ammoniacam guttam ex aceto tritam jejuno exhibe cyathi menſura. *Aliud.* Muris lienem et piperis grana ſeptem in ſico torreas et clam epulanda exhibe.

[*Epithema ad lienoſos.*] Lapidem aſium in veſicam bubulam conjicito et aceto acri madeſactam lieni ſuperimponito; ipſum comminues. *Aliud.* Myrobalanum ex aceto maceratum et ad cerati craſſitudinem redactum imponito. *Aliud.* Vulpis lienis ſuper locum alligatus lienoſos morbo liberat. *Aliud.* Hoedi lienis impoſitus lienem digerit. *Aliud.* Silveſtris braſſica ſi ex ea cataplasma fiat, lienoſis medetur. *Aliud.* Perſici arboris folia eodem modo impoſita bene faciunt. *Aliud.* Myricae ſemen aceto incoctum, tritum atque ſuperdatum juvat. *Aliud.* Ammoniacam guttam aceto maceratam linteolo illitam impone. *Aliud.* Crocomagma aceto maceratum et ad cerati craſſi-

Ed. Chart. X. [627.]

τῆς πάχος ἐπίθες. οὐκ ἀφίσταται μέχρις οὗ ἀποθεραπεύσεται. ἄλλο. καππάρεως ῥίζαν κόψας ἐπιμελῶς εἰς ὀθόνην ἐπιτίθει, αὐθήμερον ἐπιτιθέμενον ὠφελήσει.

[Πρὸς σπληνικούς.] Καππάρεως ῥίζης φλοιοῦ μεθ' ὕδατος λίτραν α'. καὶ ὄξους λίτραν S''. ἕψει ἕως ἂν ἀποτριτωθῇ καὶ δίδου γο. α'. S''. ἄλλο. φύλλα κισσοῦ ἑψήσας σὺν ὄξει καὶ κοπανίσας ἐκπίασον τὸ ὑγρὸν καὶ τοῖς μὲν ἰσχυροτέροις δίδου ἐξ αὐτοῦ, τοῖς δὲ τρυφεροῖς ὕδωρ μιγνύων, περιπατείτω δὲ καὶ οὕτως πότιζε. ἄλλο. καππάρεως ῥίζαν κοπανήσας καὶ ζέσας μετ' ὄξους καὶ μέλιτος δίδου πιεῖν νήστει.

[Πρὸς σπλῆνα.] Λαβὼν κυπαρίσσου κώνους κόψον εὐτόνως καὶ ἄλευρον ὀρόβινον λεπτότατον βάλε εἰς ὄξος καὶ ἕψε ἕως γένηται ὡς ἔμπλαστρον. ἐπιτίθει εἰς τὸν σπλῆνα ἕως ἡμερῶν γ'. καὶ μετὰ γ'. ἡμέρας λῦσον καὶ εὑρήσεις τὸ ἔμπλαστρον πεπληρωμένον. ἄλλο. Ἀμμωνιακοῦ θυμιάματος ἐναποβρέξας ὄξει σκιλλητικῷ ἐπὶ ἡμέρας γ'. καὶ λειώσας εἰς ῥάκος ἐπιθὲς καὶ μὴ λύσῃς, ἕως τὸ ἔμπλαστρον ἀποπέσῃ.

tudinem redactum imponito; non amovetur, quoad ex toto ſanaverit. *Aliud.* Capparis radix curioſe trita et linteolo illita ac loco impoſita eodem die opem tulit.

[*Ad lienoſos.*] Radicis capparis corticem in aquae libra et aceti ſemilibra incoquito usque ad tertias et potandam praebe ſesquiunciam. *Aliud.* Hederacea folia aceto inſerveſacta contunde et humorem exprime ac robuſtioribus ipſum praebeto; delicatioribus autem aquam admisceto; ſed prius ipſe ambulato atque ita bibito. *Aliud.* Capparis radicem tuſam et aceto mulſo incoctam jejuno potandam praebeto.

[*Ad ſplenem.*] Accipe cypreſſi baccas et valde conteras; et ervi farinam quam tenuiſſimam in acetum mitte et usque ad emplaſtri conſiſtentiam decoque; lienique per triduum impone; poſt tertium diem ſolve et emplaſtrum aquae plenum invenies. *Aliud.* Ammoniacam guttam in ſcillino aceto per triduum demerſam ac laevigatam panniculo illine atque impone, neque amove, quoad emplaſtrum

Ed. Chart. X. [627.]
ἄλλο. φύλλα συκαμίνου χλωρὰ ψύξας ἐν σκιᾷ καὶ τρίψας ποίησον ξηρίων γραμμάρια δ'. καὶ μετὰ ὀλίγου πεπέρεως καὶ καρυοφύλλων μετὰ οἴνου ἀκράτου θερμοῦ εἰς ἔμβασιν δίδου πιεῖν.

Κεφ. κβ'. [Πρὸς ὑδρωπικοὺς πόμα ὥστε ἐξουρεῖν τὸ παρακείμενον ὑγρόν.] Χαλκοῦ κεκαυμένου ὅσον κυάμου Αἰγυπτίου, κόπρου περιστερᾶς γο. α'. οἴνου κυάθους γ'. δίδου. ἔστω δὲ μία πόσις. ἄλλο πεπειραμένον ἡμῖν ἐπὶ πολλῶν. τιθυμάλλου χαρακίου τὴν ῥίζαν δίδου ἐσθίειν πρὸς δύναμιν καὶ παραχρῆμα κενοῖ. ἄλλο. κόκκον Κνίδιον κεκομμένον καὶ σεσησμένον ἀναλάμβανε μέλιτι, ποιῶν πάχος γλοιοῦ καὶ δίδου κοχλιάριον α'. πλῆρες δ' οἰνομέλιτος κυάθων γ'. καὶ ὀλίγου θερμοῦ ὕδατος, ὡς εἶναι γαλακτῶδες ἢ διὰ ᾠοῦ ῥοφήτου. ὑδραγωγὸν κάλλιστον πάνυ. χαμαιάκτης τὸν χυλὸν τὸν ἐκ τῆς ῥίζης κυάθων β'. καὶ οἴνου κυάθους β'. ἀπαλλάσσει δίχα τοῦ τὸν στόμαχον ἀνατρέπειν. ἄλλο. ἀγρώστεως ἀφέψημα πινόμενον ἔστι διουρητικόν. ἄλλο. στρύχνου

decidat. *Aliud.* Folia ſycamini mori viridia reſrigerata et arefacta in umbra terito, et aridum medicamentum ſacito ſcrupulorum quatuor pondere et cum pauco pipere et cariophyllis et ex vino mero calido, quum deſcendit in balneum, potui praebeto.

Cap. XXII. [*Ad hydropicos potio, ut humor incluſus per lotium ejiciatur.*] Recipe aeris uſti quantum fabam Aegyptiam aequat, fimi columbini unc. j, vini cyathos iij, exhibe; eſto autem una potio. *Aliud* nobis in multis uſu comprobatum. Tithymalli characiae radicem pro aegroti viribus eſui dato; ſtatim enim evacuat. *Aliud.* Granum Cnidium tuſum et cribratum melle comprehende, ut ſordium craſſitudo fiat, et cochlearium plenum ex vini mulſi cyathis tribus et modico aquae calidae ad lactis conſiſtentiam aut ex ovo ſorbili propinato; plurimum enim aquae dejicit. *Aliud.* Hebuli radicum ſucci cyathi duo, vini cyathi duo in unum mixti et exhibiti liberant absque ſtomachi ſubverſione. *Aliud.* Graminis decoctum potui datum urinam citat. *Aliud.* Solani ſucci cyathi

Ed. Chart. X. [627. 628.]
χυλοῦ κυάθους δ'. μέλιτος κυάθους ιστ'. δὸς πιεῖν. ἄλλο. ὕσσωπον καὶ γλυκεῖ τράγου οὖρον ποτιζόμενον διουρητικόν ἐστιν. ὁμοίως ἐὰν αἴγειον ἔχῃς.

['Επίθεμα πρὸς ὑδρωπικούς.] Κισσὸν κεκαυμένον ἐπιμελῶς κατάπλασσε. ἄλλο. ῥαφάνους καθεψήσας δι' ὕδατος ἕως τακεραὶ γένωνται, κομισάμενος κρίθινον ἄλευρον μίξας ἕψει καὶ κατάπλασσε.

[628] Κεφ. κγ'. [Πρὸς πρόπτωσιν ὀμφαλοῦ.] Τινὲς διὰ φαρμακείας εἰς τὸ κατὰ φύσιν ἐπανῆλθον οὕτως. κηκίδας καύσας ἢ τρίψας καὶ διαμίξας σὺν φλοιῷ λιβάνου καὶ ὠοῦ λευκῷ κατάπλασσε. ἄλλο. στυπτηρίας σχιστῆς < ε'. τρυγὸς οἴνου Ῥοδίνου < ι'. κηκίδων ὀμφακίνων < β'. οἴνου διεὶς καὶ μέλιτος ποιήσας πάχος ἐπίβρεχε, ἔξωθεν ἐπιῤῥίπτων σπογγάριον ὀξυκράτῳ δεδευμένον καὶ ταινιδίῳ καταλάμβανε. ἄλλο. ἐρεγμοῦ λεπύρων καὶ κηκίδων καὶ βαλαυστίου τὸ ἴσον· ἕψε ἐν ὕδατι. ὅταν δὲ διαλυθῇ τρίψας ἐπιμελῶς ἐπιτίθει σὺν τῷ σπόγγῳ, καθάπερ προείρηται.

quatuor, mellis cyathi ſexdecim in potum ſumpti benefaciunt. *Aliud.* Hyſſopum et hirci lotium ex paſſo potum urinam movet; perinde et ſi caprini copiam habueris.

[*Epithema ad hydropicos.*] Hederam crematam diligenter in modum cataplasmatis impone. *Aliud.* Raphanos aquae incoctos quoad teneritate flaccescant, accipe; deinde hordeacea ſarina adjecta misce, decoque et cataplasma facito.

Cap. XXIII. [*Ad umbilici prolapſum.*] Quidam medicamentis ad naturalem ſtatum ita reverſi ſunt. Gallas ure vel tere et permisce cum cortice thuris et albo ovi et appone. *Aliud.* Recipe aluminis ſciſſi drach. v, faecis vini Rhodii drach. x, gallarum omphacinarum drach ij, vino diluta et ad mellis craſſitudinem redacta impone, extrinſecusque ſpongiolam posca imbutam ſuperpone et faſcia deliga. *Aliud.* Recipe corticum fabae freſae, gallarum, balauſtii ana aequales partes in aqua eoquito. Ubi vero diſſoluta fuerint, diligenter trita imponito cum ſpon-

Ed. Chart. X. [628.]

ἄλλο. μολίβδου ῥινήματος < ιστ΄. κωνίου, μάννης, ψιμυθίου ὑποκυστίδος χυλοῦ ἀνὰ < α΄. οἴνῳ διαλύσας χρῶ καθὼς προείρηται.

Κεφ. κδ΄. [Πρὸς τὰ γαστρὸς πάθη καὶ πρῶτον πρὸς στρόφον καὶ ὀδύνην γαστρός.] Ἀριστολοχίας ῥίζαν ἐν οἴνῳ δὸς πιεῖν. πρὸς στρόφον καὶ λυγμὸν καὶ κεφαλαλγίαν καὶ δυστοκίας καλῶς ποιεῖ. ἁρμόζει πταρμὸς πρὸς στρόφον καὶ πάντα τὰ ἐντὸς πάθη. ἄλλο. τῆς λυχνίτιδος ἡ ῥίζα πλυθεῖσα καὶ ἑψηθεῖσα μετὰ γλυκέος, εἶτα διυλισθεῖσα καὶ ποθεῖσα ποιεῖ καλῶς. εἰ δὲ μὴ, βρώματι σεαυτοῦ πρόσβαλλε ὀλίγην κασσίαν καὶ ὀλυρίδα μὴ κόψας.

[Πρὸς στρόφον ἐντέρων καὶ κοιλίας.] Κυμίνου πεφρυγμένου καὶ κεκομμένου κοχλιάριον α΄. ἢ β΄. μεθ᾽ ὕδατος κυάθων τριῶν δίδου πιεῖν· καὶ πρὸς ἐμπνευματώσεις ὄξος ζέσας καὶ ψύξας. ἔπειτα σελίνου σπέρματος τρῖβε, παραζέων τὸ ὄξος καὶ ἐκ τοῦ αὐτοῦ δίδου πιεῖν. ἄλλο. ἐρύσιμον βοτάνην μετὰ ὕδατος τρίψας δίδου πίνειν. ἄλλο. ἐκ τοῦ λαμπροῦ τὸ ἀρκοῦν τρίψας μετ᾽ ὄξους δίδου πίνειν νήστει.

gia, ut dictum eſt. Recipe ramenti plumbi drach. xvj, cicutae, mannae thuris, ceruſae, ſucci hypocyſtidis ana drach. j, vino diſſoluta utere ut dictum eſt.

Cap. XXIV. [*Ad ventris affectus ac primum ad tormina et ventris dolores.*] Ariſtolochiae radicem in vino potui dato: ad tormina, ſingultum, capitis dolorem et partus difficultatem bene facit. Sternutatio ad tormina et omnes internas affectiones proficit. *Aliud.* Lychnitidis radix lota, dulci vino incocta, deinde percolata et pota magnifice prodeſt; ſin minus autem, cibis tuis adjice modicum caſſiae et olyrae non contuſae.

[*Ad tormina inteſtinorum et ventris.*] Cumini fricti et contriti cochlearium unum, duove ex aquae cyathis tribus potandum eſt. Et adverſus inflationes acetum ferveſacito ac refrigerato; poſtea apii ſemen tuſum admiſceto ac iterum acetum ferveſacito, ex eoque potionem dato. *Aliud.* Irionem herbam ex aqua tritam potandam dato. *Aliud.* Ex lampro quod ſatis eſt tritum ex aceto jejuno

Ed. Chart. X. [628.]
ἄλλο. δάφνην μασησάμενος νῆστις τὸν χυλὸν καταπινέτω. καὶ τὸ μάσημα ἐπιτιθέτω ἐπὶ τὸν ὀμφαλὸν καὶ παραχρῆμα παύσεται.

[Πρὸς κάθετον δακτύλιον καθαρτικὸν κοιλίας.] Εἰς χολὴν ταύρου κροκίδα βρέξας ἐντίθει εἰς τὸν δακτύλιον. ἄλλο. σαπῶνα Γαλλικὸν εἰς ἔριον ἐνδύσας ὑπόθου ἢ μάλιστα στυπτηρίαν ὑγράν.

[Πρὸς δυσεντερικούς.] Φακὸν ἑψήσας σὺν βάτου ῥίζῃ τρυφερὸν κεκομμένον ἐπίβαλε καὶ δὸς φαγεῖν. ἄλλο. κυτίνους καθεψήσας, εἰς ὀξύγαλα λειοτριβήσας ἔμβαλλε ἔλαιον τὸν αὐτὸν τρόπον καὶ δίδου φαγεῖν. ἄλλο. κέγχρον κεκομμένον ἑψήσας βάλε στέαρ μόσχειον. καὶ ποιήσας λιπαρώτατον δὸς ῥοφῆσαι θερμότατον, εἶτα ψυχρότατον τὸ ὕδωρ ἐπιῤῥοφείτω καὶ παραχρῆμα ὑγιὴς ἔσται. ἄλλο. κηκίδος τὸ ἐντὸς λαβὼν τρῖψον λεῖον καὶ μίξας ἄλευρον καὶ ὠοῦ τὸ λευκὸν φυράσας ποίησον ἀρτίσκον καὶ ὀπτήσας κατάκλα καὶ ἔγχει εἰς οἶνον ἀπαράχυτον καὶ δὸς φαγεῖν.

exhibe. *Aliud.* Laurum commanducans jejunus ſuccum devorato; partem commandueatam umbilico imponito; illico tormina ſinientur.

[*Medicamentum ano immittendum alvi purgatorium.*] In ſel tauri lanae lapſum intingito anoque immittito. *Aliud.* Gallicum ſaponem lana involutum ſubmittito, aut liquidum alumen potiſſimum.

[*Ad inteſtinorum tormina.*] Lentem teneram contuſam cum rubi radice elixam imponito ac eſui dato. *Aliud.* Flores mali punicae domeſticae acido lacti incoctos contere et oleum eodem modo inſunde et edendos appone. *Aliud.* In milium contuſum elixum vitulinum adipem inſunde et quam pinguiſſimum calidiſſimumque ſorbendum exhibe, poſtea gelidiſſimam aquam ſorbeto et confeſtim erit incolumis. *Aliud.* Gallae interiorem partem tritam ac laevigatam accipito farinaque admixta et ovi albo paſtillos eſſingito atque aſſos frangito, vinoque ſimplici madeſacito et eſui dato.

[629] [Ἔκλειγμα πρὸς δυσεντερικοὺς καὶ κοιλιακοὺς καὶ λειεντερίαν.] Σιλφίου ξύσματα μέλιτι παραμίξας δὸς ἐκλείχειν. ἄλλο. ὠὸν, μέλι, οἶνον, σίδια ἴσα διαβάλλων τηγάνιζε καὶ πεπέρεως μικρὸν ἐπιπάσσων δίδου πιεῖν ἄκρως. ἄλλο. ὠὰ τρία βαλὼν εἰς ὄξος ἔα ἐμβρέχεσθαι ἐπὶ ἡμέρας τρεῖς καὶ λαβὼν σεμιδάλιον φύρασον τοῖς ὠοῖς τοῖς τρισὶ καὶ ὀπτήσας καὶ ἐμβάψας εἰς ἄκρατον δός.

[Πότημα πρὸς δυσεντερικοὺς καὶ κοιλιακοὺς καὶ λειεντερίαν.] Ῥοῦν καθεψήσας δι' οἴνου στύφου εἰς τρίτον, δίδου πιεῖν, οἷς ἡ κοιλία οὐ καλὰ φέρει. ἄλλο. κηκίδα δι' οἴνου αὐστηροῦ καθεψήσας πότιζε τοὺς ῥευματισμένους τὴν κοιλίαν πρὸς δύναμιν.

[Πρὸς στρόφον καὶ ὀδύνην γαστρός.] Δίδου κύμινον μασώμενον καὶ καταπινόμενον. ἄλλο. κνίκον καὶ τῆλεα τρίψας καὶ ἑψήσας δίδου ἀφέψημα πίνειν. ἄλλο. δαφνίδας ξηρὰς καὶ φλοισθείσας τρίψας δίδου πίνειν κοχλιάρια θ'. ἄλλο.

[*Linctus ad dyſentericos, coeliacos et lienteriam.*] Laſerpitii ramenta melli commiscens linctui dato. *Aliud.* Ovum, mel, vinum, mali punici putamina pari portione in unum miscens frigito et piperis modicum inſpergito ac potionem dato; vehementer facit. *Aliud.* Ova tria accipiens in aceto conjicito ac ita per triduum macerari ſinito; deinde ſimilaginis modicum capiens cum tribus ovis ſubigito; mox aſſans et meraco vino madefaciens exhibeto.

[*Potiones ad dyſentericos, coeliacos et lientericos.*] Vinum aſtringens, cui rhus obſoniorum usque ad tertias incoctus ſit, potandum jubeto quibus ventriculus male ſe habet. *Aliud.* Vinum auſterum cui galla incocta ſit illis potui pro viribus concedito, quorum ventriculus fluxione vexatur.

[*Ad tortiones et dolores ventris.*] Da cuminum mandendum et devorandum. *Aliud.* Cnicum et foenumgraecum tere et coque et da decoctum bibendum. *Aliud.* Baccas lauri ſiccas et exeorticatas tere et da bibenda cochlearia novem. *Aliud.* Serpyllum terens da cum vino

Ed. Chart. X. [629.]

ἕρπυλλον τρίψας δίδου σὺν οἴνῳ πίνειν. ἄλλο. ἀφέψημα σαμψύχου δίδου πίνειν σὺν οἴνῳ. ἄλλο. ἠρυγγίου ῥίζαν δίδου σὺν οἴνῳ πίνειν ἢ ἀφέψημα σταχύος ἢ καστόριον. πρὸς τὴν δὲ ὀδύνην τῶν δυσεντερικῶν κυδώνια σὺν κηρωτῇ ῥοδίνῃ ἢ μυρσινίνῃ τὰ ἴσα τῇ γαστρὶ ἐντίθετι.

[Πρὸς κωλικήν.] Γῆρας ὄφιος ἐν ἀγγείῳ χαλκείῳ φρύξας σὺν ἐλαίῳ μέχρι τοῦ καίεσθαι, αὐτὸ δὲ διαλύσας ἐν ἐκείνῳ ἐλαίῳ καὶ ἐξ αὐτοῦ σὺν δακτύλῳ σου κατάχριε. ἄλλο. βάλανον ὀπίῳ ἐν χυλῷ τῆς θρίδακος τετηγμένῳ περιχρίσας εἰς δακτύλιον ἐντίθετι.

[Πρὸς διάῤῥοιαν γαστρός.] Καλλίτριχον ἑψήσας ἐν ὕδατι δίδου πιεῖν. ἄλλο. στοιβὴν τὴν εἰς τὰ κεράμια, τὴν ἀκανθώδη κόψον εἰς ὅλμον καὶ ἕψει δι' ὕδατος καὶ δίδου πιεῖν τὸ ὕδωρ κοιλιαλγοῦντι, ἀπυρέτῳ δι' οἴνου, πυρέττοντι χωρὶς οἴνου. ἄλλο. καρύων φλοιὸν τὸν περικείμενον περὶ τὰ τρωγόμενα, λεῖον δι' ὕδατος, δίδου πιεῖν κοχλιάρια γ'. ἄλλο. κέρας ἐλάφειον τρυφερὸν καύσας δίδου μετὰ κηκίδος ἴσης πιεῖν. ἄλλο. λαπάθου σπέρμα λειώσας καὶ ἐπιπάσας

bibendum. *Aliud.* Decoctum ſampſuci da cum vino in potum. *Aliud.* Eryngii radicem da cum vino potui vel decoctum ſpicae vel caſtoreum. Ad dolorem autem dysentericorum cotonea cum cerato roſeo aut myrteo aequis portionibus ventri impone.

[*Ad colicam.*] Spolium ſerpentis in vaſe aeneo frigens cum oleo quousque comburatur, diſſolve ipſum in illo oleo et unge ex eo cum tuo digito. *Aliud.* Glandulam opio in ſucco lactucae liquato obline et ano indito.

[*Ad ventris profluvium.*] Gallitrichi ex aqua decoctum potui dato. *Aliud.* Stoeben, qua ad teſtacea vaſa uti ſolent, ſpinis asperam in pila contundito et aquae incoquito et aquam in dolore ventris absque vino propinato quum febrem habent; quum febre vacant, vinum commisceto. *Aliud.* Nucum putamen, quod nucleos includit tritum, ex aqua potui dato cochleariorum trium menſura. *Aliud.* Cornu cervinum mollius uſtum cum

εἰς τὸν ποτὸν δίδου ἢ εἰς τὸ βρωτόν. ἄλλο. καρύων τὸ ἐντὸς τὸ ὡσανεὶ κιόνιον καὶ μήκωνος κωδειῶν τὸ ἐπικείμενον ὡς πῶμα, ἴσον δίδου δι' οἴνου. ἄλλο. δρυὸς βαλάνους κόψας καὶ σήσας πλεῖον ἐπίπασσε εἰς οἶνον αὐστηρὸν ὡς ἄλφιτα καὶ δίδου πιεῖν. ἄλλο. καράβου τὰ ὄστρακα φρύξας λεῖα διὰ ὕδατος. ἄλλο. στρουθιοκαμήλου κοιλία πινομένη καὶ ὀρνίθων ὁμοίως ὅσον κοχλιάρια β'. ἀπυρέτοις δι' οἴνου, πυρέσσουσι δὲ δι' ὕδατος. ἄλλο. λιβάνου χόνδρον κυαμιαῖον διεὶς οἴνῳ μέλανι κυάθον α'. καὶ στρύχνου χυλοῦ κυάθους β'. δίδου πιεῖν. ἄλλο. κόμμι τὸ λευκὸν κόψας μετ' οἴνου μέλανος κυάθων ϛ'. δίδου γο. α'. πίνειν, ποιεῖ ὑπόθετον τοῖς αὐτοῖς. ἄλλο. κοχλιάριον Ἀφρικανὸν λαβὼν βάλλε εἰς αὐτὸ πίσσαν ὑγρὰν καὶ θερμάνας ἔξελε τὸ κρέας καὶ ὑπόθες εἰς τὸν δακτύλιον δὶς ἢ τρίς. ἄλλο. ὄφεως γῆρας ἐν χαλκώματι μετὰ ἐλαίου φρύξας ἕως ἀνθρακωθῇ, συλλειώσας, τῷ ἐλαίῳ διάχριε τὸ δακτύλιον [630] τῷ δακτύλῳ.

gallae pari portione in potum dato. *Aliud.* Rumicis semen contritum et potioni cibove inſperſum optime facit. *Aliud.* Nucum internum illud, quod inſtar columellae eſt, et capitum papaveris, quod veluti operculum eſt, pari portione ex vino exhibeantur. *Aliud.* Quernas glandes contuſas et diutius cribratas ut polentam in vinum auſterum ſpargito potionemque concedito. *Aliud.* Carabi teſtas frictas et tritas ex aqua porrigito. *Aliud.* Struthiocameli ventriculus et gallinarum ſimiliter cochleariorum duum menſura ex vino potus febri abſente, praeſente vero ex aqua. *Aliud.* Thuris grumus ſabae magnitudinis in vini nigri cyatho uno, ſolani ſucci cyathis duobus eliquatus in potum detur. *Aliud.* Gummi albi contuſi unciam ex vini nigri cyathis ſex bibito, ad idem ano impoſitum facit. *Aliud.* Cochleam Africanam ſumens in eam liquidam picem infunde et calefactae carnem exime et in anum bis aut ter immitte. *Aliud.* Serpentis ſenium in vaſe aeneo ex oleo frigens quoad in carbonem vertatur contere et digito in oleum intincto anum perunge. *Aliud.* Herba ſacra inſerius ſoveto, aquam ne attingito.

Ed. Chart. X. [630.]

ἄλλο. βοτάνη ὑποκάτω ὕδατος μὴ ἁπτόμενος. ἄλλο. σεῦτλιον κεκομμένον μετ᾽ ὄξους καταπλαττόμενον ἀπ᾽ ἄνωθεν μέχρι κάτω καλῶς ποιεῖται δυσεντερικοῖς. ἄλλο. κερατίων ὀστᾶ κόψας κατάπλασσε τὴν κοιλίαν.

[Πρὸς ἀλγήματα δυσεντερικῶν.] Μῆλον κυδώνιον ὀπτὸν μετὰ κηρωτῆς ῥοδίνης ἑκάστου τὸ ἴσον μίξας κατάπλασσε. παραχρῆμα ἄπονον ποιεῖ.

[Πρὸς κωλικούς.] Ὀστρέων ὄστρακα καύσας καὶ λεάνας δίδου πιεῖν κοχλιάρια β'. δι᾽ ὕδατος θερμοῦ κυάθων γ'. ἄλλο. θύμον Κρητικὸν καθεψήσας διὰ ὕδατος ἕως εἰς τρίτον καταστῇ μέρος, μετὰ μέλιτος Ἀττικοῦ δὸς πιεῖν. ἄλλο. ἱερὰν ῥίζαν λεπτὴν κόψας βάλε εἰς ὕδωρ καὶ ἕψει εἰς ἥμισυ καὶ δίδου πιεῖν τὸ ἀφέψημα ἐπὶ ἡμέρας ε'. καὶ ἰᾶται. ἐπὶ πολλῶν δεδοκίμασται. ἄλλο. ἡδύοσμον χλωρὸν καθεψήσας δὸς ἐπὶ τρεῖς ἡμέρας καὶ οὐδέποτε πονήσει. ἄλλο. τῆς δάφνης οἱ ἀκρέμονες τρυφεροὶ ξύλοι τρωγόμενοι ἐπὶ ἡμέρας ἰῶνται. τὸ δὲ πολταρίδιον, ἐν ᾧ ἑψεῖς τὸ ἡδύοσμον, βλέπε μὴ γῆς ἅψηται ἐπὶ τὰς τρεῖς ἡμέρας.

Aliud. Beta ex aceto contusa et cataplasmatis more a superioribus ad inferiora usque imposita dysentericis magnifice prodest. *Aliud.* Cornorum ossa contusa ventri illinito.

[*Ad dolores dysentericorum.*] Malum cotoneum assum cum cerati rosei pari portione impositum illico dolorem levat.

[*Ad colicis doloribus vexatos.*] Ostreorum testae crematae et tritae potui dentur cochlearia duo ex calentis aquae cyathis tribus. *Aliud.* Thymum Cretense aquae usque ad tertias incoctum ex Attico melle propinetur. *Aliud.* Sacram radicem tenuem contusam in aquam mitte et ad dimidias elixa; decoctum per quinque dies potui detur et morbo liberat: hoc in multis probatum est. *Aliud.* Viridis menta elixa per triduum exhibeatur et nunquam dolebit. *Aliud.* Lauri summitates tenerae ligneae esae per triduum liberant, ollula vero, ubi mentha incocta sit, cave ne per triduum illud terram attingat.

Ed. Chart. X. [630.]

[*Πρὸς διάφραγμα.*] *Φραξίνου ξύλου κύαθον δὸς ἐπὶ ἡμέρας γ΄. πιεῖν ξύσματα καὶ ὑγιὴς ἔσται. ἄλλο πολύχρηστον. κολοκυνθίδα Ἀλεξανδρεινὴν τρήσας μὴ σιδήρῳ καὶ ἐκκενώσας βάλε εἰς οἴνου Κώου κοτύλην α΄. καὶ ἀναζέσας καὶ εὔκρατον ποιήσας δὸς πιεῖν καὶ περιπατείτω καὶ ἀνάλγητος ἔσται. κατάγει ἀπολύματα πολλὰ τουτὶ πότημα. κατέχειν δὲ ἅλας ἐν τῷ στόματι, ἵνα μὴ ναυτιάσῃ. ποιεῖ δὲ καὶ πρὸς ἰσχιάδας.*

[*Πρόσθετον κωλικοῖς.*] *Ὄπιον Σπανὸν ἀναλάμβανε θρίδακος καὶ πεσσὸν ποιῶν ἐντίθει τῷ δακτυλίῳ. ἄλλο. σκορόδου σκελιδόνιον α΄. κονίᾳ θερμάνας θὲς εἰς τὸν δακτύλιον καὶ σκύβαλα κατασπάσας ὑγίασται. ἄλλο. ἐὰν κῶλον πονῶν κύνα κοιμώμενον ἐγείρει, κατὰ δὲ αὐτὸν τόπον οὗ ἐκοιμᾶτο ὁ κύων, οὐρήσῃ, εὐθέως ἄπονος ἔσται, ὁ δὲ κύων ἀποθανεῖται.*

[*Ἐπίθεμα κωλικοῖς καὶ ἐμπνευματουμένοις.*] *Κηρωτῇ Κυπρίνῃ σίλφιον ἀναλάμβανε πολὺ καὶ ἐπιτίθει· ἐγὼ δὲ σμήγω καὶ καστόριον ὀλίγον καὶ γίνεται ἐνεργέστερον.*

[*Ad interſeptum.*] Fraxini ligni ramentorum cyathus triduum potui datus ſanitatem reſtituit. *Aliud ad multa faciens.* Colocynthidem Alexandrinam excavatam non ferro et expurgatam in vini Coi ſextarium mitte et fervefacito; vinum poſtea ad temperatum calorem reverſum bibito et deambulato, et dolore ſolutus eris. Detrahit multa excrementa haec potio; ſalem autem, ne nauſeet, ore contineto. Bene facit et ad coxendicis dolores.

[*Medicamentum ad coli dolores ano immittendum.*] Opium Hispanum lactuca excipe et in peſſum redactum ſedi immitte. *Aliud.* Allii nucleolum lixivio calefactum in anum indito et arido ſtercore detracto ſaneſcit. *Aliud.* Si coli dolore tentatus dormientem canem expergefecerit et in locum ubi canis dormiebat mejerit, ſtatim dolore levabitur et canis moritur.

[*Epithema colicis et inflatis.*] Cerato liguſtrino laſerpitium comprehende et impone; ego vero et modicum caſtorei admiſceo et efficacius redditur.

[Πρὸς στρόφον.] Κύμινον Ἑλληνικὸν μασάσθω καὶ καταπινέτω. ἄλλο. κνίκον κόψας καὶ τῆλιν ἑψήσας πότιζε τῷ χυλῷ. ἄλλο. κτένα εἰς θερμὸν ὕδωρ ἐμβρέξας καὶ ἀποκλύσας πότιζε. ἄλλο. δαφνίδων ξηρῶν λεπισμάτων ὅσον κοχλιάρια θ'. δίδου πιεῖν. ἄλλο. ἕρπυλον λειώσας μετὰ ἀκράτου δίδου πιεῖν.

[Πρὸς πάντα τὰ ἐντὸς ἀλγήματα.] Ἔντερα ἀλγοῦντι εἴ τις τοὺς πόδας νίψῃ, δὸς πιεῖν τὸ ἀπόνιμμα, ἄπονος ἔσται παραχρῆμα.

[Πρὸς διακοπὴν ἐντέρων.] Λαβὼν ἀκάνθης Αἰγυπτίας ῥίζαν καὶ κρέα ἐρίφεια σὺν ταῖς θριξὶ καὶ τῷ δέρματι, ἢ αἴγεια λείωσον καὶ ἐκ σεμιδάλεως γενομένων κρομμύων καὶ ἐν οἴνῳ συγκεράσας δίδου πίνειν. αὐτὴ ἡ ῥίζα ἐπειράθη καὶ ἐπὶ πνευμονιακοῖς πινομένη· ἡ δὲ αὐτὴ καὶ περιαπτομένη ποιεῖ πρὸς τριταῖον καὶ ἀμφημερινὸν καὶ μετὰ ἐλαίου πινομένη ἐστὶ τραυματική.

[631] [Πρὸς νεφρῶν καὶ ἰσχιάδος ἀλγήματα.] Λαβὼν ἄλευρον ἴρεως καὶ τὸ ἰσχυρὸν ὄξος αὐτοῖς διαμίγνυθι

[*Ad tormina.*] Graecum cuminum manducato ac devorato. *Aliud.* Cnici contuſi et foenigraeci elixi ſuccum potui offer. *Aliud.* Pectinem in aqua calida madefactum et ablutum propina. *Aliud.* Baccarum lauri aridarum corticis cochlearia novem in potum dato. *Aliud.* Serpillum tritum cum mero da potui.

[*Ad omnes inteſtinos dolores.*] Ex inteſtinis dolenti ſi quis pedes laverit et ex aqua ea potui dederit, dolor confeſtim evanescit.

[*Ad inteſtinorum ſciſſuram.*] Aegyptiae ſpinae radicem et carnes hoedi capraeve cum pilis et corio capiens terito et ſimilagini commixtas caepas vinó temperatas potionem facito. Eadem radix et phlegmone pulmonum laborantibus in potu auxiliatur. Eadem ſuſpenſa tertiana febre et quotidiana liberat et ex oleo pota vulneribus medetur.

[*Ad renum et coxendicis dolores.*] Accipe farinam iridis et acetum potens, permisce eis reſinam pini et lu-

ῥητίνην πιτυίνην καὶ θερμοὺς καὶ πύρεθρον καὶ τερεβινθίνην καὶ θεῖον καὶ νίτρον καὶ δαφνίδας, πάντα μίξας σὺν μέλιτι πρόσθες.

[Ἰσχιάδος καθαρτικόν.] Τιθυμάλλου τοῦ ὀποῦ ἐνστάξας σταλαγμοὺς ε'. εἰς τὸ σῦκον δίδου φαγεῖν, καθαίρει.

[Ἐπίθεμα κοιλίας λυτικόν.] Κόκκον Κνίδιον σαλεπὶς ἀναλάμβανε κηρωτῇ καὶ ἐπιτίθει ἐπὶ τῆς κοιλίας τοῖς παιδίοις ἐπὶ τὸν ὀμφαλόν. ἄλλο. χολῇ ταύρου διάχριε τὸν ὀμφαλόν. ἄλλο. ἀστράγαλον χοίρειον καύσας καὶ λειοτριβήσας δὸς πιεῖν διὰ ὕδατος. ἄλλο. τὴν ἄνθεμιν βοτάνην τρίψας μετὰ ἐλαίου ἄλειψον καὶ παύσεται. ἄλλο. κροκοφάντιον λαβὼν οἷον θέλεις ἀπὸ κεφαλῆς γυναικὸς ἐπίθες ἐπὶ τὴν κεφαλὴν τοῦ πάσχοντος καὶ ἰάσῃ. κάλλιον δὲ ἐὰν θερμάνας αὐτὸ, οὕτως ἐπιθῇς. ἄλλο. κορίαννον καύσας καὶ διεὶς ἐλαίῳ ἐπίθες ἐπὶ τὸν ὀμφαλὸν καὶ ἐπάνω ἔρια.

Κεφ. κε'. [Πρὸς δυσουριῶντας καὶ λιθιῶντας] Σκορπίοι ὠπτημένοι τρωγόμενοι· πρὸς δὲ τοὺς ἀπροθύμως ἔχον-

pinos et pyrethrum et terebinthinam et fulfur et nitrum et baccas lauri; miſcens omnia cum melle appone.

[*Ad coxendicis dolores purgatorium.*] Tithymalli ſucci guttas quinque in ficum inſtillato et eſui dato; purgat.

[*Epithema ventris ſolutivum.*] Granum Cnidium cortice liberatum cerato comprehende et ventri puerorum ſuper umbilicum imponito. *Aliud.* Felle tauri umbilicum perungito. *Aliud.* Suillus talus uſtus tritusque ex aqua potui detur. *Aliud.* Herbam chamaemelum ex oleo terito et inungito; ſtatim dolor finietur. *Aliud.* Reticulum cujusmodi volueris de mulieris capite detractum capiti laborantis imponito, ſanitatem ei reſtitues; melius fuerit autem, ſi prius caleſactum reticulum impoſueris. *Aliud.* Coriandrum uſtum, oleo maceratum, umbilico ſuperimponito et lana contegito.

Cap. XXV. [*Ad urinae difficultatem et calculos.*] Scorpii uſti edantur; illis autem, qui forſitan abhorrerent,

Ed. Chart. X. [631.]

τας στέατι ἐμφυράσας καὶ ὀπτήσας δίδου φαγεῖν ἀνυπόπτως. παραδόξως ποιεῖ. καὶ οὐρηθεὶς δὲ λίθος, πυρίνῃ ὁμοίως ἐλαίας τριβόμενος ἂν εἴη ἔμπυρον λευκὸν, οὗτος ποτιζόμενος τοὺς ἐν κύστει λίθους τήκει. καὶ αἰλούρου δὲ ἧπαρ καυθὲν καὶ τριβὲν ὥστε ποθῆναι τοὺς λιθιῶντας ἰᾶται. καὶ ὁ ἴασπις λίθος πινόμενος θρύπτει τοὺς ἐν κύστει λίθους. ἄλλο. κοτυληδόνος ῥίζα ποθεῖσα καὶ λεῖα, πινομένη καθ' ἡμέραν ὁλκὴ μία κατὰ κράματος, ποιεῖ πρὸς τοὺς ἐν νεφροῖς λίθους λίαν καλῶς. ὀμφακίου καὶ κισσοῦ πυῤῥοῦ τῶν κορύμβων μετ' οἴνου λευκοῦ τετριμμένων τὸν ὄμφακα περίχριε τοὺς δυσουροῦντας.

[*Πεσσὸς πρὸς λιθιῶντας.*] Ὅταν οὐρήσῃ, βούτυρον παλαιὸν μαλάξας περίχριε τὸ αἰδοῖον· εἰς δὲ τὴν κοίτην ἐρίῳ προστεθείσθω ἡμέρας γ'.

[*Ἐπίθεμα διουρητικὸν, ποιεῖ δὲ καὶ πρὸς νεφριτικούς.*] Καλαμίνθην μετ' ὄξους καὶ πεπέρεως κηρωτῇ ἀναλάμβανε καὶ τῷ ὀμφαλῷ ἐπιτίθει. ἄλλο. εἰς ἕψημα σαμψύχου ἐγ-

cum adipe mixti toſtique clam et citra ſuſpicionem exhibeantur; miriſice proſunt. Calculus etiam urina redditus olivae nucleo ſimilis, contritus et igne candens ſi bibatur, eos qui in veſica ſunt calculos exerit. Felis jecur uſtum tritumque ita, ut bibi poſſit, calculoſis remedio eſt. Jaspis quoque lapillus potui datus veſicae calculos diſſipat. *Aliud.* Umbilici verris radix elixa et trita unciae pondere in diem ex diluto vino bibatur: ad renum calculos vehementer proſicit. *Aliud.* Succi uvae immaturae et ruſae hederae corymborum par modus ex albo vino teratur, ſucco illinito mictus difficultate male habitos.

[*Topicum calculoſis imponendum.*] Urina reddita butyro veteri remollito penem oblinito et cubitum eunti lana apponatur per triduum.

[*Epithema urinam proritans; prodeſt et calculoſis renibus.*] Calaminthям cum aceto et pipere cerato colligito et umbilico ſuperdato. *Aliud.* In ſampſuci decocto

κάθιζε. ἄλλο. βοτάνην περδίκιον καθεψήσας δι' ἐλαίου κατάπλασσε τὰ περὶ τὴν κύστιν καὶ παραχρῆμα οὐρήσει.

[Πρὸς λιθιῶντας.] Χαμαίδρυν ὀρεινὴν καθεψήσας δι' ὑδρομέλιτος δίδου πιεῖν· τούτῳ ἐχρήσατο Σάμιος Πρίσκος. ἄλλο. κισσοῦ λευκοῦ κορύμβους πότιζε ἐν οἴνῳ, τήκει λίθους. ἄλλο. φύλλα ἰτέας λειοτριβήσας ἐν οἴνῳ αὐστηρῷ πότιζε ἕως ὑγιάσῃς.

[Πρὸς ἐνουροῦντας ἀπροαιρέτως.] Ἀλέκτορος λαρύγγια καύσας δίδου πιεῖν νήστει ἐν ὕδατι κοχλιάριον α'. ἄλλο. ἄνθη λευκανθέμου τῇ ζ'. πότιζε ἐν ὕδατι τρίψας. ἄλλο. λαγωοῦ ὄρχιν ξηρὸν ξύων εἰς οἶνον εὐώδη δίδου πιεῖν. ἄλλο. κόρεις γ'. θλάσας μετὰ οἴνου αὐστηροῦ δὸς πιεῖν ἐπὶ [632] ἡμέρας θ'. ἄλλο. καλαμίνθην καὶ σμύρναν ἐν ὕδατι δὸς πιεῖν πρὸ τοῦ δειπνῆσαι. ἄλλο. χηνείας γλώσσας ἑφθὰς δὸς φαγεῖν ἐπὶ ἡμέρας γ'. ἀνὰ μίαν. ἄλλο. πηγάνου ἀγρίου σπέρμα δὸς φαγεῖν ἐπὶ ἡμέρας γ'. ἄλλο. καταχριέσθω αὐτοῦ τὸ αἰδοῖον κιμωλίαν μετὰ περδικίου χυλοῦ.

desideat. *Aliud.* Herbam parietariam oleo incoctam super locum vesicae imponito; illico urina decurret.

[*Ad calculosos.*] Montana trixago mulsae incocta potanda offeratur; hoc remedio Samius Priscus utebatur. *Aliud.* Albae hederae corymbi ex vino poti lapillos confringunt. *Aliud.* Salicis solia tusa ex vino austero tantisper accipiatur, dum sanitas restituatur.

[*Ad eos qui nolentes urinam reddunt.*] Galli guttur ustum cochlearii mensura jejuno ex aqua propinato. *Aliud.* Leucanthemi flores septem tritos ex aqua potui dato. *Aliud.* Leporis testiculum aridum minutatim concisum ex vino odorato potandum praebe. *Aliud.* Cimices tres contusos ex vino austero propinato per novem dies. *Aliud.* Calamintham et myrrham ex aqua ante coenam potui dato. *Aliud.* Anserinas linguas per triduum, quoque die unam, edendas apponito. *Aliud.* Rutae silvaticae semen per triduum esui dato. *Aliud.* Ipsius penis cimolia ex muralis herbae succo oblinatur.

Ed. Chart. X. [632.]

[Πρὸς δυσουρίαν.] Ῥοῦν καὶ τοὺς κισσοῦ ἐρυθροῦ κορύμβους τρίψας σὺν οἴνῳ λευκῷ κατάχριε μόρια τὰ τῶν δυσουριώντων ὀμφάλῳ ὑποκειμένων.

[Ὡς διαβήτης ἵσταται.] Λαβὼν ὑμένια τὰ τῆς ἀλεκτορίδων κοιλίας ἔσωθεν καὶ ξηράνας ἐν ἡλίῳ ἀναλάμβανε ἐξ αὐτῶν < α΄. ἄλλο. λαβὼν σταγονίου καὶ βαλάνου ξηρᾶς καὶ βαλαυστίου καὶ κηκίδων ἀνὰ < γ΄. τρίψας δίδου ἐξ αὐτῶν νήστει σὺν μέλιτι ῥοδίνῳ ἐν ὕδατι ψυχρῷ.

Κεφ. κστ΄. [Πρὸς γυναικεῖα πάθη.] [α΄. Πρὸς σύλληψιν.] Ἰσχάδας νήστει μετὰ φύλλων ἐλαινῶν δὸς φαγεῖν. ἄλλο. προβάτου μηρυκωμένου ἄρας τῷ δακτύλῳ τὸν ἀφρὸν δὸς πιεῖν μετὰ οἴνου. ἄλλο. κάρδαμον λεῖον μετ' ὄξους δίδου φαγεῖν ἐπὶ ἡμέρας δ΄. μετὰ τὴν κάθαρσιν. ἄλλο. ἀλώπεκος ἀφόδευμα ἐν πεσσῷ παρατιθέμενον καὶ ὑποχριόμενον συγγιγνέσθω. ἄλλο. ἀρτεμισίαν λείαν πρόσθες καὶ συλλήψεται. χριέσθωσαν δὲ τὴν φύσιν κόμμι, ὅταν ᾖ ἀπὸ τῶν ἐμμήνων τρίτη, καὶ συλλήψεται.

[*Ad difficultatem mingendi.*] Rhum et corymbos hederae rubrae tere ex vino albo et unge partes, quae ſunt ſub umbilico patientium dyſuriam.

[*Ad ſiſtendam exuberantiam urinae exeuntis.*] Accipe pelliculas, quae ſunt in ventre gallinarum et ſicca in ſole et ſume ex eis drachmam. *Aliud.* Recipe thuris masculi et glandis ſiccae et floris punici ſilveſtris et gallarum ana drach. iij, tere et da ex eis jejuno cum melle roſaceo ex aqua frigida.

Cap. XXVI. [*Ad foeminarum affectiones.*] [1. *Ad conceptum.*] Caricas jejunae cum oleae ſoliis eſui dato. *Aliud.* Ruminantis pecudis ſpumam digito ſumens ex vino in potum exhibe. *Aliud.* Naſturtium tritum ex aceto per quatriduum edito paſt purgationem. *Aliud.* Vulpinum ſtercus in peſſo apponatur et loci muliebres ſublinantur, atque ita venere utatur. *Aliud.* Artemiſiam tritam apponito et concipiet. Inunge autem muliebre pudendum gummi, quum a purgatione menſtrua tertius fuerit dies et concipiet.

Ed. Chart. X. [632.]

[β'. Πρὸς σύλληψιν.] Ὑστέραν λαγωοῦ ξηράνας καὶ τρίψας δίδου πίνειν μετὰ τὴν ἀπὸ τῶν ἐμμήνων κάθαρσιν.

[γ'. Ἐὰν γυνὴ ἄῤῥενα γεννῆσαι θέλει.] Φασκίᾳ λευκῇ παιδικῇ δῆσον τὸν δεξιὸν πόδα καὶ συγίνου.

[δ'. Ἐὰν δὲ θῆλυ.] Φασκίᾳ μελαίνῃ τὸν ἀριστερόν.

[ε'. Πρὸς γνῶναι ἢ ἄῤῥεν ἢ θῆλυ τὸ ἐν γαστρί.] Σέλινον μὴ γινωσκούσης ἐπὶ τὴν κεφαλὴν ἐπίθες καὶ ὃ ἂν φωνήσῃ πρῶτον, εἴτε ἄῤῥεν, εἴτε θῆλυ, ἐκεῖνο τέξεται· ἀπαράβατόν ἐστιν. ἄλλο. λαβὼν τῆς ἐν γαστρὶ ἐχούσης οὖρον ὄρυξον βοθρίσκους δύο καὶ εἰς τὸν ἕνα βάλε κριθὰς καὶ εἰς τὸν ἕτερον πυροὺς καὶ ἐπίχεε γῆν μετὰ τὸ ἐμβαλεῖν τὸ οὖρον αὐτῆς, καὶ ἐὰν πρῶτον ἐκβλαστήσουσιν οἱ πυροὶ, ἄῤῥεν τέξεται· ἐὰν δὲ αἱ κριθαὶ, θῆλυ.

[στ'. Πρὸς σύλληψιν ἀῤῥενοτόκιον.] Χηνὸς στέαρ καὶ ῥητίνην τερεβινθίνην διαχριέσθω ἐπὶ ἡμέρας β'. τῇ δὲ γ'. συγγινέσθω καὶ συλλήψεται. ἄλλο. ἀνὴρ τὸν δεξιὸν ὄρχιν ἀποδήσας συγγενέσθω· ἐὰν δὲ θῆλυ, τὸ ἀριστερόν.

[ζ'. Κατόχιον ἐμβρύων.] Ἀετίνην λίθον περίαπτε·

[2. *Ad conceptionem.*] Uterum leporis ſicca et tere et da potui quando a menſtruis fuerit purgata,

[3. *Ut mulier marem generet.*] Alba fascia puerili dextrum pedem ligato et coëat.

[4. *Ut feminam.*] Nigra ſascia ſiniſtrum pedem.

[5. *Notae maris et feminae in utero.*] Apium inſcia muliere ſuper caput imponito quodque primum voce protulerit, aut marem, aut ſeminam, illud pariet; comprobatum eſt. *Aliud.* Gravidae mulieris urinam accipiens duas ſoveolas ſacito, in unam hordeum, in alteram triticum conjicito; deinde urina conſpergito atque ita demum terram ſuperjacito; ſi prius triticum expullulaverit, mas pariet; ſin vero hordeum, femina.

[6. *Ut mas concipiatur.*] Anſerino adipe et reſina terebinthi loci perungantur per biduum; tertio die cum viro conjungatur et marem concipiet. *Aliud.* Vir ſiniſtro teſte ligato venere utatur; ut femina dextro.

[7. *Ut foetus retineatur.*] Lapis Aëtites appenda-

Ed. Chart. X. [632. 633.]
κατέχει δὲ ἔμβρυον λίθος ὁ βλαστήσας εἰς ἀχράδα καὶ περιμείνας, εἶτα περιαπτόμενος. καὶ μαλάχης δὲ ἀγρίας ῥίζαν ἁπτόμενος καὶ ἐπίβοσκον λέγουσι· κατέχει καὶ σαρδὰ ἔμβρυα μέχρι τέλους. χρὴ δὲ τῇ κοιλίᾳ περιάπτειν. ἔστι δὲ καὶ ἡ σιδηρῖτις βοτάνη τῶν ἐμβρύων, τηρητικὴ περιαπτομένη.

[633] [η'. Πρὸς δυστοκίαν.] Χαμαιπίτυν καὶ ἄσφαλτον ἐπὶ τῶν ἀνθράκων θεὶς ὑποκάπνιζε ἢ αὐτὰ πρόσθες.

[θ'. Ἐκβόλιον ἐμβρύου τεθνηκότος.] Χολῆς ταύρου τὸ μέγεθος ἀμυγδάλου διεὶς οἴνῳ ὕδατι κεκραμένῳ, κοχλιάρια β'. δὸς πιεῖν, ἐκβαλεῖ παραχρῆμα. ἄλλο. λύκιον ὠμὸν καυλίσκου συγκεκομμένῳ κεδρίᾳ χρίσων καὶ θέρμανον καὶ δὸς πίνειν νήστει. ἄλλο. ἀρτεμισίαν ἑψήσας μετὰ μελικράτου δὸς πίνειν. ἄλλο. λίθον κυνόδηκτον πρὸς κύνα ἀπεῤῥιμμένον, ἐν γῇ τεθειμένον μεταβαινέτω δυστοκίαν ἡ φέρουσα γυνή.

[ι'. Πρὸς ἐξάγειν καταμήνια.] Λαβὼν πρασίου, νε-

tur. Foetum quoque et lapis ille retinet, qui in piraſtro adnatus inhaereſcit, iſte ſimiliter penſilis geſtetur. Et malvae agreſtis radix, quam epiboscon nominant, appenſa. Sardonius etiam lapis retinet foetus usque in finem; ventri autem eum deligare oportet. Eſt herba quoque ſideritis, cujus appenſu foetus cuſtodiuntur.

[8. *Ad difficultatem partus.*] Ajugam et bitumen pone ſuper carbones et ſuffumiga vel ipſa appone.

[9. *Ad extrahendum foetum mortuum.*] Fellis tauri magnitudinem amygdalae diſſolvens in vino aquato da cochlearia ij, potui et emittet conſeſtim. *Aliud.* Lycium crudum trito caule junge cum cedria et calefacias et da bibendum jejuno. *Aliud.* Artemiſiam coque in mulſa et propina. *Aliud.* Super lapidem, quem mordet canis, quando projicitur in eum, poſitum in ſole tranſeat mulier quae patitur difficultatem partus.

[10. *Ad educenda menſtrua.*] Marrubium, nepetam,

Ed. Chart. X. [633.]

πέτης, πηγάνου καὶ καππάρεως φλοιοῦ ἀνὰ < γ'. ἐν οἴνῳ ἑψήσας ἢ ὕδατι δίδου πιεῖν. ἄλλο. τὸ τὶ ὕδατος, ἐν ᾧ διαλύεται ἡ ζύμη παλαιὰ ὅτε ποιεῖται ἄρτος, δὸς πίνειν.

[ια'. Πρὸς πόνον ὑστέρας.] Παιονίας ῥίζαν πότιζε· ἢ ἴριδος ῥίζαν ἢ παιονίας σπέρματος κόκκους ιε'. ἢ ψυλλίου ἢ ἀκαλήφης χυλὸν πρόσθες. ἢ τὰ φύλλα μελισσοφύλλου ἀφηψήμενα ἐν οἴνῳ. ἄλλο. λαβὼν πήγανον χλωρὸν καὶ κόψας σὺν βουτύρῳ καὶ στέατι χοιρείῳ ποίει χρῖμα.

[ιβ'. Ὡς γυνὴ ἡ βεβιασμένη παραφαίνηται παρθένος.] Λαβὼν ὀμφακιτίδων, κύπρου, ξυλοκασσίας, ῥόδων ξηρῶν, πεπέρεως λευκοῦ καὶ κόκκου γνιδίου ἀνὰ ἐξάγιον α'. προλελουμένη ὑστέρᾳ προσθέτω ταῦτα· ὠφελεῖ δὲ καὶ σπέρμα ὀξυλαπάθου τετριμμένον καὶ πρόσθετον.

[ιγ'. Ὠκυτόκιον.] Βολβοὺς πικροὺς τρίψας διὰ γλυκέος δὸς πιεῖν καὶ παραχρῆμα τέξεται. ἄλλο. δίκταμνον διὰ οἴνου ἢ ὕδατος πότιζε. ἄλλο. ὕειον γάλα ἐν μέλιτι πινέτω. ἄλλο. χαλβάνην τρίψας ἐν ὕδατι δὸς πιεῖν καὶ τέξεται παραχρῆμα.

rutam, corticem capparis, ana drachmas iij, coque in vino aut aqua et da bibenda. *Aliud.* De aqua, qua diſſolvitur ſermentum vetus quando fit panis potui dato.

[11. *Ad dolores uteri.*] Paeoniae radicem propina; vel radicem iridis vel ſeminis paeoniae granula xv, vel pulicariae aut urticae ſuccum appone vel folia apiaſtri cocta in vino. *Aliud.* Accipe rutam viridem et tere et cum butyro et adipe porci fac unguentum.

[12. *Ut mulier violata appareat virgo.*] Accipe gallarum immaturarum, liguſtri, xylocaſiae, roſarum ſiccarum, piperis albi, grani gnidii ana exagium unum; tere et prius lotae vulvae apponat iſta. Confert autem et ſemen rumicis acidi tritum et appoſitum.

[13. *Ut partus acceleretur.*] Bulbi, amari triti ex vino dulci potui dentur, illico pariet. *Aliud.* Dictamnum ex vino aut aqua propinatum idem facit. *Aliud.* Suillum lac ex melle bibitum. *Aliud.* Galbanum ex aqua tritum potumque confeſtim educit foetum.

Ed. Chart. X. [633.]

[ιδ'. Ὑποθυμίαμα δυστοκούσαις.] Χαμαιπίτυν ἐπὶ τῶν ἀνθράκων θεὶς ἢ ἄσφαλτον οἷον οἱ χαλκεῖς χρῶνται β'. προστιθέσθω καὶ εὐθέως ποιεῖ. ἄλλο. γλήχωνος δεσμίδιον εἰς ὕδωρ θερμὸν βαλὼν ποίει περικαθίσαι τὴν γυναῖκα καὶ λέγε εἰς τὸ οὖς αὐτῆς, χοῦ. κᾶ. μῖ. δοῦς. ἄλλο. λαβὼν ἔλαιον εἰς τὰς χεῖρας ἀνάτριψον αὐτῆς τὰ ἰσχία ἐπιλέγων· χορίον στῆθι σῶμα, ὅτι ἐπιτάσσει σοι μεγάλη ἡ θεοτόκος.

[ιε'. Γάλα κατασπάσαι.] Ῥαφανῖδας μετὰ πυρῶν ἀναζέσας ἐν οἴνῳ καὶ διηθήσας δὸς πιεῖν. ἄλλο. πίτυρα μετὰ μαράθρων ῥιζῶν ἑψήσας τὸ ὕδωρ δὸς πιεῖν. ἄλλο. μελάνθιον διεὶς ἐν μελικράτῳ οἷον ὁλκὴν δίδου πιεῖν. ἄλλο. κισσοῦ φύλλα διεὶς ἐν μελικράτῳ δὸς πιεῖν.

[ιστ'. Γάλα σβέσαι.] Κατάντλει θαλάσσῃ καὶ κατάπλασσε τοῖς στύφειν δυναμένοις καὶ ἀναξηραίνειν. ἄλλο. ἅλμην ποιήσας θερμὴν καὶ σπόγγοις ἐκθλίβων καὶ μάννα ἐπιπάσσων ἐπίδει καὶ χάρτας ὁμοίως.

[ιζ'. Ἐὰν δὲ σκληροὶ ὦσι καὶ φλεγμαίνωσι.] Κατάπλασσε

[14. *Suffitus ad aegre parientes.*] Ajuga ſuper carbones poſita aut bituminis, quo fabri ferrarii utuntur, duplum carbonibus injectum mirifice prodeſt. *Aliud.* Pulegii fasciculum in aquam calidam mittito, in eaque mulierem deſidere jubeto ipſique in aurem dicito Chy. ca. mi. dus. *Aliud.* Oleum manibus continens ejus ilia perfricato atque ita dicito: ſecundae ſiſtite corpus, quoniam praecipit vobis magna dei genitrix.

[15. *Ad lac attrahendum et creandum.*] Radiculas cum tritico vino incoctas percola et vinum potui offeras. *Aliud.* Aquam, cui furfures cum foeniculi radicibus incoctae ſint, propinato. *Aliud.* Nigellae drachmam in mulſa mixtam da potui. *Aliud.* Mulſa hederae folia contuſa habens potui detur.

[16. *Ad lac reſiccandum.*] Aqua maris foveto et aſtringere ſiccareque valentia ſuperimponito. *Aliud.* Muriam calidam ſpongiis exprimens et thuris pulvisculum inſpergens deligato et chartas eodem modo.

[17. *Quodſi mammae durae inflammataeque fuerint.*]

Ed. Chart. X. [633. 634.]

λινοσπέρμῳ δι' ὀξυμέλιτος ἑφθῷ, ἢ τήλει ὁμοίως ἑψηθείσῃ ἢ σησάμῳ ἀπλύτῳ, ψυχθέντι καὶ λειωθέντι μίξας μέλιτι ἢ σύκοις κατάπλασσε. ἄλλο. κύμινον τρίψας μετ' οἰνομέλιτος καὶ κηρωτῆς πάχος ποιήσας ἔμπλασσε εἰς ὀθόνιον ἐπιθείς.

[634] [ιη'. Πότημα ἐκβόλιον ἐμβρύου τεθνηκότος ἢ μὴ φερομένου κατὰ φύσιν.] Χολῆς ταύρου τὸ μέγεθος ἀμυγδάλου διεὶς οἴνῳ παλαιῷ κεκραμένῳ κοχλιάρια β'. δὸς πιεῖν, ἐκβάλλει παραχρῆμα. ἄλλο. ᾠὸν ὠμὸν κεδρίᾳ χρῖσον καὶ θέρμανον καὶ δὸς ῥοφῆσαι νήστει. ἄλλο. ἀρτεμισίαν ἑψήσας μετὰ μελικράτου δὸς πιεῖν. ἄλλο. ὁ φοινικίτης λίθος ἐγχριόμενος ἐκβόλιόν ἐστιν· ἀτελὲς δὲ ἔμβρυον ἐκβάλλει λίθος κυνόδηκτος ἂν τεθῇ καὶ ὑπερβῇ αὐτὸν ἡ κύουσα, ὡς τάχος ἐκβάλλει τὸ κατὰ γαστρός.

[ιθ'. Γυναῖκα γνῶναι εἰ ἐκτρώσει τὸ ἐν γαστρί.] Ἐὰν οἱ μαστοὶ ἰσχναίνοιντο, σημαίνει ἔκτρωσιν.

[κ'. Κατάπλασμα φθόριον.] Ἐρεγμοῦ καθαροῦ κύαθοι δύο ἕψει ἐν πολταρίῳ μετ' ὄξους· μετὰ δὲ τὸ ἡμίεφθον

Lini ſemine aceto mulſo incocto illine; aut foenogracco ſimiliter elixo aut ſeſamo non loto refrigerato, trito et melli admixto aut ex ſicis cataplasma facito. *Aliud.* Cuminum tritum mulſo temperatum ad cerati craſſitudinem linteolo illitum impone.

[18. *Potio foetum mortuum aut non ritu naturali exeuntem ejiciens.*] Fellis tauri quanta eſt nux amygdala vini veteris diluti ligulis duabus temperatum potandum offeras; ſtatim foetum excludit. *Aliud.* Ovum crudum cedri lacryma illinito, calefacito et jejunae ſorbendum dato. *Aliud.* Mulſam artemiſiam incoctam habentem propinato. *Aliud.* Lapis phoenicites vocatus illitu foetum detrahit. Item lapis demorſus a cane foetum nondum perfectum evocat, ſi praegnans mulier ſuper ipſum tranſeat; nam quod in ventre eſt valde cito expellit.

[19. *Ut cognoscatur, mulier an abortum fecerit.*] Mammae gracileſcentes abortum ſignificant.

[20. *Cataplasma ad abortum impellens.*] Fabae freſae mundae cyathi duo in ollula ex aceto decoquan-

Ed. Chart. X. [634.]
γενέσθαι ἀλόης γο. α'. καὶ μαλαγματῶδες ποιήσας ἐπιτίθει κατὰ τοῦ ὀμφαλοῦ μέχρι κτενὸς καὶ ἐπίδει.

[κα. Κατάπλασμα ὥστε φθεῖραι ἄνευ πάσης βλαβῆς καὶ βασάνου.] Κυπαρίσσου φύλλων ἑψήσας μέρος ὕδατι λείανον ἐπιμελῶς ὡς μαλαγματῶδες γενεσθαι καὶ ἐπίθες ἐπὶ τὸν ὀμφαλόν καὶ τὸ ἐπιγάστριον καὶ κατάδει φασκίᾳ· κέλευον ἐπικαθίσαι ὑπτίαν ἢ ἐπὶ κουρικοῦ βάθρου καθίσαι καὶ κοιμωμένη ἀπόνως ἐκβάλλει.

[κβ'. Ἐκβόλιον ἀκίνδυνον ὥστε μηνῶν τριῶν ἢ δ'. ἐκβάλλειν.] Ὀποπάνακος ὀβολοῦ κολλύριον ποιήσας ὑπόθες. ἀκίνδυνόν ἐστι καὶ πεπείραται ἐπὶ πολλῶν. ἄλλο. στρουθίον λεῖον μετὰ μέλιτος ἀναλαβὼν ἀνάπλασσε πεσσοὺς μικροὺς καὶ ὑποτίθει. ἄγει καὶ τὰ δεύτερα καὶ καταμήνια. ἄλλο. ἀρτεμισίας τῶν φύλλων λειοτριβήσας μετὰ ῥοδίνου καὶ ποιήσας γλοιοῦ πάχος προστίθει· καταμηνίων ἀγωγόν. ἄλλο. ἰσχάδας β'. S''. νίτρου ὀβολὸν πεσσὸν ποιήσας ἐπιτίθει. ἄλλο. ἀρτεμισίαν τρίψας ἐπιτίθει. ἄλλο. πηγάνου ἀγρίου

tur; quum ad dimidium conſumptum fuerit, aloës uncia adjiciatur, ut malagmatis inſtar reddatur; deinde illinito ab umbilico ad pectinem usque et adalligato.

[21. *Cataplasma ad necandum foetum citra noxam ullamque ſuſpicionis notam.*] Cupreſſi foliorum partem aqua elixam curioſe terito ad malagmatis temperaturam atque umbilico et abdomini imponito fasciaque deligato; deinde ſupinam jacere jubeto aut in ſella ſedere, qua in partu mulieres uti ſolent: et ſopita ſine dolore foetum emittet.

[22. *Medicamentum periculi expers, ut trimeſtris aut quadrimeſtris foetus ejiciatur.*] Opopanacis obolum accipe et collyrium fac et locis muliebribus ſubmitte; tutum eſt atque multis expertum. *Aliud.* Radiculam tritam melle exceptam peſſis illine parvis et eos mulieris genitalibus impone; educit hoc ſecundas et menſtrua purgamenta. *Aliud.* Artemiſiae folia teras ex roſeo et ſordium craſſitudinem faciens appone; menſes citat. *Aliud.* Caricas duas et ſemiſſem, nitri obolum accipe; peſſum

Ed. Chart. X. [634.]

σπέρμα προστίθει. ἄλλο. γαγάτης λίθος ὑποθυμιώμενος τὰς μὴ καθαιρομένας καθαίρει.

[κγ'. Ἐὰν τεκούσῃ αἷμα μὴ ἐκκριθῇ.] Ἄρου σπέρμα τρίψας ἐν οἴνῳ λευκῷ νηστικῇ δίδου πιεῖν.

[κδ'. Πρὸς τὰς ἐκ τοκετοῦ χλωράς.] Πάνακος ῥίζας τρίψας ἐν οἴνῳ γλυκεῖ δίδου πιεῖν νηστικῇ. ἄλλο. κυτίνων ἄνθος ῥοῶν μετὰ μύρων ἑψημένων δὸς πιεῖν. ἄλλο. λαβὼν τρύγα οἴνου παλαιοῦ καὶ ῥίζαν κρίνου καὶ σκόροδα λεάνας κατάχριε πρόσωπον δείλης καὶ πρωῒ ἀπόπλυνε καὶ τοῦτο ἕως ἂν τὸ πρόσωπον ἐρυθρὸν γένηται.

[κε'. Πρὸς κοιλίαν κατεῤῥωγυῖαν καὶ μαστοὺς καὶ μηροὺς καὶ ἰσχία.] Κοχλίου θαλασσίου τὸν ὑπόμακρον καύσας καὶ λειοτριβήσας πρόσβαλε ὠοῦ τὸ λευκὸν ἢ ὄνειον γάλα καὶ κατάχριε. ἄλλο. διαφανὲς κόψας καὶ τρίψας ὅταν εἰς βαλάνειον εἰσέρχεται καὶ κατάχριε πρὶν ἀλείψασθαι. ἐπὶ ἡμέρας κ'. ἀφανίζονται.

[κστ'. Πρὸς τὸ κοιλίαν, ἢ ὑποχόνδριον, ἢ μηροὺς

facito et submitte. *Aliud.* Artemisiam tritam impone. *Aliud.* Rutae agrestis semen immitte. *Aliud.* Gagates lapis suffitus non purgatis mulieribus menses ducit.

[23. *Ad mulierem, quae a partu non purgetur.*] Ari semen tritum ex vino albo jejuna bibito.

[24. *Ad pallorem mulieris a partu.*] Panacis radices contusae ex dulci vino a jejuna potae pallorem discutiunt. *Aliud.* Flores mali punici domesticae odorato oleo incocti potui dentur. *Aliud.* Accipe faecem vini antiqui et radicem lilii et allia et lenias et unge faciem vespere et mane lava et hoc quousque facies rubefiat.

[25. *Ad ventris, mammarum, femorum coxendicumque scissuras.*] Marinam cochleam oblongam cremato et conterito, deinde ovi albo aut asinino lacte adjecto illinito. *Aliud.* Lapidem diaphanes contere contritumque in ingressu balnei, antequam inungatur, illinito et vicesimo die scissurae evanescent.

[26. *Ad sudores ventris, hypochondriorum, femo-*

ἱδροῦσθαι ἐκ τοκετῶν.] Κιμωλίας καὶ μάννης ἑκάστου ἴσον ἀναλάμβανε ὠοῦ λευκῷ καὶ κατάχριε μετὰ κηρωτῆς κυπρίνης.

[635] [κζ'. Πρὸς τὰ ἐν τοῖς ἰσχίοις ἐμφυσήματα.] Ἄρτου τὸ ἐντὸς καὶ μελαντηρίαν συμφυράσας ἐπιτίθει· τοῦτο καθίστησιν.

[κη'. Πρὸς ἐξομφάλους.] Κηκίδας καύσας, τρίψας μετὰ ὕδατος κατάπλασσε.

[κθ'. Ὀμφαλὸν ἐκ τοκετοῦ μέγαν καὶ καλὸν ποιῆσαι.] Λαβὼν βύσμα ἀπὸ ληκύθου βίβλινον περιείλησον ὀθονίῳ, ἔπειτα μάνναν ὠοῦ τῷ λευκῷ ἀναλαβὼν κατάχρισον καὶ ἔνθες εἰς τὸν ὀμφαλὸν καὶ ἐπίδει προστύπως.

[λ'. Πρὸς ὑστερικὰς πνίξεις.] Χελώνης χερσαίας ἧπαρ λεῖον ἐν πεσσῷ ὑποτίθει, ἀπαράβατόν ἐστι, μηδενὶ μεταδίδου.

[λα'. Πόμα πρὸς πόνον ὑστέρας.] Λαγωοῦ καρδίαν ξηράνας ἐπιξύων δίδου πιεῖν.

[λβ'. Πρὸς τοὺς γενομένους στρόφους ἀπὸ τοκετοῦ

rumque a partu.] Cimoliae et pulveris thuris par modus ovi albo exceptus cum liguſtrino cerato illinatur.

[27. *Ad inflationes in coxendicibus.*] Panis medullam et melanteriam una ſubigito et imponito; bene facit.

[28. *Ad prominentes umbilicos.*] Gallas uſtas tritasque ex aqua ſuperdato.

[29. *Ut umbilicus a partu magnus ac elegans fiat.*] Operculum urcei chartaceum ſumens panniculo involve, deinde thuris pulvisculum ovi albo comprehendens illine et in umbilicum mitte tenaciterque alligato.

[30. *Ad uteri ſtrangulatus.*] Teſtudinis terreſtris jecur tritum in peſſo naturalibus imponito; perpetuo reſpondet, cuiquam ne communices.

[31. *Potio ad uteri dolorem.*] Leporis cor aridum et in ramenta conciſum potui detur.

[32. *Ad tormina uteri a partu, corruptiones et*

Ed. Chart. X. [635.]

καὶ φθορὰς καὶ πνιγμούς.] Λεπτοσφαίρους ὀβολοῦ S″. ὀρεσίνημα καλοῦσι, τοῖς τρισὶ δακτύλοις μετὰ γλυκέος πινέτω.

[λγ′. Πρὸς ὑστέρας πόνους.] Γλυκείας ῥοᾶς ῥίζαν ἐν οἴνῳ πινέτω.

[λδ′. Πρὸς τὰς ἐκ μήτρας σκληρίας.] Κύμινον λεῖον καὶ πηγάνου φύλλα ἀναλάμβανε πίσσῃ ὑγρᾷ καὶ βουτύρῳ καὶ πεσσὸν ποιήσας δι᾽ ἐρίου ἐντίθει.

[λε′. Πόμα πρὸς ὑστερικὰς γυναῖκας.] Καστόριον μετὰ ἀνίσου πότιζε. ἄλλο. κύμινον τρίψας καὶ μελανθίου μέρος S″. μετὰ ὀξυμέλιτος πότιζε.

[λστ′. Πόμα πρὸς ῥοῦν γυναικεῖον.] Πευκεδάνου ῥίζαν καὶ κυπαρίσσου σφαιρίων ἴσα ἑκάστου ἐν οἴνῳ λευκῷ δίδου πιεῖν. ἄλλο. γίγαρτα σταφυλῆς μελαίνης ξηρὰ λειώσας ἐν οἴνῳ μελαυστηρῷ δίδου πίνειν. ἄλλο. πιτυὰν ἐρίφου λαβὼν λεῖανον σὺν ὄξει δριμυτάτῳ καὶ δίδου νήστει πιεῖν. ἄλλο. κοράλλιον δίδου ἐν οἴνῳ μέλανι καὶ παραχρῆμα στήσεται. ἄλλο. νάρθηκος σποδὸν καὶ μήκωνος κονίαν ἐν ὕδατι δίδου πίνειν πρὸς ὀλίγον· εἰ δὲ εἴη πλέον φερόμενον, σπόγ-

ſtrangulatus.] Leptoſphaeros accipito ad oboli ſemiſſem, oreſinema vocant, tribus digitis et ex dulci bibito.

[33. *Ad uteri dolores.*] Mali punici dulcis radicem ex vino propinato.

[34. *Ad uteri duritias.*] Cuminum tritum et rutae folia pice liquida excepta et butyro in peſſu ex lana facto impone.

[35. *Alia potio ad mulieres in utero laborantes.*] Caſtoreum cum aniſo propina. *Alia.* Cuminum tritum et nigellae ſemiſſem ex aceto mulſo propina.

[36. *Potio ad muliebre profluvium.*] Peucedani radicis et cupreſſi baccarum pares portiones ex vino albo potentur. *Alia.* Uvae nigrae acinorum arida ſemina ex vino nigro auſtero potui dentur. *Alia.* Hoedi coagulum acerrimo aceto maceratum jejuno propinato. *Alia.* Corallium ex nigro vino dato et confeſtim ſupprimetur profluvium. *Alia.* Ferulae cinerem et papaveris pulverem ex aqua pauxillum exhibeto; quodſi largis effluat, ſpon-

Ed. Chart. X. [635.]

γον καύσας δίδου ὅσον < γ'. ἄλλο. κέρας ἐλάφειον καύσας δὸς πιεῖν.

[λζ'. Πρόσθετα.] Ῥοιὰν σὺν ἐρίῳ καταπλάσας προστίθει. ἢ σίδια ἑψήσας καὶ τρίψας ἐν ἐρίῳ δεῖ προστίθεσθαι ἐν πεσσῷ. ἄλλο. κηκίδος τὸ ἐντὸς καὶ λιβάνου ἀναλαβὼν ἐν πεσσῷ προστίθει διὰ ὕδατος. ἄλλο. γλήχωνα λεῖον ἀναλαβὼν ἐρίῳ καθαρῷ προστίθει· βοηθεῖ δὲ ὄξει ζεστῷ σπόγγος βαπτόμενος καὶ ἐκθλιβόμενος συμμέτρως καὶ μηρῶν δὲ συναγωγὴ καὶ δέσις ἄκρων καὶ κατάκλισις ἐπὶ κεφαλήν.

[λη'. Πρὸς τὸ μὴ καθυγραίνεσθαι τὸ αἰδοῖον ἐν ταῖς συνουσίαις τῶν γυναικῶν.] Κηκίδος ὀμφακίνης κόκκους δ'. σποδίου, ᾧ χρῶνται εἰς τὰ ὀφθαλμικὰ, μύστρα δύο τρῖψον καὶ μῖξον εἰς τὸ αὐτὸ καὶ ἀπόθου εἰς ἀγγεῖον καθαρὸν καὶ τούτου λαμβάνουσα μύστρον οἴνῳ παλαιῷ διεῖσα καὶ τούτῳ ὑποποτιζέσθω ταῖς πρώταις ἡμέραις, ἡ γαμηθεῖσα καθ' ὅλου τοῦ βίου διαμενεῖ τοὺς τόπους μὴ καθυγρουμένη. ἄλλο. κηκίδας ἐμβρέχων εἰς ὕδωρ ἡμέρας η'. εἶτα βρέχε ἔριον

giae combuſtae drachmas iij exhibeto. *Alia.* Cornu cervinum uſtum potui dato.

[37. *Medicamenta naturalibus imponenda.*] Malum punicum in lana more cataplasmatis appone. Aut mali punici coria elixa in lanaque trita in peſſo apponenda ſunt. *Aliud.* Gallae interiora et thuris tantundem in peſſo accipiens ex aqua appone. *Aliud.* Pulegium tritum lana munda comprehendens naturalibus impone. Opitulatur etiam ſpongia ferventi aceto madida et mediocriter expreſſa; femorum praeterea coitio, extremorum deligatio atque in caput decubitus.

[38. *Ut mulierum naturalia in concubitu non humescant.*] Gallae immaturae grana quatuor, cinerulae, qua in oculorum vitiis uti conſueverunt, myſtra duo terito, in unum misceto et in nitido ut vitreo vaſe reponito; ex hoc myſtrum ſumens veteri vino dilutum eo primis diebus nupta naturalia ſublinat, ac per totam vitam lo-

Ed. Chart. X. [635. 636.]

τεθυωμένον τρυφερὸν τῷ ἀποβρέγματι καὶ μὴ ἐκπιέζων ἔα ξηρανθῆναι καὶ πεσσὸν ποιῶν τοῦ ὁρίου δίδου ὑποτίθεσθαι· [636] καὶ ἔσται ὡς παρθένος ἐν τῇ συνουσίᾳ. αἱρείτω τὸ ἔριον καὶ ξηραινέτω καὶ πάλιν χρήσθω εἰ θέλει. ἄλλο. ὀξυλαπάθου σπέρμα τρίψας δίδου ὑποτίθεσθαι καὶ ἔσται ὡς παρθένος. ἄλλο. κηκίδας κόψας εἰς ὕδωρ ἔμβαλε καὶ δίδου προσκλύζεσθαι καὶ θερμοτέρας ποιεῖ τὰς γυναῖκας. ἄλλο. ὀθόνια ἰσχνὰ ἀποβρέχειν εἰς στυπτηρίαν μετὰ ὕδατος ἀνειμένην καὶ ξηραίνειν· εἶτα κυπέρου καὶ κασσίας καὶ κηκίδος ἴσον ἑκάστου τρῖβε ἐν οἴνῳ παλαιῷ πάχος ποιεῖν μέλιτος. τούτῳ τὰ ὀθόνια βρέχων ἀναξήρανον καὶ δίδου προστίθεσθαι καὶ κέλευε συνέχειν ὥραις δυσὶ ταμιευομένην πρὸς τὴν χρείαν· ὅταν δὲ ὁμιλεῖν μέλλῃ, τότε ἀφαίρετο ἐκεῖνα. ἄλλο. λαβοῦσα δὲ μέλι καὶ νίτρον καταχριέτω τὸ μόριον μέχρι τοῦ ἐφηβαίου. οὕτως συγγίνου.

Κεφ. κζ΄. [α΄. Πρὸς τὸ ἀνέντατόν τινα γενέσθαι.]

corum illorum humiditatem non praecipiet. *Aliud.* Gallas per octo dies in aqua macerato; deinde lanam mollem sulfure suffumigatam aqua illa madefacito et non expressam siccescere sinito; ex lana pessum faciens naturalibus immittito; in congressu venereo virgo putabitur; deinde lanam tollito exsiccatoque atque iterum, si lubet, utitor. *Aliud.* Acidi rumicis semen tritum submittendum exhibeto et erit ut virgo. *Aliud.* Gallas contusas in aquam demitte, ex qua subluantur mulierum naturalia: angustiora enim reddentur. *Aliud.* Panniculos tenues in aquam alumen liquatum habentem demergito et exsiccato; deinde quadrati junci, cassiae, gallarum, singul. parem modum ex vino veteri conterito, donec mellis crassitudo fiat; in hoc panniculos madefaciens resiccato utque imponant concedito, atque ita per duas horas retineant vel prout requirit necessitas; et cum venere uti volent, eximant. *Aliud.* Melle et nitro usque ad putem naturalia oblinito atque ita concubito.

Cap. XXVII. [1. *Ut ne cui penis arrigi possit.*]

Ed. Chart. X. [636.]

Κήρυκα καύσας σβέσον οὔρῳ βοὸς τομίου καὶ λάμβανε ἀπὸ τούτου ἢ ἐν ποτῷ ἢ ἐν βρωτῷ. τὸ δὲ ἄλλο εἰς ἀγγεῖον ἀπόθου. ἄλλο. λύσις. ἄναψον τὸ ξυλάριον καὶ παύεται. ἄλλο. ὀξύσχοινος ἐντεθεῖσα καὶ γενομένη κηρύκου σχῆμα τοῦ ὄξεως ἐκκριθέντος εἰς τὴν κοίτην ἐπιτίθει ὑπὸ τὰ στρώματα καὶ κατέχει τὰς ἐπὶ τὰ ἀφροδίσια ὁρμάς. ἄλλο. κορίαννον ἢ γλήχων ἐσθιόμενος πολλάκις ἀνέντατον ποιεῖ. ἄλλο. χολὴ νάρκης ἐάν τις τὸ μόριον ἀνέντατον ἔσται. ἄλλο. ἀπὸ λύχνου αὐτομάτως σβεσθέντος λαβὼν πομφόλυγα τὴν ἔτι ζῶσαν βάλλε εἰς τὸ πόμα καὶ δὸς πιεῖν, γενήσεται γὰρ ἀνέντατος ὅλην τὴν νύκτα ὁ πιών.

[β΄. Ἐντατικὰ τοῦ αἰδοίου.] Αἰδοῖον ἐντείνουσι καὶ ἐξορμάουσι πρὸς ἀφροδίσια τάδε· κωναρίων, πεπέρεως, πετροσελίνου, ἐλαφίου αἰδοίου ῥινήματος τερεβινθίνης ἀνὰ ἴσα μέλιτι ἀναλάμβανε καὶ σὺν οἴνῳ δίδου πίνειν. ἄλλο. λαβὼν ἐρεβίνθων ὠμῶν, κωναρίων γο. β΄. εὐζόμου σπέρματος, πεπέρεως λευκοῦ ἀνὰ γο. α΄. μέλιτος τὸ ἀρκοῦν, δίδου δι-

Buccinum ustum lotio bovis castrati extinguito; hoc in cibis aut potionibus utitor; quod remanet, in vase reponito. *Aliud.* Parvulum lignum appendito, et desinit. *Aliud.* Acutus juncus impositus, ut in figuram cyrici redactus illius qui cito semen excernit, sub stragulis vestibus positus, impetum in venerem cohibet. *Aliud.* Coriandrum aut pulegium si frequentius edatur, penem flaccidum reddit. *Aliud.* Fel torpedinis si quis potui det, genitale membrum minime rigebit. *Aliud.* Lucernae sponte exstinctae scintillam adhuc vivam si in poculum conjeceris et potui dederis, per totam noctem penis arrigi non poterit.

[2. *Ad arrectionem pudendi.*] Pudendum intendunt et movent ad coitum ista: nucum pinearum, piperis, petroselini, scobis pudendi cervini aridi, terebinthinae, singulorum partes aequales excipe melle: et ex vino bibendas praebe. *Aliud.* Recipe cicerum crudorum, nucum pinearum singulorum unc. ij, seminum erucae, piperis albi ana unc. j, mellis quod sufficit, da drach. ij

δραχμον σὺν οἴνῳ. ἄλλο. αἰδοῖον κατάχριε τῷ μέλιτι προ ἀφροδισίας. ἄλλο. εὐζόμου σπέρμα σὺν μέλιτι δίδου πίνειν. ἄλλο. χυλοῦ τοῦ εὐζόμου κυάθους β΄. μετὰ πεπέρεως λευκοῦ τὸ ἀρκοῦν δίδου διὰ τριῶν ἡμερῶν τῶν ἐπαλλήλων ἡμερῶν. ἢ χυλοῦ εὐζόμου καὶ πεπέρεως λευκοῦ δίδου κοχλιάριον α΄. νήστει. συμφέρει καὶ ὄστρακον ἐχίνου θαλασσίου πινόμενον καὶ τὸ γάλα βόειον πιόν. ἄλλο. πολυγόνου βοτάνης σπέρμα καὶ σάρκα ἰχθύων ποταμίων ξηρὰν τρίψας δίδου πίνειν· ἐντατικὸν γάρ ἐστι. ὁμοίως σπέρμα τῆς ἀνδράχνης ἑψηθὲν μετὰ γάλακτος βοείου δίδου· πάνυ βοηθέει. ὁμοίως ᾠὰ πέρδικος ἐσθιόμενα. ἄλλο. σπέρμα πράσου σὺν ἀκράτῳ οἴνῳ δὸς πίνειν. ἄλλο. χυλὸς πολυγόνου βοτάνης πινόμενος ποιεῖ ἀφροδίσια ἑτοιμοτέρους. ἄλλο. τὸ ὕδωρ ἐν ᾧ σβεσθῇ ὁ σίδηρος πῖνε σὺν οἴνῳ. ἄλλο. ὀρχιδίου ξηροῦ ἀλώπεκος κοχλιάριον α΄. πῖνε. ἄλλο. χυλὸν ἀσφοδέλου ῥίζης ἐκπιέσας δίδου πίνειν. ἄλλο. ὅταν ὁ ταῦρος μετὰ συνουσίαν οὐρήκῃ, γῆν συμμίξας τῷ πηλῷ ἐξ οὔρου καταπλασσομένῳ αἰδοῖον κατάχριε. ἄλλο. κόπρῳ τῇ βοείᾳ προσφάτῳ αἰδοῖον κατά-

cum vino. *Aliud.* Unge pudendum melle antequam coëas. *Aliud.* Semen erucae bibendum exhibeto cum melle. *Aliud.* Succi erucae cyathos ij, cum pipere albo quod ſufficit da tribus diebus alternis diebus. Vel ſucci erucae et piperis albi da cochlear unum jejuno. Confert etiam teſta marini erinacei bibita et lac bubulum bibitum. *Aliud.* Sanguinalis herbae ſemen et carnem piscium fluvialium ſiccam terens bibendam praebe; tentiginem enim facit. Similiter ſemen portulaceae coctum cum lacte bubulo mire prodeſt. Item ova perdicis ſi comedantur. *Aliud.* Semen porri cum vino mero bibendum exhibe. *Aliud.* Succus ſanguinalis herbae bibitus facit promptiores ad coctum. *Aliud.* Aquam, in qua exſtinguitur ferrum, bibe cum vino. *Aliud.* Teſticuli vulpis ſicci bibe cochlear unum. *Aliud.* Succum expreſſum e radice haſtulae regiae da bibendum. *Aliud.* Quando taurus, poſtquam coiverit, minxerit, terram commisce et luto, quod ſit ex urina, unge pudendum. *Aliud.* Stercore bovis recenti unge pudendum.

χρίε. ἄλλο. κόκκον γνίδιον τρίψας καὶ σὺν ἐλαίῳ ῥοδί-
[637] νῳ διαμίξας κατάχριε. ἄλλο. χυλῷ περιστερεῶνος αἰδοῖον κατάχριε.

[γʹ. Πρὸς ὕπνον.] Εἰς φύλλον δάφνης ἐπίγραφε καὶ ὑποτίθει ἐπὶ τὴν κεφαλὴν λεληθότως, ὀνομάζων κόνκοφον βραχερέον.

[δʹ. Πρὸς τοὺς μὴ δυναμένους συνουσιάζειν.] Σκαμμωνίαν μεθ᾽ ὕδατος χρίου.

Κεφ. κηʹ. [Πρὸς τὸ δῆγμα τῶν ἰοβόλων ζώων.] Πρὸς δῆγμα τῶν ἰοβόλων θηρίων τὰ μελίας φύλλα κόψας χυλοῦ δίδου κοχλιάρια γʹ. ἀπυρέττουσι μετὰ τῶν νʹ. κυάθων τοῦ οἴνου. ἄλλο. φλοῖον δένδρου βαλάνου ἢ εὔζυμον τὸ ἐν τοῖς λαχάνοις γιγνόμενον, ἢ χαμαιπίτυα, ἢ σκόροδον, ἓν ἐξ αὐτῶν τρίψας σὺν οἴνῳ ἀκράτῳ νήστει δίδου πίνειν. ἄλλο. αἷμα τῆς νήττης ἐναντιοῦται πᾶσι τοῖς δηλητηρίοις καὶ θανασίμοις. τοῦτο μὲν αὐτὸ ποιοῦσιν αἱ σάρκες τῆς ὄρνιθος προσφάτως ἀναιρεθείσης τοῖς δήγμασιν ἐντιθέμεναι· ἐναντιοῦνται γὰρ τοῖς ἰοβόλοις ἅπασι καὶ ἰαοῦνται

Aliud. Granum gnidium tere et permifce cum oleo rofaceo et unge. *Aliud.* Succo verbenacae unge pudendum.

[3. *Ad fomnum conciliandum.*] Lauri folia infcripta capiti clanculum fubjicito, nominans concophon brachereon.

[4. *Ad eos, qui coïre nequeunt.*] Scammoniam ex aqua illinito.

Cap. XXVIII. [*Ad morfum venenoforum animalium.*] Ad morfum venenoforum animalium fraxini folia tere et fucci da cochlearia tria non febricitantibus cum tribus cyathis vini. *Aliud.* Corticem arboris glandis vel erucam, quae in oleribus nascitur, vel ajugam, vel allium, unum ex his terens da cum vino non aquato jejuno bibendum. *Aliud.* Sanguis anatis adverfatur omnibus venenofis et mortiferis. Hoc idem etiam faciunt carnes gallinae nuper occifae, fi morfibus imponantur; obfiftunt enim omnibus venenofis et medentur praeter aspidis

Ed. Chart. X. [637.]
πλὴν δήγματος τοῦ ἀσπίδος. ἄλλο. πήγανον σὺν οἴνῳ δίδου πίνειν. ἄλλο. ἐγκέφαλος τῆς ὄρνιθος πινόμενος ὠφελεῖ.

[Πρὸς τὰ τῆς ἔχεως δήγματα.] Τὴν χαλβάνην σὺν κυπρίνῳ πρόσθες. ἄλλο. ἕρπυλλον σὺν ὄξει ὁμοίως κατάχριε.

[Ὑποθυμιάματα τῶν ἰοβόλων φευτικά.] Τὸ πύρεθρον καὶ θεῖον ἐμπύριζε καὶ φευξοῦνται. ἄλλο. ταυτὸ ποιεῖ τὸ κέρας ἐλάφου καὶ τὸ στέαρ αὐτοῦ· ἔτι καὶ τὸ σκύτος καὶ πόδες, τὰ μὲν ταῖς πύλαις ἐμπηγνύμενα τὴν ἅπαντος ἰοβόλου εἴσοδον κωλύουσιν. ἄλλο. πνεύμων ὄνου ὑποθυμιαζόμενος ἅπαν ἰοβόλον φυγαδεύει.

[Ὡς ἔχιδνα μὴ δήκῃ.] Δρακόντιον τρίψας τὴν χεῖρά σου κατάχριε καὶ μὴ δηχθήσῃ. σπέρμα δὲ ταύτης βοτάνης τετριμμένον σὺν ὕδατι καὶ τιθὲν ἐν τοῖς ὕδασι τῶν ἀποδημεόντων αὐτὰς φυγαδεύει. ἄλλο. χυλῷ στρύχνου χεῖρας κατάχριε.

[Ἐπίθεμα πρὸς τὰ δήγματα τῆς ἐχίδνης.] Ἐχίδνης κεφαλὴν ἀποκόψας τὸ μόριον αἱματηρὸν τῷ τόπῳ ἀποδηχθέντι προστίθετι καὶ ἐπίδει καὶ οὕτως ἐᾳ.

morſum. *Aliud.* Rutam da cum vino bibendam. *Aliud.* Cerebrum gallinae bibitum juvat.

[*Inunctio ad morſus viperae.*] Galbanum cum cyprino unge. *Aliud.* Serpyllum cum aceto ſimiliter illine.

[*Suffitus fugantes venenoſa animalia.*] Pyrethrum et ſulſur incende et fugient. *Aliud.* Cornu cervi et ejus pinguedo idem facit; pellis etiam et pedes dextri ſi inſigantur januae, prohibent ingreſſum cujuslibet venenoſi. Pulmo aſini ſi fumigetur, omne venenoſum fugat.

[*Ut vipera non mordeat.*] Dracunculum tere et obline manum et non mordeberis. Semen vero ipſius herbae tritum cum aqua et poſitum in aquis peregrinantium ſugat eas. *Aliud.* Ex ſucco ſolani manus illine.

[*Epithema in morſis a vipera.*] Viperae caput abſcindens applica partem cruentam loco demorſo, liga et dimitte ſic.

Ed. Chart. X. [637.]

[*Πυρία πρὸς τὸ δῆγμα τῆς ἐχίδνης καὶ μυγάλης.*] *Τρίφυλλον ἀσφάλτιον ἕψε καὶ ἀφεψήματι θερμῷ τόπον ἀποδηχθέντα πυρίᾳ. οὐδεὶς δὲ πυρίᾳ ταύτῃ χράσθω ὁ μὴ πάσχων. μεταβαίνει γὰρ ἡ διάθεσις εἰς αὐτὴν, ὡς νομίζῃ ἑαυτὸν ἀπὸ τῆς ἐχίδνης ἢ μυγάλης ἀποδηχέντα.*

[*Fomentum ad morſum viperae et muris aranei.*] Trifolium bituminoſum coque et decocto calido locum demorſum fove. Nullus autem fomento illo utatur, qui non patitur: tranſit enim affectus in eum, ut putet ſe a vipera vel araneo mure demorſum.

ΓΑΛΗΝΟΥ ΠΕΡΙ ΕΥΠΟΡΙΣΤΩΝ ΒΙΒΛΙΟΝ ΤΡΙΤΟΝ ΠΡΟΣΓΕΓΡΑΜΜΕΝΟΝ.

Ed. Chart. X. [638.]

[638] [*Περὶ τῆς σταφυλῆς πασχούσης θεραπείας.*] Θεραπεύσῃς σταφυλὴν οὕτως· ἐν ἀρχῇ μὲν αὐτῆς τῆς φλεγμονῆς δίαιτα λεπτὴ καὶ εὔχυμος ἔστω καὶ ῥοφήματα καὶ ἀναγαργαρίσματα δι' οἰνομέλιτος, ἢ μελικράτου, ἢ ἑψήματος χλιαροῦ, ἢ ὀξυμέλιτος ἀναγαργαριζομένου καὶ ἀποχεομένου καὶ μὴ καταπινομένου· καὶ μασήματος διὰ πυρέθρου ἢ πεπέρεως, ἢ σταφίδας ἀγρίας λειώσας μετὰ

GALENI DE REMEDIIS PARABILIBUS LIBER TERTIUS ADSCRIPTITIUS.

[*De uvae affectibus curandis.*] Sic uvam laborantem curaveris: per inflammationis initia victus tenuis et boni fucci instituatur; sorbitiones et gargarismata fiant ex mulso vel ex mulsa vel sapa tepida vel aceto mulso quod gargarizetur et effundatur nec sorbeatur. Manducetur autem pyrethrum vel piper vel staphisagria, quae

νίτρου καὶ ἁλὸς παράτριβε τὸν οὐρανίσκον καὶ τὴν σταφυλὴν, καὶ παύει τὴν φλεγμονήν· ἔξωθεν δὲ ἐπίθετα τὰ αὐτὰ καὶ τὰ ὁμοίως θερμαίνοντα καὶ τὴν φλεγμονὴν παρηγοροῦντα καὶ τὴν ὀδύνην παύοντα· ἐπιθέματα δὲ καὶ καταπλάσματα ἐπιτήδεια.

[*Περὶ τῆς ἀνακρεμασθείσης σταφυλῆς*] Ὑσσώπου ῥίζαν καὶ ἰσχάδων χυλὸν μίξας ἀναγαργάριζε, ὁμοίως καὶ εἰς παρίσθμια καὶ σταφυλὴν ὁμοῦ ζέσας ἀναγαργάριζε φοίνικας δηλονότι καὶ φακήν.

[*Εἰς τὸ τηρεῖν ἀδίψους ἀεί ποτε.*] Γλυκυῤῥίζης χυλὸν πότιζε ἢ ἀνδράχνης ὅσον κύαθον καταπιεῖν. ἄλλο. ἀνίσου γο. α΄. γλυκυῤῥίζης χυλοῦ γο. β΄. τραγακάνθης βεβρεγμένης γο. β΄. ἀνάπλασον τροχίσκους καὶ ξήρανον ἐν σκιᾷ καὶ ἐκ τούτων δίδου κατέχειν ὑπὸ τὴν γλῶτταν ἕνα τροχίσκον καὶ τὸν χυλὸν καταπίνειν καὶ οὐ διψήσει.

[*Πρὸς δυσηκοΐας καὶ κωφώσεις.*] Χολὴν αἰγείαν πρόσφατον ἴσα μίξας μέλιτι ἀκάπνῳ χλιαρὸν ἔνσταζον εἰς τὸ οὖς. ἄλλο. λαγωοῦ χολὴν νεαρὰν μέλιτι μίξας ἐπίσης καὶ

cum ſale et nitro trita, palato uvaeque aſſricta phlegmonem ſedat; ea itidem exterius appoſita et id genus alia caleſacientia et phlegmonem mitigantia doloremque ſedantia; epithemata vero et cataplasmata idonea ſunt.

[*Ad pendentem uvam.*] Hyſſopi radicem et caricarum ſuccum ſimul mixta gargarizato; ita etiam ad tonſillas, columellam, palmulas et lentem ſimul fervefactas gargarizato.

[*Ut diu ſine ſiti quis ſervetur.*] Radicis dulcis ſuccum bibat aut portulacae cyathum devoret. *Aliud.* Recipe aniſi unc. j, ſucci radicis dulcis unc. ij, tragacanthae madeſactae unc. ij, ex his trochiscos confice eosque in umbra exſicca et trochiscum unum ſub lingua contineat ſuccumque ejus devoret nec ſitiet.

[*Ad gravem auditum et ſurditatem.*] Fel caprinum recens cum pari portione mellis ſine fumo cocti mixtum in aures tepidum inſtillato. *Aliud.* Leporis fel recens cum

χλιάνας ἐν φλοιῷ κρομμύου ἐπίσταζον εἰς τὸ οὖς· καὶ γὰρ καὶ τοὺς μηδ᾽ ὅλως ἀκούοντας ποιεῖ ἀκούειν. ἄλλο. συὸς ἡμέρου χολὴν ἴσα μέλιτι ἀκάπνῳ ἑνώσας χλιαρὸν ἐγχωμάτισον· ἢ σκίλλης χυλὸν καὶ ῥόδινον μίξας χρῶ. ἄλλο. ὀρόβου χυλὸν ἔνσταζον, ἐπίθες στυππίῳ μετὰ ῥοδίνου.

[*Πρὸς κοιλιακοὺς ἐργαλεῖον.*] *Μύρτων χλωρῶν, ῥόδων ξηρῶν, σιδίων ῥοιᾶς, βαλαύστια, κηκίδας ε΄. οἰνομέλιτι φυράσας διὰ γα-* [639] *στρὸς παράπεμψον, ἢ κυάμου λέπυρα σὺν οἴνῳ ἀποζέσας ἔνιε διὰ κλυστῆρος· ἢ φακὴν ἀποζέσας τὸν χυλὸν χλιάριον ὁμοίως ποίει· ἢ ὀρύζης μὴ κεκαθαρισμένης τὸν χυλὸν ὁμοίως, ἢ σιδηρίτιδος βοτάνης τὸν χυλὸν χλιαρὸν ὁμοίως, ἢ ἀκακίας χυλὸν ἔνιε, ἢ ψιμύθιον καὶ λιθάργυρον λειώσας μετὰ μέλιτος καὶ οἴνου παράπεμψον.*

[*Εἰς στρόφον κοιλίας.*] *Κύμινον μετὰ μέλιτος δίδου φαγεῖν καὶ θαυμάσεις· ἢ καλάμου ῥίζαν καύσας πότισον μετὰ οἴνου κύλικος ἑνός.*

[*Εἰς τὸ στῆσαι κοιλίαν.*] *Ὀρίγανον μετὰ ὕδατος ἑψή-*

mellis portione pari in cortice caepae tepefactum in aures inſtillato, hoc enim eis etiam qui nihil prorſus audiunt, auditum reſtituit. *Aliud.* Domeſtici ſuis fel cum melle non fumoſo ad pares portiones mixtum tepidum in aures inſtillato; aut ſcillae ſuccum cum roſaceo mixtum in uſu ſit. *Aliud.* Ervi ſuccum inſtilla et ſtuppam roſaceo imbutam deſuper appone.

[*Ad coeliacos.*] Myrteas baccas virides, roſas aridas, malicoria, balauſtia, gallas v, mulſo ſubactas in ventriculum demitte; vel fabae cortices in vino ferveſactas clyſteri ſupponito; vel lentis inferveſactae ſuccum tepidum per clyſterem imponito; ſimili modo et oryzae non purgatae vel ſideritis herbae ſuccum vel acaciae pariter ſuccum injice, vel ceruſam et argenti ſpumam tritam ex melle et vino per clyſteres impone.

[*Ad ventris tormina.*] Cuminum ex melle eſui dato et miraberis; vel calami radicem uſtam potui dato ex vino calicis unius menſura.

[*Ad ſiſtendum alvi profluvium.*] Aquam in qua

Ed. Chart. X. [639.]

σας δίδου πιεῖν. ἄλλο. σηπίας ὄστρακον καύσας καὶ τρίψας μετὰ οἴνου παλαιοῦ δὸς πιεῖν· ἢ βάτου καρπὸν σὺν τοῖς φύλλοις ἀποτριτώσας δὸς πιεῖν. ἄλλο. κύμινον Ἑλλαδικὸν καὶ κηκίδα ἄτριπτον καῦσον καὶ μετὰ οἴνου παλαιοῦ δὸς πιεῖν μετὰ τὸ ἀποτριτωθῆναι ἐπὶ ἡμέρας τρεῖς.

[Πρὸς ἐσωχάδας, ῥαγάδας καὶ συκάμινα.] Ἀρσενικοῦ σχιστοῦ γο. γ'. σφέτλης δρυΐνης γο. δ'. λειώσας πάντα ὁμοῦ ἔχε ξηρίον, ἐπὶ δὲ τῆς χρείας ἀπονίψας οὔρῳ παιδὸς ἀφθόρου τοὺς τόπους ἐπίπασον.

[Πρὸς ἐσωχάδας καὶ ἐξωχάδας.] Ῥίζαν σιλφίου κόψας καὶ λειώσας κατάπλασον.

[Ξηρίον πρὸς βεβρωμένας οὔλας καὶ ὀδόντας σειομένους.] Μαστίχης γο. α'. λιβάνου γο. β'. σμύρνης, ῥόδων ξηρῶν ἀνὰ γο. γ'. σαρκοκόλλης, κηκίδος ἀνὰ γο. δ'. ὁμοῦ λειώσας ἐπίπασον τὰ οὖλα, προδιακλύσας ἀειζώου, ἢ μύρτων, ἢ σχοίνου, ἢ ἄγνου, ἢ ἐλαίας τῶν φύλλων τῶν χλιαρῶν.

fuerit incoctum origanum bibendam dato. *Aliud.* Sepiae teſtam et capillamentum uſta et trita ex veteri vino da potui. Vel fructus rubi cum foliis ad tertias decoctos potui dato. *Aliud.* Cuminum Graecum et gallam non tritam urito et ex veteri vino bibendum dato per triduum; prius tamen ad tertias redigito.

[*Ad internas eminentias, fiſſuras ficosque in ſede.*] Auripigmenti ſiſſi unc. iij, cariei quercus unc. iv, ex his ſimul tritis aridum medicamentum conſice, quum vero uſus occaſio ingruerit, urina pueri impubis locum detergito ac medicamentum inſpergito.

[*Ad eminentias tam internas quam externas.*] Laſerpitii radicem tuſam et tritam in modum cataplasmatis apponito.

[*Aridum medicamentum ad gingivas corroſas et labantes dentes.*] Maſtiches unc. j, thuris unc. ij, myrrhae, roſarum aridarum, utriusque unc. iij, ſarcocollae, gallarum utriusque unc. iv, omnia ſimul terito et gingivas conſpergito; eas tamen prius decocto ſedi aut myrti aut lentisci aut viticis aut foliorum oleae tepido colluito.

Ed. Chart. X. [639.]

[Πρὸς ὀδονταλγίας.] Ὕσσωπον ἢ ὀρίγανον μετὰ ὄξους ἑψήσας δὸς διακλύζεσθαι· ἢ πύρεθρον καὶ πέπερι καὶ ζέμμα καὶ μαστίχην ἐξ ἴσου δίδου διαμασᾶσθαι. ἄλλο. σταφίδας ἀγρίας κόκκους δ'. μαστίχης κόκκους η'. δίδου διαμασᾶσθαι.

[Εἰς πεσόντας ὀδόντας ἀπὸ πληγῆς.] Σταφίδας ἐν ἐλαίῳ ζέσας πυρίαζε τὸν τόπον καὶ γῆν ἑξῆς τῷ ὄξει, τῆς ὀδύνης δηλονότι ἐρεθιζούσης, ἐπὶ ἡμέρας δὲ τρεῖς ποίει, οὕτως καὶ πάλιν ἀναφύουσιν οἱ ὀδόντες.

[Πρὸς οὖλα βιβρωσκόμενα.] Ἀριστολοχίας τρίψας μετὰ μέλιτος ἐπίπασον τὰ οὖλα, ἢ κέρας ἐλάφειον κεκαυμένον ἕως ἂν γένηται λευκὸν καὶ ψιμύθιον καὶ λιθάργυρον καὶ νάρδον καὶ κίσσηριν κηρωτῇ ἀναλάβου καὶ κατάχριε· ἢ χελώνης ὄστρακον καύσας καὶ τρίψας μίξας τε μετ' ἐλαίου ἔνσταζον εἰς τὸ οὖλον. ἄλλο. εὐζώμου σπέρμα σὺν τῷ χυλῷ καὶ χολὴ αἰγὸς ἢ μελάνθιον μέλιτι κατάχριε.

[Πρὸς ὀφθαλμοπονίαν.] Μυελὸν αἴγειον περίχριε καὶ ἰᾶται· ἢ στέαρ αἴγειον ἢ προβάτειον ἀποβρέχων εἰς ὕδωρ

[*Ad dentium dolores.*] Aceto cui incoctum ſuerit hyſſopum aut origanum colluat; aut pyrethrum et piper et zemma et maſtichem pari pondere data commanducet. *Aliud.* Uvae taminiae grana iv, maſtiches grana viij, offer manducanda.

[*Ad dentes ab ictu decidentes.*] Paſſulis oleo incoctis locum foveto ac deinde aceto, dolore nimirum ingravescente, poſt triduum id ipſum facito et iterum renascentur dentes.

[*Ad corroſas gingivas.*] Ariſtolochia cum melle trita gingivas inſpergito; aut cornu cervinum uſtum quoad album reddatur et ceruſſam et argenti ſpumam et nardum et pumicem cerato excipe et illine, aut teſtam teſtudinis exuſtam et tritam et oleo mixtam in gingivam inſtillato. *Aliud.* Erucae ſemen cum ſucco et fel caprae aut nigellam eodem modo cum melle illinito.

[*Ad dolores oculorum.*] Medulla caprina illinito et curabitur, aut caprinam ovillamve adipem aqua calida

θερμὸν ἐπιτίθει, ἢ λινοσπέρμου χυλὸν, ἢ γάλα γυναικεῖον ἐπίχριε.

[Πρὸς λεύκωμα καὶ οὔλας παλαιὰς ἐν ἐλαχίσταις ἡμέραις· ἔστι δὲ καὶ ὀξυδορκικὸν θαυμαστόν.] Ἰοῦ ξυστοῦ γο. δ'. ἀμμωνιακοῦ γο. δ'. ψιμυθίου γο. β'. κόμμεως γο. α'. τὸ δὲ ὑγρὸν ἔστω σικύου ἀγρίου χυλὸς ὁ τῆς ῥίζης. ἄλλο. δαφνοκόκκων κεκαθαρισμένων καὶ λελειωμένων, κόμμεως τὸ [640] ἀρκοῦν πρόσπλεξον καὶ ποίει κολλύρια, ἐπὶ δὲ τῆς χρείας λειώσας οὔρῳ παιδὸς ἀφθόρου ἀναλάμβανε καὶ οὕτως χρῖε. πεπείραται γάρ.

[Πρὸς αἰγίλωπας.] Κόπρου περιστερᾶς ξηροῦ γο. δ'. σὺν λιβάνῳ ἄῤῥενι λειώσας ἐπίπασον ἕως οὗ παύσῃ. ἐδοκιμάσθη γάρ.

[Πρὸς λευκώματα δόκιμον· καὶ γὰρ πολλοὺς ὤνησεν.] Πέρδικος ἄῤῥενος χολὴν μετὰ μέλιτος χρῖε. ἄλλο. λαδάνου γο. β'. λειώσας μετὰ καλλίστου οἴνου καὶ ἐλαίου ἀφ' ἱκανοῦ χρῖε τοὺς ὀφθαλμούς.

madentem admove aut ſuccum ſeminis lini aut lac muliebre illine.

[*Ad oculorum albuginem; veteres cicatrices curandas; idem etiam viſum mirifice acuit.*] Aeruginis raſae unc. iv, guttae ammoniaci unc. iv, ceruſſae unc. ij, gummi unc. j. Sit autem liquidum medicamentum; ſuccus radicis cucumeris ſilveſtris. *Aliud.* Recipe baccarum lauri mundatarum laevigatarumque gummi quod ſatis ſit, ex eis permixtis confice collyria, at ubi eis uti volueris terito et ex lotio pueri impubis illinito, medicamentum probatum eſt.

[*Ad aegilopas i. e. oculorum fiſtulas.*] Recipe fimi columbini aridi unc. iv, tritas cum thure masculo inſpergito, quoad morbus tollatur; experientia comprobatum eſt.

[*Ad albugines medicamentum comprobatum, quod multos juvit.*] Perdicis masculi felle ex melle illinito. *Aliud.* Recipe ladani unc. ij, terito ex optimo vino et oleo quantum ſit ſatis et oculos illinito.

Ed. Chart. X. [640.]

[*Πρὸς ὑπόχυσιν ὑπερφυῶς παραχρῆμα τὸ βλέπειν ποιῶν.*] *Αἷμα μυὸς καὶ χολὴν ἀλέκτορος καὶ γάλα γυναικεῖον ἴσα μίξας καὶ λειώσας χρῶ· ἐδοκιμάσθη γὰρ καὶ ἄκρως ὠφέλησεν.*

[*Ἄλλο πρὸς ὑποχύσεις παλαιάς τε καὶ νέας καὶ ἀμβλυωπίας καὶ πᾶν ἐπισκοτοῦν τὴν ὅρασιν.*] *Δαφνίδας ἐκλελεπισμένας ἀριθμὸν κοκκίων ι'. κόμμεως γο. β'. ὕδατι ὀμβρίῳ ποιήσας κολλύρια χρῖε τοῖς ὑποκεχυμένοις μετὰ οὔρου παιδίου ἀφθόρου, τοῖς δὲ ἀμβλυωποῦσι μετὰ ὕδατος ὀμβρίου.*

[*Πρὸς πόνον ὀφθαλμῶν καὶ ἀγρυπνίας.*] *Μελίκρατον ἐγχυματίσας καὶ προβρέξας ὠὸν καὶ περικαθάρας καὶ τεμὼν εἰς β'. δῆσον ἐπάνω τῶν ὀφθαλμῶν καὶ ὑπνώσει.*

[*Πρὸς ἄνθρακας ὀφθαλμῶν καὶ παντὸς τοῦ σώματος.*] *Περδικιάδα βοτάνην μετὰ ψιχίων λειώσας, προβρέξας τὰ ψίχια ὀξυκράτῳ χρῶ.*

[*Ad ſuffuſiones admirabile, quod confeſtim viſum reſtituit.*] Sanguinem muris, galli fel et muliebre lac paribus portionibus misce et tritis utere; probatum eſt et mirum in modum profuit.

[*Aliud ad ſuffuſiones, novas veteresque, ad viſus etiam hebetudinem et ad omnia tandem, quae viſum obtenebrant.*] Recipe baccas lauri a cortice mundatas numero decem, gummi unc. ij, ex aqua pluviali facito collyria et illine; ſuffuſos quidem ex urina pueri nondum experti venerea; quibus autem hebes eſt viſus, ex aqua pluviali.

[*Ad oculorum dolores et vigilias.*] Mulſam facito ovumque a cortice mundatum et in duas partes diſpertitum, in ea madefacito ac ſuper oculum deligato, a ſomno corripietur.

[*Ad oculorum totiusque corporis carbunculos.*] Parietariam herbam cum panis micis prius posca madefactis terito ac utitor.

Ed. Chart. X. [640.]

[Ὀξυδερκικόν.] Μαράθρου ξύλον τρίψας καλῶς μετὰ μέλιτος πωλίου νεαροῦ ἀκάπνῳ χρῶ ἐπιχρίων.

[Περὶ τῶν ἐν βλεφάροις κριθῶν.] Ἀκακίαν σὺν οἴνῳ χρῖε.

[Πρὸς ῥευματισμοὺς τῶν ὀφθαλμῶν.] Ἐπὶ δὲ τῶν ῥευματιζομένων τοὺς ὀφθαλμοὺς ἐν ἀρχῇ μὲν ἁρμόζει ὀλιγοσιτία καὶ ὑδροποσία καὶ ἀποχὴ συνουσίας καὶ ἡ κοιλία ὑποσυρέσθω καὶ πολλῷ ψυχρῷ πρῶτον καὶ ὀλίγου μιγνυμένου ὄξους συνεχῶς τὸ πρόσωπον νιπτέσθω καὶ ἐν τῇ κλίνῃ ὀσφραινέσθω, κονιορτοῦ τε καὶ καπνοῦ καὶ τὴν ἀφ' ἡλίου καὶ λύχνου αὐγὴν ἀποφευγέτω· ἔπειτα ῥόδα χλωρὰ ἢ ξηρὰ βρέξας ἐν γλυκεῖ λείανε καὶ μίξας ὠοῦ λεκίθῳ κατάπλαττε ἢ κριθίνου ἀλεύρου σὺν γλυκεῖ ἑψηθέντος· ἐὰν δὲ ἡ ὀδύνη μεγίστη ᾖ, πρόσμιξον καὶ ὑοσκύαμον.

[Κατάπλασμα εἰς ῥευματιζομένην κεφαλήν.] Τοῦτο τὸ μίγμα οὐκ ἐᾷ κεφαλὴν ῥευματισθῆναι οὔτε ὀφθαλμὸν ἀδικηθῆναι ποτέ. κιμωλίας, νίτρου, βρυωνίας ῥίζης ξηρᾶς, σι-

[*Medicamentum quod viſum acuit.*] Foeniculi caulem probe ex melle alvearii novi cocto ſine fumo terito et illinito.

[*Ad ordeolos in palpebris exortos.*] Acacia cum vino inunge.

[*Ad oculorum fluxiones.*] Oculi fluxione laborantibus inter initia confert parcitas cibi, aquae potus, abſtinentia a venere, alvus cieatur primumque multa frigida pauco permixto aceto aſſidue facies lavetur, eam etiam in lectulo olſaciat, a pulvere, fumo, ſolis lucernaeque ſplendore caveat; roſas deinde virides aut aridas paſſo madefactas terito mixtasque ovi vitello ut cataplasma imponito aut ex farina hordei ex paſſo cocta facito cataplasma. At ſi dolor maximus fuerit, altercum quoque admisceto.

[*Cataplasma ad caput fluxione vexatum.*] Haec compoſitio caput a fluxione ſervat, oculos etiam ab omni injuria. Recipe cimoliae, nitri, radicis bryoniae aridae, cucumeris ſilveſtris radicis, farinae fabarum ſingulorum

κύου ἀγρίου ῥίζης, κυάμου ἀλεύρου ἀνὰ γο. β'. λειοτριβήσας ὁμοῦ καὶ ἑνώσας εἰς γλοιοῦ πάχος χρῶ ἐν βαλανείῳ ὡς κάλλιστον.

[Ἀποφλεγματισμὸς κατασπῶν ἐκ τοῦ κρανίου φλέγμα.] Ἀγριοσταφίδας μετὰ μαστίχης δίδου μασᾶσθαι ἢ μαστίχην καὶ ζίγγιβερ, εἰ δὲ ἡ μαστίχη σκληρὰ εἴη, πρόπλεξον καὶ ὀλίγον κηρόν.

[Πρὸς κεφαλαλγίαν.] Πήγανον κόψον ἐπιμελῶς καὶ σὺν ὄξει καὶ ῥοδίνῳ κατάχριε τὸ μέτωπον.

[Πρὸς ἡμικρανίαν.] Πράσου κεφαλὴν καὶ κόμην ἑψήσας ἐλαίῳ βρέχε τὴν κεφαλὴν καὶ παύεται εὐθὺς ἡ ὀδύνη. ἄλλο. κισσοῦ ἀκρέμονας ἐλαίῳ ἑψήσας [641] βρέξον τὴν κεφαλὴν καὶ θαυμάσεις. ἄλλο. ἀμύγδαλα πικρὰ λειοτριβήσας κατάχριε τὸ μέτωπον.

[Πρὸς ἥλους δόκιμον, κἂν ἐν κεφαλῇ εἰσίν.] Σανδαράχης, σχιστῆς, χαλκάνθου, μίσυος καὶ ἀσβέστου ζῶντος καὶ σάπωνος ὅλα μίξας ἐξ ἴσου, τὸ ἄσβεστον διπλοῦν λειώσας μετὰ πρωτείου ζωμοῦ τοῦ σάπωνος χρῶ. θαυμάσιον γάρ ἐστι.

[Πρὸς ἡμικρανίαν.] Λαβὼν εὐζώμου σπέρμα γο. γ'.

unc. ij, his ſimul tritis et ad ſordium craſſitudinem deductis in balneo utere, praeſtantiſſimum remedium eſt.

[*Apophlegmatismus pituitam e capite detrahens.*] Staphiſagriam cum maſtiche manducandam exhibe; vel maſtichem et zingiber; quod ſi dura maſtiche ſit, cerae modicum admisceto.

[*Ad capitis dolorem.*] Ruta probe trita ex aceto et roſaceo frontem illinito.

[*Ad hemicraniam.*] Porri caput cum coma decoquito eoque caput imbuito, ſtatim namque dolor ſedatur. *Aliud.* Hederae ſummitatibus oleo incoctis caput perfundito et miraberis. *Aliud.* Amaris amygdalis tritis frontem delinito.

[*Probatum ad clavos, ſi etiam in capite ſint.*] Recipe ſandarachae, aluminis ſciſſi, atramenti ſutorii, miſyos, calcis vivae, ſaponis, caeterorum omnium parem modum, calcis tantummodo duplum ex primo ſaponis jure laevigato et utere. Admirabile eſt.

[*Ad hemicraniam.*] Accipe ſeminis erucae unc. iij,

Ed. Chart. X. [641.]
πηγάνου χλωροῦ γο. ζ'. πεπέρεως κόκκους λα'. ὠῶν τριῶν τὸ λευκὸν, ὄξους τὸ ἀρκοῦν χρῖε τὸν τόπον.

[Τροχίσκος ὁ ἔνδοξος Σωκράτους πρὸς κεφαλαλγίαν καὶ ἡμικρανίαν καὶ πρὸς πάντα τὰ ῥευματικὰ πάθη θαυμάσιος.] Εὐφορβίου < δ'. θαψίας χυλοῦ < στ'. ζιγγιβέρεος < α'. ὀπίου < γ'. ὀποπάνακος < β'. λῦσον τὰ πάντα ὁμοῦ μετὰ ὄξους καὶ ποίει τροχίσκους, ἐπὶ δὲ τῆς χρήσεως ἀναλαβὼν ὄξει χρῖε τὸ μέτωπον. ἔστι δὲ καὶ καπνιστικὸν καὶ τοῖς μόριόν τι ῥευματιζομένοις ποιεῖ θαυμαστῶς.

[Περὶ ἥλων καὶ μυρμηκιῶν.] Ἀρίθμησον τοὺς ἥλους καὶ λαβὼν τοσούτους μύρμηκας δῆσον ἐν λίνῳ πανίῳ καὶ κοχλίαν ἕνα μετ' αὐτῶν καὶ καύσας αὐτοὺς λείωσον σὺν ὄξει καὶ ἐπίχριε, ἢ κόπρον βόειον μετὰ ὄξους λειώσας ἐπίχριε, ἐπὶ ἡμέρας τρεῖς κατάπλασον, καὶ πεσοῦνται οἱ ἧλοι.

[Πρὸς ἥλους καὶ μυρμηκιασμούς.] Ὀστέα φοινίκων καύσας καὶ τρίψας μετὰ ἅλατος καὶ θυμιάματος καὶ μίξας ἐν ἡλίῳ ἐπίθες καὶ θεραπεύσεις.

rutae viridis unc. vij, piperis grana xxxj, albumina ovorum trium, aceti quod ſatis ſit, misce et locum illine.

[*Paſtillus celebris Socratis ad capitis dolorem et hemicraniam, ad omnesque capitis affectus ex fluxione obortos mirabilis.*] Recipe euphorbii drach. iv, ſucci thapſiae drach. vj, zingiberis drach. j, opii drach. iij, opopanacis drach. ij, omnia ſimul ex aceto diſſolvito, indeque paſtillos fingito, quum in uſum ducere volueris, aceto excipe et frontem delinito; poteſt praeterea ſuffiri et partibus fluxioni obnoxiis mirum in modum conſert.

[*Ad clavos et verrucas i. e. formicas.*] Clavos numera totidemque formicas accipe easque in linteo deliga atque cum his cochleam unam ac urito et ex aceto terito atque illinito; vel accipe fimum bubulum cum aceto laevigatum, per triduumque apponito, quia cadent clavi.

[*Ad clavos et formicantes verrucas.*] Palmularum oſſa uſta tritaque cum ſale et ammoniaci gutta in ſole mixta imponito et curabis.

[*Πρὸς ἡμικρανίαν δόκιμον.*] *Λαβὼν γῆς ἔντερα ιέ. κόκκους πεπέρεως ιέ, ὄξους τὸ ἀρκοῦν· λειώσας ὁμοῦ χρῖε.*

[*Πρὸς θηριοδήκτους πληγάς.*] *Θηριοδήκτους καὶ λυσσοδήκτους ἴᾶται καρκίνου τῶν ἐντὸς ἡ τέφρα σὺν ὕδατι πινομένη ἅπαξ καὶ δὶς ἀνὰ δρακὸς μιᾶς.*

[*Πρὸς τὰς ἐξ οἴνου κεφαλαλγίας.*] *Πολυγόνου κλῶνας β'. πλέξας στεφάνωσον.*

[*Πρὸς πόνον ἡμικρανίου.*] *Καρδάμου σπόρον τρίψας μῖξον μετ' ὠοῦ λευκῷ καὶ κατάχριε τὸ μέτωπον καὶ ἐπάνω θὲς στυπία, ἢ τοῦ ἀετοῦ τῆς κεφαλῆς τὸ ὀστοῦν τὸ ὅμοιον τῷ ὁμοίῳ περίαπτε ὁμοίως καὶ τοῦ γυπός. ἄλλο. οἱ ἐν τῇ κεφαλῇ τοῦ λάβρακος εὑρισκόμενοι λίθοι κεφαλαλγίαν ἰῶνται καὶ εἰς ἡμικρανίαν περιαπτόμενοι δεξιὸς δεξιᾷ καὶ ἀριστερὸς ἀριστερᾷ.*

[*Πρὸς τρίχας ῥεούσας ἀπὸ κεφαλῆς καὶ πώγωνος.*] *Σεῦτλον μετὰ μυρσινελαίου καὶ πολυτρίχων τρίχας κατάχριε ἢ ἀδίαντον καὶ λάδανον ἴσα λειώσας μετ' ἐλαίου ὀμφακίνου*

[*Ad hemicranium dolorem celebre medicamentum.*] Accipe terreſtres lambricos xv, piperis grana xv, aceti quod ſufficiat; ſimul tritis oblinito.

[*Ad morſus et ictus ferarum venenoſarum.*] Morſus ferarum venenoſarum rabidorumque canum ſanat interiorum cancri cinis ex aqua ſemel aut bis pota, quantum manus una capere poteſt.

[*Ad dolorem capitis ex vini potu.*] Sertum ex duobus coliculis ſanguinalis herbae contextum imponito capiti.

[*Ad hemicranium dolorem.*] Naſturtii ſemen tritum albumineque ovi exceptum fronti adhibeto, ſtupa deſuper appoſita; aut os capitis aquilae appende ſimile ſimili, eodem modo et vulturis. *Aliud.* Lapilli qui in capite lupi piscis reperiuntur, capitis dolorem ſanant appenſique hemicraniae conſerunt, dexter parti dextrae et ſiniſter ſiniſtrae.

[*Ad capillos tum ei capite tum e barba defluentes.*] Betam cum myrteo oleo et polytrichis capillis illinito; vel adiantum et ladanum paribus portionibus trita ex oleo

ἢ μυρσινίνου, ἢ σχίνινου ἐπίχριε. ἄλλο. λάδανον ἀποβρέξας σὺν οἴνῳ Ἀμιναίῳ καὶ μυρσινελαίῳ λειώσας ἄμφω πάχος μέλιτος καὶ χρῖε τὴν κεφαλὴν ἐν βαλανείῳ· βέλτιον δ' ἐστὶ καὶ τὸ ἀδίαντον, ὅ τινες καλοῦσι πολύτριχον, τὸ ζ'. μέρος λαδάνῳ πρόσβαλλε καὶ χρῖε.

[Πρὸς τρίχας ῥεούσας, ἵνα δὲ καὶ πλέον γένωνται.] Μυοχόδων < γ'. καλάμων κονατήλων κεκαυμένων < δ'. ἀμύγδαλα πικρὰ οβ'. ὀπὸν βαλσάμου, λά- [642] δάνου ἀνὰ < δ'. πολυτρίχων < ζ'. νάρδου Κελτικῆς < α'. ἐν ὑγροπίσσῳ βρέξας τὸ λάδανον καὶ οἴνῳ καὶ ἐλαίῳ λειώσας. τὰ δὲ ξηρὰ κόψας εἰς χνοῦν, μετὰ τῶν ὑγρῶν μίξας χρῶ ἀλειφόμενον καθ' ἡμέραν. ἐμοὶ δοκεῖ καὶ φαλακροὺς τριχῶσαι.

[Βηχὸς θεραπεῖαι διάφοροι.] Ἀρκευθίδος ὁ καρπὸς ἐσθιόμενος καὶ πινόμενος· ἢ βδέλλιον πινόμενον, ἢ δαῦκος Κρητικὸς σὺν οἴνῳ πινόμενος· ἢ δρακοντίου ῥίζα ὁμοίως ἑψηθεῖσα καὶ λειωθεῖσα μέλιτι· ἢ ἑλενίου βοτάνης καὶ περδικιάδος χλιαρὸς νηστικῶς καταῤῥοφούμενος ὁ χυλὸς σὺν

immaturo vel myrteo vel lentiscino illinito. *Aliud.* Ladanum ex Aminaeo vino et oleo myrteo terito ad ſpiſſitudinem mellis caputque in balneo inungito. Sed adiantum, quod polytrichum quidam vocant, melius eſt, ſi ejus pars ſeptima ladano adjiciatur et inungatur.

[*Ad profluvium capillorum et ut plures ſuboriantur.*] Accipito muris ſtercoris drach. iij, cannarum, quas conatelos vocant, uſtarum drach. iv, amygdala amara lxxij, ſucci balſami, ladani utriusque drach. iv, polytrichi drach. vij, nardi Gallici drach. j, immerſum ladanum in picem liquidam vinumque et oleum laevigato; arida vero trita in pulverem redigito et cum liquidis miſceto et utere quotidie inungens; mihi quidem viſum eſt etiam calvis capilles reſtituiſſe medicamentum.

[*Ad tuſſim varia remedia.*] Fructus juniperi comeſtus et potus valet; aut bdellium potu ſumptum; aut daucus Creticus ex vino potus; aut radix dracunculi elixa et ex melle trita; aut helenii aut herbae perdicialis ſuccus tepidus ante cibum potus ex aqua. Aut ſuccus her-

ὕδατι πινόμενος, ἢ ἀρκείου βοτάνης ἡ ῥίζα, ἢ στροβιλίου σὺν ὕδατι πινόμενον, ἢ πρόπολις θυμιωμένη καὶ ῥητίνη πινομένη· καὶ τερεβινθίνη θυμιωμένη, ἢ ἀρσενικὸν σχιστὸν μετὰ χαλβάνης θυμιωμένης· καὶ ὁ καπνὸς καταπινόμενος, ἢ ἄσφαλτον καὶ λίβανον καὶ στύραξ καὶ κύμινον θυμιαζόμενα, ἢ κιννάμωμον σὺν μέλιτι χλιαρῷ πινόμενον, ἢ κυπαρίσσου σφαιρία τριβέντα μετὰ γλυκέος καὶ σμύρνης νηστικῶς λαμβανόμενα, ἢ μαράθρων ῥίζας καὶ σπέρμα σὺν οἴνῳ ἑψηθέντα καὶ πινόμενα, ἢ νάρθηξ χλωρὸς σὺν οἴνῳ ἑψηθεὶς καὶ ποθείς· ἢ ὀρίγανον σὺν μέλιτι ἑψηθὲν καὶ ποθέν· ἢ μυρίκης ἄνθος καὶ ὁ καρπὸς καὶ τὰ φύλλα σὺν οἴνῳ ἑψηθέντα καὶ πινόμενα· ἢ πευκίου ὁ φλοιὸς σὺν ὕδατι πινόμενος· ἢ λεύκης φύλλα καὶ τὰ κλωνία σὺν ὕδατι ἢ οἴνῳ πινόμενα, ἢ φλόμου ῥίζα σὺν οἴνῳ πινομένη ἐν βαλανείῳ, ἢ σκόροδον ὠμὸν καὶ ἡψημένον ἐσθιόμενον, ἢ στρουθίου βοτάνης ἡ ῥίζα σὺν μέλιτι ἀναλαμβανομένη τοὺς πάνυ ἐσχάτως ἔχοντας ἐν τῷ πάθει· λαγωοῦ κόπρος λεία σὺν οἴνῳ θερμῷ ποθεῖσα ὠφελεῖ. ἀρτηριακοὺς καὶ κιονικοὺς καὶ δυσπνοϊκοὺς

bae ſanguinalis eodem modo acceptus. Aut perſonatae herbae radix. Aut nuclei pineae ex aqua bibiti. Aut propolis ſuffita. Aut reſina pota et terebinthina ſuffita. Aut arſenicum ſciſſile cum galbano ſuffitum et fumus devoratus. Aut bitumen, thus, ſtyrax, cuminum, haec omnia ſuffita. Aut cinamomum ex tepido melle potum. Aut cupreſſi baccae tritae cum paſſo et myrrha jejuno exhibeantur. Aut foeniculi radix et ſemen ex vino decocta et bibita. Aut decoctum viridis ferulae ex vino bibitum. Aut origanum cum melle decoctum et potui datum. Aut flos myricae cum foliis et fructu ex vino elixus et bibitus. Aut piceae cortex ex aqua bibitus. Aut populi albae folia et ramuli ex aqua aut vino bibantur. Aut verbasci radix ex vino bibita in balneo. Aut allium crudum vel elixum comeſtum. Aut lanariae herbae radix accepta ex melle peſſime affectos liberat. Leporis ſtercus tritum et ex vino calido potu aſſumptum prodeſt affectibus gurgulionis, arteriae ac difficile ſpirantibus.

Ed. Chart. X. [642.]
μεγάλως θεραπεύει ἀετοῦ γλῶσσα περιαπτομένη· ἢ στροβίλιον ἀκέραιον καύσας καὶ τρίψας μετὰ πεπέρεως ὀλίγου καὶ ἀναλαβὼν μέλιτι δίδου τῷ πάσχοντι κοχλιάριον ἕν.

[Πρὸς χρόνιον βῆχα.] Θεῖον ἄπυρον τρίψας καλῶς, ἐμβαλὼν ὠὸν ῥόφησον ἐν βαλανείῳ· ἢ σίνηπι τρίψας καὶ μίξας μέλιτι δίδου δακόλους τρεῖς· ἢ καρδαμόσπορον λεῖον σὺν ὕδατι πινόμενον εἰς κοίτην, ἢ λίβανον τριβόμενον μετὰ μέλιτος καὶ ἐκλειχόμενον πρωῒ καὶ εἰς κοίτην· ἢ ῥαφάνου χυλὸς μετὰ μέλιτος καταῤῥοφούμενος τῷ πρωΐ. ἄλλο. ἀρκευτίδες ε΄. ἢ ζ΄. μετὰ μέλιτος πινόμεναι. ἄλλο. πεπέρεως < δ΄. καρύων < β΄. στροβίλου ὑσσώπου ἀνὰ < α΄. γλήχωνος < δ΄. ἴρεως < δ΄. κνίδης σπέρμα < δ΄. μέλιτος ἡ δόσις κοχλιάριον α΄. ἄλλο. σίνηπι καὶ κύμινον, μελάνθιον, κάρδαμον ἴσα ὁμοῦ κόψας ἀναλάμβανε οἴνῳ καὶ δίδου. ἄλλο. γλήχωνα δίδου μασᾶσθαι συνεχῶς καὶ συντρίψας μετὰ οἴνου καὶ λεάνας δίδου πιεῖν. ἄλλο. κυμίνου πεφρυγμένου < α΄. μελανθίου πεφρυγμένου < α΄. πεπέρεως κοκ-

Magnopere prodeſt lingua aquilae appenſa collo; aut nucleus pineus integer uſtus, tritus, cum pauco pipere melleque exceptus detur ad cochlearium laboranti.

[*Ad veterem tuſſim.*] Sulfur ignem inexpertum probe terito ac ovo injectum in balneo ſorbelo. Aut ſinapi tritum cum melle misce et da tres dacolos. Aut tritum naſturtii ſemen eunti dormitum da potui ex aqua. Aut ſummo mane thus tritum cum melle lingendum dato vel eunti cubitum. Aut raphani ſuccus ex melle diluculo ſorbeatur. *Aliud.* Juniperi baccae quinque aut ſeptem ex melle bibantur. *Aliud.* Recipe piperis drach. iv, nucum drach. ij, nucleorum pinearum, hyſſopi, utriusque drach. j, pulegii drach. iv, iridis drach. iv, ſeminis urticae drach. iv, mellis quod ſatis ſit, detur cochlearium unum. *Aliud.* Sinapi, cuminum, nigella, naſturtium ſimul paribus portionibus terantur, ex vino excipiantur et offerantur. *Aliud.* Pulegium adſidue commanducetur; praeterea vero tritum ex vino potui detur. *Aliud.* Recipe cumini fricti

κία μ'. συντρίψας καὶ ζυμώσας μέλιτι δίδου νήστει καὶ εἰς κοίτην.

[Κάπνισμα.] Ἀρσενικὸν σχιστὸν, πέπερι, πράσιον, κριθῆς ἄλευρον, χαμαίδρυν, ἀμπέλου ῥίζης δέρμα, χαμαιλεύκην, μαστίχην κόστον, κρόκον ὠῶν, πάντα ἑνώσας πλάττε κολλούρια καὶ κάπνιζε νήστει καὶ εἰς κοίτην. ἄλλο. πέπερι, κάρυα, ἀρσενικὸν σχιστὸν συντρίψας καὶ μίξας μέλιτι [643] κάπνιζε. ἄλλο. βούτυρον, στέαρ χηνὸς, ῥητίνην μέλιτι συντρίψας δίδου νήστει καὶ εἰς κοίτην. ἄλλο. ῥάβδον μαράθρου καὶ σπέρμα πεπέρεως συντρίψας καὶ μετὰ μέλιτος ζυμώσας δίδου. ἄλλο. φυσαλίδας ἑψήσας σὺν ταῖς ῥίζαις δὸς πιεῖν.

[Βηχικὸν καὶ εἰς ἀναγωγὴν αἵματος.] Κόστον, κιννάμωμον, ῥῆον βάρβαρον ἀνὰ < α'. συντρίψας καὶ ἑνώσας μετ' οἴνου χλιαροῦ πότισον.

[Ἄλλο ποιῶν καὶ ἐκτηκομένοις.] Λαβὼν λιβάνου, πε-

drach. j, nigellae drach. j, piperis grana xl, haec ſimul trita et melle fermentata jejuno et cubitum eunti dato.

[*Suffimentum.*] Accipe auripigmentum ſciſſum, piper, marrubium, farinam hordei, triſſaginem, corticem radicum vitis, chamaeleucen, maſtichen, coſtum, ovorum croccum, omnia ſimul miſce et collyria confice, quibus ſuffumigato ante cibum et quum cubitum iturus eſt. *Aliud.* Accipe piper, nuces, auripigmentum ſciſſile eaque una terito, ac melli immiſceto et potui dato. *Aliud.* Butyrum adipem anſeris, reſinam, omnia ſimul trita ex melle da jejuno et cubitum ituro. *Aliud.* Virgulam foeniculi ſemenque et piper una trita et ex melle fermentata exhibeto. *Aliud.* Herbam veſicariam una cum radicibus elixam potui dato.

[*Ad tuſſim et ſanguinis rejectionem.*] Recipe coſti, cinnamomi, rhabarbari, ſingulorum drach. j, ſimul omnia contrita et in unum redacta ex vino tepido bibenda praebeto.

[*Aliud quod et tabescentibus benefacit.*] Thuris,

Ed. Chart. X. [643.]

πέρεως, ἀρσενικοῦ σχιστοῦ, καρυοφύλλου πάντα ὁμοῦ συντρίψας μετὰ μέλιτος καὶ ζυμώσας δίδου πρωῒ καὶ εἰς κοίτην· ἢ ἀρσενικὸν σχιστὸν ἀντὶ ἅλατος εἰς ᾠὸν ῥυτὸν καὶ ῥόφησον νῆστις· ἢ ἀρσενικὸν συντρίψας μετ᾽ οἴνου χλιαροῦ πότισον ἐν λουτρῷ· ἢ ἀρσενικὸν σχιστὸν καὶ κρόκον ᾠοῦ μίξας ἐπάλειφε εἰς βάμβηκα καὶ κάπνιζε διὰ κιχώνης, ὅταν δὲ ὀλιγωθῇ ὁ καπνιζόμενος, δίδου αὐτῷ καὶ καταπιεῖν βούτυρον, ὅσον λεπτοκαρύου μέγεθος καὶ πάλιν καπνιζέσθω, ποίει δὲ ἑπτάκις. ἄλλο. στύρακος καλοῦ καὶ κράμβης χυλὸν συντρίψας καὶ ζυμώσας δίδου νήστει καὶ εἰς κοίτην· ἢ δαφνελαίου καὶ οἴνου καλοῦ ἀνὰ < γ'. μίξας χλιαρὸν πότιζον ἐν λουτρῷ καὶ οἰνέλαιον θερμὸν κέραμον πυρίαζε τὸν στόμαχον, τὸ οἰνέλαιον μὴ δίδου φθισικῷ πίνειν, ἀλλὰ τὴν σκευασίαν τοῦ οἰνελαίου ἀκριβῶς σκευάσας καὶ χλιάνας πυρίαζον μετὰ σπόγγων τὸν στόμαχον. ἄλλο. θέρμων ἀφέψημα θερμὸν στακτὴν βρέξας πυρίαζε τοὺς πόδας βήσσοντος καὶ ἀποσπογγίσας αὐτοὺς ἐπάλειφε βούτυρον καὶ

piperis, auripigmenti fciffilis, cariophylli par pondus, omnia fimul mixta, trita et cum melle fermentata exhibe jejuno et cubitum eunti. Aut auripigmentum fciffile pro fale in ovum injicito et forbendum praebeto. Aut auripigmentum tritum ex vino tepido bibat in balneo. Aut auripigmento fciffili cum croco trito et cum ovo mixto bombicem imbue et per cichonem fuffumigato. Quum vero qui fuffumigatur deficere videbitur, da illi devorandum butyrum quanta eft nux avellana, ac deinde iterum fuffumigato idque fepties faciendum eft. *Aliud.* Styracem optimum et brafficae fuccum fimul terito et fermentatum da jejuno et domitum ituro: aut oleum laurinum et vinum optimum accipe utriusque drach. iij tmisce et tepidum in balneo bibendum dato et vino oleoque mixtis et in olla calefactis ftomachum foveto; ne dato oenoleum bibendum phthifico; fed oenoleum probe paratum calefacito et fpongia madefacta ftomachum foveto. *Aliud.* Lupinorum decocto myrrham ftactem macerato tuffientisque pedes foveto et fpongia deterfos butyro illinito iterumque

Ed. Chart. X. [643.]
πυρίαζε, τοῦτο τρισέσας ἰαθήσεται. ἄλλο. κισσοῦ κόκκους ἢ ξύλα, ἢ φύλλα κάπνισον τὸν βήσσοντα· ἢ ῥητίνην σὺν οἴνῳ παλαιῷ συντρίψας πότισον νήστει· ἢ ἀγριοκανάβης σπέρμα τρίψας πότισον μετὰ ὕδατος· ἢ κεδρίαν πότισον νηστικῷ, ἢ ὕσσωπον καὶ γλήχωνα μετὰ ὀξυκράτου δὸς πιεῖν προεψήσας· ἢ βερονίκην φυράσας μετὰ μέλιτος δίδου φαγεῖν· ἢ ῥάφανοι ὀπτοὶ ἐσθιόμενοι πρωῒ καὶ ὀψέ· ἢ χαμαιλεύκη θυμιωμένη. ἄλλο. δαφνίδας μετὰ πεπέρεως καὶ στροβίλους μετὰ μέλιτος δίδου πρωῒ καὶ εἰς κοίτην.

[*Εἰς βήσσοντας, τετραχωμένους τὴν ἀρτηρίαν, ἀποκεκομμένους τὴν φωνὴν καὶ ἀναφορικούς.*] Λαβὼν τραγακάνθης, κόμμεως ἀνὰ < α΄. σμύρνης καλῆς < α΄. γλυκυῤῥίζης χυλοῦ καὶ γλυκέος τὸ ἀρκοῦν, κόψας πάντα καὶ ἑνώσας, ἐπειδὰν λειωθῶσι, τὰ ξηρία μῖξον μετὰ τῶν λοιπῶν.

[*Ἄλλο πρὸς βήχιον καὶ ἑλκομένην ἀρτηρίαν.*] Λαβὼν τερεβινθίνης, κόμμεως, καλοῦ μέλιτος ἀνὰ < α΄. τὸ μέλι καὶ τὴν τερεβινθίνην προεψήσας βάλλε τὸ κομμίδιον καὶ δίδου

foveto; hoc ter facto curabitur. *Aliud.* Hederae granis aut lignis aut foliis ſuffumigato tuſſientem. Aut reſina ex veteri vino laevigatum ante cibum bibita; aut canabis ſilveſtris ſemen tritum et ex aqua potum; aut liquorem cedri potui jejuno datum aut hyſſopus et pulegium ex posca cocta bibenda dentur; aut beronicen melle ſubactam edendam praebe. Vel raphani toſti quum mane ac vespere eduntur, conferunt. Chamaeleuce quoque ſuffita. *Aliud.* Lauri baccas cum pipere, pineos etiam nucleos cum melle dato mane et cubitum eunti.

[*Ad tuſſientes, arteriae aſperitate laborantes, voce captos et ſanguinem expuentes.*] Recipe tragacanthae, gummi, utriusque drach. j, myrrhae optimae drach. j, ſucci radicis dulcis et paſſi quantum ſatis ſit, omnia contere ſimul et ubi fuerint laevigata, arida cum aliis misce.

[*Aliud ad tuſſim et exulceratam arteriam.*] Recipe terebinthinae, gummi, mellis optimi, ſingulorum drach. j, mel et terebinthinam ſimul coquito, mox gummi indito

ὅσον ἐλαίας μέγεθος διακρατεῖν ἐν τῷ στόματι. ἄλλο. κόμμεως, λυκίου ἀνὰ γο. δ'. βάλλε εἰς ὕδωρ καὶ ἔασον τακῆναι, εἶτα βάλλε κοτύλην Κρητικοῦ γλυκέος μίαν καὶ ἕψε ἕως οὗ γένηται γλοιῶδες καὶ χρῶ ἐν ἐκλεικτῷ.

[Ἄλλο εἰς βηχία καὶ βρόγχους καὶ αἵματος ἀναγωγάς.] Λαβὼν τραγακάνθης < β'. λινοσπέρμου πεφρυγμέ- [644] νου < δ'. ἀμύγδαλα λελεπισμένα ι'. στροβίλου ὠπτημένης στέατι < γ'. τὴν τραγάκανθαν ἐν ὕδατι βρέχε χλιαρῷ καὶ τὰ λοιπὰ μῖξον γλυκὺ καὶ παραχέας λειοτρίβει. πρὸς δὲ τὰς ἀνακοπὰς τῆς φωνῆς καὶ ἐὰν ἀνάγῃ αἷμα, χρῶ μέλιτι ἀντὶ τοῦ γλυκέος. ἄλλο. ῥάφανον κατακόψας καὶ στρογγύλα ποιήσας ὄπτησον ἐπ' ἀνθράκων καὶ μετὰ μέλιτος φάγε νῆστις.

[Πρὸς βῆχα χρόνιον.] Λαβὼν πεπέρεως < α'. θέρμων ἀλεύρου γο. γ'. καὶ μέλιτος κοχλιάριον α'. δὸς ῥοφεῖν. ἄλλο. τῆς ἀκοῆς τοῦ χοίρου τὸ τετριμμένου ὀστοῦν περιαφθὲν τραχήλῳ προφυλακτικόν ἐστι βηχός.

[Βηχικὸν καὶ κιονικὸν καὶ ἐν φλεγμονῇ παρισθμίων.]

et praebe oleae magnitudinem ore continendam. *Aliud.* Recipe gummi, lycii utriusque unc. iv, ea in aquam injice donec liquescant, poſtea adde heminam paſſi Cretici et coque quoad acceperit ſordium ſpiſſitudinem et delingendo ſumatur.

[*Aliud ad tuſſiculas, raucedines et ſanguinis rejectionem.*] Recipe tragacanthae drach. ij, ſeminis lini fricti drach. iv, amygdala decorticata decem, nucleorum pineorum adipi incoctorum drach. iij, tragacantham aqua calida macerato ac caetera misceto paſſumque infundito et laevigato; ad abſciſſam vero vocem ſanguinisque ſcreatum pro paſſo melle utere. *Aliud.* Raphanum in taleas rotundas concidito et ſuper prunas torreto et jejuno comedendum ex melle praebeto.

[*Ad tuſſim diuturnam.*] Recipe piperis drach. j, farinae lupinorum unc. iij, mellis cochlearium unum, ſorbendum praebeto. *Aliud.* Os perforatum auriculae porci collo appenſum a tuſſi praeſervat.

[*Medicamentum quod tuſſi et columellae affectibus*

Ed. Chart. X. [644.]

Οἱ ἐν ταῖς καλιαῖς τῶν νοσσιῶν τῶν χελιδόνων εὑρισκόμενοι λίθοι περιαπτόμενοι προφυλακτικόν ἐστι βηχός.

[*Βηχικοῖς καὶ ἐν ῥίζῃ σταφυλῆς καὶ εἰς κατάῤῥουν.*] *Λαβὼν ζιγγιβέρεως < α'. χαλβάνης, ὀπίου, στύρακος ἀνὰ < α'. γλυκεῖ ἀναλαβὼν ποίει ὀροβιαῖα καὶ ἀντὶ καταποτίου πάρεχε ἐν κοίτῃ δύο καὶ ἐπιῤῥόφα καὶ τὸ γλυκὺ κεκραμένον. ἄλλο. ζιγγιβέρεως < δ'. στύρακος < δ'. γλυκεῖ ἀναλάμβανε καὶ ποίει ὀρόβια καὶ ἀντὶ καταποτίου δίδου εἰς κοίτην γ'. ἐπιῤῥοφῶντι γλυκὺ κεκραμένον.*

[*Εἰς κατάῤῥουν καὶ βῆχα δόκιμον.*] *Λαβὼν ὀπίου < β'. καστορίου < α'. ποίει ὀροβιαῖα καὶ δίδου εἰς κοίτην πρὸς δύναμιν.*

[*Ἄλλο ᾧπερ ἐχρήσατο ὁ σοφώτατος Ἀλέξανδρος.*] *Πυρέθρου < β'. κόστου < α'. κόψας καὶ σήσας ἐν δὲ τῇ χρήσει κέλευε ἅπτεσθαι τῶν μυκτήρων καὶ στέλλε εὐθύς.*

[*Πρὸς τοὺς ἐκ κατάῤῥου τὴν ἀρτηρίαν ῥευματισθέντας*

et inflammationi tonſillarum medetur.] Lapilli, qui reperiuntur in nidis pullorum hirundinum appenſi a tuſſi tuentur.

[*Ad tuſſientes et uvae radice laborantes et ad deſtillationes.*] Recipe zingiberis, galbani, opii, ſtyracis, ſingulorum drach. j, eaque paſſo excepta in globulos ervi magnitudine redigito et ex his duos loco catapotiorum da dormituro; ſorbeat etiam paſſum dilutum. *Aliud.* Recipe zingiberis drach. iv, ſtyracis drach. iv, excipe paſſo et fac orobia et ex his tres cubitum eunti da pro catapotiis, qui ſorbeat paſſum dilutum.

[*Ad deſtillationem et tuſſim probatum.*] Recipe opii drach. ij, caſtorii drach. j, confice trochiscos ervi magnitudine et pro viribus dormituro exhibe.

[*Aliud quo uſus eſt ſapientiſſimus Alexander.*] Recipe pyrethri drach. ij, coſti drach. j, terito et cribrato; in uſu jube nares tangere ac ſtatim conſtringe.

[*Ad eos quibus in arteriam fluit catarrhus et ad*

Ed. Chart. X. [644.]

καὶ βήσσοντας.] Λαβὼν στύρακος < η'. καστορίου < δ'. ζιγγιβέρεως < δ'. χαλβάνης < δ'. ἑνώσας ποίει ὀροβιαῖα καὶ πάρεχε εἰς νύκτα β'. ἢ γ'. καὶ μὴ ἐπιπινέτω ὁ πίνων παραχρῆμα καὶ ὠφεληθήσεται.

[Πάσμα κρανίου παύων ῥεῦμα αὐτοῦ.] Λαβὼν ὑπερικοῦ, σχοίνου ἄνθους, ἴρεως, ξυλοβαλσάμου γο. α'. κόψας καὶ σήσας χρῶ ἐπιπαύων τῷ κρανίῳ.

[Πάσμα κρανίου ἀναξηραντικόν.] Λαβὼν κόστου φύλλων μαλαβάθρου, κηκίδων, ναρδοστάχυος, ἴρεως, νάρδου Κελτικῆς, ῥόδων ξηρῶν, ἀνὰ γο. α'. κόψας καὶ σήσας ἐπίπασον.

["Αλλο πάσμα.] Λαβὼν ἐρείκης καρποῦ, κηκίδων, σχοίνου ἄνθους, σαμψύχου, κόστου, ἴρεως, ξυλοβαλσάμου, ἀνὰ γο. α'. κόψας καὶ σήσας ἐπίπασον τὴν κεφαλήν.

[Ἀποφλεγματισμὸς χειμερινός.] Λαβὼν ὑσσώπου < δ'. ὀριγάνου < δ'. γλήχωνος < β'. καλαμίνθης < α'. σταφίδος ἀγρίας < α'. πυρέθρου < β'. πρασίου < α'. σινή-

tuſſientes.] Recipe ſtyracis drach. viij, caſtorii drach. iv, zingiberis drach. iv, galbani drach. iv, ex his unitis facito pilulas ad ervi formam; duas autem vel tres eunti dormitum praebe neque ſtatim poſt bibat; juvabitur etenim.

[*Pulvis cephalicus rheuma ſedans.*] Recipe hyperici, junci odorati, iridis, ligni balſami, ſingulorum drach. j, trita et cribrata calvariae inſperge.

[*Alius qui caput exſiccat.*] Recipe coſti, foliorum malabathri, gallarum, ſpicae nardi, iridis, nardi Celtici, roſarum aridarum, ſingulorum drach. j, ea trita et cribrata inſperge.

[*Alius pulvis.*] Recipe ericae fructus, gallarum, junci odorati, ſampſuchi, coſti, iridis, ligni balſami, ſingulorum drach. j, trita et cribrata capiti inſpergito.

[*Apophlegmatismus hiemalis.*] Recipe hyſſopi drach. iv, origani drach. iv, pulegii drach. ij, calaminthae drach. j, ſtaphiſagriae drach. j, pyrethri drach. ij, marrubii drach. j,

πεως ∠ α'. ἑψήματος ξέστην α'. ὄξους ξέστην α'. ἑνώσας ἕψει ἕως οὗ ἀποτριτωθῇ καὶ ἀποφλεγμάτιζε.

[*Ἀποφλεγματισμὸς ἐαρινός.*] *Λαβὼν* ὑσσώπου γο. δ'. ὀριγάνου γο. γ'. γλήχωνος γο. β'. καλαμίνθης γο. α'. ἑψήματος ξέστην α'. ὄξους ξέστας τρεῖς.

[645] [*Ἀποφλεγματισμὸς θερινὸς καὶ φθινοπωρινός.*] *Λαβὼν* ὑσσώπου γο. δ'. ὀριγάνου γο. γ'. γλήχωνος γο. β'. καλαμίνθης γο. α'. ναρδοστάχυος γο. α'. καρυοφύλλου γο. α'. κινναμώμου γο. γ'. πρασίου γο. δ'. ἴρεως γο. γ'. κυπέρου γο. β'. πυρέθρου γο. α'. ἑψήματος ξέστην μίαν, ὄξους ξέστην α'. ἕψει ἕως ἀποτριτωθῇ καὶ ἀποφλεγμάτιζε.

[*Εἰς κατάῤῥουν.*] *Λαβὼν* ὀριγάνου δεσμίδια β'. γλήχωνος δεσμίδιον α'. μετὰ ὄξους βαλὼν εἰς χύτραν καθαρὰν καὶ ἰσχάδας στ'. καὶ σταφίδας ὡσεὶ ιβ'. ἕως ἀποτριτωθῇ καὶ σακκέλισον καὶ βάλλε εἰς ποτήριον καὶ λαβὼν ἀναγαργάριζε.

[*Πρὸς τοὺς ἐν τῷ θώρακι χυμούς.*] *Κνίδης* τὰ φύλλα συνεψηθέντα πτισάνῃ δίδου, λύει δὲ καὶ ἐμπνευματώσεις καὶ ἀνάγει τὰ ἐν τῷ θώρακι.

ſinapis drach. j, ſapae ſextarium j, aceti ſextarium j, omnia ſimul ad tertias coquito et gargarizet.

[*Apophlegmatismus vernus.*] Recipe hyſſopi unc. iv, origani unc. iij, pulegii unc. ij, calaminthae unc. j, ſapae ſextarium, aceti ſextarios tres.

[*Apophlegmatismus aeſtivus et autumnalis.*] Recipe hyſſopi unc. iv, origani unc. iij, pulegii unc. ij, calaminthae unc. j, ſpicaenardi unc. j, caryophyllorum unc. j, cinnamomi unc. iij, marrubii unc. iv, iridis unc. iij, cyperi unc. ij, pyrethri unc. j, ſapae ſextarium j, aceti ſextarium j, ad tertias coquito et gargarizandum praebeto.

[*Ad deſtillationem.*] Recipe origani fasciculos ij, pulegii fasciculum j, injice in ollam mundam cum aceto et adjicito caricas vj et paſſulas xij, decoquito ad tertias et deinde percolato ac id in calicem conjectum gargariza.

[*Ad humores in pectore reſidentes.*] Urticae folia ptiſanae incocta offerto; diſcutit inflationes et quae in pectore ſunt educit.

Ed. Chart. X. [645.]

[*Πρὸς βῆχα καὶ δύσπνοιαν ἐν στομάχῳ καὶ ἀναγωγὰς αἵματος.*] Λαβὼν σπόγγον λευκὸν καὶ κενὸν καὶ καύσας καὶ λειοτριβήσας μῖξον τὴν σποδιὰν σὺν μέλιτι καὶ πεπέρει τῷ ἀρκοῦντι, καὶ ποιήσας ὡς ἔκλειγμα λάμβανε ὀψὲ μετὰ τὸν δεῖπνον, ὅσον αἴροις τοῖς τρισὶ δακτύλοις.

[*Πρὸς συνάγχην.*] Χολὴν βοὸς ἄῤῥενος χρῖε τὸν τράχηλον.

[*Πρὸς βῆχα ξηραντικόν.*] Τῆλιν ἑψήσας ἕως ὅτου ἀποτριτωθῇ καὶ τὸ ζεμμάτιον λαβέτω πρωῒ μετὰ μέλιτος.

[*Τροχίσκος βηχικὸς τοῖς τὸν θώρακα ῥευματιζομένοις.*] Γλήχωνος, ὑσσώπου, πεπέρεως, καρδάμου ἀνὰ γο. α΄. μέλιτι ἀναλαβὼν ποίει τροχίσκους ἀνὰ < α΄. καὶ χρῶ.

[*Περὶ παρισθμιῶν.*] Ἰτέας φύλλα καὶ καρπὸν ἑψήσας ὕδατι ἐπιπολὺ δίδου ἀναγαργαρίζεσθαι. τοῦτο ἀποσπᾷ τὰ παχέα τῶν δερμάτων μάλιστα καὶ εἰς συναγχικοὺς ποιεῖ. ἄλλο. μυρσίνην καὶ φακὴν ἑψήσας δίδου ἀναγαργαρίζεσθαι.

[*Ad tuſſim et ſpirandi difficultatem a ſtomacho et ſanguinis excreationes.*] Acceptam ſpongiam albam novamque urito et terito, cinerem illum cum melle miscelo et piperis quod ſatis ſit adjicito indeque linctum componito, atque ſero a coena quantum tribus digitis capi poteſt aſſumito.

[*Ad anginam.*] Collum felle bovis masculi obline.

[*Exſiccatorium ad tuſſim.*] Foenum graecum ad tertias elixato jusculumque id ſummo mane cum melle exhibeto.

[*Paſtillus tuſſi commodus, in quibus fluxio ad pectus deſtillat.*] Recipe pulegii, hyſſopi, piperis, naſturtii ſingulorum drach. j, ex his melle exceptis confice paſtillos pendentes ſingulos drachmam et eis utere.

[*Ad tonſillarum vitia.*] Salicis folia et fructus plurimum ex aqua decocta gargarizentur; hoc medicamentum craſſam pituitam maxime a pelle evellit; probe etiam facit ad anginam. *Aliud.* Decoctum myrti et lenticulae gargarizandum praebe.

[Πρὸς συνάγχην.] Αἰγεία κόπρος σὺν μέλιτι ἀναγαργαριζέσθω, ἢ πηγάνου χυλὸν ἀνοίξας τὸ στόμα ἐπίκλυζε τὸν φάρυγγα.

[Πρὸς κατάῤῥοιαν.] Ὕσσωπον ἑψήσας μετὰ σύκων καὶ μέλιτος καὶ πηγάνου μετὰ ὕδατος δὸς ἀναγαργαρίζεσθαι.

[Εἰς καλλιφωνίαν.] Τραγάκανθα ἀποβραχεῖσα ἐν οἴνῳ καὶ ποθεῖσα φωνὴν λαμπρύνει.

[Πρὸς ἀποκοπὰς φωνῆς.] Στύρακα λειώσας μετὰ ὕδατος ποίει καταπότια ἴσα ἐρεβίνθου καὶ δίδου τρία καὶ εὐθέως λαλήσει.

[Πρὸς φλεγμονὴν ἐρυσιπέλατος.] Ἀγχούσης φύλλα σὺν ἀλφίτοις καταπλασσόμενα, ἢ ἀνδράχνης φύλλα σὺν ἀλφίτοις καταπλασσόμενα, ἢ κράμβης φύλλα καταπλασσόμενα, ἢ καλάμου φύλλα χλωρὰ λέανον καὶ κατάπλασον· ἢ βάτου φύλλα καταπλασσόμενα, ἢ ῥάμνου καὶ ῥόδων φύλλα καταπλασσόμενα.

[Πρὸς ἕλμινθας.] Πολυποδίου ῥίζα μιγνυμένη μετὰ ἑψήματος καὶ ἐσθιομένη, ἢ ῥαφάνου σπέρμα σὺν ὕδατι πι-

[*Ad anginam.*] Caprinum ſtercus gargarizetur aut ore hianti fauces ſucco rutae illinito.

[*Ad deſtillationem.*] Hyſſopum, ficus, mel et ruta ex aqua coquantur, id decoctum gargarizetur.

[*Ad clarificandam vocem.*] Tragacantha vino macerata et epota vocem claram praeſtat.

[*Ad abſciſſam vocem.*] Styracem aqua macerato, catapotia fingito ciceris magnitudine, ex illis tria dato, ſtatim loquetur.

[*Ad inflammationem eryſipelatis.*] Anchuſae folia in cataplasma redacta cum polenta impoſita. Aut portulacae folia etiam cum polenta. Aut braſſicae aut cannarum virentia folia trita et impoſita. Aut rubi aut rhamni et roſarum folia in modum cataplasmatis impoſita.

[*Ad lumbricos.*] Polypodii radicem cum ſapa miſtam edat. Aut raphani ſemen ex aqua bibat. Aut allium

Ed. Chart. X. [645. 646.]

νόμενον, ἢ σκορόδου τρωγόμενον, ἢ πτελέας ῥίζα σὺν μελικράτῳ πινομένη, ἢ συκαμίνου ῥίζης ὁ φλοιὸς σὺν ὕδατι ἑψηθεὶς καὶ [646] ποθεὶς, ἢ μελάνθιον πινόμενον καὶ καταπλασσόμενον, ἢ κράμβης σπέρμα σὺν ὕδατι πινόμενον, ἢ ἡδυόσμου χυλὸς πινόμενος, ἢ κάρδαμος μετὰ ἡδυόσμου πινόμενος.

[*Ἰδία πεῖρα.*] *Καννάβεως σπέρμα ξηρὸν κόψας καὶ σήσας, ὕδατι μίξας καὶ χυλῶδες ποιήσας καὶ ῥάκει καθαρῷ ἀποπιάσας δὸς πιεῖν· ἢ βόλβιτον ξηρὸν καύσας καὶ ποιήσας ξηρίον ἐξ αὐτοῦ δὸς πιεῖν* < *α΄. μετ᾽ οἴνου.*

[*Πρὸς ἕλμινθας πλατείας καὶ ἀσκαρίδας.*] *Λαβὼν νίτρου, καρδάμου, πεπέρεως ἀνὰ γο. α΄. ποιήσας ξηρίον δίδου κοχλιάριον α΄. μετ᾽ οἴνου.*

[*Εἰς τὸ κινεῖν ἱδρῶτας καὶ ἀποπαύειν πυρετούς.*] *Κάγχρυος σπέρμα μετ᾽ ἐλαίου συγχριόμενον, ἢ πύρεθρον μετὰ ἐλαίου θερμανθὲν καὶ ἐπιχρισθὲν πρὸ μιᾶς ὥρας τῆς ἐπισημασίας.*

[*Ἄλλο πρὸς πυρετὸν δόκιμον.*] *Ἔλαιον κινναμομέλαιον,*

rodat. Aut ulmi radicem ex mulſa epota. Aut cortex radicis ſycamini ex aqua decocta et epota valet. Aut nigella in potu accepta et in cataplasmate adminiſtrata. Aut braſſicae ſemen ex aqua bibitum. Aut ſuccus menthae epotus. Aut naſturtium cum mentha potum.

[*Proprium experimentum.*] Semen cannabis aridum tritum cretumque et aqua miſtum ut ſucci habeat ſpiſſitudinem ac linteo mundo percolatum potui detur. Aut ſimum bubulum aridum et tritum potandum dato pondere drachm. j, ex vino.

[*Ad lumbricos latos et teretes.*] Recipe nitri, naſturtii, cardamomi, piperis, ana unc. j, in pulverem redigito, da cochlearium ex vino.

[*Ad proritandos ſudores finiendamque febrem.*] Semen canchryos ex oleo illitum benefacit. Item pyrethrum ex oleo calefactum et per horam ante invaſionem inunctum.

[*Aliud ad febrem probatum.*] Oleum cinnamome-

Kk 2

Ed. Chart. X. [646.]
χαμαιμήλινον, ὄξος, νίτρον ἅμα φύλλοις δάφνης καλῶς συνεψήσας χρῖε τὸν κάμνοντα καὶ σκεπάσας ἐπιεικῶς αὐτίκα ἱδρώσει.

[Σύγχρισμα πυρέσσουσιν.] Λαβὼν βουτύρου μέτρα δύο, μέλιτος μέτρον α'. μίξας καὶ χλιάνας χρῶ. ἄλλο. λαβὼν θρίδακος φύλλων χυλοῦ μέτρον α'. ἐλαίου κοινοῦ μέτρα β'. μίξας καὶ ἀνασκέψας ἐπιμελῶς σύγχρισον ὅλον τὸ σῶμα. δόκιμον γάρ ἐστιν. ἄλλο. λαβὼν ἀρτεμισίας χυλοῦ μέτρον α'. ῥοδίνου μέτρα β'. μίξας χρῶ.

[Πρὸς πόνον ἡμικρανίον.] Στρύχνου χυλὸς μετ' ἐλαίου συγχριόμενος πάνυ ὠφελεῖ. ἄλλο. σινήπεως σπέρμα μετὰ μέλιτος κατάπλασον. ἄλλο. πηγάνου ἡμέρου σὺν ὄξει καὶ ῥοδίνῳ ἑψηθέντος καταχριομένου.

[Πρὸς κυνοδήκτους.] Κνίδης σπέρμα καταπλασσόμενον, ἢ πρασίας μελαίνης τὰ φύλλα καταπλασσόμενα, ἢ μελισσόφυλλον σὺν οἴνῳ πινόμενον καὶ τοῖς δήγμασιν ἐπιτιθέμενον, ἢ σκόροδα καταπλασσόμενα καὶ ὀπτὰ ἐσθιόμενα καὶ πινόμενα.

laeum, chamaemelinum, acetum, nitrum cum lauri foliis coquito et febricitantem illinito probeque tegito, ſtatim enim ſudabit.

[*Illitus ad febricitantes.*] Recipe butyri partes duas, mellis partem unam, miſce et tepido utere. *Aliud.* Recipe ſucci foliorum lactucae partem unam, olei communis partes duas, misce et eis probe agitatis univerſum corpus illine, probatum eſt medicamentum. *Aliud.* Artemiſiae partem unam, roſacei partes duas miſce et utere.

[*Ad hemicranium dolorem.*] Solani ſuccus cum oleo illitus plurimum confert. *Aliud.* Ex ſinapis ſemine et melle confectum cataplasma adminiſtra. *Aliud.* Ruta domeſtica ex aceto et roſaceo cocta et illita valet.

[*Ad canis morſum.*] Urticae ſemen in modum cataplasmatis appoſitum confert. Aut folia nigri marrubii. Aut apiaſtri folia ex vino pota et morſibus appoſita. Aut allia in cataplasmatis modum appoſita atque etiam toſta, comeſta et bibita.

[Πρὸς τοὺς φοβουμένους τοὺς κύνας.] Ῥοδοδάφνης ῥίζαν περίαψον τὸν τράχηλον καὶ ἀπαλλαγήσεται. ἐὰν δὲ θέλῃς πειρᾶσαι, ὅταν κύων μανῇ, ἐπίθες περὶ αὐτὸν καὶ εὐθέως ἀφίσταται τῆς μανίας.

[Πρὸς λυσσοδήκτους.] Λυσσοδήκτων τοῖς τραύμασι κράμβης φύλλα λεῖα μετὰ σιλφίου καὶ ὄξους ἐπιτιθέσθω. καθ' ἑαυτὴν γὰρ λυττῶντος κυνὸς δῆγμα ὠφελεῖ καὶ τὸ ἀφέψημα αὐτῆς πινόμενον, ἑφθὴ δὲ κράμβη προτρωγομένη φθισικοὺς θεραπεύει καὶ τὰς περὶ τὴν ἀρτηρίαν διαθέσεις ἰᾶται. λειοτριβηθεῖσα δὲ καὶ καταπλασθεῖσα ἐπὶ σπληνὸς τοῦτο ὑπεκτήκει.

[Πρὸς συνάγχην καὶ πόνον τραχήλου.] Λεύκη ξηρὰ μέλιτι λειωθεῖσα καὶ ἐπιχρισθεῖσα τῷ τραχήλῳ, ἢ καρδάμου σπόρον καὶ κόπρον περιστερᾶς σὺν μέλιτι ἐμπλασσόμενα σὺν μέλιτι χλιαρῷ ἀναγαργάριζε, ἢ κυνείαν λευκὴν λεάνας μετὰ ὄξους ἐπίχριε εἰς τὸν τράχηλον.

[Πρὸς δυσωδίας μυκτήρων.] Κισσοῦ τῶν φύλλων ὁ χυλὸς χλιαρὸς ἐγχυματιζόμενος τοῖς ῥώθωσιν, ἢ καλαμίνθης

[*Ad timentes canem irruentem.*] Radicem nerii collo appendito et liber evadet; id vero ſi experiri volueris, furenti cani radicem circumponito, illico enim furor mitescet.

[*Ad morſus rabidi canis.*] Vulneribus ex morſu rabidi canis factis folia braſſicae cum laſſere et aceto trita apponito: braſſica enim per ſe valet ad morſus rabidi canis ejusque decoctum in potu acceptum. Elixa etiam braſſica ſi eſtur ante alios cibos, phthiſicos ſanat; etiam affectus arteriae curat. Sed et contuſa et in modum cataplasmatis lieni appoſita ipſum attenuat.

[*Ad anginam collique dolores.*] Populus alba arida et ex melle trita et cervici illita. Aut naſturtii ſemen cum columbino fimo ex melle appoſitum aut tepidum cum melle gargarizatum. Aut canino ſtercore albo ex aceto illine collum.

[*Ad foetidos narium odores.*] Valet ſuccus foliorum hederae tepidus naribus inſtillatus. Aut calaminthae

χυλὸς ὁμοίως χλιαρὸς ἐγχεόμενος, ἢ σμύρνα λειωθεῖσα σὺν γάλακτι γυναικείῳ καὶ ἐγχεομένη.

[*Πρὸς αἱμοῤῥοΐαν μυκτήρων.*] Ἀκακίαν σὺν ὄξει λειώσας ἔγχεε τοῖς ῥώθωσιν. [647] ἄλλο. λαβὼν ὄξος σὺν ἅλατι βάλλε ἐν χύτρᾳ ἢ ἐν τρυβλίῳ καὶ βαλὼν ἔρια ἔμβρεχε ἐν αὐτῇ καὶ χλιάνας αὐτὰ ὅσον ἔχει δέχεσθαι ἐπίθες εἰς τὴν κεφαλὴν καὶ συντόμως κέλευε σκεπάζεσθαι πλείστοις σκεπάσμασι.

[*Καθάρσιον ῥινῶν.*] Θύμον καὶ ὀρίγανον ἀναλαβὼν μέλιτι ποίει τροχίσκους καὶ δίδου διαμασᾶσθαι.

[*Πρὸς πλευριτικούς.*] Βδέλλιον σὺν οἴνῳ πινόμενον ὁμοίως καὶ ὕδατι, ἢ καρπὸς βαλσάμου σὺν ὕδατι πινόμενος, ἢ σὺν μέλιτι ἐκλειχόμενος, ἢ ἀριστολοχίας ῥίζα σὺν ὕδατι πινομένη, ἢ πήγανον σὺν μελικράτῳ πινόμενον.

[*Πρὸς ὀξὺν πυρετόν.*] Πέπονος ἡμέρου ὁ χυλὸς συγχριόμενος, ἢ κολοκύνθης ξυσμάτων ὁ χυλὸς συγχριόμενος καὶ ῥόδα μετ᾽ ἐλαίου, ἢ ἀρνόγλωσσον καταπλασσόμενον.

ſuccus ſimili modo tepidus inſtillatus. Aut myrrha ex muliebri lacte laevigata et infuſa.

[*Ad profluvia ſanguinis e naribus.*] Acacia ex aceto laevigata naribus infundatur. *Aliud.* Accipe acetum cum ſale idque in ollam aut mortarium mittito lanamque acceptam illis imbuito tepefactamque quantum laborans ferre poteſt capiti imponito, pluribus deinde veſtibus ſtatim tegi jubeto.

[*Medicamentum nares expurgans.*] Thymum et origanum melle excepta in paſtillos redigito et eos commanducandos exhibeto.

[*Ad pleuriticos.*] Bdellium ex vino potum valet; itemque ex aqua. Aut fructus balſami ex aqua bibitus aut delinctus ex melle. Aut radix ariſtolochiae ex aqua epota. Aut ruta ex mulſa etiam pota.

[*Ad acutam febrem.*] Conſert ſuccus peponis illitus. Aut ſuccus ramentorum cucurbitae inunctus. Aut roſa ex oleo aut cataplasma ex plantagine appoſitum.

Ed. Chart. X. [647.]

[Πρόγνωσις ἐπὶ πυρεσσόντων.] Ῥόδινον ἀλείψας κατάπλασον, σελινόκοκκον τριπτὸν καὶ ἐπίθες εἰς τὴν καρδίαν αὐτοῦ στυππεῖον ὡς τροχὸν καὶ ἐπίχεε τὸν κρόκκον τοῦ ὠοῦ καὶ σκέπασον αὐτὸν νεφελίᾳ, καὶ ἐὰν γένηται σκορπισμὸς τοῦ ὠοῦ, γίνωσκε θάνατον. τοῦτο λέγεται αὐτὴ ἡ ψυχὴ ποιεῖν.

[Πρὸς τραῦμα παρακολλᾷν.] Ἀγρώστεως ῥίζα λεία καταπλασσομένη ὡς ξηρίον, ἢ σιδηρίτιδος βοτάνης τὰ φύλλα ἐπιπλασσόμενα.

[Θεραπεία ὠταλγίας.] Ἀμυγδαλέλαιον ἐνσταζόμενον εἰς τὸ οὖς, ἢ καρέλαιον ἐνσταζόμενον, ἢ δαφνέλαιον, ἢ βαλσαμέλαιον, ἢ δρακοντίου βοτάνης τοῦ καρποῦ ὁ χυλὸς μετ' ἐλαίου ἐγχεόμενος, ἢ περδικιάδος ὁ χυλὸς μετ' ἐλαίου ῥοδίνου χλιαρὸς ἐνσταζόμενος, ἢ πήγανον χλωρὸν σὺν ἐλαίῳ ἑψηθὲν καὶ χλιαρὸν ἐνσταζόμενον, ἢ σμύρνα καὶ μέλι χλιαρῶς ἐνσταζόμενα, ἢ πήγανον μετὰ γυναικείου γάλακτος ἀῤῥενοτόκου περιχλιάνας ἔνσταξον, ἢ σκόροδον χυλώσας ἔνσταξον εἰς τὸ οὖς, ἢ πράσον χυλώσας χλιαρὸν ἢ ἕψημα χλιαρὸν,

[*Praeſagium in ſebricitantibus.*] Roſaceo inunge primum, mox ſemen apii tritum impone ſtuppamque rotundam in modum rotae cordi impone ovique luteum affunde et reticulo contegito; ſi fiat ovi diſſipatio, mortem inſtare noveris; nam anima hoc ſacere dicitur.

[*Ad vulnera conglutinanda.*] Radix graminis trita ut aridum medicamentum imponatur. Aut ſideritidis herbae folia ſuſpendentur.

[*Curatio dolorum auris.*] Amygdalinum oleum in aures inſtillatum confert. Aut oleum ex nucibus confectum; item inſtillatum. Aut laurinum aut balſaminum oleum. Aut ſuccus fructus dracontii herbae infuſus. Aut ſuccus herbae perdiciadis cum roſaceo tepidus in aures inſtillatus. Aut oleum in quo ruta incocta ſit tepidum inſtillatum. Aut myrrha et mel tepefacta et inſtillata. Aut rutam cum lacte muliebri ejus quae masculum pepererit tepidam inſtillato. Aut expreſſum ex allio ſuccum in aures inſtillato. Aut porri ſuccum vel ejusdem deco-

Ed. Chart. X. [647.]
ἢ πράσου χυλὸν σὺν μέλιτι μίξας ἔνσταξον, ἢ βαλὼν ἔλαιον εἰς τὸ στόμα εἰς τὸ ὠτίων ἔμπτυε, ἢ κολοκύνθης χυλὸν μετὰ ῥοδίνου ἔνσταξον.

[*Πρὸς ψώρας καὶ κνησμούς.*] *Πτελέας φύλλα ξηρὰ λειωθέντα καὶ ἐπιπλασσόμενα ἐν βαλανείῳ, ἢ θεῖον ἄπυρον καὶ σταφυλὴ ἀγρία καὶ ἀρσενικὸν καὶ σανδαράχη σὺν ἐλαίῳ καὶ ὄξει ἐπιχριόμενα ἐν βαλανείῳ. ἄλλο. σμύρναν μετὰ γάλακτος γυναικείου ἐπίχριε, ἢ γλυκυῤῥίζης χυλὸν μετὰ γλυκέος δὸς πιεῖν, ἢ ὠὰ ὄρνιθος ὁλόκληρα βάλλε εἰς ὄξος δριμύτατον ἡμερονύκτιον καὶ ἐμβαλὼν αὐτὰ, τριῶν δηλονότι ὄντων τῶν ὠῶν, τρῖβε αὐτὰ μετὰ τῶν ὀστράκων ἐν τῷ αὐτῷ ὄξει καὶ θεῖον ἄπυρον γο. α΄. καὶ ἀρσενικὸν σχιστὸν γο. α΄. σταφίδα ἀγρίαν γο. α΄. ψιμύθιον γο. α΄. λιθάργυρον γο. α΄. ῥοδοδάφνης χυλὸν γο. α΄. ἔλαιον παλαιὸν τὸ ἀρκοῦν, λειοτριβήσας χρῖε ἐν βαλανείῳ.*

[*Κατάπλασμα στομαχικοῖς.*] *Καλαμίνθης φύλλα χλωρὰ σὺν κριθίνῳ ἀλεύρῳ κατάπλασον.*

ctum tepidum. Aut porri ſuccum cum melle mixtum inſtillato. Aut ore aſſumptum oleum in aures inſufflato. Aut cucurbitae ſuccum cum roſaceo infundito.

[*Ad ſcabiem et pruritum.*] Ulmi folia arida trita in balneo inſpergantur. Aut ſulfure ignem non experto, uva taminia, arſenico et ſandaracha ex aceto et oleo inungatur in balneo. *Aliud.* Myrrha ex muliebri lacte illinito. Aut radicis dulcis ſuccum ex paſſo potui dato. Aut gallinae ova integra in acetum acerrimum injice per diem et noctem, ſint autem ova tria, ea in eodem aceto cum putaminibus trita, quibus deinde adde ſulfuris ignem non experti unc. j, arſenici ſciſſilis unc. j, uvae taminiae unc. j, ceruſſae unc. j, ſpumae argenti unc. j, ſucci nerii unc. j, olei veteris quod ſit ſatis; his omnibus tritis obline in balneo.

[*Cataplasma ſtomachicis.*] Ex calaminthae tritis foliis viridibus cum hordeacea farina cataplasma factum apponito.

Ed. Chart. X. [647. 648.]

[*Πρὸς ἀπεψίαν καὶ ἐμπνευματώσεις στομάχου. ὅστις γὰρ λάβοι ταύτην παρ' αὐτὰ πεινάσει.*] Πεπέρεως λευκοῦ < στ'. ἀνίσου < ιβ'. λιβυστικοῦ < στ'. ἄμμεως, πετροσελίνου, μαράθρου ἀνὰ < στ'. ταῦτα κόψας καὶ σήσας ἀναλάμβανε μέλιτι ἑφθῷ καὶ δίδου < α'.

[*Πρὸς καυσούμενον στόμαχον καὶ μὴ κατέχοντα τὴν τροφήν.*] Θρίδακος χυλὸν μετὰ γλυκέος δὸς πιεῖν καὶ οὐκ ἔτι ἐμέσει.

[*Πρὸς πόνον στομάχου.*] Ἄνθρακα δρυὸς εἰς γάλα σβέσας πότιζον τῷ πάσχοντι.

[*Πρὸς ὀξυσμὸν στομάχου.*] Χαμαίδρυον μετὰ οἴνου πινόμενον παύει ὀξυσμόν.

[*Πρὸς ἐμπνευμάτωσιν στομάχου.*] Πεπέρεως, δαφνίδων, κυμίνου, ἀνίσου ἴσα κόψας καὶ σείσας δίδου νήστει μετὰ εὐκράτου κοχλιάριον α'. ἐπὶ ἡμέρας τρεῖς, ἢ ἄνισον νηστικὸς μασοῦ.

[*Πρὸς ὀφθαλμοὺς ῥευματιζομένους.*] Μαράθρου χυλὸς ἐπὶ ἡμέρας τρεῖς ἐπιτιθέμενος, ἢ λίβανον σὺν μέλιτι καὶ

[*Ad ventriculi cruditatem inflationemque; quisquis enim eousus fuerit, statim famescet.*] Recipe aniſorum drach. xij, piperis albi drach. vj, libyſtici drach. vj, ammeos, petroſelini, foeniculi ana drach. vj, haec omnia contuſa et creta excipe cocto melle; exhibe drach. j.

[*Ad aestuantem ventriculum nec cibum continentem.*] Succum lactucae da bibendum ex paſſo, nec amplius evomet.

[*Ad ventriculi dolorem.*] Lac in quo querni ſint extincti laboranti potui dato.

[*Ad acorem ventriculi.*] Triſago, ſi ex vino bibatur, acorem removet.

[*Ad inflationem ventriculi.*] Recipe piper, baccas lauri, cuminum, aniſum paribus portionibus, eaque trita et creta ex vino temperato dato ad unum cochlearium per tres dies. Aut aniſum commanducato jejunus.

[*Ad oculos fluxione laborantes.*] Foeniculi ſuccus per tres dies impoſitus confert. Aut thus ex melle et

γάλακτι ἐπιχριόμενον, ἢ κενταυρίου χυλὸς σὺν μέλιτι ἐπιχριόμενος, ἢ πενταδακτύλου φύλλα σὺν μέλιτι ἐπιτιθέμενα.

[*Πρὸς ἀχλὺν ὀφθαλμῶν.*] *Κολοκύνθης* ξυσμάτων ὁ χυλὸς ἐπιπλασσόμενος.

[*Πρὸς λεύκωμα.*] Ὑοσκυάμου φύλλα μετὰ ἀλφίτου καταπλασσόμενα, ἢ ξυλοβάλσαμον σὺν γυναικείῳ γάλακτι ἐπιχριόμενα, ἢ πήγανον χλωρὸν καταπλασσόμενον, ἢ ψύλλιον σὺν γάλακτι γυναικείῳ ἐπιχριόμενον, ἢ καλάμων χλωρῶν τῶν φύλλων ὁ χυλὸς ἐπιχριόμενος.

[*Πρὸς ὀφθαλμῶν ἀπόκρουσμα περίδνωμα.*] *Λαβὼν* φύλλα ἐλαίας, κόψον καὶ ἐκπιάσας τὸν χυλὸν ἐπίχριε καὶ θαυμάσεις.

[*Πρὸς ῥεῦμα κατάπλασμα.*] Ἀνδράχνην λείωσον μετὰ κρόκου καὶ στέατος χηνείου, ἢ σελίνου φύλλα μετὰ ἀλφίτων· ἐπὶ δὲ τῶν μεγάλων ῥευμάτων ῥόδα καὶ μελίλωτα ἑφθὰ μετὰ ἀμύλου τοὺς ὀφθαλμοὺς κατάπλασον.

[*Πρὸς ὀδονταλγίαν.*] *Μελάνθιον* σὺν ὄξει διακλυζόμενον, ἢ κηκίδες σὺν ὀμφακίνῳ διακλυζόμεναι, ἢ πλατάνου

lacte illitus. Aut centaurii ſuccus ex melle illitus. Aut quinquefolii herbae folia trita ex melle appoſita.

[*Ad caliginem oculorum.*] Ramentorum cucurbitae ſuccus appoſitus valet.

[*Ad albuginem.*] Alterci folia cum polenta imponito. Aut lignum balſami ex muliebri lacte illitum. Aut ruta viridis in modum cataplasmatis impoſita. Aut pulicaris herba ex muliebri lacte illita. Aut connarum foliorum ſuccus illitus.

[*Ad oculorum vertiginem tollendam.*] Accipe folia olivae et contunde, ſuccoque ex eis expreſſo inunge et miraberis.

[*Ad oculorum fluxionem cataplasma.*] Portulacam cum croco terito et anſerino adipe. Aut folia apii cum polenta. In magnis autem fluxionibus cataplasma ex roſis et meliloto elixis cum amylo oculis apponito.

[*Ad dolorem dentium.*] Nigella ex aceto, ſi os colluatur, juvat. Aut gallae in oleo immaturo incoctae.

Ed. Chart. X. [648.]
σφαιρία σὺν ὄξει ἑψηθέντα καὶ διακλυζόμενα, ἢ πενταφύλλου ῥίζα σὺν ὄξει διακλυζομένη, ἢ πευκεδάνου ῥίζα λεία καυθεῖσα ἐπιπλασσομένη, ἢ σίδια καὶ ῥόδα ἑψήσας τὸ ἀφέψημα διακλυζόμενον.

[Πρὸς ὀδόντων τραῦμα.] Λαβὼν νίτρον, σηπίας ὄστρακον, σμύρναν, ἀνὰ γο. α΄. λειώσας χρῶ.

[Ξηρίον πρὸς ὀδόντας, πλαδαρὸν στόμα καὶ αἱμῶδες σμῆξαι καὶ οὖλα σαρκῶσαι καὶ ὀδόντας λευκᾶναι.] Λαβὼν νίτρου κεκαυμένου γο. α΄. σμύρνης τρογλιτίδος γο. α΄. σηπίας ὀστράκου γο. α΄. ῥόδων ξηρῶν γο. δ΄. κόψας καὶ σήσας χρῶ. πρόσβαλλε δὲ καὶ ἴρεως γο. α΄. τούτῳ χρώμενος θαυμάσεις.

[Πρὸς πόνον πλευροῦ.] Κράμβης χλωρᾶς καυλοὺς σὺν ταῖς ῥίζαις κατακαύσας ἀναλάμβανε στέατι χοιρείῳ καὶ χρῶ· θαυμάσιον τὸ βοήθημα. ἢ σελίνου σπέρμα ἀποτριτώσας πότιζον, πάνυ γὰρ ὠφελεῖ.

[Πρὸς ἐσωχάδας.] Ἀμάραντον ἀποβρέξας ὀψὲ καὶ πρωῒ πότιζον.

Aut platani fructus aceto incocti, ſi eo os colluatur. Aut decoctum radicis quinquefolii ex aceto, ſi os colluatur. Aut radix peucedani uſta et trita impoſita. Aut malicorii roſarumque decocto fiat collutio.

[*Ad dentium vulnus.*] Recipe nitri, teſtae ſepiae, myrrhae ſingulorum drachmam j, tritis utere.

[*Aridum medicamentum ad humidum cruentumque os detergendum, carnem gingivarum inſtaurandam et dentes dealbandos.*] Recipe nitri uſti unc. j, myrrhae troglodyticae unc. j, teſtae ſepiae unc. j, roſarum aridarum drach. iv, his tritis et cretis utitor; ſed ſi addideris unciam iridis, miraberis.

[*Ad lateris dolorem.*] Viridis braſſicae caulem cum radicibus uſtum excipe adipe ſuillo et utere; id remedium mirabile eſt. Aut ſemen apii ad tertias decocti in potum exhibeto; efficax remedium eſt.

[*Ad internos ani tumores.*] Amarantum aqua madefactum bibendum dato mane et vesperi.

[*Εἰς σπλῆνα κατάπλασμα πάνυ καλόν.*] *Σελίνου, σινήπεως δαφνίδων κατὰ λόγον κοπανήσας, εἶτα ἐξελὼν φλοῦν καρύας, νέας, κόψον μικρὰ καὶ βαλὼν ἐν ὄλμῳ, κόψον ἰσχυρῶς καὶ ἐκβαλὼν ἀπόβρεξον ἐν ὄξει δριμεῖ ἡμέρας γʹ. καὶ ἑνώσας ἀμ-* [649] *φότερα μετὰ χυλοῦ τιβεριάδος ἕψει ἕως γένηται κατάπλασμα καὶ τίθει ἐπάνω τοῦ σπληνὸς ἀπὸ πρωῒ ἕως ὥρας ηʹ. προρρήξας τὴν γαστέρα καὶ θαυμάσεις.*

[*Ἄλλο σπληνικὸν διὰ πείρας.*] *Φλοῦν συκέας ἐκδείρας χλωρὰν νέου δένδρου τάραξον σὺν σποδιᾷ θερμαίνων.*

[*Πρὸς τριταῖον.*] *Μέλι μετὰ σκαμμωνίας πινόμενον ἅπαξ ἰᾶται.*

[*Περὶ τεταρταίου.*] *Πέπερι τετριμμένον, δαφνόκοκκα καὶ κύμινον καὶ μαστίχην καὶ σμύρναν καὶ λίβανον καθαρὸν κοπανήσας καθ᾽ ἓν ἕκαστον καὶ ἕνωσον αὐτὰ καὶ βάλλε μέλι καλὸν τὸ ἀρκοῦν καὶ ἐπίθες ἕως ἡμέρας τέσσαρας.*

[*Πρὸς αἷμα ῥέον ἐκ μυκτήρων.*] *Ὠοῦ φλοῦν ἀκέραιον*

[*Cataplasma ad lienem praeſtans admodum.*] Accipe apium, ſinapi, lauri baccas bene contritas; deinde nuces novas dempto cortice parum tundito, poſtea ea omnia in pilam conjecta valide contundito et extracta in acetum acre demergito per tres dies, quae ubi in unum redacta fuerint, ſucco tiberiadis incoquito, donec factum ſit cataplasma, quod lieni ſuperpoſitum a ſummo mane usque ad horam octavam, prius tamen alvus excernat: effectum miraberis.

[*Aliud ad lienem experientia probatum.*] Corticem ficus viridem a nova arbore decorticatum cum cinere misceto et calefacito.

[*Ad febrem tertianam.*] Mel ſemel cum ſcammonio potum ſanat.

[*Ad quartanam.*] Accipe tritum piper, lauri baccas, cuminum, maſtichem, myrrham, thus purum, ſingula ſeparatim terito et in unum deinde redigito mellisque quod ſatis ſit adjicito ac per quatriduum imponito.

[*Ad ſanguinem e naribus profluentem.*] Ovi puta-

Ed. Chart. X. [649.]
καύσας καὶ ποιήσας στακτὴν μῖξον σὺν σχιστῷ ἀρσενικῷ καὶ βάλλε εἰς τὰς ῥῖνας τοῦ πάσχοντος· εἰ δὲ οὐκ ἔστιν ἀρσενικὸν, ἔστω ἡ στακτὴ μόνη τοῦ ὠοῦ. ἄλλο. τρίχας αἰγὸς θηλείας καύσας καὶ τρίψας, ὁμοίως καὶ σμύρναν τρίψας καὶ μίξας τὰ ἀμφότερα ἐμφύσησον εἰς τὰς ῥῖνας, εἰ μὲν ἀνδρὸς εἴη μετὰ χάρτου, εἰ δὲ γυναικὸς εἴη, μετὰ ἄλλου τινός. οἷον δὲ μέρος ἐκβάλει τὸ αἷμα, τὸ βυζὶν δῆσον.

[*Πρὸς βιασμοὺς καὶ αἱμοῤῥοίας.*] Κηκίδας ἀλέσας καὶ ῥοιᾶς φλοιὸν, τοὺς δὲ κόκκους κοπανήσας καὶ μίξας ἐλαίῳ σχιστῷ καὶ μέλιτι καὶ φυράσας, δὸς πρωῒ καὶ ὀψὲ ὡς κηκίδων μέλιτος.

[*Πρὸς κοιλίας στρόφους καὶ ἐμπνευματώσεις.*] Λαβὼν πηγάνου, πεπέρεως, ζιγγιβέρεως, ἴσα λειώσας μεθ' ὕδατος θερμοῦ δίδου, ἢ ἀρτεμισίαν κόψας καὶ σήσας δίδου, ἢ νίτρον καύσας καὶ λειώσας ἐγχυμάτισον.

[*Εἰς τὸ μὴ νοσεῖν βόας.*] Ἐλάφου κέρας θὲς ἐπάνω πανίου καὶ ἐπάνω ἅψον κανδήλαν καὶ μὴ ἐπιλάθου τὴν

men integrum urito, liquorem facito et cum arſenico ſciſſili mixtum in nares aegrotantis injicito; quod ſi arſenicum non ſit, ſolo liquore ex ovi confecto utitor. *Aliud.* Caprae foeminae villos uſtos terito pariterque et myrrham tritam et cum pilis caprinis miſtam naribus inſufflato; ſi viri fuerit, cum charta, ſi foemellae, cum alio quopiam; qua autem parte ſanguis effluit, ſtrictiſſime ligato.

[*Ad ſanguinis violentas eruptiones.*] Gallas in mola tuſas, corticem mali punici ejusdemque grana tuſa et miſta cum oleo ſciſſili, melle ſubacta, exhibe mane et vesperi, ut mel gallarum.

[*Ad ventris tormina et inflationes.*] Recipe rutae, piperis, zingiberis pares portiones, terito et ex aqua calida propinato. Aut artemiſiam tuſam et cretam exhibeto. Aut nitrum uſtum et tritum ex humore aliquo praebeto.

[*Ut ne boves aegrotent.*] Cornu cervi ſuper panis dei ſacellum imponito et deſuper candelam accendito et

Ed. Chart. X. [649.]
ἡμέραν καὶ κατὰ χρόνον ἐπικαλοῦ τὸν ἅγιον Δημούσαριν καὶ Ἄρσον, φυλάξοντας τὰ κτήνη καὶ τὸν βίον σοῦ.

[*Εἰς τὸ μὴ νοσεῖν χοίρους.*] Ῥάσδου ῥίζαν κοπανήσας βάλλε εἰς τὸ πλύμμα αὐτῶν.

[*Εἰς τὸ ποιῆσαι σαρκόκολλαν.*] Τρίψας σκώληκας ἐκ γῆς, μετὰ τὸ φρύξαι ἐπίπασον.

[*Θεραπεία πληγῶν.*] Σμύρναν καὶ ἀλόην τρίψας ἐπίπασον, ἢ ῥητίνην πεύκης, ἢ καὶ μαστίχην καὶ κισσοῦ δάκρυον ποιήσας ἔμπλαστρον ἐπίθες, ἢ τράγειον ἀξούγγιον ἄλειφε τὴν πληγὴν καὶ κέρας αἰγὸς μελαίνης ἐπίπασον. ἄλλο. κόστον στάχυν, κιννάμωμον, ζιγγίβερ, κύμινον ἐξ ἴσου τρίψας καὶ πίσσῃ φυράσας ἐπίθες, ἢ ὄψιν ἄρτου ξηρὰν τρίψας καὶ σὺν οἴνῳ καὶ ἐλαίῳ φυράσας ἐπίθες ἐπὶ ἡμέρας καθ' ἑκάστην ἀλλάσσων.

[*Εἰς ψώραν ἵππου.*] Σχίσας ὄφιν καὶ λαβὼν τὸ στέαρ αὐτοῦ ἄλειψον μετὰ ξύλου τὸ στεφάνιον τῶν ὀνύχων αὐτοῦ.

[*Εἰς τὸ κοιμηθῆναι τὸν ἀγρυπνοῦντα.*] Γράψον εἰς

ne interdiu illam accenſam oblivioni tradito et in tempore ſanctum Demuſarim invocato et Arſum; armenta et tuam cuſtodient vitam.

[*Ut porci non aegrotent.*] Rhamni radicem tritam in aquam ubi ſe proluunt, projicito.

[*Ad carnem conglutinandam.*] Vermes terrae frixos et tritos inſpergito.

[*Curatio plagarum.*] Myrrham et aloën tritas inſpergito. Aut reſinam piceam vel maſtichen et hederae lacrimam emplaſtro ex his facto imponito. Aut hircina axungia plagam illinito cornuque caprae nigrae inſpergito. *Aliud.* Coſtum, ſpicam, cinnamomum, zingiber, cuminum ſingulorum parem portionem terito et pice ſubactam imponito. Aut aridam cruſtam panis vino oleoque ſubactam imponito, eam quotidie per vices immutato.

[*Ad ſcabiem equorum.*] Anguem diſcindito et adipe ejus oras ungularum ligno inungito.

[*Ad ſomnum conciliandum.*] Foliis lauri infra ſcri-

Ed. Chart. X. [649. 650.]

φύλλα δάφνης τὰ στοιχεῖα ταῦτα καὶ θὲς ὑποκάτω τῶν σωγιῶν αὐτοῦ μὴ νοοῦντος τοῦ ἀνακειμένου. ξστ'. χστστ'. φθ'.

[*Εἰς τὸ μὴ φαντάζεσθαι ἄνθρωπον τὴν νύκτα.*] Πηγάνου σπέρμα κρέμασον εἰς τὸ προσκεφάλαιον αὐτοῦ μὴ νοοῦντος καὶ οὐ φαντάζεται.

[650] [*Πρὸς θώρακα.*] Ὠῷ ἀρσενικὸν μίξας σχιστὸν καὶ πέπερι, κριθάλευρον καὶ δαφνόκοκκα καὶ κωνάρια καὶ δίδου. ἄλλο. σκόροδος κοκκία ζ'. ἀρσενικοῦ σχιστοῦ καὶ πεπέρεως ἀνὰ κοκκία ιγ'. βάμβικα, κωνάριον, κηρὸν ὀλίγον μίξας μετὰ κρόκου ὠοῦ λάβε συχνόν.

[*Πρὸς ὀδόντας βεβρωμένους.*] Ἀρσενικὸν, πέπερι, τυρὸν, ἄσβεστον ζῶσαν ζυμώσας μετ' ὄξους πρόπλασον.

[*Ἐργαλεῖον νεφριτικόν.*] Γλήχωνος, ὀριγάνου, σαμψύχου, ἑρπύλλου, χαμαιμήλου, ἀψινθίου, κενταυρίου, δάφνης φύλλων, συκῆς ἀγρίας, πέπονος ὁμοῦ ἑψήσας μέλιτι σὺν ὕδατι, προανακόψας μέλιτι σὺν ἐλαίῳ καὶ ἅλατι ἐπίβαλλε ἐκ τοῦ ἀποζέματος τὸ ἀρκοῦν.

pta elementa inſcribito et cubantis ſtragulis eo ignorante ſupponito. ξστ. χστστ. φθ.

[*Ut noctu homo non ſomniet.*] Rutae ſemen cervicali ipſo neſciente ſuſpendito, nec dormiens ullas videbit imagines.

[*Ad pectus.*] Ovo arſenicum ſciſſile miſceto et piper et farinam hordeaceam et lauri baccas nucleosque pineos adhibeto. *Aliud.* Allii nucleos ſeptem, arſenici ſciſſilis, piperis utriusque grana xiij, bambacem, pineos nucleos, cerae parum miſce et ſaepe cum ovi luteo accipe.

[*Ad corroſos dentes.*] Arſenicum, piper, caſeum, calcem vivam cum aceto fermentata apponito.

[*Ad renum affectus clyſter.*] Accipe pulegium, origanum, ſampſuchum, ſerpillum, chamaemelum, abſinthium, centaurium et lauri folia, cucumerem ſilveſtrem, peponem, prius contuſa ſimul decoquito ex aqua et melle et hujus decocti quantum ſatis ſit cum oleo et ſale injicito.

Ed. Chart. X. [650.]

[*Ἐργαλεῖον ἰσχιαδικόν.*] Σικύου ἀγρίου ῥίζας, δάφνης φύλλα, πηγάνου φύλλα, ἀψινθίου, πεντανεύρου, χαμαίδρυος, πρασίου, καλαμίνθης, γλήχωνος, ὀριγάνου, θύμου, θρίδακος, εὐφορβίου, ἀνήθου, πυρέθρου, σταφίδος ἀγρίας· ταῦτα πάντα ἑψήσας ἐν ὕδατι καὶ μίξας μετὰ μέλιτος, ἐλαίου καὶ ἅλατος δίδου εἰς ἐργαλεῖον.

[*Εἰς τὸ λευκᾶναι ὀδόντας σαθροὺς καὶ μέλανας.*] Λαβὼν ἅλατος λείου μέρος α'. ῥόπου μέρος α'. σηπίας ὀστράκου μέρος α'. λειώσας ὁμοῦ ἀνάτριβε, προδιακλύσας ὄξει καθαρῷ.

[*Κατάπλασμα εἰς ῥευματιζομένην κεφαλήν· τοῦτο τὸ σμῆγμα οὐκ ἐᾷ κεφαλὴν ῥευματισθῆναι οὔτε ὀφθαλμὸν ἀδικηθῆναι ποτέ.*] Λαβὼν μαστίχης γο. α'. σμύρνης γο. α'. σαρκοκόλλης γο. α'. λιβάνου γο. α'. λαδάνου γο. α'. νίτρου γο. α'. ψιμυθίου γο. α'. κιμωλίας γο. α'. στύρακος γο. α'. ῥόδων γο. α'. σάπωνος σάγκου λίτρ. α'. μέλιτος λίτρ. α'. θέρμων πικρῶν ἀπόζεμα τὸ ἀρκοῦν, ἑνώσας ἀντὶ σάπωνος ἐν λουτρῷ.

[*Clyſter qui benefacit coxendicis doloribus.*] Cucumeris ſilveſtris radices, folia lauri, rutae folia, abſinthium, plantaginem, triſſaginem, marrubium, calamintham, pulegium, origanum, thymum, lactucam, euphorbium, anethum, pyrethrum, uvam taminiam; haec omnia ex aqua decoquito et cum melle, oleo et ſale miſceto, in clyſterem adhibeto.

[*Ad dentes putridos et nigros dealbandos.*] Recipe ſalis triti partem j, ropi partem j, teſtae ſepiae partem j, his ſimul tritis frica dentes, ſed collue prius aceto puro.

[*Cataplasma ad capitis fluxionem; idem etiam praeſtat, ne caput a fluxione unquam tentetur oculumque ab omni injuria tuetur.*] Recipe maſtiches unc. j, myrrhae unc. j, ſarcocollae unc. j, thuris unc. j, ladani unc. j, nitri unc. j, ceruſſae unc. j, cimoliae unc. j, ſtyracis unc. j, roſarum aridarum unc. j, ſaponis ſanci lib. j, mellis lib. j, decocti amarorum lupinorum quod ſit ſatis; his in unum mixtis pro ſapone in balneo utitor.

Ed. Chart. X. [650.]

[*Τροχίσκος ὁ διὰ σπερμάτων εἰς βηχικούς.*] *Λαβὼν ἀνίσου πικροῦ γο. α'. μαράθρου σπέρμα, ὑοσκυάμου σπέρμα, ἄμμεως ἀνὰ* < *α'. σελίνου σπέρμα* < *γ'. ὀπίου* < *α'. λειοτρίβει ἕκαστον καὶ παράχεε ὕδωρ χλιαρὸν μέχρις ἂν γένηται γλοιῶδες καὶ ποίει τροχίσκους, κυάμου τὸ μέγεθος ἡ δόσις α'. ὠφελεῖ γὰρ τοῖς βήσσουσιν.*

[*Ἡπατικὰ ἐκλελεγμένα διὰ πείρας.*] *Κηκίδας ἑψήσας κατὰ λόγον τὸν ζωμὸν δὸς πιεῖν μετὰ κωδείας, ἐν βαλανείῳ σκεπαζόμενος καὶ πίπτων ἐπὶ τὸ πάσχον μέρος· ἢ κισσοῦ ῥίζαν ἑψήσας μετὰ οἴνου δὸς πιεῖν. ἄλλο. δάφνης κόκκους ζ'. πεπέρεως κόκκους κ'. λειώσας μετὰ οἴνου δίδου πιεῖν. ἄλλο. ἀλόης* < *δ'. ἀσάρου, κόστου, εὐπατορίου, ἡδυσάρου, μελιλώτου, μαστίχης, κρόκου, ὠκίμου σπέρμα ἀνὰ* < *β'. κόψας καὶ σήσας δίδου μετὰ εὐκράτου.*

[*Ἄλλο εἰς ἧπαρ ἐνεργὲς καὶ εὐστόμαχον.*] *Δαφνίδων, κινναμώμου καλοῦ, καρυοφύλλου, ἀλόης, ἡδυσάρου, κόστου ἀνὰ* < *α'. κόψας καὶ μέλιτι ἑνώσας μετὰ οἴνου παλαιοῦ*

[*Paſtillus ex ſeminibus ad tuſſientes.*] Recipe aniſorum amarorum unc. j, ſeminum foeniculi, ſeminis ammeos, ſeminis alterci, ſingulorum drach. j, ſeminis apii drach. iij, opii drach. j, omnia terito, paulatim tepidam aquam inſtillando donec ſordium ſpiſſitudinem aſſequatur, paſtillosque conficito fabae magnitudine, unum exhibeto, tuſſientibus confert.

[*Medicamenta experientia ſelecta ad jecoris affectus.*] Gallarum elixatarum cum capitibus papaveris jus in balneo bibendum dato, et ſit tectus ac in affectum latus decumbat. Aut decoctum radicis hederae ex vino elixatae potui dato. *Aliud.* Lauri baccas vij, piperis grana xx, trita in potum ex vino praebeto. *Aliud.* Recipe aloës drach. iv, aſari, coſti, eupatorii, edyſari, meliloti, maſtiches, croci, ſeminis ocimi, ſingulorum drach. ij, omnia tuſa et creta exhibe ex vino temperato.

[*Aliud ad jecur efficax et ventriculo commodum.*] Recipe baccarum lauri, cinnamomi optimi, caryophyllorum, aloës, hedyſari, coſti, ſingulorum drach. j, haec omnia

πότισον. ἄλλο. ἀκόρου < α'. λινοσπέρμου < α'. ζιγγιβέρεως < α'. ἀνίσου < δ'. πηγάνου φύλλων τῶν ἁπαλῶν < α'. σὺν μελικράτῳ δίδου. ἄλλο. ἀρτόμελι κατάπλαττε θερμὸν ὡς ἔμπλαστρον, ἢ ἀψινθίου κοχλιάριον α'. μίξας [651] σὺν εὐκράτῳ μέλιτι, δὸς πιεῖν καὶ ἀναπαυθήτω ἐπάνω τοῦ ἥπατος.

[Πρὸς γλῶσσαν ῥευματιζομένην.] Φύλλα κυνάρων τρίψας μετὰ μέλιτος, ἄλειφε τὴν γλῶσσαν, ἢ φλεβοτόμησον τὴν φλέβα τοῦ μέρους, οὗ ῥέῃ, καὶ ὠφεληθήσεται.

[Πρὸς ξηρότητα στόματος.] Σῦκα ἑψήσας ἐν ἑψήματι φοινίκων πτερῷ διάχριε καὶ διακρατείτω.

[Πρὸς χείλη ῥηγνύμενα.] Λινόσπερμα κοπανήσας μετὰ μέλιτος ἐπίθες.

[Πρὸς τοὺς λιποτριχοῦντας τὸ γένειον, οὓς καλοῦσι σπανοπώγωνας.] Πεπέρεως, εὐφορβίου, πυρέθρου ἀνὰ γο. α'. καλάμων φύλλων ἁπαλῶν χυλὸν, μυοχόδου, ἐλαίου ἐξ ἀποκαύματος λειώσας πρόστριβε καὶ συνεχῶς ἐπιξύρα.

trita melleque excepta in potum ex veteri vino dato. *Aliud.* Acori drach. j, ſeminis lini drach. j, zingiberis drach. j, aniſi drach. iv, rutae mollium foliorum drach. j ex mulſa bibendum praebeto. *Aliud.* Ex melle et pane cataplasma imponito in modum emplaſtri. Aut abſinthii cochlearium j mixtum cum melle temperato potui detur; deinde ſuper jecur aegrotus decumbat.

[*Ad fluxionem linguae.*] Foliis cinarae ex melle tritis linguam illine. Aut vena ejus partis unde fluit humor ſecetur; conferet.

[*Ad oris ariditatem.*] Ficus in palmularum decocto elixato et penna illinito et contineto in ore.

[*Ad labia ſciſſa.*] Lini ſemen cum melle tritum imponito.

[*Ad eos quibus menti pili decidunt, quos ſpanopogonas vocant.*] Recipe piperis, euphorbii, pyrethri, ana unc. j, ſuccum foliorum tenerorum cannarum, ſtercoris muris, oleum per combuſtionem expreſſum; ea omnia ſimul trita aſſrica et aſſidue rade.

Ed. Chart. X. [651.]

[Ἐμετικὸν ὃ παρείληφα ὡς μύστρον.] Ἀφρόνιτρον λευκὸν βάλλε εἰς χλιαρὸν ὕδωρ, ἕως οὗ λυθῇ, καὶ βραχύ τι ἐλαίου ἐπίβαλλε καὶ παράσχου πιεῖν.

[Σταλτικὰ ἐμέτων.] Ἡδύοσμον κόψας καὶ σήσας καὶ μίξας ἐλαίῳ ῥοδίνῳ χρῖε τὰς ῥῖνας καὶ τὸ στῆθος. ἄλλο. φοίνικας Θηβαϊκὰς καὶ ἡδυόσμου κλῶνας ἑψήσας μεθ' ὕδατος ὡσεὶ ποτηρίων β'. μέχρι γλοιώδους συστάσεως, τὸ ἥμισυ πότισον. ἄλλο. φοινίκων βαλάνων λειῶν τὸ αὔταρκες κατ' ὀλίγον παράσταξον οἴνου μυρτίνου καὶ ἀναλαβὼν δίδου μετ' οἰνομέλιτος καὶ ὕδατος κοτύλης μιᾶς.

[Πρὸς τοὺς ἐμοῦντας αἷμα.] Σχοίνου ἄνθος ἑψήσας μεθ' ὕδατος πότισον.

[Ἐμετικὰ φλέγματος.] Ἡδύοσμον χλωρὸν, ἢ ξηρὸν μετὰ εὐκράτου πινέτω. πρὸς δὲ τὸ ἀλύπως σαμψύχου φύλλα δὸς πιεῖν καὶ ῥαφάνου σπέρμα δὸς φαγεῖν. ἐμέσει δὲ πλῆθος φλέγματος.

[Σύνθεσις κοκκίων καθαρτικῶν κενούντων φλέγμα.]

[*Medicamentum vomitorium, quod myſtri menſura accipitur.*] Aphronitrum album in aquam tepidam injectum donec fuerit diſſolutum, adjecto aliquantulum olei, bibendum exhibeatur.

[*Reprimentia vomitum.*] Menta trita et creta roſaceoque miſta nares et pectus inungito. *Aliud.* Palmulas Thebaïcas et menthae ramulos duobus aquae ſcyphis incoquito quoad ſordium ſpiſſitudinem habeat; hujus partem mediam bibendam dato. *Aliud.* Palmulas quod ſatis ſit tundito, paulatim vinum myrteum inſtillans, deinde exceptas ex mulſo et aquae hemina praebeto.

[*Ad ſanguinem vomentes.*] Florem junci odorati aquae incoctum potui dato.

[*Vomitorium pituitam detrahens.*] Mentha viridis vel arida ex aqua temperata bibatur. Ut facile autem vomat, ſampſuchi folia bibat, ſemen vero raphani comedat; multam evomet pituitam.

[*Compoſitio granorum purgantium pituitam vacuan-*

Ed. Chart. X. [651.]

Λαβὼν ἀλόης γο. στ'. μαστίχης γο. β'. ἀψινθίου χυλοῦ γο. β'. κολοκυνθίδος γο. δ'. ἡ δόσις κοκκία κθ'.

[Πρὸς καρδιακούς.] Φακὴν σὺν σπατητοῖς φοίνιξι καὶ οἴνῳ Μενδησίῳ πότισον ἑψητόν.

[Πρὸς δὲ τοὺς ὀδυνωμένους τὴν καρδίαν.] Πολύγονον λειώσας εὖ μάλα, ἢ μῆλα, ἢ κυδώνια σὺν ὄξει ἑψηθέντα καὶ λειωθέντα μετὰ κηρωτῆς ῥοδίνης ἀναλαβὼν κατάπλασσε, ἢ ἀνδράχνην μετὰ κηρωτῆς ῥοδίνης ἀναλαβὼν, ἢ μυρσινίνης ἐπίθες.

[Ἕτερον θαυμάσιον διὰ πείρας.] Λινοσπέρμου κοτύλας δ'. ὕδατος κοτύλας ζ'. ἑψήσας χρῶ, τοῦτο δὲ τὸ φάρμακον ποιεῖ ὑγείαν. οὐδὲν γὰρ ὁ ἀσθενὴς ἐπὶ τὸ χεῖρον ἀπέλθοι, ἀλλὰ ἐπὶ τὸ κρεῖττον.

[Τροχίσκος δυσπνοϊκοῖς καὶ τοῖς βήσσουσι πολλοῦ χρόνου εἰς κάπνισμα.] Καρδάμου γο. α'. σινήπεως γο. α'. ἀβροτόνου γο. α'. πηγάνου ἀγρίου γο. α'. σανδαράχης γο. α'. λειώσας ὕδατι ποίει τροχίσκους καὶ χρῶ σπουδαίως.

[Πρὸς δύσπνοιαν καὶ αἵματος ἀναγωγάς.] Θύμον

tium.] Recipe aloës unc. vj, maſtiches unc. ij, abſinthii ſucci unc. ij, colocynthidis unc. iv, dentur xxix grana.

[*Ad cardiacos.*] Lentem cum paſſis palmulis vino Mendeſio incoctam potui dato.

[*Ad eos autem qui dolent cor.*] Sanguinariam probe tritam vel mala vel cotonea ex aceto cocta tritaque et cerato roſaceo excepta ponantur in modum cataplasmatis. Aut portulacam cerato roſaceo vel myrteo exceptam imponito.

[*Aliud admirabile experientia probatum.*] Recipe lini ſeminis heminas iv, aquae heminas vij, ſimul coquito et utere. Medicamentum hoc ſanitatem facit; non enim aegrotus in deterius labetur, ſed in melius mutabitur.

[*Paſtillus dyſpnoea laborantibus diuque tuſſientibus ſuffitus prodeſt.*] Recipe naſturtii unc. j, ſinapis unc. j, abrotoni unc. j, rutae ſilveſtris unc. j, ſandarachae unc. j, terito et ex aqua in paſtillos redigito; eis ſedulo utitor.

[*Ad difficilem reſpirationem et ſanguinis rejectionem.*]

Ed. Chart. X. [651. 652.]

μετὰ πεπέρεως κόψας καὶ λειώσας μέλιτι ποίει ἔκλειγμα καὶ χρῶ σπουδαίως. πάνυ γὰρ κα- [652] λόν ἐστι. ἄλλο. πράσων κεφαλὰς μέλιτι συνεψήσας δίδου νήστει ἐσθίειν, ἢ πηγάνου ξηροῦ γο. δ'. ἡδυόσμου ξηροῦ γο. δ'. λῦσον μετὰ μέλιτος καὶ λάμβανε κεράτια β'. εἰς κοίτην μετὰ εὐκράτου· ὠφελεῖ δὲ δυσπνοϊκοὺς καὶ πιστάκια ἐσθιόμενα.

[*Πρὸς αἱμοπτοϊκούς.*] Λαβὼν συμφύτου < δ'. μαστίχης κιῤῥᾶς < δ'. λημνίας σφραγῖδος < β'. βαλαυστίων < β'· κόψας καὶ σήσας δίδου κοχλιάριον ἓν σὺν ὀξυμέλιτι πίνειν.

[*Ἄλλο διὰ πείρας.*] Λαβὼν λημνίας σφραγῖδος γο. α'. γῆς ἀστέρος γο. β'. κοραλλίου γο. β'. δίδου μετὰ ὀξυμέλιτος ἀκράτου κοτύλην α'. πρωῒ καὶ ἑσπέρας τοῦτο χρῶ. ἄλλο. ἀκακίας κιῤῥᾶς, ἀμύλου ἰατρικοῦ ἴσα λειώσας δίδου πιεῖν μετὰ εὐκράτου κοχλιάρια ε'.

[*Ληξοπύρετον τοῖς ἐκ πυρετοῦ καυσουμένοις.*] Λαβὼν ἀειζώου καὶ ἀνίσου φύλλα ε'. ἢ ζ'. ἀπόζεσον ἐλαίῳ ῥοδίνῳ καὶ χρῖε ἀπὸ κεφαλῆς ἕως πέλματος καὶ θαυμάσεις· ἢ πυ-

Thymum cum pipere tuſum et tritum, in eclegma cum melle redactum, ſedulo delingendum offerto; praeſtans remedium eſt. *Aliud.* Porrorum capita melli incocta dentur jejuno comedenda. Aut rutae ſiccae unc. iv, menthae unc. iv, ex melle terito, hujus duo ceratia accipiat iturus cubitum ex aqua temperata. Spirantes aegre juvant et piſtacia ſi edantur.

[*Ad eos qui ſanguinem ſpuunt.*] Recipe ſymphyti drach. iv, maſtiches ruffae drach. iv, ſigilli lemnii drach. iv, balauſtiorum drach. ij, trita et creta da bibendum ad cochlearium unum ex aceto mulſo.

[*Aliud experientia probatum.*] Recipe ſigilli lemnii unc. j, terrae ſtellaris unc. ij, corallii unc. ij, ex his dato heminam ex aceto mulſo puro mane et veſpere, hoc utere. *Aliud.* Acaciae ruffae, amyli medicinalis pares portiones terito et potui dato cochlearia v ex aqua temperata.

[*Ad eos qui ardente febre tenentur.*] Recipe ſempervivi et aniſi folia v vel vij, et ea fac ut in oleo roſaceo ferveant, ac deinde a capite usque ad pedis veſtigium

Ed. Chart. X. [652.]
ρέθρου ῥίζαν λεάνας σὺν ἐλαίῳ σύγχρισον. τοῦτο γὰρ ἱδρῶτας κινεῖ καὶ τὰ χρόνια ῥίγη παύει καὶ τὰ κατεψυγμένα μέρη τοῦ σώματος, ἢ παρειμένα ἰᾶται. ἄλλο. δαφνίδας καὶ θύμον ἐν οἴνῳ τὰ ἀμφότερα λειώσας ἐπίχρισον καὶ περίβαλλε ἱματίοις καὶ ἱδρώσει.

[*Πρὸς ἰσχὺν αἰδοίων καὶ χρονίας διαθέσεις.*] *Λαβὼν* καλαμίνθην καὶ κόψας καὶ σήσας ἐπίβαλλε ἐν τρυβλίῳ καὶ ἀναλαβὼν μέλιτι ἕψει ἕως δίκην καταπλάσματος καὶ ἐπιπλάσας λεπτῇ ὀθόνῃ ἐπίθες φασκιῶν, πεπείραται γὰρ παρὰ πολλοῖς.

[*Ἄλλο πρὸς ἰσχὺν αἰδοίων καὶ νεφρῶν· μὴ γοῦν τινὰ θεραπεύσεις πρὸ τοῦ τὸν μισθὸν ἆραι, πεπείραται γὰρ παρὰ πολλοῖς.*] Ζιγγιβέρεως < δ'. βράθυος < α'. πεπέρεως λευκοῦ < α'. δίδου μετ' οἰνομέλιτος. ἄλλο. πίσσης ξηρᾶς, τηλεφίου, κολοφωνίας, μαστίχης, ὑέλου λευκοῦ ἴσα λείου καὶ ποίει ξηρίον καὶ προλούσας ἔτι θερμῶς ἔχοντος τοῦ χρωμένου ἐπιχρίσας ὑγρᾷ πίσσῃ, ἐπίπασον τὸ ξηρίον καὶ ἄνωθεν ἐπίθες καὶ δέσμει καλῶς.

inungito et mirabere. Aut radice pyrethri trita ex oleo inunge. Hoc medicamentum ſudores excitat, veteres rigores tollit, partes corporis refrigeratas reſolutasve ſanat. *Aliud.* Lauri baccas et thymum ex vino terito et illinito veſtibusque contegito, quia ſudabit.

[*Ad vim genitalium et veteres affectus.*] Recipe calaminthan eamque tuſam et cretam projice in pilam, melleque exceptam dicoque ad conſiſtentiam cataplasmatis, id linteolo illitum tenui imponito et fascia deligato; hoc a multis expertum eſt.

[*Aliud ad robur genitalium et renum; ſed neminem curato, niſi prius mercede accepta; expertum enim eſt in quamplurimis.*] Recipe zingiberis drach. iv, herbae ſabinae, piperis albi drach. j, exhibe cum mulſo. *Aliud.* Recipe picis aridae, telephii, colophoniae, maſtiches, nitri albi, portiones pares, laevіga et effice aridum medicamentum; locum prius lavato et calido adhuc permanente inunge liquida pice; deinde aridum medicamentum inſpergito ſuperque imponito et probe obligato.

[*Εἰς τὸ σκορπίσαι τὰ ἐν τοῖς γόνασι ῥεύματα.*] Ἀγριοσύκην κοπανήσας ἐκ τοῦ χυλοῦ τριβέσθω ἢ τῆς ῥίζης τὸν χυλὸν ἀνατριβέσθω ἐν βαλανείῳ. καὶ ἅλας καὶ περιστερᾶς κόπρον λειώσας μετ' ἐλαίου ἐπίχριε.

[*Κατάπλασμα πρὸς πόνον ποδῶν ἀπὸ προσκρούσματος ἢ ἀπὸ καταπτώσεως, ἢ ἄλλης τινὸς δριμείας ὀδύνης.*] Ἅλατος ὀπτοῦ, ὀριγάνου, σποδὸν κληματίδων ἴσα λεκίθους ὠῶν β'. ἢ γ'. σὺν οἴνῳ μίξας κατάπλασον.

[*Πρὸς λεπριῶντας ὄνυχας θειότατον βοήθημα.*] Ὄνυξιν ἀποσπασθεῖσιν ἀπὸ προπτώματος καὶ εἰς παρωνυχίαν ὄχαρ λειώσας καὶ ξηρίον ποιήσας ἐπίπασον. ὄνυχας δὲ λεπρώδεις καθαρίσεις, εἰ θεῖον ἄπυρον καὶ κρόκον ὠοῦ ἴσα μίξας μετ' ὄξους καὶ ἐπιθήσεις.

[*Πρὸς πυρίκαυστα.*] Λιθαργύρου γο. β'. κρόκου γο. β'. ὠῶν ὀπτῶν λεκίθους γο. δ'. ῥοδίνου τὸ ἀρκοῦν. ἄλλο. ὀθόνιον καύσας τὴν σποδιὰν ῥοδίνῳ μίξας καὶ κηρῷ καὶ ἀγχούσῃ ἑνώσας χρῶ.

[*Πρὸς αἱμοῤῥοίας ἐκ παντὸς φερομένας.*] Σώρεως,

[*Ad discutiendas genuum fluxiones.*] Caprifici tritae succo fricetur aut ejus radicis succo perfricetur in balneo. Aut sal et fimum columbinum tritum ex oleo illine.

[*Cataplasma ad pedum laborem ex offensione vel ex casu vel aliquo alio acri dolore.*] Recipe salis tosti, origani, cineris sarmentorum vitis pares portiones, ovorum vitellos ij aut iij, omnia cum vino mixta imponito.

[*Ad scabros ungues remedium divinissimum.*] Unguibus ex casu revulsis et in reduviam delapsis sachar laevigatum et in aridum medicamentum redactum inspergito. Scabros vero ungues mundabis, imposito sulfure ignem non experto et croco aequis partibus, idque cum vitello ovi mixtis ex aceto impones.

[*Ad ambusta.*] Recipe argenti spumae unc. ij, croci unc. ij, ovorum tostorum vitellos ponderis unc. iv, rosacei quantum satis sit. *Aliud.* Cinere usti linteoli oleo mixto, addita cera et anchusa utere.

[*Ad sanguinis eruptionem undecunque fluat.*] Re-

χαλκάνθου, στυπτηρίας, χαλκίτεως, μίσυος, γύψου [653] κόμμεως, ἀνὰ < η'. λειώσας χρῶ. πάνυ γὰρ καλόν ἐστι καὶ πεπείραται. ἄλλο. χαλκίτεως < στ'. ῥητίνης φρυκτῆς < δ'. μάννης < β'. ξηρῷ χρῶ.

[Πρὸς λειχῆνας δόκιμον.] Λιβάνου ἄῤῥενος, ζιγγιβέρεως, ἀλόης, θείου ἀπύρου, ἀνὰ < β'. ὄξει ἀναλαβὼν χρῖε πτερῷ, προτρίψας ῥάκει ἐξ ἐρίου. ἄλλο. ἀμμωνιακοῦ θυμιάματος, ἀλκυονίου, θείου ἀπύρου ἴσα λειώσας χρῶ.

[Εἰς τὸ λευκᾶναι πρόσωπον.] Ἀλκυονίου κεκαυμένου καὶ λειωθέντος σὺν μέλιτι καὶ ἀλεύρῳ μίξας σμῆχου. ἄλλο. λυσσομούμουδον λειώσας μετ' ὄξους χρῖε ἐν ἡλίῳ, ἢ ἄνθος κεράμων λειοτριβήσας μετ' ὄξους, εἶτα τρίψας τὸν τόπον ῥάκει, ἕως ἐρυθρὸν γένηται, χρῖε ἐν ἡλίῳ.

[Εἰς τὸ καθᾶραι πρόσωπον.] Βούτυρον σαπωνίῳ μίξας κατάχριε.

[Πρὸς πόνον μήτρας τῶν ἁγίων ἀναργύρων.] Λαβὼν ἄσαρον μετὰ γλήχωνος δὸς πιεῖν.

cipe ſoreos, atramenti ſutorii, aluminis, chalcitidis, miſyos, gypſi, gummi, ſingulorum drach. viij, tritis utere; praeſtans remedium eſt, experientia probatum. *Aliud.* Chalcitidis drach. vj, reſinae friotae drach. iv, mannae drach. ij, arido utere.

[*Ad impetiginem probatum.*] Recipe thuris masculi, zingiberis, aloës, ſulſuris ignem inexperti, ana drach. ij, aceto excipito et loco prius panniculo perfricato illine. *Aliud.* Guttae ammoniaci, alcyonii, ſulſuris ignem non experti pares portiones tere et utere.

[*Ad dealbandam faciem.*] Alcyonio uſto et trito cum melle et ſarina mixto ſaciem deterge. *Aliud.* Lyſſomumudon tere ex aceto et illine in ſole. *Aliud.* Florem ollarum ex aceto terito locumque panno prius donec rubeſcat affricato, deinde in ſole illinito.

[*Ad faciem mundam efficiendam.*] Illine butyro cum ſapone mixto.

[*Ad dolorem uteri remedium ſanctorum argentum non deferentium.*] Aſarum cum pulegio potui dato.

Ed. Chart. X. [653.]

[*Παξαμάδων καθαρτικά.*] *Λαβὼν σκαμμωνίας* < *β'. ἢ τρία, μαστίχης* < *γ'. σελίνου σπέρμα* < *β'. πολυποδίου* < *δ'. κινναμώμου* < *α'. ζύμης καθαρᾶς λίτραν μίαν, τὰ ξηρία ἐπίβαλλε καὶ μάλασσε ἐπιμελῶς.*

[*Εἰς τὸ ἀποκτεῖναι κώνωπας.*] *Μελάνθιον καὶ χάλκανθον θυμίασον.*

[*Εἰς τὸ διῶξαι ὄφεις.*] *Χαλβάνην καὶ κέρας ἐλάφου καὶ ὄνυχας αἰγὸς καὶ ῥίζαν κρίνου θυμίασον· ἐπὶ δὲ τοῦ δήγματος τοῦ ὄφεως ἅλας καὶ πράσον κατάπλασον.*

[*Εἰς τὸ διῶξαι ψύλλας.*] *Σικύου ἀγρίου φύλλα ζέσας ῥαῖνε εἰς τὴν οἰκίαν.*

[*Πρὸς δυσουρίαν κτηνῶν.*] *Ὄστρεα κολυμβάδων ἐλαιῶν θλάσας περιϊστάμενος κάπνιζε ἐπὶ ἡμέρας ε'.*

[*Πρὸς πληγὴν καλάμου.*] *Καλάμου ῥίζαν παύσας τὴν τέφραν ἐπίθες.*

[*Πρὸς ἐπιληπτικοὺς πάνυ καλόν.*] *Ὀρτύγων ἐγκέφαλον μετὰ μυρσίνου μύρου λειώσας ἀπόθου ἐν ἀγγείῳ κασσι-*

[*Biſcoctus panis purgatorius.*] Recipe ſcammoniae drach. ij aut iij, maſtiches drach. iv, ſeminis apii drach. ij, polypodii drach. iv, cinnamomi drach. j, fermenti mundi libram j, arida permiſce et curioſe ſubige.

[*Ad necandos culices.*] Suffito nigellam cum atramento ſutorio.

[*Ad fugandos ſerpentes.*] Galbanum, cervi cornu, ungulas caprae et lilii radicem ſuffito. Ad ſerpentis vero morſus beneſacit cataplasma ex porro et ſale.

[*Ad fugandos pulices.*] Folia cucumeris ſilveſtris coquito et domum conſpergito.

[*Ad difficultatem urinae jumentorum.*] Salſarum olivarum interior pars lignea conteratur et per quinque dies tecta ſuffumigetur.

[*Ad ictum calami.*] Radicis cannae uſtae cinerem ſuperapponito.

[*Ad comitiales praeſtantiſſimum remedium.*] Coturnicum cerebrum ex myrteo unguento tritum repone in

τερινῷ, καὶ ὅταν ἴδῃς πεσόντα ἀπὸ τῆς ἐπιληψίας, περίχριε τὸ πρόσωπον, καὶ θαυμάσεις τὴν ἐνέργειαν τοῦ φυσικοῦ τούτου βοηθήματος· καὶ γὰρ ἀναστήσεται ὁ νοσῶν παραυτίκα.

[Πρὸς ἀνορεκτοῦντας.] Σμύρναν, λίβανον, ἀμμωνιακὸν, μαστίχην μετὰ λευκοῦ ὠοῦ λειώσας ἐπὶ πλείστην ὥραν περίχριε τὸ στῆθος καὶ τὰ σπλάγχνα καὶ ἐπίθες στυππεῖα.

[Περὶ βδελλῶν.] Τοὺς βδέλλας καταπιόντας χρὴ στῆσαι πρὸς τὸν ἥλιον καὶ κατανοῆσαι ἐν ποίῳ τόπῳ κρέμανται καὶ ἐπιστάξαι αὐταῖς γάρος καὶ εὐθέως ἀφίστανται τοῦ τόπου καὶ ἀποπτύονται· ἢ ὄξος καὶ βούτυρον μίξας καὶ πυρώσας σίδηρον καὶ σβέσας ἐν αὐτοῖς δὸς πιεῖν καὶ βάλλει τὰς βδέλλας, ἢ βάλλε τὸν καταπιόντα τὴν βδέλλαν εἰς θερμὸν ὕδωρ ἕως τοῦ πώγωνος καὶ γεμώσας φιάλην ὕδατος ψυχροῦ στόματι πρόσαγε ταῖς χερσὶν αὐτοῦ, μὴ δὸς δὲ πιεῖν καὶ εὐθέως ἡ βδέλλα ἐξελεύσεται. ἄλλο. βδέλλας καταποθείσας ἀνάγει ὄξος θερμὸν καταῤῥοφούμενον, ἢ ὀπὸς συριακὸς καταῤῥοφούμενος, ἢ κόριδες ὑποθυμιώμεναι.

vas ſtanneum et quum videris cadentem aliquem ex comitiali morbo, faciem oblinito, miraberisque hujus naturalis remedii efficaciam; nam ſtatim aegrotus aſſurget.

[*Ad eos qui cibum non appetunt.*] Myrrham, thus, ammoniacum, maſtichem cum albumine ovi terito diutius, pectusque et viscera illinito, ſtupam ſupra addito.

[*Ad devoratas hirudines.*] Qui hirudines devoraverit, ad ſolem conſtituatur locumque ubi affixae ſunt animadvertito garumque inſtillato, nam ſtatim ab eo loco cadent et expuentur. Aut in butyrum aceto mixtum candens ex igne ferrum exſtinguito et potui dato; ille enim hirudines rejiciet. Aut eum qui hirudines devoraverit, in aquam calidam mento tenus demergito, phialam vero frigidae ori admove ejus manibus nec illi potui dato; egredietur namque hirudo. *Aliud.* Acetum calidum abſorptum hirudines educit. Aut ſuccus ſyriacus bibitus. Aut ſuſſiti cimices.

[*Περὶ μελισσῶν δήγματος.*] Χυλὸς μαλάχης τοὺς ὑπὸ μελισσῶν πληγέντας ἀπόνους ποιεῖ.

[*Πρὸς ὀφίτην.*] Κέρας αἴγειον καύσας καὶ μετὰ ὄξους λειώσας κατάπλασον, ἢ [654] καπνέαν φούρνου μετὰ μέλιτος κατάχριε, ἢ καλάμου ῥίζας καὶ ἐρεβίνθην καὶ φαιρία κυπαρίσσου καὶ κέρας ἐλάφου, κεκαυμένα τὰ πάντα λειώσας καὶ κενώσας πότισον σὺν ὄξει καὶ πράσῳ.

[*Πρὸς τὰς ἀπὸ φλεβοτόμου γινομένας φλεγμονὰς καὶ σκληρίας τῶν βραχιόνων καὶ πυρακτώσεις καὶ θρομβώσεις.*] Ζύμην σιτίνην μετὰ ἀξουγγίου μαλάξας ἐπιμελῶς χρῶ, δόκιμον γάρ ἐστι.

[*Πρὸς ὑδρωπικούς.*] Λαβὼν βόλβιτον, ἐὰν ἀνὴρ πάσχῃ, ἄῤῥενος· εἰ δὲ θήλεια, θηλείας καὶ βαλὼν εἰς χύτραν καινὴν καὶ πωμάσας περίπλασον πηλὸν τῷ πόματι, ὥστε μὴ διαπνεῖν, εἶτα λαβὼν τὴν χύτραν θὲς ἐπὶ τέφραν ἀσβέστου ἐπὶ ἡμέρας ζ'. περὶ δὲ τὴν ὀγδόην ἀνοίξας ἔξελε τὸν βόλβιτον καὶ ποιήσας ξηρίον ἀπόθου ἐν ὑελίνῳ ἀγγείῳ, ἐπὶ δὲ τῆς χρείας δίδου κοχλιάρια γ'. μετ' οἴνου ἐπὶ ἡμέρας

[*Ad ictus apum.*] Malvae ſuccus ictos ab apibus a dolore liberat.

[*Ad ictus ſerpentum.*] Cornu caprinum uſtum ex aceto terito et in modum cataplasmatis imponito. Aut furni fuliginem ex melle illinito. Aut radices cannarum, cicer, baccas cupreſſi et cornu cervi, omnia uſta et trita ſimulque miſta, bibenda dato cum aceto et porro.

[*Ad inflammationes a ſectore venae factas humerorumque durities et ſanguinis grumos.*] Fermentum triticeum cum axungia diligenter ſubige ac utere, probatum remedium eſt.

[*Ad hydropicos.*] Recipe ſtercus bovis et ſiquidem vir ſit qui laboret, masculi, ſin foemina, foeminae et in ollam injice, atque operi, luto illinens operculum, ne perſpiret; ollam autem imponito ſuper cinerem non exſtinctam per dies ſeptem, octava vero olla aperta exime ſtercus et ex eo facto arido medicamento ſerva in vitreo vaſe; quum vero uſurus es, da tria cochlearia ex vino

ζ΄. δέον δὲ τὸν οἶνον εἶναι ἀπεζεσμένον ἐν πηγάνῳ. τοῦτο τὸ πόμα ποιεῖ καὶ ἐὰν ὦσιν ὄγκοι καὶ οἰδήματα, ξηραίνει καὶ κενοῖ διὰ τῶν οὔρων· ὁ δὲ πάσχων μὴ πινέτω δι᾽ ὅλης τῆς ἡμέρας, εἰ μὴ τρία μόνον· δόκιμον γάρ ἐστι.

[Πρὸς τὸ μισῆσαι τὸν οἶνον, τοῦ μὴ μεθύσαι.] Ἐγχέλυς ἰχθὺς πνιχθεὶς ἐν οἴνῳ καὶ δοθεὶς ὁ οἶνος εἰς πόμα μῖσος οἴνου ποιεῖ. ὁμοίως καὶ σταφυλὴ ἀπεζεσμένη. ἀμέθυσος διατηρηθῆναι εἰ θέλεις καὶ ἄνοσος, φύλλα πηγάνου ἔσθιε· παύει δὲ καὶ κεφαλαλγίαν τὴν ἐξ οἴνου. ὁμοίως καὶ ἡ ἄκορος ἐσθιομένη καὶ ἡ Θηβαία. ἀμέθυσος διατηρεῖται ὁ προφαγὼν ἀμύγδαλα πικρὰ τὸν ἀριθμὸν ζ΄. ἢ θ΄. ἢ ια΄. ἀμέθυστος διατηρεῖται ὁ πνεύμονα προβάτου νήστης ἐσθίων ἑφθὸν, ὅσα γὰρ πίῃ, οὐ μεθύσει.

[Εἰς τὸ μεθύειν ἐξ ἑνὸς ποτηρίου.] Κληματίδων ἀμπέλων χλωρῶν ἢ ξηρῶν μικρὸν καύσας ἀπόσβεσον ἐν τῇ φιάλῃ ἔνθα ἐστὶν ὁ οἶνος, καὶ εὐθέως μεθύσει.

[Πρὸς φακοὺς ἐν προσώπῳ.] Δαφνίδων τὸ ἐντὸς λει-

ad dies ſeptem; ſit autem vinum in quo ruta ſerveſacta fuerit. Valet haec potio, etiamſi adſint tumores et oedemata: exſiccat etenim et per urinam evacuat; aegrotus vero non bibat per totum diem, niſi ter tantum; probatum namque eſt.

[*Ut vinum odio ſit et ad cavendam ebrietatem.*] Si anguilla vino ſuffocata ſit vinumque id detur potui, efficit odium vini. Simili modo ex uſu eſt uva inſerveſacta. Si tutus ab ebrietate et morbo eſſe volueris, folia rutae edito; tollunt etiam dolorem capitis ex ebrietate; idem et acorus comeſta facit et palmula Thebaïca. Ebrietatem non ſubit, qui amara amygdala ſeptem numero praecomederit vel novem vel undecim. Qui etiam jejunus pulmonem ovis elixum comederit, quantumvis bibat, nulli erit ebrietati obnoxius.

[*Ut quis vel uno vini poculo hauſto ebrius evadat.*] Sarmentorum vitis aut aridae vitis parum comburens exſtinguito in phiala ubi vinium eſt, ſtatim ebrius erit.

[*Ad lenticulas in facie.*] Quod interius eſt lauri

Ed. Chart. X. [654.]

ώσας μετὰ μέλιτος ἐπίχριε, ἢ στρόβιλον μέλιτι συνεψήσας ἐπίχριε τοὺς ὀφθαλμούς.

[Πρὸς τὰς ἐκπιπτούσας ἕδρας τῶν βρεφῶν.] Τὸ τῶν χαλκέων ὕδωρ, εἰς ὃ τὸν σίδηρον ἀποσβεννύουσι, θερμάνας πρόκλυζε. εἶτα οὕτως κοχλίαν καύσας καὶ ποιήσας ξηρίον ἐπίπασον.

[Πρὸς οὖλα παιδὸς καὶ ὀδόντας φυομένους.] Ῥόδων ἄνθη λεάνας μετὰ μέλιτος ἔγχριε, ἢ ἐγκέφαλον προβάτου μετὰ μέλιτος ἔγχριε, ἢ βούτυρον μετὰ μέλιτος.

[Εἰς τὸ πλεονάσαι γάλα.] Σήσαμος λειωθεὶς μετὰ γλυκέος καὶ πινόμενος, ἢ πτισάνη ἑφθὴ σὺν μαράθρῳ ῥοφουμένη, ἢ κάρδαμον μετὰ κράμβης πινόμενον.

[Πρὸς τὰ ἀπὸ χειμῶνος ἀποκαύματα.] Ἅλμην κατάντλα καὶ φακὴν ἑφθὴν καὶ ψίχια καὶ ῥόδινον λειώσας κατάπλαττε.

[Πρὸς ὑδροκήλην.] Μολίβδιν ἑψήσας μετὰ θείου καὶ ὄξους ὀλίγου καὶ ἐλαίου περίχριε τὸν τόπον. ἄλλο. κάρυα παλαιὰ σεσηπότα λειώσας ἔμβαλλε εἰς τρυβλίον καὶ χρῖε.

baccarum tritum ex melle illinito. Aut nucleum pini melli incoctum illinito oculos.

[*Ad procidentem anum in pueris.*] Aqua fabrorum qua ferrum exſtinguunt calida ablue, deinde cochleam urito et pulvisculum facito et inſpergito.

[*Ad puerorum gingivas et dentes exorientes.*] Roſarum floribus tritis ex melle illine; aut cerebro ovis ex melle, aut butyro et melle illine.

[*Ad lac plurimum gignendum.*] Seſami ſemen tritum et ex paſſo potum; aut ptiſanae cum foeniculo elixa et abſorpta; aut naſturtium cum braſſica potum.

[*Ad exuſtiones per hiemem.*] Muria locum foveto et cataplasma ex lenticula cum micis panis elixa confectum imponito.

[*Ad aquoſam ramicem.*] Plumbagine cum ſulfure et aceto modico et oleo elixa locum illinito. *Aliud.* Nuces veteres putridas in mortario terito et illine. *Aliud.* Ace-

Ed. Chart. X. [654. 655.]

ἄλλο. ὄξος πότιζε καὶ ἐλάφου κέρας καύσας κατάπλασον, ἢ λιθάργυρον καὶ ὄξος καὶ ἔλαιον μίξας χρῖε εἰς ἥλιον.

[*Πρὸς τραῦμα ἀνιάτως ἔχον ἐν οἵῳ δήποτε μέρει τοῦ σώματος.*] *Βούγλωσσον βοτάνην ἀνάσπασον καὶ κόψας τὰς ῥίζας πλῦνον καλῶς καὶ ὁλμοκοπήσας πρόσπλεξον χοίρειον ἀξούγγιον καὶ μαλάξας καλῶς ἐπίθες τῷ τραύματι.*

[655] [*Πρὸς ἔμετον.*] *Σελίνων ῥίζας ε΄. μαράθρου ῥίζας τρυφερὰς δ΄. ἀνίσου* < *α΄. ὄξος καὶ μέλι καὶ κρόκος ἀληθινὸς, ἑψείσθωσαν πάντα χωρὶς τοῦ κρόκου καὶ μετὰ τὴν ἕψησιν ἐμβληθήτω ὁ κρόκος καὶ δοθήτω ἥμισυ φιάλης.*

[*Πρὸς ἄφθας.*] *Ἐλαῖαι μαῦραι διαμασώμεναι, ἢ ἀγριοσταφίδες ἐν ὄξει ἑψηθεῖσαι καὶ διακλυζόμεναι.*

[*Πρὸς ἀσφαλακίας.*] *Πλῦνον αὐτὰς πρῶτον μετ᾽ οἰνομέλιτος, εἶθ᾽ οὕτως ἔμβαλλε χολὴν βοείαν καὶ λαγωοῦ ἀφόδευμα, ἢ τὸ διὰ σάπωνος, ἢ πηγάνου χυλὸν ἔνσταξον εἰς τὰς ὀπὰς, ἢ ἀριστολοχίαν τρίψας γέμισον ἐν αὐταῖς τὰς τρυπὰς μετ᾽ ὄξους.*

tum bibat et cervinum cornu uſtum in cataplasma redactum imponito. Aut argenti ſpuma cum aceto et oleo mixta inunge ad ſolem.

[*Ad vulnus incurabile in quavis parte corporis.*] Bugloſſum herbam evellito, radices vero bene lotas contundito, illisque ſuillam axungiam adjicito probeque emollitam vulneri imponito.

[*Ad vomitum.*] Recipe apii radices v, foeniculi radices teneras iv, aniſi drach. j, acetum, mel et crocum verum; omnia praeter crocum decoquantur et facta decoctione injiciatur deturque phialae dimidium.

[*Ad aphthas i. e. oris ulcera.*] Olivae molles manducentur; aut ſilveſtrium paſſularum decocto ex aceto os colluatur.

[*Ad capitis tumores, talpas vocatos.*] Eas primum mulſo lavato, deinde fel bovis cum leporino ſtercore injice. Aut conſectum ex ſapone medicamentum. Aut ſuccum rutae inſtilla in foramina; aut trita ariſtolochia foramina in ipſis cum aceto impleto.

Ed. Chart. X. [655.]

[*Περὶ πηγάνου.*] *Τὸ πήγανον πρῶτον μὲν ἐσθιόμενον καὶ πινόμενον ὀξυδορκίαν ποιεῖ καὶ συνουσίας ἀποστρέφει, πόνον δὲ κεφαλῆς ἰᾶται, εἴ τις τοῖς ἁπαλοῖς τῆς κεφαλῆς τὰ ὀστᾶ ἐμφράσσει. ἑνωθεὶς δὲ χυλὸς τοῦ πηγάνου μετὰ χυλοῦ μαράθρου καὶ μέλιτος καὶ καταχριόμενος ἀμβλυωπίας ἰᾶται· τὸ αὐτὸ ποιεῖ καὶ ὁ χυλὸς τοῦ καρποῦ τῆς ῥάμνου μετ' οἰνομέλιτος χριόμενος, καὶ ἡδύοσμον μετ' ἀλφίτου καταπλασθὲν ἰᾶται ἀποστήματα.*

[*Πρὸς τὸ στῆσαι αἷμα.*] *Βερονίκην μέλιτος ἀκάπνου πληρώσας δὸς φαγεῖν· καὶ κράμβης σπέρμα καὶ βασιλικοῦ σπέρμα τρίψας ἀνὰ κόκων στ'. μετὰ οἴνου δὸς πιεῖν γυναικὶ ὑπὸ πολλοῦ αἵματος πασχούσῃ.*

[*Προγνωστικὸν ἀῤῥώστου.*] *Ἰτέας ἁπλᾶ φύλλα κόψας ἐπίχριε. καὶ ἐὰν ῥόδινον γένηται, ζῇ· εἰ δὲ χλωρὸν, τελευτᾷ.*

[*Πρὸς τὸ μὴ δύνασθαι συνουσιάζειν.*] *Τὸ εὔζωμον οἱ ἱερεῖς ἐσθίουσι καὶ τὸ πήγανον καὶ τὸ ἄγνον· τὸ οὖν σπέρμα τοῦ εὐζώμου σὺν μέλιτι, νήστει καὶ σὺν τήλει χριόμενον οὐκ ἐᾷ ὀρθοῦσθαι.*

[*De ruta.*] Ruta primum quidem comesta et bibita visum acuit, venerem arcet, capitis dolorem sanat, si teneris ejus soliis capitis ossa contegas; succus rutae cum foeniculi succo et melle mixtus et inunctus hebetudinem visus tollit; hoc idem praestat et feminis rhamni ex melle illitus. Mentha etiam facto cum polenta cataplasmate abscessibus medetur.

[*Ad sistendum sanguinem.*] Beronicem mellis sine fumo costi plenam comedendam offerto. Brassicae et ocimi semen utriusque grana sex terito et ex vino potui mulieri dato multi sanguinis profluvio laboranti.

[*Praesagium de aegrotante.*] Teneris salicis foliis tritis inungito. Quod si roseus reddatur, vivet: sin viridis, obibit.

[*Ut quis nequeat uti venereis.*] Eruca sacerdotes vescuntur, rutaque et vitice. Erucae igitur semen cum foenograeco illitum jejuno facit ut arrigi non possit.

Ed. Chart. X. [655.]

[*Πρὸς πόνον ὀφθαλμῶν.*] *Κρόκον συντρίψας καὶ ἀναζυμώσας μετὰ ῥοδοστάγματος ἐπάλειφε.*

[*Πρὸς πόνον κεφαλῆς ἀνθρώπου.*] *Ἐὰν γένηται τὰ σημεῖα ταῦτα, σκοτισμὸς ὀφθαλμῶν καὶ πόνος αὐτῆς τῆς κεφαλῆς, ὤτων ἦχος καὶ ῥινῶν ἔμφραξις καὶ ὀφθαλμοὶ δακρύουσι τῷ πρωΐ, τινὲς δὲ καὶ ἀμβλυωποῦσιν· ὅτε ταῦτα γίγνονται, τὴν κεφαλὴν καθάρισον τρόπῳ τοιῷδε, λαβὼν ὀρίγανον καὶ ὕσσωπον καὶ ἅλας τὰς ῥῖνας ἀνάτριψον καὶ οὐκέτι ἀλγήσει κεφαλή· εἰ δ' ἀμελὴς γένοιο, παρέπονται αἱ νόσοι αὗται, ἀμβλυωπία, ὤτων ἦχος, τριχῶν ἔκρυσις καὶ πόνος ὀδόντων.*

[*Περὶ στήθους ἀνθρώπου.*] *Ἡνίκα ἐπὶ τὸ στῆθος μέλλει πάθος γενέσθαι, τὸ πρῶτον φαίνεται ἐν αὐτῷ ὑγρότητα ἔχειν καὶ εἰς τὰς πλευρὰς ὠμοὺς χυμοὺς, ἔκκαυσιν καὶ δίψαν ἔχων, καὶ ἡ γλῶσσα αὐτοῦ τραχεῖα, ἀφρὸν ἔχουσα, καθ' ἑκάστην ὥραν πτύων, ἔξεστι δ' αὐτὸν μετὰ τὸ δειπνῆσαι ἐμέσαι, εἴτε τῷ πρωῒ ξεράσαι, προλαμβάνων λεπτοῤῥίζα ῥαφάνου, εἴτε σίνηπι χλωρὸν, ἢ εὔζωμον, ἢ κάρδαμον μετὰ*

[*Ad dolorem oculorum.*] Crocum tritum fermentatum cum liquore a rofis deftillante illinito.

[*De humani capitis dolore.*] Si haec figna affuerint, oculorum obtenebratio, dolor ipfius capitis, aurium ftrepitus, narium obftructio oculique illacrimaverint fummo mane, fed et nonnullis caligant oculi; quibus itaque haec omnia adfunt, hoc modo caput purgato, origano, hyffopo, fale nares fricato, nec amplius caput dolebit. Sed fi negligens fueris, hi morbi fequentur: vifus obtufus, aurium ftrepitus, capillorum defluxus et dentium dolor.

[*De pectore humano.*] Quum affectus aliquis pectus occupaturus eft, primum videtur humiditatem habere in fe ipfo; crudos praetere ad coftas habet humores, aeftuationem fitimque, linguam asperam, fpuma redundantem, fingulis horis expuit. Poteft autem is a prandio evomere aut fummo mane ftomachum purgare, praefumptis tenuibus raphani radicibus aut finapi viridi aut eruca aut na-

Ed. Chart. X. [655. 656.]

χλιαροῦ ὕδατος καὶ ἐμέσας εὐθέως σωθήσεται· εἰ δ' ἀμελήσῃ, γίνεται αὐτῷ δύσπνοια καὶ πλευροῦ πόνοι καὶ πυρετοὶ ὀξεῖς καὶ πάντοτε ἄϋπνος γίνεται.

[*Περὶ κοιλίας.*] Ὁπόταν δὲ περὶ τὴν κοιλίαν μέλλῃ πάθος τι συνίστασθαι, τὸ πρῶτον γίνονται αὐτῷ στρόφοι καὶ πόνοι περὶ αὐτὴν τὴν κοιλίαν [656] καὶ στένωσις γαστρὸς καὶ ἀνάδοσις καὶ ταράσσονται ἐν αὐτῷ τὰ σιτία καὶ τὰ ποτὰ πικρὰ φαίνονται καὶ βάρος ἐπὶ τῶν γονάτων καὶ ἐπὶ τὰς ψόας καὶ τοὺς νεφροὺς πόνοι καὶ πυρέσσει πάντοτε· τούτου οὖν οὕτως γινομένου, δεῖ τοῖς ἁπλοῖς φαρμάκοις καθαίρειν. λαβὼν κνίκον, κόψας καὶ διαλύσας ὕδατι θερμῷ δίδου πίνειν· ἢ κράμβης ἢ σεύτλου χυλὸν μετὰ μέλιτος γλυκάνας πρόσβαλλε καὶ ἅλας ὀλίγον καὶ δὸς πιεῖν καὶ θαυμάσεις. εἰ δ' ἀμελὴς γένηται, ἐπέρχεται, αὐτῷ δυσεντερία καὶ τεινεσμοὶ καὶ ἁρμοπονίαι.

[*Πρὸς βαρυηκοΐαν καὶ ἦχον ὤτων.*] Ἀφρὸν νίτρου εἰς ὄξος ἐμβαλὼν ἐπίσταξον ῥοδέλαιον καὶ οἶνον καὶ ἄλειφε

ſturtio ex aqua tepida: quum enim vomuerit, ſtatim ſanus evadet; quod ſi id neglexerit, a ſpiritus difficultate corripietur laterisque doloribus, acutis febribus, omninoque ſomno carebit.

[*De ventre.*] Quotiescunque autem affectus quispiam ventri ſuperventurus eſt, primum in ipſo ſuboriuntur tormina doloresque circa ipſum ventriculum, alvi praeterea adſtrictio et excretio, cibi etiam in ipſo potusque perturbantur et amari videntur, gravitas in genibus, in lumbis ac renibus dolor et omnino febricitabit. Igitur qui ſic ſe habuerint, purgandi ſunt medicamentis ſimplicibus. Itaque accipe cnicum tritum et aqua calida diſſolutum, potui dato. Aut braſſicae aut betae ſuccum melle conditum, pauco adjecto ſale, in potum dabis et miraberis. Quod ſi id neglexerit, ſuperveniet dyſenteria, tenesmi et humerorum dolores.

[*Ad gravem auditum et aurium ſonitus.*] Spumam nitri in acetum conjice et oleum roſaceum vinumque in-

τὰ ὀπίσθια τῆς κεφαλῆς. ἄλλο. ἐλλεβόρου μέλανος ῥίζαν ἔμβαλλε εἰς τὸ οὖς καὶ ὑγιαίνει. δόκιμον γάρ ἐστι.

[Πρὸς τὸ φυλαχθῆναι ἄμπελον.] Κενταυρίου τὸ ἀπόζεμα ῥαινόμενον τοῖς κλήμασι. τοῦτο καὶ κύνας καὶ ἀλώπεκας καὶ πετεινὰ τοῦ οὐρανοῦ ἀποδιώκει.

[Περὶ ὑστερικῶν πνίγων.] Ὀστοῦν ἐλάφου ὃ ἔχει ἐν τῇ καρδίᾳ αὐτοῦ, λαβὼν τρῖψον καὶ πότισον τὴν γυναῖκα καὶ ὄψει τὴν δόξαν τοῦ θεοῦ.

[Πρὸς ἕλμινθας θαυμαστόν.] Μελάνθιον τρίψας μετὰ γάρους δὸς πιεῖν.

[Εἰς τὸ γνῶναι ἐκ τοῦ ἀνδρὸς καὶ γυναικὸς ὁποῖός ἐστιν ἄπαις.] Φακὴν ἀπόρεξον εἰς τῶν ἀμφοτέρων τὸ οὖρον χωρὶς καὶ ὁποῖον φύσει, ἐκεῖνός ἐστιν ὁ ποιῶν παῖδα, καὶ τὸ μὴ φύων ἄπαις.

[Πρὸς ῥῖγος.] Γράψον εἰς μῆλα τρία ἢ πεπώπουλα οὕτως, φησὸν, σαὸς δράος δάνονος δανάβιος, καὶ δίδου τρώγειν.

[Κατασκευὴ γάρους Ἰωάχου τοῦ μαρτυροπολίτου.] Λα-

ſtillato et his occiput oblinito. *Aliud.* Nigri veratri radicem in aures imponito et ſanus erit: probatum enim eſt.

[*Ad cuſtodiendam vitem.*] Decocto centaurii vitis palmites conſpergito: hoc canes, vulpes caelique volucres fugat.

[*Ad ſtrangulatus uteri.*] Os quod cervus in corde habet, terito et mulieri potandum dato et videbis gloriam dei.

[*Ad lumbricos remedium mirabile.*] Nigellam tritam cum garo bibendam dato.

[*Ad cognoſcendum uter, maſculusne aut foemina ſterilis ſit.*] Lentem in utriusque urinam ſeorſim conjice et utrius lens germinabit, ille filios creare poteſt; cujus vero non germinabit, ſterilis erit.

[*Ad rigorem.*] Scribe in tribus malis vel pepolis ſic, aut ita dicas, ſanus, dravus, danonus, danabius, et eſui dato.

[*Confectio gari Joachi Martyropolitae.*] Recipe

Ed. Chart. X. [656.]

βῶν ψωμίον ἄζυμον ἀνάρτυτον, σεσημμένον λίτρ. α'. μελάνθιον τζιαρίκην α'. ἡμίκλου συγκεκομμένον ἡδύοσμον, καλαμίνθην, βουνίσην ἄνυδρον, ἀνὰ ἡμίλιτρον· πήγανον τράμια μ'. ἀγριοθύμβρον τράμια μ'. μάραθρον τράμια μ'. ἄνισον τράμια λ'. ναναχουὰν τράμια μ'. σταφίδας, μαύρας λιπαρὰς ἡμίλιτρον· φοινίκια καθαρὰ τζιαρίκην α'. μέλι ἀληθινὸν, ἱλαροῦ μελισίου ἡμίλιτρον, σάκχαρ κάντιον τζιαρίκην α'. ῥόδα ξηρὰ ἢ ῥοδόσταγμα τράμια ρ'. ταῦτα δεῖ τίθεσθαι ἐν πίθῳ μετὰ ὕδατος καὶ τίθεσθαι ἐν ἡλίῳ ἡμέρας μ'. σὺν αὐτοῖς δὲ δεῖ βάλλειν ἐν ὀθονίῳ καθαρῷ ξυλαλόην τράμια ε'. στάχυν τράμια ζ'. καρυόφυλλα τράμια β'. κρόκον τράμια γ'. μαστίχην τράμια ι'. λίβανον τράμια ι'. τρουτζίον φλοιὸν τράμια ιε'. μόσχου τράμιον α' ἄμβαρ τάγκια β'. βάλλε ὁμοῦ ὅλα ἐν τῇ ὀθόνῃ καὶ θὲς μέσον τοῦ χυλοῦ ἐν τῷ πίθῳ καὶ τὰς μ'. ἡμέρας καθ' ἑκάστην τρῖβε καὶ ἀποπιάνειν κρεμάμενον δηλονότι ἐν τῷ πίθῳ μέσον τοῦ χυλοῦ καὶ μετὰ μ'. συνάγειν τὸ ὕδωρ τὸ ἐπάνω τοῦ χυλοῦ καὶ τιθεῖν εἰς ἕτερον ἀγγεῖον· τῷ δὲ χυλῷ τιθεῖν ἕτερον ὕδωρ ἡλιαζόμενα ἀμφό-

frustuli panis non fermentati, non conditi, putrefacti lib. j, nigellae tziaricam j, semicontusae menthae, calaminthae, bunisae aridae, singulorum semilibram; rutae, thymbrae silvestris, foeniculi, singulorum tramia quadraginta, anisi tramia triginta, nanachuam tramia xl, uvarum passarum, pinguium maurarum semilibram, palmularum mundatarum tziaricam j, mellis veri, hilari melisii semilibram, sacchari cantii tziaricam j, rosarum siccarum aut liquoris ab eis per ignem extracti tramia c. haec in dolio ponenda sunt cum aqua et per xl dies soli exponenda; ipsa praeterea dejicienda sunt in linteo mundo deligata ligni aloës tramia v, spicae tramia vij, caryophyllorum tramia ij, croci tramia iij, masticbes tramia x, thuris tramia x, corticis struthii tramia xv, musci tramium j, ambrae tramium j, haec omnia linteolo inclusa in dolioli medium succum demittito et per xl dies quotidie terito et exprimito, suspendens videlicet in dolio in medio succo, et post quadragesimum diem aquam succo

τερα. μετὰ δὲ τὸ συναχθῆναι τὸν ζωμὸν ὅλον εἰς ἕτερον ἀγγεῖον, βαλὼν ἐν κακκαβίῳ γανωτῷ ἢ ἐν χύτρᾳ, καὶ ἀποτριτώσας, κυδώνια ὥριμα πληροῖς, τὴν δὲ ὀθόνην μηδέποτε ἄρῃς ἐκ μέσου τοῦ γάρους καὶ λάβῃς γάρος ἄριστον καὶ ὠφέλιμον ἐν πᾶσιν ἀνθρώποις.

[Περὶ κεφαλαλγίας Βαρλαμὰ μοναχοῦ.] Ἄλευρον κυάμινον λεῖον χειροπληθὲς καὶ μαστίχης ὁμοίως ὀλίγον σὺν κυμίνῳ ὀλιγοστῷ· δεῖ ἑνῶσαι μετὰ τοῦ ζωμοῦ τῶν κυδω-
[657] νίων μήλων καὶ ποιῆσαι ἔμπλαστρον καὶ ἐπιθεῖναι τῷ μετώπῳ ἀπὸ μήνιγγος.

[Περὶ δυσουρίας.] Μύρον χριστὸν βάλλε εἰς τὸν οὐρητῆρα καὶ εὐθέως οὐρήσει· ἢ μέλι καὶ ἀγριοκάνναβον ἑνώσας ποίησον ὑπόθεμα καὶ θὲς ὑπὸ τὸν ἀφεδρῶνα, ἢ μόσχον θὲς ἐν τῷ οὐρητῆρι.

[Πρὸς αἷμα ἐκ ῥινῶν.] Καννάβου φύλλα ξηράνας καὶ τρίψας ἐμφύσα εἰς τὸν ῥόθωνα, ἢ πάνην λινὸν καύσας μετ' ὄξους δριμέος ἐμφύσα εἰς τὰς ῥῖνας.

ſupernatantem projice in aliud vas et ſucco aquam alteram impone atque utraque illa iterum ſoli expone; poſtquam autem totum jus coactum fuerit, imponito in altero vaſe, in cacaboque nitido, aut olla decoquito ad tertias maturisque cotoneis impleto, neque ex medio garo unquam linteolum eximas, ſic enim optimum garum habeas et omnibus hominibus utile.

[*Ad capitis dolorem Barlamae monachi.*] Recipe fabaceae farinae pugillum, maſtiches parum cum modico etiam cumino; haec in unum miſcenda ſunt indeque cum ſucco malorum cotoneorum emplaſtrum faciendum eſt, quod membranae illitum fronti apponendum eſt.

[*Ad dyſuriam.*] Optimum unguentum injice in urinarium meatum et ſtatim minget; aut mel cum canabi ſilveſtri in unum mixtum perinaeo impone: aut muſcum impone urinario meatui.

[*Ad ſanguinem e naribus profluentem.*] Canabis folia arida et trita in narem inſufflato. Aut lineum pannum uſtum et ex acri aceto tritum in nares inſufflato.

Ed. Chart. X. [657.]

[*Περὶ ὑστέρας γυναικός.*] *Ὄψον ψωμίου καὶ ἀμανητάριον ἀληθινὸν καὶ καρδὶδ, καύσας μετὰ οἴνου παλαιοῦ δὸς πιεῖν.*

[*Περὶ τοῦ μὴ ἀπολλύειν τὸ δένδρον τὸν καρπόν.*] *Κρίνου ῥίζαν κρέμασον εἰς τὸ δένδρον καὶ στήκει ὁ καρπὸς αὐτοῦ καὶ μὴ πίπτει.*

[*Πρὸς τραῦμα γλυκύ.*] *Καρδίαν μετὰ τοῦ φλοιοῦ καὶ κέρας ἐλάφου καύσας μετὰ ἐλαίου ἄλειφε.*

[*Πρὸς στόμαχον.*] *Πήγανον καὶ θύμβραν μετὰ ὠοῦ καὶ κύμινον καὶ ἡδυόσμου τὰς ῥίζας δὸς πιεῖν.*

[*Πρὸς λειχῆνας.*] *Πέπερι τρίψας μετὰ γυναικείου γάλακτος ἐπάλειφε καὶ ἴαται.*

[*Πρὸς πόνον ὀδόντων.*] *Λεπίδια ὠῶν καὶ σηπίαν καὶ ἔλαιον μίξας ἀποτρίτωσον καὶ χλιάνας βάλλε εἰς τὸν τόπον.*

[*Πρὸς ἕλμινθας.*] *Κέρας ἐλάφου ῥηνίσας μετὰ οἴνου παλαιοῦ δὸς πιεῖν ἀπὸ λουτροῦ.*

[*Ad muliebres uteros.*] Obſonium ex juſculo et verum amanetarium et cardid uſtum ex vino veteri bibendum dato.

[*Ut fructus arbor non amittat.*] Lilii radicem arbori ſuſpendito fructusque ſtabilis manebit nec decidet.

[*Ad vulnus dulce.*] Cor cum pelle et cornu cervi comburito et ex oleo illinito.

[*Ad ſtomachum.*] Rutam et thymbram cum ovo et cuminum et menthae radices potui dato.

[*Ad impetigines.*] Piper ex muliebri lacte terito et illinito, curabitur etenim.

[*Ad dolores dentium.*] Ovi putamina, ſepiae teſtam et oleum ſimul miſceto et ad tertias decocta tepida dolenti loco apponito.

[*Ad lumbricos.*] Cornu cervi ramenta ex vino veteri a balneo potui dato.

Ed. Chart. X. [657.]

[*Πρὸς δυσουρίαν.*] *Κορίανδρον καὶ ἡδύοσμον καὶ ὕδωρ μετὰ μέλιτος ἀποτριτώσας δός.*

[*Πρὸς τραῦμα γλυκύ.*] *Ἀφόδευμα χοίρου μετ᾽ ἐλαίου καὶ ὄξους δριμέος μίξας καὶ τὸν τόπον ἐκδείρας μετὰ τρίχινον πάνην ἐπάλειφε.*

[*Πρὸς πόνον πλευροῦ.*] *Παλιουρέας ῥίζαν μετὰ οἴνου ἀποτρίτωσον καὶ δὸς πιεῖν ἀπὸ λουτροῦ.*

[*Πρὸς ἧπαρ καὶ στόμαχον.*] *Ἀλόην καὶ στάχυν ἀνὰ μιλιαρίου ἑνὸς μίξας μετὰ οἴνου ἀπὸ λουτροῦ πότισον καὶ ἴαται.*

[*Πρὸς ὕπνον.*] *Αἰγὸς κοπρίαν μετὰ χαμαιδρύος πηλὸν ποιήσας ἄλειφε τὸ πρόσωπον.*

[*Πρὸς βῆχα.*] *Ῥαφάνου σπόρον καὶ μάραθρον μετὰ μέλιτος δὸς πιεῖν.*

[*Πρὸς καρδιόπονον.*] *Πήγανον καὶ λινόσπερμα καὶ μάραθρον κατὰ τὴν καρδίαν θές.*

[*Πρὸς ἕλμινθας.*] *Λυπινάρια καὶ δαφνόκοκκα καὶ χολὴν ταύρου μίξας ἐπίθες εἰς τὸν ὀμφαλόν.*

[*Ad urinae difficultatem.*] Coriandrum menthamque ex aqua et melle ad tertias decoque et bibenda dato.

[*Ad vulnus dulce.*] Suillum ſtercus cum oleo et aceto acri miſceto et locum panno ſetaceo excoriatum prius illinito.

[*Ad laterum dolores.*] Paliuri radicem donec tertia pars remaneat ex vino coctam a balneo bibendam dato.

[*Ad jecur et ſtomachum.*] Aloës et ſpicae utriusque miliarium unum ex vino potandum exhibeto a balneo et curabis.

[*Ad ſomnum conciliandum.*] Luto facto ex ſtercore caprae et triſagine faciem illine.

[*Ad tuſſim.*] Semen raphani foeniculique ex melle potui dato.

[*Ad cordis dolorem.*] Rutam, lini ſemen et foeniculi cordi imponito.

[*Ad lumbricos.*] Lupinos, baccas lauri et fel tauri ſimul mixta umbilico imponito.

Ed. Chart. X. [657. 658.]

[Περὶ αἱμοῤῥοούσης.] Χελώνης καύκαλον ὑποκάπνισον.

[Πρὸς καύστραν.] Ὠὰ ὀπτὰ, τοὺς κρόκους καύσας εἰς τηγάνην καὶ ἀποπλάσας ἄλειφε.

[658] [Περὶ κνησμονῆς.] Γάρος καὶ θεῖον ἄπυρον καὶ ἔλαιον ἄλειφε καὶ θαυμάσεις.

[Πρὸς ἴκτερον.] Χρυσολαχάνου σπόρον καὶ μέλι καὶ κρόκον ταράξας εἰς τὸ κραββάτιον χρῖε καὶ ὠφελεῖ.

[Περὶ σκωλήκων.] Χαμαιλέοντος τὴν ῥίζαν βάλλε καὶ κνίδης τὰς κορυφὰς λειώσας ἐπίβαλλε.

[Περὶ βηχός.] Μαράθρων τὰς ῥίζας τρίψας δὸς πιεῖν νήστει ἐπὶ ἡμέρας θ'. καὶ θαυμάσεις.

[Πρὸς κεφαλίου πλοκάμους.] Μολόχην καὶ ἐλελισφάκου τὴν ῥίζαν λειώσας κατὰ λόγον καὶ βάλλε εἰς ἀγγεῖον μετὰ οἴνου καλοῦ καὶ ἀπὸ λουτροῦ χρῖε τοὺς πλοκάμους.

[Πρὸς ὤτων πόνους.] Τοῦ βάτου ὁ χυλὸς ἐκπιεζόμενος καὶ χλιαινόμενος καὶ ἐνσταζόμενος εἰς τὸ οὖς παύει τὸν πόνον.

[Πρὸς ἴκτερον.] Χρυσολάχανον κοπανήσας κοχλιά-

[*Ad haemorrhoïdas.*] Teſtudinis teſtam ſuffito.

[*Ad exuſtionem.*] Vitellos ovorum toſtos in ſartagine in modum emplaſtri impone.

[*Ad pruritum.*] Garo et ſulfure ignem non experto et oleo illinito et miraberis.

[*Ad morbum regium.*] Chryſolachani ſemen, mel et crocum confundito et lectulo cubantem illinito, bene ſaciet.

[*Ad vermes.*] Chamaeleontis radicem tritam adjectis ſummitatibus urticae tritis imponito.

[*Ad tuſſim.*] Foeniculi radices tritas da per novem dies jejuno bibendas et mirabere.

[*Ad comam.*] Malvam et ſalviae radicem diligenter tritas cum vino optimo in vas conjice, poſt ablutionem comam illinito.

[*Ad aurium dolores.*] Rubi expreſſus ſuccus, tepeſactus, in aurem inſtillatus dolorem ſedat.

[*Ad regium morbum.*] Recipe chryſolachani triti

ριον ἓν καὶ μέλι κοχλιάριον ἓν καὶ οἶνον θερμὸν δὸς νήστει.

[Ἄλλο πάνυ καλόν.] Εἰς τὸ δεξιὸν ὠτίον τοῦ ἐπικειμένου λεπτὴν φλέβα κόψον καὶ ἐξερχομένου τοῦ αἵματος θαυμάσεις, ἐὰν δὲ πονήσῃ σπλῆνα, ποίησον ὁμοίως εἰς τὸ ἀριστερόν.

[Πρὸς ἡπατικοὺς, σπληνικοὺς καὶ στομαχικοὺς ἀπαράβατον.] Ἀγνοκούκκια δίδου ἐσθίειν καὶ πίνειν καὶ οἴνου πρωῒ καὶ ὀψέ. ἄλλο. σελίνου σπόρον καὶ μακεδονίου καὶ ἐρεβίνθην καὶ ἀγνόκοκκα πάντα συντρίψας μετὰ οἴνου θερμοῦ δὸς πιεῖν.

[Βοήθημα πρὸς νεφριτικούς.] Εὐζώμου σπέρμα, καρδάμου σπέρμα, ῥαφάνου σπέρμα λειώσας ἕνωσον μετὰ μέλιτος Ἀττικοῦ καὶ δίδου < α΄. μετὰ οἴνου παλαιοῦ.

[Βασιλείου ἰκτοῦ τοῦ μελιτινιώτου δίαιτα πρὸς βασιλέως νοτάριον τὸν γραμματικόν. σκευασία οἴνου εἰς τὸ ποιῆσαι εὔγνωστον καὶ κόκκινον.] Οἶνον ὡσεὶ μέτρα εἴκοσι πληροῖς γέμισον πίθον καὶ ἆρον ἐξ αὐτοῦ μέτρα β΄. καὶ

cochlearium j, mellis cochlearium j, da jejuno calidum ex vino.

[*Aliud admodum bonum.*] Tenuem venam auriculae dextrae decumbentis ſecato et ſanguine effluente, effectum mirabere; quod ſi lien male habeat, idem facito in ſiniſtra aure.

[*Ad hepaticos, lienoſos et ſtomachicos remedium quod non fallit.*] Viticis grana in potum et in cibum dentur cum vino mane et veſperi. *Aliud.* Apii et petroſelini macedonici ſemen et cicer et viticis grana omnia trita ex vino calido dentur bibenda.

[*Remedium ad renum vitia.*] Erucae ſemen, naſturtii ſemen, raphani ſemen trita ſimul in unum miſce et cum melle Attico exhibe drach. j ex vino veteri.

[*Baſilii icti melitinoti victus ratio ad notarium Regis Grammaticum. Confectio vini perſpicui et coccini.*] Dolium quod viginti menſuras capiat vino reple et ex eo exime menſuras duas et in ollam lapideam injice et

Ed. Chart. X. [658.]

βάλλε ἐν χύτρᾳ λιθίνῃ, ἐπίβαλλε μαράθρου μιλιάρια ρ'. σελινόσπορον μιλιάρια ρ'. ἄνισον μιλιάρια ν'. μετὰ τούτων δεῖ βράσαι καλῶς καὶ σακκελίζειν καὶ ξέστου ὄντος ἐνστρέφειν ἐν τῷ πίθῳ, εἶτα ἔπαρον τριψίδιον μιλιάρια ρ'. καρυοφύλλων μιλιάρια ε'. κρόκου μιλιάριον α'. μαστίχης μιλιάρια γ'. κύπερον μιλιάρια ε'. ξυλαλόην μιλιάρια ε'. τρίψας ὅλα ὁμοῦ καὶ σήσας ἔμβαλλε ἐν ὀθόνῃ λινῇ καὶ θὲς μέσον τοῦ πίθου καὶ χρῶ.

[*Τοῦ αὐτοῦ περὶ ἐνδυναμούμενα στομάχου διὰ τὸ πληθυνθῆναι τὰ φλέγματα ἐν αὐτῷ καὶ ἀνενέγκαι κεφαλαλγίαν.*] Δεῖ σε λαβεῖν ῥοδόμελι καθ' ἑκάστην ἡμέραν μιλιάρια κ'. σελινόσπερμον μιλιάριον ἓν, ἄνισον μιλιάριον τὸ S''. καὶ ἐπινηστεύειν τὸν μεσημερίον καὶ τότε γεύεσθαι. καὶ γὰρ διὰ τοῦτο ὡρίσαμεν ποιεῖν σε οὕτως, διὰ τὸ εἶναι τὸ ῥόδον ἐνδυναμοῦντα τὸν στόμαχον, τὸ δὲ μαστίχην θερμαῖνον τὸ μάραθρον καὶ τὸ σέλινον, διὰ τὸ ἐὰν εὕρωσιν ἐν τῷ ἥπατι καὶ τῷ σπληνὶ πλῆθος χυμῶν μελανικῶν, αἴρωσι καὶ κατάγωσι διὰ τῶν οὔρων ἀνωδύνως, τὸ ἄνισον, διὰ τὸ διώκειν τὰ πνεύματα

adde ſeminum foeniculi, apii, utriusque miliaria centum, aniſi miliaria l, poſtea vero oportet ut ferveat bene, deinde ut coletur et quum ſextarium fuerit, in dolium infunde, deinde accipe tripſidii miliaria c, caryophillorum miliaria v, croci miliarium j, maſtiches miliaria iij, cyperi miliaria v, ligni aloes miliaria v, trita omnia ſimul et creta impone in lineum linteolum et in medio dolio collocato et utere.

[*Ejusdem ad roborandum ventriculum pituita refertum et capiti dolorem afferente.*] Oportet ut mellis roſacei quotidie accipias miliaria xx, ſeminis apii miliarium, aniſi ſeminis miliarium ſemis et usque ad meridiem a cibo te contineas, deinde comedas, nam ſic te facere inſtituimus, quia roſa ſtomachum roborat, maſtiche calefacit, foeniculum et apium ſi in jecore aut liene repererint copiam atrorum humorum, detrahunt ac per lotium vacuant absque ulla moleſtia, aniſum, quia e ventre flatus propellit atque ſtomachum ſirmat et propterea juſſi-

ἀπὸ τῆς γαστρὸς καὶ ῥωννύειν τὸν στόμαχον καὶ διὰ [659] τοῦτο ὡρίσαμεν νηστεύειν ἐς τὸ μεσημέριον, ἵνα μὴ φανῇ ἕτερον νόσημα, καὶ ἀπομείνῃ ἡ δύναμις τῶν βοτανῶν· μετὰ δὲ τὸ διαβιβάσαι τὰς ι'. ἡμέρας τὴν αὐτὴν ἀκολουθίαν ἀεί ποτε ποίει μετὰ ῥοδοσάκχαρος διὰ τὸ ῥωννύειν τὸν στόμαχον καὶ ζῆν ἀνωδύνως. ὡρίσαμεν δὲ καὶ περὶ τροφῆς δεκάλογον τρόπῳ τοιῷδε.

[*Διαγωγὴ ἐν κρέασι καὶ νηστείαις.*] Τὴν πρώτην ἡμέραν δεῖ σε φαγεῖν ἀμύγδαλα πικρὰ τὸν ἀριθμὸν ι'. σὺν ἄρτῳ καὶ οἴνῳ τὸ ἀρκοῦν· τῇ δευτέρᾳ ἡμέρᾳ φάγε μέλι μετὰ ἄρτου καὶ οἴνου τὸ ἀρκοῦν· τῇ τρίτῃ ἡμέρᾳ κρέας ἀμνοῦ ἐνιαυσιαίου ὠμοπλάτην κοπανήσας καὶ ἑψήσας, ὄπτα πυρὶ καὶ τρέφου σὺν οἴνῳ τῷ ἀρκοῦντι καὶ ἄρτῳ καὶ παξαμαδίῳ· τῇ τε τετάρτῃ ἡμέρᾳ ὀρύζην μόνον ἕψει ἐν ὕδατι καὶ τίθει μέλι καὶ τρέφου μετὰ ἄρτου καὶ οἴνου τὸ ἀρκοῦν· τῇ ε'. ἡμέρᾳ ῥοΐδια καὶ ἀμύγδαλα καὶ σκόροδον μετὰ δαύκων καὶ σύκων, ἰσχάδων, σταφίδων καὶ μέλιτος ἕψει καὶ τρέφου μετὰ ἄρτου καὶ οἴνου τοῦ ἀρκοῦντος· τῇ στ'. ἡμέρᾳ

mus ut a cibo ad meridiem ſe contineat, ne morbus quispiam alius appareat et ut herbarum vis in ventriculo permaneat: poſtquam autem decem pertranſierint dies, eundem ordinem ſervato aſſidue cum roſaceo ſaccharo, ut robur ſtomacho addatur et ſine dolore vivas. Sed et alimenti rationem in hunc definivimus modum.

[*Ratio victus in cibo et jejunio.*] Primo die amygdala amara decem comedas cum pane et vino quantum ſit ſatis, oportet. Secundo vero die comede mel cum pane et vino quantum ſatis eſt. Tertio die agni aniculi carnem comedito ejusque ſcapulam elixam igne torreto, cum biscocto pane et vino quod ſatis ſit edito. Quarto die oryzam ſoli aquae incoctam appoſito melle comede cum pane et vino quantum ſit ſatis. Quinto die grana mali punici, amygdala, allium cum dauco, ſicis aridis et paſſis uvis melleque coquito et cum pane et vino quantum ſufficiat comede. Sexto die eodem modo anicu-

Ed. Chart. X. [659.]

κρέας ὅμοιον ἐνιαυσιαῖον τίθει ἐν τηγάνῳ μετὰ δαύκων καὶ ἕψει καὶ τρέφου μετὰ ἄρτου καὶ οἴνου τὸ ἀρκοῦν, διὰ τὸ τὴν δύναμιν τῶν ῥοιῶν σε σβέσαι· ψυχραὶ γὰρ ὄντως εἰσὶ καὶ διὰ τοῦτο ὡρίσθησαν αἱ ῥοιαὶ πρὸς ψυχρασίαν, δηλονότι τῶν προωρισθέντων ἔμπροσθεν εἰς τὰς ε'. ἡμέρας. θερμὰ γὰρ ὄντως. τῇ ἑβδόμῃ ἡμέρᾳ κρέας κοπανιστὸν μετὰ ἐρεβίνθων καὶ ἀρτυμάτων ἕψει, τρέφου τὸ ἀρκοῦν· τῇ ὀγδόῃ ἡμέρᾳ κρέας σὺν μέλιτι καὶ ὄξει, συκάδων, ἀμυγδάλων, καρύων συρικῶν, κρόκου, δαύκου, σταφίδων σὺν ἑτέροις κρέασι κοπανιστοῖς ἕψει μετὰ μέλιτος ἱκανοῦ καὶ τρέφου σὺν οἴνῳ τὸ ἀρκοῦν· τῇ ι'. ἡμέρᾳ ἐν κρέασι καὶ ἐν νηστείαις ῥοὸς κόκον ὁμοίως τοῖς προειρημένοις ἕψει καὶ τρέφου σὺν οἴνῳ τὸ ἀρκοῦν. αὕτη ἐστὶν ἡ δίαιτα τῶν τροφῶν. ἐν τῇ ὥρᾳ τοῦ δείπνου ἀεὶ χρῶ ἡδυοσμόμελι, διὰ τὸ τὰς τροφὰς χωνεύειν καὶ οὐκ ἐᾷν πληθυνθῆναι φλέγμα ἐν τῷ στομάχῳ· καὶ ὡς ἂν ὑγιὴς μένῃς, μηκέτι φλεβοτόμει ἄνευ πάθους. ὅταν δέ σοι συμβῇ νόσημα περὶ τὴν κεφαλὴν,

Iam carnem in ſartagine cum dauco coque et cum pane comede vinoque quantum ſatis ſit, ut videlicet punici mali facultas reprimatur, quae frigida eſt et propterea inſtitutum eſt, ut adminiſtraretur malum punicum, ut ea refrigerarentur quae prioribus quinque diebus ſunt aſſumpta: erant enim revera calida. Die ſeptimo carnem minutim conciſam cum ciceribus et condimentis coque et quantum videatur ſatis comede. Octavo die carnem cum aceto, caricis, amygdalis, nucibus ſyriacis, croco, dauco, uva paſſa, cum aliis carnibus conciſis coquito ex melle ſufficienti quantitate et comedito cum ea vini portione quae ſit ſatis. Sed decimo die in eſu carnium et jejunio ea ſit ratio, ut mali punici grana quemadmodum et praedicta decoquas et edas cum vino quae ſint tibi ſatis. Haec ſit victus ratio quantum ad ſumendos cibos pertinet. In hora coenae utere mentha ex melle, ut cibos concoquas, ne multa in ventriculo gignatur pituita. Dum autem ſanus degis, ne citra affectum venam ſeces. At quum morbus aliquis caput invadit, venam ſecato cephalicam et

Ed. Chart. X. [659.]

φλεβοτόμησον τὴν κρανιακὴν φλέβα καὶ ἔμβαλε ὅσον μιλιάρια ι'. συσκεύαζε δὲ τὸν χρόνον δὶς τὸν Ἀπρίλλον μῆνα καὶ τὸν Σεπτέμβριον ποιῶν ἀποχὴν ἡμέρας γ'. ἔμπροσθεν καὶ ὄπισθεν πίνειν καὶ βοήθημα τὸν χρόνον δὶς τοῖς προειρημένοις μησί. καὶ κωδείαις χρῶ διὰ τὸν ὕπνον· δεῖ σε ἀπέχεσθαι τῶν συνουσιῶν, εἰ δὲ βούλει, ἅπαξ τὴν ἑβδομάδα μετὰ τὸ διαβῆναι τὸ μεσόνυκτον· τὸν δὲ Ἰούλιον μῆνα καὶ τὸν Αὔγουστον δεῖ σε ἐμεῖν ἡμέρας β'. ἄμφω, διὰ τὸ εἰς μίαν ἡμέραν ὁ στόμαχος κάθαρσιν οὐ λαμβάνει· ὅταν δὲ ἐμεῖς, βλέπε μήποτε πίῃς ὕδωρ ἢ ἔμπροσθεν ἢ ὄπισθεν· ὅταν δὲ ἐμεῖς, τοὺς ὀφθαλμοὺς σκέπασον καὶ δῆσον καὶ ἱστάμενος ἔμει ἐν ὑψηλῷ τόπῳ ἢ ἐν ποταμῷ. μετὰ τὸ ἐμέσαι εἰ διψεῖς πιέζου λαβὴν καὶ ἐπινήστευσον· δεῖ σε λούεσθαι τὸν Ἀπρίλλον μῆνα μέχρι καὶ ὅλου τοῦ Νοεμβρίου μηνὸς καὶ τοὺς ἀπηγορευμένους μῆνας ἀπέχου τοῦ λούεσθαι· ὅταν δὲ λούεσθαι τὴν ἑβδομάδα ἅπαξ, ἀεὶ δὲ πότε νήστης λοΐου. καὶ ἐὰν δίψῃς, πίε εὔκρατον ὕδωρ καὶ μετὰ τὸ ἐξελθεῖν ἄλειφε τὴν κεφαλὴν ἔλαιον ἢ γάλα γυναικεῖον θηλυ-

detrahes ſanguinem ad miliaria decem, quod ſane bis feceris, menſe videlicet Aprili et Septembri, atque per tres dies antea et per tres poſtea abſtinentiam inſtitue auxiliumque aſſumito bis praedictis menſibus. Utere praeterea propter ſomnum capitibus papaveris et a venere te contineto, niſi forte ſemel in hebdomada, ſi ita volueris, et poſt mediam noctem. Julio autem menſe et Auguſto per duos dies ciendus eſt vomitus, et utrumque, quia unico die non videtur ſtomachus poſſe purgari: quum vero vomueris, cave ne ante neve poſt aquam bibas. Quum etiam vomis, oculos vela et deliga, ſtansque ex loco edito aut ſuper flumen vomito. A vomitu ſi ſitias, ſitim tolera et jejuna. Oportet autem a menſe Aprili usque ad Novembrem univerſum balneo utaris; menſibus autem quibus id vetatur, a balneo abſtineto; quod ſi lavari volueris, id in hebdomada ſemel fiat, ſemper vero jejunus lavator. Sed ſi ſitias, temperatam aquam bibito, atque poſtquam exieris, caput oleo vel lacte muliebri

τρόφου, τοὺς δὲ πόδας κατὰ νύκτα ἄντλει θερμῷ ὕδατι σὺν πιτύροις.

[660] [Περὶ κεφαλαλγίας.] Ἀμύγδαλα λίτρ. γ'. σπόρον κολοκύνθης λίτρ. α'. ἔκβαλον τὸ ἔλαιον τῶν ἀμφοτέρων καὶ ἄλειφε τὴν κορυφὴν καὶ τοὺς μυκτῆρας, τας χεῖρας καὶ τοὺς πόδας.

[Πρὸς βλαβὴν οἴνου βοήθεια.] Ἔπαρον κυδώνια ὥριμα καὶ γλυκέα καὶ καθαρὰ καὶ ἄρον τὸν ζωμὸν καὶ ἔνιε τῷ οἴνῳ.

[Ἄλειμμα δόκιμον πρὸς ἁρμοπονίαν καὶ πρίσμα χειρῶν καὶ ποδῶν καὶ ἀποφθορὰς καὶ ἀπόκαυσιν χειμῶνος καὶ ἀνέμου καπουλίων χειρῶν τε καὶ ποδῶν, λεγομένου Σαρακινιστὶ τλεν. ἡ σκευασία αὕτη.] Ἔπαρον ἀξούγγιον χηνὸς μοίρας β'. μυελὸν ἐλάφων ἐκ τῶν ἀτζῶν καὶ μαρτασάγκην ταπαρὴν καὶ μέλι ἄκαπνον ὑλιστὸν καὶ τίθει ἐν πετρίνῳ τηγάνῳ καὶ βράσον, ὥστε λυθῆναι τὰ ῥηθέντα ἀλείμματα καὶ θερμοῦ ὄντος ἔμβαλλε τὸ μαρτασάγκην, καὶ ὅταν ψυχρανθῇ τελικῶς, βάλε τὸ μέλι καὶ μάλαξον καλῶς δίκην μα-

quae foemellam pepererit, pedes vero per noctem aqua calefacta cum furfuribus ablue.

[*Ad capitis dolorem.*] Recipe amygdalarum lib. iij, seminis cucurbitae lib. j, et oleo ex utrisque expresso inunge capitis verticem, nares, manus et pedes.

[*Ad vini noxam remedium.*] Recipe cotonea mala matura dulcia et mundata et succum ex ipsis expressum vino inde.

[*Inunctio experta ad artuum dolores et intertrimenta manuum pedumque et corruptiones, adustiones hiemis et venti manus pedesque laedentis, qui lingua Saracenica dicitur Tlen. Confectio se habet in hunc modum.*] Recipe anserini adipis partes ij, medullam cervi juvenis et martasancem raparum et mel coctum sine fumo et percolatum, eaque in lapideam sartaginem imposita fervefacito, quoad praedicta pinguia liquescant, quibus adhuc calidis martasancem injice, et ubi prorsus refrixerint, mel addito et perinde ac malagmata subigito, ad ignemque aut in

λάγματος καὶ ἄλειφε ἐν πυρὶ ἢ ἐν κλιβάνῳ καὶ τύλιξον καλῶς, ἄλειφε δὲ ἕως ὅτι ἀπέλθῃ ὁ πόνος.

[Περὶ αἰγίλωπος.] Χολὴν βοὸς καὶ ὑγρόπισσον καὶ ὄξος ἑνώσας ποίει ἔμπλαστρον καὶ ἐπίθες· ἢ πηγάνου φύλλα μετὰ χωρυγίου ἐπίθες εἰς τὰς ὀπάς.

[Πρὸς τραύματα ἀνίατα.] Ἀριορεπανίου ῥίζαν βάλλε μετ᾽ οἴνου γλυκέος καὶ δὸς πιεῖν τῷ κάμνοντι.

[Πρὸς περιπνευμονίας.] Τρῖψον πέπερι κόκκους ιε'. καὶ ἅλας ὁμοίως βάλλε ἄπλυτον καὶ τεάφην καὶ ἑνώσας μετὰ ἀφοδεύματος ὀρνιθίου ξανθοῦ, σὺν ἐλαίῳ ἄλειφε· ἢ δαύκου σπέρμα καὶ μελάνθιον καὶ πράσον λειώσας πότισον.

[Πρὸς ἀσπάλακας.] Λαβὼν χαμαίδρυν καὶ κριθάλευρον καὶ ζυμώσας ταῦτα μέλιτι ἐπίχριε καὶ κατάπλαττε.

[Πρὸς πόνον κοιλίας καὶ στομάχου.] Βάλλε δενδρολίβανον εἰς τζουκάλιον μετὰ οἴνου παλαιοῦ καὶ ἀποτριτώσας ἐν λουτρῷ πότισον· ἢ ἔλαιον καὶ οἶνον ὁμοίως ποίησον καὶ πότισον ἐν λουτρῷ χλιαρόν.

furno inungito et bene perfricato; inungito autem donec dolor abierit.

[*Ad aegilopas i. e. fistulas angulorum oculi.*] Fel bovis et picem liquidam cum aceto in unum misceto, fac emplastrum et imponito. Aut folia rutae cum chorygio in foramina imponito.

[*Ad vulnera incurabilia.*] Ariorepanii radicem in vinum dulce imponito et bibendum dato aegrotanti.

[*Ad pulmonum inflammationes.*] Terito xv grana piperis, totidemque micas salis et teaphen addito, simulque cum fimo gallinaceo flavo ex oleo illinito. Aut dauci semen et nigellam et porrum omnia trita in potum dato.

[*Ad talpas.*] Recipe trisaginem et hordeaceam farinam et haec cum melle fermentata illine et cataplasma impone.

[*Ad dolorem ventris et stomachi.*] Conjice thus in cacabum cum vino antiquo, idque decoquito donec tertia pars reliqua sit, quod bibendum in balneo dato. Aut oleum et vinum eodem modo coquito et in balneo propinato.

Ed. Chart. X. [660. 661.]

[Πρὸς στομαχικούς.] Κύμινον καὶ κιννάμωμον κοπανήσας ἀμφότερα καὶ βαλὼν σμύρναν καὶ μαστίχην καὶ βλυσκούνην ὀλίγον καὶ ἑψήσας καὶ προσμίξας δὸς πιεῖν· ἢ ἡδυόσμου κλῶνας γ'. καὶ ῥοΐδιον καὶ φοινίκια πότισον.

[Πρὸς ἀδυναμίαν γονάτων.] Φέρε ὕδωρ καὶ βράσον λινόσπερμα μετὰ μέλιτος καὶ κατάπλασον εἰς τὴν καρδίαν.

[Πρὸς πόνον πλευροῦ.] Κύμινον καὶ σίτινον ἄλευρον καὶ οἶνον παλαιὸν ποίησον κατάπλασμα καὶ τίθει ἐπάνω τῆς καρδίας.

[Πρὸς σπληνικούς.] Κράμβης φύλλα καὶ ἀμμωνιακὸν καὶ ὄξος δριμὺ τρῖψον καὶ μίξας ἐπίχριε τὸν τόπον ἡμέρας γ'. ἢ πλατάνου φύλλα ἕψησον μεθ' ὕδατος, ἕως οὗ ἀποτριτωθῇ, καὶ πότισον· ἢ κραμβίου φύλλα φλόγισον ἐν πυρὶ καὶ λειώσας μετὰ οἴνου πότισον.

[Πρὸς αἱμόῤῥοιαν γυναικός.] Ταύρου κέρατα ξυόμενα καὶ μετὰ ὕδατος πινόμενα αἱμοῤ- [661] ῥοίας ἴαται, ἢ λουλάκην καὶ κραμβόσπερμα καὶ σκαμμωνίας, ἑνώσας τὰ τρία, δὸς πιεῖν.

[Πρὸς βιασμούς.] Κηκίδας τετριμμένας καὶ ῥοὸς

[*Ad ſtomachicos.*] Cuminum et cinnamomum conterito et myrrham, maſtichen et blyſcunae modicum adjicito, deinde cocta et mixta potui offerto. Aut menthae ramulos tres et grana punici mali et palmulas propinato.

[*Ad debilitatem genuum.*] Lini ſemen et mel in aqua fervefacito et cordi cataplasma imponito.

[*Ad dolorem lateris.*] Ex cumino, triticea farina et vino veteri cataplasma facito et cordi ſuperdato.

[*Ad lienoſos.*] Braſſicae folia, ammoniacum, acre acetum miſceto, conterito et locum per triduum oblinito. Aut platani folia aquae incoquito, quoad tertia pars ſuperſit, et potui dato. Aut braſſicae folia igne torreto et trita ex igne propinato.

[*Ad profluvium ſanguinis muliebre.*] Taurini cornu ramenta ex aqua pota ſanguinis profluvium ſanant. Aut lulacem et braſſicae ſemina et ſcammoniam in unum miſceto et potanda exhibeto.

[*Ad ſtomachi compreſſionem.*] Recipe gallas tritas

ἄνθη. ἢ τὰ σίδια μετ᾽ οἴνου ἀποτριτώσας δὸς πιεῖν ἢ τῆλιν ἑψήσας μετὰ μέλιτος δὸς πιεῖν τὸν ζωμόν.

[Πρὸς κοιλιακούς.] Βάλλε καρδαμοσπόρον εἰς καινὸν τζουκάλιον ἕως ἑψηθῇ, καὶ λαβὼν ὠὸν ἔκζεσον χωρὶς καὶ ἐκλέπισον καὶ ἔπαρον τὸ ὄσπρον αὐτοῦ χωρὶς καὶ κόψον αὐτὸ λεπτῶς καὶ ἔμβαλον τῷ ἑψηθέντι καρδαμοσπόρῳ καὶ βρασάτωσαν μίαν καὶ εἰ θέλει ὁ νοσῶν φαγέτω αὐτὸ, εἰ δὲ οὐχὶ, ἕως γένηται ὕδωρ καὶ ἀσπίει αὐτό· ἢ ταύρου νεφροὺς φρύξας πότισον, ἢ τυρὸν παλαιὸν ἑξέσας μετ᾽ ὄξους δριμέος δὸς φαγεῖν νήστει.

[Πρὸς δυσουρίαν.] Πάγουρον ποτάμιον κοπανήσας καὶ εἰς πανίον ἀποπιάσας δὸς πιεῖν· ἢ μαράθρων ῥίζας ἀποτριτώσας δὸς πιεῖν τῷ πάσχοντι.

[Πρὸς ἐξωχάδας.] Ἄσβεστον καὶ ἀρσενίκιον νέον ἑνώσας, ἐπίθες.

[Πρὸς ἀρμοπονίας.] Πεντάνευρον καὶ σκορπίδιον καὶ ὄξυς βραχὺ ἄλειφε τὸν τόπον, ἢ βαλλε σίνηπι καὶ ἰσχάδας καὶ κοπάνησον καὶ ἐπίπλασον ἐν λουτρῷ.

et rhoi flores aut malicoria et usque ad tertiam partem decocta potui dato. Aut foenigraeci melli incocti jus potui dato.

[*Ad coeliacos i. e. ventriculoſos.*] Naſturtii ſemen in novam ollam conjice et decoque, deinde ovum ſeparatim elixa et ejus putamen detrahito et ipſum diligenter conterito et naſturtii ſemini elixo adjicito et una fervefacito atque, ſi velit aegrotans, edito; ſi id non poſſit, aquam potato. Aut taurinos renes frictos potui dato. Aut veterem caſeum acri aceto incoctum jejuno eſui dato.

[*Ad urinae difficultatem.*] Pagurum fluviatilem conterito et panniculo expreſſum potui exhibeto. Aut foeniculi radices ad tertiam partem decoctas laboranti propinato.

[*Ad exterius prominentes ani tumores.*] Vivam calcem et recens arſenicum in unum mixta imponito.

[*Ad artuum dolores.*] Quinquenervium et ſcorpidium et acetum modicum misceto et locum oblinito. Aut ſinapi et caricas in unum conterito et in balneo ſuperdato.

Ed. Chart. X. [661.]

[*Πρὸς πόνον γονάτων.*] *Μαλάχην καὶ κριθάλευρον καὶ λινόσπορον κοπανίσας καὶ τηγανίσας μετ' ἐλαίου ἐπίθες τῷ τόπῳ.*

[*Πρὸς κλάσμα ὀστέων.*] *Λαβὼν πίσσαν καὶ κόνιν τοῦ λιβάνου καὶ φοινίκια καὶ ἄνθος μαλάχης καὶ τοῦ ᾠοῦ τὸ λευκὸν ἐπίθες καὶ ἐπάνω στυππεῖα καὶ καλάμωσον καὶ φασκίωσον, καὶ ἴαται.*

[*Ἄλλο πρὸς τεταρταῖον.*] *Χαμαίδρυν ἑψήσας μετ' οἴνου παλαιοῦ δὸς πιεῖν τρίτον.*

[*Πρὸς δῆγμα σκορπίου.*] *Ὄστρακον πυρωθὲν ἐπίθες, ἢ πτερύγιον μετὰ μέλιτος δὸς πιεῖν, ἢ κύψας οἷον λίθον πιάσῃς ἐπίθες.*

[*Πρὸς φαρμακείας.*] *Καρίδιον καὶ πλατυκύμινον καὶ ζωχίου ῥίζαν ἀποτριτώσας δὸς πιεῖν μετ' οἴνου παλαιοῦ καὶ φορείτω καὶ γλανέων ὀστᾶ, καὶ γὰρ καπνιζόμενα δαίμονας διώκει.*

[*Εἰς σύλληψιν γυναικός.*] *Λαγωοῦ μήτραν φρύξας καὶ λειώσας πότισον συνεχῶς. ἐχέτω δὲ καὶ τὸ αἷμα αὐτοῦ, ἢ*

[*Ad dolorem genuum.*] Malvam, hordei farinam, lini ſemen una contere et in ſartagine cum oleo fricta loco impone.

[*Ad oſſa fracta.*] Recipe picem, thuris pulverem, palmulas, malvae florem, ovi album, mixta imponito et ſtupa ſuperaddita, calamis ac fascia deligato, ſanabitur.

[*Ad quartanam aliud.*] Vinum vetus triſaginem incoctam habens ter potui dato.

[*Ad morſum ſcorpii.*] Teſtam igne candentem impone. Aut alam ex melle potui dato. Aut humum reſpiciens, quem lapidem premebas, eum imponito.

[*Ad veneficia et praeſtigia.*] Caridion et latum cuminum et zochii radicem ad tertiam partem decoque et ex vino vetere potui da. Geſtet et glanorum oſſa; haec enim ſuffita daemonas abigunt.

[*Ut mulier concipiat.*] Leporis uterum frige tritumque aſſidue propina; habeat autem et leporis ſangui-

ἀλώπεκος κόπρον μίξας μετὰ βοείου ἀλείμματος ἄλειφε τὸ αἰδοῖον τῆς γυναικὸς ὁμοίως καὶ τοῦ ἀνδρός.

[*Περὶ τεθνηκότος ἐμβρύου ἐν τῇ μήτρᾳ.*] Γάλα γυναικεῖον μετὰ μέλιτος καὶ ῥίζας ἀμαράνθου δὸς πιεῖν καὶ ἐξέρχεται.

[*Εἰς τὸ πλεονάσαι γάλα.*] Μάραθρον καὶ ἄνηθον μετὰ μέλιτος ἑψήσας καὶ οἴνου χρῖε καθ' ἡμέραν τοὺς μασθοὺς, καὶ ποιεῖ γάλα ἡ γυνή.

[*Πρὸς ὑστέρας.*] Ὄρνιθα σφάξας καὶ καρφίον τυλίξας πανην λινοῦν καὶ βάλλε ἔσωθεν τῆς ὄρνιθος καὶ ὡς ἑψηθῇ καὶ δὸς πιεῖν τὸν ζωμὸν, ῥάψον δὲ τὴν ὄρνιν, ἢ ὄψιν ψωμίου καὶ μαντηάρην ἀληθινὸν, καὶ καρίδιον καύσας δὸς πιεῖν.

[662] [*Περὶ τῶν ἀκουσίως ἐνουρούντων.*] Κόψον γούλαν ἀλέκτορος καθώς ἐστι μετὰ τοῦ λάρυγγος καὶ καύσας καὶ τρίψας καλῶς μετ' οἴνου παλαιοῦ δὸς πιεῖν.

[*Περὶ ἐνδυναμώσεως αἰδοίου.*] Ῥεπαπόσπορον τρίψας ἕνιε μετὰ μέλιτος καὶ τίθου εἰς ῥάκος καὶ τύλιξον τὸ αἰδοῖον.

nem. Aut vulpis ſtercus cum ſevo bubulo miſce et muliebris virique genitalia inunge.

[*Ad foetum in utero mortuum.*] Muliebre lac cum melle et radicibus amaranthi potui dato et exibit.

[*Ut lac abundet.*] Foeniculum et anethum cum melle et vino decoque et quotidie mammas obline; lacte mulier affluet.

[*Ad uteros.*] Gallinam jugulato et feſtucam lineo panniculo involutam intra avem condito atque ita elixato et jus potui dato; ſuito vero avis oculos et manetarem verum et caridion ure et propina.

[*De involuntario mictu.*] Gallinae gulam gutturi annexam conterito et urito ac iterum diligenter terito et ex vino vetere potui dato.

[*Ad roborandum penem.*] Rapi ſemen tritum melli admisceto et panniculo attrito illitum peni circundato.

Ed. Chart. X. [662.]

[*Πρὸς λεπριῶντας ὄνυχας.*] *Σίνηπι καὶ ἡδύοσμον ἕψει μετ' ὄξους καὶ τίθει.*

[*Εἰς πρίσματα.*] *Ὕδωρ θαλάσσιον, βρύον θαλάσσης ἐκζέσας καὶ ὑποπιάσας ἐπίθες.*

[*Περὶ ποδαλγίας.*] *Σμύρναν λεγόμενον μοὺρ καὶ ψύλλιον ἤτοι πυζουρκατοῦν μύστρον μετ' ὄξους ἄλειφε τοὺς πόδας.*

[*Περὶ ἐνδυναμώσεως στομάχου*] *Λαβὼν ξυλαλόην καὶ ἄκαρον, κύπερον καὶ μαστίχην, λίβανον, μελάνθιον, μάραθρον καὶ σπάντως, τρῖψον λίαν καὶ ἕνωσον μεθ' ὕδατος ῥοιᾶς καὶ μέλιτος ἀκάπνου, δίδου νήστει.*

[*Περὶ πτύσεως.*] *Ῥοσάτον τοῦ ζουφὰ ἤτοι τοῦ ὑσσώπου, ὅπερ ὠφελεῖ εἰς τὸν βῆχα καὶ τὴν στένωσιν καὶ εἰς τὸν πόνον τοῦ στήθους, ἡ σκευασία. μανουσιάκων < β'. οὐνάπια ἤτοι ξύντζιφα κ'. ζεπιστάνια ἤτοι μύξία κ'. συκάδια ἄσπρ. γλυκέα ιε'. ἤτοι γλυκύῤῥιζαν μεσότριπτον < α'. χασχάσιν κεκοπανισμένον ἤτοι κωδείαν < ε'. παρήσαυσα*

[*Ad ſcabiem unguium.*] Sinapi menthamque ex aceto coctam imponito.

[*Ad intertrigines.*] Muscum marinum aquae marinae incoquito et expreſſo humore imponito.

[*Ad podagram.*] Accipe myrrham mur vocatam, herbamque pulicarem aut pyzurcatum myſtri menſura ex aceto, pedes illinito.

[*Ad roborandum ſtomachum.*] Accipe lignum aloës, acorum, cyperum, maſtichem, thus, nigellam, foeniculum et ſpantos, valde conterito et in unum corpus redigito et ex ſucco punici mali et melle ſuper carbones cocto, potui jejuno offeras.

[*Ad ſputum.*] Roſaceum zupha aut hyſſopi, quod ad tuſſim facit et anguſtiam et dolorem pectoris; compoſitio haec eſt. Recipe manuſiacorum drach. ij, unapia vel zinzipha xx, zepiſtania vel myxia xx, ficos aſpr. dulces xv, aut dulcem radicem ſemitritam menſura drach. j, chaſchaſis contuſi vel papaveris capitulorum drach. v,

Ed. Chart. X. [662.]
ἤτοι πολύτριχον < β'. ἀνησούεν ἤτοι γλυκάνισον < β'. τόλμη καραὺς ἤτοι σελινόσπερμον < β'. σταφίδας, κοκκία καλὰ λογαρικῆς S''. ζουφὰν ἤτοι ὕσσωπον < γ'. ῥαζανὸν ἤτοι μαραθρόσπορον < β'. σταφίδας κόκκια, τὰ ἀμφότερα ἀναμίξας πλῦνον καὶ αἱμοσχάσουν μεθ' ὕδατος κρύου ἡμέραν α'. καὶ τῷ πρωΐ, ἵν' ἑψηθῇ μετὰ τοῦ ῥηθέντος δηλονότι λογαρικύου γο. δ'. καὶ ἀνεψηθῇ ἕως γένηται τὸ ὕδωρ λογαρικὴ αS''. καὶ τότε σακκελισθῇ καὶ ἵνα κατασταθείη μὴ ἔχειν ὕλην καὶ ἔπειτα βάλλε σάκχαρ λογαρικὴν α'. ἵνα γένηται ζουλάπιον καὶ καθ' ἑκάστην ἡμέραν α'. πίε ἐξ αὐτοῦ ἕως ἡμέρας η'. ἐπίσταξον ἀμυγδαέλαιον.

[*Περὶ χολεμεσίας.*] Τοῖς χολὴν ἐμοῦσι κατάπλασμα προσεκτέον διὰ φοινίκων, συκιδίων, κηκίδων ἡψημένων ἐν οἴνῳ, ἢ ὀξυκράτῳ συνελεομένων ἄρτῳ· καὶ ἀκακία δὲ καὶ ὑποκυστὶς καὶ βαλαύστιον καὶ ῥοῦς συμπλεκέσθω τῷ καταπλάσματι καὶ σικύα δὲ προσβαλλομένη μεγάλη ὠφελεῖ μετὰ φλογὸς πολλῆς. τὴν δὲ τροφὴν πολλάκις κατὰ βραχὺ δώσα-

parefaufa vel polytrichi drach. ij, anefuen vel dulcis anifi drach. ij, tolme caraus vel apii feminis drach. ij, uvas paffas, grana bona logarices S. zupha vel hyffopi drach. iij, rhazani vel feminis foeniculi drach. ij, uvas paffas granaque mixta lavato et emofchafum ex aqua refrigera per diem unum et fummo mane; et elixatum cum praedicto videlicet logaricyon unc. iv et tantisper decoquatur, donec aquae remaneat logarica una et femis; et tunc percoletur, ut certe fciatur in ipfa nullam remanere materiam, deinde facchari logaricam unam addito, ut zulapion fiat; et quotidie unum potato per dies viij et oleum amygdalinum inftillato.

[*Ad vomitum biliofum.*] Bilem vomentibus cataplasma adhibendum eft, quod ex his conftat: palmulis, ficis, gallis in vino aut posca incoctis et pane exceptis; acacia praeterea, hypocyftis et balauftia et rhus cataplasmati adjiciantur; item cucurbitula magna cum multa flamma ftomacho fi affigatur, benefacit; cibus paucus et crebro exhibendus eft; verum ad atram bilem vomentes et

Ed. Chart. X. [662. 663.]

μεν. ἐπὶ δὲ τῶν χολὴν μέλαιναν ἐμούντων καὶ φυσωμένων τὸν στόμαχον σπόγγους ὄξει δριμυτάτῳ θερμῷ βεβρεγμένους ἐντίθει· ἢ κισσοῦ φύλλοις ἑφθοῖς ἐν οἴνῳ κατάπλασσε.

[*Περὶ λυγμοῦ.*] Λυγμὸς γίνεται ἤτοι διὰ πλήρωσιν ἢ διὰ κένωσιν, ἢ δριμέων χυμῶν δακνόντων τὸν στόμαχον, ὧν ἐμεθέντων παύεται· πολλοὶ δὲ καὶ τὸ διὰ τριῶν πεπέρεων λαβόντες, εὐθέως ἂν ἐπιπίνωσιν οἶνον, λύζουσιν. ὅτι δὲ καὶ διαφθείροντες τινὲς λύζουσιν, ἔμετον [663] μὲν ἂν εὕρομεν αὔταρκες ἴαμα τῶν διὰ πλῆθος ἢ δῆξιν λυζόντων, θερμασίαν δὲ τῶν διὰ ψύξιν· ὅταν δὲ ὑπὸ πληρώσεως ὑγρῶν γένηται λυγμὸς, βιαίας δεῖται κενώσεως. τοῦτο δὲ ὁ πταρμὸς ἐργάζεται. τοὺς δ' ἐπὶ κενώσει λυγμοὺς οὐκ ἰᾶται πταρμὸς, διδόναι δὲ τοῖς λύζουσι πήγανον μετ' οἴνου, ἢ νίτρον ἐν μελικράτῳ, ἢ σέσελι, ἢ δαῦκον, ἢ κύμινον, ἢ ζιγγίβερ, ἢ καλαμίνθην, ἢ νάρδον Κελτικήν· ταῦτα τῶν ἐπὶ διαφθορᾷ σιτίων, ἢ ἐπὶ ψύξεσιν, ἢ ἐπὶ πληρώσει, βοηθήματα. τοῖς δὲ ὑπὸ πλήθους λύζουσιν ἐπὶ ψυχροῖς, ἢ

ſtomachum inflatum ſpongias aceto acerrimo calido imbutas adhibeto, aut ex hederae foliis vino incoctis cataplasma facito.

[*De ſingultu.*] Singultus aut ex repletione aut ex inanitate aut ob acres humores ſtomachum mordentes excitatur, quibus vomitu rejectis deſinit. Plerique autem, ſi compoſitione ex tribus piperibus devorata mox vinum biberint, ſingultire ſolent. Cibo praeterea immordacem qualitatem corrupto quidam ſingultiunt; vomitum ſane ob plenitudinem aut morſum ſingultientibus remedio eſſe invenimus; caliditatem iis, qui ex reſrigeratione; ſi vero ex humorum copia ſingultus fiat, evacuare vehementius oportet: id ſternutatio praeſtabit: ſi ab evacuatione ſingultus ſternutatio non curat. Singultientibus autem ruta ex vino danda eſt aut nitrum ex mulſa aut ſeſeli aut daucum, aut cuminum, aut zingiber, aut calamintha, aut nardum Gallicum; haec ſingultibus ex cibi corruptela; aut ex frigore aut ex multitudine ciborum auxilia ſunt. Ad eos vero qui ob frigidorum aut craſſorum ſuccorum mul-

Ed. Chart. X. [663.]

γλισχροῖς χυμοῖς καστόριον δίδου πίνειν δι' ὀξυκράτου. καὶ κατὰ τοῦ δέρματος δὲ ἐπιτιθέμενον ὠφελεῖ ἅμα σικυωνίῳ παλαιῷ ἐλαίῳ. ἁρμόζει καὶ τὸ σκιλλητικὸν ὄξος, ἢ ὀξύμελι πινόμενον, καὶ κατοχὴ πνεύματος μεγάλως ὀνίνησι.

[Πρὸς πρήσματα ποδῶν καὶ ῥαγάδας καὶ πτέρνας.] Μιλτάριον ἤτοι συνωπίδα καὶ κιμωλίαν τὸ ἴσον μετὰ χυλοῦ ἀγριοσύκης χρῖε. ἄλλο. κισσὸν καὶ καλαμίνθην καὶ ἅλας συνεψήσας ὕδατι καλῶς νίπτε τοὺς πόδας ἅπαξ καὶ δὶς καὶ ἀποπρίσκονται. ἄλλο. ποιήσας ἅλμην δασεῖαν μετὰ θερμοῦ ἄντλει τοὺς πόδας καὶ τὰς πτέρνας τρίτον, ἅλας καὶ κύμινον καὶ ἐμβαλὼν ἔλαιον ἀνάλαβε, καὶ προαλείψας τοὺς πόδας κατάχρισον καλῶς· καὶ διὰ τῶν ἀδήλων πόρων ἐξέρχεται ἡ ὕλη.

[Πρὸς ποδαλγίαν.] Ἀειζώου τὸν χυλὸν ἕψει καλῶς καὶ χρῶ. ἄλλο. οἴνου χυλὸν μίξας ὀνείῳ γάλακτι καὶ γλυκεῖ οἴνῳ κατάχριε. ἄλλο. φώκης δέρμα, ἢ λέοντος, ἢ λύκου, ἢ ἀλώπεκος, ἐάν τις ἐργάζηται καὶ φορῇ ὑποδήματα, οὐκ ἀλγήσει τοὺς πόδας. ἄλλο. νυκτερίδας πιάσας ἕψει ἐν ὕδατι

titudinem ſingultiunt, caſtorium ex posca potui datum benefacit; cuti quoque ex oleo vetere cucumerino illitum prodeſt, ſcillinum quoque aut mulſum acetum potum juvat: item ſpiritus retentio magnifice ſingultum discutit.

[*Ad pedum inflationes, ſciſſuras et perniones.*] Rubricae vel ſynopidis et cimoliae paribus portionibus ex caprifici ſucco illinito. *Aliud.* Hederam, calamintham et ſalem in aqua ſimul incoquito diligenter ac pedes ſemel atque iterum lavato et ſanitatem recuperant. *Aliud.* Muriam craſſam calidae aquae admisceto, ex ea pedes ac perniones foveto tertium, ſal, cuminum oleumque misceantur et prius inunctos pedes illinito curioſe; nam materia elabitur per inſenſiles meatus.

[*Ad podagram.*] Sempervivi ſuccum diligenter coque et utere. *Aliud.* Vini ſuccum aſinini lacti ac paſſo misceto et illinito. *Aliud.* Phocae aut leonis aut lupi aut vulpis corium, ſi quis elaboret et calceos geſtet, pedes non dolebit. *Aliud.* Tres vespertiliones pluviali aquae inco-

ὀμβρίμῳ ὡσεὶ γ'. εἶθ' οὕτως ἐν αὐτῷ τῷ ὕδατι βάλλε λινόσπερμον τριπτὸν γο. δ'. εἶτ' ὠὰ ὠμὰ γ'. καὶ ἐλαίου κύαθον, βοείαν κόπρον γο. δ'. κηροῦ γο. δ'. ἑνώσας ἀμφότερα καὶ μαλάξας, χρῶ εἰς κοίτην ἅπαξ καὶ δίς.

[*Γαλήνου σκευασία σκιλλητικοῦ ὄξους.*] Ὑγιεινὸν κάλλιστον τὸ περὶ σκίλλης Πυθαγόρᾳ γραφέν, ᾧ πᾶς μὲν αὐτοκράτωρ κέχρηται, λέγεται δὲ παρὰ τοῦ δεδωκότος ὅτι μακροβίους ποιεῖ τοὺς τοῦτο λαμβάνοντας καὶ τὰ ἄκρα ἄρτια ὑπάρχει ἕως τέλους. καὶ αὐτὸς μὲν ὁ Σάμιος γέρων (οὐκ ἀγνοεῖς γὰρ ὅσον χρόνον προέκοψεν) μέμνηται ἐν τῷ συντάγματι, ὡς τῷ κατ' αὐτὸν γένει μεταδεδωκὼς τὴν δύναμιν. ὅταν δὲ ἤρξατο τούτῳ χρῆσθαι, πεντηκονταετὴς ὑπῆρχεν. καὶ ἐβίωσεν εἰς ἑπτακαιδέκατον καὶ ἑκατοστὸν ἔτος ἄρτιος καὶ ἄνοσος διατελέσας. καὶ ταῦτα μὲν ὁ πατὴρ τοῦ φαρμάκου καὶ τάχ' ἀνὴρ φιλόσοφος καὶ ψεύσασθαι μὴ δυνάμενος. ἡμεῖς δὲ τῆς τοῦ ἀνδρὸς πίστεως πεῖραν ἐπιθέντες βεβαίαν καὶ ἀδιάπτωτον τὴν δύναμιν ἐπιφαίνομεν. χρὴ

quito et deinde huic aquae sic imponito, lini seminis triti unc. iv, ova cruda iij, olei cyathum unum, bubuli stercoris unc. j, cerae unc. iv, omnia in unum corpus redacta subigito et eunti cubitum semel atque iterum applicato.

[*Confectio aceti scillini ex Galeno.*] Salubre ac optimum est quod a Pythagora de scilla scriptum est, quo Imperatores omnes usi sunt. Ab auctore fertur diuturnam iis vitam reddere qui illud assumunt, eorumque extrema integra ad finem usque perduratura. Et ipse quidem senex Samius, neque enim ignoras quanto ille tempore vixerit, in suo de hac re libro narravit, se suos congeneres hujus medicamenti participes fecisse; quumque hoc medicamento uti coepit, quinquagesimum agebat annum et ad centesimum decimum septimum pervenit integer et absque morbo. Haecque auctor medicamenti, qui vir philosophus erat et mentiri nescius. Nos autem de hujusce viri fide facto periculo affirmamus facultatem hujus

τοίνυν λαβόντα σκίλλαν ὀρεινὴν λίτρ. α'. περιελεῖν τὰ σκληρὰ καὶ κατατεμεῖν τὰ ἁπαλὰ καὶ βαλεῖν ὄξους δριμυτάτου ξέστας η'. εἰς ἄγγος ὑέλινον. εἶθ' οὕτως καταδύσας ἔασον ἀποβρέχεσθαι ἐν τοῖς τοῦ ἀπὸ κυνὸς καύμασιν ἡμέρας λ'. εἶτα ἐξελὼν τὴν σκίλλην καὶ ἀποπιάσας, ἐκ τούτου δεῖ τῷ πρωῒ μικρὸν καταῤῥοφεῖν. συμβήσεται δέ σοι περὶ τὸν φάρυγγα, ἢ τὸ στόμα μηδέποτε μαλακισθῆναι. καὶ τὰ περὶ τὸ στόμα τῆς κοιλίας ὑγιαίνειν. εὔπνους τε ὑπάρ- [664] ξεις καὶ τὰ περὶ τὴν φωνὴν εὐεκτεῖν, σπουδαῖον καὶ τὰ περὶ ὄμματα ὀξυδερκέστατον καὶ περὶ τὴν ἀκοὴν ὀξύκοον. οὐδὲν γὰρ πνεῦμα ἐν κοιλίᾳ ποτὲ συστήσεταί σοι οὔτε σπλάγχνον μετέωρον ἕξεις. εὔπνους τε καὶ εὔχρους διαμεῖνεις καὶ πρὸς τὰ ἀστεῖα πάντοτε εὖ διακείμενος. οὐκ ὀξυρεγμίσεις, οὐ λύξεις ἁλυκῶς. ἐὰν πᾶς τίς τι δὸς ἐξ αὐτοῦ καὶ κελεύω μετὰ τὸ ῥοφῆναι τοῦτον νηστικὸν ὄντα κινεῖσθαι σταδίους ζ'. καὶ διαλυθήσεται. ὁ δὲ τούτῳ χρώμενος περὶ τὴν δίαιταν παῤῥησίαν ἀγέτω ἥντινα βούλεται, πάντα γὰρ κατεργάζεται ταῦτα, ὡς ἀπὸ μηδενὸς βλαβῆναι ποτὲ, μήτε

medicamenti firmam eſſe et quae minime fallat. Oportet itaque ſcillam montanam ponderis librae unius accipere duraque circumcidere, mollia vero minutim concidere atque in vitreum vas injicere aceti acerrimi ſextarios octo, et id obturare et ita per triginta dies canicularibus caloribus macerari ſinere. Deinde vero exemptam ſcillam exprimito, ex hoc parum mane ſorbeto. Hoc enim aſſequeris, ut faucium et oris partes nunquam molles reddantur et ut os ventriculi bene valeat utque reſpiratio facilis ſit; bene etiam vox habebit, oculi acutiſſime cernent auresque audient; nullus flatuoſus ſpiritus in ventre conſiſtet; viſcera non habebis ſuſpenſa; bene ſpirans bonique coloris eris; ad civilia negotia ſemper bene affectus; non acidum ructabis, non ſalſum; ſi jejunus aliquid aceti acceperit quiſpiam, eumque inſtitueris ut ſeptem ſtadia perambulet, nam ſic diſſolvetur. Qui praeterea eo uſus fuerit, ea abutatur victus licentia quam voluerit, nam omnia conficiet, ut a nullo unquam laedatur; ad nimiam

Ed. Chart. X. [664.]
εἰς πλησμονὴν ἔλθοντα μήτ' ἐφ' ᾧ δοκοῦμεν συμφέρειν, περισσὸν δὲ οὐδὲν καταλειφθήσεται ἐν τῷ σώματι, οὐ πνεῦμα, οὐ χολὴ, οὐ σκύβαλον, οὐκ οὖρον. ἀλλὰ πάντα εὐέκκριτα καὶ εὐανάγωγα ποιεῖ, κοιλία διὰ πάντος εὔλυτός ἐστι. καθαρτικὸν δὲ τοῦ σώματος τὸ βοήθημα, κᾂν ἐν τοῖς ὀστέοις ᾖ ῥυπαρία. φθισικοὺς δὲ τοὺς ἐκ πάντων ἀπηγορευομένους ἀπὸ τοῦ φαρμάκου τούτου θεραπευθέντας εἴδομεν. ἐπιληψίας τὰς μακρὰς ὤνησεν ἱκανῶς, ὥστε ἀπὸ διαλειμμάτων χρόνου πολλοῦ γίνεσθαι. τὰς δὲ ἀρχομένας καὶ νέας εἰς τέλος ἰᾶται. καὶ τὸ πάθος γίνεσθαι οὐκ ἐᾷ, ποδάγρας τε καὶ ἀρθριτίδας καὶ σκληρίας ἥπατος καὶ σπληνὸς ἐθεράπευσε. καὶ αἱ μὲν κατὰ μέρος ἐνέργειαι αὗται· αἱ δὲ κοιναὶ καὶ πλεῖσται καὶ ὑφ' ὧν κινηθέντες ἐκδεδώκαμέν σοι τὸ ὑγιεινὸν φάρμακον τοῦτο, ὑγείας καὶ ἀρτιότητος ἕνεκα ἀποτελεοῦται.

[*Γαλήνου σκευασία οἴνου τοῦ σκιλλητικοῦ.*] Οὗτος ὁ οἶνος πινόμενος πάσης ὑγείας ἐστὶ παροχηκώς. λεπτύνει

plenitudinem nunquam deveniet, ſed in melius ſemper tendet; nullum in corpore excrementum acervabit, non flatum, non bilem, non ſtercus, non lotium. Id enim omnia ad excretionem et eductionem prompta reddit, alvus omnino lubrica evadit; eſt enim hoc medicamentum corporis purgatorium, quamvis oſſibus ſordes infixae ſint. Saepe vidimus phthiſicos ab omnibus deſtitutos hoc medicamento priſtinae valetudini reſtitutos; comitiales praeterea morbos diuturnos non parum juvit, ut nonniſi per longa intervalla invadant; incipientes autem et novos perfecte curat; hominem etiam ab hoc morbo tuetur; podagras quoque et articulares dolores, jecoris lienisque duritias tollit. Particulares effectus hujusce aceti hi ſane ſunt; communes vero plurimi unde commoti ſumus, ut hujus medicamenti te faceremus participem, ſanitatis nimirum ac integritatis gratia.

[*Confectio vini ſcillini ex Galeno.*] Vinum hoc epotum omnem ſanitatem elargitur; attenuat enim humores, praecipue vero pituitam, quam nec in ſtomacho

γὰρ τοὺς χυμοὺς καὶ ἐξαιρέτως τὸ φλέγμα καὶ οὐκ ἐᾷ συστῆναι ἐν τῷ στομάχῳ, ἢ ἐν τῇ κοιλίᾳ, ἢ ἐν κεφαλῇ, ἢ ἥπατι, ἢ σπληνὶ, ἢ νεύροις, ἢ ὀστέοις, ἤ τι τοιοῦτον γλίσχρον χυμὸν καὶ ποιοῦντα τὰς ἐμφράξεις· ἀλλὰ πάντα λύει καὶ γαστέρα μαλάσσει καὶ οὕτως ὑπάγει καὶ οὖρα κινεῖ καὶ δι' αὐτῶν τὰς αἰτίας λεπτομερεῖ καὶ ἐκκρίνει. οὕτως δὲ καθαίρει κεφαλὴν, ὡς μηδὲ τοὺς μυξωτῆρας ὑγρότητα ἔχειν. πεποίηται δὲ ποδαγρικοῖς, ἀρθριτικοῖς, ἐπιληπτικοῖς, οὕτως γὰρ πάσης ὑγείας ἐστὶ περιποιητικός. ἔχει δὲ οὕτως. λαβὼν σκίλλαν ἐξ ὀρέων λευκὴν περὶ τὴν κυνὸς ἐπιτολὴν λίτρ. α'. διάψυξον ἐν σκιᾷ ἡμέρας ι'. καὶ δι' ἐμβάλλας εἰς ὕελον τὰ φύλλα τὰ διαψυχθέντα τῆς σκίλλης, βάλλε οἴνου λευκοῦ παλαιοῦ ξέστας ιβ'. καὶ κρεμάσας ἡμέρας μ'. ἔπαγον τὴν σκίλλην ἐκ τοῦ οἴνου καὶ ῥῖψον καὶ τὸν οἶνον χρῶ πρὸς τὰ ἐπαγγελθέντα καὶ εὑρήσεις αὐτοῦ τὴν δύναμιν, χρώμενος ἑκάστοτε πρὸ σιτίων ἐκ τοῦ οἴνου γο. β'. εἰ δ' ἀπὸ κοίτης γο. S''. εἰ δὲ βούλει πρὸς πόμα αὐτὸ ποιῆσαι, διὰ τὴν ἡδύτητα πρόσμιξον καὶ μέλιτος ξέστας δύο, ἢ γ'.

neque in ventre neque in capite neque in jecore aut liene neque in offibus nervisve confiftere permittit, neque alium praeterea viscidum humorem, qui obftructiones poffit efficere; imo omnia folvit et alvum mollit et fubducit; fed et lotia ciet et per ipfa caufas attenuat et educit; fic etiam caput purgat, ut nares humiditate careant; confert podagricis, arthriticis, epilepticis et tandem omnis fanitatis elargitor eft; conficitur autem hoc pacto. Accipe fcillam albam montanam circa canis ortum librae pondere et per dies decem in umbra refrigera; deinde refrigerata folia in vas vitreum conjice, defuperque vini albi veteris fextaria duodecim infunde, fufpenfumque vas per dies xl, fervato, mox fcillam extrahe ex vino et abjice vinoque ad jam enarrata utere, et vim ejus percipies, quotidie ante cibum affumptis unciis duabus vini hujus; fin a cibo, unciam mediam: quod fi velis ipfum gratius ad bibendum parare, ut magis delectet, fextarios duos aut tres mellis addito.

[Ἀποφλεγματισμὸς ἀνασπῶν ἐκ τοῦ στομάχου φλέγμα ἐσθιόμενος· ἀπὸ δὲ τῆς κεφαλῆς, ἀναγαργαριζόμενος.] Ὀριγάνου, κόμμεως, ὑσσώπου, σαμψύχου, γλήχωνος, θύμου, ταῦτα ἕψει μετὰ γλυκέος γο. γ'. ἕως οὗ γένηται α'. καὶ δίδου ἀναγαργαρίζεσθαι. ἐκτινάσσει γὰρ καὶ τὰ ἐν τῷ πνεύμονι ἐσθιόμενος. ποιεῖ δὲ τοῦτο ἐπὶ ἡμέρας, πεπείραται γάρ.

[Πρὸς δυσουριῶντας καὶ μὴ δυναμένους οὐρῆσαι.] Κόριδας ἀπὸ κλίνης λειώσας κατάχριε τὸν οὐρητῆρα καὶ εὐθέως οὐρήσει. τοῦτο δὲ καὶ παιδίοις μὴ δυ- [665] ναμένοις οὐρῆσαι ποιεῖ.

[Πρὸς λιθιῶντας καὶ διουρητικὸν δόκιμον.] Δαφνίδων καὶ πεπέρεως ἴσα κόψας καὶ σήσας μετὰ ὑδρομέλιτος μέτρον α' δίδου. ἑκάστῳ δὲ τὸ ὑδρόμελι θερμόν.

[Ἄλλο θρύπτον λίθους καὶ παρασκευάζον οὐρεῖν ἄνδρας καὶ γυναῖκας.] Δάφνης φλοιὸν ἀναζέσας ὕδατι συμφύρα καὶ δίδου ἐκ τούτου ῥοφᾷν. ἐνεργεῖ γὰρ λίαν.

[Πρὸς αἷμα οὐροῦντας.] Ζιγγιβέρεως < β'. κράμ-

[*Gargarismus, quo qui ſumptus e ſtomacho pituitam gargarizatus e capite detrahit.*] Origanum, gummi, hyſſopum, ſampſucum, pulegium, thymum, haec omnia unciis tribus paſſi incoquito quatenus una remaneat et gargarizandum dato; ſi manducetur, materias e pulmone excutit: quotidie id facito, probatum enim eſt.

[*Ad eos qui urinandi difficultate laborant aut etiam eam reddere nequeunt.*] Lectuli cimices terito et eis urinarium meatum illine, ſtatim urinam reddet; id ipſum pueris mingere nequeuntibus confert.

[*Ad calculoſos et lotium ciendum celebre.*] Lauri baccas et piper aequis portionibus terito et cribrato atque ex menſura una mulſae praebeto; ſit vero mulſa calida.

[*Aliud quod lapides atterit, mulieribus ac viris urinam provocat.*] Lauri corticem aquae incoctum et ſubactum ſorbendum exhibeto; efficax remedium eſt.

[*Ad ſanguinis mictum.*] Recipe zingiberis drach. ij,

βης σπέρμα < δ'. μήκωνος < α'. χυλὸν ἀναλαβὼν ποίει καταπότια καὶ δίδου τῷ πάσχοντι.

[*Οὐρητικὸν στραγγουριῶσιν.*] Θύμου καὶ μαράθρου ἐξ ἴσου κόψας ἐν εὐκράτῳ θερμῷ δὸς πιεῖν.

[*Πρὸς πόνον οὐρητῆρος καὶ δυσουρίαν καὶ δύσπνοιαν καὶ οὐροῦντας αἷμα καὶ λιθιῶντας.*] Ἀσάρου, μίσυος, νάρδου Κελτικῆς ἴσα ἀναλάμβανε μέλιτι Ἀττικῷ ἀπηφρισμένῳ καὶ δίδου καρύου Ποντικοῦ τὸ μέγεθος, εὐρωστεῖν γὰρ ποιεῖ καὶ πρεσβύτας, τοὺς ξηρὰν ἔχοντας ῥύσιν καὶ εὐτονωτέραν ποιεῖ.

[*Πρὸς ἐνουροῦντας.*] Ῥίζαν κρίνου δὸς πιεῖν προαναζέσας, ἢ ὑοσκυάμου χυλὸν ἢ καρπὸν μετὰ οἰνογάλακτος φυράσας ἔμβαλλε εἰς δέρμα ἐλάφου καὶ περίαπτε τὸν δεξιὸν μηρὸν καὶ θαυμάσεις. *ἄλλο.* συάγρου ὄνυχας ὀπτήσας μετ' οἴνου πότισον, ἢ ἀλέκτορος ὄρχιν ὀπτήσας δὸς φαγεῖν. *ἄλλο.* κοχλίαν καύσας μετὰ τοῦ ὀστράκου καὶ λειώσας δίδου πιεῖν μετὰ οἴνου εἰς κοίτην.

[*Εἰς δυσουρίαν καὶ λιθίασιν.*] Λινοσπέρμου, πεπέ-

ſeminis braſſicae drach. iv, papaveris drach. j, haec ſucco excipe et facito catapotia et da laboranti.

[*Ad urinae ſtillicidium.*] Thymi et foeniculi aequales partes terito et ex aqua temperata calida potui dato.

[*Ad dolorem urinarii meatus, urinae et ſpirandi difficultatem, mictum ſanguinis et calculos.*] Recipe aſari, miſyos, nardi Celticae pares portiones et melle Attico cocto et deſpumato excipe et magnitudinem nucis Ponticae exhibe; nam et ſeniores convalescere facit, quibus etiam ſiccior ſit effluxus, validiorem efficit.

[*Ad eos qui mingunt involuntarie.*] Lilii radicem elixam da potui. Aut alterci ſuccum vel fructum in vino et lacte maceratum inde in corium cervi dextroque femori alligato et effectum miraberis. *Aliud.* Apri ungulas uſtas ex vino bibendas dato. Aut galli teſtem toſtum dato edendum. *Aliud.* Cochleam cum teſta uſtam et tritam potui exhibe eunti cubitum.

[*Ad difficultatem urinae et calculum.*] Lini ſemen,

Ed. Chart. X. [665.]
ρεως, πετροσελίνου κόψας καὶ σήσας μετὰ κονδίτου λάμβανε κοχλιάριον α'.

[Λίθων θρυπτικὸν δόκιμον.] Σκορπίδια θαλάσσια τρία μικρὰ καύσας ὁλόκληρα τὴν τέφραν πότιζε μετὰ κονδίτου.

[Ἐς τὸ στῆσαι κοιλίαν.] Ῥοῦν μετὰ οἴνου καὶ ὀρύζης ἑψήσας καὶ ἀποτριτώσας ἔνιε, ἢ τράγου ἧπαρ ἑψήσας μετὰ οἴνου αὐστηροῦ δὸς πιεῖν, ἢ κηκίδας καύσας λείωσον καλῶς καὶ μίξας στέαρ χοίρειον καὶ τηγανίσας μετὰ ὄξους δὸς φαγεῖν τῷ πάσχοντι, ἢ λαβὼν πεπέρεως < α'. θερμίνου ἀλεύρου ἤτοι λουπιναρίου < γ'. καὶ μέλιτος κοχλιάριον α'.

[Πρὸς τὸ κινεῖν ἱδρῶτας καὶ ἀποπαύειν πυρετούς.] Κάχρυος σπέρμα μετ' ἐλαίου συγχριόμενον, ἢ πύρεθρον μετ' ἐλαίου θερμανθὲν καὶ ἐπιχρισθὲν μετὰ μίαν ὥραν τῆς ἐπισημασίας.

[Πρὸς κυνοδήκτους.] Κνίδης σπέρμα καταπλασσόμενον, ἢ πρασίας μελαίνης τὰ φύλλα καταπλασσόμενα, ἢ μελισσόφυλλον σὺν οἴνῳ πινόμενον, ἢ τοῖς δήγμασι ἐπιτιθέ-

piper, petroſelinum, tuſa et cribrata ex condito accipe cochlearium unum.

[*Expertum ad exterendos calculos.*] Scorpiones marinos tres integros parvos urito et cinerem ex condito in potum dato.

[*Ad ſiſtendam alvum.*] Rhum oryzamque vino incoquito ad tertias et per clyſteres immittito. Aut jecur hirci ex vino auſtero coctum in potum dato. Aut gallas uſtas probe terito et adipem ſuillam commisceto frixasque ex aceto laboranti da edendas: vel recipe piperis drach. j, farinae lupinorum drach. iij, mellis cochlearium.

[*Ad ſudores ciendos et febrem tollendam.*] Cachryos ſemen ex oleo inunctum. Aut pyrethrum ex oleo calefactum et inunctum poſt horam unam inſultus acceſſionis.

[*Ad morſum canis.*] Urticae ſemen cataplasmate appoſitum. Aut nigri marrubii ſolia cataplasmate appoſita. Aut apiaſtrum ex vino potum vel morſibus impoſitum.

μενον, ἢ σκόροδα καταπλαττόμενα καὶ ὀπτὰ ἐσθιόμενα καὶ πινόμενα.

[Πρὸς λυσσοδήκτους.] Λυσσοδήκτων τοῖς τραύμασι κράμβης φύλλα λεῖα μετὰ σιλφίου καὶ ὄξους ἐπιτιθέσθω· καθ' ἑαυτὴν γὰρ λυττῶντος κυνὸς δῆγμα ὠφελεῖ. καὶ τὸ ἀφέψημα αὐτῆς πινόμενον. ἑφθὴ δὲ κράμβη προτρωγομένη φθισικοὺς θεραπεύει. καὶ τὰς περὶ ἀρτηρίαν διαθέσεις ἰᾶται. λειοτριβηθεῖσα δὲ καὶ καταπλασθεῖσα ἐπὶ σπληνὸς τοῦτο ὑπεκτήκει.

[666] [Πρὸς συνάγχην καὶ πόνον τραχήλου.] Λεύκη ξηρὰ μέλιτι λειωθεῖσα καὶ ἐπιχρισθεῖσα τῷ τραχήλῳ, ἢ καρδάμου σπόρον καὶ κόπρον περιστερᾶς σὺν μέλιτι ἐμπλασσόμενον.

[Πρὸς ἐσωχάδας.] Ἀμάραντον ἀποβρέξας μεθ' ὕδατος ὀψὲ καὶ πρωῒ πότισον.

[Εἰς σπλῆνα κατάπλασμα πάνυ καλόν] Ἑλενίου, σινήπεως, δαφνίδων κατὰ λόγον κοπανίσας, εἶτα ἐξελὼν γλοῦν καρύας νέας κόψον μικρά. εἶτα βάλλε ἐν ὅλμῳ καὶ κόψον αὐτὸν ἰσχυρῶς καὶ ἐκβαλὼν ἀπόβρεξον ἐν ὄξει δριμεῖ ἡμέ-

Aut allia cataplasmate impoſita aut aſſa eſui potuique data.

[*Ad morſus rabidi canis.*] Vulneribus a rabido cane illatis imponito folia braſſicae trita cum laſſere et aceto; nam et ea per ſe conferunt morſui rabioſi canis, et ejus praeterea decoctum bibitum; ſed et elixa et aliis cibis praeaſſumpta phthiſicos curat ſanatque affectus arteriae; trita vero et facto ex ea emplaſtro lienique impoſita illum extenuat.

[*Ad anginam et colli dolorem.*] Alba populus arida ex melle trita ex illita confert. Aut naſturtii ſemen et fimum columbinum ex melle imponito.

[*Ad internas ani prominentias.*] Amarantum aqua maceratum coque et ſummo mane bibendum offer.

[*Ad lienem cataplasma valde bonum.*] Inulam, ſinapi, baccas lauri ſecundum proportionem accipe et tere; ac deinde exime corticem novae nucis et parum contundito, deinde in pilam conjice et validius contunde ac

ρας τρεῖς καὶ ἑνώσας ἀμφότερα μετὰ χυλοῦ τιβεριάδος ἕψει ἕως γένηται κατάπλασμα καὶ τίθει ἐπάνω τῆς σπληνὸς ἀπὸ πρωῒ ἕως ἡμέρας η'. προκενώσας τὴν γαστέρα καὶ θαυμάσεις.

[Ἄλλο πρὸς τῆξιν σπληνός.] Καππάρεως ῥίζης γο. γ'. ἀσβέστου γο. δ'. κόψας καὶ σήσας καὶ ὄξει μίξας ἐπίθες μὴ πλέον ὥρας μιᾶς καὶ ὅλον τήκεται. ἄλλο. κράμβης ζωμὸν ἕψει μόνον, μετὰ δὲ ὀξυμέλιτος πότισον νηστικῷ, ἢ βάτου ῥίζαν μετ' ὄξους ἀποτριτώσας δίδου πιεῖν ἡμέρας τρεῖς. ἄλλο. φλοῦν καρύας μετ' ὄξους καὶ μέλιτος ἑψήσας πότισον νηστικῷ, ἢ σίδηρον πυρώσας ἐν οἰνομέλιτι σβέσας ἐν ποτηρίῳ δὸς πιεῖν καὶ θαυμάσεις.

[Πρὸς ὀδόντας μέλανας.] Φοινίκων ὀστᾶ καὶ μαστίχην καὶ μέλι τρῖβε, τοὺς ὀδόντας ἐπὶ ἡμέρας ζ'. καὶ λευκαίνονται.

[Πρὸς ἕλμινθας.] Θέρμους καὶ δάφνης φύλλα καὶ χολὴν ταύρου μίξας ἐπίθες ἐπὶ τὸν ὀμφαλὸν τῆς κοιλίας καὶ ὠφελεῖ.

extractum in aceto per triduum macerandum ponito, atque in unum cum ſucco herbae tiberiadis redige et coque quoad fiat cataplasma et lieni impone ſummo mane per dies octo, corpore prius evacuato, et mirabere.

[*Aliud ad attenuandum lienem.*] Capparis radicum unc. iij, calcis vivae unc. iv contunde et cribra et ea cum aceto mixta appone lieni, nec ultra horam ſinito, univerſum lienem abſumet. *Aliud.* Decoctum braſſicae ſolum ex aceto mulſo da jejuno bibendum. Aut rubi radicem usquequo tertia pars remaneat decoquito et decoctum per triduum dato. *Aliud.* Corticem nucis et aceto et melle coctum jejuno potui dato. Aut candens ferrum in mulſum extinguito et potui dato et mirabere.

[*Ad dentes nigros.*] Palmularum oſſa, maſtichen et mel terito et dentes per dies ſeptem fricato et candidi reddentur.

[*Ad alvi lumbricos.*] Lupinos, lauri folia et fel tauri misceto et umbilico imponito, nam proderit.

Ed. Chart. X. [666.]

[Πρὸς ἐσωχάδας καὶ ἐξωχάδας.] Ἄμυλον καὶ πίσσαν καὶ ὕδωρ ζεννύμενα δὸς πιεῖν ἐπὶ ἡμέρας ἑπτὰ μετὰ τὸ ἀποτριτωθῆνα τὸ εἰς τὸ ἕψημα.

[Πρὸς πόνον ὀδόντων.] Ἀμπελοβόθρακα κρατήσας τηγάνισον μετ' ἐλαίου καὶ ἔμβαλλε τῷ ὠτίῳ καὶ ὑγιαίνει.

[Πρὸς βδέλλας.] Τρίψας ἀριστολοχίαν ἀλάτιζε.

[Πρὸς λιθιῶντας διουρητικά.] Δαφνίδων πεπέρεως ἴσα δίδου μύστρον α'. μετὰ ὑδρομέλιτος.

[Ἄλλο θραῦον λίθους.] Δάφνης φλοιὸν ἀνάζεσον ὕδατι ἕως ἀποτριτώσεως καὶ δίδου ῥοφεῖν. ἄλλο ὅμοιον. τρυγόνος ὀρνέου κόπρον καύσας πάρεχε μετὰ μελικράτου, ποιεῖ γὰρ ἐξουρεῖσθαι τοὺς λίθους.

[Πεπειραμένον εἰς λιθιῶντας.] Στρουθίου, ῥέου Ποντικοῦ, καππάρεως, ἀνὰ < α'. δίδου σὺν οἴνῳ λευκῷ καθ' ἡμέραν < α'. καὶ οὐρήσεις ὑπόστασιν ἐν τῷ οὔρῳ λιθώδη. ἄλλο. ὀρίγανον ἀποζέσας ἕως ἀποτριτώσεως μεθ' ὕδατος πάρεχε κύαθον ἐκ τοῦ ἀποζέματος πιεῖν.

[*Ad interiores et exteriores ani prominentias.*] Amylum, picem et aquam fervefacito donec tertia pars relinquatur et per dies ſeptem potui dato.

[*Ad dentium dolorem.*] Vitis racemum in ſartagine frigito ex oleo et in aurem inſtillato et bene habebit.

[*Ad hirudines.*] Ariſtolochiam tritam inſperge.

[*Ad calculoſos diuretica.*] Baccarum lauri et piperis partes aequales misceto et ex eis da myſtrum unum ex mulſa.

[*Aliud quod calculos frangit*] Corticem lauri aquae incoque donec ad tertiam partem deveniat et ſorbendum exhibe. *Aliud ſimile.* Turturis avis ſtercus uſtum ex mulſa praebeto, calculos enim per urinam ejicit.

[*Aliud expertum ad calculoſos.*] Recipe ſtruthii, rheu pontici, capparis, ana drach. j et ex his dato quotidie drach. j ex vino albo et minget ſedimentum lapidoſum. *Aliud.* Origanum ad tertias decoquito ex aqua, ex eo decocto in potum dato cyathum unum.

[*Εἰς στραγγουρίαν.*] *Μαράθρου σπέρμα, δαφνίδων Θηβαϊκῶν ἐξ ἴσου κόψας σὺν εὐκράτῳ δίδου θερμόν.*

[*Πρὸς δυσουρίαν καὶ στραγγουρίαν.*] *Κόστου, μέλιτος, ὕδατος κυάθους θ'. δίδου πιεῖν κρατῆρα, τὸν μισθὸν προαπαιτῶν. ἄλλο. Κυπέρου Ἀσιατικοῦ κο-* [667] *χλιάριον α' μετὰ ἀκράτου δίδου λεῖον ἢ μετὰ μέλιτος· ἔστι γὰρ δόκιμον.*

[*Πρὸς δυσουρίαν.*] *Πετροσελίνου Μακεδονικοῦ κόψας δίδου κοχλιάριον α'.*

[*Πρὸς στραγγουρίαν.*] *Κολοκύνθην κοπάνισον ξηρὰν ὡς ἀλεύρου καὶ κοχλιάριον μικρὸν μεθ' ὕδατος δὸς πιεῖν.*

[*Πρὸς τοὺς ἐνουροῦντας εἰς τὰ σάγια.*] *Λαγωοῦ ἐγκέφαλον σὺν οἴνῳ πότισον. ἄλλο. φῦσαν ὀπτήσας δὸς φαγεῖν ἐπὶ ἡμέρας γ'. ἢ κύπερον λειώσας πότισον, ἢ λαγωοῦ ὄρχιν ἐν οἴνῳ εὐώδει χλιαρῷ δὸς πιεῖν.*

[*Πρὸς στραγγουρίαν.*] *Δενδρολίβανον λαβὼν βράσον μετ' οἴνου πλεῖστον ἐπὶ ἡμέρας τρεῖς πάρεχε πίνειν. λαβὼν ῥαφίδα τὸ θαλάσσιον ὀψάριον καύσας καὶ τὴν σποδιὰν δὸς πιεῖν.*

[*Ad urinae ſtillicidium.*] Foeniculi ſemen, palmulas Thebaïcas ad portiones pares conterito et ex aqua temperata calida bibenda dato.

[*Ad urinae difficultatem et ſtillicidium.*] Recipe coſti, mellis, aquae cyathos ix, ex his in potum da craterem, mercede tamen prius expetita. *Aliud.* Cyperi Aſiatici triti cochlearium j ex vino meraco aut ex melle exhibe: probatum eſt.

[*Ad urinae difficultatem.*] Petroſelini Macedonici triti da cochlearium.

[*Ad ſtillicidium.*] Cucurbitam aridam tritam inſtar farinae da ex aqua quantitate cochlearii parvi ad bibendum.

[*Ad mingentes in ſtragulis.*] Leporis cerebrum ex vino bibat. *Aliud.* Veſicam aſſam comedendam dato per triduum. Aut cyperum tritum bibendum dato, vel teſtem leporis ex vino odorato tepido potui dato.

[*Ad ſtillicidium.*] Arborem thuris diutius ferveſacito in vino et per triduum potui dato. Accipe raphida marinum pisciculum, urito et cinerem bibendum offerto.

[*Περὶ λειχήνων.*] *Κέρας ἐλάφου ῥινήσας μετ' ὄξους δριμυτάτου ἀποτριτώσας ἐπάλειφε.*

[*Πρὸς ἀγρίου λειχῆνας.*] *Κριθάλευρον μετ' ὄξους δριμέος ἐμμίξας ἄλειφε, ἢ ἀκροσφοδείλου ῥίζαν σὺν ὄξει λειώσας χρῖε συχνῶς, ἢ καῦσον λινοῦν πανίον ἐπάνω σιδήρου καὶ ἄλειφε, ἢ φύλλα καρύας χλωρὰ ἀποζέσας κατάπλαττε. τοῦτο καὶ ἐπὶ ψώρας.*

[*Πρὸς αἰδοίου πόνον καὶ φλεγμονήν.*] *Κύμινον ἑψήσας πολλὰ καὶ λέπυρα ᾠῶν ἐπάντλει, καὶ θαυμάσεις.*

[*Πρὸς λειχῆνας.*] *Σκόροδον καὶ θεάφην, ὕδωρ καὶ ἔλαιον σμήξας ἄμφω ἄλειφε.*

[*Κατάπλασμα πρὸς τραύματα πρόσφατα ἀπὸ ξίφους ἢ ξύλου.*] *Ἰτέας φύλλα τρίψας ἐπίθες καὶ τὸ αἷμα στήσεις καὶ τὰ τραύματα παρακολλᾷ καὶ ὑγιαίνει. ἢ βολβοὺς προβάτων ἅμα ἐλαίῳ λειώσας κατάπλασον.*

[*Πρὸς δηλητήρια φάρμακα.*] *Πήγανον καὶ σῦκον καὶ κάρυον τρίψας πότισον μετ' οἴνου, ἢ τῆς νύσσης τὸ αἷμα*

[*Ad impetigines.*] Cornu cervi ramenta ad tertias ex acerrimo aceto coquito ac illinito.

[*Ad ferinas impetigines.*] Hordeaceam farinam acri aceto misce et illine. Aut haſtulae regiae radicem ex aceto terito et inungito frequenter. Aut linteum lineum urito ſuper ferro candenti et illinito. Aut ſolia virentis nucis coquito et facto cataplasmate apponito; hoc valet etiam ad ſcabiem.

[*Ad dolorem et inflammationem penis.*] Cuminum et ovi putamina plurimum decoquito et foveto, et mirabere.

[*Ad impetigines.*] Allium et theaphen, aquam et oleum ſimul misce et illine.

[*Cataplasma ad recentia vulnera ex enſe vel ligno.*] Salicis folia trita imponito et ſanguinem reprimes et vulnera conglutinabis, ſanitatemque reſtitues. Aut fimum ovillum ex oleo tritum in modum cataplasmatis imponito.

[*Ad medicamenta pernicioſa.*] Rutam, ficum et nucem terito et ex vino da in potum. Aut fulicae ſanguis

Ed. Chart. X. [667.]
ὑγρὸν σὺν ἐλαίῳ πινόμενον σώζει τοὺς πιόντας δηλητήριον φάρμακον καὶ τοὺς ὑπὸ ἐχίδνης δηχθέντας.

[*Πρὸς ῥεῦμα ἐν τῷ λαιμῷ.*] Χελιδόνος νεοττιὰν λειώσας μετ᾽ ὄξους κατάχριε.

[*Πρὸς μαστῶν γυναικῶν ὄγκους.*] Αἰγὸς ἀφόδευμα ξηρὸν μετὰ οἴνου ἀκράτου ἐπίθες καὶ λύει τὴν φλεγμονήν.

[*Εἰς λυκοκεφαλίαν.*] Χοίρου ἀφόδευμα καύσας καὶ λαβὼν σποδὸν, μίξας μετὰ μέλιτος, ξυρήσας τὴν κεφαλὴν ἄλειφε καὶ ἐπίθες ἐπάνω κράμβης φύλλα.

[*Βηχικοῖς καὶ ἑκτικοῖς.*] Στύρακος καὶ κράμβης χυλοῦ συντρίψας καὶ ζυμώσας δίδου νήστει καὶ εἰς κοίτην, ἢ δαφνελαίου καὶ οἴνου καλοῦ, ἀνὰ < γ΄. σμήξας καὶ χλιάνας ἐν λουτρῷ ἔσωθεν καὶ οἰνελαίου θερμοῦ κέρα καὶ συμπυριάσας τῷ στομάχῳ. ἄλλο. θερμῶν πυρίαν στακτὴν βρέξας, πυρία πόδας τοῦ βήσσοντος καὶ ἀποσπογγίσας αὐτοὺς ἐπάλειφε καὶ πυρίαζε. τοῦτο δὲ βῆχας ἰαθήσεται.

[*Εἰς βῆχας.*] Ῥητίνην συντρίψας μετὰ οἴνου παλαιοῦ

liquidus cum oleo bibitus eos ſervat qui medicamentum venenoſum auferunt et eos quos momordit vipera.

[*Ad fluxionem gutturis.*] Hirundinis nidum ex aceto terito et illinito.

[*Ad tumores mammarum mulierum.*] Si caprinum ſtercus aridum teras ex vino meraco et imponas, inflammationem ſolves.

[*Ad lupinum capitis dolorem.*] Stercus ſuillum urito cineremque cum melle miſceto et caput prius raſum illinito, appoſitis deſuper braſſicae foliis.

[*Ad tuſſim et febrem hecticam.*] Styracem et braſſicae ſuccum ſimul terito et ea fermentata jejuno et eunti cubitum exhibeto. Aut recipe olei laurini et optimi vini utriusque drach. iij et miſce et tepeſac in balneo interius, et vinum oleumque calidum temperato et ſtomachum ſoveto. *Aliud.* Lixivio collato calido pedes ſoveto et ſpongia deterſos illinito et foveto; hoc tuſſes curat.

[*Ad tuſſes.*] Reſinam tritam ex vino veteri jejuno

πότισον νήστει. καὶ γλήχωνα μετ᾽ ὀξυκράτου προεψήσας δὸς πιεῖν, ἢ βερονίκην ζυ- [668] μώσας μετὰ μέλιτος δίδου φαγεῖν, ἢ ῥαφανὴν ὀπτὴν ἐσθιομένην δίδου πρωΐ καὶ ὀψὲ, ἢ βούτυρον ἄναλον καπινέτω βασιλικοῦ καρύου μέγεθος.

[Πρὸς τοὺς ἐν τῷ θώρακι χυμούς.] Κνίδης τὰ φύλλα συνεψηθέντα πτισάνῃ δίδου πίνειν. ποιεῖ δὲ καὶ πρὸς πνευματώσεις καὶ ἀνάγει τὰ ἐν τῷ θώρακι.

[Πρὸς βῆχας.] Τῆλιν ἑψήσας ἕως ὅτου ἀποτριτωθῇ, τὸ ζεμάτιον λάβε τῷ πρωΐ μετὰ μέλιτος.

[Εἰς καλλιφωνίαν.] Τραγάκανθα ἀποβραχεῖσα ἐν οἴνῳ καὶ ποθεῖσα φωνὴν λαμπρύνει.

[Πρὸς ἀποκοπὰς φωνῆς.] Στύρακα λειώσας μετὰ ὕδατος ποίει καταπότια ἴσα ἐρεβίνθοις καὶ δίδου τρίτον καὶ εὐθέως λαλήσει.

[Αὐξητικὰ πλοκάμων καὶ πώγωνος, εἰ ἐπιῤῥέουσι.] Τεῦτλον μετὰ μυρσινελαίου καὶ πολυτρίχου μίξας κατάχριε τὰς τρίχας, ἢ ἀδίαντον καὶ λάδανον ἴσα λειώσας μετ᾽ ἐλαίου

bibendam dato. Et decoctum pulegii ex poſca bibatur. Et beronicem cum melle fermentatam edendam dato. Aut raphanum toſtum comedendum offerto mane et vesperi. Aut butyrum ſine ſale quantitate nucis avellanae devoret.

[*Ad humores in pectore detentos.*] Urticae folia ptiſanae incocta potui dato; ſed ad inflationes benefaciunt materiamque ex pectore educunt.

[*Ad tuſſes.*] Foenum graecum decoctum quousque tertia pars ſuperſit et ejus jusculum ſummo mane ex melle bibat.

[*Ut vox canora fiat.*] Tragacantha vino madefacta et epota vocem claram efficit.

[*Ad amiſſam vocem.*] Styracem terito, ex qua catapotia ex aqua formato magnitudine ciceris et ter dato, ſtatimque loquetur.

[*Ad augendos capillos et barbam, ſi decidant.*] Betam cum oleo myrteo et polytrichum misce et illine capillos. Aut adiantum et ladanum paribus portionibus te-

Ed. Chart. X. [668.]

ὀμφακίνου ἢ μυρσίνου ἢ σχινίνου ἐπίχριε. ἄλλο. λάδανον ἀποβρέξας σὺν οἴνῳ Ἀμιναίῳ καὶ μυρσινελαίῳ, λειώσας ἄμφω, ποίει πάχος μέλιτος καὶ ἐπίχριε τὴν κεφαλὴν ἐν βαλανείῳ. βέλτιόν ἐστι καὶ τὸ ἀδίαντον, ὅ τινες καλοῦσι πολύτριχον, τὸ ἕβδομον μέρος λαδάνῳ ἐπίβαλλε καὶ χρῖε.

[Πρὸς ὀδύνας νεφρῶν.] Γλήχωνι συνεψείσθωσαν πίτυρα ἐξ ἀλεύρων καὶ σακκελίσας τὸν ζωμὸν καὶ σπόγγῳ τοῦτο βρέξας, πυριαζέσθω οὕτως.

rito ex immaturo oleo vel myrtino vel lentiscino et illine. *Aliud.* Ladanum madefactum in vino Aminaeo et oleo myrtino terito ambo ad mellis ſpiſſitudinem, et in balneo caput illinito; melius autem eſt adiantum, quod nonnulli polytrichum vocant, ſi ſeptimam partem ladano indideris et inunxeris.

[*Ad dolorem renum.*] Pulegium cum farinae furfuribus decoquito et in jus collatum demiſſa ac imbuta ſpongia foveto.

ΓΑΛΗΝΟΥ ΠΕΡΙ ΤΩΝ ΠΑΡΑ ΤΗΝ ΛΕΞΙΝ ΣΟΦΙΣΜΑΤΩΝ.

Ed. Chart. II. [73.] Ed. Bas. IV. (32.)

[73] (32) *Κεφ. α΄.* [*Παρὰ τρόπους ἓξ τὸν ἀριθμὸν γίνεσθαι τὰ παρὰ τὴν λέξιν σοφίσματα, τῇ τοῦ Ἀριστοτέλους ἀξιοπιστίᾳ.*] Ἀριστοτέλης ὁ φιλόσοφος διδάσκων ἡμᾶς ἐν τῷ περὶ σοφιστικῶν ἐλέγχων συγγράμματι παρ᾽ ὅσους τρόπους γίνεται τὰ παρὰ τὴν λέξιν σοφίσματα, τρόπους μὲν ἓξ τὸν ἀριθμὸν εἶναί φησι, ἐκτίθεται δὲ αὐτοὺς οὕτως. παρ᾽ ὁμωνυμίαν, ἀμφιβολίαν, προσῳδίαν, σύνθεσιν, διαίρεσιν,

GALENI DE SOPHISMATIS SEU CAPTIONIBUS PENES DICTIONEM.

Cap. I. [*Sex modis sophismata in dictione contingere, Aristotelis auctoritate.*] Aristoteles philosophus docens nos in libro de sophisticis elenchis (*captiosis argumentis*) quot modis in dictione sophismata seu captiones contingant, modos sex quidem numero esse asserit, eosque ita exponit: in aequivocatione, in ambiguitate, in accentu, in compositione, in divisione, in dictionis figura. So-

σχῆμα λέξεως. καλεῖ δὲ παρ' ὁμωνυμίαν μὲν ὅταν διὰ τῶν ὀνομάτων ἐν τῷ λόγῳ πλείω σημαίνηται, καθάπερ ἐν τῷ κύνα τεθήρακα· πλείω γὰρ οὗτος ὁ λόγος σημαίνει διὰ τοὔνομα τὸν κύνα. παρ' ἀμφιβολίαν δὲ, ὅταν παρ' αὐτὸν τὸν λόγον ἐν αὐτῷ τὸ διττὸν ᾖ. καθάπερ ἔχει τὸ, γένοιτο καταλαβεῖν τόνδ' ἐμὲ, ἐνταῦθα τῶν μὲν ὀνομάτων οὐδὲν διττὸν, αὐτὸς δὲ ὁ λόγος ἐφ' ἑαυτοῦ σημαίνει τὸ, ἑλεῖν τε καὶ ἀναιρεθῆναι. παρὰ δὲ τὴν προσῳδίαν, ὅταν διττὸν γίγνηται. καθάπερ ἐν τῷ [74] Ορος ἕστηκε. τὸ γὰρ διπλοῦν, παρὰ τὴν διττὴν προσῳδίαν τιθεμένην κατ' ἀρχὰς, ἢ περιαιρουμένην· παρὰ δὲ τὴν σύνθεσιν καὶ διαίρεσιν, ὅταν αὐτὴ ποιῇ τοῦ σημαινομένου τὴν διαφορὰν, ὥσπερ

Πεντήκοντ' ἀνδρῶν ἑκατὸν λίπε δῖος Αχιλλεύς.

ἡ γὰρ διαφορὰ τοῦ ἀνδρῶν, τοῦ ἢ συντιθεμένου, ἢ διαιρουμένου ἀπὸ τῶν ν' ἐστί. παρὰ δὲ τὸ σχῆμα τῆς λέξεως, ὁπόιαν ἕτερον τῷ ὄντι σημαίνῃ, ἕτερον δὲ διὰ τὸ εἶδος καὶ τὸ σχῆμα. δοκεῖ δὲ οἷον τὸ ἀκούω. ἔστι μὲν τοῦ πάσχειν

phismata in aequivocatione vocat, ubi nomina in oratione posita plura significant, ut canem venatus sum: plura enim haec oratio significat ob id vocabulum, canem. Sophismata vero in ambiguitate, quum orationi ipsi in se duplex sensus est, ut haec se habet, hunc licet capere me: hic nominum quidem nullum ambiguum, sed oratio ipsa per se capere et capi significat. At in accentu, quum duplex contingit, ut hac in dictione, *Ορος ἕστηκε*, mons aut terminus stabat; ipsum enim nomen duplex ob duplicem accentum, qui in principio ponitur aut tollitur. Sophisma autem in compositione et divisione quum ipsae significationis differentiam faciunt, ut

Quinquaginta virum centenos liquit Achilles.

Differentia namque est dictioni, virum, aut compositae cum quinquaginta aut a quinquaginta divisae. Denique in dictionis figura quum aliud *dictio* vere significat, aliud vero propter speciem et figuram significare videtur, ut

δόξης ἂν τοῦ ποιεῖν, διὰ τὴν προφορὰν, ὅπερ ἐστὶ τὸ σχῆμα παραπλήσιον κρατεῖσθαι τοῖς τοῦ ποιεῖν, τοῦ τρέχω καὶ νοῶ. ἑλκύσει γὰρ ἂν ὁ σοφιστικὸς πρὸς ἑκάτερον. πρὸς μὲν τὸ πάσχειν ὅτι ἐστί. πρὸς δὲ τὸ ποιεῖν ὅτι φαίνεται. τούτους δ' ἐξηριθμημένους τοὺς τρόπους ἐφεξῆς δείκνυσιν, ὅτι μηδεὶς ἐστιν ὃν παραλέλοιπε, μηδὲ οἷόν τέ ἐστι τῶν παρὰ μὲν τὴν λέξιν τι σοφισμάτων, ἔξω πεσεῖν τῶν εἰρημένων. ὁ δὲ λόγος δι' οὗ ταῦτα δείκνυσίν ἐστιν οὗτος. τούτου δὲ πίστις ἥ τε διὰ τῆς ἐπαγωγῆς καὶ συλλογισμὸς, ἄν τε ληφθῇ τις ἕτερος καὶ ὅτι τοσαυταχῶς ἂν τοῖς αὐτοῖς ὀνόμασι καὶ λόγοις, μὴ ταὐτὸν μέντοι δηλώσαιμεν. τὸ μὲν οὖν τῆς ἐπαγωγῆς γνώριμον. εἰ γὰρ καθ' ἕκαστον εἰπόντι καὶ λαβόντι τῶν παρὰ τὴν λέξιν σοφισμάτων φαίνοιτο μηδὲν πίπτειν ἔξω τῶν εἰρημένων τρόπων, δῆλον ἤδη ταύτῃ γε, ὅτι μηδεὶς παραλέλειπται τρόπος· τὸ δ' ἐφεξῆς παντάπασιν ἀσαφές ἐστι, τί ποτε βούλεται λέγειν ἐν τῷ καὶ συλλογισμὸς, ἄν τε ληφθῇ τις ἕτερος καὶ ὅτι τοσαυταχῶς ἂν τοῖς αὐτοῖς ὀνόμασι καὶ λόγοις οὐ ταὐτὰ δηλώσαιμεν,

verbum audio: eſt quidem paſſionis cum actionis eſſe videatur, propter prolationem, id eſt figuram ſimilem iis quae verborum actionis ſunt, ut curro et intelligo. Trahet enim ad utramque partem ſophiſticus *homo;* ad paſſionem, quoniam *ita* eſt; ad actionem, quia ita videtur. His vero ſex enumeratis modis deinceps oſtendit nullum eſſe ab eo praetermiſſum, neque poſſe aliquod in verbo ſophisma extra *modos* propoſitos cadere. Verba vero, quibus id oſtendit, haec ſunt: Hujus rei fides eſt et ea, quae per inductionem fit et ſyllogismus et ſi alius aliquis ſumatur et quod tot modis, nominibus iisdem et orationibus non eandem rem ſignificamus. Ea igitur, quae de inductione loquitur, contextus pars manifeſta eſt: ſi enim ſingula in verbo ſophismata percurras ſumasque nec ullum horum appareat extra praedictos modos cadere, perſpicuum jam ita eſt, nullum praetermiſſum eſſe modum: quod vero ſequitur, omnino obſcurum eſt quid velit quum dicit et ſyllogismus et ſi alius aliquis ſumatur et quod tot

οὐδέ γε ὅπως ἂν ἕτερόν τινα λάβοιμεν συλλογισμὸν εἴρηται· τὸ δὲ καὶ ὅτι τοσαυταχῶς ἂν τοῖς αὐτοῖς ὀνόμασι καὶ λόγοις οὐ ταὐτὰ δηλώσαιμεν, συλλογισμοῦ συμπεράσματι μᾶλλον ἔοικεν ἢ συλλογισμῷ. σύνηθες δὲ τὸ τοιοῦτο τάχος τῷ φιλοσόφῳ καὶ καθάπερ ἐπὶ σημείων ἐκφέρειν τὰ πολλὰ καὶ διὰ τὸ, πρὸς τοὺς ἀκηκοότας ἤδη γράφεσθαι. τῶν οὖν ἐξηγησαμένων αὐτὸν οἱ μὲν οὐδ' ἐπεχείρησαν ταῦτ' ἀκριβῶσαι τὸν προσήκοντα τρόπον· οἱ δ' οὐκ ἔτυχον. ἡμεῖς δὲ πειραθῶμεν οὐκ Ἀριστοτέλους ἕνεκεν, οὐδ' ὡς τῷ λόγῳ βοήθειάν τινα πορίζοντες, ἀλλ' ἡμῶν αὐτῶν. φιλοσόφου γὰρ οὐ μόνον τὰς προτάσεις λαβόντα συλλογίσασθαι, καθάπερ τοῖς πλείστοις εἴωθεν, ἀλλὰ καὶ τοῦ συμπεράσματος κειμένου τὰς προτάσεις κατασκευάσαι.

Κεφ. β'. [Παρὰ τὸ διττὸν πάντα τὰ παρὰ τὴν λέξιν σοφίσματα γίνεσθαι.] Ἐπεὶ δὲ δεῖξαι πρόκειται τοσαυταχῶς γίνεσθαι τὰ παρὰ τὴν λέξιν σοφίσματα, ὁσαχῶς Ἀριστοτέλης ἔφη, τὰ παρὰ τὸ διττὸν, δῆλον ὡς δύο δεικτέον

modis, nominibus iisdem et orationibus non eandem rem ſignificamus, ſiquidem nec quonam modo alium aliquem ſumamus ſyllogismum dictum eſt: id vero et quod tot modis, nominibus iisdem et orationibus non eandem rem ſignificamus, ſyllogismi concluſioni magis ſimile eſt quam ſyllogismo: conſueta vero eſt haec huic philoſopho dicendi brevitas et veluti per ſigna expromere multa, quia ad hos qui jam adiverant, ſcribebantur. Qui igitur eum expoſuerunt, alii haec accurate tractare, quod decebat ne tentarunt quidem: alii non conſequuti ſunt: nos vero tentemus non Ariſtotelis cauſa, neque ut orationi ejus opem feramus, ſed cauſa noſtra. Philoſophi enim eſt non ſolum aſſumptis propoſitionibus ratiocinari, ut multorum mos eſt, ſed etiam concluſione poſita propoſitiones ipſas conſtruere.

Cap. II. [*Penes ipſum duplex omnia in dictione ſophismata accidere.*] Quoniam vero monſtrare propoſitum eſt, tot modis in verbo ſophismata fieri, quae penes ipſum duplex ſunt, quot modis Ariſtoteles dixit, patet duo

ἡμῖν, ἓν μὲν ὅτι πάντα τὰ παρὰ τὴν λέξιν παρὰ τὸ διττόν ἐστιν, ἕτερον δ' ὅτι παρὰ τὸ διττὸν τοσαῦτα. δῆλον δ' ἐκεῖνό γε πᾶσιν, ὅτι πάντα τὰ παρὰ τὴν λέξιν σοφίσματα παρὰ κακίαν αὐτῆς ἀνάγκη συμβαίνειν· ταύτης γὰρ ὥσπερ ἀρχῆς ἐχόμενοι ἐξαπατῶσιν οἱ σοφισταὶ τοὺς ἀπειροτέρους ἐν τούτοις καὶ μὴ συνορῶντας τὸ κίβδηλον. εἰ δὴ ὅσα βουλοίμεθα καλῶς λαβεῖν πόσα παρὰ τὴν λέξιν συμβαίνει σοφίσματα, ληπτέον πόσαι πότ' εἰσὶν αἱ κακίαι ἐν αὐτῇ· ὃ ἂν συνοφθείης τῆς ἀρετῆς ληφθείσης, εἴπερ ἐστὶ μία εἴ τε πλείους ἁπασῶν· ἁμαρτία γὰρ τῆς ἀρετῆς ἔοικεν εἶναι [75] καὶ ταύτης ὀρθῶς ληφθείσης εὐθὺς κἀκείνην γνωρίζεσθαι. ἐπεὶ δὲ, καθάπερ ἐν ἑτέροις ἀποδέδεικται λόγοις, τὸ εὖ τε καὶ ἡ ἀρετὴ, ἐν ἐκείνῳ πρὸς ὃ πέφυκεν, ἢ γέγονεν, ἀνθρώπου μὲν τὸ ζῆν, μαχαίρας δὲ τὸ τέμνειν, ληπτέον ἂν εἴη τὸ πρός τι πέφυκεν ἢ γέγονεν ἡ λέξις. φαίνεται δὲ πρὸς ἓν τὸ σημαίνειν· δῆλον οὖν ὅτι καὶ εὖ καὶ κακῶς ἐν τούτῳ· δῆλον δὲ ὅτι καὶ μόνη τῶν ἀρετῶν αὕτη καθ' αὑτὴν τῆς λέξεως, αἱ δ' ἄλλαι κατὰ συμβεβηκὸς καὶ ἔξωθεν καὶ οὐ

haec a nobis demonſtranda eſſe, alterum, omnia in verbo ſophismata penes ipſum duplex eſſe, alterum tot eſſe numero penes ipſum duplex. Perſpicuumque illud omnibus eſt, omnia in verbo ſophismata ex vitio hujus contingere neceſſe eſſe: hoc enim tanquam principium ſequentes ſophiſtae decipiunt in ea re minus verſatos et qui captionis fraudem non animadvertunt. Si vero recte volumus quot in verbo ſophismata contingunt accipere, quot vitia ſunt, ſumendum eſt: quod cognoveris, ſi virtutem ſumas unicam eſſe aut plures: error enim a virtute eſſe vitium videtur: qua recte cognita ſtatim hoc quoque cognoscitur. Quoniam vero, ut alibi demonſtratum eſt, ipſum bonum virtusque in eo eſt, ad quod nata aut facta res eſt, ut hominis in vivendo, gladii in ſcindendo, idcirco ad quod nata aut facta eſt dictio ſumendum eſt: manifeſtum vero eſt ad unum hoc, ut ſignificet. Patet igitur, in hoc et bonum et vitium eſſe; patet quoque ſolam e virtutibus hanc in dictione eſſe per ſe: reli-

τοῦ πράγματος, οἷον εὐαρμοστία καὶ εὐγραμματία. τοῦτο γὰρ εἰ καὶ φαίνεταί τισιν εὖ, ἀλλ' οὐ κατὰ τὸ πρᾶγμα· ἀλλ' ὥσπερ εἰ ξίφος ἐλεφαντόκωπον εἴη, ἢ ὀφθαλμὸς ὑπογεγραμμένος· καὶ γὰρ τούτοις ταῦτα ἔξωθεν, τὰ δὲ καθ' αὐτὰ, ἐν τῷ τέμνειν τε καὶ ὁρᾶν καὶ τὴν ἀρετὴν ἑκάστου τυγχάνειν, εἶθ' ὡς λέγεται καθ' ἣν ἕδραν ἔχειν, πρὸς ὃ πέφυκεν, ἢ γέγονεν· δῆλον ὡς καὶ τὸν ἀριθμὸν τῶν ἀρετῶν ἐντεῦθεν ἄν τις γνοίη ὁπόσος ἐστίν· εἰ μὲν γὰρ πρὸς πολλὰ, πλείους, εἰ δὲ πρὸς ἕν, μία. φαίνεταί γε μὴν ἡ λέξις πρὸς ἓν τὸ σημαίνειν· εἴπερ τὸ καλῶς πρὸς τοῦτο μὴ σημαίνειν ἢ μὴ εὖ σημαίνειν κακία ἔσται καίτοι ἴσως δεῖται σκέψεως, εἰ θετέον εἶναι λέξιν ἔτι, τὴν μὴ σημαίνουσαν. οὐδὲ γὰρ αὐλητὴς ὁ μὴ πεφυκὼς αὐλεῖν ὅλως· οὐκοῦν οὐδὲ κακὸς αὐλητής· οὐδὲ λέξεως ἄρα κακία τὸ μὴ σημαίνειν· τοῦτο δὲ εὐθὺς καὶ σημεῖον τοῦ μόνην τὴν ὑφ' ἡμῶν δὲ λεγομένην ἀρετὴν εἶναι τῆς λέξεως καθ' αὑτήν· ἐν ᾧ γὰρ ἑκάστου τὸ εἶναι, ἐν τούτῳ καὶ ἡ ἀρετή· ἡ δὲ λέξις ἐν τῷ

quas vero per accidens extrinfecusque effe, nec rei ipfius, ut concinnitas et apta literarum formatio; haec enim et fi quibusdam fe bona oftendant, non tamen fecundum rem fe habent: fed perinde ac fi enfis manubrio eburneo fit aut fucatus oculus: haec etenim his extrinfeca funt: quae vero funt per fe, ea in fcindendo et in cernendo funt. Si igitur uniuscujusque rei virtus eft, five ut dicitur in eo pofita eft, ad quod nata res aut facta eft, patet quod et virtutum numerum hinc quis noverit quantus fit; fi enim ad multa res genita fit, plures illae funt: fi ad unum, una virtus eft. Apparet fane dictio ad unum nata, hoc eft ad fignificandum. Si igitur bonum ipfum in hoc pofitum eft, hoc ipfum non fignificare aut non recte fignificare, vitium erit: nam confiderandum videtur, an, quae non fignificat, ea dictio ftatuenda fit: non enim tibicen is eft, qui tibia natura non aptus eft ullo modo canere, nec malus igitur tibicen eft: fic nec dictio eft, quae non eft ad fignificandum apta: quare nec vitium dictionis erit non fignificatio. Hoc vero protinus fignum, folam eam

σημαίνειν· τούτου γέ τοι διαφθαρέντος, οὐδὲ λέξις, οὐκοῦν ἐν τούτῳ καὶ ἡ ἀρετὴ, διὸ καὶ μόνη συναποβάλλεται· αἱ δ' ἄλλαι, διὰ τὸ μὴ κατ' αὐτὸ τὸ πρᾶγμα εἶναι, οὐδὲν κωλύονται καὶ περὶ τὴν μὴ σημαίνουσαν ὑπάρχειν, οἷον ἡ εὐαρμοστία καὶ ἡ εὐγραμματία. κρείττω γοῦν διὰ ταῦτα καὶ τῶν βαρβαρικῶν διαλέκτων ἑτέραν ἑτέρας φαμὲν, οἷον τὴν Περσίδα τῆς Αἰθιοπικῆς, καίτοι μὴ σημαίνουσαν ἡμῖν· τὸ δ' αἴτιον, ὅτι φωνὴ μᾶλλόν ἐστιν ἢ λέξις. ἀλλ' εἴ τῳ καὶ δοκεῖ τοῦτο κακία τὸ μὴ σημαίνειν καὶ πλανᾶταί τις διὰ τὴν ὁμοιότητα τοῦ καλεῖσθαι. ἀλλ' ἐκεῖνο δὲ δῆλον, ὡς οὐδ' ἂν διὰ ταύτην κακίαν σόφισμα συμβαίνοι. τίς γὰρ ἂν ὁμολογήσειεν, ἢ συνθείη τίς πρὸς ἄσημον καὶ ἀσαφῆ λέξιν. λείπεται δὴ διὰ τὸ μὴ εὖ σημαίνειν· τοῦτο δὲ, ὅτι διττόν. ἐν τούτῳ γὰρ ὑπάρχει μόνῃ τῇ λέξει, σημαίνειν μέν τι, μὴ εὖ δὲ σημαίνειν. τὸ γὰρ κύων ὄνομα σημαίνει μέν τι, οὔπω δὲ τόδε τι, οὐδὲ ἀφωρισμένον ὅπερ ἦν (33) τὸ εὔληπτον·

quae nunc a nobis dicta eſt, virtutem eſſe dictionis per ſe: in quo enim unaquaeque res eſſe habet, in hoc ipſa virtus eſt: dictio autem habet in ſignificando eſſe, eoque corrupto, neque dictio eſt: igitur in hoc ipſo virtus eſt. Quare haec una cum ſignificatione deperditur, reliquae vero, propterea quod non ſecundum rem ipſam ſunt, non impediuntur circa hanc eſſe, quae non ſignificat, ut concinnitas et apta ſcriptura. Has ob res, quae linguae barbarae ſunt, earum alteram meliorem altera dicimus, ut Perſicam Aethiopica, quanquam nihil nobis ſignificantem: cauſa vero eſt, quia potius vox eſt quam dictio; ſed etſi vitium videatur, non ſignificatio, cum propter ſimilitudinem nominis decipiantur, patet non propter hoc vitium ſophisma contingere. Quis enim eſt, qui conſentiat aut quis eſt, qui proponat dictionem ſignificatione privatam et ignotam? Reſtat igitur, ut propterea contingat ſophisma, quia non recta ſignificatio ſit: haec vero talis eſt, quia duplex; in hoc enim ſolo dictio habet quidem quod ſignificet, verum non recte: canis enim nomen aliquid ſignificat, non tamen hoc aliquid, neque definitum quid-

κἀκεῖνο δὲ λέγεται καλῶς ὑπὸ Πλάτωνος, ὅτι πάντα ὅσα φθαρτὰ τῇ σφετέρᾳ κακίᾳ, φθείρει δὲ καὶ τούτων τὴν λέξιν. ἄγει γὰρ πρότερόν τινα εἰς ἀσάφειαν, ἀλλ' οὐχὶ ἁπλῶς ὥσπερ τὰ μηδὲν σημαίνοντα· ἡ δ' ἀσάφεια καὶ πρόσθεν ἐλέγετο διαφθορά τις εἶναι παντελὴς τῆς λέξεως· ὥσπερ πᾶν καὶ διὰ τοῦτο, μόνη κακία τὸ διττὸν, χωρὶς εἰ μή τις οἴεται κἀκεῖνα κακίας, οἷον ἔνδειαν, ἢ μακρολογίαν, ἢ πριττολογίαν· λανθάνειν τοῦτον νομίζω, ἀπατώμενον καὶ μὴ συνιέντα τούτων οὐδὲν ἁπλῶς κακὸν τῆς λέξεως, εἰ μὴ τὴν ἀσάφειαν, ἢ τὸ διττὸν ἐργάζοιτο· εἰ δὲ μόνη κακία λέξεως αὕτη καὶ καλῶς τὰ πρόσθεν εἴρηται. πάντα δὲ τὰ παρα τὴν λέξιν σοφίσματα παρὰ τὴν κακίαν ταύτην γίγνεται· πάντα τὰ παρὰ τὴν λέξιν ἔσται παρὰ τὸ διττόν.

[76] Κεφ. γ'. [Τὸ παρὰ τὸ διττὸν παρ' ἓξ τρόπους παρὰ τὴν λέξιν γενέσθαι. ὅ τι ποτέ ἐστι λόγος.] Δεικτέον δὲ τὸ μετὰ τοῦτ' ἂν εἴη, διὰ τί τὸ παρὰ τὸ διττὸν τοσαυταχῶς, ὁσαχῶς Ἀριστοτέλης φησὶ, συνίσταται· εἰ δὲ καὶ

quam, quod erat recte ſignificare. Illud vero recte a Platone dicitur, quaecunque proprio vitio corrupta ſunt, horum omnium dictionem corrumpit: ducit enim in obſcuram ſignificationem quodam modo, ſed non ſimpliciter, ut ea quae nihil ſignificant: obſcura vero ſignificatio prius dicta eſt perſecta eſſe dictionis corruptio: quapropter ſolum vitium eſt ipſum duplex: niſi quis ea quoque vitia putet, deſectum, longitudinem, ſuperfluitatem dicendi: latere autem hunc arbitror deceptum et ignarum, nullum horum eſſe ſimpliciter dictionis vitium, niſi obſcuritatem aut duplicitatem efficiat: ſi vero ſolum hoc dictionis vitium eſt et recte ſupra dictum eſt omnia, quae in verbo ſophismata ſunt, ex ejus vitio fieri, propter ipſum duplex erunt omnia, quae in verbo ſophismata contingunt.

Cap. III. [*Ipſum duplex ſex tantum modis in dictione fieri. Quid ſit oratio.*] Poſt vero demonſtrandum eſt, propter quid tot modis ipſum duplex accidat, quot Ariſtoteles ſcribit: id vero ſi recte inveniri debet, ſumen-

τοῦτο μέλλει καλῶς εὑρεθήσεσθαι, ληπτέον πρότερον, ὅ τί ποτέ ἐστι λόγος τε καὶ ἐκ λόγων· λόγοι γὰρ καὶ αἱ προτάσεις· τούτων τινὶ ἢ τισι διττὸν ζητοῦμεν· ἔσται δὴ λόγος, ὡς πρὸς τὸ παρὸν ἀποχρώντως εἰπεῖν, σύνθεσις ὀνομάτων· καλῶ δὲ ὀνόματα κἂν καὶ τὰ ῥήματα καὶ ὅλως τι σημαίνει διὰ τὸ γνωριμώτερα· ἀνάγκη τὸ διττὸν, ἢ ἔν τινι τούτων εἶναι τῶν ὀνομάτων, ἢ ἐν αὐτῷ τῷ λόγῳ· τρίτον γὰρ οὐδὲν ἔχομεν ὅπως συσταίη· ὁπόταν ὥσπερ οὐδ' ἄν τις ἔχοι παρ' ἕκαστα τῶν λίθων, ἢ τὸ συγκείμενον· καὶ τοῦτο, ἢ ἐνεργείᾳ, ἢ δυνάμει, ἢ φαντασίᾳ. παρὰ ταῦτα γὰρ οὐδὲν ἕτερόν τις εὕροι ὑπάρχον, ἢ λεγόμενον, καθάπερ ἐν ἄλλοις ἀποδέδεικται· πάντα δὲ ταῦτα συλλαβόντες ἔχουσιν οἱ εἰρημένοι τρόποι· ἐνεργείᾳ μὲν γὰρ τὸ διττὸν ἔχουσι παρά τε τὴν ὁμωνυμίαν καὶ τὴν ἀμφιβολίαν καὶ ἐν ὀνόματι μὲν ὁ παρὰ τὴν ὁμωνυμίαν, ἐν λόγῳ δὲ ὁ παρὰ τὴν ἀμφιβολίαν· ἐνεργείᾳ δὲ, ὅτι τῷ ὄντι δύο σημαίνουσι· δυνάμει δ' ὁπότε τῇ προσῳδίᾳ γίγνονται διττοὶ καὶ παρὰ τὴν σύνθεσιν καὶ διαί-

dum prius eſt, quid ſit oratio et ex orationibus orationem eſſe, etenim et ipſae propoſitiones orationes ſunt: harum alicui aut aliquibus quaerimus ipſum duplex. Oratio ſane erit, quod in praeſenti dicere ſat eſt, nominum compoſitio: voco vero nomina, etſi verba ſint ſignificentque omnino aliquid, propterea, quod ſic notius vocabulum eſt; neceſſe eſt ipſum duplex aut in aliquo horum nominum eſſe, aut in oratione ipſa: nullum enim habemus tertium quomodo conſtituatur: quemadmodum neque in lapidibus praeter aut ſingulos ſeorſum aut illorum ſimul compoſitionem, eamque aut actu aut potentia aut apparentia nihil aliquis excogitare poteſt: praeter haec enim nihil eſt, quod eſſe aut dici quispiam inveniat, ut alibi demonſtratum eſt. Omnia vero haec comprehendentes modi praedicti habent. Ipſum enim actu duplex modus habet, et qui ſecundum aequivocationem eſt et qui ſecundum ambiguitatem: ſed in nomine duplicitatem is habet qui ſecundum aequivocationem eſt, in oratione qui ſecundum

ρεσιν· οὗτοι γὰρ οὐ σημαίνουσι πλείω, ἀλλὰ πάντως ἕν. διά τε τὸ ἑκάτερον ἐνδέχεσθαι διττοὶ λέγονται· διὸ καὶ δυνάμει φαμὲν αὐτοὺς, τοιοῦτο γὰρ τὸ δυνάμει οἷον τοῦτο αὖ πάλιν, ὥσπερ καὶ πρόσθεν διῄρητο, ἢ ἐν ὀνόμασιν, ἢ ἐν λόγῳ· ἐν μὲν οὖν ὀνόμασιν ἡ προσῳδία ποιεῖ τὸ διττόν· αὕτη γὰρ ἐφ' ἑκάτερον ἕλκει τοὔνομα, ὥσπερ ἐν τῷ Ορος ἕστηκεν, ἡ δασεῖα κατ' ἀρχὰς τεθεῖσα, ἢ μή· ἐν δὲ λόγῳ, διότι σύνθεσις καὶ διαίρεσις διττὸν ποιεῖ, δύναται δὲ κἀν τοῖς συνθέτοις τῶν ὀνομάτων αὕτη, διὰ τὸ προσεοικέναι λόγῳ, καθάπερ ἐν τῷ Νεάπολις καὶ καλὸς κἀγαθός· μεταβάλλοι δ' ἀντὶ τῶν ἁπλῶν· ἀλλ' οὐκ εἰς ἕτερον ὄνομα. τοῦτο γὰρ ἡ προσῳδία μόνη ποιεῖ· ἀλλ' εἰς λόγον, ὥσπερ τὸ αὐλητρὶς δηλονότι, καὶ τὸν λόγον συνθείη πότ' ἂν εἰς ὄνομα, ὥσπερ τὸ προκείμενον· δόξει δ' οὐδὲν ἧττον ἄτοπον ἴσως τὸ φάσκειν, διὰ τὴν προσῳδίαν τε καὶ τὴν σύνθεσιν συμβαίνειν τὰ σοφίσματα· εἴπερ ταῦτα μὲν διὰ τὸ διττὸν, κα-

ambiguitatem: actu vero eſſe dicuntur, quoniam revera res duas ſignificant. Potentia vero, dum accentu duplices fiunt, compoſitioneque et diviſione; hi enim non plura ſignificant, ſed prorſus unum: propterea vero quod ad utrumque verti licet duplices dicuntur: quare hos potentia dicimus: tale enim eſt hoc ipſum potentia eſſe. Id ipſum vero rurſus, ut ſupra quoque diviſum eſt, vel in nominibus vel in oratione eſt: in nominibus accentus duplicitatem efficit: trahit enim ad utramque partem nomen accentus, ut in oratione, hoc *Ορος ἕστηκεν*, hoc eſt mons *vel* terminus ſtabat, accentus aſpiratus facit, in principio cum aut ponitur aut abeſt. In oratione vero compoſitio et diviſio duplicitatem facit: in compoſitis quoque nominibus eandem facere poteſt, quia orationi ſimilia ſunt, ut in nomine Neapolis et *καλὸς κἀγαθὸς*, id eſt probus, mutaret ea quis loco ſimplicium non in nomen, hoc enim ſolus accentus facit, ſed in orationem ut in hac voce *αὐλητρὶς* videlicet, id eſt tibicina, ſicut rurſus et ipſam orationem in nomen componeret, ut eſt in propoſito nomine; videbitur autem nihilominus abſurdum fortaſſis id,

θάπερ ἐλέγετο πρόσθεν· εἰ δὲ προσῳδία τε καὶ τὰ ὁμογενῆ καὶ τῶν δυνάμει διττῶν ἐξαιρεῖ τὸ διττὸν, ποιεῖ γὰρ ἤδη ταῦτα, θάτερον σημαίνειν καὶ λέγεται ἀληθῶς συμβαίνειν οὐδὲν ἧττον τὰ σοφίσματα διὰ ταῦτα· τῷ γὰρ τὸν λόγον ἐπιδέχεσθαι διὰ τούτων τὸ διττὸν, λαβόντες θάτερον κατ' ἀρχὰς οἱ σοφισταὶ, θάτερον συνάγουσι, μεταβάλλοντες μὲν διὰ τούτων τὸν λόγον, πάντως γὰρ οὐκ ἂν ἄλλως τὸ σόφισμα συμβαίη, συλλογιζόμενοι δὲ ὡς ταὐτὸ λαμβάνοντες, ὥσπερ ἕν τι λογικὸν ὄνομα καὶ ἴδιον ἀνθρώπου, τὸ λογικὸν ἄρα ἓν ἴδιον ἀνθρώπου· καὶ εἰ ὅρος ἐνταῦθα εἱστήκει ὁ τὸ χωρίον, ὄρος δ' ἐνταῦθα οὐχ [77] ἕστηκε καὶ λάθοι μὲν οὐδένα τὸ κίβδηλον· αὐτὰρ οὐκ ὀκνοῦσιν οἱ σοφισταὶ πανταχῇ σμικρὸν φροντίζειν τοῦ εὐλόγου· ἐπεὶ κἂν τοῖς ἐνεργείᾳ διττοῖς οὗτοί γε ταὐτὸν τοῦτο ποιοῦσι. λαβόντες γὰρ ἕτερον συλλογίζονται· ἀλλ' ἐκεῖ μὲν ἀφανέστερον ὅτι καὶ ὁτιοῦν σημαίνῃ ἂν ὁ λόγος, ὁμολογηθείη· ἐνταῦθα δὲ προδήλως,

quod propter accentum compoſitionemque et diviſionem ſophismata contingere dicamus: ſiquidem haec propter ipſum duplex, ut ſupra dictum eſt, contingunt: accentus vero et quae ejus generis ſunt ipſum duplex iis quae facultate duplicia ſunt eripiunt: etenim ut haec alterum ſignificent efficiunt: ſed tamen nihilominus vere dicuntur propter haec ſophismata contingere: quia enim oratio per eadem haec ipſum duplex accipit, alterum in principio ſophiſtae ſumunt, alterum concludunt, orationem per ea ipſa mutantes, prorſus enim non aliter ſophisma contingeret, ratiocinantes vero tanquam idem accipientes: quale eſt unum quid rationale nomen eſt: proprium hominis eſt ipſum rationale: igitur unum proprium hominis eſt. Praeterea ſi ὅρος, hoc eſt terminus, hic ſtabat is qui agros ſeparat, ὄρος autem, hoc eſt mons, hic non ſtabat: ſed neminem lateret id quod ſic adulterinum eſt: verum ut ubique etiam ad minimum apta oratio ſit ſophiſtae ſtudent: nam et in iis, quae actu duplicia ſunt, hi illud idem faciunt, ut aliud ſumentes aliud concludentes ratio-

διὸ καὶ αὐτοῦ τοῖς ὀνόμασι καὶ λόγοις Ἀριστοτέλης ἔφη· οἱ μὲν γὰρ κἀκεῖ εἰσιν οἱ τὸ εἶδος σοφισταὶ βιαζόμενοι· ἐπεὶ δὲ ἔχομεν τὸ ἐνεργείᾳ τε καὶ δυνάμει, λείπεται φαντασίᾳ· τοῦτο δέ ἐστι τὸ παρὰ τὸ σχῆμα τῆς λέξεως, καθάπερ ἐλέγετο ἔμπροσθεν· φαίνεται γὰρ καὶ τὸ ὄνομα διττὸν οὐχ οὕτως ἔχον καὶ ὁ λόγος ὁμοίως καὶ οὐ τοσοῦτον καθ' ἕκαστον τῶν προειρημένων· τὰ παραδείγματα λάβοι τὶς ἂν ἔκ τε τῶν καὶ Εὐδήμου κἀξ ἄλλων· ἐπεὶ δ' οὖν ἔχομεν πάντας κατειλεγμένους τοὺς τρόπους, ἂν γένοιτό τι διττὸν, ἔχομεν πάντα τὰ παρὰ τὴν λέξιν σοφίσματα. ταῦτα γὰρ οὖν ἐστι, ἢ παρὰ τὸ διττόν· ἐχόμενον δὲ καὶ τὸ τοσαυταχῶς αὐτοῖς τοῖς ὀνόμασι καὶ λόγοις οὐ ταὐτὸν δηλώσαιμεν, ὅτι ἢ ἐνεργείᾳ, ἢ δυνάμει, ἢ φαντασίᾳ. δῆλον δ' ὅτι καὶ συλλογισμοῦ τρόπον, ὁποῖόν τις ἂν προέλοιτο, δυνατὸν ποιεῖν, ἅπαξ γε τὴν διαίρεσιν ἔχοντα καὶ ἐξ εὐθείας καὶ εἰς τὸ ἀδύνατον ἀπάγοντα. εἰ γὰρ τὸ δυνατὸν, ἀλλ' ἔσται οὔτ' ἐν ὀνόματι

cinentur: ſed ibi obſcurius, quoniam quicquid ſignificet ſermo, ipſe ſibi conſentiat: hic vero maniſeſte: quare ſuis nominibus et orationibus Ariſtoteles dixit: Etenim ii ſophiſtae ſunt, qui ſpeciem violant. Cum jam habeamus id ipſum, quod actu dicitur, itemque quod potentia, quod reliquum eſt, ad apparentiam attinet: quae ſecundum ſiguram dictionis eſt, ut eſt ſupra dictum: oſtenditur enim ipſum nomen, ſimiliterque oratio, non aliud duplex adeo habere, nec in ſingulis, quae praedicta ſunt; adeo quis exempla ex Eudemo ex aliisve caperet. Cum igitur jam collectos modos omnes habeamus, quibus duplex ipſum fieri poſſit, habemus omnia in dictione contingentia ſophismata: haec enim penes ipſum duplex ſunt: ſequitur vero id, quod tot modis nominibus ipſis et orationibus non eandem rem ſignificamus: nam aut actu aut potentia aut apparentia id facimus: maniſeſtum vero eſt et ſyllogismi modum, modo habita diviſio ſit, fieri poſſe, utrumvis quis eligat aut e directo aut ad impoſſibile ducentem: ſi enim poſſibile eſt alium haberi modum, is erit ne-

οὔτ' ἐν λόγῳ, οὔτ' ἐνεργείᾳ, οὔτε δυνάμει, οὔτε φαντασίᾳ· παρὰ ταῦτα δ' οὐδὲν ὁ λόγος ἐδείκνυ· κατ' αὐτὸ μὲν ἀφωρίσθω τὸν τρόπον τοῦτον· ὅτι δ' οὐ κατ' αὐτὸν τὴν διαίρεσιν εὑρήκαμεν, οὐ γὰρ Ἀριστοτέλει χαριζόμεθα νῦν. ἀλλὰ ταῦτα ἅπαντα κατὰ τὴν μέθοδον γέγραπται, δῆλον· τὸ μὲν γὰρ ἢ ἐν ὀνόματι δεῖν, ἢ ἐν λόγῳ τὸ διττὸν εἶναι σαφῶς αὐτὸς εἴρηκεν ἐν οἷς φησιν ὅτι τοῖς αὐτοῖς ὀνόμασι καὶ λόγοις τὸ ἐνεργείᾳ, ἢ δυνάμει, ἢ φαντασίᾳ γνώριμον ἐκ τῆς τάξεως· γέγραπται γοῦν ἀφωρισμένα καθ' ἕκαστον εἶδος ἢ γένος τὰ ὁμογενῆ, καὶ πρῶτα μὲν τὰ ἐνεργείᾳ, δεύτερον δὲ τὰ δυνάμει, τρίτον δὲ τὰ φαντασίᾳ, καθάπερ δίκαιον, ἢ διὰ τί ποτ' οὐ συγκέχυται ταῦτα· ἀλλ' ὡς γελοῖον ἴσως καὶ τὸ τῶν τοιούτων ἑτέραν πίστιν πειρᾶσθαι φέρειν, μὴ τὴν ἐκ τοῦ πράγματος: εἰ γὰρ οὕτως ἔχει καθάπερ ἡ τέχνη φησὶ δηλονότι καὶ γέγονε κατ' αὐτὴν, ὥσπερ ἡ ἰατρικὴ, τομήν τινα οὐκ ἂν τύχῃ οὐδὲ ταὐτόματα ἐργάσαιτο· ταῦτα μὲν οὖν ὑπὲρ τούτων ἱκανὰ πρὸς τὸ παρόν ἐστιν.

que in nomine neque in oratione neque actu neque potentia neque apparentia: praeter haec autem nihil ſermo oſtendit: ſecundum igitur ipſum definitum ſit in hunc modum: quod vero non ex ejus diviſione invenimus, non enim Ariſtotelis gratia nunc ſcribimus, ſed omnia haec methodo ſcripta ſunt, perſpicuum eſt: nam aut in nomine aut in oratione ipſum duplex eſſe oportere aperte ipſe dixit, cum dixit, quod ipſis nominibus et orationibus: ipſum vero actu eſſe aut potentia aut apparentia notum ex ipſo ordine eſt: ſcripta igitur ſeparatim ſunt in ſingulis generibus, quae ejusdem ſunt generis, primaque quae ad actum attinet: ſecunda quae ad potentiam: tertio loco quae ad apparentiam, ut decuit: aut cur haec non fuere confuſa? ſed fortaſſe ridiculum eſt his fidem aliam afferre conari, quam eam quae a re deducitur: etenim ſi ſic ſe habent, ut Ars, qualis Medicina eſt, artisque ſunt, diviſionem ullam fortuito aut caſu factam non reciperent. Sed de his ſatis haec in praeſenti ſint.

Κεφ. δ'. [Οἱ τῆς ἀμφιβολίας καὶ τῶν ἄλλων σοφισμάτων τρόποι.] Εἴρηται δέ τινα καὶ τοῖς Στωϊκοῖς περὶ τῶν τοῦ μέρους δικαίων ἐπελθοῦσιν ἰδεῖν, εἴ τις ἔξω πίπτει τρόπος εἶναι εἰρημένων. εἴη γὰρ ἐπαγωγή τις αὕτη πίστις καὶ δίκαιον ἄλλως, μηδεμίαν δόξαν ἀνδρῶν εὐδοκίμων πάρεργον τίθεσθαι· τὸν μὲν οὖν τῆς ἀμφιβολίας ὅρον, εἰ καὶ πρὸς πολλὰ τῶν ἡμετέρων μάχεσθαι δοκεῖ, τό γε νῦν ἐατέον, ἑτέρας γὰρ καὶ ὑπὲρ τούτων σκοπεῖν πραγματείας ἐστὶ, τὰς δὲ διαφορὰς τῶν λεγομένων ἀμφιβολιῶν αὐτὰς ληπτέον· εἰσί γε πρὸς τῶν χαριεστέρων λεγομένων τὸν ἀριθμὸν η'. μία μὲν, ἣν κοινὴν ὀνομάζουσι τοῦ τε εἰρημένου καὶ τοῦ διαιρετοῦ, οἷα ἐστὶν ἡ αὐλητρὶς παῖς οὖσα· κοινὴ γὰρ αὕτη τοῦ τε αὐλητρὶς ὀνόματος καὶ τοῦ εἰρημένου. δευτέρα δὲ, παρὰ τὴν ἐν τοῖς ἁπλῶς, οἷον ἀνδρεῖος, ἢ γὰρ χιτὼν, ἢ ἄνθρωπος. [78] τρίτη δὲ, παρὰ τὴν ἐν τοῖς συνθέτοις ὁμωνυμίαν, οἷον ἄνθρωπός ἐστιν, ἀμφίβολος γὰρ ὁ λόγος, εἴτε τὴν (34) οὐσίαν εἴτε τὴν πτῶσιν εἶναι σημαίνει.

Cap. IV. [*Ambiguitatis et reliquorum ſophismatum modi.*] Dictum quoque a ſtoicis aliquid eſt de partitionis dignitate, noſſe, ſi quis modus extra propoſitos cadat tentantibus: erit enim inductio fides haec. Et alias aequum eſt nullam probatorum virorum opinionem obiter ponere: ambiguitatis igitur definitionem, quanquam cum multis noſtris pugnare videtur, in praeſentia tamen praetermittemus: de his enim conſiderare alterius negotii eſt: quae vero ambiguitates dicuntur, harum differentiae ſumendae ſunt. Sunt quidem apud graviores viros numero octo. Una eſt, quam communem et ei quod dictum eſt et diviſibili nominant, qualis eſt, quae *αὐλητρὶς*, id eſt tibicina, puella exiſtens, communis enim haec et ipſius *αὐλητρὶς* nominis eſt atque ejus quod dictum eſt. Altera, quae in ſimplicibus eſt, ut virilis: aut enim tunica aut homo. Tertia vero ad ipſam in compoſitis aequivocationem attinet, ut homo eſt: ambiguus enim ſermo eſt, utrum ſubſtantiam an caſum eſſe ſignificat. Quarta ex deſectu eſt, ut tui

τετάρτη δέ ἐστι παρὰ τὴν ἔλλειψιν, ὡς ὅ ἐστί σου· καὶ γὰρ ἐλλείπει τὸ διὰ μέσου, οἷον δεσπότου, ἢ πατρός. πέμπτη δὲ παρὰ τὸν πλεονασμὸν, ὥσπερ ἡ τοιαύτη, ἀπηγόρευσεν αὐτῷ μὴ πλεῖν· τὸ γὰρ μὴ προσκείμενον ἀμφίδοξον ποιεῖ τὸ πᾶν εἴτε τὸ πλεῖν ἀπηγόρευσεν εἴτε τὸ μὴ πλεῖν. ἕκτην φασὶν εἶναι τὴν μηδὲν σαφοῦσαν τί μετὰ τίνος ἄσημον μόριον τέτακται, ὡς ἐν τῷ, καὶ νῦν καὶ μὴ παρήλασε. τὸ γὰρ στοιχεῖον ἂν μὴ γένοιτο διαζευκτικόν. ἑβδόμη δέ ἐστιν ἡ μὴ δηλοῦσα τί μετὰ τίνος τέτακται σημαντικὸν μόριον, ὡς ἐν τῷ

Πεντήκοντ' ἀνδρῶν ἑκατὸν λίπε δῖος Ἀχιλλεύς.

ογδόη ἡ μὴ δηλοῦσα τί ἐπὶ τί ἀναφέρεται, ὡς ἐν τῷ, Δίων Θέων ἐστίν· ἄδηλον γάρ ἐστιν εἴτε ἐπὶ τὴν ἀμφοτέρων ὕπαρξιν ἀναφέρεται, εἴτε ἐπὶ τοιοῦτον, οἷον ὁ Δίων Θέων ἐστὶν, ἢ πάλιν· οἱ μὲν δὴ τρόποι πρὸς τῶν χαριεστέρων οὗτοι κατηρίθμηνται. δῆλόν δέ γε, ὅστις μὴ παρέργως τῶν ἔμπροσθεν ἤκουσεν, ὅτι πάντες πίπτουσιν εἰς τοὺς

eft: deeft enim quod ad medium locum attinet, ut domini aut patris. Quinta ex fuperabundantia, quale eft, ei ut non navigaret denegavit: adjecta enim ea negatio, non, ambiguam orationem facit, utrum navigare negavit an non navigare. Sextam effe dicunt eam, quae haud notum facit, quae cum qua fignificatione carens pars ordinata fit, ut illud eft, et nunc et non appulit: pars enim ea non disjunctiva effe poteft. Septima eft, quae ignotum reliquit, quae cum qua fignificativa pars conftructa fit, quale eft:

Quinquaginta virum centenos liquit Achilles.

Octava eft, quae non declarat quid ad quid referatur, quale eft, Dion Theon eft: incertum enim eft utrum ad utriusque exiftentiam verbum, eft, referatur, an ad id, ut Dion fit Theon: aut contra. Hi funt a graviffimis viris numerati modi. Quicunque vero non obiter, quae fupra dicta funt audivit, manifeftum eft ei, eos omnes in hos cadere

κατειλεγμένους ὑφ' ἡμῶν τρόπους, τὸ δ' ἀμέθοδόν τε καὶ ἄτεχνον πρόδηλον· οὔτε γὰρ ἐκ τῶν εἰρημένων ἀπόδειξίν τις λάβοι τοῦ κατ' οὐδένα τρόπον ἕτερον ἀμφίβολόν τι δύνασθαι συστῆναι, τό τε κᾂν τοῖς πεπλεγμένοις ὁμωνυμίαν φάσκειν συμβαίνειν, παντελῶς οὐδ' ἀκουόντων ἐστὶν ὀνομάτων· πῶς δὲ οὐκ ἔστι ταῖς γενικαῖς διαφοραῖς εἰδικὰς καταριθμεῖσθαι, καθάπερ ἐπὶ τῶν τὴν διαίρεσιν ποιουσῶν ἀσήμαντον μόριον σημαῖνον διαιρούμεναι. λάβοι γὰρ ἂν οὕτως πλείους τὰς εἰδικὰς διαφοράς· ἔτι δ' ἂν τοῦτον τὸν τρόπον τὰς καὶ τῆς ὁμωνυμίας τις ποιήσειε πλείους εἰδικὰς λεγομένας διαφορὰς, ὅτι αὐτὸς παρὰ τὸ ἀπὸ τύχης, αἱ δὲ παρὰ τὴν ἀναλογίαν, ἢ ὁμοιότητα, ἢ ἄλλον τινὰ τρόπον συνίστανται· καὶ μὴν καὶ τῆς ἐν λόγῳ ὁμωνυμίας ἀπ' αὐτῶν λεγομένης πλείους οἱ τρόποι, οἱ μὲν γὰρ τῇ παραθέσει τῶν ὁμοίων πτώσεων γίγνονται, ὡς ἐν τῷ, εἴη μέλλει τὸν Σωκράτην νικῆσαι· οἱ δ' ἄλλοι τρόποι· ταῦτα μὲν ἐλάττω, ἐκεῖνο δ' ἄξιον ἀπορίας, πῶς τὰ περὶ τὰς φαντασίας διττὰ, πολὺ δὲ μᾶλλον ἔτι, πῶς τὰ τῆς προσῳδίας· οἱ γὰρ τιθέμενοι διτ-

modos, qui a nobis numerati ſunt: carereque methodo et arte perſpicuum eſt: neque enim ex iis, quae dicta ſunt, demonſtrationem quis ceperit, nullum alium modum ambiguum conſtitui poſſe: in connexisque aequivocationem contingere dicere, hominis eſt in nominis intelligentia parum verſati: non ineptum vero eſt generalibus differentiis ſpeciales enumerare, ut ea, quae ad diviſionem attinet, per partem ſignificatione carentem et per ſignificantem dividatur: ſic enim quis ſpeciales differentias plures acciperet: quin etiam ad hunc modum quis aequivocationis differentias ſpeciales dictas plures faceret: quia ille ſecundum id, quod a ſortuna: hae vero ſecundum analogiam aut ſimilitudinem, aut alium aliquem modum conſtituantur: quin et aequivocationis ejus, quam ipſi in oratione dicunt plures modi caſibus ſimilibus appoſitis fiunt, quale illud eſt, ſuturum eſt Socratem vincere: caeteri vero modi minores ſunt. Id vero dubitatione dignum eſt, quo modo quae ad apparentiam attinent duplicia ſunt: magisque

τοὺς τοὺς παρὰ τὴν θέσιν, πῶς οὐχὶ καὶ παρὰ τὴν προσῳδίαν; ὥσπερ γὰρ ἐκείνη τῇ διαλήψει τοῦ ὅλου καὶ τῇ μὲν σιωπῇ δύναται πρὸς τὸ διττὸν ἕλκεσθαι, οὕτω δὴ καὶ τὸ ὄνομα τῇ προσῳδίᾳ· καθάπερ ἔξωθεν ὂν ὁ κενὸς χρόνος τοῦ λόγου καὶ οὐ μόριον αὐτοῦ, διττὸν ποιεῖν αὐτὸν πέφυκεν, οὕτω δὴ καὶ ἡ προσῳδία· ἔτι δὲ καὶ οἱ σοφισταὶ καθάπερ ἐκείνῳ χρῶνται πρὸς τὰς ἔριδας καὶ τούτῳ· καὶ μὴν αὐτὸ ἄν τις ἐφ' ἑαυτοῦ σκοπούμενος, ὥσπερ ἂν παρὰ τὴν σύνθεσιν ἢ διαίρεσιν ἀμφισβητοῦσιν, οὕτω δὴ καὶ παρὰ τὴν προσῳδίαν· δῆλον δὲ ἐπὶ τῶν γεγραμμένων λόγων, οἷς μὴ πρόσκειται τὰ διακρίνοντα σημεῖα, δεῖται γὰρ ὥσπερ ἐκείνων εἰς τὴν διάκρισιν, οὕτω καὶ τῆς προσῳδίας, οὐκ ἀεί γε μὴν καὶ δι' αὐτὴν γένοιτο διττὸς ὁ λόγος.

quo modo quae ad accentum: qui enim ſecundum compoſitionem duplex ponunt, quo modo non ſecundum accentum? ut illa per continuationem totius et per ſilentium ad ipſum duplex trahi poteſt, ſic ipſum nomen per accentum: quemadmodum orationis extrinſecum, inane tempus cum ſit, nec ejus pars, eam tamen facere duplicem poteſt, ſic accentus quoque: itemque ſophiſtae ut illo, ſic hoc ad contentiones utuntur: et quis ſecum cogitans, quemadmodum ſecundum compoſitionem et diviſionem contendunt, ſic ſecundum etiam accentum idem fieri poſſe cognoscet. Manifeſtum vero in ſcriptis orationibus eſt, cum non adjecta ſunt dividentia puncta: ut enim his egent ad diviſionem, ſic accentu quoque, non ſemper tamen etiam propter hunc duplex oratio fuerit.

ΓΑΛΗΝΟΥ ΠΕΡΙ ΤΟΥ ΠΡΟΓΙΝΩΣΚΕΙΝ ΠΡΟΣ ΕΠΙΓΕΝΗΝ ΒΙΒΛΙΟΝ.

Ed. Chart. VIII. [829.] Ed. Baf. III. (451.)

[829] Κεφ. α'. Ὅσον μὲν ἐπὶ τοῖς πολλοῖς τῶν ἰατρῶν, ὦ Ἐπίγενες, ἀδύνατόν ἐστι προγινώσκειν τὰ τοῖς κάμνουσιν ἐσόμενα καθ' ἑκάστην νόσον. ἀφ' οὗ γὰρ οἱ τὸ δοκεῖν μᾶλλον ἢ εἶναι σπουδάσαντες οὐ κατὰ τὴν ἰατρικὴν μόνον, ἀλλὰ καὶ κατὰ τὰς ἄλλας τέχνας ἐπλεόνασαν, ἠμέληται μὲν τὰ κάλλιστα τῶν τεχνῶν, ἤσκηται δ' ἐξ ὧν

GALENI DE PRAENOTIONE AD POSTHUMUM LIBER.

Cap. I. Ut fane vulgus medicorum eft, o Pofthume, nemo poteft ea, quae aegris per fingulos morbos eveniunt, praenofcere. Ex quo enim ii, qui videri potius quam effe docti non in medica tantum, fed etiam aliis artibus ftuduerunt, numero vicere, optima quaeque artium neglecta funt: ea yero in ufu habita, unde aliquis fermone

ἄν τις εὐδοκιμήσειεν παρὰ τοῖς πολλοῖς, εἰπεῖν τι καὶ πρᾶξαι πρὸς ἡδονὴν, κολακεύεσθαι, θωπευτικῶς προσαγορεύειν ἑκάστης ἡμέρας, τοὺς πλουτοῦντάς τε καὶ δυναμένους ἐν ταῖς πόλεσι συμπροέρχεσθαι, παραπέμπειν προερχομένους οἴκαδε, δορυφορεῖν ἐν τοῖς δείπνοις, βωμολοχεύεσθαι. τινὲς δ᾽ αὐτῶν οὐ ταῦτα μόνον, ἀλλὰ καὶ τῇ τῶν ἱματίων καὶ δακτυλίων πολυτελείᾳ καὶ τῷ πλήθει τῶν ἀκολουθούντων καὶ σκευῶν ἀργυρῶν παρασκευῇ τοὺς ἰδιώτας ἀναπείθουσιν, ὡς ἀξιοζήλωτοί τινες ὄντες. ἐκ τούτων οὖν ἁπάντων τὰ μὲν ἥδοντες, τὰ δ᾽ ἐκπλήττοντες ἀνθρώπους ἀπείρους ἀληθινῆς κρίσεως πραγμάτων, ὡς μὲν οὗτοι νομίζουσιν, ἀγαθῶν πολλῶν τυγχάνουσιν, ὡς δ᾽ ἐγὼ φαίην ἂν οὕτως ὄντων ἀγαθῶν ἄλλων, αὐτοὶ ψευδῆ ὑπειλήφασιν. ἅτε δ᾽ ὄντες τοιοῦτοι, τἄλλα παρανομεῖν οὐκ ὀκνοῦσιν, ἐλαχίστῳ τε χρόνῳ τὰς τέχνας ἐπαγγελλόμενοι διδάσκειν ἀθροίζουσι πλῆθος μαθητῶν, ἐξ ὧν καὶ αὐτοὶ προσλαμβάνουσι τὸ δύνασθαι κατὰ τὰς πόλεις, ἐν αἷς διατρίβουσιν. αὕτη μὲν οὖν κοινὴ τῶν τεχνῶν ἁπασῶν δυστυχία κατείληφε τὸν νῦν βίον. ἡ δὲ τῆς

hominum celebretur; nempe apud vulgus dicere aliquid et facere ad gratiam: item adulari blande, opulentos ac potentes in civitatibus quotidie ſalutare et ſimul cum eis incedere ac domum redeuntes deducere, in coenis latus eorum cingere et ſcurriliter nugari. Quidam ipſorum non haec modo, ſed etiam veſtium et annulorum ſumptu, comitum multitudine et vaſorum argenteorum apparatu idiotis perſuadent, magni ſe pretii eſſe homines et imitatione dignos. Ex his igitur omnibus partim allicientes partim attonitos reddentes homines veri in rebus judicii imperitos, ut quidem hi exiſtimant, multis bonis fruuntur: ut autem ego dixerim, quum vere bona non ſint, ipſi falſo opinantur. Quum itaque tales exiſtant, praeter alia contra leges facere non dubitant breviſſimoque tempore artes ſe docturos polliciti complures diſcipulos comparant, a quibus etiam ipſi poteſtatem in civitatibus, in quibus degunt, accipiunt. Haec igitur communis omnium artium infelicitas praeſentem vitam occupavit. Medicinae autem

ἰατρικῆς ἐστι μὲν πολυειδὴς, ἀλλ' ἕν τι τῶν κατ' αὐτὴν ἔγνωκα προχειρίσασθαι τῶν ἐμοὶ μάλιστα διαφερόντων. ὅταν γάρ τις ἰατρὸς τῷ νόμῳ μεμαθηκότων αὐτὴν, ἢ παραφροσύνην ἐσομένην ἐπινοσοῦντος, ἢ ῥῖγος, ἢ καταφορὰν, ἢ αἱμοῤῥαγίας, ἢ παρωτίδας, ἢ ἀπόστασιν ἄλλην ἐς ὁτιοῦν μέρος, ἢ ἔμετον, ἢ ἱδρῶτας, ἢ κοιλίαν ταραχθησομένην, [830] ἢ συγκοπὴν, ἤ τι τῶν τοιούτων προείπῃ ἄλλο, ξένον τε καὶ τέρας τοῖς ἰδιώταις ὑπ' ἀηθείας φαίνεται καὶ τοσοῦτον ἀποδεῖ τοῦ θαυμάζεσθαι παρ' αὐτοῖς ὁ προειπὼν, ὥστε ἀγαπήσειεν ἂν, εἰ μὴ καὶ γόης τις εἶναι δόξειεν. ὀλίγοι δέ τινες αὐτῶν οὐκ ἀπογινώσκουσι μὲν, ὡς ἀδυνάτου τῆς τοιαύτης θεωρίας· ἐρωτῶσι δ' εὐθέως καὶ αὐτὸν τὸν προειπόντα καὶ τοὺς ἄλλους ἰατροὺς, εἰ καὶ τοῖς ἔμπροσθεν εὕρηταί τι τοιοῦτον, ἢ μόνον αὐτοῦ τοῦ προειπόντος ἐστὶν εὕρημα. τοὐντεῦθεν οὖν ἀναγκαῖον γίγνεται τοὺς μὲν ἰατροὺς ἀποκρυπτομένους σφετέραν ἀμαθείαν, ἴσως δέ τινας καὶ ὄντως ἀγνοοῦντας, οὐδενὶ φάναι τῶν ἔμπροσθεν οὐδὲν

varia quidem eſt, ſed unum aliquod ex iis, quae in illa accidunt, ſtatui promere, ut quod ad me potiſſimum pertineat. Quando enim medicus aliquis ex iis, qui legitime eam didicerunt, aut delirium futurum in aegrotante, aut rigorem, aut cataphoram, aut ſanguinis profluvium, aut parotidas, aut abſceſſum aliquem in quacunque parte, aut vomitum, aut ſudorem, aut alvi perturbationem, aut ſyncopen, aut aliud quid hujusmodi praedixerit, et peregrinum et monſtrum prae diſſuetudine idiotis apparet: ac tantum abeſt, ut qui praedixerit in admirationem apud illos veniat, ut bene actum ſecum putaverit, ſi non etiam praeſtigiator aliquis eſſe videatur. Pauci autem quidam ipſorum hujusmodi ſpeculationem non damnant quidem, ceu quae haberi nequeat: ſed interrogant ſtatim et ipſum, qui praedixit et alios medicos, num etiam tale quid a majoribus inventum ſit, an ſolum ipſius praedicentis ſit inventio? Hinc itaque neceſſarium eſt quosdam ſane medicos inſcitiam ſuam occultantes, forſan autem nonnul-

τοιοῦτο γεγράφθαι, γόητα δ' εἶναι τὸν ἐπιδεικνύμενον τοιαύτην πρόῤῥησιν. αὐτὸν δὲ τὸν προειπόντα, μήθ' ὅτι γέγραπται πολλοῖς τῶν ἔμπροσθεν καὶ μάλιστα τῷ Ἱπποκράτει, τῷ πάντων ἡμῖν τῶν καλῶν ἡγεμόνι, τολμᾷν εἰπεῖν αἰδοῖ τε ἅμα τῶν παρόντων ἰατρῶν καὶ μίσους ὑποψίᾳ, μήθ' ὡς αὐτὸς εὑρηκὼς εἴη, ψεύδεσθαι γὰρ οὕτως καὶ μᾶλλον μισηθήσεσθαι πρὸς αὐτῶν. ἄπορον δὴ πανταχόθεν ἐρώτημά τις ὑπεχόμενος, ὀκνῶν οἶμαι καὶ διαβουλευόμενος, αὐξάνει μὲν τὴν τῆς γοητείας ὑποψίαν αὐτῷ τῷ μέλλειν ἀεὶ, τελευταῖον δὲ φθόνον ὑπ' ἑαυτὸν ἤγειρεν, ὥστ' ἐπιβουλεύεσθαι πρὸς αὐτῶν. πρώτη μέντοι τῆς φαρμακείας ἐνέδρα· δευτέρα δὲ ᾗ Κόϊντος ἥλω, βελτίων μὲν ὢν ἰατρὸς τῶν καθ' ἑαυτὸν, ἐκβληθεὶς δὲ τῆς πόλεως, ὡς ἀναιρῶν τοὺς νοσοῦντας, ὥστε δυοῖν θάτερον ἀναγκαῖον γίνεται παθεῖν τὸν φιλοσόφως τὴν τέχνην μετιόντα καὶ τῶν Ἀσκληπιαδῶν ἀξίως ἢ παραπλησίως Κοΐντῳ φαγαδευθέντων, λαμπρὰ τῆς αἰσθήσεως τὰ ἐπίχειρα κομίσασθαι ἢ διαβαλλόμενόν γε φα-

los etiam vere ignorantes, dicere, a nullo majorum tale quid esse proditum: sed praestigiatorem esse, qui hujusmodi praedictionem ostendit. Ipse vero praedicens neque quod a pluribus majoribus scriptum sit et praesertim ab Hippocrate, omnium nobis bonorum auctore et duce, audet fateri, metu simul praesentium medicorum et odii suspicione, neque quod ipse invenerit: mentiretur enim ita et magis odio ab ipsis haberetur. Quaestionem itaque sustinens, ad quam quid prorsus respondere debeat, ambigit, si detrectet et deliberandum censeat, meo judicio augebit sane praestigii suspicionem in futurum: postremo autem invidiam in se concitabit, ut insidias ab iis experiatur: primum sane per pharmaca, deinde quibus Quintus captus fuerat, praestantissimus quidem sui temporis medicorum, urbe autem ejectus, tanquam aegrotantes interimeret. Quare necesse est ut ei, qui artem philosophice et ut Asclepiadis dignum est exercet, alterutrum contingat, aut ut Quinto similiter in exilium relegatus praeclara sensus praemia reportet: aut calumnias sustinens

νερῶς, εἰ μὲν ἀτολμηρότερος εἴη, τὰ δὲ ἀπολογούμενον, τὰ δὲ ὑποπτήσσοντα, λαγῶ βίον ζῆν, ἀεὶ τρέμοντα καὶ τί πείσεσθαι προσδοκῶντα, πρὸς τῷ καὶ τὴν τῆς γοητείας ὑποψίαν αὐξάνειν. εἰ δ' εὐτονώτερος ὢν ὁμόσε χωρεῖ καὶ διαμάχεται μόνος πολλοῖς πανούργοις ἀνθρώποις καὶ πολλοὺς ἀδοκιμωτάτους τρόπους ἠσκηκόσιν αὐτὸς ἐκ παιδείας καὶ μαθημάτων ὁρμώμενος καὶ τῶν τοιούτων ἄπειρος κακῶν, ἤτοι κατὰ κράτος ἁλόντα, γενέσθαι τὸ λοιπὸν ἐπ' ἐκείνοις, ὅ τι ἂν αὐτῷ χρῆσθαι βουληθῶσιν, ἢ εἴπερ ἐπὶ πλέον ἀντέχοι καὶ διαγωνίζοιτο, τύχῃ τινὶ χρησάμενος θαυμαστῇ. τὸ μὲν οὖν ἀεὶ πολεμεῖν τε καὶ πολεμεῖσθαι τὸν χείριστον τῶν πολέμων, ὃν ὀνομάζουσιν ἐμφύλιον, ἐκφεύγειν μὴ δύνασθαι. συμβαίνειν οὖν ἀναγκαῖον πολλοῖς τῶν οὕτως παρεσκευασμένων καὶ τῶν ἄλλων ὅσοι τετιμήκασιν ἀλήθειαν εἰλικρινῶς, οὐ διά τι τῶν ἔξωθεν, ἀλλ' αὐτὴν δι' ἑαυτῆς, ὅταν ἅπαξ πειραθῶσι τῆς κατεχούσης τὸν νῦν βίον ἀδικίας καὶ γνῶσι σαφῶς, οἷς οὐδὲν ἔσονται τοῖς ἀνθρώποις ὄφελος, ἐξαναχωρεῖν τοῦ τῶν πολλῶν συρφετοῦ καὶ ὥσπερ χειμῶνι μεγάλῳ

et manifefto, fiquidem timidior fuerit, partim refpondens partim fubticens leporis vitam degat, femper tremens et ut patiatur aliquid exfpectans, praeterquam quod praeftigii fufpicionem augeat. Sin autem animofior cominus procedat folusque cum multis verfutis hominibus ac in plerisque improbatiffimis fraudum generibus exercitatis decertet, ipfe eruditione et difciplinis fretus ac talium malignitatum imperitus vel omnino victus obtemperet in pofterum ad omnia illa, in quibus illo uti voluerint: et fi diutius refiftat certetque, mirabili quadam fortuna ufus femper certe bellum longe deterrimum, quod inteftinum nominant, gerere cogetur, cum effugere non poffit. Accidet igitur neceffario, multos ita fraudibus oppreffos et alios qui veritatem fincere non propter aliquod exterius, fed ipfam propter fe honorant, ubi femel iniquitatem praefentis feculi fuerint experti noverintque manifefto, quam nulli fint mortalium commodo futuri, ex vulgi confortio difcedere, tanquam in tempeftate magna et agita-

καὶ ζάλη πνευμάτων, ἑαυτοὺς γοῦν σῶσαι σπεύδοντας. οὗτοι δὲ τοῖς πολλοῖς μὲν ἄγνωστοι, γνώριμοι δὲ καὶ φίλοι μάλιστα μὲν καὶ πρῶτον θεοῖς, εἶτα τῶν ἀνθρώπων τοῖς ἀρίστοις ἐν ἡσυχίᾳ βιοῦσιν, ἐπιτρέψαντες τοῖς πανούργοις εὐδοκιμεῖν παρὰ τοῖς πολλοῖς ἀνθρώποις. ἁπάντων δὲ τούτων τὰ αἴτια τοῖς ἀνθρώποις ἐστὶ, τῶν πλουτούντων ἐν ταῖς πόλεσι καὶ δυναμένων ἡ τρυφή. οἱ περαιτέρω ἡδονὴν ἀρετῆς τετιμηκότες ἐν οὐδενὶ λόγῳ τίθενται τούς τι καλὸν ἐγνωκότας, τοῖς δὲ ἄλλοις ὑφηγήσασθαι δυναμένους. ὅλοι δ' ἐπὶ τοῖς τὰς ἡδονὰς ἐκπορίζουσίν εἰσι καὶ τούτους πλουτίζουσι καὶ θαυμάζουσι καὶ ὑψηλοὺς αἴρουσιν, ὥστε τῶν μὲν ὀρχηστῶν καὶ τῶν ἡνιόχων εἴκονας ποιοῦνται, τοῖς τῶν θεῶν ἀγάλμασι συνέδρους. [831] τοὺς δ' ἀπὸ τῶν μαθημάτων τοσαῦτα τιμῶσιν, ὅσα τῆς χρείας αὐτῶν δέονται. τὸ γὰρ ἐν ἑκάστῳ καλὸν οὐ θεωροῦσιν, οὔτε τῶν δεινῶν αὐτῶν ἀνέχονται, ἀλλὰ γεωμετρίας μὲν καὶ ἀριθμητικῆς ὅσον εἰς ἀναλωμάτων λογισμοὺς καὶ οἰκίας κατασκευὴν, ἀστρονομίας δὲ καὶ μαντικῆς ὅσον εἰς τὸ προγνῶναι τίνων κλη-

tione ventorum fe ipfos faltem fervare conantes. Hi fane vulgo quidem incogniti, noti vero et amici maxime quidem et primum diis ipfis, deinde hominum praeftantiffimis in quiete vitam agentibus, permittentes fraudulentis iftis gloriam apud vulgus aucupari et inclarefcere. Omnium horum caufa hominibus divitum in urbibus et potentum deliciae exiftant; qui voluptatem virtuti praeponentes in nullo honore habent eos, qui aliquid honefti noverunt quique alios docere quid poffunt. Toti autem illis dediti funt, qui voluptates fuppeditant, hos ditant, hos admirantur et in coelum efferunt, nec non hiftrionum et adulatorum imagines deorum ftatuis affeclas conftituunt eruditos autem tanti faciunt, quantum opera ipforum indigent. Nam in unoquoque honeftum non refpiciunt, neque peritos ipfos fuftinent, fed geometriam quidem et arithmeticen, quantum ad impenfarum rationem et domus conftructionem attinet, aftronomiam vero et divinatoriam, quantum ad praenofcendum quorum heredes futuri

ρονομήσουσι χρήζουσιν, ὥσπερ γε καὶ μουσικῆς· ὅσον εἰς ἡδονὴν ἀκοῆς. τὴν δὲ τούτων συμπάντων τὸ κῦρος ἔχουσαν φιλοσοφίαν, ἀποδεικτικῆς θεωρίας οὐδὲν αὐτοῖς μέλει, πλὴν ὅσον ἡ χρεία προσάγει τινὰς τῶν ῥητορικῶν ἀνδρῶν, ὀργάνῳ πανούργῳ, τῇ σοφιστικῇ καλουμένῃ χρῆσθαι θεωρίᾳ. φιλοσοφίας γὰρ αὐτῆς οὐδὲν ἐπαΐουσιν, ἀλλὰ πάντων (452) μαθημάτων ἀχρηστότατον τοῦτο νενομίκασιν ὁμοίως τῷ κέγχρον τρυπᾷν. οὗτοι τοίνυν εἰσὶν οἳ καὶ τῆς ἰατρικῆς τὴν ἀναγκαίαν χρείαν ὁρῶσι μόνην, οὐδὲ ταύτην ὀρθῶς. ἀλλ' ὡς Πλάτων πού φησιν, εἰ δέοι κρίνεσθαι παρὰ παισὶν, ἢ ἀνθρώποις ἄφροσιν ἰατρὸν καὶ μάγειρον, ὁ μάγειρος ἂν οὐκ ὀλίγῳ δή τινι πλέον ἐνέγκαιτο.

Κεφ. β'. Ταῦτ' οὖν ἐγὼ ἀγνοῶν, κατὰ τὴν προτέραν ἐπιδημίαν ἐν Ῥώμῃ μοι γενομένην οὐδὲν ὑφορώμενος ἐπεδεικνύμην οὐ διὰ λόγων ψιλῶν, ἀλλὰ τοῖς ἔργοις τάς τε τῶν ἐσομένων προγνώσεις καὶ τὰς θεραπείας ἄχρι τοῦ γενέσθαι τι τοιοῦτον, ὡς ἐπίστασαι σὺ ὁ μάλιστα παρὼν τῇ νόσῳ πάσῃ, μέχρι τέλους ἀπ' ἀρχῆς Εὐδήμου τοῦ περιπα-

ſint opus eſt, uſurpant; quemadmodum et muſicen, quatenus auditum oblectare velint. Philoſophiae autem, quae horum omnium praecipuum continet, demonſtratoriae ſpeculationis nullam habent rationem, niſi quantum uſus cogit, quosdam rhetoricorum virorum inſtrumento ſubdito ſophiſtica dicta ſpeculatione uti. Philoſophiae enim ipſius nulla mentio, ſed omnium diſciplinarum inutiliſſimam hanc inſtar milii perſorati arbitrantur. Hi igitur ſunt, qui etiam medicinae uſum neceſſarium vident duntaxat, neque hunc recte, ſed, ut Plato alibi dicit, ſi de medico et coquo a puero aut ſtultis hominibus ſententia ferri debeat, coquus utique non paulo plus laudis reportabit.

Cap. II. Haec igitur ego ignorans in priori meo Romam adventu nihilque ſuſpicans indicavi non verbis nudis, ſed operibus futurorum praenotionem curationemque; donec tale quippiam accideret, ut tu noviſti, qui potiſſimum per totius morbi Eudemi peripatetici philoſophi

τητικοῦ φιλοσόφου. ἤρξατο μὲν γὰρ ἡμέρᾳ τινι μετὰ λουτρὸν ἀνωμαλία τις αὐτῷ, φρίκη δ' ἀπὸ ὥρας ὀγδόης, δι' ἧς ἀναγκασθεὶς ἀσιτῆσαι, κατὰ τὴν ὑστεραίαν ἀμέμπτως διάγων ὑπέλαβεν ἀσφαλέστερον εἶναι τὴν ὀγδόην ὥραν ὑπερβάλλειν. ὡς δ' οὐ κατ' αὐτὴν ἀπήντησέ τι δυσχερὲς ἀντήσαντί γε μέχρι τῆς ἐνάτης καὶ πρόσω οὐδεμία παραλλαγή τις ἐφαίνετο, λουσάμενός τε καὶ βραχέα προσενεγκάμενος ἐπὶ τῇ τρίτῃ ἡμέρᾳ συνεγένετο μὲν, ὡς ἔθος, ἡμῖν. ἀσφαλείας δ' ἕνεκεν ἔδοξεν αὐτῷ καὶ κατ' ἐκείνην ὑπερβάλλειν τὰς ὑπόπτους ὥρας. ἐλούσατο οὖν μετὰ τὴν ὀγδόην καὶ τραφεὶς εὐφόρως ἐπέπειστο μηδὲν αὐτῷ γενήσεσθαι δυσχερές. ἐν τῇ τετάρτῃ δὲ τῶν ἡμερῶν, ἐν ᾗ συγγενόμενος ἡμῖν ἐπὶ τὸ βαλανεῖον ἐστέλλετο, μειδιάσας τε ἅμα καὶ ἀποβλέψας πρός σε, πότερα, ἔφη, καὶ κατὰ τήνδε τὴν ἡμέραν τετάρτην οὖσαν ἀσφαλέστερόν ἐστιν ὑπερβάλλειν τὴν ὀγδόην ὥραν ἢ τῷ λουτρῷ χρηστέον ἤδη; σὺ μὲν οὖν, ὡς οὐδενὸς ἐσομένου δυσχεροῦς, ἐκέλευσας ἐπιέναι λουσόμενον, οἵ τ' ἄλλοι πάντες οἱ παρόντες, ἐγὼ δ' ἐσιώπων μόνος. ἐρομένῳ

curriculum adfuifti. Itaque die quodam nonnulla ipfum invafit inaequalitas, horror autem ab hora octava; propter quem a cibo abftinere coactus, poftridie inculpate agens, putavit tutius effe eum poft octavam horam differre. Quum autem nihil eadem hora moleftum occurreret inedia ufo usque ad nonam, ac ulterius nulla permutatio appareret, lotus et modico cibo affumpto tertio die pro confuetudine nobiscum verfabatur. Securitatis autem gratia vifum ei eft etiam in illo die cibum poft horas fufpectas differre. Lavit itaque poft octavam et cibo affumpto levi credidit nihil ei moleftum acceffurum. Quarto die, quo nobiscum verfatus ad balneum difceffit, ridens fimul et refpiciens te: utrum, inquit, in hoc quarto die tutius eft octavam horam inedia excedere, an balneo utendum jam eft? Tu igitur tanquam nihil molefti futurum effet, lavacrum accedere juffifti aliique omnes qui aderant, ego autem folus fubticebam. Roganti vero ipfi cur

δέ αὐτῷ περὶ τῆς σιωπῆς ἀπεκρινάμην οὐκ εἶναί μοι τελέως ἀνύποπτον ἀρχὴν γεγονέναι τεταρταίας περιόδου κατὰ τὴν πρώτην ἡμέραν, ἡνίκα με τὸν σφυγμὸν ἐκέλευσας ἅψασθαι. τὸ δὲ μὴ προεγνωκέναι μέ ποτε τὸν κατὰ φύσιν σου σφυγμὸν ὁποῖός τις ἦν, οὗ χωρὶς οὐχ οἷόν τε τὰς βραχείας αὐτοῦ μεταβολὰς εἰς τὸ παρὰ φύσιν ἐπιγνῶναι, σαφῶς οὐδὲν ἀπεφηνάμην, ὥσπερ οὐδὲ νῦν πλέον ἔχω τι τῆς τότε μοι γενομένης ὑποψίας εἰπεῖν. ἐλούσατό τε οὖν εὐφόρως καὶ ἐτράφη μετρίως, εἶτα περὶ τὴν ἑσπέραν μετακαλεσάμενός με καὶ πάλιν τὸν σφυγμὸν αὐτοῦ κελεύσας ἅψασθαι, τὴν αὐτὴν ἀπόφασιν ἤκουσεν ἣν πρὸ τοῦ λουτροῦ, [832] καὶ μᾶλλον ἔτι θαῤῥαλεώτερον, ἢ τότε. διὰ τοῦτο οὖν ἔδοξε τὴν ἑξῆς ἡμέραν, ἑβδόμην μὲν ἀπὸ τῆς ἀρχῆς ἐσομένην, τετάρτην δὲ ἀπ᾽ ἐκείνης, ἀκριβέστερον παραφυλάξαι καὶ διατρίψας ἐπὶ τῆς οἰκίας ἐλούσατό τε καὶ σιτίων προσηνέγκατο πλειόνων, ὡς οἶσθα, τελέως ἀπύρετον αὐτὸν εἶναι φάντων. ἐγὼ μὲν οὖν ἐρομένῳ σοι, μέμνησαι γὰρ πάντως καὶ τοῦτο, τὴν ὑποψίαν μοι νῦν φήσας, ὡς μικροτάτης τινὸς αὐτῷ τε-

tacerem, refpondi, non omnino me citra fufpicionem effe, initium quarti circuitus fecundum primi diei rationem, quo me pulfum tangere juffifti, accidiffe. Quum autem praenoviffem naturalem tuum pulfum qualis erat, fine quo non licet exiguas ipfius mutationes in ftatum praeter naturam deprehendere, manifefto nihil pronuntiavi; quemadmodum neque nunc magis poffum aliquid de fufpicione tunc mihi oborta proferre. Lavit igitur ex facili et mediocriter nutritus eft. Deinde cum circa vefperam vocaffet me ac rurfus pulfum ejus tangere juffiffet, idem quod ante balneum pronuntiavi audivit, ac magis adhuc confidentius quam tunc. Iccirco vifum eft fequentem diem, qui feptimus ab initio futurus erat, quartus autem ab illo, exactius obfervare: ac cum domi fuiffet commoratus, lavit cibosque affumpfit, quum plures, ut nofti, omnino absque febri ipfum effe dicerent. Ego igitur quaerenti tibi, meminifti enim omnino et hoc, fufpicionem mihi nunc effe

ταρταίας περιόδου προοίμιον εἴη συμβαῖνον. ἐχωρίσθην ἔχων ἐπισκοπεῖσθαί τινα περὶ τὴν ἑσπέραν ἄῤῥωστον οὐκ ἐγγὺς οἰκοῦντα. λουσάμενος δ' Εὔδημος ἐτράφη μὲν εὐθέως, οὐ μετὰ πολὺ δὲ θερμασίας ἤσθετο δι' ὅλου τοῦ σώματος, ἣν ἐν τῷ ποθέντι πόματι γεγονέναι νομίσας. οἴνου γὰρ παλαιοῦ προσηνέγκατο κατὰ τὴν ὑστεραίαν αὐτὸ τοῦτο διηγήσατο τοῖς συνήθεσιν ἰατροῖς, αἰτιασαμένων τε κᾀκείνων ἑτοίμως τὸν οἶνον, οὐδὲν ἔτι νομίσας ἔσεσθαι δυσχερὲς ἐν τῇ τετάρτῃ μετὰ τὴν γενομένην θερμασίαν, ἐλούσατό τε καὶ διῃτήθη τῷ συνήθει τρόπῳ, σαφῶς δὲ πυρέττειν ἀρξάμενος, ἐπείσθη τεταρταίου μὲν εἶναι περίοδον. ἐπῄνει δὲ τοὐντεῦθεν ἐμὲ μόνον, ὡς ἀκριβῶς ἁπτόμενον σφυγμοῦ κατὰ τὸν ἔμπροσθεν χρόνον, ἐν φιλοσοφίας θεωρίᾳ μόνῃ πεπεισμένος ἀξιόλογον ἕξιν εἶναί μοι, τῶν δὲ κατὰ τὴν ἰατρικὴν ἐν παρέργῳ πεφροντικέναι. καὶ γὰρ ἐπέπειστο τοῦ πατρὸς ἐπὶ φιλοσοφίαν ἄγοντός με, προσταχθὲν αὐτῷ δι' ὀνείρων ἐναργῶν, ἐκδιδάξαι καὶ τὰ τῆς ἰατρικῆς, οὐχ ὡς πάρεργόν τι μάθημα τοῦτο. συνέβη μοι γεγονέναι τότε κατά τινα τύχην,

dixi, minimae fcilicet cujusdam quartanae circuitionis initium ei oboriri. Difceffi igitur vifitaturus quendam circa vefperam aegrotum non prope habitantem. Interim lavatus Eudemus ftatim quendam cibum fumpfit, non multo poft calorem per totum corpus fenfit, quem ex potu haufto proveniffe ratus, vinum enim vetus poftridie affumpferat, hoc ipfum confuetis medicis recenfuit: quumque et illi ftatim vinum caufarentur, nihil hic adhuc molefti in quarto die poft calorem obortum fore ratus, lavit et confueto more cibo ufus eft, manifefto autem febricitare orfus, perfuafum habuit quartanae effe circuitum. Me vero folum inde commendavit, tanquam exacte pulfum priore tempore tangentem, perfuafus mihi foli habitum effe in philofophica fpeculatione mentione dignum, medicinae vero obiter rationem habuiffe. Etenim audierat quum pater me ad philofophiam duceret, injunctam ei per fomnia evidentia, ut me medicinam edoceret, non ut fuperfluam quandam difciplinam mihi futuram. Con-

ὡς οἶσθα καὶ αὐτὸς, νενοσηκότος τινὸς ἀνθρώπου κατὰ τὴν ἀρχὴν τοῦ φθινοπώρου νόσον ὀξεῖαν, εἶτα κατὰ τὴν ἀνάληψιν, ἀρξαμένου περὶ πέμπτην ὥραν πυρέττειν, θεασάμενον τὸν ἄνθρωπον ἀποφήνασθαί σοι παρόντι σαφεστάτην εἰσβολὴν εἶναι τεταρταίου περιόδου. ὁπότε γὰρ κατὰ τὴν ἀναλογίαν ἡ διὰ τὴν τετάρτην ἀνταπόδοσις ἐγένετο, πυθόμενος παρὰ σοῦ τὴν γενομένην πρόῤῥησιν ὁ Εὔδημος, ἔτι μᾶλλον ἐπείσθη προσέχειν ἐμοί· ὥστε ἐπειδὰν προύβαινεν ὁ κατὰ τὴν περίοδον παροξυσμὸς εἰς μέγεθος, ἀθροίσας τοὺς ἀρίστους τῶν κατὰ τὴν πόλιν ἰατρῶν ἠξίωσε σκέψασθαι περὶ τῆς θεραπείας τοῦ νοσήματος. ἐγὼ δὲ ἑκὼν ἀπελείφθην, οὐ βουλόμενος ἁμιλλᾶσθαι διὰ λόγων αὐτοῖς. ὡς δὲ τοῖς ἐνδοξοτάτοις αὐτῶν ἔδοξε τῆς θηριακῆς αὐτὸν πιεῖν, ἕωθεν ἐκείνῃ τῶν ἡμερῶν, ἐν ᾗ προσδοκώμενος ἦν ὁ διὰ τῆς τετάρτης παροξυσμὸς ἔσεσθαι, χωρισθέντων αὐτῶν, ὡς οἶσθα, σοῦ παρόντος, ἐπυνθάνετό μου τίνα τὴν ἐλπίδα τῆς τοῦ φαρμάκου χρήσεως ἔχοιμι. γινώσκεις οὖν ὅπως ἀπεκρινάμην αὐτῷ μηδὲν ἀμφιβάλλων ὡς οὐ μόνον οὐδὲν ὀνήσει τὸ φάρ-

tigit etiam tunc forte fortuna, ut novifti et ipfe, laborante quodam homine per initia autumni morbo acuto, deinde per tempus refectionis, circa horam quintam febricitare exorfo, pronuntiaffe me tibi praefenti, quum hominem illum vidiffem, manifeftiffimum effe quartani circuitus infultum. Quum enim juxta proportionem per quartum diem repetitio fieret, Eudemus factam praedictionem abs te audiens multo magis attendere mihi perfuafus eft; quare cum fecundum circuitum acceffio in magnitudinem procederet, convocatis praeftantiffimis quibusque urbis medicis de morbi curatione confiderandum cenfuit. Ego autem fponte relictus fum, ut qui nollem verbis cum ipfis contendere. Quum vero celeberrimis ipforum theriacen aegro propinare vifum effet mane eo die, quo acceffio quarto repetens futura exfpectaretur; digreffis illis, ut nofti, te praefente interrogabat me quam fpem de medicamenti ufu haberem. Nofti igitur quomodo ei refponderim, nihil ambigens, medicamentum fcilicet non

μακον, ἀλλὰ καὶ διπλοῦν ἐργάσεται τὸν τεταρταῖον. καὶ τὴν γ' αἰτίαν ἐρωτήσαντος αὐτοῦ, δι' ἣν οὕτως ἀπεκρινάμην, ἄπεπτον ἔφην ἔτι εἶναι τὸ νόσημα, τό τε φάρμακον τοῦτο κακοχυμίαν ἄπεπτον καὶ μάλιστα ἐν χειμῶνος ἀρχῇ, μέχρι μὲν τοῦ ταράξαι δύνασθαι προσαγαγεῖν, οὐ μὴν οὔτε πέψαι τελέως οὔτε διαφορῆσαι. ταῦτα μὲν οὖν ἀπεκρινάμην ἐγὼ τῷ Εὐδήμῳ. κατὰ δὲ τὴν ὑστεραίαν ἕωθεν ἀφικόμενοι πρὸς αὐτὸν, οὐδέπω παρόντων ἡμῶν, ἔδοσαν τὸ φάρμακον αἰδεσθέντος διηγήσασθαι τὰ ὑπ' ἐμοῦ λεγόμενα αὐτῷ καὶ ἅμα θεασάμενος μετ' ἐνστάσεως, ὡς ὑποσχομένους τοὺς ἀφικνουμένους ἰατροὺς ἅπαντας, ὀνήσειν αὐτὸν οὐ σμικρὰ τὴν τοῦ φαρμάκου προσφοράν. γενομένου δὲ τοῦ παροξυσμοῦ κατὰ τὴν αὐτὴν ὥραν, ἐνίοτε συμβαίνειν οὕτως ἔφασαν ἐπὶ τῆς πρώτης πόσεως, ὡς κινεῖσθαι καὶ μοχλεύεσθαι τὸ νόσημα. [833] δεύτερον δὲ πιόντα ἀπαλλάττεσθαι τελέως, εἰ κατὰ τὴν ἡμέραν, ἐν ᾗ προσδοκᾶται γενησόμενος ὁ διὰ τετάρτης παροξυσμὸς, ὁμοίως ἕωθεν αὐτοῦ προσενέγκαιτο. ἐκεῖνοι μὲν οὖν οὕτως εἰπόντες ἐχωρίσθησαν εὐέλπιδες. οὐ

modo nihil praefidii illaturum, fed etiam duplicem effecturum quartanam. Ac quum ipfe caufam quaereret cur ita refponderem, crudum adhuc effe morbum dixi; ac medicamentum hoc adhiberi, quatenus vitiofum humorem crudum, praefertim per hiemis initia, perturbare poffit, non tamen vel perfecte concoquere vel difcutere. Haec igitur ego Eudemo refpondi. Subfequenti die mane venientes ad ipfum medici, nobis nondum praefentibus, medicamentum propinarunt reverito narrare eis, quae ego ipfi dixeram: ut qui fimul omnes medicos difcedentes confidenter promittere videret, medicamentum affumtum non parum ipfi profuturum. Quum autem eadem hora acceffio invaderet, dicebant ita nonnunquam accidere in prima potione, ut morbus moveretur agitareturque, fecundo autem potu in totum difcuti, fi die, quo acceffio quarto repetens futura expectatur, fimiliter mane ex eo affumeret. Illi quidem ita locuti cum bona fpe difcefferunt. At

περιμείνας δὲ τὴν ἑξῆς περίοδον ὁ τεταρταῖος ἀπροσδοκήτως ἐνέβαλε τὴν ὀγδόην ὥραν, ἰσχυρότερος ἢ κατὰ τὴν προτέραν ἡμέραν ἐγεγόνει. ἐλθοῦσιν οὖν ἕωθεν αὐτοῖς, ὡς οἶσθα, δεύτερον ἐδόκει διδόναι τοῦ φαρμάκου. καὶ δὴ καὶ δόντες ἐπὶ τῆς ἡμέρας ἀνάλογον τῷ προτέρῳ παροξυσμῷ τὸ φάρμακον ἐχωρίσθησαν. ὁ γοῦν ἀνάλογος τῷ προτέρῳ παροξυσμῷ κατ᾽ αὐτὸν ἀπήντησε καὶ ὁ μετ᾽ αὐτὸν ἐπιγενόμενος δεύτερον· ἐφ᾽ ᾧ κατὰ τὴν ἑσπέραν ἐπυνθάνετό μου τίνα προσδοκίαν ἔχοιμι τῶν μελλόντων. ἐγὼ δὲ, ὡς οἶσθα, καταμαθὼν αὐτοῦ τὴν κίνησιν τῶν ἀρτηριῶν, νῦν μὲν, ἔφην, ἀποκρίνασθαί σοί τι πρὸς τὴν ἐρώτησιν ἀσφαλῶς ἀδύνατος ὑπάρχω, ἕωθεν (453) δὲ τάχα ἂν δυνηθείην, θεασάμενος ἅπαντα τὰ διὰ τῆς νυκτὸς οὐρηθησόμενα. παραγενόμενος οὖν ὑπὸ τῆς ἕω καὶ θεασάμενος αὐτὰ, ἐαθῆναί τε κελεύσας αὖθις, ἐὰν οὐρήσῃ τι μεταξὺ, περὶ τετάρτην ὥραν ἔφην ἀφίξεσθαι. καὶ μὴν καὶ παραγενόμενος, ὡς ἐθεασάμην τε τὰ οὖρα καὶ τῶν σφυγμῶν ἐπὶ πλέον ἡψάμην, ἀπεφηνάμην αὐτῷ τρίτον τεταρταίου γενήσεσθαι παροξυσμὸν, ὡς περὶ τὴν αὐτὴν ὥραν. ἐγὼ μὲν οὖν ἐχωρίσθην· ὀλίγον δ᾽ ὕστερον

quartana, non exſpectato proximo circuitu, praeter opinionem hora octava invaſit, idque fortior quam die primo fuerat. Venientibus itaque mane medicis, ut noſti, iterum ex medicamento propinare viſum eſt. Quumque pro proportione prioris acceſſionis exhibuiſſent, diſceſſerunt; ac quae ſecundo poſt ipſam ſupervenit acceſſio priori in ipſa reſpondebat; cujus rei gratia circa veſperam me rogabat, quid exſpectarem futurum. Ego, ut noſti, arteriarum motum ipſius explorans, nunc ſane, dicebam, reſpondere tibi quippiam ad quaeſtionem tuto non poſſum; mane autem forſan potero, intuitus omnem quae noctu redditur urinam. Reverſus itaque ſub auroram intuitusque lotium, ſinere juſſi, ac rediturum me dixi circiter horam quartam, ſi quid interea mingeret. Ac ſane jam eo profectus, poſtquam urinas inſpexiſſem pulſumque diutius tetigiſſem, pronuntiavi ei tertiam quartanae acceſſionem circiter eandem horam adfuturam, quo dicto jam diſceſſi. Paulo poſt

ἐπισκεψόμενοι τὸν Εὔδημον ἀφίκοντο Σέργιός τε καὶ ὁ Παῦλος, ὃς οὐ μετὰ πολὺν χρόνον ὕπαρχος ἐγένετο τῆς πόλεως, καὶ Φλάβιος ὑπατικὸς μὲν ὢν ἤδη καὶ αὐτὸς, ἐσπευκὼς δὲ περὶ τὴν Ἀριστοτέλους φιλοσοφίαν, ὥσπερ καὶ ὁ Παῦλος, οἷς διηγησάμενος ἅπαντα ὁ Εὔδημος τὰ κατ' ἐμὲ, λυπεῖν ἔφη τὴν σήμερον ἐσομένην πρόῤῥησιν ἐπὶ τοῦ μέλλοντος παροξυσμοῦ, παραφυλάττειν δ' ὅπως ἀποβήσοιτο. γενομένου δὲ κἀκείνου περὶ τὴν αὐτὴν ὥραν τοῖς προγεγενημένοις ὁ μὲν Εὔδημος ἐθαύμαζέ τε καὶ τοῖς ἐπισκοπουμένοις αὐτὸν ἅπασιν ἐδήλου τὰς ἐμὰς προῤῥήσεις. ἦσαν δὲ οὗτοι σχεδὸν ἅπαντες οἱ κατὰ τὴν Ῥωμαίων πόλιν ἀξιώματί τε καὶ παιδείᾳ προὔχοντες. ὁ δ' οὖν Βοηθὸς, ἀκηκοὼς εἰς ἄκρον ἠσκῆσθαί με τὴν ἀνατομικὴν θεωρίαν, ἔτυχεν ἤδη παρακαλῶν ἐπιδεῖξαί τι περὶ φωνῆς τε καὶ ἀναπνοῆς, ὅπως τε γίγνοιτο καὶ διὰ τίνων ὀργάνων. ὡς οὖν ἐγνώρισέ μου τὸ ὄνομα καὶ τοῦτ' αὐτὸ τῷ τε Παύλῳ διηγήσατο καὶ μετὰ τὴν πεῖραν ἔφη παρακαλεῖν με, δεῖξαί τε καὶ αὐτῷ· πᾶν γὰρ ἔφη δεῖσθαι τῆς θέας τῶν κατὰ τὰς ἀνατομὰς φαι-

Sergius et Paulus, qui non multo poſt urbis praefectus creatus eſt, et Flavius conſularis, jam et ipſe in Ariſtotelis philoſophia exercitatus, ſicut et Paulus Eudemum viſitatum venerunt: quibus ille omnia, quae a me audierat, recenſens triſtitia ſe afficere dicebat factam de futura acceſſione praedictionem, obſervare autem quomodo eveniret. Quum jam et illa circa eandem horam ut praeteritae accideret, Eudemus ſane admirabatur et inviſentibus ipſum omnibus meas praedictiones indicabat. Erant autem hi prope omnes, qui Romae et dignitate et eruditione praecellebant. Quum igitur Boëthus in anatomica ſpeculatione me ſumme eſſe exercitatum audiviſſet, rogabat jam me, ut aliquid de voce et reſpiratione, quomodo fieret et per quae inſtrumenta, oſtenderem. Ut igitur cognovit nomen meum, etiam hoc ipſum Paulo narravit, qui et ipſe poſtquam innotuiſſet me rogabat ut etiam ſibi quid oſtenderem; dicebat enim omnino ſe ſpeculatione

νομένων ὁ Παῦλος. ὁμοίως δὲ καὶ Βάρβαρος ὁ θεῖος τοῦ βασιλεύοντος Λευκίου, κατὰ τὴν Μεσοποταμίαν ὀνομαζομένην ὄντος ὑπάρχου, ἐδεῖτο τοῦ μαθήματος καὶ αὐτὸς, ὥσπερ ὁ Παῦλος. ὕστερον δὲ καὶ Σεβῆρος ὕπατος μὲν ὢν, ἐσπουδακὼς δὲ καὶ περὶ τὴν Ἀριστοτέλους φιλοσοφίαν. ὅπως μὲν οὖν τὰ κατὰ τὰς ἀνατομὰς ἐγένετο, γινώσκοντί σοι βραχείας ἀναμνήσεως δεήσει, μικρὸν ὕστερον ἐσομένης.

Κεφ. γ΄. Ἐπὶ δὲ τὰ κατὰ Εὔδημον ἐπάνειμι. καταπονούμενος γὰρ ὑπὸ τῶν τριῶν τεταρταίων ἀπήλπιστο πρὸς τῶν ἰατρῶν ὄντος ἤδη που μέσου χειμῶνος. ἐγὼ δὲ οἷα διδασκάλῳ μὲν, ἀλλὰ καὶ κατὰ τύχην οἰκῶν αὐτοῦ πλησίον, ἀνάγκην [834] εἶχον ὑπακούειν δὶς τῆς ἡμέρας καλοῦντι. καταγελῶν δέ μου κατὰ τὸν καιρὸν ἐκεῖνον Ἀντιγένης εἷς τῶν Κοΐντου μαθητῶν, συγγεγονὼς δὲ καὶ Μαρίνῳ, πρωτεύειν τε τῶν ἰατρῶν πεπιστευμένος, ἅπαντάς τε τοὺς πολὺ δυναμένους ἰώμενος, οὐκ οἶδ᾽ ὅ τι δόξαν αὐτῷ τοῖς ἐπαινοῦσι καταγελῶν ἔφασκεν, ὀλίγον ὕστερον αὐτοὺς γνώσεσθαι τίνα τυγχάνουσιν ἐπαινοῦντες, ὅταν ἐκφερόμενον ἴδωσιν Εὔ-

eorum, quae in diſſectionibus apparent, indigere. Similiter et Barbarus avunculus regis Lucii, qui Meſopotamiae dictae praeerat, ipſe quoque ſicut Paulus diſciplinam deſiderabat. Poſtea et Severus conſulatum tunc gerens, in Ariſtotelis philoſophia etiam verſatus. Quomodo igitur diſſectiones ſucceſſerint quum ipſe ſcias, paucis commemorare opus erit et breviter paulo poſt repetemus.

Cap. III. Nunc autem ad Eudemum revertor. Quum enim tribus quartanis laboraret, medici de ejus ſalute deſperarunt, hieme jam fere media. Ego vero primum tanquam praeceptori meo, deinde quod forte fortuna prope ipſum habitabam, neceſſe habui obtemperare bis die vocanti. At Antigenes me eo tempore deridebat, unus ex Quinti diſcipulis, qui et Marino convixerat principatumque inter medicos obtinere creditus omnes potentes medicabatur; haud ſcio qua opinione ductus laudantibus me ridendo dicebat, paulo poſt ipſos cognituros quem commendarent, cum Eudemum efferri viderint. Atque haec

δημον καὶ ταῦτα λέγων πρὸς τοὺς παρόντας ἰδιώτας, ἀποστρέφων ἐνίοτε μὲν τὸν λόγον, ἀποβλέπων τε πρὸς τοὺς ἰατροὺς ἔφασκεν, Εὔδημον ἑξηκοστὸν καὶ τρίτον ἔτος ἄγοντα, τρεῖς ἔχοντα τεταρταίους ἐν μέσῳ χειμῶνος, θεραπεύειν ὑπισχνεῖται Γαληνός. σὺ μὲν οὖν, Ἐπίγενες φίλτατε, τάς τε μετὰ ταῦτα γενομένας προῤῥήσεις ἐπ᾽ αὐτοῦ καὶ τὴν θεραπείαν οἶδ᾽ ὅτι κηρύττων διετέλεσας. ἐμοὶ δ᾽ ἀρχὴ φθόνου τότε πρῶτον ἐγένετο, θαυμαζομένῳ ἐπί τε βίου σεμνότητι καὶ τοῖς κατὰ τὴν τέχνην ἔργοις. ἐκ γὰρ τῶν τριῶν τεταρταίων τὸν μὲν πρῶτον ἀρξάμενον ἐν τῇδε παύσασθαι τῇ ἡμέρᾳ προειπὼν ἐθαυμάσθην· ἐπεὶ δὲ καὶ τοῦ δευτέρου τὴν προθεσμίαν τῆς λύσεως ἠλήθευσα, ἅπαντες μὲν ἐξεπλάγησαν· ἐπὶ τοῦ τρίτου γοῦν ἀποτυχεῖν με τοῖς θεοῖς ηὔχοντο. παυσαμένου δὲ κἀκείνου κατὰ τὴν ὑπ᾽ ἐμοῦ προῤῥηθεῖσαν ἡμέραν, οὐκ ἐπὶ ταῖς προῤῥήσεσι μόνον, ἀλλὰ καὶ τῇ θεραπείᾳ δόξαν ἔσχον οὐ σμικράν. ὁ οὖν Ἀντιγένης μονονοὺ κατὰ γῆς ἐδύετο διὰ τὰς προπετῶς αὐτῷ γενομένας εἰς ἐμὲ βλασφημίας· ὁμοίως δ᾽ αὐτῷ καὶ Μαρτιανὸς, οὗ καὶ

ad praefentes idiotas dicens, nonnunquam fermone averfo refpiciensque ad medicos ajebat, Eudemum fexagefimum et tertium annum agentem, tribus laborantem quartanis in media hieme Galenus fe curaturum promittit. Tu igitur, Pofthume cariffime, et praedictiones de eo poftea factas et curationem novi quanto praeconio extuleris; mihi autem primum tunc invidiae initium obortum eft, ut qui tum propter gravitatem vitae tum artis opera effem admirationi. Etenim ex tribus quartanis quum primam quidem exorfam hoc finitum iri die praefagiiffem, vifus fum admirabilis; quum autem et fecundae ftatum folutionis tempus vere protuliffem, omnes fane fuerunt attoniti; in tertia certe deos precabantur ut fucceffu fruftrarer. Cum autem et illa in die a me praedicto ceffaret, non ob praedictiones tantum, fed etiam curationem, haud mediocrem gloriam fum confecutus. Antigenes igitur fere in terram fe coram me dimifit propter temerarias ipfius in me oblocutiones habitas; fimiliter et Martianus, qui ipfe quoque

αὐτοῦ κατά τε τὸν χρόνον ἐκεῖνον ἔτι δὲ πρότερον ὡς ἀνατομικωτάτῳ δόξα μεγάλη παρὰ τοῖς ἰατροῖς νεανίσκοις ἦν. ἐσπουδάζετο δὲ δύο βιβλία τῶν ὑπ᾽ αὐτοῦ γεγραμμένων ἀνατομῶν. ἀνιαθεὶς δὲ καὶ αὐτὸς ἐφ᾽ οἷς Εὔδημος οὐ μόνον ἐπαινεῖσθαι χρῆναί με πρὸς ἅπαντα δικαίως, ἀλλὰ καὶ θαυμάζεσθαι δεῖν ἔφασκεν, οὐκ ἐξ ἰατρικῆς τὰς προῤῥήσεις, ἀλλ᾽ ἐκ μαντικῆς γίνεσθαι ταύτας ὑπ᾽ ἐμοῦ διέβαλε. καὶ τήν γε μαντικὴν ἥντινα λέγοι ἂν πυνθανομένων τινῶν, ἐνίοτε μὲν οἰωνιστικὴν ἔφασκεν, ἐνίοτε δὲ θυτικὴν, ἔστι δ᾽ ὅτε συμβολικὴν, ἢ μαθηματικήν. ὕστατον δέ τι παρὰ τῷ Εὐδήμῳ τοιοῦτον ἐγένετο, τοῦ τρίτου τῶν τεταρταίων τῆς ἡμέρας ἐνστάσεις, ἐν ᾗ τελείαν ἀπαλλαγὴν αὐτῷ προειρήκειν ἔσεσθαι. παραγενόμενος ὁ Μαρτιανὸς πρὸς τὸν Εὔδημον ὥρας ἐνάτης, οὐ σμικρῷ σφοδρότερον, ἀλλὰ καὶ πάνυ πολλῷ τοῦ προγεγενημένου παροξυσμοῦ τὸν νῦν ὄντα φήσας ὑπάρχειν, ἐχωρίσθη παραχρῆμα φαιδρῷ τῷ προσώπῳ, φανερῶς ἐνδεικνύμενος ἐπιχαίρειν, ὡς ἀποτετευγμένης τῆς προῤῥήσεως. αἰσθανόμενος δὲ ὁ Εὔδημος εὐφορίας ὁποίας

tum per illud tempus tum antea adhuc ceu maximus anatomicus in magno honore et gloria apud adolefcentes medicos extitit. Legebantur autem duo ejus libri de diffectionibus fcripti. Is ipfe quoque dolore affectus, eo quod Eudemus non modo jure in omnibus laudari me oportere, fed etiam pro miraculo haberi dicebat; non ex medicina praedictiones, fed ex vaticinatoria has a me fieri calumniabatur. At vaticinatoriam quam tandem diceret quum nonnulli quaererent, interim auguratricem dicebat, interim e facrificio petitam, aliquando fymbolicam aut mathematicam. Poftremo tale quid apud Eudemum accidit, tertiae quartanae die inftante, qua perfecte eum liberatum iri dixeram. Martianus hora nona ad Eudemum profectus praefentem acceffionem non paulo, fed etiam multo vehementiorem praeterita effe dixit ac ftatim abit vultu laeto, manifefto indicans fe gaudere, tanquam praedictio non fucceflerit. Eudemus autem fentiens facilitatem morbi

οὔπω πρότερον ᾔσθετο, καὶ μέντοι καὶ θαῤῥῶν, ὡς οὐ σφαλησομένῳ μοι κατὰ τὴν πρόῤῥησιν, ἀναμείνας ἀφικέσθαι τινα καὶ ἄλλον ἰατρόν· ἀφικομένου δὲ οὐχ ἑνὸς μόνον, ἀλλὰ καὶ δυοῖν καὶ τριῶν (ἐπετήρουν γὰρ ἅπαντες ὅπως ἀποβῇ τὰ κατὰ τὴν πρόῤῥησιν, εὐχόμενοι κἂν ἐπί γε τοῦ τρίτου τῶν τεταρταίων ἀτυχῆσαί με τῆς τε προῤῥήσεως καὶ τῆς ἀπ' αὐτοῦ θεραπείας) ὁ μὲν Εὔδημος ἠξίωσε κἀκείνους ἀποφήνασθαι πῶς ἔχειν αὐτοῖς τὰ κατ' αὐτὸν δοκοίη, τὴν δ' αὐτὴν ἀπόκρισιν ἀκούσας, ἣν ὁ Μαρτιανὸς πεποίηται, καὶ προσχὼν ὁμοίως κἀκείνοις, ὡς Μαρτιανῷ, φαιδροτέροις γεγονόσιν, ἐνόησε μὲν καὶ αὐτὸς ἐπιχαίρειν αὐτοὺς, ὡς ἀποτετευγμένης τῆς προῤῥήσεώς τε καὶ θεραπείας. ἐπεὶ δ' ἐχρόνιζον ἐγὼ παρὰ τὸ ἔθος ἐν ἐπισκέψει τινὶ κατεχόμενος, ἔπεμπε συνεχῶς πρός με πλησίον οἰκοῦντα, καθάπερ ἔφην, ἐπι- [835] κριθῆναι τὴν εὐφορίαν ἣν εἶχεν ὑπ' ἐμοῦ βουλόμενος. ὡς δ' οὖν ἀφικόμην, οὐδὲ καθίσαι με περιμείνας ἐξέτεινε τὴν χεῖρα, κελεύων ἅψασθαι τῶν σφυγμῶν. ἁψαμένου δὲ μετὰ σπουδῆς ἐπυνθάνετο τί ποτε ἀγγέλλοιμι.

tolerandi, qualem necdum antea perceperat, quin etiam confidens mihi tanquam non erraturo in praedictione, exſpectans dum alius etiam quidam medicus accederet; quumque non unus tandem adveniret, ſed duo et tres (obſervabant enim omnes quomodo praedictio ſuccederet, optantes ſaltem in tertia quartana fruſtrari me et praedictione et curatione ipſius), Eudemus ſane voluit et illos pronuntiare quam ipſi de morbo ſuo opinionem haberent. Quumque eandem reſponſionem audiviſſet, quam Martianus protulerat, et attendens ſimiliter etiam illis ceu laetioribus Martiano redditis, intellexit ſane et ipſe gaudere illos quaſi et praedictio et curatio improſpere ſucceſſerit. Quoniam autem diutius morabar praeter conſuetudinem in viſitando quodam occupatus, miſit continue ad me juxta habitantem, ut dixi, cupiens, ut de facilitate ipſius, quam habebat, ferrem judicium. Ut igitur acceſſi, ne ſedere quidem me permittens manum exporrexit, jubens ut pulſum tangerem. Quum autem exploraſſem ſtudioſe, quae-

κἀγὼ μειδιάσας, τί ἄλλο, ἔφην, ἢ ἀγαθά; ποῖα, εἶπε, ταῦτα ἰδικῶς μοι φράσον. ἐγὼ δ', οὐκ ἀρκέσει, ἔφην, σοὶ τὸ κεφάλαιον αὐτὸ ἀθρόως ἀκηκοότι χαίρειν ἐπὶ τοῖς ἐσομένοις; οὐδαμῶς, εἶπεν. ἀκοῦσαι γὰρ ποθῶ καὶ τὰ κατὰ μέρος. ἄκουε δή· ἀπαλλαγήσῃ τῇ νυκτὶ ταύτῃ τελέως ἁπάσης τῆς νοσώδους διαθέσεως, ἧς ἀπαλλαγείσης, τῶν τ' ἐπιγενομένων καὶ τῶν ἐσομένων αὐτῇ συμπτωμάτων ἁπάντων ἡ λύσις ἀκολουθήσει. καὶ τοῦτ' ἔφην ἄρτι μοι διὰ σφυγμῶν δεδηλωκέναι τὴν διοικοῦσάν σου τὸ σῶμα φύσιν ἐπεγηγερμένην ἤδη καὶ κινουμένην, ὡς ἐκβαλεῖν ἐκ τοῦ σώματος ἅπασαν οὖσαν ἔν σοι μοχθηρίαν τὴν ἐν τοῖς κατὰ τὸ σῶμα χυμοῖς. πῶς οὖν δὴ παρὰ τῆς φύσεως τοῦτο λέγεις σοι δεδηλῶσθαι; οὐ γὰρ δὴ φθεγξαμένη γε ταῦτ' εἶπε, ἀπόκριναί μοι, πάντως γὰρ οἶσθα παρακολουθήσαντά με τῷ λόγῳ μᾶλλον ἁπάντων τούτων ἰαλέμων ἰατρῶν. ὅτι τὴν (454) κίνησιν, ἔφην, τῶν ἀρτηριῶν εἰς ὕψος ἀνήγαγεν, ἐπὶ πλέον τῆς ἐφ' ἑκάτερον διαστάσεως, ὅπερ ἀεὶ ποιεῖν εἴωθεν ἐγχειροῦσα τὸ λυποῦν ἐκκρίνειν τοῦ σώματος. ἐπὶ τούτοις ῥηθεῖσιν ὁ Εὔ-

rebat quidnam nuntiarem. Ac ego ridens, quid aliud, inquam, quam bona? qualia, ait, haec particulatim mihi edicito. Ego rurfus, non fatis, inquam, erit tibi fummam ipfam univerfim audienti, gaudere ob ea, quae futura funt. Nequaquam, inquit; audire enim defidero particulatim. Audito jam. Hac nocte tota difpofitione morbofa perfecte liberaberis; quibus factis etiam fymptomatum omnium et fupervenientium et futurorum folutio comitabitur. Atque hoc dicebam nuper mihi ex pulfibus indicaffe naturam, quae corpus tuum difpenfat, excitatam jam motamque, ut omnem humorum corporis pravitatem ex corpore tuo expellat. Quomodo igitur jam a natura hoc tibi indicatum effe dicis? non enim loquens haec tibi dixit; refponde. Omnino enim novifti me quae dices intellectu magis affecuturum quam omnes hos miferabiles medicos. Quoniam motum, dixi, arteriarum elatius extulit quam ad alteram dimenfionem: quod femper facere confuevit, ubi id quod noxium eft excernere e corpore

δημος ὑπολαβὼν ἔφη, ἀλλ' ἐπεὶ πολλαὶ τῆς ἐκκρίσεως ὁδοὶ τετάχαται τῇ φύσει· καὶ γὰρ ἔμετος καὶ γαστὴρ καταῤῥήξασα, τάχα δὲ καὶ οὔρων πλῆθος, ἱδρώτων τε πολλῶν ἐκκρίσεις, αἱμοῤῥαγία τε καὶ συνήθης αἱμοῤῥοῒς ἀναστομωθεῖσα κένωσιν ἀθρόαν ἐργάζεται· τῆς σῆς ἂν εἴη τέχνης ἔργον οἰκεῖον ἑρμηνεῦσαί μοι τὸ τῆς κενώσεως εἶδος. αἱμοῤῥαγίας μὲν οὖν, ἔφην, ἐσομένης τάδε καὶ τάδε προηγεῖται σημεῖα, καθάπερ γε καὶ ἱδρώτων ταυτί. προσέθηκα δ' ἐν τῷ λόγῳ καὶ τὰ τῶν ἐμέτων προηγούμενα. τῆς δὲ διὰ τῆς κάτω γαστρὸς κενώσεως ἀθρόας κριτικῆς οὐδὲν ἔχομεν ἴδιον ἐξαίρετον σημεῖον, ἀλλ' ἐκ τοῦ μηδὲν τῶν ἄλλων παρεῖναι καταλείποιτ' ἂν ἐλπίζειν ἐπὶ σοῦ γενήσεσθαι τοῦτο. διαλεκτικῶς, ἔφη, συνελογίσω τὴν εὕρεσιν τοῦ γενησομένου. ταῦτα μὲν ἑσπέρας οὔσης ἤδη διελέχθημεν ἀλλήλοις. παραγενόμενος δ' ἕωθεν ἤκουσας αὐτὸς σὺ τοῦ κεφαλαίου τῆς προῤῥήσεως, οὐχ ὑπομένοντος μετρίως φθέγγεσθαι τοῦ φιλοσόφου, καθάπερ εἴωθεν· κεκραγότος δὲ πρὸς ἅπαντας ἡμᾶς τοὺς εἰσιόντας φίλους, ὡς ὁ Πύθιος Ἀπόλλων, διὰ τοῦ

nititur. Poſt haec dicta Eudemus iterato ſermone intulit. Verum quia multae excretionis viae a natura diſtributae ſunt (etenim vomitus, alvus profluens, forſan et urinarum copia, ſudorum multorum eruptiones, ſanguinis profluvium et conſueta haemorrhois adaperta vacuationem ſubitam efficit) proprium artis tuae munus fuerit vacuationis ſpeciem interpretari. Sanguinis igitur profluvium futurum haec et illa ſigna praecedunt, quemadmodum etiam ſudores haec. Adjeci autem inter dicendum et ea quae vomitus praecedunt. At vacuationis per ventrem ſubitae criſin fatentis nullum peculiare eximium ſignum habemus. Verum ſi nullum ex aliis adſit, reliquum eſt ut ſperemus in te hoc futurum. Dialectice, inquit, collegiſti ejus quod fiet inventionem. Haec ſane cum adveſperaſceret jam inter nos differebamus. Quum itaque mane accederem, tu ipſe audiviſti ſummam praedictionis a philoſopho, qui non ſuſtinebat moderate loqui, ut conſueverat; ſed vociferabatur ad omnes nos ingredientes amicos, Py-

Γαληνοῦ στόματος, ἐβουλήθη θεσπίζειν τοῖς νοσοῦσι μετὰ τοῦ θεραπεύειν αὐτοὺς, ἀπαλλάττειν τε τελέως αὐτοὺς ἐν ἡμέρᾳ τῇ προῤῥηθείσῃ. τὴν γοῦν γεγενημένην λύσιν τοῦ νοσήματος, πέπεισμαι γὰρ ἤδη τελέως ὑγιαίνειν, ἐπαγγειλάμενος ἐκ πολλοῦ καὶ τῆς θεραπείας καὶ τῆς προῤῥήσεως ἔτυχον. ἀπήλλαξε δέ με τριῶν τεταρταίων, οἷς ἀκαίρου πόσεως τοῦ θηριακοῦ φαρμάκου περιπεσὼν, ὁπότε καιρὸς αὐτῆς ἐγένετο, μηδὲν ἐκείνων φθεγγομένων δοὺς τοῦτο ἀπήλλαξέ με καταγελώμενος ὑπ᾿ αὐτῶν, εἴ γε νομίζει γέροντα χειμῶνος ὥρᾳ κάμνοντα τρισὶ τεταρταίοις ἀπαλλάξειν.

Κεφ. δ'. Οἱ μὲν οὖν ἰδιῶται τῆς ἰατρικῆς τέχνης ἀκούοντες ταῦτα, κοινὸν ἀγαθὸν ἡγούμενοί με τοῖς ἐν Ῥώμῃ γενήσεσθαι, πάντες ἔχαιρον. ὁ δ᾿ οὐκ ἰατρὸς μόνον, ἀλλὰ καὶ φίλος εἶναι μαρτυρούμενος Μαρτιανὸς, ἀκούσας τήν τε κατὰ τὴν γεγονυῖαν ἡμέραν [836] ἀπόφασίν μου, περὶ τῆς ἐν ταῖς ἀρτηρίαις κινήσεως, ἣν ἐκεῖνοι θορυβώδη νομίζοντες, οὐ κριτὴν ἐδεδίεσαν, εὑρόντες κατὰ φύσιν ἀκριβῶς ἔχοντα τὸν Εὔδημον, ἐπαινέσαι μὲν οὐδ᾿ ἄχρι ῥήματος

thium Apollinem per Galeni os voluiſſe oracula aegrotantibus dicere nec non curare ipſos liberareque in totum die praedicto. Nam cum factam morbi ſolutionem (perſuaſum enim habeo jam ex toto me eſſe ſanum) longo tempore antea praenuntiaſſet et curationem et praedictionem ſum conſecutus. Liberavit autem me tribus quartanis, in quas ex intempeſtivo theriacae medicamenti potione incidi, quando tempus ipſius eſſet non illis eloquentibus; hic propinans me liberavit, deriſus ab iis, quod ſenem hiberno tempore laborantem tribus quartanis levaturum ſe putaret.

Cap. IV. Imperiti ſane artis medicae quum haec audirent, commune bonum me Romae degentibus futurum exiſtimantes omnes gaudebant. At Martianus, qui non medicum modo, ſed etiam amicum eſſe ſe teſtabatur, quum audiviſſet, quid ſuperiori die pronuntiaſſem de arteriarum motu, quem illi turbulentum, non decretorium nominantes extimuerunt, etſi Eudemum ſecundum natu-

ἑνὸς ὑπέμεινέ με. καταβὰς δὲ εἰς τὸ Σανταλάριον ἀπήντησέ μοι κατὰ τύχην, εὐθέως δὲ μήτε προσαγορεύσας, ὡς ἔθος εἶχεν, ἐπύθετο πότερον ἀνεγνωκὼς εἴην τὸ δεύτερον τῶν Ἱπποκράτους προῤῥητικῶν, ἢ ὅλως ἀγνοοῖμι τὸ σύγγραμμα, κᾄπειτα ἀκούσας ὡς ἀνεγνωκὼς εἴην καί μοι δοκοῖεν ὀρθῶς, ἔνιοι τῶν ἰατρῶν οὐκέτι εἶναι τῶν γνησίων Ἱπποκράτους βιβλίων αὐτὸ καὶ προσηκόντως ἀποφήνασθαι. πάντως γοῦν γινώσκεις, ἔφη, τῶν γεγραμμένων ἐν αὐτῷ; ἐγὼ δὲ τοιαῦτα οὐ μαντεύομαι· πρὸς τί δὲ, ἔφην, εἴρηταί σοι νῦν τοῦτο; καὶ ὡς ἄρτι κεχωρίσθαι παρ' Εὐδήμου θαυμάζοντος ἔλεγεν ἐπὶ τοῦ χθὲς ἑσπέρας, ἁψάμενόν σε τὸν σφυγμὸν προειπεῖν ἔκκρισιν ἔσεσθαι διὰ τῆς κάτω γαστρὸς, ἐφ' ἧς μηκέτι πυρέξειν. εἰπόντος οὖν αὐτοῦ ταῦτα, μόνον ἀποκρινάμενος ἐγὼ, παρ' Εὐδήμου ταῦτ' ἀκήκοας, οὐ παρ' ἐμοῦ, παρῆλθον αὐτίκα. πορευθείς τε πρὸς τὸν Εὔδημον ἀπήγγειλα τὸ γεγονὸς, ἐθαύμαζόν τε τὴν κακόνοιαν τῶν εὐδοκιμούντων ἰατρῶν ἐν τῇ Ῥωμαίων πόλει. ὁ δὲ κατὰ λόγον ἔφη μοι τοῦτο πεπονθέναι, ἀπεικάζων τοῖς ἐν πατρίδι

ram prorfus habere offenderent, ne verbo quidem uno laudari me fuftinebat. Digreffus autem in Sandalarium forte mihi occurrit ac ftatim neque falutans, uti folebat, rogavit, num fecundum Hippocratis Prorrheticorum librum legiffem, an omnino mihi effet incognitus. Ac deinde ubi audiviffet me legiffe, ac mihi videntur, inquit, nonnulli medicorum recte ac convenienter pronuntiaffe ex germanis Hippocratis libris ipfum non effe. Omnino igitur novifti, inquit, quae in eo fcripta funt? Ego vero hujusmodi non vaticinor; quorfum autem hoc nunc dictum ab eo effet quaefivi. Quod cum ab Eudemo te admirante digreffus effes, ajebat, heri vefperi ex pulfus tactu praedixeris excretionem per alvum futuram, poftquam non amplius febricitaret. Quae ubi ipfe protuliffet, ego tantum refpondens, ab Eudemo haec audivifti, non a me, ftatim difceffi; profectusque ad Eudemum quid accidiffet nunciavi, demirabarque medicorum in Romanorum urbe celebrium malevolentiam. Ille fecundum rationem hoc

τοὺς τῇδε, κατὰ πλείους αἰτίας εἰς ἄκρον ἥκοντας κακοηθείας, καὶ διῆλθεν ἁπάσας ἑξῆς ὧδέ πως. μὴ νόμιζε τοὺς ἀγαθοὺς ἄνδρας ἐν ταύτῃ τῇ πόλει γίνεσθαι πονηροὺς, ἀλλ' ὅσοι φθάνουσιν εἶναι πονηροὶ, πραγμάτων ὕλην εὑρόντες ἐνταῦθα καὶ κέρδη πολὺ μείζονα τῶν ἐν ταῖς ἔξω πόλεσιν ἔχουσιν. ὁρῶντές τε πεπλουτηκότας ὁμοίους αὐτοῖς πολλοὺς, ἐμιμήσαντο τὰς πράξεις αὐτῶν πολυειδεῖς οὔσας καὶ ἐκ πλειόνων αἰτιῶν εἰς ἔσχατον ἥκουσιν πονηρίας. ἐρῶ δέ σοί τινας αὐτῶν, ὡς ἂν ἐκ πολλοῦ χρόνου πεπειραμένος. οὐ γὰρ μόνον ἡ φύσις, οὐδὲ ἡ τῶν κερδαλέων πραγμάτων ὕλη τὴν πονηρίαν ηὔξησε τῶν φύσει πονηρῶν, ἀλλὰ καὶ μάθησις ἠκολούθησε πανουργίας ὁδῶν, ἃς ἑώρων ὁσημέραι γινομένας ὑπὸ τῶν ὁμοίων ἑαυτοῖς· εἶτα ἐν τῷ μιμεῖσθαι ταύτας διετρίβησαν. κἂν φωραθῶσιν ὑπό τινος πανουργοῦντες, ἐπ' ἄλλους ἔχειν ἀγνῶτας ἑαυτῶν μεταβαίνειν, οἷς ἐκ τῆς πρώτης πείρας ὧν πράττοντες κακῶς ἐγνώσθησαν ἀσφαλέστερον προσφέρονται, οὐ σμικρὰν ἔχει δύναμιν οὐδ'

mihi accidere dixit, conferens cum patriae noftrae medicis eos, qui in hac urbe verfantur, pluribus de caufis ad fummum malitiae tendentes; ac deinde mihi omnes in hunc modum recenfuit. Ne arbitreris bonos viros hac in urbe fieri malos, fed qui mali jam funt, rerum materiam hic et quaeftum multo uberiorem quam ii, qui in externis urbibus agunt, inveniunt. Ac dum multos ipfis fimiles locupletatos vident, actiones eorum varias imitantur atque hinc ex pluribus caufis in extremam pravitatem delabuntur. Dicam autem tibi nonnullas ipforum pravitates ceu longo tempore expertus. Non enim folum natura, neque quaeftuofarum rerum materia malitiam eorum, qui natura pravi funt, adauxit; fed etiam difciplina viarum impofturae fecuta eft, quas quotidie a fui fimilibus iniri confpiciebant: deinde in his imitandis tunc verfantur. Et fi ab aliquo maleficii arguantur, ad alios ignotos transgrediuntur; quibus illa, quae prima experientia perperam facere funt deprehenfi, tutius offeruntur; id quod non

αὐτὸ πρὸς τὸ μηδέποτε παύεσθαι πανουργοῦντας. οἱ δ' ἐν ταῖς σμικραῖς πόλεσιν οὔθ' ὑπὸ μεγέθους κερδῶν δελεαζόμενοι, καθάπερ οἱ τῆσδε, γινωσκόμενοί τε ῥᾳδίως ὑπὸ τῶν πολιτῶν, εἰ καὶ μικρὸν ἁμάρτοιεν, ἀγύμναστον ἔχουσι τὴν θεωρίαν. ἐνταυθοῖ δὲ καὶ τὸ μὴ γιγνώσκεσθαι πρὸς ἁπάντων, ἃ πράττουσιν ἑκάστοτε πανουργοῦντες, αὐξάνει τὴν κακίαν τῆς φύσεως αὐτῶν. ἐπιτίθενται γὰρ τοῖς ἀγνοοῦσιν αὐτοὺς ἀπροοράτοις, καὶ μάλισθ' ὅταν ἀντιδακεῖν αὐτοὺς οἱ δι' ἁπλότητα γνώμης μὴ δύνανται, καθάπερ αὐτοὶ δάκνουσιν ἀλλήλους, ἐάν τι καὶ σμικρὸν ἀδικηθῶσιν. ὡς οὖν οἱ παρ' ἡμῶν λῃσταὶ βοηθοῦσι μὲν ἀλλήλοις ἐπὶ τῇ τῶν ἄλλων ἀδικίᾳ, ἑαυτοῖς δὲ φείδονται, κατὰ τὸν αὐτὸν δὴ τρόπον οἱ τῇδε καθ' ἡμῶν ποιοῦντες τὰς συνωμοσίας, μόνῳ τούτῳ διαφέροντες τῶν λῃστῶν τῷ κατὰ τὴν πόλιν, οὐκ ἐν τοῖς ὄρεσι κακουργεῖν. ἀλλὰ τό γέ μοι προκείμενον, ἔφην, ἀκήκοας ἤδη πολλάκις, ὡς ἐπειδὰν ἡ κατὰ τὴν πατρίδα μου στάσις παύσηται, παραχρῆμα θεάσῃ με τῆς πόλεως τῆσδε χωριζόμενον, καὶ ὀλιγοχρόνιον ἔτι ποιήσω τὴν ἐνταῦθα δια-

parum eos movet ut nunquam a maleficiis deſiſtant. Qui autem parvas urbes inhabitant, neque magnitudine quaeſtus alliciuntur, quemadmodum hujus incolae, cognoſcunturque facile a civibus, et ſi etiam parum deliquerint, inexercitatam habent ſpeculationem. Hic autem et quod non ab omnibus cognoscantur, quae frequenter maleficia moliuntur, naturae ipſorum malignitatem auget. Nam ingerunt ſe ignorantibus ex improviſo, et praeſertim iis, qui propter animi ſimplicitatem ipſos contra mordere nequeunt, ſicut ipſi ſe invicem conviciis lacerant, ſi quam etiam parvam injuriam intulerint. Ut igitur latrones apud nos ob maleſicium aliquod ſe mutuo juvant ſibique parcunt, eodem modo qui hic agunt adverſus nos conjurati ſola hac re a latronibus differunt, quod in urbe, non in montibus facinora ſua perpetrent. Sed jam quod propoſueram, ajebam, ſaepe audiviſti: quare quamprimum ſeditio ac belli tumultus in patria mea ceſſaverit, conſpicies me ex hac urbe diſceſſurum et brevem adeo hic moram factu-

τριβὴν, ὥστε θᾶττον ἀπαλλαγῆναι τῆς πανουργίας τῶν μοχθηρῶν τούτων ἀνθρώπων. ἀλλ' οὔτε γινώσκουσιν, ὁ Εὔδημος ἔφη, δεδογμένον σοι τοῦτο· [837] καὶ εἰ γνῶσιν, ὥσπερ αὐτοὶ ψεύδονται, πάντες σε νομιοῦσιν ὁμοίως αὐτοῖς ψεύδεσθαι. καὶ ὥσπερ αὐτοὶ τῶν ἀπόρων τε καὶ ἀπαιδεύτων ὄντες ἐν ταῖς πατρίσιν οὐ δύνανται διαμένειν, διὰ τὸ γινώσκεσθαι τἄλλα ὅσα προείρηκα πανουργοῦντες μαθεῖν, εἰς τήνδε τὴν πόλιν ἧκον, οὕτω καὶ τοὺς ἄλλους οἴονται παραγεγονότας εἰς αὐτὴν καὶ οὐκ ἂν ἐθελῆσαι πρὶν ἀθροίσουσιν ἀργύριον ἀπαλλαγῆναι. κἂν ἀκούσωσιν ὑπὸ τῶν πολιτῶν σου τὸ γένος καὶ τὴν κτῆσιν, ὡς οὐκ ἐκ τῶν ἀπόρων εἴης, κατεσκευάσθαι πάντως ὑπὸ σοῦ φήσουσιν, ἕνεκα τῆς τῶν ἀκουσόντων ἀπάτης· ἃ γὰρ αὐτοὶ πεπράχοιεν, περὶ πάντων ὑπονοοῦσιν. εἰπόντος οὖν Εὐδήμου ταῦτα καὶ τοιαῦθ' ἕτερα καὶ προσθέντος ὡς εἰ μὴ ταῖς πανουργίαις ἡμᾶς βλάψαι δυνηθεῖεν, ἐπὶ τὴν διὰ τῶν φαρμάκων ἐπιβουλὴν ἔρχονται· καὶ φάντος γε ἐν τῇ διηγήσει νεανίσκον τινὰ πρὸ ἐτῶν ὡς δέκα παραγενόμενον εἰς τὴν πόλιν, ἐπιδεικνύντα τε δι'

rum, quo citius ab improbis iftis nebulonibus liberer. Sed ignorant, Eudemus ait, hoc tibi inftitutum effe et fi noverint, quemadmodum ipfi mentiuntur, omnes te fimiliter ut ipfos mentiri cenfebunt. Et quemadmodum ipfi rerum indigi et imperiti quum in patria manere nequeant, eo quod praeter alia, quae dixi, vafritiam fubdolam improbamque exercere cognoscuntur, in hanc urbem migrarunt, ita quoque alios huc profectos arbitrantur et nolle prius discedere quam pecuniam acervaverint. Et fi a civibus genus tuum poffeffionemque audiant, quod non fis ex eorum numero, qui rerum inopia laborent, effictum omnino abs te effe dicent, ut auditoribus imponas; quae enim ipfi fecerint, ea de omnibus fufpicantur. Quum igitur haec aliaque id genus Eudemus dixiffet, addidiffetque eos, nifi improba vafritie nos laedere potuerint, ad infidias per pharmaca defcendunt, quumque retuliffet idem inter narrandum, adolescentem quendam ante annos circiter decem in hanc urbem profectum, qui operibus fimi-

ἔργων ὁμοίως ἐμοὶ τὴν ἐν τῇ τέχνῃ παρασκευὴν, ὑπὸ φαρμάκων ἀναιρεθῆναι μεθ' ὧν (455) ἧκε δυοῖν ἱκετῶν· χάριν, ἔφην, γινώσκω σοὶ, φίλτατε διδάσκαλε, πάντα μοι διηγησαμένῳ τὰ τῆς πονηρίας αὐτῶν. ἐγὼ γὰρ ἀσφαλῶς ἐμαυτὸν φυλάξω, χωρήσας αὐτοῖς ὁμόσε, κατάφωρόν τε τὴν ἀμαθίαν αὐτῶν ἐργασάμενος ἀπαλλάξομαι τῆς μεγάλης τῆσδε καὶ πολυανθρώπου πόλεως εἰς τὴν ὀλιγάνθρωπόν τε καὶ σμικρὰν, ἐν ᾗ πάντες ἴσμεν ἀλλήλους ἐκ τίνων τε γεγόναμεν ὅπως τε παιδείας ἔχομεν καὶ κτήσεως καὶ τρόπου καὶ βίου. τραπόμενος οὖν ἐπὶ τοῦτο τὴν ἀμαθίαν αὐτῶν καὶ τὴν πονηρίαν αὐτῶν ἐλέγχειν οὐκ ἐφρόντισα.

Κεφ. ε'. Ἀλλὰ τόν τε προειρημένον νεανίσκον, ᾧ παραγενόμενος εὐθέως κατὰ τὴν πρώτην ἡμέραν ἔφην εἰσβολὴν παροξυσμοῦ τεταρταίου πυρετοῦ γεγονέναι παραλαβὼν, ἐθεράπευσα, τὴν προθεσμίαν τῆς λύσεως τοῦ νοσήματος ὡς ἐπ' Εὐδήμου προειπὼν, ὑπὸ σοῦ τε παρακληθεὶς, ἄνθρωπόν τινα Χαριλαμποῦς τοῦ κοιτωνητοῦ μὲν, ὡς ἅπαντες οἱ νῦν Ἕλληνες ὀνομάζουσι, σωματοφύλακος δὲ, ὡς οἱ περιέρ-

liter ac ego tractationem artis indicabat, pharmacis fuiſſe ſublatum cum famulis duobus, qui una cum ipſo advenerant. Gratiam tibi habeo, dixi, praeceptor cariſſime, qui omnem ipſorum pravitatem mihi recenſueris. Ego enim ſecure me ipſum tuebor, digreſſus ab eis procul; claraque inſcitia eorum facta, a magna hac et populoſa civitate in parvam paucorumque hominum migrabo, ubi omnes inter nos novimus ex quibus orti ſimus, quam eruditionem habeamus, poſſeſſionem et mores, quamque vitae rationem ineamus. Eo igitur animum convertens inſcitiam ipſorum et vafritiem redarguere non ſtudui.

Cap. V. Sed commemoratum adoleſcentem ad quem profectus primo ſtatim die dixi quartanae febris acceſſionis inſultum fore, ubi accepiſſem curavi, ſtatum morbi ſolutionis tempus, ut in Eudemo, praefatus; quumque a te vocatus eſſem, ut hominem quendam inviſerem Charilampi cubicularium quidem, ut omnes nunc Graeci nominant, corporis vero cuſtodem, quemadmodum et ii qui

γως ἀττικίζοντες, νευρότρωτον γενόμενον ἐθεράπευσα, μηδενὸς τῶν κατὰ τὴν αὐλὴν ἰατρῶν δυναμένου τοῦτο ποιῆσαι· καὶ μετὰ αὐτὸν ἐν τῷ Σανδαλαρίῳ ῥήτορος Διομήδους, οὗ μηδ᾽ αὐτοῦ τῶν ἐκ τῆς αὐλῆς οἱ εὐδοκιμώτατοι τὴν διάθεσιν τοῦ νοσήματος εὕρισκον, ἀλλὰ διὰ τῶν ἐναντίων ἢ προσῆκεν ἐποιοῦντο τὴν θεραπείαν, ἡμέραις ὀλίγαις προνοησάμενος ἰασάμην τελέως χρόνιον τὸ νόσημα. καὶ τοῦ θέρους ἐπιστάντος ἐπὶ τῶν πρωτευόντων ἐν τῇ Ῥώμῃ προῤῥήσεις τε καὶ θεραπείας ἐποιησάμην ἀξίας ἐπαίνου μεγάλου καὶ ἐν πολλῇ δόξῃ παρὰ πᾶσιν ἦν, ὡς οἶσθα, καὶ μέγα ἦν τοὔνομα Γαληνοῦ. συνηυξάνετό τε τῇ δόξῃ φθόνος ἐκ τῶν οἰομένων εἶναί τι καὶ αὐτῶν, ὡς ἂν ἐν παντὶ μέρει τῆς τέχνης ὑπ᾽ ἐμοῦ νικωμένων, ἔλεγόν τε περιθέοντες τὴν πόλιν ἄλλος ἄλλο τι διαβάλλων, ὁ μὲν ὡς κατὰ τύχην ἰασάμην τόνδε τινα ῥιψοκινδύνῳ τρόπῳ θεραπείας χρησάμενος, ὁ δ᾽ ὡς ἐκ μαντικῆς αἱ προῤῥήσεις καὶ οὐκ ἐκ θεωρίας ἰατρικῆς γίγνοιντο. προσεγένετο δὲ καὶ τὸ κατὰ τὴν ζήτησιν, ἣν πρὸς τοὺς Στωϊκούς τε καὶ Περιπατητικοὺς ἐποιησάμην,

perperam Atticos imitantur, in nervo vulneratum perfanavi, id quod nullus aulicorum medicorum praeftare potuerit. Ac poft ipfum in Sandalario Diomedem rhetorem, cujus nec ipfius quoque morbi affectionem celeberrimi inter aulicos medicos inveniebant, fed etiam fecus quam decens erat curationem moliebantur, paucis diebus quum morbum admodum diuturnum praenoviffem, reftitui. Ac aeftate appetente in primatibus Romae et praedictiones, ut curationes magna laude dignas molitus fum; ac in multo honore et gloria apud omnes eram, ut fcis, nomenque Galeni celebre. Ac cum gloria crescebat invidia eorum, qui et ipfi putabantur effe aliquid, tanquam in omni artis parte a me vincerentur, adhibebantque urbem circumcurrentes alius aliam calumniam; hic, quod cafu illum curaverim, periculofo curationis modo ufus; ille, quod e vaticinatrice, non ex medica fpeculatione praedictiones fierent. Acceffit etiam his quaeftio, quam cum Stoïcis et Peripateticis habebam, quos Boëthus ipfe convocarat.

[838] ἀθροίσαντος αὐτοῦ τοῦ Βοηθοῦ. καὶ μετὰ ταῦτα τῆς Ἰουστοῦ γυναικὸς, ἧς συντηκομένης ἄνευ τοῦ φαίνεσθαί τι μόριον πεπονθέναι ἐξεῦρον οὐ μόνον ἐρῶσαν, ἀλλὰ καὶ τίνος ἤρα, καὶ μικρὸν ὕστερον ὅθεν εὗρον τοῦτο λεχθήσεται. τὸν δὲ κατὰ τὸν πρὸς τοὺς Στωϊκούς τε καὶ Περιπατητικοὺς ἀγῶνα, παρόντων καὶ ἄλλων τινῶν ἅμα μετ' αὐτοῖς ἰατρῶν τε καὶ φιλοσόφων, ἀναμνήσω σε πρῶτον ὅθεν ἤρξατο διελθὼν, ἵν', εἴ καί τινων τῶν ἀξίων κοινωνίας τοιούτων λόγων ἐθελήσαις μεταδοῦναι τουτὶ τὸ γράμμα, τὴν ἀκολουθίαν ἅπασαν ἴδοις τῶν γενομένων καὶ μὴ διὰ παντὸς ἀσχολίαν ἔχοις αὐτὸς διηγούμενος, ὅσα διά τε τῶν ἔργων τῆς ἰατρικῆς τέχνης, ἀνατομῶν τε καὶ τῶν ἐπ' αὐταῖς λόγων ἐπράχθη μοι τοὺς φθονεροὺς ἰατρούς τε καὶ φιλοσόφους ἐλέγχοντι. προπηλακιζόμενος γὰρ ὑπ' αὐτῶν ἐπὶ τοῦτ' ἦλθον, Ὁμήρου με παιδεύσαντος

Ἄνδρ' ἐπαμύνασθαι, ὅτε τις προτέρως χαλεπήνῃ.

τοιαύτην οὖν ἀρχὴν ἔσχεν ἡ πρὸς αὐτοὺς συνουσία. Φλά-

Adde quae in Jufti uxore fecerim, quam contabescentem citra ullius partis affectum evidentem non folum amare deprehendi, fed etiam quem amaret; et paulo poft quomodo invenerim aperiam. Sed primum certaminis, quod cum Stoïcis et Peripateticis gelli, praefentibus etiam aliis fimul cum ipfis et medicis et philofophis, mentionem fum facturus, fimulatque unde incepit, percenfuero, ut fi etiam alicui ex iis, qui hujusmodi fermonum communicatione digni funt, librum hunc voles impertire, omnem jam factorum ordinem habeas; et ne femper narrando occuperis, quae in artis medicae operibus diffectionibusque et in disputationibus ipforum fecerim, invidos et medicos et philofophos redarguens. Quum enim provocarer ab eis, ad hoc descendi, Homerum imitatus, qui me docuerit

Hominem viciffim impetere, quum quis prior molestus fuerit.

Tale igitur initium converfatio cum eis habuit. Flavius

βιος Βοηθὸς ὑπατικὸς ἀνὴρ, ὅπως μὲν ἦν φιλόκαλός τε καὶ φιλομαθὴς οἶσθα καὶ σύ. διδασκάλῳ δ' ἐχρῆτο τῶν Περιπατητικῶν δογμάτων Ἀλεξάνδρῳ τῷ Δαμασκηνῷ, γινώσκοντι μὲν καὶ τὰ τοῦ Πλάτωνος, ἀλλὰ τοῖς Ἀριστοτέλους προσκειμένῳ μᾶλλον. ὁπότ' οὖν παρεκάλεσέ με, διδάξαι διὰ τῶν ἀνατομῶν ὅπως ἀναπνοή τε καὶ φωνὴ γίνεται, παρεσκεύασεν ἐρίφους τε καὶ χοίρους πλείονας· πιθήκων γὰρ οὐδὲν ἔφην δεῖσθαι τὴν ἀνατομὴν, ὁμοίως τε τὴν κατασκευὴν ἐχόντων οὐ μόνον τούτων τῶν ζώων, ἀλλὰ καὶ πεζῶν σχεδὸν ἁπάντων· ὅσα δὲ φωνὴν ἔχει μεγάλην, ἐπιτηδειότερα τῶν μικροφώνων εἶναι, παρασχεῖν ἀποδεικτικὰ λήμματα πρὸς τὴν τοῦ προκειμένου πίστιν. παρῆσαν δ' ἐν τῇ μελλούσῃ γενήσεσθαι δείξει καὶ ἄλλοι μέν τινες, ἀτὰρ οὖν καὶ Ἀδριανὸς ὁ ῥήτωρ, οὔπω σοφιστεύων, ἀλλ' ἔτι συνὼν τῷ Βοηθῷ· καὶ ὁ Δημήτριος Ἀλεξανδρεὺς ἑταῖρος Φαβωρίνου, δημοσίᾳ λέγων ἑκάστης ἡμέρας εἰς τὰ προβαλλόμενα κατὰ τὴν ἰδέαν τῆς Φαβωρίνου λέξεως. ἐμοῦ δὲ πρὶν ἀνατέμνειν εἰπόντος ὡς αὐτὸς μὲν δείξαιμι τὰ ἐκ τῆς ἀνατομῆς φαι-

Boëthus, vir conſularis, quam fuerit et honeſti ſtudioſus et doctrinae cupidus, tu quoque noſti. Utebatur autem praeceptore ſectae Peripateticae Alexandro Damasceno; qui quidem et Platonis ſcita noverat, ſed Ariſtotelicis magis adhaerens. Quum igitur rogaſſet me ut per ſectiones docerem quomodo reſpiratio et vox fieret, comparavit et hoedos et porcos complures; ſimias enim dicebam non deſiderare diſſectionem, quum non ſolum haec animalia ſimilem habeant conſtructionem, ſed etiam pedeſtria fere omnia, quae autem magnam edunt vocem, aptiora exili voce praeditis eſſe, quae ſumptiones demonſtratorias ad fidem de re propoſita faciendam praebeant. Advenerant ſpectatum quae oſtenſurus eſſem cum alii quidam, tum et Adrianus rhetor, nondum rhetoricas inſtitutiones docens, ſed cum Boëtho adhuc agens; item Demetrius Alexandreus, Favorini familiaris, quotidie publice exponens ea, quae ſecundum Favorini dictionis ſpeciem proponebantur. Quum autem ego ante diſſectionem dicerem, me quidem ea, quae in

νόμενα, συλλογίσασθαι δὲ τὰ ἐξ αὐτῶν περαινόμενα, οὐκ ἐμοῦ μόνον, ἀλλὰ καὶ τῶν ἁπάντων μᾶλλον ἐλπίζοιμι δύνασθαι τὸν διδάσκαλον Ἀλέξανδρον· οἱ μὲν ἄλλοι πάντες ὡς ἐπιεικῆ τὸν λόγον ἀπεδείξαντο, τιμὴν εἰς τὸν Ἀλέξανδρον ἔχοντες καὶ ἅμα προτροπὴν εἰς τὴν ὅλην οὐσίαν ἄνευ φιλονεικίας γενέσθαι. γινώσκεις γὰρ ὡς ἐπὶ τούτῳ τῷ πάθει πρὸς ἁπάντων καὶ Ἀλέξανδρος ἐγινώσκετο, καθάπερ καὶ τότε σαφῶς ἐδήλωσε. δείξειν γὰρ ὑποσχομένου μου νευρίων λεπτοτάτων, ὡς εἶναι τριχοειδῆ συζυγίαν τινὰ τοῖς τοῦ φάρυγγος μυσὶν ἐκφυομένην, τοῖς μὲν ἐκ τῶν ἀριστερῶν μερῶν, τοῖς δὲ ἐκ τῶν δεξιῶν· ἐφ' οἷς βρόχῳ διαληφθεῖσιν, ἢ τμηθεῖσιν ἄφωνον γίνεται τὸ ζῶον, οὔτ' εἰς τὴν ζωήν τι βλαπτομένου, οὔτ' εἰς τὴν ἐνέργειαν· ὁ Ἀλέξανδρος ὑπολαβὼν πρὶν δειχθῆναι, τοῦτο πρῶτον, ἔφη, ἄν σοι συγχωρηθῇ, τοῖς διὰ τῶν αἰσθήσεων φαινομένοις πιστεύειν ἡμᾶς δεῖν. ἀκούσας δ' ἐγὼ ταῦτα, καταλιπὼν αὐτοὺς ἐχωρίσθην ἓν μόνον φθεγξάμενος, ὡς ἐσφάλην οἰόμενος οὐκ εἰς τοὺς ἀγροικοπυῤῥωνείους ἥκειν, ἢ οὐκ ἂν ἀφικνεῖσθαι.

diſſectione apparerent, oſtenſurum, quae vero inde ſequantur, non meum eſſe tantum colligere, ſed etiam omnium praeceptorem Alexandrum magis poſſe ſperare; omnes ſane reliqui tanquam modeſtum ſermonem receperunt, honorem Alexandro deſerentes; ac ſimul adhortabantur eum ut toti negotio citra contentionem incumberet. Quippe non latet te, Alexandrum hoc affectu ab omnibus nosci, quemadmodum et tunc manifeſto indicavit. Quum enim oſtenſurum me pollicerer nervulorum tenuiſſimorum, quaſi capillarem conjugationem quandam gutturis musculis inſeri, aliis ex ſiniſtris partibus, aliis ex dextris, ob quos funiculo interceptos vel ſectos animal mutum redditur, ita ut nec vita neque actio ipſius offendatur; Alexander commodum reſpondens priusquam oſtendatur, hoc primum, inquit, utique tibi concedetur, ſed iis, quae ſenſu apparent, credere nos oportet. Quae ubi ego audiviſſem, relictis ipſis diſceſſi, unum hoc locutus, erraſſe me, qui putarem ad ruſticos Pyrrhoneos me

ἐμοῦ δὲ χωρισθέντος οἵ τ' ἄλλοι τοῦ Ἀλεξάνδρου κατέγνωσαν ὅ τ' Ἀδριανὸς καὶ ὁ Δημήτριος, ἐχθρῶς ἀεὶ διακείμενοι πρὸς τὴν φιλονεικίαν αὐτῷ, πιθανὴν ἀφορμὴν εἶχον ἐπιτιμῆσαι σφοδρῶς. ἐπεὶ δὲ καὶ τοῖς φιλολόγοις ἅπασιν, ὅσοι κατὰ τὴν τῶν Ῥωμαίων πόλιν ἦσαν, ἐγνώσθη τοῦτο καὶ τῷ Σεβήρῳ καὶ τῷ [839] Παύλῳ καὶ τῷ Βαρβάρῳ, πάντες οὖν σφοδρῶς ἐπετίμησαν αὐτῷ καὶ παρόντων αὐτῶν ἠξίωσαν γενέσθαι τὰς ἀνατομὰς, ἀθροίσαντες εἰς αὐτὸ τοὺς ἄλλους ἅπαντας, ὅσοι κατὰ τὴν ἰατρικήν τε καὶ φιλοσοφίαν ἦσαν ἔνδοξοι. γινομένης δὲ πλείοσιν ἡμέραις τῆς συνουσίας καὶ δείξαντος ἐμοῦ τὴν μὲν εἰσπνοὴν γίνεσθαι διαστελλομένου τοῦ θώρακος, τὴν δὲ ἐκπνοὴν συστελλομένου, δείξαντος δὲ καὶ τοὺς μῦς, ὑφ' ὧν τε διαστέλλονται καὶ πρὸς τοῦτό γε τὰ εἰς αὐτοὺς κατεσχημένα νεῦρα, τὴν ἔκφυσιν ἐκ τοῦ νωτιαίου μυελοῦ ποιούμενα καὶ ὡς μὲν ἀβίαστος ἔξω φορὰ τοῦ πνεύματος ἐκπνοὴν ἄψοφον ἐργάζοιτο, βιαίαν δ' εἶναι τὴν ἑτέραν αὐτῆς γινομένην μετὰ ψόφου, ἣν ἐκφύσησιν ὀνομάζομεν· ἐπιδείξαντος δὲ καὶ ὡς ἡ

non venire, aut certe non venturum fuiſſe. Poſtquam jam diſceſſiſſem, cum alii Alexandrum increpabant, tum Adrianus Demetriusque, male ſemper erga contentionem affecti, probabilem occaſionem habebant, qua vehementer eum corriperent. Quum vero ſtudioſi etiam omnes, qui in urbe Romanorum erant, et Severus Paulusque et Barbarus id reſciverunt, omnes certe graviter ipſum accuſarunt, voluerantque praeſentibus ipſis fieri diſſectiones, congregatis ad hoc aliis univerſis, qui in medicina et philoſophia erant celebres. Durante igitur conventu pluribus diebus, oſtendi inſpirationem fieri thorace dilatato, exſpirationem vero contracto; praeterea muſculos indicavi, a quibus dilatatur; ad haec nervos, qui in ipſos inſeruntur, ex ſpinali medulla proficiſci: inſuper quomodo non coacta ſpiritus foras dilatio exſpirationem ſine ſtrepitu efficiat; violentam vero eſſe diverſam ab ea cum ſtrepitu accidentem, quam efflationem nominamus. Quum autem

τοιαύτη μόνη κατὰ τὴν διὰ τοῦ φάρυγγος ἔξοδον ὑπὸ τῶν κατὰ τὸν χόνδρον πληττομένη τὴν φωνὴν ἐργάζοιτο, καὶ ὡς ὑπὸ μυῶν οὗτοι κινοῖντο καὶ ὡς τὰ νεῦρα τὰ τούτους κινοῦντα κακωθέντα, τὴν ἀφωνίαν ἐργάζοιτο καὶ τῶν παραφθεγξαμένων ὁπότε ἐδείκνυον ταῦτα πάντων ἐλεγχθέντων, ὁ Βοηθὸς ἐδεήθη μου σχεῖν αὐτῶν ὑπομνήματα. καὶ πέμψαντός γε αὐτοῦ τοὺς διὰ σημείων ἠσκημένους ἐν τάχει γράφειν, ὑπηγόρευσα πάντα τὰ δειχθέντα καὶ λεχθέντα μὴ προορώμενος εἰ μέλλει δώσειν αὐτὰ πολλοῖς. καὶ μέχρι δὲ νῦν, ὦ Ἐπίγενες, οὐδὲν ἐτόλμησέ τις ἀντειπεῖν (456) αὐτοῖς ἐτῶν ἐν τῷ μεταξὺ γεγονότων ιε΄. καίτοι γε διαβουλευομένων γε πολλῶν ἀντειπεῖν, ὅπως ἀκουσθῶσιν αὐτὸ τοῦτο μόνον, ὡς ἀντειρήκασιν, οὐ μὴν τολμώντων γε εἰς κρίσιν ἐπὶ φιλολόγων ἀνδρῶν ἀγαγεῖν τὰ γραφέντα.

Κεφ. στ΄. Λοιπὸν οὖν ὅπερ ὑπεσχόμην ἐφεξῆς σοι διηγήσομαι, ἣν λέξιν καὶ προσθεῖναι δὲ τῷ παρόντι λόγῳ, μάλιστ᾽ ἐπειδὰν καὶ τῶν σοφιστῶν ἰατρῶν ἔνιοι, ἀγνοούμενοι τίνι λόγῳ τὸν ἔρωτα τῆς παλλακῆς τοῦ πατρὸς Ἐρα-

monſtraſſem etiam talem ſolam, dum per arteriam aſperam exit, a cartilaginibus ictam, vocem efficere et a musculis has moveri, nervosque hos moventes affectos vocis abolitionem moliri; et oblocutoribus haec ubi indicaſſem, omnibus convictis, Boëthus rogavit me ut eorum commentaria ſibi darem. Ac cum miſiſſet ipſe, qui notis celeriter ſcribere noverunt, dictavi omnia et oſtenſa a me et dicta, non praevidens, an ea multis eſſet communicaturus. Et hactenus, o Poſthume, nemo auſus eſt refragari, quindecim interea annis praeteritis; quamvis multi contradicere nitantur, ut hoc ſolum apud vulgus audiant, nempe Galeno ſe contradixiſſe, non tamen audent ſcripta ad doctorum hominum judicium referre.

Cap. VI. Reliquum igitur, quod pollicitus ſum, deinceps tibi enarrabo, modo et hoc apponere ſermoni praeſenti oporteat; praeſertim quum et ſophiſtarum medicorum nonnulli, ignorantes qua ratione Eraſiſtratus adoleſcentis

σίστρατος ἐγνώρισεν, ἔγραψαν τῶν ἀρτηριῶν τοὺς σφυγμοὺς τοῦ νεανίσκου, σφυζουσῶν ἐρωτικῶς ἐξευρεῖν αὐτὸν, οὐκέθ᾽ ὑπομείναντες εἰπεῖν ἐκ τῶν σφυγμῶν εὑρεθῆναι. ἐγὼ δ᾽ ὅπως μὲν Ἐρασίστρατος ἔγνω, τοῦτο λέγειν οὐκ ἔχω. ὅπως δὲ αὐτὸς ἔγνων ἤδη σοι φράσω. παρεκλήθημεν εἰς τὴν ἐπίσκεψίν τινος γυναικὸς, ὡς ἀγρυπνούσης ἐν ταῖς νυξὶ καὶ μεταβαλλούσης ἑαυτὴν ἄλλοτε εἰς ἄλλο σχῆμα κατακλίσεως, εὗρον δ᾽ ἀπύρετον, ἐπυθόμην ὑπὲρ ἑκάστου τῶν κατὰ μέρος αὐτῇ γεγονότων, ἐξ ὧν ἴσμεν ἀγρυπνίας συμβαινούσας. ἡ δὲ μόγις, ἢ οὐδ᾽ ὅλως ἀπεκρίνετο, ὡς μάτην ἐρωτωμένην ἐνδεικνυμένη καὶ τὸ τελευταῖον ἀποστραφεῖσα, τοῖς μὲν ἐπιβεβλημένοις ἱματίοις ὅλῳ τῷ σώματι σκεπάσασα πᾶσαν ἑαυτὴν, ἄλλῳ δέ τινι μικρῷ ταραντινιδίῳ τὴν κεφαλὴν ἔκειτο καθάπερ οἱ χρήζοντες ὕπνου. χωρισθεὶς οὖν ἐγὼ δυοῖν θάτερον αὐτὴν ἐνόησα πάσχειν, ἢ μελαγχολικῶς δυσθυμεῖν, ἤ τι λυπουμένην οὐκ ἐθέλειν ὁμολογεῖν. εἰς τὴν ὑστέραιαν οὖν ἀνεβαλλόμην ἀκριβέστερον διασκέψασθαι περὶ

erga ancillam patris cognovit amorem, fcribant arterias pulfus juvenis amatorios edentibus ipfum inveniffe, nunc autem non amplius, ut quis ex pulfibus inventum effe dicat, fuftinent. Ego fane quomodo Erafiftratus id deprehenderit, dicere non poffum; quomodo autem ipfe cognoverim, jam tibi aperiam. Vocatus fum ad mulierem invifendam, quae noctu vigiliis torquebatur et alias in aliam decubitus figuram fe transmutabat. Hanc dum febri carentem invenio, rogo de fingulis particulatim ei obortis, unde vigilias accidere deprehendimus. Ipfa autem vix aut nequaquam refpondebat, ceu fruftra interrogaretur indicans; denique vultu averfo veftimentis fuperinjectis univerfo corpori, totam fe contegit, ac alteri cuipiam exiguo pulvino caput inclinabat, quemadmodum ii, qui fomno indigent. Digreffus itaque ego, inde alterutrum ipfam pati exiftimabam, aut melancholice animo torqueri, aut qua triftitia afficeretur, nolle fateri. Differebam itaque in fubfequentem diem exactius de ipfa confiderare, ac quum

αὐτῶν καὶ πορευθεὶς τὸ μὲν πρότερον ἤκουσα τῆς παραμενούσης οἰκέτιδος ὡς ἀδύνατον αὐτὴν ἄρτι θεάσασθαι· δεύτερον δ' ἐπανελθὼν ὡς ἤκουσα πάλιν ταυτὸ, τρίτον πάλιν ἧκον. εἰπούσης δέ μου τῆς θεραπαίνης ἀπαλλάττεσθαι, μὴ βούλεσθαι γὰρ ἐνοχλεῖσθαι τὴν γυναῖκα, καὶ γνοὺς αὐτὴν ἐμοῦ χωρισθέντος λελουμένην τε καὶ τὰ συνήθως προσενεγκαμένην [840], ἧκον τῇ ὑστεραίᾳ καὶ μόνος διαλεχθεὶς τῇ θεραπαίνῃ πολυειδῶς, ἔγνων σαφῶς τίνι λύπῃ τειρομένην, ἣν ἐξεῦρον κατὰ τύχην, ὁποίαν οἶμαι καὶ Ἐρασιστράτῳ γενέσθαι. προεγνωσμένου γάρ μοι τοῦ μηδὲν εἶναι κατὰ τὸ σῶμα πάθος, ἀλλὰ ἀπὸ ψυχικῆς τινος ἀηδίας ἐνοχλεῖσθαι τὴν γυναῖκα, συνέβη κατὰ τὸν αὐτὸν καιρὸν ὃν ἐσκόπουν αὐτὴν βεβαιωθῆναι τοῦτο, παραγενομένου τινὸς ἐκ τοῦ θεάτρου καὶ φάντος ὀρχούμενον ἑορακέναι Πυλάδην· ἠλλάγη γὰρ αὐτῆς καὶ τὸ βλέμμα καὶ τὸ χρῶμα τοῦ προσώπου, κἀγὼ θεασάμενος τοῦτο, τῷ καρπῷ τῆς γυναικὸς ἐπιβαλὼν τὴν χεῖρα, τὸν σφυγμὸν εὗρον ἀνώμαλον ἐξαίφνης πολυειδῶς γενόμενον, ὅστις δηλοῖ τὴν ψυχὴν τεθορυβῆσθαι· ὁ αὐτὸς οὖν καὶ τοῖς ἀγωνιῶσι περί τι πρᾶγμα

veniſſem, primum audivi ab ancilla aſtante fieri non poſſe ut ipſam viderem. Iterum reverſus poſtquam idem audiviſſem, tertio redii: ac cum famula mihi diceret ut discederem, nolle enim mulierem moleſtari, quumque noviſſem, ipſam me egreſſo et lotam et ſolita aſſumpſiſſe, veni poſtridie, ac ſolus cum ancilla multiſariam diſſerens cognovi manifeſto triſtitia quadam affectam, quam caſu inveni, ut etiam Eraſiſtrato accidiſſe puto. Nam cum certus eſſem nullum in corpore affectum exiſtere, ſed animali quadam moleſtia mulierem torqueri, contigit eodem tempore, quo ipſam inviſebam, id confirmari, adventante quodam ex theatro et nuntiante ſe Pyladem vidiſſe ſaltantem: mutatus enim ipſius viſus eſt et faciei color: quod ego contemplatus manu mulieris brachiali injecta pulſum deprehendi inaequalem, ſubito ac multis modis agitatum, qui animam turbatam eſſe indicat: idem igitur et de re quadam contendentibus obvenit. Poſtridie dixi

συμβαίνειν. κατὰ τὴν ὑστεραίαν οὖν εἰπὼν ἀκολούθῳ τινὶ τῶν ἐμῶν, ὅταν ἐπισκεψάμενος ἔλθω πρὸς τὴν γυναῖκα, μετ' ὀλίγον ἀφικόμενος ἀνάγγειλόν μοι, Μόρφον ὀρχεῖσθαι σήμερον, εἶθ' ὡς ἤγγειλεν, ἄτρεπτον εὗρον τὸν σφυγμόν. ὁμοίως δὲ καὶ κατὰ τὴν ἑξῆς ἡμέραν ποιήσας ἀγγελθῆναι περὶ τοῦ τρίτου τῶν ὀρχηστῶν, ὁμοίως μείναντος ἀτρέπτου τοῦ σφυγμοῦ. κατὰ τὴν τετάρτην ἠκρίβωσα νύκτα πάνυ παραφυλάξας, ἡνίκα Πυλάδης ὀρχούμενος ἠγγέλθη, ταραχθέντα πολυειδῶς αὐτὸν ὁρῶν, εὗρον οὕτως ἐρῶσαν τοῦ Πυλάδου τὴν γυναῖκα καὶ τοῦτο παραφυλαχθὲν ἀκριβῶς ἐν ταῖς ἐφεξῆς ἡμέραις εὑρέθη βεβαίως. καθάπερ γε καί τινος ἄλλου τῶν πλουσίων δοῦλος οἰκονόμος ὁμοίως κάμνων ἐγνώσθη μοι. λυπούμενος γὰρ ἐν τῷ μέλλειν ἀποδιδόναι λογισμοὺς ὧν διῴκησεν, ἐν οἷς ἠπίστατο λεῖπον οὐκ ὀλίγον ἀργύριον, ὑπὸ τῆς φροντίδος ἠγρύπνει τε καὶ λυπούμενος ἐτήκετο, προειπὼν δὲ αὐτοῦ τῷ δεσπότῃ μηδὲν εἶναι σωματικὸν πάθημα τῷ πρεσβύτῃ, σκέψασθαι συνεβουλευσάμην, ὅτι φοβοῖτο μέλλοντος αὐτοῦ τοὺς λόγους, ὧν ἐνεχείρισεν

cuidam ex iis, qui fequebantur me, quum mulierem vifitatum accederem, ut paulo poft adveniens nuntiaret mihi Morphum hodie faltare; id ubi factum eft, pulfum nihil offendi mutatum. Similiter et fequenti die quum curaffem ut de tertio faltatore nuntiaretur, fimiliter pulfus haud mutatus eft. Quarta rem diligenter examinavi nocte; qua obfervans pulfum, quum Pylades faltare nuntiaretur, turbatum ipfum multifariam ipfum videns, deprehendi ita mulierem Pyladem amare, atque hoc exacte obfervatum diebus fubfequentibus confirmatum eft. Quemadmodum etiam divitis cujusdam fervus oeconomus fimiliter cognitus eft mihi aegrotare. Quum enim angeretur de reddendis rationibus eorum, quae difpenfarat, in quibus non parum argenti defiderari fciens, prae curis vigilabat et triftitia contabefcebat. Quum autem praedixiffem domino ipfius nullum effe affectum corporeum feni, infpicere confului, qui timeret, quum ipfe rationes eorum, quae adminiftra-

ἀπαιτεῖν, καὶ διὰ τοῦτο λυποῖτο, γινώσκων οὐκ ὀλίγον ἐν αὐτοῖς εὑρήσεσθαι λεῖπον. ἐπειδὴ καλῶς ἔφη με στοχάζεσθαι, τοῦτο συνεβούλευσα βεβαίας ἕνεκεν διαγνώσεως, εἰπεῖν αὐτῷ ὅσον ἔχει παρακείμενον ἀργύριον αἰτῆσαι τοῦτο, μή πως ἐξ αἰφνιδίου τελευτήσαντος ἀπόληται, μεταστάσης εἰς ἄλλον οἰκέτην τῆς διοικήσεως, οὗ μήπω πεῖραν ἔχει· παρὰ γὰρ ἐκείνου μὴ χρήζειν ἀπαιτήσεως λογισμῶν. ὡς δὲ ὁ δεσπότης αὐτῷ ταῦτα διελέχθη, πεισθεὶς οὐκ ἐξετασθήσεσθαι καὶ διὰ τοῦτο γινόμενος ἄλυπος ἐν τῇ τρίτῃ τῶν ἡμερῶν τὴν κατὰ φύσιν ἕξιν τοῦ σώματος ἀνεκτήσατο. τί δή ποτ᾽ οὖν ἐλάνθανε τοὺς ἔμπροσθεν ἰατροὺς τήν τε προειρημένην γυναῖκα καὶ τὸν προειρημένον οἰκέτην ἐπισκοπουμένους; ἐκ γὰρ κοινῶν ἐπιλογισμῶν εὑρίσκεται τὰ τοιαῦτα, κἂν βραχεῖαν ἐπιστήμην ἔχῃ τῆς ἰατρικῆς θεωρίας. ἐγὼ μὲν ἡγοῦμαι διότι μηδεμίαν ἔχουσι διάγνωσιν, ὧν τὸ σῶμα διὰ τῆς ψυχῆς πάθη πάσχειν εἴωθει. ἴσως δὲ ὅτι οὐδὲ διὰ τοὺς ἀγῶνας καὶ τοὺς φόβους ἐξαίφνης τὴν ψυχὴν ταράξαντας οἱ σφυγμοὶ τρέπονται γινώσκουσιν. ὅπερ Ἐρασίστρατος ἐπι-

vit, esset repetiturus, nam idcirco tristitia afficiebatur, quod sciret non exiguum in eis desideratum iri. Quoniam recte conjecisti hoc, inquit, consului firmae agnitionis causa ut ei diceret quantam haberet famulus repositam pecuniam, hanc postularet, ne derepente eo mortuo periret, dispensatione in alium domesticum translata, quem nondum esset expertus; ab illo enim non desideraret rationes. Postquam dominus haec servo dixisset, is persuasus se non examinatum iri postea, eoque evadens laetior, tertio die naturalem corporis habitum recuperavit. Curnam igitur priores medicos et praedictam mulierem praedictumque famulum visitantes haec latebant? Nam ex communibus ratiocinationibus hujusmodi inveniuntur; etiam si exiguam speculationis medicae scientiam habeant. Ego sane puto, eo quod nullam habent cognitionem eorum, quae corpus propter animi affectus pati consuevit; forsan etiam, quod neque ob contentiones et metus subito animum turbantes pulsus mutari cognoscunt. Quod Erasistra-

στάμενος ἐπὶ τῆς αὐτῆς οἰκίας τῷ νοσοῦντι τῆς γυναικὸς υπαρχούσης εὐκολώτερον ἐξεῦρεν, ὡς ἂν δυναμένου αὐτοῦ συνεχέστερον ὁρᾶσθαι τὸν νεανίσκον, μὴ διὰ πλειόνων ἡμερῶν καθάπερ ὁ Πυλάδης· οὐδ' οὖν οὐδὲ τότε φαινομένου, ἀλλ' ἀκουομένου ἐκταράττειν τὴν γυναῖκα. λῆρος οὖν μακρὸς ἐρωτικῶς κινούμενοι σφυγμοὶ τῶν οὐ γινωσκόντων ἔρωτος μὲν οὐδένα δηλωτικὸν σφυγμὸν εἶναι, θορυβουμένης δὲ ψυχῆς τοὺς σφυγμοὺς ἀλλοιοῦσθαι, μήτε τὴν κατὰ φύσιν ὁμαλότητα μήτε τὴν τάξιν ἀποσώζοντας.

[841] Κεφ. ζ'. [Διὰ τίνων τεχνῶν τὸν Κύριλλον τὸν Βοηθοῦ υἱέα κατέλαβε ἐσθίειν λάθρα.] Ἓν οὖν ἔτι προσθεὶς, ἐφ' οὗ παραχρῆμα μὲν ἐξεπλάγη Βοηθὸς, ἀκούσας δ' ὅπως εὑρέθη θαυμάζειν οὐκέτι ἔφασκεν, ἀλλὰ τῶν ἀγνοούντων τὸ θεώρημα καταγινώσκειν ὡς ἀμαθῶν, ἐπ' ἄλλο τι μεταβήσομαι. νοσήσαντος γὰρ αὐτῷ θατέρου τῶν υἱῶν, εἶτα ῥωσθέντος ὑποστρέψαντός τε τοῦ νοσήματος, εἶτ' αὖθις παυσαμένου καὶ μετὰ ταῦτα πάλιν ἐπιπυρέξαντος τοῦ παιδὸς, ἐμοῦ τε λέγοντος ἐσθίειν αὐτὸν λάθρα· τὰ γὰρ ἐν τῷ φα-

tus intelligens, quando mulier in eadem domo cum aegrotante eſſet, facilius invenit, ut quae ab adoleſcente frequentius videri poterat, non pluribus diebus quemadmodum Pylades, qui neque tunc apparens, ſed auditus tantum mulierem turbaret. Nugae igitur ſunt pulſus amatorie moti eorum qui ignorant nullum quidem pulſum amoris eſſe indicem, ſed anima turbata ob quamcunque rem pulſus alterari, neque naturalem aequalitatem neque ordinem conſervantes.

Cap. VII. [*Quibus artibus Cyrillum Boëthi filium clam cibum ſumere deprehendit.*] Itaque quum unum adhuc adjecero, ob quod ſtatim ſane obſtupuit Boëthus, ubi autem quomodo eſſet inventum audiſſet, admirari non amplius ſe dicebat, ſed ignorantes ſpeculationem tanquam indoctos damnare, ad aliud quid digrediar. Quum itaque alter filiorum ipſius aegrotaſſet, deinde convaluiſſet, quumque mox recidivam morbus feciſſet iterumque ceſſaſſet et poſt haec rurſus puer febricitaſſet, dixi eum clancu-

νερῷ διδόμενα πρὸς τῷ ταῖς ποιότησιν ὑπάρχειν ἐπιτήδεια καὶ τῇ ποσότητι σύμμετρα εἶναι, τὴν μητέρα τοῦ παιδὸς ὑποσχομένην ἀκριβῶς αὐτὸν φυλάξαι ἐπέστησε φύλακα παρακαθημένην τε δι' ὅλης τῆς ἡμέρας, ἀποκωλύουσάν τε τοὺς εἰς τὸν οἶκον ἐκεῖνον εἰσιόντας, κατὰ τὸν οἶκον αὐτοῦ κοιμωμένου, ἀποκεκλεισμένον ἔνδοθεν ἀκριβῶς ἀπ' αὐτῆς. ἐπεὶ δὲ τέτρασιν ἡμέραις οὕτω φυλαττόμενος ἐθερμάνθη διὰ τῆς νυκτὸς, ὁ *Βοηθὸς* ἀναρτήσας με καὶ παραλαβὼν ἦγεν εἰς τὴν οἰκίαν ἐπὶ τὸν παῖδα, συνηκολούθησαν δ' αὐτῷ καὶ οἱ κατὰ τὴν ὁδὸν ἀπαντῶντες, ἐν οἷς ἦσθα καὶ σύ. κατέλαβον δὲ ἐκ μὲν τοῦ κοιτῶνος ἅμα τῇ μητρὶ προεληλυθότα τὸν παῖδα πρὸς ἕτερον οἴκημα, ἐν ᾧ καὶ κλίνη, καθ' ἧς ἡ μήτηρ τοῦ παιδὸς ἐκαθέζετο· σκίμπους δέ τις ἔζευκτο μικρὸν τῶν μέσων αὐτοῦ κατωτέρω, καθ' οὗ τὸν παῖδα κατακλίνασα παρεφύλαττεν, ὡς μηδεὶς αὐτῷ προσέρχοιτο. καθέδρα δὲ ἦν μία τοῦ σκίμποδος, οἷα σύμμετρον ἐφ' ἑαυτῇ ἐπ' αὐχένι ἔχουσι. κατάντικρυς δὲ τοῦ σκίμποδος πρὸς τοῖς ἄνω πέρασι τῆς κλίνης ἐφεξῆς ἀλλήλων ἔκειντο δύο βάθραι,

lum comedere. Nam quae manifesto ei dabantur, praeterquam quod qualitatibus essent idonea, etiam quantitate moderata fuerant. Quapropter matrem pueri, ubi diligenter se ipsum observaturam promitteret, constituit custodem, quae toto die assideret, prohiberetque domum illam ingredientes, in qua ipse dormiebat, occlusam interius ab ipsa exacte. Posteaquam quatuor jam diebus ita observaretur, noctu incaluit; ob quod Boëthus mihi indignatus et acceptum domum suam deduxit ad puerum; sequuti autem sunt ipsum etiam qui in via occurrebant, inter quos et tu eras. Puerum deprehendi ex cubiculo una cum matre ad aliud domicilium digressum, ubi etiam lectus erat in quo mater pueri decumbebat; lectica vero quaedam exigua inter duos lectos inferius, juncta, in quam puerum collocans observabat ne quis eum accederet. Porro sedile unum lecticae mediocre ad cervicem ejus habebatur. E regione juxta superiores lecti terminos duo ordine sedilia

καθ᾽ ὧν ὁ Βοηθὸς ἡμᾶς καθίσας αὐτὸς, τῇ γυναικὶ παρακαθε (457) σθεὶς, ἤγαγον Γαληνὸν, ἔφη, τοῦτον ὅπως ἀκούσῃ παρὰ σοῦ περὶ τῆς ἀκριβοῦς φυλακῆς ἐν ταύταις ταῖς ἡμέραις γεγενημένης τοῦ παιδὸς, ὡς οὐδὲν ἐν τῇ διαίτῃ πλημμελοῖτο· θεασάμενός τε πότερον ὄντως ἐπύρεξε διὰ τῆς νυκτὸς, ἢ σὺ φάσκουσά μοι θερμότερον αὐτὸν γεγονέναι παρελογίσθης ὑπὸ δειλίας, ὡς οἰηθῆναι πυρετὸν εἶναι τὴν θερμότητα δι᾽ ἄλλην ἴσως αἰτίαν γενομένην· ἵνα μὲν ὅπως διάγει σαφῶς ἡμῖν δηλώσειεν, ἅμα δὲ καὶ τὰ τῆς διαίτης αὐτῷ πάντα σε διδάξειεν. ἁψάμενος οὖν ἐγὼ τῆς κατὰ τὸν καρπὸν ἀρτηρίας τοῦ παιδὸς ἀπύρετον μὲν αὐτὸν ἔφην εἶναι, παρέχειν δέ μοι σκωμμάτων ἀρχὴν τοῖς ὀνομάζουσί με μάντιν. ὑπολαβὼν οὖν ὁ Βοηθὸς ἔφη· κἀγὼ πρὸς ἐκείνους, ὡς οἶσθα, καλεῖν εἴωθά σε μάντιν ὄντα, ὅταν τοιοῦτον εἴπῃς, ὁποῖον οἱ ἀντίτεχνοί σου φάσκουσιν ἀδύνατον εἶναι, διὰ τῶν τῆς ἰατρικῆς θεωρημάτων γνωσθῆναι. ἀλλά τοι μέχρι δεῦρο πάντ᾽, ἔφην, ἔδειξά σοι τὰ τοιαῦτα διὰ θεωρίας ἰατρικῆς εὑρισκόμενα καί τινάς τε τῶν ἰατρῶν

vicina erant: fuper quae Boëthus nos collocans, ipfe uxori aflidens, adduxi Galenum, inquit, hunc, ut audiat abs te quam diligenter hisce diebus puerum cuftodieris, ne quicquam in victus ratione peccaretur; videatque num revera nocte febricitarit, an tu, quum calidiorem ipfum factum effe diceres, defipueris prae timore, quae putaris febrem effe calorem ob aliam forte caufam obortum; ut deinde quomodo habeat manifefto nobis indicet, fimulque omnem ipfius victus rationem te doceat. Quum itaque arteriam pueri in brachiali tetigiffem, absque febri ipfum effe dixi, fed praebere me convitiorum occafionem iis, qui me vaticinatorem appellant. Interloquens itaque Boëthus ait: et ego apud illos te vocare, ut nofti, confuevi vatem, quum hujusmodi diceres, quale hoftes tui fieri non poffe dictitant, ut ex medicinae fpeculationibus cognofcatur. Atqui hactenus omnia (dicebam) oftendi tibi talia ex fpeculatione medica inveniri et quosdam medicorum ea fcri-

αὐτὰ γεγραφότων. λέγειν οὖν ἐκελεύετε πάντες ἤδη τὸ μάντευμα· κἀγὼ δεηθεὶς ἅπαξ ἔτι συγχωρήσειν μοι τῶν σφυγμῶν ἅψασθαι τοῦ παιδὸς, ἐπειδὴ τοῦτ᾽ ἔπραξα, μαρτυρήσεις, ἔφην, ὦ Βοηθὲ, μηδένα μοι παραγιναμένῳ μετὰ σοῦ διαλεγομένων ἡμῶν δι᾽ ὅλης τῆς ὁδοῦ προσεληλυθότα τὸ μέλλον λέγεσθαι μάντευμα μεμηνυκέναι. φάντος οὖν αὐτοῦ μαρτυρήσειν, οἶσθα ὅπως γελάσας ἐγὼ προσέχειν τε καὶ ἀκούειν ὑμᾶς ἐκέλευσα τὸ τοῦ μάντεως θέσπισμα τοιόνδε τι φήσας εἶναι· τῷ Κυρίλλῳ τούτῳ κατὰ τὸν οἶκον τοῦτον ἀποκέκρυπταί τι τῶν ἐδωδίμων, ὅπως ὅταν εἰς τὸ βαλανεῖον ἡ μήτηρ αὐτοῦ πορευομένη κλείσῃ τὸν οἶκον, [842] εἶτα ὑπὲρ ἀσφαλείας εἰς γλωττόκομον ἐμβάλλουσα τὴν κλεῖν κατασημήνηται, τοῦτο γὰρ ἀκούω ποιεῖν αὐτὴν ἑκάστοτε, κατακεκρυμμένον ἀνελόμενος ὁ υἱὸς αὐτῆς οὕτως προσενέγκηται. ταῦτ᾽ ἀκούσας Βοηθὸς εὐθέως ἐξορμήσας πρὸς τὸν παῖδα συναρπάζει τε καὶ μετακομίσας ἐπὶ τὴν κλίνην, ἀναστορεθῆναι τὸν σκίμποδα κελεύσας, ἐπειρᾶτο τὸ κατακεκρυμμένον ὡς αὐτίκα φανησόμενον. ἐπειδὴ τά τ᾽ ἐπιβλήματα πάντα καὶ τὸ ὑπεστορεσμένον αὐτοῖς ἀνετινάχθη, τὸ γνάφαλον ἑξῆς

pfiffe. Dicere igitur jam vaticinium omnes mihi juffiftis; ac ego precatus vos femel adhuc ut permitteretis mihi pueri pulfum tangere, pofteaquam hoc feciffem, teftaberis, dixi, o Boëthe, nullum mihi proficiscenti tecum, quum tota via nos differeremus acceffiffe, qui futurum vaticinium praedicaverit. Poftquam itaque ipfe dixiffet fe atteftaturum, Novifti, inquam, quomodo ridens ego advertere et audire vos juffi vatis oraculum, tale quoddam effe loquutus. Cyrillo huic in domo ifta aliquid ex esculentis occultatum eft, quod quum mater ipfius ad balneum proficiscens domum claufetit, deinde fecuritatis gratia clavi ferae injecta obfignaverit, hoc enim audio ipfam frequenter facere, abfconfum filius accipiens, ita ingerat. Poftquam hoc Boëthus audiviffet, ftatim profiliens ad puerum corripit ipfum et in lectum transferens lecticamque fterni jubens fperabat occultatum quamprimum appariturum. Ubi operimenta omnia et fubfternicula excuffa effent, pannum

ἀνετίναξεν. εἶτα τὴν καθέδραν ἐπάρας ἐπεσκοπεῖτο μή τι κατακεκρυμμένον ὑπ᾽ αὐτῇ φανείη. ὡς δ᾽ οὐδὲν οὐδ᾽ οὕτως ἐφάνη, μετακομίσας ἀπὸ τῆς κλίνης τὸ παιδίον ἐπὶ τὸν σκίμποδα τὴν κλίνην ὅλην ἀναστορέσας, ἐκέλευσεν αὖθις στρώννυσθαι. γελάσας τε, τί, φησὶν, ὁ μάντις λέγει; θαυμάσας δ᾽ ἐγὼ διότι μηδὲν εὗρεν ἐφ᾽ ὧν ᾤετο κατακεκρυμμένον, ὃ μόνον ἀζήτητον, ὡς οὐδενὸς ὑποπτεύοντος ἐν αὐτῷ περιέχεσθαι τὸ ζητούμενον ἐπάρας ἀνέσειον· ἦν δὲ τοῦτο παντελῶς σμικρὸν τῆς μητρὸς αὐτοῦ ταραντινίδος ἐπικείμενον τῇ καθέδρᾳ, σεισθέντος δ᾽ αὐτοῦ μέρος ἄρτου τὸ περιεχόμενον ὑπ᾽ αὐτοῦ κατὰ γῆς ἔπεσε καὶ ὑμεῖς πάντες ἀνακεκράγατε μέγιστον ἅμα τῷ Βοηθῷ γελῶντες καὶ τὴν μαντικὴν ἐπαινοῦντες. ὁ δ᾽ οὖν Βοηθὸς ὑπὲρ πάντας γελῶν ἐθαύμαζε πῶς ὁ σφυγμὸς, εἰ καὶ τὸ κατακεκρυμμένον ἐδώδιμον, ἱκανός ἐστι δηλοῦν. ἀλλὰ τό γε μέλλον ὑπὸ τοῦ παιδὸς ἔσεσθαι λουομένης τῆς μητρὸς ἐμήνυσα· κἀγὼ πρὸς αὐτὸν ἔτι ἔφην, ὦ δριμύτατε, μὴ δηλωσάντων τοῦτο τῶν σφυγμῶν ὁ Γαληνὸς ἐτεκμήρατο. κλεισθείσης γὰρ ἀκριβῶς

deinde perſcrutatus eſt. Poſtea ſedili ſublato obſervabat num aliquid ſub eo occultatum appareret. Quum autem nihil ita apparuiſſet, translato puero a lecto ad lecticam, lectum totum iterum ſterni juſſit, ac in riſum ſolutus, quid, ait, vaticinator dicit? Ego autem admiratus quod nihil inveniſſet, ubi occultatum putabatur, id quod ſolum indiscuſſum remanſerat, tanquam nullo quod quaerebatur in eo contineri ſuſpicante, in altum attollens commovebam; erat autem hoc exiguum matris ipſius velamentum ſedili impoſitum, quo discuſſo pars panis in eo contenta in terram decidit, ac vos omnes altiſſime clamaſtis, una cum Boëtho ridentes, vaticinatoriamque commendantes. Boëthus vero ſupra omnes ridens admirabatur, quomodo pulſus esculentum reconditum indicare poſſit. Sed quid puer facturus eſſet, matre lavante, indicavi; dixique praeterea, o vir acerrime, pulſibus hoc non indicantibus, Galenus conjecit. Nam oſtio exacte clauſo puerum ſine metu

τῆς θύρας κατὰ πολλὴν σχολὴν, τὴν ἐδωδὴν αὐτῷ τῷ παιδὶ γενέσθαι δυναμένην ἀδεῶς, οὐ χαλεπὸν ἦν τεκμήρασθαι, ἀλλὰ καὶ ὅτι κατακέκρυπταί τι καὶ τὸ κατακεκρυμμένον ἐδώδιμόν ἐστιν, ὁ μὲν σφυγμὸς οὐκ ἤγγειλέ μοι· τεταραγμένον δ' αὐτὸν θεασάμενος ἐνόησα, καθάπερ ἐπὶ τῆς ἐρώσης γυναικὸς καὶ τοῦ φοβουμένου δούλου τὴν ταραχὴν ἐπὶ ψυχικῷ τινι πάθει γενέσθαι, ἀπυρέτου τελέως γε ὄντος τοῦ παιδός. ἐρωτήσεις οὖν ἴσως ἐκ τίνος ἐτεκμηράμην ἐδώδιμον εἶναι τὸ κατακεκρυμμένον· ἄκουε δὴ καὶ περὶ τούτου τὴν ταραχὴν τῆς ψυχῆς. οὔτε δίκην μέλλων ἐρεῖν ὁ παῖς οὔτε παλαίειν, ἢ παγκρατιάζειν, ἢ ὅλως ἐπιδείκνυσθαι πλεονέκτημά τι σωματικὸν, ἢ ψυχικὸν, οὐχ ὅλως ἐγκαλούμενός τι διαμένουσιν ἴσχειν. ἀκούσας οὖν ὁ Βοηθὸς ταῦτα, νὴ τοὺς θεοὺς ἔφη θαυμάζειν, εἰ οὕτως εὔγνωστα φάρμακα τῶν ἰατρῶν οὐδεὶς οἶδεν. εὔδηλον γὰρ ὅτι μήτ' αὐτοὶ τοιοῦτον ἔργον ἐπεδείξαντο πώποτε, καὶ σὲ πάντα μᾶλλον ἢ ἐξ ἰατρικῆς αὐτὰ πράττειν φασίν. ἐοίκασι δ', ἔφη, μὴ μόνον ἀγνοεῖν ὁποῖός ἐστι τῶν ἀγωνιώντων ὁ σφυγμὸς, ἀλλὰ μηδ' εἴπερ

comedere potuiſſe, haud erat difficile conjectu. Imo etiam quod aliquid occultatum eſſet, idque esculentum, pulſus ſane non indicavit; verum turbatum ipſum puerum conſpicatus intellexi ut in muliere amante et ſervo timente, turbationem ex animali quodam affectu obortam, quum puer omnino febri vacaret. Rogabis igitur forſan, unde id quod occultatum erat esculentum eſſe conjecerim. Audi jam de hoc quoque turbationem animi. Quum puer neque cauſam eſſet dicturus in judicio, nec luctaturus neque certamen ſolemne initurus, aut denique a quoquam reprehenſus fuiſſet, ob rem corpoream magis quam animalem turbari eum ratio indicat. Quae quum audiviſſet Boëthus, per deos, inquit, mirandum eſt tam nota medicamenta nullum medicorum cognoviſſe. Unde clare conſtat et ipſos hujusmodi opus nunquam oſtendiſſe; ac te omnia aliunde potius quam ex medicina facere dictitant. Videntur autem, ajebat, non modo ignorare qualis ſit contendentium pulſus, ſed neque ſi forte aliquis ipſorum no-

ἔγνω τις αὐτῶν κατὰ τύχην ἃ προσελογίσω, προσεπιλογίσασθαι δύνασθαι. διὰ τὸ μήτε φῦναι συνετοὶ μήτε μαθήσει γεγυμνάσθαι τὸν λογισμόν. ἀλλά γε τῆς κακοηθείας ἔφην ἔργα γεγυμνασμένοι τέ εἰσι καὶ σοφοί.

Κεφ. η΄. [*Τὴν γυναῖκα τοῦ Βοηθοῦ τῷ γυναικείῳ ῥῷ περιπεσοῦσαν ἰᾶται παρὰ τὴν ἄλλων δόξαν.*] Τούτων μὲν οὖν, ὦ Ἐπίγενες, αὐτὸν ἔχω μάρτυρά σε, πολλῶν δ' ἄλλων ἑτέρους ἁπάντων τῶν πραχθέντων μοι κατὰ τὴν πρώτην ἐπιδημίαν. ἤκουες δ' αὐτὸ παρ' αὐτῶν τῶν ὑπ' ἐμοῦ θεραπευθέντων. ἓν οὖν ὄντως θαυμάσιον πραχθὲν, ὃ οὐ μόνον με παραδοξολόγον ὡς ἔμπροσθεν οἱ πολλοὶ τῶν ἰατρῶν ὠνόμαζον, ἀλλὰ καὶ παραδοξοποιὸν ἐποίησε κληθῆναι σιωπήσω. ἡ γὰρ τοῦ Βοηθοῦ γυνὴ τῷ καλουμένῳ ῥῷ γυναικείῳ περιπεσοῦσα κατ' ἀρχὰς μὲν [843] αἰδουμένη τοὺς ἀξιολόγους ἰατροὺς, ὧν εἷς ἤδη κἀγὼ πᾶσιν ἐδόκουν εἶναι, ταῖς συνήθεσι μαίαις ἀρίσταις οὔσαις τῶν κατὰ τὴν πόλιν ἑαυτὴν ἐπέτρεπεν. ὡς δ' οὐδὲν ὠφελεῖτο, πάντας ἡμᾶς ὁ Βοηθὸς ἀθροίσας ἐπεσκοπεῖτο τί χρὴ ποιεῖν. ὡς δὲ συν-

vit, quae tu ratione disquifieris, posse disquirere: eo quod nec natura prudentes, nec disciplina mentem exercuerunt. At in malignitatis, ajebam, operibus et exercitati et sapientes sunt.

Cap. VIII. [*Boëthi uxorem uteri profluvio laborantem praeter spem aliorum sanat.*] Horum igitur, o Posthume, teipsum testem habeo; aliorum autem multorum, quae in prima profectione omnia a me gesta sunt, alios. Audivisti autem ea ab illis, qui a me sunt curati. Unum igitur revera mirabile, non tantum me praeter omnium opinionem dicentem, ut antea plerique medicorum nominabant, sed etiam praeter opinionem facientem, appellari effecit. Nam Boëthi uxor fluore muliebri ut appellant infestata, quum per initia celebres medicos, e quorum numero et ego jam unus esse omnibus videbar, revereretur, consuetis obstetricibus optimis quibusque in urbe seipsam concredidit. Postquam vero nihil juvaretur, Boëthus congregatos nos omnes consulebat quid esset fa-

ωμολογήθη, κατὰ τὴν γεγραμμένην ὑφ' Ἱπποκράτους τε καὶ τῶν ἀρίστων μετ' αὐτὸν ἰατρῶν θεραπείαν, ἅπαντα πράττειν ἀξιώσαντος αὐτοῦ καὶ συνεχῶς ἐπιφαίνεσθαί με ταῖς ὑπηρετούσαις αὐτῇ γυναιξὶν, ὁρᾷν τε τὰς ὕλας τῶν κατὰ μέρος βοηθημάτων πρὸς τὸν καθόλου σκοπὸν ἀποβλέποντα, κεφάλαιον ἔχοντα, ξηραίνειν μὲν οὐ μόνον τῆς μήτρας τὰ χωρία, ἀλλὰ καὶ σύμπαν τὸ σῶμα, προσφέρειν τε καὶ ἀλειμμάτων στυφόντων τοῖς γυναικείοις τόποις, ἐποίουν οὕτως. ἐπεὶ δὲ ταῦτα πραττόντων ἐφαίνετο χείρων ἡ διάθεσις ἀποτελουμένη, κατὰ τὸ εἰκὸς ἀπορία πᾶσιν ἡμῖν ἐγίνετο καὶ ζητοῦσιν ἑτέραν ἀγωγὴν θεραπείας, ἐφ' ἣν μεταβῶμεν, οὔτ' ἐκ λογισμοῦ τις εὕρισκεν οὔτ' ἐκ πείρας ἀνεμιμνήσκετο βέλτιον τῆς ὑπὸ τῶν ἀρίστων ἰατρῶν ὁμολογουμένης. ἐν τούτῳ δὲ καὶ ὄγκος τις ὤφθη κατὰ τὴν γαστέρα παραπλήσιος τῷ γινομένῳ ταῖς κυούσαις, ὃν ἔνιαι τῶν θεραπευουσῶν αὐτὴν γυναικῶν ᾠήθησαν ὄντως ἐπὶ κυήσει γενέσθαι, οὐ μὴν τῶν γε ἄλλων ἰατρῶν τις ἐπείθετο. τὰ γὰρ ἐκκρινόμενα γνωρίσματα ὄντα τοῦ ῥοῦ τοῦ γυναικείου καθ' ἑκάστην ἡμέραν

ciendum. Quum itaque inter nos conveniffet ut fecundum fcriptam ab Hippocrate et praeftantiffimis poft ipfum curationem univerfa fierent, quumque ipfe Boëthus cuperet me frequenter famulantibus ipfi mulieribus adeffe, ac materias particularium praefidiorum univerfalem fcopum refpicientium intueri, quae huc potiffimum fpectabant, ut ficcarent quidem non modo uteri regiones, fed etiam totum corpus, ita ut et unctiones aftrictoriae muliebribus locis adferrentur, fic faciebam. Verum quum haec agendo difpofitio deterior fieri appareret, dubitatio ut verifimile eft, omnes nos invafit; ac quaerentibus aliam curationis rationem ad quam digrederemur, non ex ratione aliquis invenit, neque ab experientia fuggerebat meliorem ea, quae apud optimos medicos in confeffo eft. Interea et tumor aliquis in ventre vifus eft fimilis ei, qui gravidis accidit, quem nonnullae mulieres ex iis, quae ipfi inferviebant, exiftimarunt revera ob conceptum accidiffe, non tamen aliorum medicorum quisquam arbitrabatur.

ἀντιμαρτυρήσει τῇ δόξῃ ταύτῃ. τῆς φυλαττούσης οὖν αὐτὴν, ἣν ἐπεπιστεύκειμεν ἀρίστην εἶναι, τά τ' ἄλλα πραττούσης ὡς ἐπὶ κυούσης λουούσης τε καθ' ἑκάστην ἡμέραν, συνέβη κατὰ τὸν πρῶτον οἶκον τοῦ βαλανείου σφοδροτάτης ὠδίνης γενομένης, οἷαι ταῖς τικτούσαις εἰώθασι συμπίπτειν, ὑδατῶδες ὑγρὸν ἐκκενωθῆναι τοσοῦτον ὡς λειποθυμήσασαν ἐξενεχθῆναι τοῦ βαλανείου τὴν γυναῖκα. καλουσῶν δὲ καὶ κεκραγυιῶν τῶν ἀμφ' αὐτὴν, οὐδεμιᾶς δὲ (458) οὐδὲ πόδας οὐδὲ χεῖρας οὐδὲ τὸ στόμα τῆς γαστρὸς, ὃ δὴ καὶ στόμαχον ὀνομάζουσι κατὰ τὸ σύνηθες, ἀνατριβούσης, ἐγὼ κατὰ τύχην ἑστὼς πρὸ τῆς ἔξω θύρας τοῦ βαλανείου, κραυγῆς ἀκούσας, εἰσεπήδησα καὶ θεασάμενος ἀπεψυγμένην αὐτὴν, εἰς χεῖρας λαβὼν ναρδίνου μύρου τὸν στόμαχον ἀνατρίβειν ἐγκελευσάμενος ταῖς παρούσαις, μὴ μάτην ἑστάναι κεκραγυίας, ἀλλὰ τὰς μὲν τοὺς πόδας ἐκθερμαίνειν, τὰς δὲ τὰς χεῖρας, ἐνίας δ' ὀσφραντὰ προσφέρειν τῇ ῥινί· τότε μὲν ἀνεκτησάμεθα ταχέως αὐτήν. ἥδετο δὲ μεγάλως ἡ μαῖα, προσταλείσης ἐπὶ τῇ κενώσει τῆς γαστρὸς, οὐχ οὕτως ἐπὶ τῷ σφαλῆναι ἐπὶ τῇ τοῦ τίκτειν

Nam muliebris fluxus notae, quae quotidie excernebantur, opinioni huic repugnabant. Quum itaque mulier eam obſervans, quam praeſtantiſſimam eſſe crediderat, tum alia faceret, ut in gravida tum quotidie lavaret, accidit in prima balnei domo ut vehementiſſimo dolore oborto, quales parientibus accidere conſueverunt, aqueus humor evacuaretur tantus, ut animo defecto mulier e balneo exportaretur. Dum autem famulae ipſius lugerent clamarentque omnes, nulla vero nec pedes nec manus nec os ventriculi, quod ſane et ſtomachum conſueto vocabulo appellant, perſricaret, ego ſorte fortuna ante externum balnei oſtium ſtans clamore exaudito inſilii; ac intuitus ipſam perſrixiſſe, nardino unguento in manus ſumpto ſtomachum fricui, juſſique praeſentibus ne fruſtra vociferantes otioſae conſiſterent, ſed aliae pedes excaleſacerent, aliae manus, nonnullae odoramenta naribus offerrent, atque his tunc ſtatim ipſam recollegimus. Laetabatur autem mirifice obſtetrix, ventre ob evacuationem compreſſo, non adeo

δόξῃ, ἀλλ' ἐπὶ τὸ διατεταγμένον ἀπιστοῦσιν ἡμῖν ἀντιλέγειν, ὡς ἐπιστημονικῶς εἰδυῖα τὸ πρᾶγμα. ἀποροῦντος δ' ἑκάστου ὅ τι δεῖ πράττειν καὶ μὴ κατὰ τὸν αὐτὸν σκοπὸν τῷ πρόσθεν ἰᾶσθαι τὴν γυναῖκα, κατατολμῶντας ἐφ' ἕτερον μεταβῆναι, φροντίζοντι νύκτωρ ἐπῆλθε τοιόνδε τι. λειποψυχίας αὐτῇ γεγενημένης, ὡς ἔφην, ὁπότε καὶ τὰς γυναῖκας εἶπον οὐδὲν μὲν βοηθεῖν, ἑστάναι δὲ κλαιούσας, ἐμαυτόν τε μύρον νάρδινον εἰς τὰς χεῖρας λαβόντα τὸ στόμα τῆς γαστρὸς καὶ τὸ ὑποχόνδριον παρατρίβειν, ἀνεμνήσθην ὅτι τοσαύτην εὗρον ἐν τοῖς χωρίοις τούτοις μαλακότητα τῶν ὑποχονδρίων μυῶν, ὡς ἐμὲ γοῦν ἐν ἀρχῇ βιαιότερον ἀνατρίβειν αὐτὰ διεγνωκότα, φοβηθέντα μὴ θλίψας τὴν σάρκα πελιδνὸν ἐργασαίμην τι μόριον, ἀποστῆναι τοῦ βιαίου. ὡς γὰρ ἄν τις ἄκρως εἰκάσαι βουληθείη παραπλήσια γάλακτι μὲν πηγνυμένῳ εἰς τυροῦ γένεσιν, οὐ μὴν ἤδη γε πεπηγότι, κατεφάνη μοι κατὰ τὸ ὑποχόνδριον ἅπαντα. τοῦ μὲν οὖν ξηραίνειν τὴν ἄμετρον ὑγρότητα τοῦ πάθους ὑδατώδους ὄντος τυροῦ πάντες ἔχεσθαι διεγνώκαμεν, ἐξευρεῖν δὲ τρόπον ἰάσεως,

quod falfa effet quae parere ipfam opinaretur, fed quod difpofitioni nobis non credentibus contradixerit, ceu rem fcientifice nofcens. Porro dum ambigimus quid faciendum effet, fimiline, ut prius, fcopo mulierem medicari auderemus, an ad alium tranfire, folicito mihi per noctem tale quid in mentem venit: ac memini, deliquio animi ut dicebam orto, quando etiam mulieres nihil quidem auxiliari dicebam, aftare autem plorantes, ego vero unguento nardino in manus fumpto os ventriculi et praecordia perfricarem, tantam in his regionibus mollitiem musculorum per praecordia inveniffe, ut quum per initia violentius ea infricare ftatuiffem, timens poftea ne carne preffa partem quandam lividam efficerem, a violentia deftiti. Ut enim quis per fumma voluerit affimilare omnia praecordiorum loca, fimilia lacti fane in cafei generationem coalescenti, non tamen jam concreto mihi apparuerunt. Itaque immoderatam affectus cafei modo aquofi humiditatem ficcare omnes ftatuimus, ac curationis modum invenire, ex ma-

[844] οὐ διὰ ξηραινούσης ὕλης μόνον, ἀλλὰ καὶ θερμαινούσης, ὅπως μὴ τήκοιτο τὸ σῶμα, ψυχρᾶς κράσεως ἀμέτρως ὑπάρχον· καὶ μάλιστ' ἐπειδὴ θέρους ὥρᾳ κατ' ἐκεῖνον τὸν καιρὸν ἡμεῖς τοὐναντίον ἐπράττομεν, ἐν θαλαττίᾳ ψάμμῳ θερμῇ κατακλίναντες αὐτήν· λογισάμενος δέ τι καὶ ἄλλο κοινότερον ἁμάρτημα κατὰ τὰ πλεῖστα τῶν παθῶν ἑκάστοτε γιγνόμενον ὑπὸ τῶν ἰατρῶν κενούντων μὲν τὸ περιττὸν, ὅπως δὲ μὴ γεννῷτο παραπλήσιον τῷ κενωθέντι παραλειπόντων, ἐνενόησα τὸν σκοπὸν τῆς διαίτης ποιήσασθαι διά τε πόματος ἐλαχίστου καὶ τρίψεως ὅλου τοῦ σώματος, ἔτι τε χρίσεως οὕτω σκευαζομένης, οὐ διὰ πίττης τε καὶ ῥητίνης, ἀλλὰ διὰ μέλιτος μόνου μέχρι πλείονος μὲν ἑψηθέντος, ἀποψυχθέντος δ' εἰς τοσοῦτον, ὡς τούτῳ δὴ τῷ κατὰ τὰς κρήνας ὕδατι θέρους ὥρᾳ παραπλήσιον εἶναι. καθάπερ δὲ διὰ τοῦ δέρματος ἔγνων ἄμεινον εἶναι διαφορεῖν τὴν περιττὴν ὑγρότητα, τὸν αὐτὸν τρόπον οὐρητικοῖς τε φαρμάκοις ἐπὶ τὴν κύστιν αὐτὴν ποδηγεῖν· ἐπιμελεῖσθαι δὲ τοῦ καὶ διὰ κάτω γαστρὸς ὑπάγεσθαι. πειραθεὶς δ' ἐν ταῖς μετὰ

terie quae non tantum ficcet, fed etiam calefaciat ne corpus contabescat frigida temperie immoderate praeditum; praefertim quum aeftivo tempore contrarium tunc nos moliamur maritimae arenae calidae eam immittentes. Ratiocinatus autem etiam aliud quoddam communius peccatum in plerisque affectibus frequenter a medicis committi, qui fuperfluum quidem inaniunt, ut autem inanito fimile generetur, dicere omittunt; cogitavi victus rationis confilium inftituere ex potione paucillima, totius corporis frictione, praeterea unctione ita praeparata, non ex pice et refina, fed ex melle folo largius quidem cocto, fed refrigerato tantum, ut aquae fontanae aeftivis horis fit perfimile. At quemadmodum fatius effe novi fuperfluam humiditatem per cutem diffipare, eodem modo urinam moventibus medicamentis ipfam ad veficam deducere; caeterum ut alvus fubducatur cura habenda eft. Facto autem diebus poft fubitam excretionem circiter feptem fubfequen-

τὴν ἀθρόαν ἔκκρισιν ἡμέραις ἐφεξῆς ὡς ἑπτὰ, καθ' ἃς ὁ μὲν Βοηθὸς ἅπαντας ἡμᾶς ἰδίᾳ τε καὶ κοινῇ παρεκάλει σκοπεῖσθαί τινα θεραπείας τρόπον, ἀπαγαγὼν αὐτὸν ἀπὸ τῶν παρόντων οἰκετῶν τε καὶ φίλων ἰδίᾳ ἐπὶ τῆς οἰκίας διελέχθην, οὐδὲν, εἰπὼν, ἄχρι τήμερον οὐδὲ καθ' ἓν με σφαλέντα τῶν ἰατρικῶν ἔργων ἐπιστάμενος ἐπίσκεψαι κατὰ σαυτὸν εἰ συγχωρεῖς δέκα ταῖς πάσαις ἡμέραις, ὡς βούλομαι πρᾶξαι περὶ τὴν γυναῖκά σου· κᾂν μὲν ἄμεινον ἴσχειν ἑκάστοτε φαίνηται, μετὰ ταῦτα ἄλλαις τοσαύταις ἐπιτρέψεις μοι πράττειν τι περὶ αὐτήν· εἰ δὲ μὴ, τότε κᾀγὼ χωρισθήσομαι τελέως αὐτῆς. ἑτοίμως δέ μοι συγχωρήσαντος αὐτοῦ, πρῶτον μὲν ὑδραγωγῷ φαρμάκῳ διὰ τῆς κάτω γαστρὸς ἐκένωσα, μετὰ ταῦτα δὲ πίνειν ὕδωρ ἐναφεψηθέντος ἀσάρου τε καὶ σελίνου. ἐπεὶ δὲ ταῖς πρώταις ἡμέραις δύο τούτων γενομένων οὐδὲν ἐφάνη τοῦ ῥοῦ, κατὰ τὴν τρίτην ἔδωκα πάλιν οὐ πολὺ τοῦ διὰ τῆς κάτω γαστρὸς ἐκκενοῦντος τὸ ῥέπον ἔμπροσθεν εἰς τὴν μήτραν, οὐ μόνον δι' οὔρων, ἀλλὰ καὶ διὰ τῆς κάτω γαστρὸς παροχετεύειν βουλό-

tibus experimento, ſecundum quos Boëthus omnes nos et privatim et communiter rogabat, ut aliquem curationis modum proſpiceremus, abduxi tum eum a praeſentibus et familiaribus et amicis in domo ſeorſim ac cum eo diſſerui, In nullo, inquiens, ne in uno quidem opere medico hactenus erraſſe me quum ſcias, tu conſiderato apud te an decem in totum diebus permiſſurus ſis ea quae circa uxorem tuam facere inſtituo; et ſi melius habere quolibet die videatur, poſtea aliis totidem diebus aliquid ei facere concedes; ſin minus, tunc et ego prorſus ab ea discedam. Quod quum prompte ille annuiſſet, primum ſane medicamento aquam ducente per alvum evacuavi; poſtea bibere aquam, in qua decoctum ſit aſarum et apium. Ubi vero primis diebus duobus his adminiſtratis nihil ex fluore apparuiſſet, tertio rurſus exhibui, non copioſe per alvum evacuans id quod prius in uterum vergebat, non modo per urinas, ſed etiam per ventrem inferiorem derivare cupiens. Poſt haec corpus melle ſingulis diebus il-

μενος. καὶ μετ᾽ αὐτὸ ἔχριόν τε τῷ μέλιτι καθ᾽ ἑκάστην ἡμέραν, ἀνέτριβόν τε τὸ σῶμα τὰ μὲν πρῶτα διὰ σινδόνων μαλακωτάτων, εἶτα διὰ σκληροτάτων· ἐδίδουν τε κρέα τῶν ὀρείων ὀρνίθων, ἰχθύων δὲ πετραίων. ὡς δὲ διὰ τούτων ἡμέραις πεντεκαίδεκα τῆς θεραπείας γινομένης οὐδὲν ὅλως ἐφάνη τοῦ πάθους γνώρισμα, γνοὺς ὁ Βοηθὸς μεῖζον ἢ κατὰ τὴν ὑπόσχεσιν εἰργασμένον με, τελέως ἐκθεραπεῦσαι τὴν διάθεσιν ἐδεῖτο, ὑποθήκας τε δοῦναι πρὸς τὸν λοιπὸν χρόνον, ὅπως μηκέθ᾽ ὁμοίως νοσήσειε. ἐπεὶ δὲ πληρωθέντος τοῦ μηνὸς εὔχρους τε ἦν ἀκριβῶς, ὡς μηδὲν ἀποδεῖν ἀκριβῶς τῆς κατὰ φύσιν ἕξεως, οὐδὲν δὲ τοῦ ῥεύματος ἐπεφάνη, τετρακοσίους μὲν ἔπεμψέ μοι χρυσοῦς, ηὔξησέ τε τὸν φθόνον τούτων τῶν γενναίων ἰατρῶν ἐφ᾽ οἷς ἐτύγχανεν ἐπαινῶν με. καὶ μέντοι καὶ αὐτὸς ἕτοιμος ἦν, ὥσπερ ὅ τε Σεβῆρος, τὸ μηνῦσαι τὰ κατ᾽ ἐμὲ τῷ τε κατὰ τὴν τῶν Ῥωμαίων πόλιν ὄντι Μάρκῳ Αὐρηλίῳ Ἀντωνίνῳ αὐτοκράτορι. Λεύκιος γὰρ ἀπεδήμει τῆς πόλεως ἕνεκα τοῦ Παρθικοῦ πολέμου γενηθέντος ὑπὸ Βολογέσου.

levi ac perfricui, primum ſane linteis molliſſimis, deinde duriſſimis; dedique carnes avium montanarum et piſces ſaxatiles exhibui. Poſtquam vero his remediis quintodecimo curationis die adveniente nulla prorſus aſſectus nota appareret, Boëthus intelligens plus a me quam eſſem pollicitus praeſtitum, rogabat ut in totum diſpoſitionem perſanarem, praeceptiones darem in reliquum tempus ne amplius ſimiliter aegrotaret. Quoniam vero menſe completo colorata exacte erat, ut nihil plane a naturali habitu deſideraretur, nihil quoque ex fluore conſpiceretur, quadringentos aureos ad me miſit, auxitque generoſorum horum medicorum invidiam, inde quod me laudibus extolleret. Quin etiam ipſe quemadmodum et Severus opera a me geſta haud detrectabat indicare Romanorum urbis imperatori Marco Aurelio Antonino. Lucius enim ab urbe diſceſſerat Parthici belli gratia, quod a Bologeſo ortum erat.

Κεφ. θ'. [Γαληνοῦ ἐπάνοδος εἰς τὴν πατρίδα καὶ ἡ πρὸς τῶν αὐτοκρατόρων ἐπανάκλησις αὐτοῦ.] Κἀγὼ θεασάμενος αὐτῶν τὴν ὁρμὴν καὶ δείσας μὴ φθασάντων τι πρᾶξαι κωλυθῶ τῆς ἐς Ἀσίαν ἐπανό- [845] δου, παρεκάλεσα βραχὺν ἐπισχεῖν χρόνον. ἐγὼ γὰρ ἔφην ἐρεῖν αὐτοῖς τὸν καιρὸν, ὁπόταν βουληθῶ τοῦτό μοι γενέσθαι. καὶ τοίνυν ὅταν ἐπυνθανόμην πεπαῦσθαι τὴν στάσιν, ἄφνω τῆς Ῥωμαίων πόλεως ἐξῆλθον, ὡς δῆθεν εἰς Καμπανίαν ἀπιὼν, ἕνα καταλιπὼν οἰκέτην φυλάττοντα τὰ κατὰ τὴν οἴκησιν· ᾧ προσέταξα πλοῖον ἐπιτηρήσαντι τῶν εἰς Ἀσίαν ἐξιόντων, ἡμέρᾳ μιᾷ τῶν ἐκ τῆς Βηβούρας κερκώπων παραλαβόντα τινὰ πωλῆσαί τε τὰ κατὰ τὴν οἰκίαν, ἐξελθεῖν τε παραχρῆμα καὶ τῆς νεὼς ἐπιβάντα κατὰ τὸν ἐπὶ Σικελίας πλοῦν εἰς τὴν πατρίδα παραγενέσθαι. ταῦτα μὲν οὖν ὀλίγον ὕστερον ἐπράχθη. ἐγὼ δ' ἀνὰ Καμπανίαν γενόμενος, εἶτ' ἐκεῖθεν ἔσπευσα μὲν εἰς τὸ Βρεντήσιον· ἀφικόμενος δὲ ὥρισα κατὰ τὴν πρώτην ἀναγενομένην ναῦν, εἴτ' ἐς Δυῤῥάχιον εἴτ' ἐπὶ τῆς Ἑλλάδος πλέοι, διαπεραιωθῆναι· δεδιὼς μὴ

Cap. IX. [*Galeni reditus in patriam, ejusque ab imperatoribus revocatio.*] Ac ego intellecta ipforum prompta voluntate, ac veritus ne dum hoc illi agerent a reditu in Afiam impedirent, rogavi eos ut pauco tempore id differrent. Ego enim dicebam me tempus ipfis nunciaturum, quum hoc in gratiam meam fieri vellem. Quando igitur bellum ceffaffe intellexi, ftatim ex Romanorum urbe difceffi, ceu nimirum in Campaniam iturus, famulo videlicet uno relicto, qui domum obfervaret; cui injunxi ut navigio ex iis quae in Afiam proficiscuntur inveftigato, una die adducto quodam inftitorio ex Bebura emptore venderet ea, quae in domo haberentur, exiretque protinus urbem et navim ingreffus Siciliam adiret, inde in patriam reverteretur. Haec igitur paulo poft gefta funt. Ego autem per Campaniam profectus illinc poftea ad Brundufium contendi; quo perveniens ftatui prima quaque navi, five in Dyrrhachium five in Graeciam navigaret, permeare; veritus ne quis praepotentum virorum vel etiam impera-

τις ἄρα τῶν πολὺ δυναμένων ἀνδρῶν ἢ καὶ αὐτὸς ὁ αὐτοκράτωρ γνούς μου τὴν ἔξοδον, ὡς δραπέτου πέμψας στρατιώτην εἰς Ῥώμην ἐπανελθεῖν κελεύσειεν. ἐγὼ μὲν οὖν οὕτως μετὰ μίαν ἡμέραν εἰς Κασσιόπην ἔπλευσα. ζητοῦντες δέ με οἱ ἐν Ῥώμῃ φίλοι, παρά τε τοῦ καταλειφθέντος οἰκέτου πυνθανόμενοι ποῦ ποτ' εἴην, ἀκούοντες δὲ ἐν τῇ Καμπανίᾳ διατρίβειν με, τὸ μὲν πρῶτον ὑπώπτευον τὸ γεγονός· προϊόντος δὲ τοῦ χρόνου μήθ' ὁρῶντες μήτε τὸν ἐμὸν ἄνθρωπον ἐν Ῥώμῃ, ἔγνωσαν πεποιηκότα με τὰ ἐξαρχῆς λεγόμενα· καὶ τότε μόγις ἐπείσθησαν ἅπαντες οἱ πρόσθεν ἀπιστοῦντες ὄντως προκεῖσθαί μοι καταλιπεῖν τὴν Ῥώμην, ὅτι μὴ ψευδῶς, ἀλλ' ἀληθῶς ἔφασκον τοῦτο. μετὰ χρόνον δ' οὐ πολὺν ἐπανεληλυθότος τοῦ Λευκίου, πολέμου δ' ἑτέρου τοῦ (459) πρὸς Γερμανοὺς πολεμηθέντος αὐτοῖς ἀρχὴ καθεστήκει. γενομένου δὲ λόγου περὶ τῶν ἔργοις, οὐ λόγοις ἐπιδεικνυμένων ἰατρικήν τε καὶ φιλοσοφίαν, οὐκ ὀλίγοι τῶν περὶ αὐτοὺς ὠνόμαζον ἐμὲ τοιοῦτον ὑπάρχειν. ἐξωρμηκότες οὖν ἤδη τῆς πόλεως, ὡς ἐπὶ τὸν πόλεμον, ὡρικότες τε τοῦ

tor, cognito diſceſſu, tanquam fugitivi, militem mitteret, quo me Romam juberet reverti. Ego itaque poſt unum diem Caſſiopen navigavi. Amici autem Romae dum me quaererent et a famulo relicto ſciscitarentur ubinam eſſem, audirent autem me in Campania agere, primum ſane id quod factum erat ſuſpicabantur; at procedente tempore, quum neque me neque famulum meum Romae viderent, intellexerunt ea quae ab initio dicebam eſſe facta; atque tunc vix perſuaſum habebant omnes qui prius non credebant, revera mihi inſtitutum fuiſſe Romam relinquere, quoniam non falſo, ſed vere id dicebam. Haud multo tempore poſt Lucius reverſus eſt, ſed alterius belli, quod contra Germanos ſuſceptum erat, initium conſtitutum. Porro ubi mentio de his, qui operibus, non verbis medicinam philoſophiamque oſtenderent, fieret, haud pauci ex familiaribus ipſius talem me eſſe nominabant. Egreſſi igitur jam ex urbe ad bellum ſtatuentesque per hiemem in

χειμῶνος ἐν Ἀκυληΐᾳ διατρῖψαι, παρεσκευακότες τε καὶ συγκροτοῦντες τὸ στράτευμα πέμπουσιν ὡς ἐμὲ κελεύοντες ἥκειν ὡς αὐτούς. ἀλλὰ τοῦ Λευκίου κατὰ μέσον τοῦ χειμῶνος μεταστάντος εἰς θεοὺς ὁ ἀδελφὸς αὐτοῦ κομίσας εἰς Ῥώμην τὸ σῶμα καὶ ποιήσας ἀμφ᾽ αὐτῷ τὰ νομιζόμενα, τῆς ἐπὶ τοὺς Γερμανοὺς ὁδοιπορίας εἴχετο κελεύων ἕπεσθαι κἀμέ. χρηστὸν δ᾽ ὄντα καὶ φιλάνθρωπον αὐτὸν ἐδυνήθην, ὡς οἶσθα, πεῖσαι καταλιπεῖν ἐν τῇ Ῥώμῃ με· καὶ γὰρ διὰ ταχέων ἐπανήξειν. παντὶ δ᾽ οὖν τῷ τῆς ἀποδημίας αὐτοῦ χρόνῳ μεμνημένος τῆς συνήθους κακοηθείας τῶν κατὰ τὴν πόλιν ἰατρῶν τε καὶ φιλοσόφων ἔγνων ἀναχωρεῖν αὐτῆς ἄλλοτε εἰς ἄλλο χωρίον, ἐν ᾧπερ ἂν ὁ υἱὸς αὐτοῦ Κόμμοδος, ὑπὸ Πειθολάῳ τρεφόμενος ἐντολὰς ἔχοντι παρ᾽ αὐτοῦ τοῦ αὐτοκράτορος Ἀντωνίνου, καλεῖν πρὸς τὴν ἐπιμέλειαν ἐπὶ παιδὸς, εἰ νοσήσειέ ποτε. παρὰ προσδοκίαν δ᾽ αὐτοῦ χρονίσαντος ἐν τῷ Γερμανικῷ πολέμῳ, παντὶ τούτῳ τῷ χρόνῳ πολλὰς πραγματείας ἔγραψα φιλοσόφους τε καὶ ἰατρικὰς, ἃς ὑποστρέψαντος τοῦ βασιλέως εἰς τὴν Ῥώμην αἰτήσασι τοῖς φίλοις ἔδωκα, παρὰ μόνοις ἐκείνοις ἐλπίσας

Aquileia degere, ac praeparato maturatoque exercitu mittunt ad me, jubentes ut ad ipſos venirem. Verum quum Lucius media hieme ſatis conceſſiſſet, frater ipſius corpore Romam translato, factisque ei juſtis, profectionem ad Germanos ſuscepit, injungens et me ipſum comitari. Quoniam autem benignus erat et humanus, potui, ut noſti, ab eo impetrare ut Romae manerem, quia ſtatim erat rediturus. Toto igitur quo ipſe aberat tempore, memor ego conſuetae urbis medicorum et philoſophorum improbitatis, decrevi inde recedere alias in alium locum, ubicunque filius ipſius Commodus eſſet, qui a Pitholao educabatur; cui imperator ipſe Antoninus injunxerat ut, ſi quando puer aegrotaret, me ad curationem ejus accerſeret. Quum autem ipſe diutius in bello Germanico quam putarat moraretur, univerſo hoc tempore multa opera conſcripſi et philoſophica et medica, quae rege Romam reverſo amicis petentibus exhibui, ſperans ipſa apud ſolos illos ſore.

αὐτὰς ἔσεσθαι. ὡς εἴ γε ἠπιστάμην ἐκδοθήσεσθαι τοῖς ἀναξίοις, οὐκ ἂν οὐδ' ἐκείνοις ἔδωκα. καλῶ δ' ἀναξίους ὅσοι μοχθηροὶ τὴν ψυχὴν, οὐχ ἕνεκα τοῦ μαθεῖν τι πρὸς τὴν ἀνάγνωσιν ἥκουσιν, ἀλλ' ὅπως ἐπηρεάσαι τινὰ δυνηθῶσιν ἐξ αὐτῶν. ἐν τούτοις οὖν τοῖς βιβλίοις ἡ θεωρία πᾶσα γέγραπται τῆς τε διὰ τῶν σφυγμῶν προγνώσεως καὶ τῶν ἄλλων προγνωστικῶν σημείων. ἣν οὖν πρόγνωσιν ἐποιησάμην ἐπὶ θατέρου τῶν Κυιντιλιανοῦ υἱῶν ἐξ αὐτῶν βουληθέντι σοι μαθεῖν [846] ἐκ τίνος θεωρίας ἐγένετο, ῥᾳδία καὶ καταφανὴς ἔσται τὴν περὶ κρίσεων πραγματείαν ἀναγνόντι, γεγυμνασμένῳ τὸν λογισμὸν ἐκ παιδὸς ἐν γεωμετρίᾳ τε καὶ διαλεκτικῇ. τοῖς πολλοῖς δὲ τούτοις ἰατροῖς, ὅσοι τῆς μὲν ἐν τοῖς ἔργοις γυμνασίας ἀπέστησαν, εἰς πανουργίαν δ' ἐκτραπόμενοι τὴν ἐπ' αὐτῇ τέχνην ἤσκησαν, οὔτε γνωσθῆναί τι τῶν γεγραμμένων δύνανται οὔτε ἀκουσθῆναι

Κεφ. ι'. [Πρόγνωσις ὑποστροφῆς πυρετοῦ καὶ λύσις αὐτῆς δι' ἱδρῶτος.] Ἔξστος οὖν Ἀντωνίνου υἱὸς ἤρξατο μὲν ὀξύτατα νοσεῖν, ὡς μὴ δύνασθαι τὴν ἑβδόμην ἡμέραν

Nam fi indignis communicatum iri fcivillem, ne illis quidem dedillem. Voco autem indignos, qui animo pravi non ut discant aliquid ad lectionem fe conferunt, fed ut quaedam ex ipfis pollint calumniari. In his igitur libris tota fpeculatio praenotionis ex pulfibus et aliorum praefagiendi modorum tradita eft. Quam igitur praenotionem in altero Quintiliani filio molitus fum, fi inde voles discere, ex qua fpeculatione facta fit, facilis et perfpicua tibi erit, quum opus de crifibus perlegeris ingeniumque a puero exercueris in geometria et dialectica. At vulgares hi medici, qui ab operum exercitio deftiterunt, ad impofturas autem converfi, artem in eis exercuere, neque intelligere quippiam ex iis quae funt fcripta poffunt, nec audire.

Cap. X. [*Recidivae febris praenotio et illius per fudorem difceffus.*] Sextus igitur Antonini filius acutiffime coepit laborare, ut feptimum diem citra crifin egredi

ὑπερβαλεῖν ἄνευ κρίσεως. ἥτις δ' αὐτοῦ τούτου πρόγνωσίς ἐστι, διὰ τῶν περὶ κρίσεως ὑπομνημάτων γέγραπται, δι' ὧν καὶ ὅτι προεκρήγνυται πολλάκις ἡ κρίσις, οὐ περιμείνασα τὴν πιστῶς κρίνουσαν δεδήλωται. συμβῆναι δὲ τοῦτο τῷ Ἔξστῳ δυνάμενον ἔγνων κατὰ τὴν τετάρτην ἡμέραν, ὡς προειπεῖν ἐρομένῳ Πειθολάῳ τῷ κοιτωνίτῃ ὅ τι θεσπίζοιμι περὶ τῶν μελλόντων. ἤρετο γὰρ οὗτος, ἐπειδὴ προεπειρᾶτό μου, πολλὰ τῶν δοκούντων τοῖς σοφωτάτοις ἰατροῖς ἀδυνάτων εἶναι προειρηκότος. ἀπεκρινάμην οὖν αὐτῷ γελάσας, τῆς μὲν ἑβδόμης ἡμέρας ἐξωτέρω μὴ δύνασθαι προελθεῖν τὸ νόσημα· κριθήσεσθαι δὲ πάντως ἢ ἑκταῖον, ἢ ἑβδομαῖον. ἑκταῖον μὲν οὖν κριθὲν ὑποστρέψειν αὐτό· ἑβδομαῖον δὲ βεβαίαν ἕξειν τὴν κρίσιν· ἔσεσθαι μέντοι τὴν κρίσιν ἐξ ἀνάγκης δι' ἱδρῶτος. ἐπεὶ δὲ κατὰ τὴν ἕκτην ἡμέραν οὕτως γε ἐκρίθη, φιλόνεικος ὢν ἐσχάτως ὁ Ἔξστος, ὅπως ἐλέγξῃ ἐμὲ μὴ γενομένης ὑποστροφῆς, ἐλούετο μὲν καθ' ἑκάστην ἡμέραν, οὔτε δ' οἶνον ἔπινεν οὔτε προσηνέγκατό τι πλὴν χυλοῦ πτισάνης, ἢ αὐτὴν, ἢ μετὰ ψίχας ἄρτου· πολλάκις

non poſſet. Quae vero hujus ipſius praenotio ſit, commentariis de criſi proditum eſt; quibus etiam criſin frequenter antevertere ac praerumpi, dum non expectat diem ſideliter decernentem, oſtendimus. Hoc autem quum Sexto poſſet accidere, ſtatui in quarto die ceu praedicere Pitholao, roganti quid de ſuturis augurarer. Interrogabat autem hic, quum praeſciret me multa ex his quae ſapientiſſimi medici ſieri non poſſe arbitrantur, praeſagiiſſe. Reſpondi igitur ipſi ridens, extra ſeptimum quidem diem morbum progredi non poſſe, ſed omnino aut ſexto aut ſeptimo criſin experturum. Quod ſi igitur ſexto ſuerit judicatus, recidivam ejus eſſe timendam; ſin autem ſeptimo, ſirmam habiturum criſin, eamque fore neceſſario per ſudorem. Poſtquam vero ſexto die criſin ita expertus eſſet Sextus, natura admodum contentioſus, ut me corriperet, recidiva non facta, lavabat ſane quotidie, neque vinum bibebat neque aliquid praeter ptiſanae cremorem vel ſolum vel cum micis panis aſſumebat; frequenter et

δὲ καὶ αὐτὸς τὸν ἄρτον ἐν ὕδατι βρέξας ἠρκεῖτο μόνον. ταῦτα ποιήσας ἄχρι τῆς δωδεκάτης ἡμέρας ἐκαυχήσατο κατ' αὐτὴν νενικηκέναι μου τὴν πρόγνωσιν. ἔπιε δὲ κατὰ τὴν τρισκαιδεκάτην ἡμέραν τρίτῃ ὥρᾳ ὑδατώδους οἴνου βραχύ τι σὺν τῷ καὶ τὴν ὅλην δίαιταν ἁδροτέραν βραχὺ ποιήσασθαι τῆς ἔμπροσθεν, ἔτι μέντοι φυλάττων λεπτήν· ἀλλὰ κατά τε τὴν ἑξῆς ἡμέραν ἀπὸ τῆς πρώτης κατακλίσεως τεσσαρεσκαιδεκάτην οὖσαν ἀρξάμενος πυρέττειν ἐκέλευσε μηδένα μοι δηλῶσαι, νομίζων μηδὲ σφοδρὸν ἔσεσθαι τὸν πυρετὸν μηδὲ πλέον ἡμέρας μιᾶς ἐκταθήσεσθαι αὐτόν. ἐπεὶ δὲ προϊούσης τῆς ἡμέρας ἀεὶ καὶ μᾶλλον ἐφαιδρύνετο, Κλαύδιος Σεβῆρος ὑποστρέφων εἰς τὴν ἑαυτοῦ οἰκίαν πλησίον οὖσαν τῆς ἐκείνου, πυθόμενος αὐτὸν πυρέττειν ἐπορεύθη πρὸς αὐτὸν, εὑρών τε σφοδρῶς ἤδη πυρέττοντα, πρῶτον μὲν ἐπύθετο τίνα γνώμην ἐγὼ περὶ τῆς ἀρχῆς τοῦ γεγενημένου πυρετοῦ νῦν [αὐτῷ φαινοίμην ἔχων, ἀκούσας δὲ παρ' αὐτοῦ τὸ ἀληθὲς, ὡς διὰ φιλονεικίαν οὐκ ἐδήλωσε πορευθῆναί τινα πρός με, ἐκέλευσε παρακαλεῖν με εἰς τὴν ἐπίσκεψιν τοῦ Ἕξστου καὶ μετὰ ταῦτα πρὸς αὐτὸν ἀφικέσθαι. τούτων

pane ipſo in aqua macerato contentus erat. His ad duodecimum usque diem factis jactitabat in eo praenotionem meam ſe viciſſe. Bibit autem tertiodecimo die hora tertia vini aquoſi pauxillulum, necnon totam victus rationem pleniorem paulo priori inſtituit, ſervans tamen adhuc tenuem. Sequenti die a primo decubitu quartodecimo febricitare orſus juſſit ut nemo mihi indicaret, putans neque vehementem fore febrem neque die diutius uno duraturam. Ubi vero procedente die ſemper etiam magis incrudeſceret, Claudius Severus revertens in ſuam ipſius domum illi vicinam, quum audiret ipſum febricitare, ad ipſum profectus eſt, ac vehementer jam affligi offendens, primum ſane rogabat quam ſententiam ego de ortae febris initio nunc habere ei viderer, auditaque ab ipſo veritate, quod ob contentionem noluerit quenquam ad me qui indicaret accedere, Claudius ipſe juſſit ut Sextum inviſerem ac poſtea ad ipſum accederem. Quibus factis roga-

γενομένων ἐπυνθάνετο τί μοι δοκεῖ περὶ τῆς ὑποστροφῆς τοῦ νοσήματος. ἀπεκρινάμην οὖν αὐτῷ ὅπερ καὶ τῷ Ἔξστῳ προειρήκειν, μετὰ τρεῖς ἡμέρας λυθήσεσθαι τὴν ἐπιβολὴν ταύτην ἱκανῶς θερμοῦ γενομένου τοῦ πυρετοῦ κατὰ αὐτάς· εἶτα κριθησομένου κατὰ τὴν ἑπτακαιδεκάτην ἀπὸ τῆς ἀρχῆς ἡμέραν. Ἔξστος οὖν ἡδέως ἀκούσας τὴν ἐν τάχει γενησομένην λύσιν ἑτοίμως ἐπίστευσεν· ὃ γὰρ ἕκαστος βούλεται δηλονότι, τοῦτο καὶ οἴεται γενήσεσθαι. Σεβῆρος δ' ὅτι οὐκ ἂν σφαλείην ὑπὲρ τοῦ [847] σωθήσεσθαι τὸν Ἔξστον ἐπίστευσέ μοι· τὸ δὲ τῆς ἡμέρας ἐν ᾗ τελέως ἀπαλλαγοῖτο τοῦ νοσήματος οὐκ ἐπίστευε, δύσκολον εἶναι νομίζων ἄνευ τοῦ περιμεῖναι κἂν τὴν ἑξῆς ἡμέραν ἀποφήνασθαί τι βέβαιον ὑπὲρ τῶν εἰς τετάρτην ἡμέραν ἐσομένων. ἅτε δ' οὕτως διακείμενος ἔπεμψεν ὄρθρου βαθέος ἐπὶ τὴν οἰκίαν Ἔξστου περιμένοντά τε καὶ πρὸς αὐτὸν ἄξοντα μετὰ τὴν ἐσομένην ἐπίσκεψιν. ὡς δὲ θεασάμενος τὸν Ἔξστον ἐπορεύθην πρὸς αὐτὸν, ἀντιφήσεις, ἔφη, οἷς χθὲς εἶπες, ἢ διαμενεῖς ἐπὶ τῶν αὐτῶν; ἐπεὶ δὲ νῦν μᾶλλον ἔφην ἢ χθὲς ἀποφήνασθαί μοι

bat quid mihi de morbi recidiva videretur. Refpondi igitur ei quod et Sexto praedixeram, poft tres dies acceffionem hanc folutum iri, febri in ipfis admodum calida reddita; deinde crifin feptimodecimo poft initia die expertura. Sextus igitur libenter audiens folutionem brevi futuram, prompte credidit: quod enim nimirum unusquisque cupit, id etiam futurum putat. Severus autem quod quidem non erraffem in Sexto fervando, fidem mihi adhibuit; veruntamen diem quo prorfus a morbo liberaretur non credidit, difficile effe autumans ut non expectato vel fequenti die certi aliquid de his, quae quarto die futura erant, pronunciarem. Atque fic affectus mifit multo mane ad domum Sexti, dicens fe expectare ut me vocet, quo poftquam illum invififfem ad fe venirem. Ut igitur invifi Sextum, ad ipfum fum profectus. Contradices, inquit, iis quae heri protulifti? aut in iisdem perfiftes? Poftquam vero nunc magis quam heri eadem ac confentanea priori-

τὰ αὐτὰ, μετ' ἄριστον αὖθίς με καλέσας ἤρετο πάλιν εἰ βεβαίως εἴην πεπεισμένος Ἕξστῳ ἐσομένην κρίσιν. ἤκουεν οὖν παρ' ἐμοῦ μᾶλλον ἢ χθὲς ἔχειν διατείνασθαι. ὡς δὲ καὶ τὴν δευτέραν ἡμέραν ἐπύθετό μου πότερον φυλάττοιμι τὴν αὐτὴν γνώμην ἐπὶ τοῖς προειρημένοις, ἤ τι καὶ μετακινοῖμι τῶν ῥηθέντων, ἤκουσεν οὐδὲν μὲν ἐκείνων κινεῖν, προστίθεσθαι δέ τι τοῖς εἰρημένοις ἔχων. καὶ ὃς αὖθις ἤρετο τί τοῦτό ἐστιν; ἤκουσεν ὅτι διελθούσης τῆς ἑπτακαιδεκάτης ἡμέρας ἄρξασθαι τὸν ἱδρῶτα περὶ δευτέραν ὥραν νυκτερινήν. ἆρ' οὖν, ἔφη, καὶ Πειθολάῳ ταῦτ' εἶπας; εἰρηκέναι τε ἔφην αὐτῷ καὶ πεπεῖσθαί γε ἐκεῖνον ὡς οὐκ ἂν σφαλείην ἐν τῇ προῤῥήσει καὶ θεραπείᾳ. πάντως οὖν ἔφη καὶ τῷ αὐτοκράτορι δεδηλωκέναι Πειθόλαον. ἴσως, ἔφην, οὗτος ἔφη· ἐμοὶ δ' οὐ μέλει τῆς ἐπὶ τοῖς τοιούτοις δόξης, οὐ γὰρ περιέρχομαι κηρύττων τὰς ἐμὰς προγνώσεις τε καὶ θεραπείας, ἵνα μᾶλλον οἱ ἰατροί τε καὶ φιλόσοφοί με μισῶσι, γόητά τε καὶ μάντιν ἕτερά τε κατ' ἐμοῦ τοιαῦτα θρυλοῦντες. ὑμῖν δὲ τοῖς φίλοις ὅσοι κατε- (460) γνώκατε

bus pronunciare me dixiſſem, a prandio rurſus advocatum interrogabat denuo, an firmiter criſin Sexto futuram perſuaſum haberem. Audivit igitur me id magis quam heri affirmare. Item ſecundo die rogabat, eandemne ſententiam cum praedictis ſervarem, an aliquid ex prolatis immutarem; imo, inquam, tantum abeſt ut quid ex illis immutem, ut etiam nonnihil commemoratis adjiciam. Quo audito ille quaerebat quid id eſſet; dixi, nocte ſeptimadecima praeterita ſudorem circa horam ſecundam noctis incepturum. Num igitur haec quoque narraſti Pitholao, ait? Reſpondi et me dixiſſe et illum habere perſuaſum nihil a me vel in praedictione vel curatione eſſe erratum. Omnino igitur, inquit ille, etiam imperatori Pitholaus haec indicavit? Ad quod ego reſpondi, pro arbitrio Pitholaus agat, gloriam ex hujusmodi non admodum venor; quippe non obambulo praenotiones meas ac curationes praeconio eſſerens, quo magis tum medici tum philoſophi me odio proſequantur, praeſtigiatorem et vatem

τῆς ἰατρικῆς τέχνης ἐκ τῆς τούτων ἀμαθίας, ἐπιδείκνυμι τὴν μὲν τέχνην ἀξίαν Ἀπόλλωνός τε καὶ Ἀσκληπιοῦ, τοὺς δὲ ἰατροὺς τούτους ὑβρίζειν αὐτήν· ὥσπερ καὶ τοὺς φιλοσόφους φιλοσοφίαν, οἵ γε μηδενὸς ἰδιώτου βέλτιον βιοῦντες ὀνομάζουσιν αὐτοὺς ὀνόματι σεμνῷ τῷ τῆς φιλοσοφίας. ταῦτα μὲν εἶπον τῷ Σεβήρῳ· σὺ δὲ, ὦ Ἐπίγενες, ἔγνως τὴν κακοήθειαν τῶν ἰατρῶν σχεδὸν ἁπάντων εὐχομένων φανερῶς ἀποτυχεῖν με πεμπόντων τε δι' ὅλης ἡμέρας τοὺς γνωσομένους τε καὶ ἀγγέλλοντας αὐτοῖς τὸ γενησόμενον· οὐ γὰρ ᾔδεσάν με τῷ Σεβήρῳ καὶ Πειθολάῳ προειρηκότα δείλης ὄψεσθαι ἐσομένην τὴν ἀρχὴν τῆς κρίσεως. ἐπεὶ δὲ περὶ τὴν ἑβδόμην ὥραν ἐπιπαροξυνθέντα τὸν Ἔξστον ἐπύθοντο, καταγελῶντες καὶ φανερῶς ἐπιχαίροντες ἅπασι τοῖς ἀπαντῶσιν ἔλεγον κερτομοῦντες ὡς ἡ θαυμαστὴ μαντεία τοῦ Γαληνοῦ κατὰ τοὐναντίον ἀπέβη. γενομένης μέντοι τῆς κρίσεως, ὡς προειρήκειν κατὰ τὴν προτεραίαν (ἔφασαν ἐπομένην ἐναλλὰξ) ἐτρέποντο πάντες αἰσχυνόμενοι, καὶ ταῦτα τῆς προγνώσεως οὐδὲν ἐχούσης θαυμαστὸν, ὡς ἔδειξά σοι

appellantes, aliaque id genus convitia in nomen meum proclamantes. Vobis autem amicis, qui artem medicam ex horum inſcitia damnaſtis, oſtendo ſane eam et Apolline et Aeſculapio dignam, medicos autem hos ipſam dehonetare; ſicut etiam philoſophos philoſophiam, qui quum ne ullo quidem idiota incorruptius vivant, venerando philoſophiae nomine ſe appellari patiuntur. Haec quidem Severo dixi. Tu autem, o Poſthume, medicorum fere omnium malitiam noviſti, qui me ſucceſſu proſpero fruſtrari maniſeſto optant, mittuntque toto die qui quid accidat indipiſcantur eisque nuncient. Non enim ſciverant me Severo et Pitholao praedixiſſe veſperi criſis futurum principium conſpectum iri. Poſtquam autem circa ſeptimam horam acceſſionem Sextum invaſiſſe intellexerunt, in cachinnos ſoluti; palamque gaviſi omnibus qui occurrebant convitioſe dixerunt mirandam Galeni divinationem contrario modo eveniſſe. Oborta vero criſi, ut praedixeram pridie, vice verſa omnes pudore ſuffuſi ſunt; quum

διά τε τῶν εἰς πρῶτον ἐπιδημιῶν ὑπομνημάτων, ἔτι τε τὴν περὶ τῶν κρίσεων πραγματείαν. τούτοις μέντοι τοῖς ἰατροῖς, οὐ μόνον ἀγνοεῖν ὑπάρχει τὰ γεγραμμένα τοῖς παλαιοῖς, ἀλλὰ μηδὲ τὰς ἡμέρας ἀριθμεῖν ἔτι μετὰ τὴν ἑβδόμην καὶ μάλιστα ἐὰν ἀπύρετος γενόμενος ὁ κάμνων, αὖθις ἐξ ὑποστροφῆς πυρέττῃ. καίτοι παρ' Ἱπποκράτους κατὰ τῶν ἐπιδημιῶν βιβλία γεγραμμένων ἁπασῶν τῶν ἡμερῶν ἐφ' ἑκάστῳ τῶν ἀῤῥώστων ἄχρι τῆς ἐσχάτης λύσεως οὐ μόνον εἰ κατὰ τὴν ιδ'. ἡμέραν ἀλλὰ καὶ κατὰ τὴν ξ'. ἢ π'. τύχῃ γεγενημένη. αὕτη μὲν οὖν ἡ πρόῤῥησις, ὡς ἔφην, εἰ καὶ θαυμαστὴ τοῖς πολλοῖς τούτοις ἰατροῖς ἔταξεν, ἀλλ' οὐ τοιαύτη γε κατ' ἀλήθειαν ἦν, ὥσπερ οὐδ' ἡ μετὰ γνώσεως τῶν ἐνεσιώτων θεραπεία τοῦ παιδὸς αὐτοῦ Κομμόδου κατὰ τὴν ἐπιδημίαν ἐκείνου γενομένη.

[848] *Κεφ. ια'.* [*Διάγνωσις τῆς κοιλίας παθούσης ὑπὸ τῆς εἰσβολῆς τοῦ πυρετοῦ.*] Θαυμαστὴ δ' ὄντως ἡ νῦν ἐπ' αὐτοῦ τοῦ βασιλέως συμβᾶσα, δόξαντος μὲν καὶ

tamen haec praenotio nihil haberet admiratione dignum, ut oftendi tibi cum in commentariis in primum de morbis publice graffantibus, tum praeterea in opere de crifibus. At hi medici non modo quae a veteribus fcripta funt ignorant, fed ne dies quidem adhuc poft feptimum numerare poffunt, praefertim fi aeger a febri immunis rurfus ex recidiva febricitet. Attamen Hippocrates in Epidemiorum libris omnes dies in fingulis aegrotantibus adusque folutionem extremam, non folum eam quae quartodecimo die, fed etiam quae fexagefimo aut octogefimo accidit, memoriae prodidit. Haec igitur praedictio, ut dixi, tamquam admiranda etiam vulgaribus iftis medicis putabatur, fed talis revera non erat; ficut nec curatio pueri ipfius Commodi, quae iis qui aderant confciis, peregre illo agente fuit adminiftrata.

Cap. XI. [*Ventriculi laborantis ab invafione febris dignotio.*] Illa porro vere admirabilis, quae in ipfo Rege accidit; dum ipfe quidem ipfiusque medici qui cum eo

αὐτοῦ καὶ τῶν ἀμφ' αὐτὸν ἰατρῶν, ὅσοι συναπεδήμησαν αὐτῷ, παροξυσμόν τινα πυρεκτικὸν ἄρξασθαι, σφαλέντων δὲ πάντων καὶ τῆς δευτέρας καὶ τρίτης ἡμέρας εωθεν καὶ περὶ τὴν ὀγδόην ὥραν. εἰλήφει δὲ τῆς προτεραίας τοῦ διὰ τῆς ἀλόης πικροῦ φαρμάκου πρώτης ὥρας, εἶτα τῆς θηριακῆς, ὡς ἔθος ἦν αὐτῷ καθ' ἑκάστην ἡμέραν προσφέρεσθαι, καὶ τότε προσενεγκαμένου περὶ ὥραν ὡς ἕκτην, εἶτα λουσαμένου περὶ δυσμὰς ἡλίου καὶ βραχὺ τραφέντος καὶ ἐπιγενομένων ὅλης τῆς νυκτὸς στρόφων ἅμα τῇ διὰ τῆς κάτω γαστρὸς κενώσει καὶ διὰ τοῦτο πυρέξαντος αὐτοῦ, καὶ τῶν ἀμφ' αὐτὸν ἰατρῶν θεασαμένων, ἡσυχάσαι τε κελευσάντων, εἶτα ῥοφήματι θρεψαμένων ὥρας ἐννάτης, ἐμοῦ δὲ μετὰ ταῦτα κληθέντος, ὅπως καὶ αὐτὸς ἐν τῷ Παλατίῳ κοιμηθείην, ἧκέ τις καλῶν ἡμᾶς ἄρτι λύχνων ἡμμένων ὑπὸ τοῦ αὐτοκράτορος στελλόμενος. ὡς δὲ τριῶν ὄντων τῶν ἕωθέν τε καὶ περὶ τὴν ἕω ἑωρακότων αὐτὸν, ἁψαμένων τε δυοῖν τῶν σφυγμῶν, ἐπισημασίας ἀρχή τις εἶναι πᾶσιν ἐφαίνετο, σιωπῶν δὲ εἱστήκειν ἐγὼ, προσβλέψας με πρῶτον ἐπύθετο,

peregrinati fuerant, acceſſionem quandam febrilem incepiſſe opinarentur; errarent autem omnes et in ſecundo et tertio die, mane et circa horam octavam. Sumpſerat pridie medicamentum ex aloë amarum hora prima, deinde Theriacen, ut conſuevit quotidie aſſumere. Ac quum circa horam ſextam ingeſſiſſet, mox ſole occiduo laviſſet, ciboque uſus eſſet modico, oborta ſunt tota nocte tormina necnon alvi inanitio; eoque ipſe febri correptus eſt. Quod quum medici ipſius vidiſſent, conquiescere juſſerunt, deinde ſorbitione ad horam nonam aluerunt; poſt illa ego vocatus ſum ut et ipſe in Palatio dormirem; quo facto ecce venit aliquis qui nos lucernis accenſis juſſu Imperatoris accerſivit. Jam circiter tribus praeſentibus, qui in diluculo ipſum inviſerant explorarantque pulſum, initium quoddam acceſſionis omnibus eſſe apparebat; ego autem tacitus aſtabam. Intuitus me Imperator, primum interrogabat, cur aliis pulſum tangentibus ego ſolus non tangerem. Reſpondi igitur tunc in hunc modum. Quum hi bis jam

διὰ τί τῶν ἄλλων ἁψαμένων ἐγὼ μόνος οὐχ ἡψάμην. εἶπον οὖν αὐτῷ, ὅτι δύο ἤδη τούτων ἡμμένων, ἤδη δὲ ἴσως καὶ κατὰ τὴν μετά σου γεγενημένην αὐτοῖς ἀποδημίαν ἐγνωσμένης τῇ πείρᾳ τῆς ἰδιότητος τῶν σφυγμῶν σου, μᾶλλον αὐτοὺς ἐλπίζω διαγινώσκεσθαι τὴν ἐνεστῶσαν ἄρτι διάθεσιν. ὡς δ' εἰπόντος μου ταῦτα καὶ αὐτὸν ἐμὲ κελεύσαντος ἅψασθαι, φανέντος μου τοῦ σφυγμοῦ περὶ τὸ κοινὸν μέτρον ἁπάσης ἡλικίας τε καὶ φύσεως ἀφεστηκέναι τοῦ δηλοῦντος ἀρχὴν ἐπισημασίας, ἀπεφηνάμην εἰσβολὴν μὲν οὐδεμίαν εἶναι πυρετοῦ, θλίβεσθαι δὲ αὐτοῦ τὸν στόμαχον ὑπὸ τῆς εἰλημμένης τροφῆς, φλεγματωθείσης μὲν πρὸ τῆς ἐκκρίσεως, ἐμφαινούσης δ' ἔπαινόν τινα τῆς διαγνώσεως αὐτῇ λέξει τῇδε, τρὶς ἐφεξῆς εἰπὼν αὐτό ἐστιν, αὐτὸ τοῦτο ὃ εἶπες ἔστιν. αἰσθάνομαι γὰρ ὑπὸ ψυχροτέρας τῆς τροφῆς βαρυνόμενος. καὶ ἤρετο τί ποιεῖν χρή. ἐγὼ δ' ἀπεκρινάμην ἅπερ ἔγνων καὶ ἐλέχθη μοι πρὸς αὐτὸν, ὡς, εἰ ἄλλος τις ἦν ὁ διακείμενος οὕτως, ἔδωκα ἂν αὐτῷ, καθάπερ εἴωθα, πιεῖν οἶνον πεπέρεως ἐπιπάσας. ἐφ' ὑμῶν δὲ τῶν βασιλέων, ἀσφαλεστάτοις βοη-

tetigerint et forte jam pulfuum tuorum proprietatem ufu ac experientia cognitam habeant, ut qui tecum peregrinati fuerint, magis ipfos fpero affectionem praefentem modo agnofcere. Quae quum dixiffem, juffiffetque ipfe me pulfum tangere, isque appareret juxta communem omnis et aetatis et naturae menfuram, plurimum abeffe ab eo qui acceffionis initium indicaret pronunciavi; invafionem quidem nullam effe febris, fed ftomachum affumpto alimento comprimi, quod in pituitam verfum effet, antequam excerneretur. Quae dignotio quum laudem aliquam mereretur, ipfis his verbis ter ordine Imperator dixit, ipfum eft, hoc ipfum quod dixifti eft, fentio enim a frigidiore alimento me gravari. Rogabat igitur quid effet faciundum. Ego fane refpondi quae fenfi, dixique ad eum: quod fi alius quispiam ita effet affectus, darem ei quemadmodum confuevi vinum potui, cui piper effet infperfum. In vobis autem regibus, quum medici praefidiis fecuriffimis uti foleant, abunde eft lanam potius nardino unguento

θήμασιν εἰωθότων χρῆσθαι τῶν ἰατρῶν, ἀρκεῖ ναρδίνῳ μύρῳ θερμῷ δεύσαντα μαλλὸν ἐρίου, θεῖναι κατὰ τοῦ στόματος τῆς κοιλίας. ὁ δὲ καὶ ἄλλως εἰπὼν ἔθος ἐκείνῳ ὅταν ποτὲ μέμψηται τὸν στόμαχον, ἀνειλημμένον πορφυρέῳ ἐρίῳ τὸ νάρδινον μύρον ἐπιτιθέναι θερμὸν, κελεύσας τε Πειθολάῳ πρᾶξαι τοῦτο καὶ ἡμᾶς ἀπολῦσαι, ἐπιθέντος δ' αὐτοῦ καὶ τῶν ποδῶν ἐκθερμανθέντων ὑπὸ τῶν ἀνατριβόντων θερμαῖς ταῖς χερσὶν, ᾔτησεν οἴνου Σαβίνου καὶ πεπέρεως ἐπιβαλὼν ἔπιε· καὶ εἰπὼν τῷ Πειθολάῳ μετὰ τὸ πιεῖν ὡς ἰατρὸν ἔχων ἕνα καὶ τοῦτον ἐλεύθερον πάνυ διετέλει τε περὶ ἐμοῦ λέγων ἀεὶ, καθάπερ οἶσθα καὶ σὺ, τῶν μὲν ἰατρῶν πρῶτον εἶναι, τῶν δὲ φιλοσόφων μόνον· ἐπεπείρατο γὰρ ἤδη πολλῶν, οὐ μόνον φιλοχρημάτων, ἀλλὰ καὶ φιλονείκων καὶ φιλοδόξων καὶ φθονερῶν καὶ κακοήθων. ὅπερ οὖν ἔφην ἐγὼ, ταύτης τῆς ἐπισκέψεως οὐδεμίαν ἄλλην ἡγοῦμαί μοι γεγονέναι θαυμαστοτέραν. ἐζητημένου γὰρ ἅπασι τοῖς ἄριστα τὴν περὶ τοὺς σφυγμοὺς τέχνην ἀσκήσασιν, ὧν εἷς καὶ Ἀρχιγένης ἐγένετο, τί σημεῖον ἴδιον ἐπι-

calido imbutam ventriculi orificio imponere. Ille alioquin etiam fibi confuetudinem effe dixit, quum aliquando de ftomacho conquereretur, nardinum unguentum calidum purpurea lana exceptum applicare. Quod quum Pitholao facere juffiffet ac nos dimitteret, impofita ea et pedibus manuum calidarum confricatu excalfactis, vinum Sabinum poftulavit pipereque injecto bibit; ac poft potionem Pitholao dicebat, fe medicum unum, eumque admodum liberum habere, ac nunquam ficut et tu novifti me praedicare deftitit; primum fane medicorum effe, philofophorum autem folum; quippe expertus erat jam multos non modo pecuniae ftudiofos, fed etiam contentiofos, gloriae cupidos, invidos et malignos. Quod igitur ego dixi, hac inveftigatione nullam puto mihi magis admirabilem obtigiffe. Quum enim quaeratur ab omnibus, qui optime in pulfuum arte exercitati funt, quorum unus etiam Archigenes extitit, fignum aliquod acceffionis peculiare; et in

σημασίας, [849] καί τινων μὲν ἐν ἀρχῇ τῆς κατὰ τὴν ἀρτηρίαν συστολῆς εὑρίσκεσθαι φάντων αὐτῶν, τινῶν δὲ μηδόλως αἰσθητὴν εἶναι τὴν συστολὴν, εὐτυχήσας ἐγὼ, τί γὰρ ἂν ἄλλο φαίη τις αἰσθητικωτάτην ἁφὴν τῆς παρὰ μικρὸν ἐν τοῖς σφυγμοῖς διαφορᾶς, ἁμαρτανόντων εἰς τοσοῦτον ἐνίων ἰατρῶν ἐπειράθην, ὡς ἀρχομένους ἐπισημαίνεσθαί τινας εἰς τὸ βαλανεῖον ἐκπέμπειν, ἢ τραφῆναι κελεύειν ἐκώλυσα. διαπαντὸς οὖν ἀκριβῶς ἐμαυτοῦ πεπειραμένος διαγνόντος ἀρχὴν παροξυσμοῦ προπετέστερον μὲν ἴσως, ὅμως δ' ἐτόλμησα βασιλεῖ διατεινάμενος εἰπεῖν, ὅτε πρῶτον ἡψάμην, ἐναντίαν ἀπόφασιν ἧς αὐτός τε καθ' ἑαυτὸν ἐδόξαζε καὶ τῶν ἰατρῶν ἤκουε. τὸ μέντοι κατὰ Κόμμοδον ἔχειν μέν φασί τι μέγιστον, τῇ δ' ἀληθείᾳ πάμπολυ λείπεται τοῦδε.

Κεφ. ιβ'. [Ἐκ τῶν σφυγμῶν διαγινώσκει τὴν φλεγμονὴν τῶν παρισθμίων.] Τῆς παλαίστρας γὰρ ἀπαλλαγέντος αὐτοῦ πρὶν σιτίων, ὥρας ὀγδόης εἰσέβαλε θερμὸς ἱκανῶς πυρετός· ἁψαμένῳ δέ μοι τῶν σφυγμῶν φλεγμαίνειν τι μόριον ἐφαίνετο· καὶ ταῦτα ἀκούσας ὁ Πειθόλαος θαυ-

quibusdam per initia arteriae ſyſtolen inveniri ipſi dicant, nonnulli vero neutiquam ſenſibilem eſſe ſyſtolen, ego bona quadam ſortuna, quid enim aliud dixeris, cui tactus etiam in exigua pulſuum differentia percipienda exactiſſimus contigerit? Medicorum aliquos adeo aberrantes ſum expertus, ut qui acceſſionem habere inciperent, relegarent in balneum, aut cibum aſſumere juberent, ego prohibui. Perpetuo igitur exacte expertus me cognoſcere acceſſionis initium, praecipitantius forſan, attamen auſus ſum aſſeveranter Regi dicere ex primo pulſus tactu aliam ſententiam, quam et ipſe apud ſe opinabatur et a medicis audierat. Quod porro in Commodo praeſtiti, maxime ajunt mirandum eſſe, at revera permultum ab hoc abeſt.

Cap. XII. [*Faucium inflammationem ex pulſu cognoſcit.*] Nam a palaeſtra reverſum, ante cibum ingeſtum, hora octava febris admodum calida invaſit; mihi autem pulſu explorato pars quaedam inflammationem ſuſtinere videbatur. Quibus auditis Pitholaus admirari ſe dixit, ſi

μάζειν ἔφησεν, εἰ τῶν παρισθμίων ἡ φλεγμονὴ τὸν σφυγμὸν ἠλλοίωσε τοῦ παιδὸς, οὐδὲν γὰρ ἄλλο μέρος αὐτοῦ φλεγμαίνει κἀν τούτῳ διανοίξας αὐτῷ τὸ στόμα κελεύει μοι θεάσασθαι. φανέντων δὲ τόπων τραχέων καὶ λίαν ἐρυθρῶν, οὐ μέντοι μέγαν ὄγκον ἐχούσης τῆς φλεγμονῆς, ἠρόμην τίς ὁ ἀνατρίψας εἴη στοματικῷ φαρμάκῳ σφοδροτέραν τῆς ἁρμοζούσης τῷ παιδὶ στύψιν ἔχοντι. τοῦ δὲ φάντος ἑαυτὸν εἶναι τὸν ἀνατρίψαντα τῷ διὰ μέλιτος καὶ ῥοῦ φαρμάκῳ, μεταβῆναι μὲν ἐπὶ μελίκρατον ἐναφεψημένων (461) ῥόδων ἐκέλευσα καὶ τούτῳ μόνῳ χρῆσθαι διά τε τῆς νυκτὸς καὶ τῆς ἐχομένης ἡμέρας ὅλης πολλάκις ἅμα τῇ μετ' αὐτὴν νυκτὶ, τῇ δὲ τρίτῃ τῶν ἡμερῶν ἕωθεν, ἐπειδὴ τά τε τῆς φλεγμονῆς ἐπέπαυτο τελέως ἀπύρετός τε ἦν μικροῦ δεῖν ὁ παῖς. ἔπεισα δ' οὖν τὸν Πειθόλαον εἰς βαλανεῖον ἐγγὺς ὂν τοῦ κοιτῶνος εἰσαγαγόντα, μεθ' οὗ πολὺ τῷ κατὰ τὴν πύελον ὕδατι χρήσασθαι, διαβρεχομένων μὲν ἁπάντων τῶν ἄλλων μορίων, μόνης δὲ τῆς κεφαλῆς καταντλουμένης δαψιλῶς. τραφέντι αὐτῷ περὶ τρίτην ὥραν ἧκεν Ἀνία Φαυστίνη

tonſillarum inflammatio pueri pulſum immutaret; nulla enim alia ipſius pars inflammatione tentabatur; atque interea ore ipſius adaperto inſpicere jubet. Ubi jam loci apparerent aſperi multumque rubentes, non tamen magnum haberet inflammatio tumorem, rogabam quis confricuerit eam medicamento ſtomatico, quod vehementiorem quam puero conveniat aſtrictionem repraeſentat. Ubi ſeipſum reſpondit fricuiſſe ex melle et rhu medicamento, juſſi ut ad mulſam, in qua roſae decoctae eſſent, digrederetur, atque hac ſola uteretur nocte et ſequenti die toto frequenter ſimul et nocte ſuccedanea. Tertio die mane poſtquam inflammatio ceſſaſſet, ac puer paulo minus tota febri careret, perſuaſi Pitholao, ut eum in balneas vicinas cubiculo, in quo decumbebat, introduceret, ita ut ſolii aqua copioſe uteretur; qua omnes quidem aliae partes irrigarentur, ſolum autem caput ſuperfunderetur abunde. Caeterum cibo ad horam tertiam aſſumpto, Ania Fauſtina cognata Imperatori e proximo acceſſit, excuſans

συγγενὴς οὖσα τῷ αὐτοκράτορι ἔγγιστα, παραιτουμένη διότι δευτεραῖον αὐτὸ οὐκ εἶδε· χθὲς γάρ ἔφη μετ' ἄριστον ἐγνωκέναι περὶ τοῦ γενομένου πυρετοῦ· καὶ τούτοις ἔτι προσετίθει δῆλον εἶναι, μέλλοντας ἡμᾶς ὑπερβάλλειν τὴν ὀγδόην, καθ' ἣν εἰσέβαλεν ὁ παροξυσμός. μειδιάσας οὖν ὁ Πειθόλαος, πῶς δὲ οὐ μέλλομεν, ἔφη, τὸν Θεσσάλειον ὑπερβάλλειν διάτριτον; ἀλλὰ Γαληνὸς οὗτος, ἔφη, θεασάμενος ἕωθεν ἰσχνόν τε καὶ ξηρὸν μὴ πυρέξειν ἔφη· καὶ μέντοι καὶ λούειν αὖθις ἑσπέρας ἐπηγγείλατο καὶ δεῖπνον παρέχειν ὁποῖον ὑγιαίνων δειπνεῖ. ταῦτα ἀκούσασα βραχύ τι χρόνου αὐτόθι διατρίψασα ἡ Φαυστίνα, λαβομένη τῆς χειρὸς αὐτῇ συνεξήγαγεν, ἰατρόν τινα τῶν συνηκολουθηκότων αὐτῇ μεθοδικῶν παίζουσα Γαληνὸν, ἔφη, τοῦτον ἴσθι μὴ λόγοις, ἀλλ' ἔργοις ὑμῖν τοῖς μεθοδικοῖς πολεμεῖν. πολλάκις γὰρ ἤδη πολλοὺς τῶν ἀρχομένων πυρέττειν ἔλουσέ τε καὶ ἔδωκεν οἴνου πιεῖν· ἐνίους δὲ καὶ κατὰ τὴν πρώτην, ἐνίους τῇ τρίτῃ τῶν ἡμερῶν ἀπέλυσεν ἐπὶ τὰς συνήθεις πράξεις· ἐν ᾗ πάντες ὑμεῖς ταῖς πρώταις ἡμέραις δύο προασιτῆσαι κελεύσαν-

ſe quod altero die ipſum non inviſerit, heri inquiens de febri oborta certior facta ſum; atque his adhuc adjiciebat, manifeſtum eſſe nos octavam horam, qua invadebat acceſſio, egredi debere. Ridens igitur Pitholaus ait, quidni Theſſalicam diatriton eramus egreſſuri? Verum Galenus hic, inquit, ſpeculatus mane gracilem ſiccumque puerum dixit non febricitaturum; quin etiam rurſus in balneum deducere veſperi juſſit, coenamque praebere, quali ſanus utebatur. Haec audiens Fauſtina pauliſper ibi morata, manu me prehendens, medicum quendam ex his qui eum erant comitati, Methodicum ſecum eduxit, jocansque Galenum inquit, hunc noviſti non verbis, ſed operibus cum vobis Methodicis pugnare. Frequenter enim jam multos ſebricitare incipientes lavit vinumque potui dedit; nonnullos etiam primo, quosdam tertio die ad conſueta munia relegavit, in quo omnes vos primis diebus duobus inediam praeſcribitis, ac ſuſpectas horas egredi decumben-

τες, ὑπερβάλλειν τὰς ὑπόπτους ὥρας κατακειμένους φυλάττεσθαι. καὶ νῦν οὖν, ἔφη, τὸ τῆς ἐπιστήμης βέβαιον ἐπιδείκνυται, βασιλικοῦ παιδὸς ἀποδημοῦντος τοῦ πατρὸς ἐν ταῖς πρώταις δύο πυρέξαντος σφο- [850] δρῶς, ὡς καὶ ὑμεῖς χθὲς ἠκούσατε, κατὰ τὴν τρίτην ἡμέραν οὐχ ὑπερβάλλειν, ὡς ὑμεῖς ἀξιοῦτε, τὴν ὀγδόην ὥραν ἀναμείνας, ἀλλ᾽ ἤδη λούσας τε καὶ θρέψας· ὅ τε τροφεὺς αὐτῷ Πειθόλαος ἀκριβέστατος ὢν περὶ τὰ τοιαῦτα, ὡς δειλίαν εἶναι τὴν ἀκρίβειαν αὐτοῦ, διὰ τὸ προπειρᾶσθαι τῆς τέχνης τοῦ ἀνδρὸς ἐπείσθη καὶ λοῦσαι καὶ θρέψαι πρὸ τῆς ὑπόπτου. ἡ μὲν τοιαῦτα ἔλεγε διαβαδίζουσα μέχρι τοῦ ὀχήματος· ἐγὼ δὲ μελλούσης αὐτῆς ἐπιβαίνειν αὐτοῦ χωριζόμενος εἶπον· ἐποίησάς με πολὺ μᾶλλον ἢ πρόσθεν ὑπὸ τῶν ἰατρῶν μισεῖσθαι. χωρισθείς τε τῷ Πειθολάῳ διηγούμην αὐτός. καὶ μέντοι καὶ ὅτι διὰ τοὺς τοιούτους ἰατροὺς ἔναγχος ἔγραψα τὰς πραγματείας, μίαν μὲν τὴν περὶ τὰς διαφορὰς τῶν πυρετῶν, ἑτέραν δὲ τὴν περὶ τῶν κρισίμων ἡμερῶν, καὶ τρίτην τὴν περὶ τῶν κρίσεων, ἐπιδεικνὺς ὑφ᾽ Ἱπποκράτους γεγράφθαι τὴν θεωρίαν, ἐφ᾽ ἧς ἄν τις προγινώσκοι τὰ γενησόμενα περὶ

tes obfervatis. Ac nunc ideo, inquit, fcientiae certitudo indicatur in regio puero, qui patre peregre agenti in primis duobus diebus vehementer febricitavit, ut etiam vos heri audiviftis; tertio die non differre cibum, ut vos praecipitis, poft horam octavam fuftinuit, fed jam lavit nutrivitque; et educator ipfius Pitholaus in hujusmodi rebus exactiffimus, ut diligentia ipfius timiditas fit, eo quod viri artem prius effet expertus, perfuafus eft ut et lavaret puerum et ante horam fufpectam aleret. Hujusmodi fane dicebat usque ad vehiculum pergens, ego vero quum illa effet ipfum confcenfura, recedens dixi: fecifti me multo magis quam antea a medicis odio haberi; ac digreffus Pitholao ipfe narravi. Quinetiam propter hujusmodi medicos opera confcripfi, unum de febrium differentiis, alterum de diebus decretoriis ac tertium de crifibus; oftendens ab Hippocrate traditam effe fpeculationem, ex qua quis ea quae aegrotis fupervenient praenoscit. Hi autem

τοὺς ἀῤῥώστους. οἱ δ' οὕτως εἰσὶν ἀφυεῖς, ὥστε μηδὲ μετὰ τῆς ἐμῆς ἐξηγήσεως δύνασθαι αὐτὰ μαθεῖν. αὐτὸς γάρ σὺ, Ἐπίγενες φίλτατε, τὰ γεγραμμένα μοι περὶ τούτων ἁπάντων ὧν ἐθεάσω με προλέγοντα γινώσκεις ἐπιδεδειγμένα πρὸς Ἱπποκράτους εἰρῆσθαι, μόνην αὐτοῖς προσθέντος τὴν περὶ τοὺς σφυγμοὺς θεωρίαν, ἥνπερ καὶ μόνην οὐκ ἐξειργάσατο, καθάπερ οἱ μετ' αὐτὸν ἄλλος ἄλλο τι προσθεὶς αὐτῇ μέχρι τοῦ καθ' ἡμᾶς χρόνου ἐπεκόσμησαν. καὶ γὰρ ἡ γνῶσις τῶν τοῦ σώματος διαθέσεων ἐκ θεωρίας γίνεται, ὥσπερ ἐκ τούτων ἀκριβοῦς γνώσεως, ἡ τῶν μελλόντων ἔσεσθαι πρόγνωσις.

Κεφ. ιγ'. [Πρόγνωσις τῆς ἐσομένης κρίσεως διὰ τῆς κατὰ τοὺς μυκτῆρας αἱμοῤῥαγίας.] Καὶ τό γε σοῦ παρόντος γενόμενον, ἡνίκα περὶ φλεβοτομίας ἐσκέπτοντο τῶν ἐν Ῥώμῃ πρωτευόντων ἔνιοι, διὰ τῶν ὑπομνημάτων ὧν ἐποίησα δείκνυται, δεδειγμένων ὑφ' Ἱπποκράτους τελεώτατα. πέμπτην γὰρ ἡμέραν ἦγε τοῦ νοσήματος ὁ νεανίσκος, ἐφαίνετο δὲ παραλελεῖφθαι τὸ τῆς φλεβοτομίας βοήθημα, δεο-

tam ſunt male nati ac rudes, ut ne mea quidem expoſitione adjuti ea poſſint intelligere. Nam tu ipſe noſti, Poſthume cariſſime, conſcripta a me de his omnibus, quae vidiſti me praedicere, fateri ab Hippocrate eſſe indicata, praeter ſolam pulſuum ſpeculationem; quam etiam unam non elaboravit; ſicut qui eum aetate ſequuti ſunt, alius aliud ei adjiciens, ad hunc usque diem exornarunt. Etenim corporis affectuum cognitio ex ſpeculatione petitur; ſicut rurſus ex accurata horum cognitione, futurorum praecognitio.

Cap. XIII. [*Futurae criſis per ſanguinis fluxum e naribus praenotio.*] Jam quod te praeſente factum eſt *in juvene quodam*, quum nonnulli medicorum, qui Romae principatum obtinent, de ſanguinis miſſione conſiderarent, commentariis quae conſcripſi indicatûr, ab Hippocrate abſolutiſſime oſtenſum. Etenim quintum jam diem morbi juvenis agebat, videbaturque medicis venae ſectionis praeſi-

μένου τοῦ πάθους ἐν ἀρχῇ γεγονέναι περὶ δευτέραν, ἢ τρίτην, ἢ πάντως γε τὴν τετάρτην ἡμέραν αὐτήν. εἶτ' ἐπειδὴ μήθ' ἡ ὥρα τοῦ ἔτους, μήθ' ἡλικία τοῦ κάμνοντος, ὥσπερ γε μήθ' ἡ κατὰ τὴν ζωτικὴν δύναμιν ἀσθένεια μήθ' ἡ προγεγενημένη δίαιτα τοῦ νοσήματος ἀντεδείκνυτο, πάντα δ' ἀλλήλοις ὡμολόγει τὴν φλεβοτομίαν ἐνδεικνύμενα, συνεβούλευσαν οἱ ἰατροὶ τέμνειν τὴν φλέβα, προσηκόντως φρονοῦντες. ἐγὼ δὲ περινοήσας ἀκριβῶς ἅπαντα τὰ φαινόμενα, τὰ πρὸς Ἱπποκράτους εἰρημένα τῶν αἱμοῤῥαγήσειν μελλόντων σημεῖα, καλῶς μὲν ἔφην αὐτοὺς ὁρίζειν τὴν ἀφαίρεσιν τοῦ αἵματος, ἔρχεσθαι δὲ ἐπὶ τοῦτο καὶ τὴν φύσιν ἐπειγομένην ἀποκρῖναι τὸ βαρῦνον αὐτήν· καὶ τοῦτο αὐτίκα μάλα γενήσεσθαι, κἂν ἡμεῖς μὴ ποιῶμεν. οἱ μὲν οὖν ἰατροὶ ταῦτ' ἀκούσαντες ἐθαύμαζον δῆθεν. ἐξαναστάντος δ' ἐπὶ τῆς κλίνης τοῦ νοσοῦντος, ὡς ἀναπηδῆσαι θέλοντος, ἐρωτηθέντος δὲ, τίνος ἕνεκεν ἀνεπήδησε μηδενὸς φοβεροῦ παρόντος, φάντος δὲ τὸν ἐρυθρὸν ὄφιν ἐξέρποντα

dium eſſe aſſumendum, quum affectus in principio eam ſecundo, aut tertio, aut ſaltem quarto die fieri deſideraret. Deinde quum neque anni tempus, neque aegrotantis aetas, quemadmodum neque facultatis vitalis imbecillitas, neque praecedens victus ratio indicationem morbo contrariam praeberet, omnia vero inter ſe conſentirent, ſanguinis miſſionem indicantia, conſuluerunt medici venam incidere, ut par eſt ſapientes. Ego autem omnibus quae apparent exacte conſideratis ab Hippocrate proditis indiciis, eorum quibus ſanguis erumpet. Recte dixi ipſos ſanguinis detractionem definire, ſed naturam eo impelli, coactam id quod ſe gravat excernere, atque hoc ſtatim adeo futurum eſſe, etiamſi nos non faciamus. Medici his auditis admirabantur nimirum. Ubi vero aegrotus in lecto inſurrexiſſet tanquam vellet exilire, rogatus autem qua de cauſa exiliret, quum nihil adeſſet metuendum, dixit rubrum ſerpentem ex tegula irrepentem, ſe videntem ti-

τῆς ὀροφῆς θεασάμενον αὐτὸν δεῖσθαι, μή πως ἀποσφαλεὶς ἐπ᾽ αὐτὸν κατενεχθείη, καὶ διὰ τοῦτο φυγεῖν τὸν τόπον, ἐν ᾧ κατέκειτο. τοῖς μέντοι οὐδέν τι συντελεῖν ἐδόκει τοῦτο πρὸς τὴν μέλλουσαν αἱμοῤῥαγίαν. ἐμοὶ δὲ τά τ᾽ ἄλλα διασκεψαμένῳ πάντα καὶ τὸ κατὰ τὸ δεξιὸν μέρος τῆς ῥινὸς ἄχρι τοῦ μήλου θεασαμένῳ τὴν τέως ἀμυδρὰν ἐρυθρότητα πολὺ δή τι νῦν ἐμφανέστερον γενομένην, ἐπίδοξον ὅσον οὔπω κατὰ τὸν δεξιὸν μυκτῆρα τὸ τῆς αἱμοῤῥαγίας ἔσεσθαι [851] σαφῶς ἐφαίνετο. καί τινι τῶν παρόντων οἰκετῶν τοῦ κάμνοντος ἠρέμα διαλεχθεὶς, ἀγγεῖον ἔχειν ἕτοιμον ὑπὸ τὴν ἐφεστρίδα τῶν ἐπιτηδείων δέξασθαι τὸ αἷμα, κᾄπειτα φθεγξάμενος εἰς ἐπήκοον πάντων ἰατρῶν, ἐὰν βραχύτατον προσμείνωσι, θεάσεσθαι τὸν ἄνθρωπον ἐκ δεξιοῦ μυκτῆρος αἱμοῤῥαγοῦντα. τῶν δὲ γελασάντων ἐν τῷ προειρῆσθαι προσκεῖσθαι κατὰ τὸν λόγον τὸν δεξιὸν μυκτῆρα, καὶ μὴν, ἔφην, ἢ ἀμφότερα δεῖ γενέσθαι, ἢ περὶ θάτερά με σφαλῆναι. ὑπὸ γὰρ τῆς θεωρίας ἀμφότερα τὴν πρόγνωσιν ἔχει, τό θ᾽ αἱμοῤῥαγῆσαι τὸν νοσοῦντα, τό τ᾽ ἐκ δεξιοῦ μυκτῆ-

mere, ne aberrans fuper ipfum dilaberetur, atque ideo locum in quo decumbebat. His fane medicis id nihil conferre ad futuram fanguinis eruptionem videbatur; mihi autem cum alia omnia fpeculato, tum in dextra nafi parte usque ad malas obfcuram tunc rubedinem, multo nunc factam illuftriorem, credibile propemodum jam videbatur ex dextra nare fanguinem profluxurum manifefto. Ac nonnulli ex his qui aderant aegroti famulis clanculum injunxi vas in promptu haberet fub vefte, fanguini excipiendo idoneum; ac deinde omnibus medicis audientibus loquutus, fi pauxillulum manferimus, hominem ex dextra nare fanguinem fundentem confpiciemus. At quum illi riderent, quod in praedicendo adjecerim dextram narem; atqui, dicebam, aut ambo oportet fieri, aut in altero me errare. Nam a fpeculatione utraque praenotionem habent, tum quod aeger fanguinem fundet, tum quod ex dextra nare, a quo me conjeciffe advertendum confului. Quum

ρος, ἐφ' ᾧ τεκμήρασθαι προσέχειν ἠξίωσα. θεασάμενος οὖν τὸν νοσοῦντα δάκτυλον ὡς κνίζοντι τῷ μυκτῆρι ἐνερείδοντα, προσέχειν ἠξίωσα τῷ γινομένῳ τὸν κρύπτοντα τὸ ἀγγεῖον, ὅπως, ἐπειδὰν ἴδῃ τὸ αἷμα τοῦ μυκτῆρος ἐκχεόμενον, προσδραμὼν ὑποθῇ τὸ σκεῦος. ἅμα τε οὖν ἔλεγον ταῦτα καὶ τὸν δάκτυλον ᾑμαγμένον ἐξείλκυσεν, ὅ τε οἰκέτης προσδραμὼν ὑπέθηκεν αὐτῷ τὸ ἀγγεῖον, ἐφ ᾧ μεγίστης κραυγῆς, ὡς οἶσθα, γενομένης οἱ μὲν ἰατροὶ πάντες ἔφυγον, ἐγὼ δ' ἐρομένῳ σοι τὴν θεωρίαν τῆς προγνώσεως ἐδήλωσα πᾶσαν ἐκ τῶν ὑφ' Ἱπποκράτους εἰρημένων δεδιδαγμένος· ἔτι δὲ καὶ τοῦτο προσέθηκα, σφοδρὰν ἔσεσθαι προσδοκᾷν τὴν αἱμοῤῥαγίαν. ἥ τε γὰρ ὁρμὴ τῆς φύσεως ἐστιν ἰσχυρὰ καὶ ἡ νόσος ἄπεπτος· εἰώθασι δὲ τοῖς τοιούτοις αἰτίοις ἄμετροι κενώσεις γίγνεσθαι. διὸ καὶ παραμεῖναι ὀλίγον χρόνον τῷ κάμνοντι κάλλιον εἶναι νομίσας ἔπεμψα τὸν ἀκόλουθόν μου παῖδα κομίσαντα σικυίαν μεγάλην ἀφανῶς τοῖς πολλοῖς· ἐν τάχει τε αἵματος πολλοῦ κατὰ τὸ ἀγγεῖον ἀθροισθέν- (462) τος ἕτερον αἰτήσας δεξάμενος τὸ αἷμα καὶ τὸν σταθμὸν

igitur viderem aegrum indicem digitum tanquam prurientem naſo demittere, famulo vas occultanti mentem ei quod accideret advertere juſſi, ut quum ſanguinem e nare erumpentem videret, accurrens vas ſupponeret. Simulatque igitur haec dicebam, digitum e nare cruentum extraxit, famulusque accurrens vas ei ſubjecit; propter quod maximo, ut noſti, clamore orto omnes medici auſugerunt. Ego autem roganti tibi praenotionis ſpeculationem indicavi univerſam, ex his quae Hippocrates memoriae prodidit edoctus; praeterea hoc adjeci, vehementem ſanguinis eruptionem eſſe expectandam. Etenim impetus naturae valens eſt et morbus non coctus, cujusmodi cauſas immoderatae ſanguinis vacuationes comitari conſueverunt. Quare morari aliquandiu apud aegrotum ſatius eſſe ratus, puerum me comitantem miſi, qui adferret cucurbitam magnam multis inſciis; ac quum ſubito copioſus ſanguis in vaſe colligeretur, aliud poſtulavi; ac accipiens ſanguinem ac pondus, vidi evacuati libras quatuor et dimidias, aegrum-

ἰδὼν τοῦ κενουμένου λιτρῶν ὄντα δ'. καὶ ἡμισείας ἀνάῤῥοπον τε τὸν κάμνοντα σχηματίσας καὶ ψυχρὸν ὀξύκρατον ἀναῤῥοφεῖν τῷ μυκτῆρι κελεύσας, ἐπιθείς τε τῷ μετώπῳ σπόγγον ἐκ ψυχροῦ βεβρεγμένον μελικράτου καὶ τὰ κῶλα διαδήσας, ὡς οὐδὲν ὅλως ἤνυσε ταῦτα, τὴν σικυίαν κατὰ τὸ δεξιὸν ὑποχόνδριον ὑποβαλὼν εὐθέως ἔστησα τὴν αἱμοῤῥαγίαν· ὅπερ ὅτι καὶ αὐτὸ τῆς Ἱπποκράτους ἐστὶ τέχνης, ἐδήλωσά σοι· καί μοι διὰ τοῦτο καὶ ταῦτα καὶ τἄλλα πάνθ' ὅσα διὰ τῶν ἔργων ἐπεδειξάμην ἐγράφη. καὶ γὰρ ῥῖγος ἐσόμενον ὅπως χρὴ προγινώσκειν ἔγραψα, καὶ διάῤῥοιαν γαστρὸς, ἔμετόν τε καὶ πλῆθος οὔρων ἀμέτρων ἢ ἐπίσχεσιν, ἱδρῶτάς τε καὶ παρωτίδας ἐσομένας, ἀποσκήμματά τε παραφροσύνην τε καὶ παραφορὰν, ἅπαντά τ' ἄλλα συμπτώματα. τινὰ δὲ, ὡς ἔφην καὶ πρόσθεν, ὁ προμαθεὶς ταῦτα προσεπιλογίζεται πρὸς ἑαυτοῦ, καθάπερ ἐπὶ τοῦ Βοηθοῦ παιδὸς προσεπελογισάμην ἐγὼ, ἐπί τε τῆς ἐρώσης καὶ τοῦ διὰ φόβου ἀθυμοῦντος.

Κεφ. ιδ'. [Διάγνωσις τοῦ διαλιπόντος μὲν, ἀλλά γε κατὰ φύσιν σφυγμοῦ.] Ἔναγχος, ὡς οἶσθα, καὶ τοιόνδε τι

que fublimem figuravi, ac frigidam pofcam nare haurire juffi, impofuique fronti fpongiam frigida mulfa imbutam, ac artubus deligatis, quum nihil haec omnino proficerent, cucurbitula in dextris praefixa praecordiis ftatim fanguinis fluorem cohibui; quod et ipfum ex Hippocratis arte fumi tibi indicavi, atque a me idcirco tum haec, tum alia omnia quae in ipfis operibus oftendi confcripta funt. Etenim rigorem futurum quomodo praenofcere oporteat, tradidi; alvi profluvium, vomitum, copiam urinarum immoderatam aut retentionem, fudores, parotidasque eventuras; humorum decubitus, delirium, mentis alienationem aliaque omnia accidentia; quibusdam autem, ut dixi, antea cognitis, haec praeterea apud fe confideret, quemadmodum ego in Boëthi filio ratione collegi, ac in amante muliere et fervo ex metu trifti ac dolente.

Cap. XIV. [*Intermittentis, fed naturalis pulfus dignotio.*] Nuper, ut nofti, etiam quum tale quippiam

προειπόντος μου, τοὺς πολλοὺς ἐξέπλησσεν ἡ πρόγνωσις. οἰκονόμος γάρ τις, ἅπαντα διοικῶν ὀρθῶς τὰ τοῦ δεσπότου καὶ διὰ τοῦτο τιμώμενος, ἑτέρων αὐτὸν ἰατρῶν ἰωμένων, ἐκρίθη μὲν ἑβδομαῖος ἱδρῶτι, τῇ δ' ὑστεραίᾳ διαλείποντα τὸν σφυγμὸν εὑρόντες αὐτοῦ κακοήθη διάθεσιν ἐν τῷ σώματι φωλεύειν ἔδοξαν, σφαλέντες μεγάλως. εἶτα τῆς οἰκίας ἐξελθόντος ἅμα τῷ δεσπότῃ τοῦ νεανίσκου, κατὰ τύχην ἀπήντησάν μοι, διηγησάμενοι τὰ προγεγονότα καὶ τὰ παρόντα συμπτώματα, τί ποτε σημαίνει τὸ κατὰ τὸν [852] σφυγμὸν ἀλόγως γεγονὸς, ἐδέοντο μαθεῖν. κἀγὼ πυθόμενος πλησίον εἶναι τὴν οἰκίαν, ἐν ᾗ κατέκειτο, συνῆλθον αὐτοῖς ἁψάμενος τὸν σφυγμὸν τοῦ νεανίσκου. κατὰ γὰρ αὐτὴν τὴν αἰσθητικὴν διάθεσιν, εἶπόν σοι, πολλάκις οὐκ ὀλίγα σφάλλονται καὶ τῶν ἀξιολόγων ἰατρῶν ἔνιοι, μέγαν ἡγούμενοι τὸν οὐ μέγαν σφυγμὸν, ὥσπερ γε ἐνίοτε καὶ ταχὺν τὸν οὐ ταχὺν, ἢ βραδὺν τὸν μὴ βραδύν. ὡσαύτως δὲ περὶ τὴν τῶν ἀμυδρῶν τε καὶ σφοδρῶν καὶ σκληρῶν καὶ μαλακῶν σφυγμῶν διάγνωσιν σφάλλονται, καὶ μᾶλλον ἔτι περὶ τὴν τῶν

praedicerem, vulgares iftos attonitos reddidit praenotio. Nam oeconomus quidam omnia domini negotia recte adminiftrans ac ideo in precio habitus, quum alii medici ipfum curarent, crifin per fudorem feptimo die expertus eft. Poftridie pulfum ipfius deficientem invenientes malignam in corpore difpofitionem latitare opinati funt, magno errore; deinde adolefcente una cum domino domum egreffo, cafu mihi occurrerunt, narratis fymptomatis quae praeceſſerant et in praefentia urgerent, quidnam id quod praeter rationem in pulfu evenerat, indicaret, poftulabant difcere. Ac ego audiens domum, in qua decubuerat, effe in propinquo, cum ipfis ingreffus fum, tetigique adolefcentis pulfum. Nam in ipfa fenfibili difpofitione frequenter etiam illuftrium medicorum nonnulli haud mediocriter, ut dixi tibi, errant, dum pulfum non magnum cenfent magnum, quemadmodum interim et citatum non citatum vel tardum non tardum. Pari modo in languidis et vehementibus, duris et mollibus pulfibus digno-

ἀτάκτων τε καὶ τεταγμένων, ὁμαλῶν τε καὶ ἀνωμάλων, ἐν ἀθροίσματί τε καὶ κατὰ μίαν διαστολὴν, δι᾽ οὓς κἀγὼ τέτταρα περὶ τῆς διαγνώσεως τῶν σφυγμῶν ἔγραψα βιβλία, προηγούμενα τεττάρων ἑτέρων, ἃ περὶ τῶν ἐν σφυγμοῖς αἰτιῶν ἐπιγέγραπται. δεῖται γὰρ ἀμφοτέρᾳ τῶν πραγματειῶν ἡ περὶ τῆς διὰ τῶν σφυγμῶν προγνώσεως, ἐν τέτρασί τε καὶ αὐτὴ γεγραμμένη βιβλίοις, δι᾽ ἣν καὶ αἱ προειρημέναι δύο τυγχάνουσιν οὖσαι. χρησιμωτάτης δὲ τῆς καθ᾽ ἕνα σφυγμὸν ἀνωμαλίας οὔσης, γυμνασίας ἰσχυροτέρας δεομένης εἰς διάγνωσιν, ὡς ἐπιδέδεικται, ὡς ἂν πολλὰς ἐχούσης διαφοράς. ὅταν ὁ σφυγμὸς ὅ τε κατὰ μίαν ἐνέργειαν ὅ τε κατὰ πλείους ἐφεξῆς ἀλλήλων μηδὲν ἔχῃ παρὰ φύσιν ἄλλο, πλὴν τοῦτο μόνον, ὃ κατὰ διάλειψιν γίνεται. γινώσκειν οὖν χρὴ τὸ τοιοῦτον ἐκ γενετῆς εἶναι σύμπτωμα, διαγινώσκεσθαι δὲ χαλεπώτατόν ἐστιν, μᾶλλον δ᾽ ἀδύνατον ἄνευ τῶν πασῶν τῶν κατὰ τοὺς σφυγμοὺς διαφορῶν ἀκριβῶς αἰσθάνεσθαι. θεασάμενος οὖν τὸν ἄνθρωπον οὕτως ἔχοντα, συνε-

ſcendis falluntur, ac magis adhuc in ordinatis et inordinatis, aequalibus et inaequalibus; tum in collectione tum in una diaſtole, propter quos ego etiam quatuor de pulſuum dignotione libros conſcripſi, alios praecedentes quatuor, qui de pulſuum cauſis titulum habent. Requirit enim utrosque commentarios opus de praenotione ex pulſibus et ipſum in quatuor libros diſtinctum, propter quod etiam commemorata duo exiſtunt. At quum quae in uno pulſu conſiſtit inaequalitas, maximum ut oſtenſum eſt uſum afferat, vehementiori exercitio ad dignotionem ſui indiget, ut quae multas habeat differentias. Pulſus autem et qui una actione et qui in pluribus ordine ſubſequentibus inaequalis eſt, nihil habet praeter naturam aliud, praeterquam hoc ſolum, quod per intermiſſionem accidit. Hujusmodi igitur ſymptoma ab origine eſſe, ſcire convenit, ſed quod difficillime dignoſci queat; imo non poteſt, niſi omnes pulſuum differentias exacte ſentias. Intuitus igitur hominem ita habentem conſului medicis, ut reſectoria vi-

βούλευσά τε τοῖς ἰατροῖς ἀναληπτικῶς ἄγειν αὐτὸν ἀσφαλῶς κεκριμένον, εἶθ' ὅταν προέρχηται ἤδη καὶ τὰ συνήθη πράττῃ, τότε τῶν σφυγμῶν ἁψάμενος αὐτοῦ διαλιπόντας εὑρήσειν ἔφην, ὡς καὶ νῦν. τοῦτο γὰρ αὐτῷ φύσει συμβεβηκέναι, οὐκ ἐξ ὑποπιπτούσης αἰτίας τινὸς νοσώδους. ἐκ μὲν οὖν τοῦ παραχρῆμα τὸ ῥηθὲν αὐτοῖς ἄπιστον ἐφαίνετο· κατὰ δὲ τὸν ἑξῆς λόγον ἅπαντα διαλιπόντα μίαν πληγὴν τὸν σφυγμὸν εὑρίσκεσθαι ἄλλοτε κατ' ἄλλον ἀριθμόν. ὕστερον δέ ποτε προσελθόντες μοι παρεκάλουν ἀκοῦσαί μου, διὰ τίνος σημείου τὴν φύσιν ἐγνώρισα τοῦ νεανίσκου τοιαύτην οὖσαν. ἀπεκρινάμην οὖν αὐτοῖς, ὅπερ ἤκουσά ποτε εἰπεῖν Ἰσοκράτην τὸν ῥήτορα τινὶ τῶν ἑταίρων πυνθανομένῳ περὶ τριῶν ἐτῶν ἀσκήσεως, εἰ δυνήσεται καὶ ἀσκήσας ἐν τοσούτῳ χρόνῳ ἕκαστον τῶν προβαλλομένων εἰπεῖν, ὡς ἑώρα λέγοντα τὸν Ἰσοκράτην, φασὶ γὰρ ἀποκρίνασθαι τῷ μειρακίῳ τὸν ἄνδρα· σὲ μὲν ἂν, ὦ παῖ, συνηυξάμην κἂν ἐν ἡμέρᾳ μιᾷ δύνασθαι μαθεῖν ὅπερ πυνθάνῃ· αὐτὸς δ' ἂν ἐμοὶ τοῦ κατὰ γνώμην ἀφυΐαν, ἔτεσι πολλοῖς ἀσκήσας αὐτόν.

ctus ratione eum ſecure criſin expertum alerent, addens quod quum jam egreditur et conſueta obit munia, pulſu ipſius tunc explorato, deficientem invenirent, quemadmodum etiamnum. Hoc enim ei natura accidiſſe non ex coincidente aliqua cauſa morboſa, ſtatim id quod dixeram ipſis incredibile videbatur; toto autem ſubſequenti tempore deficientem in uno ictu pulſum alias in alio numero inventuros affirmavi. Poſtea aliquando accedentes me poſtulabant audire quo ſigno adoleſcentis naturam talem cognoviſſem; reſpondi igitur ipſis quod Iſocratem rhetorem diſcipulo cuidam ſuo quandoque dixiſſe audivi; qui quum rogaret an tribus annis exercitatus poſſet de unaquaque re propoſita dicere, ut Iſocratem orantem videbat, reſpondiſſe virum adoleſcenti ferunt: te ſane, o puer, optarem etiam uno die poſſe diſcere quod quaeris; verum pro ingenii infelicitate pluribus ad diſcendum opus eſt. Caeterum cognoſcetis, dixi, omnes praeter naturam pulſuum differentias hoc libro perlecto. Erat autem primus

γνώσεσθαι δὲ ἔφην ὅσαι παρὰ φύσιν εἰσὶν ἐν τοῖς σφυγμοῖς διαφοραὶ, τουτὶ τὸ βιβλίον ἀναγνόντας. ἦν δὲ τὸ πρῶτον περὶ τοῦ τὰς τῶν σφυγμῶν διαφορὰς ἁπάσας διαγινώσκειν, ἐπαγομένων ἀσκήσεως τὴν ὁδὸν ἐν τέτταρσι γεγράφθαι βιβλίοις. ἃ λαβεῖν ἔξεστιν ὑμῖν, ὅταν ἀπὸ στόματός μου τὰς γεγραμμένας ἐν τῷδε τῷ βιβλίῳ διαφορὰς εἴπητε. τοῦτ' οὖν, ὦ Ἐπίγενες, ἀξιόλογον ἔργον ἰατρικῆς προγνώσεώς ἐστιν, ὥσπερ καὶ τὸ κατὰ τὸν αὐτοκράτορα τῆς δοκούσης αὐτῷ εἰσβολῆς γεγενῆσθαι τοῦ παροξυσμοῦ. τῶν δ' ἄλλων ὅσα θαυμάζουσιν οἱ πολλοὶ τῶν ἰατρῶν, οὐδὲν οὐδ' ἐγγὺς ὅμοιόν ἐστι. τοῖς δὲ θαυμαστὸν γὰρ εἶναι φαίνεται διὰ τὴν τῶν πολλῶν ἄγνοιαν, οὐ δι' ἑαυτὰ τοῖς νομίμως ἠσκηκόσι τὰ κατὰ τὴν τέχνην, οὐκ ἔχοντα δύσκολον τὴν πρόγνωσιν.

qui de omnibus pulfuum differentiis dignofcendis tractat eorum qui introducuntur exercitii viam tradens, quatuor libris comprehenfus. Inde namque vos eas difcere poteftis, quoties ex noftro fenfu depromptas defcriptasque pulfuum differentias agnofcere volueritis. Hoc igitur, o Pofthume, medicae praenotionis opus eft memoratu dignum, ficut et id quod in imperatore oftendi, cui acceffionem ipfum invafiffe videbatur; reliquorum autem quae vulgares ifti medici admirantur, nullum vel prope fimile eft. His enim admiranda effe apparent propter multorum ignorantiam, non iis, qui quae in arte difficilem habent praenotionem propter fe legitime exercuerunt.

ΓΑΛΗΝΟΥ ΕΙΣΑΓΩΓΗ Η ΙΑΤΡΟΣ.

Ed. Chart. II. [360.] Ed. Baf. IV. (371.)

[360] (371) *Κεφ. α'.* [*Πῶς εὕρηται ἡ ἰατρική.*] Ἕλληνες τῶν τεχνῶν τὰς εὑρέσεις ἢ θεῶν παισὶν ἀνατιθέασιν, ἤ τισιν ἐγγὺς αὐτῶν οἷς πρῶτοι οἱ θεοὶ πάσης τέχνης ἐκοινώνησαν. οὕτως οὖν καὶ τὴν ἰατρικὴν πρῶτον μὲν Ἀσκληπιὸν παρ' Ἀπόλλωνος τοῦ πατρὸς φασιν ἐκμαθεῖν καὶ ἀνθρώποις μεταδοῦναι, διὸ καὶ δοκεῖ εὑρετὴς γεγονέναι αὐτῆς· πρὸ δὲ Ἀσκληπιοῦ τέχνη μὲν ἰατρικὴ οὔπω ἦν ἐν ἀνθρώποις, ἐμπειρίαν δέ τινα οἱ παλαιοὶ εἶχον φαρμάκων

GALENO ASCRIPTA INTRODUCTIO SEU MEDICUS.

Cap. I. [*Quomodo inventa fit medicina.*] Inventiones artium Graeci vel deorum filiis vel quibusdam eorum propinquis, quibus dii artem primi communicaverunt omnem, referunt acceptas; hac igitur ratione medicinam primum Aefculapium ab Apolline patre didiciffe et hominibus tradidiffe dicunt et ideo primus ejus videtur inventor; porro ante illum nondum inter homines erat medicina, fed veteres medicamentorum et herbarum ex-

καὶ βοτανῶν, οἷα παρ' Ἕλλησι Χείρων ὁ κένταυρος ἠπίστατο καὶ οἱ ὑπὸ τούτου παιδευθέντες ἥρωες, ὅσα τε εἰς Ἀριστέα καὶ Μελάμποδα καὶ Πολύειδον ἀναφέρεται. παρὰ δὲ Αἰγυπτίοις ἦν μὲν καὶ ἡ τῶν βοτανῶν χρῆσις καὶ ἡ ἄλλη φαρμακεία, ὡς καὶ Ὅμηρος μαρτυρεῖ λέγων,

Αἰγυπτίη γῆ πλεῖστα φέρει, ζείδωρος ἄρουρα
Φάρμακα, πολλὰ μὲν ἐσθλὰ μεμιγμένα, πολλὰ δὲ λυγρά.

ἐκ δὲ τῆς ἐν ταῖς ταριχείαις ἀνασχίσεως τῶν νεκρῶν πολλὰ καὶ τῶν ἐν χειρουργίᾳ παρὰ τοῖς πρώτοις ἰατροῖς εὑρῆσθαι δοκεῖ. τινὰ δὲ ἐκ περιπτώσεώς φασιν ἐπινενοῆσθαι, ὡς τὸ παρακεντεῖν τοὺς ὑποκεχυμένους, ἐκ τοῦ περιπεσεῖν αἶγα, ἥτις ὑποχυθεῖσα ἀνέβλεψεν ὀξυσχοίνου ἐμπαγείσης εἰς τὸν ὀφθαλμόν. καὶ τὸ κλύζειν δὲ ἀπὸ τῆς ἴβεώς φασιν εὑρεθῆναι, πληρούσης τὸ περὶ τὸν τράχηλον δέρμα, ὡς κλυστῆρος ἄσκωμα θαλασσίου ὕδατος καὶ Νειλαίου καὶ διὰ τοῦ ῥάμφους ἐνιείσης ἑαυτῇ ὄπισθεν. φησὶ δὲ καὶ Ἡρόδοτος ὁ ἱστοριογράφος τὸ παλαιὸν ἐν ταῖς τριόδοις προτίθεσθαι τοὺς

perientiam quandam habuere, qualem apud Graecos Chiron Centaurus et ab eo heroes eruditi noverant, quae Ariſteo, Melampodi et Polyeido adſcribuntur. Apud Aegyptios ſane praeter herbas aliam quoque medicamentorum rationem in uſu fuiſſe Homerus hunc in modum teſtatur:

Fertilis Aegyptus rerum, medicamina mixta,
Optima multa, ſimul deterrima plurima, gignit.

Porro ex cadaverum diſſectione, quam in condiendis iis habere moris erat, multa etiam, quae manu adminiſtrantur, apud primos medicos inventa eſſe videntur. Quaedam dicuntur ex caſu obſervata fuiſſe, ut ſuffuſos pungere, inde quod capra quaepiam ex ſuffuſione male habens, junco aculeato in oculum impacto, viſum receperit. Quin et clyſteris uſum ab ibi profectum eſſe ſcribunt. Haec enim colli cute tanquam clyſteris utre marina Nilique aqua impleta, roſtro eam ſibi ipſi per anum indit. Scribit etiam Herodotus hiſtoricus quondam aegris per compita

νοσοῦντας, τοὺς δὲ περιπεσόντας τοῖς αὐτοῖς νοσήμασιν ὑφηγεῖσθαι οἷς χρησάμενος ἕκαστος ἐθεραπεύθη, καὶ οὕτως ἐκ τῆς τῶν πολλῶν [361] πείρας συνηρανίσθαι τὰ τῆς ἰατρικῆς. ἀλλ' αὕτη μὲν ἄλογος ἡ πεῖρα καὶ οὔπω λογική. τελείαν δὲ ἰατρικὴν καὶ τοῖς ἑαυτῆς μέρεσι συμπεπληρωμένην, τὴν μὲν ὡς ἀληθῶς θείαν Ἀσκληπιὸν μόνον εὑρεῖν, τὴν δ' ἐν ἀνθρώποις τοὺς Ἀσκληπιάδας παρὰ τούτου διαδεξαμένους τοῖς ἔπειτα παραδοῦναι, μάλιστα δὲ Ἱπποκράτης, ὃς πάντων ὑπερήνεγκε καὶ πρῶτος εἰς φῶς ἐξήνεγκε τὴν τελείαν παρ' Ἕλλησιν ἰατρικήν.

Κεφ. β'. [Τίνες ἀρχαὶ ἰατρικῆς.] Ἀρχαὶ οὖν τῆς ἰατρικῆς τρεῖς· ἡ μὲν εὑρέσεως, ἡ δὲ ἐκ τοῦ συστήσασθαι τὴν τέχνην, ἡ δὲ ὑφηγήσεως. εὑρέσεως μὲν οὖν ἁπλῶς τῆς ἐν τῇ ἰατρικῇ ἡ παλαιοτάτη καὶ ἄνευ λόγου ἀρχὴ ἡ πεῖρα, ὡς παρὰ Αἰγυπτίοις καὶ πᾶσι βαρβάροις. τοῦ δὲ εἰς σύστημα τέχνης ἀγαγεῖν, ὡς τὴν τῶν Ἀσκληπιαδῶν ἰατρικὴν, ταύτης δὲ ἀρχὴ λόγος καὶ πεῖρα. ὑφηγήσεως δὲ, ὥς φησιν

expoſitis, illos qui iisdem aliquando morbis laboraverant, referre ſolitos quibus unusquisque uſus ſanitatem recuperaſſet: atque hoc modo ex multorum uſu ac experimentis rem medicam conflatam eſſe. Sed haec quidem experientia ratione vacua nondumque rationalis fuit. Caeterum perfectam medicinam et omnibus numeris ſuis abſolutam nimirum divinam aio, Aeſculapius ſolus invenit, illam vero quae inter homines verſatur, hujus ſucceſſores Aſclepiadae poſteris acceptam tradiderunt, maxime Hippocrates, qui omnibus facile praecelluit primusque perfectam apud Graecos medicinam in lucem protulit.

Cap. II. [*Quae medicinae principia.*] Principia medicinae tria ſunt, unum inventionis, alterum conſtitutionis, tertium interpretationis. Inventionis igitur medicinae, ut ſimpliciter dicam, vetuſtiſſimum plane citraque rationem principium experientia eſt, quemadmodum apud Aegyptios et reliquos omnes barbaros. Redigendi vero in artis conſtitutionem, ſicut Aſclepiadarum medicinam, ratio

Ἀθήναιος, ἡ παραδόσεως, καθώς τινες λέγουσιν, ἀρχὴ ἡ φυσικὴ θεωρία. ἁπλῶς δὲ καὶ Ἱπποκράτης ἔφη, ἀρχὴ τοῦ ἐν ἰατρικῇ λόγου ἡ φύσις πρώτη· ἀπὸ γὰρ τοῦ φυσιολογεῖν ἄρχονται οἱ δογματικοὶ, ἐπειδὴ ἐκ τῶν κατὰ φύσιν καὶ τὰ παρὰ φύσιν δύνανται εἰδέναι, ἄνευ δὲ τοῦ γνῶναι τὸ κατὰ φύσιν τὸ παρὰ τοῦτο ἔχον, οὐχ οἷόν τε ἐπίστασθαι. καὶ ἐν τῷ θεραπεύειν ὁμοίως δέονται τῆς φυσιολογίας, ἐπειδὴ ἀπὸ τῆς φυσικῆς δυνάμεως τῶν προσφερομένων βοηθημάτων τὸ κατάλληλον αὐτῶν πρὸς τὰ πάθη λαμβάνουσιν. οἱ δὲ κατὰ τὰς ἄλλας αἱρέσεις παραιτησάμενοι τὸ φυσιολογεῖν ἄρχονται ἑκάτεροι ἀφ' ὧν τὴν ἕξιν τοῦ προσφέρειν τὰ βοηθήματα περιεποιήσαντο· οἱ μὲν μεθοδικοὶ ἐκ τῆς τῶν κοινοτήτων ἐνδείξεως, οἱ δ' ἐμπειρικοὶ ἐκ τῆς κατὰ τὴν πεῖραν τηρήσεως. ὥσπερ γὰρ τοῖς δογματικοῖς ἀρχὴ τοῦ ἐν ἰατρικῇ λόγου ἡ φύσις, οὕτω τοῖς ἐμπειρικοῖς ἀρχὴ ἡ πεῖρα, ἡ πλειστάκις καὶ ἀεὶ κατὰ τὰ αὐτὰ καὶ ὡσαύτως ἔχουσα. ἀπὸ ταύτης γὰρ καὶ ἡ ἱστορία (372) ἄρχεται καὶ

et experientia. Interpretationis, ut fcribit Athenaeus, vel traditionis, quemadmodum quidam dicunt, initium naturalis eft fpeculatio. Enimvero fimpliciter et Hippocrates dixit, *Medicinae rationis initium primum natura eft:* nam a naturae infpectione dogmatici aufpicantur, quoniam ex iis, quae fecundum naturam funt et illa quae contra habent, poffunt cognofcere, at fine naturalium cognitione illa, quae a naturali habitu recedunt, fcire nemo poteft. Quin etiam in curando naturae fpeculationem fimiliter requirunt: quandoquidem ex naturali admovendorum auxiliorum potentia, quae cuilibet morbo idonea funt, accipiunt. Qui vero ex aliis fectis naturae contemplationem afpernantur, utrique a quibus praefidia afferendi habitum finxere, incipiunt. Methodici ex communitatum indicatione, empirici ex obfervatione experimentali. Qua enim ratione dogmaticis medicae rationis natura, eadem empiricis experientia plerumque et fere femper in iisdem et pari modo contingens principium exiftit. Ab hac fiquidem hiftoriam quoque fuam exordiuntur et fecundum hanc

κατὰ ταύτην ἡ τοῦ ὁμοίου μετάβασις. τοῖς δὲ μεθοδικοῖς ἀρχὴ ἡ κατὰ τὰ φαινόμενα τοῦ ὁμοίου θεωρία, ἡ γνῶσις φαινομένων κοινοτήτων.

Κεφ. γ'. [Πόσαι αἱ αἱρέσεις ἐν ἰατρικῇ καὶ τίνα χαρακτηρίζοντα αὐτάς.] Αἱρέσεις δὲ ἐν ἰατρικῇ τρεῖς, λογική, ἐμπειρική, μεθοδική· λογικὴ μὲν ἡ φυσιολογίαν παρέχουσα καὶ τὰς αἰτίας τῶν νόσων ἐξετάζουσα καὶ σημειώσει πρὸς εὕρεσιν τῶν αἰτίων χρωμένη τήν τε θεραπείαν ἐξ ὧν ὑπαγορεύουσιν αἱ αἰτίαι, παραλαμβάνουσα καθ' ὑπεναντίωσιν. τὰ γὰρ ἐναντία τῶν ἐναντίων ἐστὶν ἰάματα. τέσσαρα οὖν ἐστὶ τὰ χαρακτηρίζοντα τὴν λογικὴν αἵρεσιν· φυσιολογία, αἰτιολογία, σημείωσις καὶ τέταρτον τὸ ὑπαγορεύειν αὐταῖς τὰ αἴτια τῆς θεραπείας. ἐμπειρικὴ δέ ἐστιν ἡ εἰς τὰς συνδρομὰς τῶν συμπτωμάτων, τῶν συνεδρευόντων ἐπὶ τῶν νοσούντων ἀφορῶσα καὶ τὴν κατάλληλον πρὸς τὰ συμπτώματα θεραπείαν τετηρηκυῖα, οὔτε δὲ πάθος εἰδυῖα οὔτε αἰτίας ἐξετάζουσα, ἀρκουμένη δὲ τῇ ἐπὶ τῶν συμπτωμάτων, κατὰ πεῖραν τῶν προσφερομένων [362] τηρήσει, χρωμένη δὲ

ab alio ad aliud ſimile tranſeunt. Sed methodicis evidentium ſimilitudinis inſpectio vel communitatum apparentium cognitio principium dicitur.

Cap. III. [*Quot ſectae medicorum, quaeque earum notae.*] Sectae medicorum tres ſunt, rationalis, empirica et methodica. Rationalis naturae rationem praebet, morborum cauſas inquirit et ſignis ad illarum inventionem utitur, curationem capit a contrario, prout cauſae exigunt. Nam contrariorum contraria ſunt remedia. Quatuor ergo ſunt, quae rationalem ſectam deſignant, naturae inſpectio, cauſarum ratio ac ſignorum aeſtimatio, et quartum, nempe quod cauſae ipſis curationem dictant. Empirica ad aſſidentium accidentium concurſus, quae aegris adſunt, reſpicit et convenientem accidentibus curationem obſervat, idque nec morbo cognito, nec cauſa inquiſita. Contenta eſt autem obſervatione in accidentibus, per eorum quae admoventur experientiam facta et hiſtoria prius expertorum utitur: tum a compertis ad incomperta, ſed

καὶ ἱστορίᾳ τῇ τῶν προπεπειραμένων καὶ τῇ τοῦ ὁμοίου μεταβάσει ἀπὸ τοῦ πεπειραμένου ἐπὶ τὸ ἀπείραστον, ὅμοιον δὲ κατὰ τὸ φαινόμενον εἶδος. ὅσων τε γὰρ αὐτοὶ διὰ τῆς τῶν αὐτῶν πείρας τῆς ἐπὶ πολλῶν καὶ πλειστάκις καὶ ἀεὶ κατὰ τὰ αὐτὰ καὶ ὡσαύτως ἐχούσης ἐπειράθησαν, ἢ περιπεσόντες κατὰ τύχην παρεφύλαξαν καὶ ταὐτὰ ἀεὶ καὶ ὡσαύτως ἔχοντα, θαῤῥοῦντες τούτοις χρῶνται, οὐ πολυπραγμονοῦντες τὰς ἐκ τῶν ποιοτήτων δυνάμεις αὐτῶν. πεπιστεύκασι δὲ καὶ τοῖς παλαιοτάτοις, ἀναγραψαμένοις τὰ διὰ πείρας αὐτοῖς τετηρημένα, ἣν καλοῦσιν ἱστορίαν. χρῶνται δὲ καὶ τῇ τοῦ ὁμοίου μεταβάσει, μεταβαίνοντες ἐπὶ τὰ μήπω εἰς πεῖραν αὐτοῖς ἐλθόντα, ὁπόταν ὅμοια φαίνηται τῇ κατὰ τὸ πρόχειρον ἰδέᾳ· ὡς μαλάχη καὶ βλίτον καὶ τεῦτλον καὶ λάπαθον. ἐπί τε τῶν δημητρίων, ὡς χόνδρος καὶ ὄρυζα· καὶ τράκτυον. καὶ πάλιν ἐν τοῖς ἀκροδρύοις, ὡς ἄπιος καὶ μῆλον κυδώνιον. χαρακτηρίζει οὖν καὶ τὴν ἐμπειρικὴν αἵρεσιν ταῦτα, τὸ εἰς τὰς συνδρομὰς ἀφορᾶν τῶν συμπτωμάτων, μήτε εἰς πάθος μήτε εἰς αἴτια. δεύτερον ἡ ἐπὶ ταῖς συνδρομαῖς τήρησις

ſimilia ſecundum apparentem ſpeciem tranſit. Quae enim ipſimet uſu ac experientia in multis et ſaepiſſime ac ſemper in iisdem et pari modo experti ſunt, aut quae caſu quopiam obſervarunt, eaque ſemper atque eodem modo habentia, haec confidenter uſurpant, non adeo curioſe facultates ex eorum qualitatibus disquirentes. Credunt et vetuſtiſſimis, qui rerum per experimenta ſibi obſervatarum hiſtoriam, quam vocant, memoriae prodiderunt. Utuntur etiam a ſimili tranſitu ad ea, quae nondum explorarunt, quum ſimilia ſpeciei, quae ad manum eſt, apparent, ut malva, blitum, beta et lapathum. Itidem in cerealibus, ut alica et oryza. Rurſus in arborum fructibus, ut pyrum et malum cotoneum. Notant igitur empiricam haereſim, ad concurſus ſymptomatum, non ad morbum, neque ad cauſas, reſpectus: deinde in concurſibus medicaminum congruentium per uſum obſervatio· tertio, expertorum ante hiſtoria: quarto a ſimili tranſitus. Methodica com-

τῶν διὰ πείρας ἁρμοζόντων. τρίτον ἱστορία τῶν προπεπειραμένων. τέταρτον ἡ τοῦ ὁμοίου μετάβασις. μεθοδικὴ δέ ἐστιν ἡ κοινότησιν προσέχουσα καὶ τῇ τοῦ ὁμοίου θεωρίᾳ. πάντα γὰρ τὰ ἐπὶ μέρους πάθη εἰς δύο καθολικὰ ἀνάγουσιν, εἴς τε τὸ στεγνὸν καὶ τὸ ῥοῶδες, ἃ καλοῦσι κοινότητας. γνωρίζουσι δὲ αὐτὰς ἀπὸ τῶν περὶ τὸ σῶμα γινομένων διαθέσεων, καθ' ἑκάτερον φαινομένων καὶ οὐκ ἀδήλων. διὸ οὐ δέονται σημειώσεως, οἷον τὸ μὲν στεγνὸν, ἐκ τοῦ πεπυκνῶσθαι τὸ σῶμα πᾶν καὶ ἐπισχέσθαι αὐτοῦ τὴν διάῤῥοιαν καὶ πᾶσαν φαινομένην ἔκκρισιν παραποδίζεσθαι. τὸ δὲ ῥοῶδες ἐκ τοῦ τήν τε ἐπιφάνειαν τοῦ σώματος ἀραιῶδες καὶ τὰς αἰσθητὰς ἐκκρίσεις ἐπιτετάσθαι καθ' ὁτιοῦν μέρος τοῦ σώματος. διττὸν οὖν θεραπείας εἶδος ἐνδείκνυται αὐτοῖς τὰ γενικὰ δύο πάθη, χαλᾷν μὲν τὰ στεγνὰ, στέλλειν δὲ τὰ ῥοώδη. ὅταν δὲ ἐπιπεπλεγμένα ᾖ, πρὸς τὸ κατεπεῖγον ἵστασθαι. κοινότητας δὲ πάσας μὲν φαινομένας λέγουσιν· τούτων δὲ τὰς μὲν παθητικὰς, ὡς τὸ στεγνὸν καὶ ῥοῶδες· τὰς δὲ θεραπευτικὰς, ὡς τὸ χαλᾷν καὶ στέλλειν· τὰς δὲ καιρι-

munitatibus et similis speculationi adhaeret. Omnes enim particulares affectus ad generales duos reducunt, astrictum et fluentem, quas communitates vocant. Cognoscunt eas per obortas circa corpus affectiones in utroque evidenter conspicuas. Quare notas non desiderant, exempli gratia astrictum inde oriri, quod totum corpus densatum sit et profluvium ipsius sistatur, omnisque evidens excretio impediatur: fluentem vero inde, quod summa corporis cutis rara evaserit et cujusque corporis partis excretiones sensibiles intensae sint. Duplicem igitur curationis speciem generales duo corporis morbi ipsis indicant, nempe si corpus astrictum est, laxandum esse: si profluvio laborat, comprimendum: si vitium mixtum habet, occurrendum ei quod urget. Caeterum communitates omnes nominant evidentes: harum autem alias passivas, ut astrictum et fluens: alias curativas, ut resolvere et tenere: quasdam temporales, initium, incrementum, vigorem seu statum et inclinationem. Porro medicinae, quae manu medetur com-

κὰς, ἀρχὴν, ἐπίδοσιν, ἀκμὴν, παρακμήν. αἱ δὲ ἐν χειρουργίαις κοινότητες κατὰ τὴν τοῦ ἀλλοτρίου ὑπεξαίρεσιν. διττὸν δὲ τὸ ἀλλότριον, ἤτοι γὰρ ἔξωθέν ἐστιν, ἢ τῶν ἐν τῷ σώματι τὸ μὲν ἔξωθεν ἁπλοῦν, τρία δὲ εἴδη τῶν ἐν σώματι. ἀλλὰ τὸ μὲν ἔξωθεν, ὡς σκόλοψ καὶ βέλος καὶ πᾶν ὅπερ ἀλλότριον, ἐνδείκνυται τὴν τελείαν ἐξαίρεσιν. τῶν δὲ ἐν τῷ σώματι τὸ μὲν τῷ τόπῳ ἀλλότριον, ὡς ὑπόχυμα καὶ ἐξάρθρημα καὶ κάταγμα, ἅπερ ἐνδείκνυται τὴν μετάθεσιν ἢ ἀποκατάστασιν εἰς τὸν ἴδιον τόπον. τὸ δὲ τῷ μεγέθει ἀλλότριον, ὡς τὰ ἀποστήματα πάντα καὶ οἱ ὄγκοι οἱ περὶ ὄσχεον, ἀκροχορδόνες τε καὶ φύματα καὶ κονδυλώματα, ἅπερ ἐνδείκνυται, τὰ μὲν διαιρέσει μόνῃ χρῆσθαι, τὰ δὲ περιαιρέσει τελείᾳ τῶν περιττῶν. τὸ δὲ τῇ ἐλλείψει ἀλλότριον οὐχ ὡς περιττεῦον, ἀλλ' ὡς ἐνδεές, οἷον τὰ κολοβώματα πάντα, ὡς ἐπὶ τῶν χειλῶν καὶ ὀφθαλμῶν, διὸ καλοῦνταί τινες λαγώφθαλμοι καὶ λαγώχειλοι. ὁμοίως δὲ καὶ αἱ σύριγγες καὶ ὅσα ὑπόφορα καὶ κόλποι καὶ ἕλκη καὶ πάντα τὰ τοιαῦτα ὅσα κατ' ἔνδειαν τὸ ἀναπληροῦσθαι ἐπιζητεῖ καὶ ἐνδείκνυ-

munitates, in ejus ablatione, quod alienum eſt, conſiſtunt. Duplex autem alienum eſt, vel extrinſecus, vel in corpore. Quod extrinſecus, ſimplex quidem: illius vero quod in corpore eſt, tres numerantur ſpecies. Atqui extrinſecus, ut ſpiculum, telum, quodcunque aliud id genus exiſtit perfectam eductionem oſtendit. Eorum quae in corpore ſunt, aliud loco alienum, ut ſuffuſio, luxatio et fractura, quae transpoſitionem vel reſtitutionem in proprium locum indicant. Aliud magnitudine, ut abſceſſus omnes, ſcroti tumores, penſiles verrucae, phymata et condylomata: quorum nonnulla diviſionem ſolam requirunt, nonnulla perfectam ſuperfluorum praeciſionem demonſtrant. Aliud defectu alienum, non ut ſupervacaneum, ſed veluti deficiens dicitur, cujusmodi mutila et curta omnia, ſicut in labris oculisque cernitur. Unde quidam leporinos oculos et leporina labra habentes nominantur. Pari modo etiam ſe habent fiſtulae et vitia profunda, ſinus, ulcera aliaque hujusmodi omnia, quae ex defectu repletionem deſiderant

ται. ἔστι δὲ παρὰ τὰς ἐν χειρουργίαις τέσσαρας κοινότητας καὶ τὸ λεγόμενον προφυλακτικὸν εἶδος, ὃ καὶ αὐτὸ εἰς κοινότητα τάττεται ἐπὶ τῶν δηλητηρίων καὶ τοξικῶν καὶ ἰοβόλων πάντων καὶ δακετῶν πτηνῶν τε καὶ χερσαίων καὶ ἐνύδρων. [363] κοινὸν γὰρ πάντων γένος τὸ εἶναι τὰ φθοροποιὰ, οὐχ ὑπαγόμενα τῷ στεγνῷ ἢ ῥοώδει, ἀλλὰ ἕτερον παρὰ ταῦτα τὸ γένος· διὸ καὶ ἡ θεραπευτικὴ αὐτῶν κοινότης ἑτέρα παρ' ἐκείνην, ἡ προφυλακτικὴ λεγομένη. χαρακτηρίζει οὖν καὶ τὴν μεθοδικὴν αἵρεσιν πρῶτον μὲν ἡ τοῦ ὁμοίου θεωρία ἐπὶ τῶν φαινομένων, ἀλλ' οὐκ ἐπὶ τῶν ἀδήλων, ὡς ἐν τῇ λογικῇ αἱρέσει. ταύτῃ γὰρ καὶ διορίζεται, ἐπεὶ καὶ ἐν ἐκείνῃ ἐστὶν ἡ τοῦ ὁμοίου θεωρία, ἀλλὰ ἐπὶ τῶν ἀδήλων. δεύτερον ὅτι ἐκ τοῦ ἐν τοῖς φαινομένοις ὁμοίου ἀνάγει εἰς τὰ καθόλου πάντα τὰ ἐπὶ μέρους, τά τε πάθη καὶ τὰ βοηθήματα καὶ τοὺς καιρούς. ἀλλ' οὐχ ὡς οἱ ἐμπειρικοὶ τοῖς φαινομένοις μόνον προσέχουσιν· ἵστανται δὲ ἐν τοῖς ἐπὶ μέρους καὶ οὐδὲν καθολικὸν ἴσασιν. τρίτον

atque indicant. Jam vero praeter quatuor chirurgorum communitates eſt et ſpecies quam praeſervatricem appel lant. Apponitur autem et ipſa, ut communitas, in deleteriis et toxicis beſtiisque omnibus quae virus emittunt, tum venenoſis volatilibus et terreſtribus aquatilibusque. Nam commune omnium genus, ut ſint exitialia, non tamen ad aſtrictum et fluens referuntur, ſed aliud eſt praeter haec genus. Quare et curatoria ipſorum communitas alia praeter illam habetur, dicta praeſervatrix. Methodicam quoque ſectam primum deſignat ſimilis in evidentibus conſideratio, ſed non in latentibus ſeu abditis, quemadmodum in rationali ſecta. Hoc unum intercedit diſcriminis, quod in illa quoque ſimilium inſpectio, ſed in obſcuris conſiſtit: ſecundum ex ſimili in evidentibus, affectus, auxilia, tempora, particularia omnia generalia reducit. Attamen non evidentia tantum empiricorum more animadvertunt, ſed particularibus, nullo generali cognito, inſiſtunt. Tertium eſt ex communitatum indicatione curationem ac-

τὸ ἐκ τῆς τῶν κοινοτήτων ἐνδείξεως τὴν θεραπείαν λαμβάνειν καὶ μήτε τὰ αἴτια αὐτοὺς ὑπαγορεύειν, ὡς τοὺς λογικοὺς, μήτε τῇ ἐπὶ ταῖς συνδρομαῖς τηρήσει τῶν διὰ πείρας ἁρμοζόντων ἀρκεῖσθαι, ὡς τοὺς ἐμπειρικούς.

Κεφ. δ'. [Τίνες προέστησαν τῶν τριῶν αἱρέσεων.] Προέστησαν δὲ τῆς μὲν λογικῆς αἱρέσεως Ἱπποκράτης Κῶος, ὃς καὶ αἱρεσιάρχης ἐγένετο καὶ πρῶτος συνέστησε τὴν λογικὴν αἵρεσιν, μετὰ δὲ τοῦτον Διοκλῆς ὁ Καρύστιος, Πραξαγόρας Κῶος, Ἡρόφιλος Χαλκηδόνιος, Ἐρασίστρατος Χῖος, Μνησίθεος Ἀθηναῖος, Ἀσκληπιάδης Βιθυνὸς, Κιανὸς, ὃς καὶ Προυσίας ἐκαλεῖτο. τῆς δὲ ἐμπειρικῆς προέστησε Φιλῖνος Κῶος, ὁ πρῶτος αὐτὴν ἀποτεμνόμενος ἀπὸ τῆς λογικῆς αἱρέσεως, τὰς ἀφορμὰς λαβὼν παρὰ Ἡροφίλου, οὗ καὶ ἀκουστὴς ἐγένετο. θέλοντες δὲ ἀπαρχαΐζειν ἑαυτῶν τὴν αἵρεσιν, ἵνα ᾖ πρεσβυτέρα τῆς λογικῆς, Ἄκρωνα τὸν Ἀκραγαντῖνόν φασιν ἄρξασθαι αὐτῆς. μετὰ Φιλῖνον ἐγένετο Σεραπίων Ἀλεξανδρεὺς, εἶτα Ἀπολλώνιοι δύο, πατήρ τε καὶ υἱὸς, Ἀντιοχεῖς. μεθ' οὓς Μηνόδοτος καὶ Σέξστος, οἳ καὶ

cipere: nec cauſas, ut rationalibus in uſu eſt, exponere, neque facta in concurſibus obſervatione eorum quae per experientiam conveniunt, ut empirici faciunt, contentos eſſe.

Cap. IV. [*Qui trium sectarum principes extiterint.*] Rationalis ſectae et auctor et princeps Hippocrates Cous fuit. Poſt hunc Diocles Caryſtius, Praxagoras Cous, Herophilus Chalcedonius, Eraſiſtratus Chius, Mneſitheus Athenienſis, Aſclepiades Bithynus, Cianus, qui et Pruſias dictus eſt. Empiricae praefuit Philinus Cous, qui primus eam a rationali ſeparavit, occaſione ab Herophilo ſuo praeceptore accepta. Quum autem ſuam vellent ſectam antiquiorem fingere, Acronem Agrigentinum, quo rationali eſſet antiquior, ei dediſſe initium dixerunt. A Philino Serapion Alexandrinus ea ſecta floruit: dein Apollonii duo, pater et filius, Antiocheni: hos ſecuti Menodotus et Sextus eam plane ſtabilierunt. Methodicen Themiſon Laodi-

ἀκριβῶς ἐκράτυναν αὐτήν. μεθοδικῆς δὲ ἦρξε μὲν Θεμίσων ὁ Λαοδικεὺς τῆς Συρίας, παρ' Ἀσκληπιάδου τοῦ λογικοῦ ἐφοδιασθεὶς εἰς τὴν εὕρεσιν τῆς (373) μεθοδικῆς αἱρέσεως. ἐτελείωσε δὲ αὐτὴν Θεσσαλὸς ὁ Τραλλιανός. οἱ δὲ μετὰ τούτους Μνασέας, Διονύσιος, Πρόκλος, Ἀντίπατρος· διεστασίασαν δὲ περί τινων ἐν αὐτῇ Ὀλυμπιακὸς ὁ Μιλήσιος καὶ Μενέμαχος ὁ Ἀφροδισιεὺς καὶ Σωρανὸς ὁ Ἐφέσιος. ἐγένοντο δέ τινες καὶ ἐπισυνθετικοὶ, ὡς Λεωνίδης ὁ Ἀλεξανδρεύς. καὶ ἐκλεκτοὶ, ὡς Ἀρχιγένης ὁ Ἀπαμεὺς τῆς Συρίας.

Κεφ. ε'. [*Εἰ ἐπιστήμη ἡ ἰατρικὴ, ἢ τέχνη.*] Τινὲς τῶν λογικῶν, ὧν ἐστι καὶ Ἐρασίστρατος, ὑπέλαβον τὸ μέν τι ἐπιστημονικὸν ἔχειν τὴν ἰατρικὴν, οἷον τὸ αἰτιολογικὸν καὶ φυσιολογικὸν, τὸ δὲ στοχαστικὸν, οἷον τὸ θεραπευτικὸν καὶ τὸ σημειωτικόν. οἱ δὲ μεθοδικοὶ καὶ δι' ὅλου ἐπιστήμην αὐτὴν ἀποκαλοῦσιν. διήμαρτον δὲ ἄμφω τοῦ ἀληθοῦς καὶ μάλιστα οἱ μεθοδικοί. ἐπιστήμη γάρ ἐστι γνῶσις ἀραρυῖα καὶ βεβαία καὶ ἀμετάπτωτος ὑπὸ λόγου. αὕτη δὲ οὐδὲ παρὰ τοῖς φιλοσόφοις ἐστὶ, μάλιστα ἐν τῷ φυσιολογεῖν·

ceus Syrius incepit, qui ab Afclepiade rationali occafiones nactus ad methodicae fectae inventionem fe contulit. Theffalus Trallianus eam abfolvit. Poft hos Mnafeas, Dionyfius, Proclus, Antipater. In ea autem de quibusdam differferunt Olympiacus Milefius, Menemachus Aphrodifeus et Soranus Ephefius. Fuerunt nonnulli etiam adjuncti, ut Leonides Alexandrinus: quidam delecti, ut Archigenes Apameus Syrius.

Cap. V. [*Medicina fcientiane fit, an ars.*] Rationales aliqui, e quorum numero eft etiam Erafiftratus, medicinam partim fcientiam, cujusmodi eft caufarum notitia, item naturae infpectio: partim conjecturam, ut curationem et figna habere cenfuerunt. Methodici et in univerfum fcientiam ipfam effe praedicant, fed utrique a vero, maximeque methodici aberrarunt. Scientia enim eft conveniens, firma et nunquam a ratione declinans cognitio: eam neque apud philofophos, praefertim dum rerum na-

πολὺ δὲ δὴ μᾶλλον οὐκ ἂν εἴη ἐν ἰατρικῇ, ἀλλ᾽ οὐδ᾽ ὅλως εἰς ἀνθρώπους ἔρχεται. διὸ τέχνη εἰκότως ἂν λέγοιτο ἡ ἰατρική. τέχνη γάρ ἐστι σύστημα ἐγκαταλήψεων [364] καὶ διανοιῶν, ποιόν τε καὶ ποσὸν συγγεγυμνασμένον, πρός τι τέλος νευουσῶν χρήσιμον τῷ βίῳ. καταλήψεις οὖν καὶ αὕτη ἔχουσα ἀνθρωπίνας καὶ ταύτας ἱκανὰς τῷ πλήθει, ὡς σύστημα αὐτῶν εἶναι, ἄλλως τε καὶ συγγεγυμνασμένας, τουτέστι προσεχεῖς ἀλλήλαις καὶ συνᾳδούσας, οὐχὶ ἀσυναρτήτους, ἰδιώτατα ἂν τέχνη ὀνομάζοιτο, ἐφαρμόζοντος αὐτῇ τοῦ ὅρου τῆς τέχνης καὶ εἴς τι χρήσιμον τῷ βίῳ νεύουσιν αἱ ἐν αὐτῇ καταλήψεις. ἐπὶ γὰρ τὸ σώζειν καὶ ὑγιάζ· τοὺς ἀνθρώπους παρῆλθεν εἰς τὸν βίον. διττῆς δὲ οὔσης τεχνῶν διαφορᾶς, αἱ μὲν γὰρ τοῦ καθ᾽ ἑαυτὰς τέλους ἀεὶ τυγχάνουσιν, ὡς τεκτονικὴ καὶ ναυπηγικὴ καὶ οἰκοδομική· αἱ δὲ ἐφίενται μὲν τοῦ ἑαυτῶν τέλους, ὡς σκοποῦ, οὐκ ἀεὶ δὲ αὐτοῦ τυγχάνουσιν, ἀλλ᾽ ὡς ἐπὶ τὸ πολὺ, διὸ καὶ στοχαστικαὶ λέγονται. τούτων ἂν εἴη καὶ ἰατρικὴ, ὡς ῥητορικὴ καὶ

turas perfcrutantur, invenias: multo fane minus in re medica: imo ut verbo expediam, ne ad homines quidem venit. Quamobrem medicina ars merito dici poteft: fi quidem artis nomine comprehenfionum et opinionum ad finem quendam vitae utilem fpectantium collectionem certa qualitate et quantitate commeditatam intelligimus. Comprehenfiones igitur humanas et quae numero conftitutionem quandam procreare queant, alioquin et commeditatas, hoc eft fibi concordes ac confonas cohaerentesque, medicina habet: quo fit ut artis vocabulum, cujus definitio ei convenit, optimo jure commereatur, comprehenfionesque in ea ad vitae commoditatem pertinent. Quippe ut fervaret homines ac fanos tueretur, in vitam prodiit. Sed artium duplex eft doctrina: quaedam enim finem fuum femper confequuntur, ut fabrilis, navium compactoria, aedificatoria. Quaedam finem fuum, ceu fcopum appetunt, contingunt autem non femper, fed plurimum. Unde conjecturales quoque dicuntur: ex quarum numero medicina

κυβερνητικὴ καὶ τοξική. ἔστι δὲ καὶ ἑτέρα διαφορὰ τῶν τεχνῶν, διττὴ καὶ αὐτή. αἱ μὲν γὰρ ἐν τῷ γίνεσθαι τὸ εἶναι ἔχουσιν, μετὰ δὲ τὸ παύσασθαι τῆς ἐνεργείας οὐδὲν αὐτῶν ἀποτέλεσμα δείκνυται, ὡς ὀρχηστικὴ καὶ κιθαριστικὴ καὶ παλαιστρικὴ καὶ πᾶσα μουσικὴ τέχνη. αἱ δὲ ἐν τῷ ἐνεργεῖν οὐδὲν ἔχουσιν ὅλως φαινόμενον ἔργον, ἀλλ' ὡς ἂν τινος μέλλοντος ἔσεσθαι παρασκευαστικαὶ, μετὰ δὲ τὸ ἀποστῆναι τῆς ἐνεργείας, τότε αὐτῶν τὸ ἀποτέλεσμα φαίνεται, ὡς ἀγαλματοποιητικὴ καὶ ζωγραφία καὶ τεκτονικὴ καὶ τῶν ἄλλων ὧν ὕστερον ἐπιμένει τὰ ἔργα. τούτων δ' ἂν εἴη καὶ ἡ ἰατρική. ἐν γὰρ τῷ θεραπεύειν οὐδέπω αὐτῆς διαδείκνυται τὸ τέλος, ἐνισταμένης ἀεὶ πρὸς τὰς νόσους· ὅταν δὲ συντελέσῃ τὰς θεραπείας, τότε ὑγιῆ τὸν ἄνθρωπον ἀπέφηνεν.

Κεφ. στ' [Τί ἐστιν ἰατρική.] Ὅροις μὲν ἐχρήσαντο οἱ λογικοί· ὑπογραφαῖς δὲ οἱ ἐμπειρικοί· τὸ δὲ περὶ τούτων ζητεῖν φιλοσόφοις μόνοις ἁρμόζει· ἁπλῶς δὲ καὶ οὕτως ὡρίσαντο οἱ παλαιοὶ ἰατροὶ τὴν ἰατρικὴν, ἢ ὑπέγραψαν.

fuerit: quemadmodum rhetorica, gubernatoria et ſagittandi ars. Eſt et alia doctrina et ipſa duplex: quoniam aliquae, dum fiunt, ſunt et ſimul atque ab actione deſtiterint, nihil quod perfecerint oſtenditur, cujusmodi ſaltatoria, cithariſtica, palaeſtrica et quaevis alia ars muſica. Nonnullae in actione evidens opus plane nullum habent, ſed tanquam futuri cujusdam praeparatoriae exiſtunt: ubi vero a functione ceſſaverint, tunc quid effecerint apparet: qualis ſtatuaria, pictura et fabrilis, tum aliae, quarum opera poſt actionem perdurant. Inter has medicinam quoque numeres licet. In medendo enim nondum ejus finis innoteſcit, quippe quae adverſus morbos ſemper laboret: at, ubi curationem abſolverit, tunc homini ſanitatem reſtituiſſe eam videre eſt.

Cap. VI. [*Quid ſit medicina.*] Definitionibus rationales uſi ſunt et deſcriptionibus empirici: de quibus quaeſtionem inſtituere philoſophis ſolum convenit: enimvero veteres etiam medici hoc modo medicinam ſimplici-

ἰατρική ἐστι κατὰ μὲν Ἱπποκράτην πρόσθεσις καὶ ἀφαίρεσις· πρόσθεσις μὲν τῶν ἐλλειπόντων, ἀφαίρεσις δὲ τῶν πλεοναζόντων ἐπὶ ἀνθρωπίνων σωμάτων. ὃν γάρ τινες ὅρον ἰατρικὸν ᾠήθησαν, οὐκ ἔστιν ὅρος· τό τε μὴ παράπαν ἀπαλλάσσειν τῶν νόσων τοὺς κάμνοντας καὶ τὸ τὰς σφοδρότητας ἀμβλύνειν καὶ τὸ τοῖς κεκρατημένοις μὴ ἐγχειρεῖν. οὐ γὰρ ἐξ ὧν μὴ δύνανται αἱ τέχναι, ἀλλ' ἐξ ὧν δύνανται οἱ ὅροι αὐτῶν εἰσιν. ἐρεῖ γὰρ αὐτῆς ὅσα μὴ δύναται, οὐ τὰ μὴ ὑπάρχοντα αὐτῇ ὁρίζει. οἱ δὲ νεώτεροι οὕτως ὡρίσαντο. ἰατρική ἐστιν ἐπιστήμη, ὑγιείας μὲν τηρητική, νόσων δὲ ἀπαλλακτική, οὐκ ὀρθῶς. οὐ γὰρ αὐτὴ ταῦτα ἐνεργεῖ, ἀλλ' ἐξ ὧν ἐνεργεῖ ταῦτα ἀποτελεῖται καὶ οὐκ ἀεί. διὸ οὐκ ἐκ τούτων συνέστηκεν, ἀλλ' ἐκ τῶν ὑπ' αὐτῆς ἀεὶ παραλαμβανομένων. ταῦτα δέ ἐστι πρόσθεσις καὶ ἀφαίρεσις. ὥσθ' ἅπερ λαμβάνει ἡ ἰατρική, ταῦτα εἶπεν αὐτὴν εἶναι ὁ Ἱπποκράτης, οἷς ἐπί τε τῶν ὑγιαινόντων χρῆται, ὅταν τὴν ὑγείαν αὐτῶν συντηρῇ, καὶ ἐπὶ τῶν νοσούντων, ἵνα τῶν

ter vel definierunt, vel defcripferunt. Medicina eft, ex Hippocratis fententia, adjectio et detractio. Adjectio quidem deficientis, detractio autem fuperantis in hominum corporibus. Quam enim definitionem medicinae nonnulli putaverunt, revera non eft; aegros videlicet morbis non prorfus liberare, dolores lenire morbique vehementiam retundere, malo victis manum non admoliri. Non enim ex iis, quae artes non poffunt, fed ex his quae poffunt ipfarum definitiones funt, quae enim ipfa non poteft dicit, non quae ipfi infunt definit. Recentiores hujusmodi definitionem ufurparunt. Medicina eft fcientia fanitatis confervatrix, morborum depultrix. Non recte habet: non enim ipfa haec efficit, fed ex illis quae efficit, haec proveniunt, idque non femper. Quapropter non ex his, fed illis, quae ab ea femper accipiuntur, conftituta eft. Haec autem funt adjectio et detractio. Proinde quae capit medicina, haec ipfam effe dixit Hippocrates, quibus et in fanis utitur, cum fecundam ipforum valetudinem confer-

νόσων ἀπαλλάττωνται· ἃ τοίνυν ἀεὶ ἐνεργεῖ, ταῦτά ἐστι τὰ συνιστάντα αὐτὴν, οὐ τὰ ἀπὸ τούτων ἀποτελούμενα. ἕτερον γάρ τί ἐστιν ἡ τέχνη καὶ ἕτερον τὸ τέλος αὐτῆς. οὗ γὰρ ἐφίεται, τοῦτο ἄλλο τί ἐστι παρὰ ταύτην, ἀμέλει καὶ οὐκ ἀεὶ τοῦτο σὺν αὐτῇ ἔχει. διὸ μέχρι μὴ τυγχάνει αὐτοῦ, οὐδὲ τὸ τέλος αὐτῆς λέγεται, ἀλλὰ σκοπὸς, ὅταν δὲ τύχῃ, τέλος. [365] οὕτως οὖν καὶ κυβερνητικὴ καὶ τοξικὴ οὐκ ἀπὸ τῶν τελῶν ὁρίζονται. οὐ γὰρ ἀεὶ τούτου τυγχάνουσιν, ἀλλ' ἐξ ὧν συνεστήκασι καὶ δι' ὧν ἐνεργοῦσιν, ἵνα τῶν τελῶν περιγίνωνται. δοκεῖ δὲ τοῖς μετὰ Ἱπποκράτην σχεδὸν ἅπασιν οὗτος ὁ ὅρος ὀρθῶς ἔχειν. Ἡροφίλῳ δὲ, ὅτι ἰατρική ἐστιν ἐπιστήμη ὑγιεινῶν καὶ νοσωδῶν καὶ οὐδετέρων. τριῶν γὰρ τούτων γνῶσιν ἔχει, ὑγιεινῶν μὲν ὅσα τῶν κατασκευαζόντων τὰ ἐν ἀνθρώπῳ οὕτως ἔχειν, ἐξ ὧν εὖ ἡρμοσμένων πρὸς ἄλληλα τὸ ὑγιαίνειν συνίσταται. νοσωδῶν δὲ τῶν τὴν ὑγιεινὴν ἁρμονίαν διαλυόντων. οὐδετέρων δέ ἐστιν ἅπαντα τὰ προσφερόμενα ἐν ταῖς νόσοις βοηθήματα καὶ ἡ ὕλη αὐτῶν.

vat et in aegrotis, ut morbis liberet. Quae igitur ſemper facit, ea ipſam conſtituunt, non illa, quae ab his efficiuntur. Aliud namque ars, aliud ejus finis eſt. Quod enim appetit, id aliud ab ipſa eſt, idque non perpetuo ſecum habet. Quo fit, ut quatenus ipſum non contingit, neque finis ejus, ſed ſcopus dicatur: quum autem contigerit, finis. Ita gubernatoria et ſagittandi ars non a fine, quem non ſemper contingunt, ſed ab aliis, quibus conſtitutae ſunt et per quae, ut finem aſſequantur, functiones obeunt, definitionem ſortiuntur. Porro definitio haec omnibus fere poſt Hippocratem proba eſſe videtur. Herophilo medicina eſt ſcientia ſalubrium, inſalubrium et neutrorum. Trium enim horum cognitionem habet. Salubrium, quae corporis humani conſtitutionem ita praeparant, ut ex eis pulchre invicem aptatis ſanitas concilietur: inſalubrium, quae ſalubrem convenientiam diſſolvunt. Neutrorum omnia ſunt auxilia, quae aegris afferuntur et eorum materia.

ταῦτα γὰρ πρὶν ἢ παραληφθῆναι ὑπὸ τοῦ ἰατροῦ, οὐδέτερά ἐστιν, οὐδὲ ὑγιεινὰ οὐδὲ νοσώδη.

Κεφ. ζ'. [Πόσα μέρη ἰατρικῆς.] Μέρη ἰατρικῆς τὰ μὲν πρῶτά ἐστι, τό τε φυσιολογικὸν καὶ τὸ αἰτιολογικὸν, ἢ παθολογικὸν καὶ τὸ ὑγιεινὸν καὶ τὸ σημειωτικὸν καὶ τὸ θεραπευτικόν. Ἀθήναιος δὲ ἀντὶ τοῦ σημειωτικοῦ τὸ ὑλικὸν τάττει, ὅ ἐστιν ἐν τῷ θεραπευτικῷ. ἄνευ γὰρ τοῦ ὑλικοῦ τὸ θεραπευτικὸν οὐκ ἂν εἴη. σημείωσις δὲ καὶ εἰς θεραπείαν μὲν ἀναγκαία, ἀλλ' οὐκ ἔστιν αὐτὴ ἡ θεραπεία. διὰ γὰρ τῆς ὕλης ἡ θεραπεία συντελεῖται καὶ τὸ μὲν ὑλικὸν ἄνευ θεραπείας οὐδὲν ἕτερον συμβάλλεται. τὸ δὲ σημειωτικὸν καὶ ἄνευ θεραπείας ἀναγκαῖον πρὸς τὸ εἰδέναι τίνα θεραπευτικὰ καὶ τίνα ἀθεράπευτα καὶ περιΐστασθαι αὐτὰ, ὅπως μὴ ἐπιβαλλόμενοι ἀδυνάτοις σφαλλώμεθα. ἔστι δὲ καὶ τῶν πέντε μερῶν τῆς ἰατρικῆς ὑποδιαίρεσις ἑκάστου. φυσιολογικὸν μὲν οὖν ἐστιν αὐτῆς μέρος, ἐν ᾧ περὶ τῆς φύσεως τοῦ ἀνθρώπου διαλαμβάνομεν. διαιρεῖται δὲ εἰς τὸν περὶ τῶν στοιχείων λόγον, ἐξ ὧν συνέστηκεν ὁ ἄνθρωπος,

Haec enim prius quam a medico excepta ſint, neutra, nec ſalubria nec inſalubria ſunt.

Cap. VII. [*Quot partes medicinae.*] Partes medicinae principes ſunt phyſiologia, aetiologia, pathologia, diaeta ſanorum, ſemeiotice, therapeutice. Athenaeus pro ſemeiotice materiam conſtituit, quae in therapeutice reperitur, nam ſine materia curatio ſieri non poteſt. Semeiotice et ad curationem quidem neceſſaria, non tamen ipſa eſt curatio: materiae enim beneſicio curatio abſolvitur et materia quidem ſine curatione nihil aliud confert. Semeiotice etiam et ſine curatione neceſſaria, ut quae curabilia quaeque ſive incurabilia cognoſcamus, ut in iis haereamus, ne quum ſuſceperimus impoſſibilia, hallucinemur. Jam vero quinque partium medicinae cujusque ſubdiviſio quaedam eſt. Phyſiologia igitur pars quidem illius eſt, in qua de hominis natura diſſerimus: dividitur autem in tractationem elementorum, quibus homo componitur, tum in eam, quae de generatione et formatione foetus, tertio in

καὶ εἰς τὸν περὶ γενέσεως καὶ διαπλάσεως ἐμβρύου καὶ τρίτον εἰς τὴν τῶν ἐκτὸς μερῶν τοῦ σώματος ἐπίσκεψιν, ὅτε ἀνατέμνομεν, ἢ ὀστεολογοῦμεν. αἰτιολογικὸν δέ ἐστιν, ὃ καὶ παθολογικὸν, ἐν ᾧ τὰ παρὰ φύσιν ἐξετάζομεν καὶ τὰς αἰτίας τῶν νόσων ἐρευνῶμεν καὶ τὰς συνδρομὰς τῶν συμπτωμάτων καὶ τὰς (374) καταστάσεις τῶν παθῶν πολυπραγμονοῦμεν. ἄνευ γὰρ τούτων οὐκ ἔστιν ὀρθῶς ἐνίστασθαι πρὸς αὐτὰ τὴν θεραπείαν. διαιρεῖται δὲ καὶ τὸ ὑγιεινὸν μέρος τῆς ἰατρικῆς εἴς τε τὸ συντηρητικὸν ὑγείας καὶ εἰς τὸ προφυλακτικὸν τῶν νόσων καὶ εἰς τὸ ἀναληπτικὸν ἀπὸ τῶν νόσων. διαιρεῖται δὲ καὶ τὸ σημειωτικὸν εἰς τρία, εἴς τε ἐπίγνωσιν τῶν παρεληλυθότων καὶ εἰς τὴν ἐπίσκεψιν τῶν συνεδρευόντων καὶ εἰς πρόγνωσιν τῶν μελλόντων. τὸ δὲ θεραπευτικὸν ὁμοίως καὶ αὐτὸ εἰς τρία διαιρεῖται, εἴς τε δίαιταν καὶ χειρουργίαν καὶ φαρμακείαν.

Κεφ. η'. [*Εἰ ἀναγκαία ἡ εἰς τὰ πέντε μέρη τῆς ἰατρικῆς διαίρεσις.*] Τὸ μὲν οὖν φυσιολογεῖν ἀναγκαῖόν ἐστιν, ὅτι οὐχ οἷόν τε τὰ παρὰ φύσιν εἰδέναι μὴ πρότερον ἐπιστάμενον τὰ κατὰ φύσιν. παρὰ γὰρ τὴν τούτων φύσιν

interiorum et exteriorum corporis partium fpeculationem, cum cadavera diffecamus offiumque rationes perfcrutamur: aetiologia quae et pathologia, in qua quae praeter naturam funt inquirimus et morborum caufas inveftigamus et fymptomatum concurfus, affectuum ftatus diligenter indagamus. His enim incognitis nemo recte noverit, quomodo morbos curare conveniat: medicinae pars ea quae diaeta fanorum dividitur in eam quae fanitatem tuetur et in eam quae morbos arcet praecavendo, ac in eam quae a morbis furgentes reficit. Semeiotice in tres partes dirimitur, in praeteritorum cognitionem, in praefentium infpectionem et futurorum providentiam. Similiter et ipfa therapeutice in tres partes dividitur, in diaetam, chirurgiam et pharmaciam.

Cap. VIII. [*An medicinae divifio in quinque partes neceffaria fit.*] Tractare igitur res quidem naturales neceffarium eft, quoniam haud poffibile eft quae praeter naturam funt, illum cognofcere, qui non prius noverit ea

συνίσταται τὰ νοσήματα. τὸ δὲ αἰτιολογεῖν καὶ παθολογεῖν καὶ αὐτὰ ἀναγκαῖα· τὸ μὲν ἵνα τὰς αἰτίας τῶν παθῶν ἴδωμεν, πρὸς ἃς δεῖ ἐνίστασθαι, [366] τὸ δὲ ἵνα καὶ αὐτὰ πάθη γνωρίζωμεν τὰ κατωνομασμένα τοῖς παλαιοῖς καὶ τὰς καταστάσεις αὐτῶν. εὔχρηστος δὲ καὶ ἡ τῶν συμπτωμάτων συνεδρευόντων τοῖς πάθεσιν ἐπίγνωσις· ἀπὸ γὰρ τῆς τούτων συνελεύσεως, ἣν συνδρομὴν καλοῦσιν οἱ ἐμπειρικοὶ, τὰ πάθη εἰδοποιοῦνται. ἀλλ' οἱ μὲν ἐμπειρικοὶ ἐπὶ ταῖς συνδρομαῖς ἐτήρησαν τὰ πρὸς ἕκαστον συμπτώματα ἁρμόζοντα· τοῖς δὲ μεθοδικοῖς τὰ πάθη ἐνδείκνυται τὴν θεραπείαν, ὡς τοῖς λογικοῖς τὰ αἴτια. ἐξετάζουσι δὲ οὐδὲν ἧττον οἱ λογικοὶ καὶ τὰ πάθη καὶ τὰς συνδρομάς. τὸ δὲ πᾶν τοῖς αἰτίοις παρέχουσιν, αἰτίων δὲ τὰ μὲν προκαταρκτικὰ, τὰ δὲ συνεκτικὰ, τὰ δὲ συνεργὰ, τὰ δὲ συναίτια, τὰ δὲ προηγούμενα. προκαταρκτικὰ μὲν οὖν ἐστιν ὅσα προκατάρχει καὶ ποιήσαντα ἀπαλλάσσεται, ὡς ψύξις, κόπος, ἔγκαυσις, ἀπεψία· συνεκτικὸν δὲ αἴτιόν ἐστιν, οὗ παρόντος πάρεστι καὶ τὸ νόσημα καὶ ἐξαιρουμένου λύεται, ὡς σκόλοψ καὶ βέλος· συν-

quae ſunt ſecundum naturam: nam praeter illorum naturam morbi conſiſtunt. De cauſis autem et morbis agere neceſſarium quoque eſt, cum ut affectuum cauſas, quibus reſiſtere convenit, intelligamus: tum ut etiam ipſos affectus a veteribus appellatos eorumque ſtatus cognoſcamus. Utilis ſane et ſymptomatum quae affectus comitantur cognitio eſt, nam ab horum congreſſu, quem empirici concurſu vocant, corporis vitia ſpeciem nanciſcuntur. Quanquam iidem empirici in concurſibus, quae cuique accidenti conveniant, obſervarunt. Methodicis autem curationem affectus indicant, quemadmodum rationalibus cauſae, licet ipſi nihilominus tum affectus tum concurſus inquirant. Totum autem cauſis attribuunt, quarum nonnullae evidentes, aliae continentes, quaedam coadjuvantes, aliquae concauſae, reliquae antecedentes dicuntur. Evidentes ſunt quae ubi adverſam valetudinem crearunt, ſeparantur, ut frigus, labor, ſolis exuſtio, cruditas. Continentes, cum praeſentes ſunt et morbi quoque adſunt:

αἴτιον δὲ τὸ καθ' αὐτὸ μὲν δυνάμενον ποιεῖν τὸ πάθος, ποιοῦν δὲ καὶ σὺν ἑτέρῳ, ὡς λίθος ἐν κύστει καὶ φλεγμονή. ἀμφότερα γὰρ ἰσχουρίας αἴτια. δύναται δὲ καὶ καθ' ἑαυτὸ ἑκάτερον τὴν ἐποχὴν τῶν οὔρων ἐπιφέρειν. συνεργὸν δέ ἐστι μέρος αἰτίου, καθ' ἑαυτὸ μὲν οὐ δυνάμενον ἐπιτελέσαι τὸ πάθος, συνεργαζόμενον δὲ ἑτέρῳ, ὡς συνεργεῖ λαγνεία πρὸς ἀρθρῖτιν καὶ εἰρεσία πρὸς αἵματος ἀναγωγήν. προηγούμενον δέ ἐστι αἴτιον τὸ ὑπὸ τοῦ προκαταρκτικοῦ ἢ κατασκευαζόμενον ἢ συνεργούμενον, οἷον πλεονασμὸς αἵματος γίνεται μὲν ὑπὸ πλήθους τροφῆς, προηγεῖται δὲ τῆς κατ' Ἐρασίστρατον παρεμπτώσεως, ἥτις ἐστὶ συνεκτικὴ αἰτία τῶν νοσημάτων πάντων· ἄνευ δὲ τοῦ προηγουμένου οὐ γίνεται. τὸ δ' ὑγιεινὸν οὐ μόνον ὡς μέρος ἰατρικῆς, ἀλλὰ καὶ ὡς κάλλιον τοῦ θεραπευτικοῦ προτάττεται αὐτοῦ. πολὺ γὰρ ἄμεινον τοῦ ἀπαλλάξαι τῆς νόσου τὸ μηδὲ τὴν ἀρχὴν ἐᾶσαι νοσῆσαι. ὥσπερ καὶ κυβερνήτῃ αἱρετώτερον τὸ πρὶν ἐς χειμῶνα ἐμπεσεῖν διαπεραιώσασθαι ἢ

cum tolluntur, morbi etiam difcedunt, ut fpina et telum. Concaufae, quae affectum fua vi poffunt generare: generant vero et alteri cohaerentes, ut lapis in vefica et inflammatio. Nam ambae urinae fuppreffionis caufae funt, etfi per fe utraque illam generare poffit. Coadjutrices caufarum partes quae fua virtute morbum efficere non poffunt, fed alteri auxiliantur, ut libido articularem morbum promovet et remigatio fanguinis eruptionem. Antecedentes, quae ab evidentibus vel praeparantur vel coadjuvantur, ut fanguinis abundantia, alimenti copiae foboles eft. Praecedit autem Erafiftrati coincidentiam, quae omnium morborum caufa eft conjuncta, verum citra antecedentem non accidit. Porro diaeta fanorum non folum ut pars medicinae, fed tanquam potior ea, quae medetur, ei praeponitur. Multo enim praeftat morbum prorfus non admittere quam morbo liberare: quemadmodum et gubernatori longe praeftabilius eft, ante quam in tempeftatem incidat, iter abfolvere, quam cum jactatus periclitatusque

χειμασθέντα καὶ κινδυνεύσαντα ἐκφυγεῖν. διαφέρει δὲ ἐν τῷ ὑγιεινῷ πάλιν τὸ ἐν ὑγείᾳ διατηρῆσαι τοῦ προφυλάξαι νόσους ἐπιούσας. τὸ μὲν γὰρ διὰ τῆς συνήθους διαίτης περιγίνεται, τὸ δὲ ἤδη δεῖται θεραπευτικῶν βοηθημάτων εἰς τὸ προκαταλαμβάνεσθαι καὶ προδιαλῦσαι, μέλλουσαν συνίστασθαι νόσον. ὅσα γὰρ ἤδη γενόμενα πάθη ἴᾶται, ταῦτα καὶ πρὶν ἢ γενέσθαι κωλύει συστῆναι. ὁμοίως δὲ καὶ τὸ ἀναληπτικὸν τούτων διαφέρει. ὁ γὰρ ἀναλαμβάνων οὐκέτι μὲν παρὰ φύσιν ἔχει, οὔπω δὲ κατὰ φύσιν, ἀλλ' ὁδεύει, ἄρτι ἀπαλλαγεὶς τοῦ παρὰ φύσιν, εἰς τὸ κατὰ φύσιν, διόπερ ἑτέρας ἀγωγῆς δεῖται, οὔτε θεραπευτικῆς, οὐ γὰρ νοσεῖ, οὔτε τῆς ἐπὶ τῶν ὑγιαινόντων, οὔπω γὰρ τελείως ὑγιαίνει. διὸ οὐ δύναται ἐπ' αὐτῶν παραλαμβάνεσθαι, οἷα καὶ ὅσα ἐπὶ τῶν ὑγιαινόντων. ὁ δὲ σημειωτικὸν μέρος τῆς ἰατρικῆς ἀναγκαιότατόν ἐστιν εἰς θεραπείαν τὴν κατὰ δίαιταν. τά τε γὰρ προγεγονότα συμπτώματα καὶ τὰ παρόντα πολυπραγμονοῦμεν εἰς τὸ εὑρεῖν τὴν αἰτίαν τῆς νόσου. ἀναγκαιότα-

fuerit evadere. Atqui differunt rurfus in falubri diaeta fanitatem tueri et morbos incellentes longius arcere. Etenim primum confueta victus ratione adminiftratur: alterum jam indiget curatoriis auxiliis, ut morbum, qui conflari debet. fupprimat ac diffolvere anticipet: liquidem quae jam ortis affectibus medentur, eadem quoque prius quam oriantur prohibent illos confiftere. Similiter pars quam refectricem appellant, differentiae cum illis nonnihil habet. Qui enim recreat vires recolligitque, ut non amplius praeter naturam, ita fecundum naturam fe nondum habet, fed ab eo, qui praeter naturam eft, nuper habitu folutus ad naturalem migrat. Quamobrem aliam victus rationem defiderat, nec curatoriam, non enim aegrotat: nec eam, qua fani utuntur, ut qui nondum abfoluta fruatur fanitate. Quo fit ut nec qualitate nec quantitate paria fanis poffit affumere: quae autem pars medicinae femeiotice dicitur, curationi morborum per victum fumme eft neceffaria: nam praeterita

τον δὲ καὶ εἰς τὸ προγνῶναι, εἴτε ὀλέθριον εἴτε περιεστηκὸς εἴη τὸ νόσημα. ὁμοίως δὲ καὶ τὰ κατὰ χειρουργίαν καὶ τὰ διὰ φαρμάκων θεραπευόμενα, οὔτε ἄνευ σημειώσεως συντελεῖται καὶ τὰ ἐπ' αὐτῶν ὁμοίως δεῖται τῆς προγνωστικῆς σημειώσεως πρὸς τὸ εἰδέναι τίνα αὐτῶν ἀθεράπευτά ἐστι καὶ τίνα θεραπευτὰ μὲν, βλάπτοντα δὲ μεγάλως, ἢ ἀναιροῦντα ἐὰν θεραπευθῇ. τοῦ θεραπευτικοῦ δὲ διαιρουμένου εἴς τε δίαιταν καὶ φαρμακείαν καὶ χειρουργίαν, [367] δίαιτα μέν ἐστιν ἀγωγὴ διαφορητικῶν καὶ προσθετικῶν καὶ συμπεπτικῶν βοηθημάτων, παραλαμβανομένη μὲν ἐπὶ τῶν νοσούντων πάντων, τὸ δὲ κῦρος ἔχουσα ἐπὶ τῶν πυρεττόντων. χειρουργία δέ ἐστι μόριον τοῦ θεραπευτικοῦ διὰ τομῶν καὶ καύσεων καὶ τῆς περὶ τὰ ὀστᾶ διορθώσεως ὑγιάζουσα τοὺς ἀνθρώπους. φαρμακεία δέ ἐστιν εἶδος θεραπείας διὰ ψιλῶν φαρμάκων τά τε ἐντὸς πάθη καὶ τὰ ἐκτὸς ἰωμένη. δεῖ μὲν γὰρ καταλλήλου διαίτης, ποτὲ δὲ καὶ χειρουργίας προσδεομένη, ὥσπερ γε ἡ χειρουργία καὶ δίαιτα

et praeſentia ſymptomata ad morbi cauſam inveniendam diligenter inſpicimus. Inſuper maxima ejus neceſſitas eſt ad praeſagiendum, mors, an ſalus expectanda ſit. Pari modo medicina, quae manu medetur, tum illa, quae medicamentis auxiliatur, ſine indiciorum obſervatione non abſolvitur: quippe praeſagia eodem modo deſiderant, quibus ſcias, quae curationem non admittunt, quaeque eam recipiunt quidem, ſed vehementer aut offendunt aegrum, ſi curentur, aut e medio tollunt. Quum vero therapeutice dividatur in diaetam, pharmaciam et chirurgiam, diaeta auxiliorum, quae digerendi, apponendi et concoquendi facultatem habent, eſt adminiſtratio: quae omnibus quidem aegrotis, ſed praecipue febrientibus in uſu eſt. Chirurgia pars curatoriae eſt: ea inciſionibus, uſtionibus et oſſium in ſuam ſedem deductione homines curat. Pharmacia nudis medicamentis interiores affectus et exteriores ſanat: victus enim convenientem rationem, quandoque vero manuum opus requirit, quemadmodum chirurgia et victus ratio medicatione utuntur. Itaque a rerum naturae

προσχρῶνται φαρμακείᾳ. ἄνωθεν οὖν ἀπὸ φυσιολογίας ἀρκτέον, ἐπειδή περ οὔτε ἐν ὑγιείᾳ συντηρεῖν, οὐδὲ ἐπὶ τῶν νοσούντων αἰτιολογεῖν, οὐδὲ σημειοῦσθαι, οὐδὲ θεραπεύειν ὀρθῶς δύναιτ' ἄν τις, μὴ ἐπεσκεμμένος ἐκ τίνων στοιχείων ὁ ἄνθρωπος συνέστηκε καὶ πῶς τρεπομένων τούτων παρὰ τὴν ἐξ ἀρχῆς φύσιν αἱ νόσοι γίνονται.

Κεφ. θ'. [Περὶ στοιχείων ἐξ ὧν ὁ ἄνθρωπος συνέστηκεν.] Συνέστηκε τοίνυν ὁ ἄνθρωπος ἀκολούθως τοῖς φυσικοῖς καθ' Ἱπποκράτην ἐκ τῶν κοσμικῶν τῶν πρώτων στοιχείων, ἐκ πυρὸς καὶ ἀέρος καὶ ὕδατος καὶ γῆς· οὐχ ὡς ἐκ τούτων αὐτῶν, ἀλλὰ ἐκ τῶν ἀναλόγων αὐτοῖς συνεστῶτος τοῦ ἀνθρώπου. ἐν δὲ τῷ διαλύεσθαι εἰς ταῦτα τὰ πρῶτα ἀναλύεται, καθὼς αὐτὸς ὁ Ἱπποκράτης ἔφη· καὶ πάλιν ἀνάγκη ἀποχωρέειν εἰς τὴν ἑωϋτοῦ φύσιν ἕκαστον, τελευτῶντος τοῦ ἀνθρώπου, τό τε ξηρὸν πρὸς τὸ ξηρὸν καὶ τὸ ψυχρὸν πρὸς τὸ ψυχρὸν καὶ τὸ ὑγρὸν πρὸς τὸ ὑγρὸν καὶ τὸ θερμὸν πρὸς τὸ θερμόν. τοιαύτη δὲ καὶ τῶν ζώων ἐστὶν ἡ φύσις καὶ τῶν ἄλλων ἁπάντων. γίνεταί τε ὁμοίως

contemplatione altius auſpicabimur: quoniam nec in ſanis ſecundam valetudinem tueri, nec in aegris morbi cauſam cognoſcere, nec ſignis quid deprehendere, nec curare recte poſſis, ignorans quibus homo elementis conſtet et quomodo his immutatis a natura quam obtinebant prius morbi naſcuntur.

Cap. IX. [*De elementis hominem conſtituentibus*] Conſtat igitur homo, quemadmodum docuit Hippocrates in libro de natura humana, ex primis mundi elementis: ex igne, aëre, aqua, terra, non quod ex his ipſis, ſed proportione ipſis reſpondentibus homo conſtituatur. Atqui ex ipſius Hippocratis ſententia, dum diſſolvitur, in haec prima reſolvitur et unumquodque rurſus in ſuam ipſius naturam, homine vita defuncto, redire neceſſe eſt, ſiccum in ſiccum, frigidum in frigidum, calidum in calidum, humidum in humidum. Hujusmodi tum animantium tum aliorum univerſorum natura eſt: omnia ſimiliter oriuntur

πάντα καὶ τελευτᾷ ὁμοίως. συνίσταται γὰρ αὐτῶν ἡ φύσις ἀπὸ τούτων τῶν εἰρημένων καὶ τελευτᾷ κατὰ τὰ εἰρημένα εἰς τὸ αὐτό· ὅθεν περ συνέστηκεν ἕκαστον, ἐνταῦθα καὶ ἀπεχώρησεν. καθὰ καὶ Ὅμηρος ἔφη,

Ἀλλ' ὑμεῖς μὲν πάντες ὕδωρ καὶ γαῖα γένοισθε.

δηλῶν τὴν εἰς ταῦτα διάλυσιν. ὡς δὲ ἐκ τῶν δευτέρων καὶ ἐγγὺς ὄντων τῇ ἀνθρωπίνῃ φύσει, ἐκ τῶν τεσσάρων χυμῶν, αἵματος καὶ φλέγματος καὶ χολῆς ξανθῆς τε καὶ μελαίνης συνεστάναι φασὶ τὸν ἄνθρωπον, διότι ἐν τῇ πρώτῃ διαπλάσει τοῦ ἐμβρύου, ἔκ τε τοῦ γόνου καὶ τοῦ παρὰ τῆς μητρὸς ἐπιῤῥέοντος αἵματος διὰ τοῦ οὐραχοῦ ἡ σύστασις γίνεται τοῦ (375) τικτομένου. ἐν δὲ τούτοις ἦσαν οἱ τέσσαρες χυμοί. οἱ δὲ ἐκ τῶν τριῶν καὶ συνθέτων τὸν ἤδη γενόμενον ἄνθρωπον ἐκ τῶνδέ φασι συγκεῖσθαι, ἔκ τε τῶν ὑγρῶν καὶ ξηρῶν καὶ πνευμάτων. καλεῖ δὲ αὐτὰ Ἱπποκράτης ἴσχοντα, ἰσχόμενα καὶ ἐνορμῶντα. ἴσχοντα μὲν οὖν ἐστιν ὅσα στερεὰ, ὀστᾶ καὶ νεῦρα καὶ φλέβες καὶ ἀρτη-

et defınunt fimiliter: conflatur enim ex his praedictis eorum natura et ex praedictis in eadem finit Unde fingula originem nacta funt, eo quoque revertuntur, quemadmodum Homerus inquit,

Vos aqua, vos tellus cunctos aliquando tenebit.

innuens diffolutionem in haec futuram. Caeterum hominem velut ex fecundis et humanae naturae vicinis quatuor humoribus, fanguine, pituita, bile tum flava tum atra conftitutum effe phyfici pronuntiant: quoniam foetus in prima fui formatione ex genitura et fanguine, qui e matre per urachum influit, aufpicium coepit: in his autem quatuor humores erant. Hi vero ex tribus et compofitis hominem jam genitum, ex hisce tribus conftare affirmant, humidis, ficcis et fpiritibus, quae Hippocrates continentia, contenta et impetum facientia appellat. Continentia igitur funt folida omnia, ut offa, nervi, venae,

ρίαι, ἐξ ὧν οἵ τε μύες καὶ αἱ σάρκες καὶ πᾶς ὁ τοῦ σώματος ὄγκος πέπλεκται, τῶν τε ἐντὸς καὶ τῶν ἐκτὸς τὰ συγκρίματα. ἰσχόμενα δέ ἐστι τὰ ὑγρὰ τὰ ἐν τοῖς ἀγγείοις ἐμφερόμενα καὶ κατὰ πᾶν τὸ σῶμα διεσπαρμένα, ἅπερ καλεῖ Ἱπποκράτης χυμοὺς τέσσαρας τοὺς προειρημένους. ἐνορμῶντα δέ ἐστι τὰ πνεύματα. πνεύματα δὲ κατὰ τοὺς παλαιοὺς δύο ἐστὶ, τό τε ψυχικὸν καὶ τὸ φυσικόν. οἱ δὲ Στωϊκοὶ καὶ τρίτον εἰσάγουσι τὸ ἑκτικὸν, ὃ καλοῦσιν ἕξιν. καὶ Ἐρασίστρατος δὲ ὡς ἀρχὰς καὶ στοιχεῖα ὅλου σώματος ὑποτιθέμενος τὴν τριπλοκίαν τῶν ἀγγείων, νεῦρα καὶ φλέβας καὶ ἀρτηρίας, παραλείπει τά τε ὑγρὰ καὶ τὰ πνεύματα. δυσὶ γὰρ ὕλαις ταῦτα διοικεῖσθαι λέγει τὸ ζῶον, τῷ μὲν αἵματι ὡς τροφῇ, [368] τῷ δὲ πνεύματι ὡς συνεργῷ εἰς τὰς φυσικὰς ἐνεργείας. οὐ παραλαμβάνει δὲ αὐτὰς ὡς ἀρχάς. πολλὰ δὲ καὶ ἄλλα τῶν σωμάτων εἴδη εὑρίσκεται, οὐκ ἐκ τῆς τριπλοκίας συγκείμενα, οἷον εὐθὺς ὁ ἐγκέφαλος καὶ ὁ μυελὸς καὶ πάντα τὰ ὀστᾶ. τὸν μὲν οὖν ἐγκέφαλον ἢ τὸν μυελὸν παρέγχυμα τροφῆς τολμᾷ λέγειν, ὡς τὴν πιμελὴν, καὶ τοῦ ἥπατος καὶ

arteriae, ex quibus et mufculi et carnes totaque corporis moles compacta eft, ad haec interiorum exteriorumque concretiones. Contenta vero humida funt, quae in vafis per totum corpus difperfa feruntur. Atque haec quatuor praedictos humores vocat Hippocrates. Impetum facientia fpiritus funt, quos veteres duos, animalem et naturalem numerant: Stoici tertium invehunt, quem hecticum nominant. Erafiftratus vafa triplicia, nervos, venas, arterias, omiffis fpiritibus et humidis, tanquam initia et totius corporis elementa conftituit. Nam duplici materia regi animal affirmat, fanguine tanquam alimento, fpiritu tanquam naturae functionibus obeundis coadjutore: non autem ea ut principia accipit. Multae fane aliae corporum fpecies non ex tribus illis compofitae inveniuntur, ut verbi gratia cerebrum, medulla atque offa omnia. Cerebrum igitur vel medullam nutrimenti affufionem audet appellare, ficut adipem, jecinoris, lienis et pulmonis confiftentiam. At offa neque nutrimenti affufionem neque

σπληνὸς καὶ πνεύμονος τὴν σύστασιν. τὰ δὲ ὀστέα οὐδὲ παρέγχυμα τῆς τροφῆς δύναιτ' ἂν λέγειν, οὐδ' ἐκ τῶν προειρημένων τριγενῶν ἀγγείων πεπλέχθαι. κατὰ δὲ Ἀσκληπιάδην στοιχεῖα ἀνθρώπου, ὄγκοι θραυστοὶ καὶ πόροι. κατὰ δὲ τὸν Ἀθήναιον στοιχεῖα ἀνθρώπου οὐ τὰ τέσσαρα πρῶτα σώματα, πῦρ καὶ ἀὴρ καὶ ὕδωρ καὶ γῆ, ἀλλ' αἱ ποιότητες αὐτῶν, τὸ θερμὸν καὶ τὸ ψυχρὸν καὶ τὸ ξηρὸν καὶ τὸ ὑγρὸν, ὧν δύο μὲν τὰ ποιητικὰ αἴτια ὑποτίθεται, τὸ θερμὸν καὶ τὸ ψυχρὸν, δύο δὲ τὰ ὑλικὰ, τὸ ξηρὸν καὶ τὸ ὑγρὸν, καὶ πέμπτον παρεισάγει κατὰ τοὺς Στωϊκοὺς τὸ διῆκον διὰ πάντων πνεῦμα, ὑφ' οὗ τὰ πάντα συνέχεσθαι καὶ διοικεῖσθαι. Ἱπποκράτης μὲν οὖν διὰ τριῶν κεχώρηκεν, εἰπὼν στοιχεῖα ἀνθρώπου ἴσχοντα, ἰσχόμενα, ἐνορμῶντα, δι' ὧν τὰ πάντα τῶν μετ' αὐτὸν περιείληφε στοιχεῖα καὶ τὴν κατὰ στοιχείων φυσιολογίαν τε καὶ αἰτιολογίαν τῶν παρὰ φύσιν· οἱ δὲ μετ' αὐτὸν οὐκ οἶδ' ὅπως μίαν οὖσαν τὴν θείαν ταύτην καὶ ἀληθῶς Ἀσκληπιοῦ ἰατρικὴν τριχῇ διανειμάμενοι καὶ διασπάσαντες τὰ ἐν αὐτῇ συμφυῆ μέρη, οἱ μὲν μόνοις

ex praedictis vafis triplicibus compofita effe dicere poffit. Afclepiadi hominis elementa funt corpuscula manantia, fragiliaque et invifibilia foramina. Secundum Athenaei fententiam non quatuor illa prima corpora, ignis, aër, aqua, terra, fed eorum qualitates, calidum, frigidum, ficcum et humidum. Ex quibus duo caufarum efficientium munere fungi, puta calidum et frigidum: duo materialium, ficcum et humidum fupponit. Quintum vero ex Stoicorum opinione introducit fpiritum cuncta penetrantem, a quo omnia contineantur et gubernentur. Hippocrates cum trifariam hominis elementa divififfet, in continentia, contenta et ea quae impetum faciunt, quibus omnia poft ipfum elementis comprehendit, nec non naturae elementorum tractationem, eorum quae praeter naturam funt caufas, haud fcio quomodo fucceffores ejus unam illam re vera divinam Aefculapii medicinam in tres partes fibi cohaerentes diftribuerint atque divulferint. Alii enim humidis tum eorum, quae fecundum naturam habent, con-

τοῖς χυμοῖς τῶν τε κατὰ φύσιν τὴν σύστασιν καὶ τῶν παρὰ φύσιν τὴν αἰτίαν ἀνέθεσαν, ὡς Πραξαγόρας καὶ Ἡρόφιλος. οἱ δὲ τὰ στερεὰ σώματα τὰ ἀρχικὰ καὶ στοιχειώδη ὑποθέμενοι, τά τε φύσει συνεστῶτα ἐκ τούτων καὶ τῶν νόσων τὰς αἰτίας ἐντεῦθεν λαμβάνουσιν, ὡς Ἐρασίστρατος καὶ Ἀσκληπιάδης· οἱ δὲ περὶ Ἀθήναιον καὶ Ἀρχιγένην μόνῳ τῷ διήκοντι δι' αὐτῶν πνεύματι καὶ τὰ φυσικὰ συνεστάναι τε καὶ διοικεῖσθαι καὶ τὰ νοσήματα πάντα, τούτου πρωτοπαθοῦντος γίνεσθαι ἀπεφήναντο, ὅθεν καὶ πνευματικοὶ χρηματίζουσι.

Κεφ. ι'. [Ὀνομασίαι τῶν ἐκτὸς μερῶν τοῦ σώματος.] Περὶ δὲ τῶν ἐκτὸς μερῶν τοῦ σώματος ἢ μορίων καὶ τίνες αἱ ὀνομασίαι αὐτῶν, πρῶτος μὲν ὁ Ἀριστοτέλης ὑπελάβετο διδάξαι τε καὶ συγγράψαι. ἀναγκαῖον δὲ καὶ τοῖς μεταγενεστέροις ἰατροῖς ἔδοξε καὶ αὐτοῖς τὰ αὐτὰ πραγματεύεσθαι, ὅπως μὴ τὴν χεῖρα ἐπιφέροντες δεικνύωσιν ἕκαστον τῶν μερῶν ἢ τῶν μορίων, ἀλλ' ἐκ τῆς ὀνομασίας αὐτάρκη ἔχωσι τὴν δήλωσιν αὐτῶν. μάλιστα δὲ τοῦτο οἱ περὶ Ἐρα-

ſtitutionem, tum cauſam eorum, quae praeter naturam, ſolis attribuere, ut Praxagoras et Herophilus: alii ſolidis corporibus initia et elementa attribuentes, ex his, tum quae natura conſiſtunt, tum morborum cauſas inde capiunt, ut Eraſiſtratus et Aſclepiades. Athenaeus vero et Archigenes ſpiritu ſolo ea penetrante tum naturalia conſiſtere ac gubernari, tum morbos univerſos hoc prius offenſo creari dixerunt. Unde et ſpiritales, veluti qui omnia ſpiritibus attribuant, nuncupantur.

Cap. X. [*Exteriorum corporis partium appellationes.*] De externis corporis partibus ſeu particulis et quae earum nomina ſint, primus Ariſtoteles docuiſſe ſimul ac conſcripſiſſe creditus eſt. Temporis autem proceſſu medicis quoque ipſis poſterioribus de iisdem tractare neceſſarium viſum eſt, ne manu allata quamque partem aut particulam oſtenderent, ſed ex appellatione ſufficientem earum notitiam haberent: quorum in numero id maxime

σίστρατον ἐζήλωσαν, ὡς Ἀπολλώνιος ὁ Μεμφίτης καὶ Ξενοφῶν ὁ πρὸ αὐτοῦ. διαιροῦσι τοίνυν τὸ ὅλον σῶμα οἱ μὲν Αἰγύπτιοι ἰατροὶ εἰς τέσσαρα, κεφαλὴν, χεῖρας, θώρακα καὶ σκέλη, οἱ δὲ ἄλλοι εἰς πλείονα καταδιαιροῦντες τὰ προειρημένα τέσσαρα εἰς ἕτερα μέρη τοῦ ὅλου, οὐχ ὡς ἐκείνων μόρια. κεφαλῆς γοῦν τὸ μὲν πᾶν κύτος μέρος ἂν λέγοιτο τοῦ ὅλου σώματος. ταύτης δὲ μόρια τὸ μὲν ἔμπροσθεν ὑπὲρ τὰς ὀφρῦς ψιλὸν τριγῶν ἀπὸ ὠτὸς ἐπὶ οὖς μέτωπον καλεῖται τὸ δὲ ἐπάνω τούτου τετριχωμένον βρέγμα. τὰ δὲ παρ᾽ ἑκάτερα τούτου ἐπάνω τῶν ὤτων κρόταφοι. τὸ δὲ ὑπὲρ τὸ βρέγμα κατὰ μέσον τῆς κεφαλῆς κορυφὴ, ἀφ᾽ ἧς καὶ δοκεῖ ἄρχεσθαι ἡ ἔκφυσις τῶν τριχῶν, ὡς ἀπὸ κέντρου κύκλος. τὸ δὲ μετὰ τὴν κορυφὴν ἐκ τῶν ὄπισθεν ὡς ἐπὶ τοὺς τένοντας καταβαῖνον ἰνίον. [369] ἐκ δὲ τῶν ἔμπροσθεν πρόσωπον μὲν τὸ ὑπὸ μέτωπον πᾶν λέγεται, περιοριζόμενον ὠσὶ καὶ ὀφθαλμοῖς καὶ ῥινὶ καὶ στόματι μέχρι γενείου. ἄρχεται δὲ ἀπ᾽ ὀφρύων· καθ᾽ ἃ γὰρ λήγει τὸ μέτωπον ἀπὸ τῶν ἄνω κατιὸν, αἱ ὀφρύες διαδέχονται, οἷον

fuerunt Erafiftrati fectatores aemulati, ut Apollonius Memphites et hoc prior Xenophon. Dividunt igitur totum corpus Aegyptii medici quadrifariam, in caput, manus, thoracem et crura. Alii has quatuor partes in plures diducunt, nempe in alias totius partes, non ut illarum particulas. Capitis igitur tota latitudo pars ipfius corporis dicetur. Hujus particulae funt hae. Anterior fuperpofita fuperciliis, pilis nuda, inter utramque aurem fita frons nominatur. Hac fuperior capillis intecta finciput. Partem ab utroque fincipitis latere fupra aures fitam tempora appellamus. In media capitis regione finciput fuperante eft vertex: unde velut a centro circulus capillorum exortus incipere videtur. Poft verticem a pofteriore capitis parte ad usque tendones, occiput defcendit. A priore fub tota fronte, auribus, oculis, nafo et ore ad mentum usque circumfcripta, a fuperciliis incipiens, facies dicitur. Ubi enim frons a fuperioribus defcendens definit, fupercilia ceu termini ejus eminentes et pilis con-

πέρατα αὐτοῦ ὑπερέχοντα καὶ τετριχωμένα. καθ' ἃ δὲ παρατείνει τὸ μέτωπον ἐπὶ τοὺς κροτάφους, ἐπὶ τοῖς πέρασιν αὐτοῦ, τὰ ὦτα τέτακται. τούτων δὲ τὰ μὲν ἀναπεπταμένα πτερυγώματα, τὰ δὲ ἀνακεκλασμένα εἰς τοὐπίσω ἐκ τῶν ἔμπροσθεν, αὐτοῖς τοῖς ἄκροις ἐπικαμπτόμενα κυβοειδῆ, ὑφ' ἃ τὸ μὲν ἡμικύκλιον ἐμπεριφερὲς εἰς ὀξὺ ἐπανεστηκὸς ξυστὴρ ὀνομάζεται, τὸ δὲ ὑπὸ τὴν τούτων ὀξύτητα κοῖλον κογχίον. τὸ δὲ κατὰ μέσον στρογγύλον τρύπημα ἀκουστικὸς πόρος, ὑφ' οὗ λοβίον μέν ἐστι τὸ ἀπηρτημένον τοῦ ὠτὸς πιμελῶδες. το δὲ ὑπερκείμενον ἀντιλόβιον. ὑπὸ δὲ τὰς ὀφρῦς οἱ ὀφθαλμοί εἰσιν, ἃ καὶ ὄμματα καλεῖται, τὸ πᾶν σχῆμα μετὰ τῶν μορίων αὐτῶν. τούτων δὲ τὰ μὲν σκέποντα τὴν ἔνδον τῶν χιτώνων σύστασιν βλέφαρα καλεῖται, τὸ μὲν ἄνω, τὸ δὲ κάτω, συμβάλλοντα ἀλλήλοις πυκνῶς καὶ ἀκρονιγῶς εἰς ἀνάληψιν τῆς ὄψεως καὶ εἰς τὸ ἀπερύκειν τὰ πληκτικῶς προσπίπτοντα τοῖς ὀφθαλμοῖς, ἐπ' ἀκριβὲς δὲ ὥσπερ ἐν τοῖς ὕπνοις, εἰς ἀποστροφὴν τῆς ὁρατικῆς δυνάμεως, πρὸς τὸ καθησυχασαι τὸν ἄνθρωπον. βλεφάρων δὲ

siti eam excipiunt. Qua autem frons ad tempora porrigitur, in ipsius terminis aures sitae sunt, quarum pars aperta ala dicitur, refracta ab anteriori in posterius ipsis summitatibus inflexis cubiformis, sub qua semicirculus rotundus in mucronem exurgens scalper appellatur. Hujus acumini concavum, quod subjacet, conchula. In hujus medio rotundum foramen meatus auditorius vocatur, sub quo particula pinguis ab aure suspensa lobus est seu auricula, superior pinna. Oculi superciliis subjacent, quae et lumina dicuntur, nempe tota figura cum ipsis particulis. Superius inferiusque interiores tunicas contegentes palpebrae appellantur, haec inferior, illa superior. Committuntur invicem crebro et extremo tactu ad visus recreationem et ad prohibendum, ne quid extrinsecus violenter oculis incidat: maxime vero, quemadmodum in somnis, visoriae virtutis avertendae gratia, quo melius homo conquiescat. Partes autem juxta oculos totos sitae, qua palpebrae invicem committuntur, tarsi nominantur: unde pili

τὰ μὲν πρὸς τοῖς ὀφθαλμοῖς ὅλοις, καθὰ ἡ συμβολὴ αὐτῶν πρὸς ἄλληλα γίνεται, ταρσοὶ ὀνομάζονται, ἐξ ὧν ἐκπεφύκασι τρίχες, αἳ βλεφαρίδες λέγονται, ἀφ' ὧν πεφύκασι τὰ ὀνόματα ἀπενεγκάμεναι. γεγόνασι δὲ πρὸς τὸ ἀπευθύνειν τὸ ὁρατικὸν πνεῦμα ἢ, ὥς τινες λέγουσι, τὰς ἔνδοθεν ἐκχεομένας ἀκτῖνας εἰς τὸ διορᾷν. ἀμέλει τούτων ἐκπεσουσῶν, κατακλωμένων, οὐκέτι ὁμοίως ἐπ' εὐθὺ, οὐδὲ ἐπὶ μακρὸν δύναται βλέπειν τὸ ζῶον. τὰ δὲ ἐντὸς τοῦ ὀφθαλμοῦ πέρατα, καθ' ἃ αἱ συμφύσεις τῶν βλεφάρων, κανθοὶ καλοῦνται, ὁ μὲν πρὸς τὴν ῥῖνα ὁ μέγας, μικρὸς δὲ ὁ πρὸς τὸ οὖς. τὸ δὲ μεταξὺ αὐτῶν, τὸ λευκὸν τοῦ ὀφθαλμοῦ, οὗ ἐν μέσῳ ἡ ἶρις κύκλος ποικίλος τοῖς χρώμασι, διὸ καὶ ἶρις ἐκλήθη, ἀπὸ τῆς πρὸς τὴν ὑπαίθριον ἶριν ἐμφερείας. ταύτης δὲ πάλιν τὸ μεσαίτατον κόρη, δι' ἧς τὸ ὁρᾷν συντελεῖται. ἡ δὲ ῥὶς μεταξὺ τῶν ὀφθαλμῶν τέτακται, ταύτης δὲ τὰ μὲν ἑκα- (376) τέρωθεν μυκτῆρες ἢ μυξωτῆρες καλοῦνται, δι' ὧν ἀναπνεῖ τε καὶ ὀσφραίνεται τὰ ζῶα. μυκτήρων δὲ τὰ μὲν ἔξωθεν πτερύγια, τὸ δὲ διορίζον αὐτὰ κίων. ἑκατέρωθεν

proveniunt, quos cilia nuncupant, a quibus orta ſunt, ducto nomine. Facti autem in hoc ſunt pili iſti, ut viſorium ſpiritum vel, ut quidam ajunt, radios interiore parte effuſos perſpiciendi gratia dirigant. His itaque elapſis vel retortis, nequaquam animans ſimiliter in rectum vel in longum videre poteſt. Interiores oculi termini, ubi palpebrae coaleſcunt, anguli dicuntur, qui quidem ad naſum magnus, qui ad aures parvus. Quod in horum medio conſiſtit, oculi candidum. Hujus rurſus medium iris circulus coloribus varius occupat: unde et a ſimilitudine, quam cum caeleſti illa Iride habet, nomen accepit. Hujus rurſus media pars, per quam viſus peragitur, pupilla eſt. Naſus inter oculos ſitus eſt: ejus partes utrinque ſitae nares vocantur, quibus animalia reſpirant et olfaciunt. Exteriores autem narium partes pinnulae ſive alae nominantur, quod autem eas diſcriminat, interſeptum vocamus. In utraque naſi parte, quae proprie concava ſunt ſub oculis ſita, concava nuncupamus:

δὲ τῆς ῥινὸς τὰ μὲν κοῖλα ἰδίως, τὰ ὑπὸ τῆς ὀφθαλμοῖς κοῖλα καλεῖται, ἐξ ὧν λέγονταί τινες κοῖλοι. διὰ νόσους δὲ ταῦτα ἐπαίρεται ἐξ ἀπεψίας, ἢ δυσαρεστήματος. τὰ δὲ τούτοις ἐπανεστῶτα μεταξὺ ῥινὸς καὶ ὤτων μῆλα ὀνομάζεται, ἃ τοῖς εὐχρουστέροις καὶ ἐλευθεριωτέροις ἐν τῷ αἰδεῖσθαι ἐρυθριᾷ. σιαγόνες δὲ τὰ ὑπὸ τούτων κατιόντα, ὡς ἐπὶ τὸ γένειον καὶ ταύτῃ εἰς τὸ ὀξὺ αὐτοῦ ἀπολήγοντα. γένειον δὲ πᾶν τὸ ὑποκάτω τοῦ χείλους ἐν περιφερεῖ παραμήκει σχήματι. μύσταξ δὲ τὸ ὑπεράνω τοῦ χείλους, ὑπὸ τοὺς μυξωτῆρας, ὅπερ Ὅμηρος ὑπήνην ἐκάλεσε. στόμα δὲ τὸ ἀνὰ μέσον τῶν χειλῶν, ὑπ᾽ αὐτῶν συνιστάμενον καὶ συνεχόμενον. ἔοικε γὰρ ταῦτα οἷον συμπεφυκότα, εἶτα ἀποσχισθέντα τὸ στόμα ποιεῖν, διὸ καὶ φαίνεται οἱονεὶ ἄρτι διῃρημένα. τὸ δὲ ἐκδεχόμενον τὴν κεφαλὴν μέχρι τῶν ὤμων τὸ μὲν πᾶν τράχηλος λέγεται. τούτου δὲ τὰ μὲν ὄπισθεν ἰδίως τένοντες ὀνομάζονται. ὑπὸ δὲ τὸν τράχηλον ἑκατέρωθεν οἱ ὦμοί εἰσιν ἐπανεστῶτες, ὧν τὸ μὲν ἀνώτατον ἀκρώμιον καλεῖται, τὸ δὲ ἀπὸ τούτου εἰς τὸ ἔμπροσθεν [370] κατακλεῖδες· μεταξὺ τούτων αἱ σφαγαί. ἀπὸ δὲ τῶν ὤμων αἱ

unde quidam concavi nominantur. Per morbum autem haec attolluntur ob hominis cruditatem vel difplicentem difpofitionem. His autem fuperiores inter nafum et aures malae, quae bene coloratis et ingenuis pudore fuffufis rubent. Hinc maxillae ad mentum usque defcendunt et hac in mucronem defınunt. Mentum id omne eft, quod labro inferiori longa orbiculari figura fubjacet. Superior pars labri fub naribus myftax Homero hypene appellatur. Quod intra labra defcribitur et ab eis conftituitur et continetur, os eft. Videntur enim haec quafi connata, poft diducta os efficere: quare etiam veluti nuper divifa apparent. Quod caput excipit et ad humeros usque pertinet, id totum cervix dicitur: hujus pofteriores partes proprie tendines appellantur. Dein fub cervice humeri utrinque prominent quorum verticem fummum humerum nominant, quod ab hoc prorfum vergit, claviculae exiftunt, inter quas jugulum habetur. Ab humeris manus incipiunt, utraque ex

χεῖρες ἔρχονται παρηρτημέναι ἑκατέρα τῇ καθ' αὑτὴν πλευρᾷ. τούτων δὲ τὸ μὲν ἀπὸ τοῦ ὤμου μέχρι ἀγκῶνος βραχίων καλεῖται. ἀγκὼν δὲ καθὰ συγκάμπτεται ἡ χεὶρ ὅλη, οὗ τὸ ἔξω μέρος κορωνὸν καὶ ὀλέκρανον ὀνομάζεται. τὸ δὲ μετὰ τοῦτο πῆχυς, ᾧ καὶ μετροῦσιν οἱ ἄνθρωποι. καθ' ὃ δὲ τελευτᾷ ὁ πῆχυς καὶ ἄρθρον ποιεῖ πρὸς ἄκραν χεῖρα, καρπὸς καλεῖται καὶ τὸ μετὰ τοῦτο μετακάρπιον. εἶτα κόνδυλοι, ὅθεν ἄρχονται οἱ δάκτυλοι. δακτύλων δὲ ὁ μὲν μέγιστος ἀντίχειρ καλεῖται, διὰ τὸ ὅλῃ τῇ χειρὶ ἄκρᾳ συνεργοῦντα ἴσον αὐτῇ δύνασθαι. ὁ δὲ μετὰ τοῦτον λιχανὸς, ὡς ἔοικεν, ἀπὸ τῆς χρείας τοὔνομα ἔχων· ἐφεξῆς ὁ μέσος καὶ μετὰ τοῦτον ὁ παραμέσος, ὁ τοῖς ἰατροῖς ἀνακείμενος καὶ ἀπ' αὐτῶν τοὔνομα κεκληρωμένος. ὁ δὲ ἐπὶ πᾶσι μικρὸς, καθ' ὃ πάντων ἠλάττωται. τὸ μὲν οὖν ἀπὸ τοῦ καρποῦ ἄκρα χεὶρ λέγεται. ὑπτιαζούσης δὲ τὸ μὲν κατὰ τὸν ἀντίχειρα ἐπανεστηκὸς θέναρ καλεῖται, τὸ δὲ ἀντικείμενον αὐτοῦ ὑποθέναρ. τὸ δὲ ὑπὸ τὰς ἐκφύσεις τῶν δακτύλων στῆθος χειρός. τὸ δὲ μεταξὺ τούτων ἁπάντων κοῖλον χειρός.

fuo latere propenfa: harum pars ab humero ad cubitum usque pertendens brachium vocatur: cubitus autem qua tota manus flectitur: cujus exteriorem partem corona et olecranum nominatur. Dein cubitus, quo et homines metiuntur. Ubi hic definit et cum fumma manu articulum facit, carpus dicitur. Succedens huic pars metacarpium. Inde nodi, a quibus digiti incipiunt. Digitorum maximus, pollex eft, quod toti fummae manui cooperans aequipolleat. Poft hunc index, nomen ab ufu, ut apparet, fortitus: dein medius: hunc medio proximus fequitur, medicis dicatus, atque ab iis nomen fortitus. Poftremus parvus dicitur, quod omnibus fit inferior. Itaque a carpo fumma manus dicitur: cujus fupinae pars juxta pollicem affurgens vola nominatur, huic pars oppofita fubvola vocatur. Verum unde digiti procedunt, pectus manus eft. Quod medium horum omnium eft, manus concavum dicitur. Supra vero thorax ea pars appellatur, quae a collo toto

ἄνωθεν δὲ τὸ ὑπὸ τὸν τράχηλον πᾶν, ἐκ τῶν ἔμπροσθεν μέχρι λαγόνων, θώραξ καλεῖται. τούτου δὲ τὸ μὲν ὑπὸ τὰς κλεῖδας ἀμφοτέρωθεν καὶ τὰς χεῖρας, αἱ πλευραὶ, ἐξ ὧν καὶ πλευρὸν ἑκάτερον λέγεται, τὸ δὲ μεταξὺ τούτων στῆθος. καὶ τὸ μεσαίτατον αὐτοῦ στέρνον, μέχρι τοῦ χόνδρου, ὑφ᾽ ὃν τὸ στόμα τῆς κοιλίας· ὁ δὲ τόπος οὕτως καὶ ἔξωθεν λέγεται. ἐντεῦθεν δὲ τὸ ἐπιγάστριον ἀνέρχεται. τὰ δὲ ὑπὸ στόμα τῆς κοιλίας· κατὰ τὴν ἐκτὸς ἐπιφάνειαν εἰκότως ὑποχόνδρια καλεῖται, ἐπεὶ κατὰ τὴν εὐθύτητα ὑπὸ τὸν χόνδρον ἐστὶ, ὡσανεὶ μετὰ τοῦτον. εἰσὶ δὲ μύες ἡπλωμένοι καὶ ὑπεστρωμένοι τῷ περιτοναίῳ, ἔξωθεν δὲ σκεπόμενοι τῷ δέρματι. ὁμωνύμως δὲ τούτοις καὶ τὰ ἔνδοθεν σπλάγχνα ὑποχόνδρια καλεῖται, ἐπειδὴ καὶ αὐτὰ ὑπὸ τοὺς χόνδρους ἐστὶ τῶν νόθων πλευρῶν καὶ οἷον ἐντὸς αὐτῶν. τὰ δὲ ἐκτὸς μέσα, τὰ κυρίως λεγόμενα ὑποχόνδρια, τὸ μὲν ἔμπροσθεν τῶν λαγόνων περιέχον τὸ ὑποχόνδριον, ἐπιγάστριον, τὸ δὲ ἑκατέρωθεν κενεών. τὸ δὲ μεσαίτατον τοῦ λαγόνος ὀμφαλός. τὸ δὲ ὑπὸ τοῦτον ἦτρον. εἶτα τὸ ἐφήβαιον, ὃ καὶ ἐπίσειον καλεῖται.

ad ilia usque ex anteriore parte protenditur. Hujus pars, quae ſub claviculis utrinque et manibus habetur, coſtae ſunt: ex quibus et latus utrumque dicitur. In harum medio pectus. Hujus rurſus medium usque ad cartilaginem, ſub qua ventriculi os deliteſcit, ſternum: idem locus etiam extrinſecus ita appellatur. Hinc epigaſtrium oritur. Quae ſub ventriculi ore ad partem exteriorem apparent, hypochondria nominamus, quoniam ſecundum rectitudinem ſub cartilagine veluti poſt ipſam habentur. Sunt autem muſculi, qui expanſi peritonaeo ſubjacent: extrinſecus vero cute conteguntur. Aequivoco autem cum his vocabulo etiam interiora viſcera vocamus hypochondria: quoniam et ipſa ſub cartilaginibus notharum coſtarum ab interiore parte exiſtunt: ſed exteriora proprio. Quod ante ilia hypochondria comprehendit, abdomen eſt: quod utrinque eſt, ilia. Ilium medium occupat umbilicus. Sub hoc ſumen. Poſtea pubes ſequitur, quae et aqualiculus dicitur, in quem thorax ſinit: ubi et maſculorum pudenda conſti-

εἰς ὃ τελευτᾷ ὁ θώραξ, ἔνθα καὶ τὰ αἰδοῖα τῶν ἀῤῥένων τέτακται καὶ τῶν θηλειῶν κατὰ τὴν διάφυσιν τῶν μηρῶν, ὅπως κρύπτηται ὑπὸ τούτων. τοῦ μὲν οὖν ἀρσενικοῦ τὸ προῦχον καυλός. τὸ δὲ ἄκρον αὐτοῦ βάλανος. καθ' ὃ δὲ τετρύπηται πρὸς ἔκκρισιν, ἀπὸ τῆς χρείας οὐρήθρα ὀνομάζεται· τὸ δὲ σκέπον τὸ ἄκρον ποσθή. τὸ δὲ κάτω μέρος τοῦ καυλοῦ κατὰ μῆκος αὐτοῦ ῥαφή. τὸ δὲ διατεῖνον μέχρι τῆς ἕδρας ταῦρος καλεῖται. δίδυμοι δὲ καὶ ὄρχεις ἔνδοθέν τε καὶ ἔξωθεν ὀνομάζονται. καὶ ὄσχεον τὸ περὶ τοὺς διδύμους. τοῦ δὲ γυναικείου αἰδοίου, οὕτω γὰρ αὐτὸ οἱ παλαιοὶ ὠνόμαζον, αὐτὸς μὲν ὁ κόλπος κτεὶς καλεῖται. τὰ δὲ περιέχοντα τὸν κόλπον πτερυγώματα. τὸ δὲ μέσον τούτων κατὰ τὴν διασχίδα ἐκπεφυκὸς σαρκίδιον, νύμφη, ὃ καὶ διὰ τὸ προκύπτειν ἐπὶ πολὺ ἐκτομῆς ἀξιοῦται παρ' Αἰγυπτίοις ἐπὶ τῶν παρθένων. κοινῶς δὲ τὸ στόμα τοῦ ἀπευθυσμένου διὰ τῆς ἕδρας ἐξερχόμενον, πρὸς τὸ ἐπέχειν ὁπότε βουλόμεθα τὰς ἐκκρίσεις, εὐχρηστεῖ· δακτύλιος δὲ ἀπὸ τοῦ σχήματος καὶ σφιγκτὴρ ἀπὸ τῆς ἐνεργείας κέκληται. τὸ δὲ ὑπὸ τὸν

tuta funt: tum foeminarum ad femoris utriusque exortum, ut fub hoc occultentur. Maris pars prominens coles vocatur, fummitas ejus glans: qua foramen habet ad excretionem, urethra ab ufu nuncupatur. Cutis quae eam contegit, praeputium dicitur. Inferior pars colis in longitudinem ejus vergens futura vocata eft. Quae vero adusque fedem producitur, taurus. Tefticuli duplici nomine didymi et teftes, intus et foris appellantur. Quod tefticulos ambit, fcrotum vocant. Muliebris autem pudendi (fic enim ipfum nominaverunt antiqui) finus ipfe pecten vocatur. At quae finum ambiunt, alae vocantur, inter has autem caruncula ad fiffuram exorta, nympha quam, quod multo promineat, Aegyptii in virginibus excidere confueverunt. Porro recti inteftini orificium per fedem prodiens, quo excretionem, quum lubet, retinemus; annulus a figura, ab officio fphincter vocatus eft. Caeterum pofteriores corporis partes, quae collo fubjacent,

τράχηλον ἐκ τῶν ὄπισθεν, οὕτως ἔχει διαθέσεώς τε καὶ ὀνομασίας. τὸ μὲν πᾶν νῶτα καλεῖται. ἐντεῦθεν δὲ τὰ μὲν ἑκατέρωθεν ὠμοπλάται, τὸ δὲ μεταξὺ αὐτῶν μετάφρενον, ᾧ καὶ στόμαχος ἔνδοθεν ὑπόκειται. [371] τὸ δὲ μεσαίτατον τοῦ νώτου παντὸς ἄνωθεν μέχρι γλουτῶν, ῥάχις. ταύτης δὲ τὸ μὲν εὐθὺ ὑπὸ τὸ μετάφρενον ἄκνηστιν εἶπεν Ὅμηρος, ὃ καὶ διασαφῶν προσέθηκεν,

— κατ' ἄκνηστιν μέσα νῶτα.

ἐπεὶ καὶ κατὰ εὐθεῖαν τοῦ μήκους μέσα εἰσὶ τὰ νῶτα καὶ τὸ μέσον ἐστὶ τοῦ μεταφρένου καὶ ὀσφύος. διαδέχεται οὖν ἡ ὀσφὺς, ἥτις ἰξὺς ὠνόμασται, καθ' ὃ ζωννύμεθα. λήγει δὲ αὕτη εἰς τὸ ἱερὸν ὀστοῦν. παρ' ἑκάτερα δὲ τούτου τὰ ἰσχία ἐστὶ, ἐφ' οἷς οἱ γλουτοί. διὰ τὸ ὀστᾶ εἶναι τὰ ὑποκείμενα μέγιστα, ἔνθεν ὑπεστρώθη αὐτοῖς σώματα σαρκώδη. ὧν τὰ κυρτώματα ἐκ τοῦ περιφερῆ εἶναι, σφαιρώματα προσαγορεύεται. ἐντεῦθεν δὲ ἡνωμένον τὸ σῶμα διχοφυὲς γίνεται. διαμερίζεται γὰρ εἰς δύο, ἃ καλεῖται σκέλη, ὧν τὴν διασχίδα, διχάλαν οἱ παλαιοὶ λέγουσιν. ταῦτα δὲ ὅλα μὲν μέ-

hunc ſitum et appellationem habent: totum dorſum vocatur: inde utroque in latere ſcapulae habentur. Media ipſarum pars inter ſcapulium, cui etiam ſtomachus intus ſubjacet. Rurſus media totius dorſi ſedes ſuperne ad clunes usque ſpina dicitur. Hujus partem, quae recto tramite ſub dorſo habetur inſcalptam Homerus nominavit, manifeſto aliis dictionibus exponens,

— κατ' ἄκνηστιν μέσα νῶτα,

quoniam et juxta rectitudinem longitudinis media ſunt dorſi, mediumque eſt interſcapulii et lumbi. Spinam lumbi, qui ilium oſſa nominati ſunt, qua cingimur, excipiunt. Hi in os ſacrum terminantur: in cujus utraque parte coxae ſunt: in quibus nates, quoniam quae his ſubjiciuntur, maxima oſſa ſunt. Inde carnoſa ipſis corpora ſubſtrata ſunt. Quorum gibbae partes, quod orbiculares ſunt, globoſae natium partes nominantur. Inde corpus unum in duos exit proceſſus. Nam in duo crura

χρι περάτων, σκέλη λέγεται, τούτων δὲ τὰ μὲν ἀπὸ τῶν ἰσχίων εὐθὺς ἐρχόμενα μηροί. καθὸ δὲ μετὰ ταῦτα συμβάλλει τὰ κῶλα τοῖς ὑποκάτω καὶ ἄρθρον ποιεῖ, γόνυ καλεῖται. οὗ τὰ κατόπιν, ἰγνύα ἢ ἀγκύλη. τὰ δὲ ἐντεῦθεν, ἐπὶ τὰ κάτω μέγιστα κῶλα κνῆμαι. ὧν τὸ μὲν ἔμπροσθεν ἀντικνήμιον, τὸ δὲ ὄπισθεν γαστροκνήμη. τὰ δὲ πέρατα τῶν τῆς κνήμης ὀστῶν εἴς τε τὸ ἔνδον μέρος καὶ εἰς τὸ ἔξω ἐξέχοντα, σφυρὰ προσαγορεύεται. τὰ δὲ ἀπὸ τῶν σφυρῶν κυρίως πόδες λέγονται. ἀφ' ὧν καὶ ἕτερον μέτρον ἑαυτοῖς οἱ ἄνθρωποι εὕραντο, τὸν πόδα ἄραντες. τῶν δὲ ποδῶν τὸ μὲν ὄπισθεν πτέρνα ὀνομάζεται. τὸ δὲ ἔμπροσθεν ἀπὸ τῶν σφυρῶν μέχρι δακτύλων ταρσὸς καλεῖται. τούτου δὲ τὸ μὲν ἔνδοθεν πρὸς ἀλλήλους ἀφορώντων τῶν ποδῶν, ὡς ἐπὶ τὸν μέγαν δάκτυλον, ἀρχόμενον ἀπὸ τοῦ ἔσω σφυροῦ, πεδίον. τὸ δὲ ὑπὸ τούτου εὐθὺς ἐν μέσῳ κατωτάτω τοῦ ποδὸς κοῖλον. τὸ δὲ κατώτατον, ἐφ' ᾧ πατοῦμεν καὶ ᾧ ἐπιβαίνομεν, πέλμα. οὗ τὸ μὲν πρὸς τοὺς δακτύλους μετὰ τὸ κοῖλον ἐπανεστηκὸς, στῆθος ποδός. εἶτα οἱ δάκτυλοι,

nominata bipartitur, quorum diviſionem veteres biſulcam nominant: atque haec tota ad extrema usque crura dicuntur: quae vero a coxis ſtatim incipiunt, femora: ubi vero artus poſtea committuntur inferioribus articulumque efficiunt, genua nominamus. Eorum partes retrorſum ſpectantes, poplites vel ancyle: inde ad ima maximi artus tibiae: quarum anterior pars ocrea, poſterior ſura nominantur. Poſtremum oſſium tibiae in utrumque latus excedens talus eſt: ab hoc profecti, pedes proprie appellantur: quibus etiam menſuram ſibi aliam homines attollentes pedem invenerunt. Pedis pars poſterior calx: prior a talo usque ad digitos tarſus vocatur. Interior autem quaſi pedibus invicem ſe aſpicientibus ab interiore talo verſus magnum digitum procedens, pedium appellatur. Quod ſub hac ſtatim in medio imi pedis habetur, concavum dicitur. Inſimum, quo terram contingimus et ambulamus, planta vocatur. Quod poſt concavum ad digitos aſſurgit, pectus

ἰσάριθμοι μὲν τοῖς τῶν χειρῶν, οὐ τυγόντες δὲ τῶν αὐτῶν ὀνομάτων, διὰ τὸ μηδὲ τὰς αὐτὰς χρείας ἐπιτελεῖν, πλὴν ὅσα ἐκ τῆς κατὰ τὸ μέγεθος διαφορᾶς, ἢ ἐκ τῆς κατὰ τὴν θέσιν τάξεως.

(377) Κεφ. ια΄. [Ἀνατομὴ τῶν ἐντός.] Ἀνατομὴ καταχρηστικῶς μὲν λέγεται καὶ ἡ τῶν ἐκτὸς μερῶν τε καὶ μορίων τοῦ σώματος διέξοδος, ἥτις ἐστὶ διὰ λόγου διήγησις ἑκάστου, μετὰ τῆς κατὰ φύσιν θέσεως αὐτῶν καὶ τάξεως καὶ χρείας, ἣν παρέχεται τῷ ζώῳ καὶ τῆς οἰκείας ἑκάστου ὀνομασίας, περὶ ὧν ἤδη διεξήλθομεν· κυρίως δὲ λέγεται ἡ ἀνατομὴ, ἡ τῶν ἐντὸς μετὰ λογου ἀνάπτυξις. οὐ γὰρ τὸ τῇ ὄψει αὐτὰ δειχθῆναι ἀνατομή ἐστιν, ἀλλὰ τὸ μετὰ λόγου ἑκάστου αὐτῶν γνῶσιν λαβεῖν, τάς τε κατὰ φύσιν ἐνεργείας, ὅπως δι᾽ αὐτῶν ἀποτελοῦνται ἐκμαθεῖν καὶ τὰς κοινωνίας ἃς ἔχει πρὸς ἄλληλα τὰ σπλάγχνα καὶ τὰ ἄλλα μέρη τοῦ σώματος διὰ φλεβῶν. ὁ μὲν οὖν ἐγκέφαλος ἐξ οὐδενὸς τῶν προειρημένων, κατ᾽ Ἐρασίστρατον ἀρχικῶν ἀγγείων φαίνεται πεπλέχθαι, διὸ καὶ παρέγχυμα τροφῆς δοκεῖ αὐτῷ εἶναι.

pedis nuncupatur. Deinde digiti numero manuum digitis pares. Non autem eadem ſortiti nomina, quoniam nec eosdem praeſtant uſus, quanquam magnitudine aut ſitus ordine conveniunt.

Cap. XI. [*Partium interiorum anatome.*] Anatome abuſive quidem dicitur etiam exteriorum corporis partium et particularum commemoratio, quae verbis uniuscujusque ipſorum naturalem ſitum, ordinem, uſum, quem animanti praebent, propriam cuique illorum appellationem, de quibus jam retulimus, percenſet: proprie vero anatome interiorum cum ſermone explicatio dicitur. Siquidem oculis eas indicatas eſſe, anatome non eſt, ſed cujusque notitiam ex ſermone ac verbis accepiſſe et naturales actiones, quomodo ipſas obeant, didiciſſe, praeterea quam invicem communionem viſcera aliaeque corporis partes per venas habeant. Cerebrum itaque ex nullo eorum, quae praediximus, principali vaſe compoſitum eſſe videtur Eraſiſtrato, eoque nutrimenti affuſio ipſi eſſe videtur. Eſt autem cor-

ἔστι δ' ἁπλοῦν σῶμα καὶ διὰ τοῦτο ἀρχικὸν καὶ κυριώτατον τῶν ἐν ἡμῖν. διὸ καὶ τὸ ἡγεμονικὸν τῆς ψυχῆς αὐτῷ πιστεύουσιν, ὡς Πλάτων καὶ Ἱπποκράτης. περιέχεται δὲ ὑπὸ μηνίγγων δύο, καὶ μιᾶς μὲν προσεχοῦς καὶ προστυποῦς αὐτῷ, ἣ καλεῖται χοροειδὴς καὶ ἔστι φλεβωδεστέρα. ἡ δὲ ἑτέρα ἐπὶ ταύτης οὖσα προσήρτηται μᾶλλον τῷ κρανίῳ κατά τινα μέρη. καὶ ἔστι νευρωδεστέρα. ἐκ μὲν οὖν τῶν ἄνω φλέβες ἀπὸ καρδίας εἰς αὐτὸν ὀχετεύουσι τὴν τροφὴν, κατὰ τὸ λεγόμενον ληχηνεῖον, ἐκ τῶν πρὸς τῇ βάσει ἀρτηριῶν. ἐντεῦθεν δὲ καὶ νεῦρα ἄρχεται ἐκφύεσθαι αὐτοῦ, ὅθεν καὶ εἰς πᾶν τὸ σῶμα ἀναδιδόασιν τὰς ψυχικὰς ἐνεργείας. νεύρων δὲ εἴδη δύο, τὸ μὲν τῶν συνδετικῶν, τῶν συνεχόντων τὰ ὀστᾶ πρὸς ἄλληλα. τὸ δὲ τῶν αἰσθητικῶν καὶ κινητικῶν, ἃ τὴν αἴσθησιν ἐμποιεῖ τῷ σώματι καὶ τὴν προαιρετικὴν κίνησιν εἰς πᾶν διαπέμπει, ἐξ ὧν καὶ τῶν μυῶν ἡ γένεσις. τῶν δὲ ὀφθαλμῶν οἱ πόροι ἐκπεφύκασι καὶ αὐτοὶ ἀπὸ τῆς βάσεως τοῦ ἐγκεφάλου, δι' ὧν τὸ ὁρατικὸν πνεῦμα εἰς τοὺς ὀφθαλμοὺς διαδίδοται. ἐντεῦθεν δὲ καὶ εἰς τοὺς μυκτῆρας

pus fimplex, atque ob id omnium, quae humano continentur corpore et praecipuum et princeps. Quapropter Plato et Hippocrates animi principatum in eo conftituunt. Comprehenditur fane membranis duabus: una contigua et affimili, quae choroeides appellatur venofiorque eft: altera quae huic fuperiacet, calvariae quibusdam partibus magis adhaerefcit. Sed haec nervofior exiftit. Ex fuperiore igitur parte venae nutrimentum a corde juxta eum locum, qui torcular dicitur, ex arteriis, quae ad bafin funt, acceptum in id derivant, inde et nervi exortus principium ex eo capiunt, unde et animales functiones univerfo corpori communicant. Nervorum autem fpecies duae funt, una mutuos offium connexus colligat continetque, altera fentiendi movendique pro arbitrio facultatem toti corpori transmittit. Atque hinc etiam musculorum proventus eft. Oculorum meatus et ipfi ab ima cerebri parte proveniunt et per eos viforius fpiritus oculis impertitur. Inde vero nares etiam proceffus habent, per

ἀποφύσεις ἤρτηνται, δι' ὧν τε ὀσφραινόμεθα καὶ δι' ὧν ἐκκαθαίρεται ὁ ἐγκέφαλος. εἰς δὲ τὰ ὦτα ἀποφύσεις μὲν οὐκ εἰσι. τέτρηται δὲ αὕτη ἡ μῆνιγξ ἐκ τῶν ὄπισθεν καὶ σκωληκοειδῆ ἀπόφυσιν ποιεῖται, δι' ἧς καὶ αὐτὰ ἀποκαθαίρεται καὶ ἐν ἀρχῇ ταύτης τὸ λεγόμενον κωνοειδές. ἐντεῦθεν δὲ καὶ ὁ ῥαχίτης μυελὸς ἄρχεται. κοιλίας δὲ ἔχει ὁ ἐγκέφαλος δύο· κατ' ἐνίους δὲ μίαν, ἔνθα τὸ ἡγεμονικὸν τῆς ψυχῆς ἵδρυται. περιέχεται δὲ καὶ τὰ τοῦ κρανίου ὀστᾶ, ἄνωθεν ὑπὸ τῷ δέρματι, τῷ περικρανίῳ λεγομένῳ ὑμένι, ἐκπεφυκότι μὲν διὰ τῶν ῥαφῶν, ἐκ τῶν μηνίγγων· ἀρχὴ δὲ οὗτος γίνεται τοῦ τε ὑπεζωκότος τὰς πλευρὰς ὑμένος καὶ τοῦ διαφράγματος καὶ τοῦ περιτοναίου καὶ παντὸς ὑμένος νευρώδους. ὁ δὲ ὀφθαλμὸς συνέστηκεν μὲν καθ' Ἱπποκράτην ἐκ χιτώνων δύο, οὓς μήνιγγας ὁ Ἱπποκράτης καλεῖ, ἐπειδὴ ἐκ τῶν μηνίγγων ἐκπεφύκασιν. κατὰ δὲ τοὺς νεωτέρους ἐκ τριῶν, κατ' ἐνίους δὲ ἐκ τεσσάρων. πρῶτος μὲν οὖν ἔξωθέν ἐστιν ὁ κερατοειδὴς, λευκὸς μὲν κατὰ τὰ ἄλλα, κατὰ δὲ τὴν ἶριν λεπτυνόμενος διαφαίνει τὸ ὑποκείμενον χρῶμα, καθ'

quos et olfacimus et cerebrum expurgatur. Ad aures processus non sunt, verum a posteriore parte tenuis membrana, quam meningem vocant, perforata est, atque in vermis speciem processum habet: per quam similiter ipsae repurgantur. In illius principio cerebri pars coniformis appellata, sedem habet. Jam vero illinc et spinalis medulla incipit. Caeterum duos habet cerebrum ventriculos, secundum aliquos vero unum, ubi animi principatus residet. At calvariae ossa superiore parte sub cute, membrana, quae per suturas e meningibus prodiit, pericranium appellata, conteguntur. Estque haec origo membranae costas succingentis et septi transversi et peritonaei et omnis membranae nervosae. Oculus ex Hippocratis sententia habet duas tunicas, quas Hippocrates meningas, quod ex illis provenerint, appellat. Recentiores tres ponunt, nonnulli quatuor. Ex quibus prima exterior est cornea vocata. Ea reliqua sui parte alba est, pupillae loco extenuatur, perspicuumque subjectum colorem reddit, qua-

ὁ μέλας, ἢ γλαυκότερος, ἢ χαροπὸς φαίνεται· δεύτερος δέ ἐστιν ὁ ῥαγοειδὴς ῥαγὶ σταφυλῆς ἐοικὼς τὰ ἔνδοθεν, τετρημένος κατὰ τὴν κόρην. τρίτος δὲ ὁ ἀμφιβληστροειδὴς, ἐγκολπούμενος ὥσπερ καὶ δεχόμενος ἐπ' ἄκρῳ τὸν ὑπό τινων εἰσαγόμενον τέταρτον χιτῶνα, ὃν καὶ ἄδηλον προσαγορεύουσιν. ἔστι μὲν γὰρ ὑμὴν σμικρότατός τε καὶ ἰσχνότατος. ἀλλ' ὁ μὲν πρῶτος καὶ ὁ δεύτερος στερεοὶ ὑμένες καὶ χιτῶνες παχεῖς εἰσιν. ὁ δὲ τρίτος καὶ τέταρτος ἰσχνότατοι. διὸ καὶ Ἱπποκράτης τοὺς πρώτους μόνους οἶδε, λέγων. ὁ δὲ ὀφθαλμὸς μήνιγγας ἔχει δύο ὑγρὰ δὲ περιέχουσιν οἱ ὑμένες οὗτοι τρισσὰ, τότε ὑδατοειδὲς καὶ τὸ ὑαλοειδὲς καὶ τὸ κρυσταλλοειδές· βλεφάρων δὲ τὰ μὲν ἔσωθεν σαρκώδη, τὰ δὲ μεταξὺ χονδρώδη. ἔξωθεν δὲ δέρματι σκέπεται. διὰ δὲ τὸ σκληρὸν τοῦ μεταξὺ χόνδρου πιμελὴ ὑπέστρωται αὐτῷ οἷον μάλαγμα, ἥτις ἐπὶ τὸ πολὺ πλεονάζουσα τὰς ὑδατίδας ποιεῖ. ἡ δὲ γλῶσσα σαρκώδεις μὲν τὰ πλεῖστα· διττὸν δὲ νεύρων εἶδος ἐμπέφυκεν εἰς αὐτὴν ἐκ τῆς τοῦ ἐγκεφάλου βάσεως, τὸ μὲν τῶν καλουμένων μαλακῶν νεύρων, δι' ὧν τὴν αἴσθη-

tenus niger vel caefius vel fulvus apparet. Secunda, qua pupilla eft, modico foramine concava, quae quod parte interiore fit acino uvae fimilis, nominatur. Tertia retis modo finum habens, retiformis nuncupatur: perinde quafi in fummo quartam tunicam a nonnullis invectam excipiat, quam minus apparentem vocant. Eft etenim membrana minima fimul et tenuiffima, fed prima et fecunda firmae membranae craffaeque tunicae funt: tertia vero et quarta tenuiffimae. Quare et Hippocrates priores folas cognovit, oculus, inquiens, membranas duas habet. Porro triplicem hae tunicae continent humorem. Hunc ab aquae fimilitudine aqueum vocant. Illum vitreum, quod vitro quiddam fimile referat. Tertium cryftallinum. Palpebrarum interiores partes carnofae: mediae cartilaginofae, exteriores cute teguntur. At quoniam cartilago media dura eft, adeps fubjecta eft lenimenti, malagmatisve inftar, quae frequenter exuperans veficulas aqua plenas parit. Lingua maxime carnofa eft, in quam duplex nervorum genus ab

σιν τὴν γευστικὴν ἐπὶ τὴν ἀρχὴν ἀναδίδωσι. τὸ δὲ τῶν σκληρῶν, δι' ὧν καὶ ἡ κίνησις, ἡ προαιρετικὴ ἐπ' αὐτὴν ἀναφέρεται. πρὸς δὲ τῇ ῥίζῃ αὐτῆς ἐμπέφυκεν ἡ ἐπιγλωττὶς, ἥτις ἐν τῷ καταπίνειν ἀνατρέχουσα ἐπιπωματίζει τὸν βρόγχον, ἵνα μή τι τῶν στερεῶν, ἢ ὑγρῶν ἐμπέσῃ εἰς αὐτόν. τῆς δὲ αὐτῆς αἰτίας ἕνεκα καὶ αἱ ἀντιάδες γεγόνασι, τέσσαρες οὖσαι τὸν ἀριθμὸν, δύο μὲν προφανεῖς πρὸς τῇ ῥίζῃ τῆς γλώττης ἑκατέρωθεν, δύο δὲ ἐχόμεναι τούτων ἐνδότεραι. λέγονται δὲ αὗται καὶ παρίσθμια, διὰ τὸ ἐοικέναι τὸ χωρίον ἰσθμῷ εἰς ὃ παράκεινται, μάλιστα δὲ ὅταν φλεγμαίνωσιν, διότι στενοῦσιν ἄγαν τὴν δίοδον ταύτην. [373] ἐπεὶ δὲ δύο ὕλαις διοικεῖται τὸ ζῶον, τροφῇ καὶ πνεύματι, πνεύματος μὲν ὁδοί τε καὶ καταδοχαὶ τάδε, ῥῖνες, στόμα, βρόγχος, τραχεῖα ἀρτηρία, πνεύμων. ῥὶς μὲν καὶ στόμα πρὸς τὸ ἀναπνεῖν, ὁ δὲ γαργαρεὼν, ἵνα μὴ ἀθρόως εἰς τὸν βρόγχον προσεμπίπτῃ ψυχρὸς ἀήρ. ἀρτηρία δὲ τραχεῖα, πάροδός ἐστιν αὐτῷ εἰς τὸν πνεύμονα ἐν τῷ στήθει κείμενον, δι' οὗ καὶ ἡ πᾶσα ἀναπνοὴ γίνεται, διαστελλομένου μὲν, ἵνα δέ-

ima parte cerebri prodiens inferitur. Alii molles appellati, guftandi fenfum ad principium: alii duri, motum arbitrarium ad ipfam deducunt. Ad hujus radicem exigua inhaeret epiglottis, quae cum deglutimus, recurrens arteriam claudit, ne quid ex folidioribus aut humidis in ipfam delabatur. Cujus rei quoque caufa tonfillae numero quatuor creatae funt: duae ad linguae radicem, utrinque confpicuae: duae his proximae, penitiores. Nominantur eaedem etiam parifthmia, quoniam locus ad quem fitae funt, ifthmo, praefertim cum per inflammationem intumuerunt, eoque tranfitum hunc arctum nimis reddunt, figura refpondent. Porro quum duabus animal materiis gubernetur, alimento et fpiritu; ad hunc quidem percipiendum nares, os, fauces, afpera arteria et pulmo, partes funt aptiffimae. Nares fane et os refpirationi ferviunt: gurgulio, ne frigidus in fauces aër cumulatim irrumpat: afpera arteria, ut eundem in pulmonem deducat cujus in pectore fedes eft: per hunc et omnis fit refpiratio, fubmittentem

ξηται συστελλομένου δὲ, ἵνα ἐκπέμψῃ. διὸ καὶ ἔοικε τῇ μὲν ἐνεργείᾳ ταῖς χαλκευτικαῖς φύσαις, τῷ δὲ σχήματι βοὸς ὁπλῇ ἐν πνεύμονι δὲ κατεργασθέντος τοῦ πνεύματος, τὸ μὲν ἀναγκαιότατον εἰς τὴν ἀριστερὰν κοιλίαν τῆς καρδίας φέρεται, τὸ δὲ ἄχρηστον ἐκπνεῖται δι' ὧν περ εἰσεπνεύσθη. τροφῆς δὲ ἀγγεῖα, τὰ πρὸς ὑποδοχὴν καὶ ὄργανα πρὸς κατεργασίαν τάδε· στόμα μὲν καὶ ὀδόντες, στόμαχος, κοιλία, νῆστις καὶ λεπτὰ ἔντερα. στόμα μὲν καὶ ὀδόντες πρὸς λέανσιν. στόμαχος δὲ πρὸς ὄρεξιν καὶ κατάποσιν. παρατέταται δὲ τῇ τραχείᾳ ἀρτηρίᾳ καὶ διατείνει μέχρι διαφράγματος. κοινὴ δὲ πρὸς πέψιν ἡ γαστήρ. ἄρχεται δὲ ὡς ἀπὸ μέσου τοῦ χόνδρου, ἔνθα στόμα κοιλίας λέγεται, ὑπιοῦσα δὲ τὸ ἧπαρ, τῷ κύτει σιγματοειδὴς οὖσα, ἐπὶ τὰ ἀριστερὰ νεύει, τῷ ἑτέρῳ ἄκρῳ, ἔνθα καὶ ὁ πυλωρός ἐστιν, ἵνα μὴ ἀθρόως διεκπίπτῃ αὐτῆς ἡ τροφή. νῆστις δὲ καὶ λεπτὸν ἔντερον πρὸς ἀνάδοσιν· πολλοὺς δὲ ἑλιγμοὺς ἡ νῆστις ἔχει καὶ συνέχεται τῷ μεσαραίῳ, ἢ μεσεντερίῳ, ὃ ἐξυφαίνουσιν αἱ εἰς

quidem fe, ut fpiritus emittatur, attollentem vero, ut idem recipiatur. Quare actione fimilitudinem quandam cum fabrorum follibus habere videtur, figuram vero ungulae bubulae fervat. Porro ex fpiritu in pulmone elaborato quicquid maxime neceffarium eft, ad finiftrum cordis ventriculum defertur, quicquid inutile eft, illac, qua infpiravimus, efflatur. Nutrimenti vafa ad excipiendum et inftrumenta ad elaborationem inftituta haec funt, os, dentes, ftomachus, ventriculus, jejunum et tenuia inteftina. Os quidem et dentes cibum extenuant moluntque. Stomachus appetit et deglutit: appenfus autem afperae arteriae ad feptum usque transverfum porrigitur. Ventriculus omnis eft ad concoctionem, incipit velut a media cartilagine, ubi ventris os fitum dicitur, fubfidet leviter jecinori, latitudine figma literam referens et altero extremo in finiftram partem vergit, ubi eft et pylorus, quoniam portae modo, ne nutrimentum ex eo confertim delabatur, prohibet. Jejunum et tenue inteftinum digeftioni dicatum eft, in finus

αὐτὸν καθήκουσαι φλέβες, δι' ὧν ἡ πλείστη ἀνάδοσις γίνεται ἐπὶ πύλας ἥπατος. συνάπτεται δὲ αὐτῇ τὸ λεπτὸν ἔντερον, ὡς μέρος αὐτῆς δοκεῖν εἶναι· ἔοικε γὰρ νήστει ἡπλωμένῃ. ἑξῆς δὲ τὸ τυφλὸν ἔντερον, πρὸς ὑποδοχὴν τῆς τροφῆς. ἐπὶ δὲ τούτῳ τὸ κῶλον πρὸς ὑποδοχὴν τῶν διακεκριμένων περιττωμάτων ἐκ τῆς ἀναδόσεως, δια- (378) βαῖνον δὲ ἐπὶ τὰ δεξιὰ ὑπὲρ ὀμφαλὸν ἐντὸς τοῦ ἥπατος καὶ τοῦ σπληνὸς εἰς τὰ κάτω πάλιν φέρεται διαζῶσαν τὸ ἐπιγάστριον ὅλον καὶ τελευτᾷ κατὰ τὸ ἀπευθυσμένον. δύο τοίνυν πόροι ἀρχόμενοι ἀπὸ τῆς τοῦ στόματος εὐρυχωρίας, ὁ μὲν κατὰ τὸ ἔμπροσθεν τοῦ τραχήλου τέτακται καὶ καλεῖται βρόγχος, ἢ τραχεῖα ἀρτηρία. ὅθεν δὲ ἄρχεται, καθ' ἃ ἀνεστόμωται φάρυγξ λέγεται, ἢ λάρυγξ. συνέστηκε δὲ ὁ πᾶς πόρος, ἐκ χόνδρων οἷον κρικοειδῶν, ἢ κυκλοτερῶν, ἵνα ἀσύμπτωτος μένῃ πρὸς τὸ ἀδιαλείπτως εἰσπνεῖν τὸ ζῶον, διὸ καὶ ἀεὶ ἀναπέπταται αὐτοῦ τὸ στόμα. τροφῆς μὲν γὰρ ἀποσχέσθαι ἐπὶ πλεῖστόν ἐστιν ὑπομένειν, μὴ εἰσπνεῖσθαι δὲ, οὐδὲ τὸ ἀκαριαῖον· διὰ τοῦτο δὲ καὶ καθαρὰν τῷ

multos implicitum: committitur autem meſaraeo ſeu meſenterio, quod venae in id deſcendentes intertexunt, per quas digeſtio plurima ſit ad portas hepatis. Ei vero tenuius inteſtinum eſt ita connexum, ut pars ejus eſſe videatur, quippe jejuno explicato perſimile eſt. *Differt tamen quod nec vacuum ſit, nec vaſorum copiam habeat.* Deinde caecum inteſtinum alimento recipiendo accommodatum. Huic adhaereſcit laxius inteſtinum, quod excrementa ex diſtributione ſegregata ſuſcipit. Pertendens autem in dextram ſupra umbilicum inter jecur et lienem, deorſum rurſus fertur, totumque amplexum abdomen in rectum inteſtinum deſinit. Quum igitur duo meatus a lato oris ſpatio incipiant, alterum juxta priorem colli partem bronchum vel aſperam arteriam nominamus: alterum ſtomachum. Unde vero initium capit arteria et ubi aperitur, pharyngem vel laryngem vocant. Caeterum totus meatus ex cartilaginibus annuli modo vel circuli compoſitis conſtat, quo firmus continuae animantis reſpirationi

πνεύματι τὴν δίοδον ταύτην παρέχει, ὅπως μηδέποτε ἐμποδίζῃ τὴν ὁδὸν τῷ πνεύματι. ἀμέλει εἴπου ἐν τῷ τρέφεσθαι λαθὸν παρεμπέσοι τι εἰς αὐτὸν, εὐθὺς βὴξ καὶ πνιγμὸς ἐπακολουθεῖ, ἄχρις οὗ ἐξωθούμενον ὑπὸ τοῦ πνεύματος ἀνενεχθῇ. διαπέμπει δὲ τὸ πνεῦμα ἡ τραχεῖα ἀρτηρία εἰς τὸν πνεύμονα καὶ περαιοῦται εἰς τὰς ἐν αὐτῷ τραχείας ἀρτηρίας, αἳ καὶ αὐταὶ καὶ βρόγχια καλοῦνται. ὁ δὲ στόμαχος ἐνδοτέρω τοῦ βρόγχου ὢν, πρὸς τοῖς σπονδύλοις τοῦ τραχήλου, συμπαρεκτείνεται μὲν τῇ τραχείᾳ ἀρτηρίᾳ ἐπὶ πολὺ, ἀλλ' ὁ μὲν βρόγχος προσκείμενος, ἐν τῷ καταπίνεσθαι τὴν τροφὴν προσανατρέχων, ἐπιπωματίζεται ἀκριβῶς τῇ ἐπιγλωττίδι, ἥτις πέφυκεν ἐκ τῆς ῥίζης τῆς γλώττης. ἡ δὲ ἐπιγλωττὶς οὐ μόνον τὸ στόμα ἐπιπωματίζει, ἀλλὰ καὶ τὴν τροφὴν τὴν ὑπὸ τῆς γλώττης, οἷον ὑπὸ πτύου ἀναλιχμωμένην διαπορθμεύει, ὥσπερ γέφυρα, ἐπὶ τὸν στόμαχον ὑπὲρ τὸ στόμα τοῦ βρόγχου ὑπερθεῖσα αὐτήν. [374] ὁ δὲ στόμαχος φυσικὴν ἐνέργειαν ἔχων τὴν ὀρεκτικὴν δύναμιν διαστέλλεται μὲν ὑπὸ

maneat nec comprimatur, quare etiam oſtium ejus ſemper pateſcit. Nam cibi abſtinentiam tolerare potes diutiſſime, non inſpirare, ne minimum quidem temporis potes. Hujus rei gratia purum hunc ſpiritui tranſitum natura dedit, ne impedimenti quid ſentiat. Enimvero ſi quid vel cibi vel potus in arteriam imprudentibus delabitur, ſtrangulationes et tuſſes ſtatim excitantur donec a ſpiritus impetu excuſſum efferatur. Jam vero aſpera arteria ſpiritum pulmoni transmittit, deſinitque in ejusdem arterias aſperas, quas ipſas quoque bronchia nominant. Stomachus interius quam arteria exiſtens, cervicis vertebris annexus, longiſſime cum aſpera arteria porrigitur. Sed bronchus illi adjunctus, cum cibum deglutimus, recurrens, exacte ipſum lingula cooperit, quae ex linguae radice trahit originem. Porro haec lingula non modo os claudit, ſed etiam cibum a lingua velut ventilabro purgatum et arteriae orificio ſuperimpoſitum ad ſtomachum, pontis modo dejicit. Stomachus pro naturali functione appetendi facultatem

τῆς ὀρέξεως καὶ καταπίνει τὰ εἰσφερόμενα. ἡ δὲ τῷ ὑποκειμένῳ στελλομένη, οἷον ἐκθλίβει καὶ ἀπωθεῖται αὐτὰ ἐπὶ τὰ ὑποκείμενα μέρη ἐκβαλὼν διὰ τοῦ διαφράγματος, συμφυεῖ τῷ στόματι τῆς κοιλίας, δι' οὗ στενοῦ πόρου ὄντος εἰς τὴν γαστέρα τροφὴ παρέρχεται γαστρὸς δὲ, ἡ μὲν φυσικὴ ἐνέργεια πέττει τὴν προσενεχθεῖσαν αὐτῇ τροφήν. πεφθεῖσα δὲ αὐτὴ, πρῶτον μὲν ἔοικεν χυλῷ πτισσάνης. διά τε τοῦ λεγομένου πυλωροῦ ὄντος ἔτι στενωτέρου, διηθεῖται εἰς τὴν νῆστιν ἡ τροφὴ, ἥτις λεπτὸν ἔντερον οὖσα, διὰ τοῦτο ὑπὸ τῆς φύσεως εἰς ἕλικας πλείστας συνετέθη, ὅπως μὴ ῥᾳδίως διακόπτηται, ἢ διασπᾶται. συνέχονται δὲ αἱ ἕλικες αὐτῆς καὶ ὑποβαστίζονται τῷ λεγομένῳ μεσαραίῳ, ἢ μεσεντερίῳ· οὐ μόνον δὲ τὴν χρείαν ταύτην παρέχει τὸ μεσάραιον, ἀλλὰ καὶ τὰς ὑπὸ τοῦ ἥπατος ἐκπεφυκυίας δύο φλέβας, ἔπειτα εἰς πολλὰς ἀποσχίδας διαιρουμένας, αἳ ἐμβάλλουσιν εἰς τὸ μεσάραιον, ὅπως καὶ αὗται μὴ διαῤῥήσσωνται. ἰσχναὶ οὖσαι. ἀλλ' ἀνέχονται ὑπὸ τοῦ ἐνυφασμένου αὐτῷ ὑπερεί-

habet. Dum appetit quidem, ſe attollit et quae offeruntur deglutit: dum autem accepta quaſi elidit et ad ſubjectas partes expellit, ac ventriculi orificio contiguo per transverſum ſeptum tradit, ſubmittitur. Per quem anguſtum exiſtentem meatum in ventrem alimenta deſcendunt. Ventriculi naturale officium eſt, ut alimentum ſibi commiſſum concoquat, quod a concoctione primum ptiſſanae cremori perſimile eſt: verum per eum quem pylorum appellari diximus, qui adhuc arctior eſt, alimentum jejuno inſtillatur, quod cum tenue ſit inteſtinum, in flexuoſiſſimos orbes natura implicavit, ne ex facili videlicet diſſecaretur divellereturque. Meſaraeum ſeu meſenterium amfractus et orbes ejus amplectitur, atque ipſos ſuſtentat: quamquam id non ſolum hunc praeſtat uſum, ſed etiam venas duas ſub jecinore emergentes *fulcit*, quae poſt in diverſas partes diducuntur et meſaraeo inſeruntur, quo et ipſae, ſunt enim tenues, ruptionis periculum effugiant. Suſtinentur autem ab intexto eidem fulcimento, huic in-

σματι, συγχρώμεναι τούτῳ καὶ οἷον διαβάθρα κουφιζόμεναι περαιοῦνται καὶ οὕτως ἐπὶ πάσας τὰς ἕλικας τῆς νήστεως ἐοικυίας βδέλλαις, ἀνεστομωμέναι εἰς τὴν νῆστιν, πᾶσαν δέχονται τὴν ἐν αὐτῷ κεχυλωμένην τροφήν. ἅμα δὲ τῷ δέξασθαι εὐθὺς ἐξαιματοῦσιν αὐτὴν χυλὸν ὄντα τὸ πρόσθεν, μέχρις ὅτε ἐν τῇ νήστει ἐστί. οὐδὲ γὰρ ἑτέρωθεν αἵματος ἀγγεῖον, οὔτε φλέγματος, ἢ ἄλλου τινὸς εἶναι περιεκτικὸν, ὁ τῆς φύσεως νόμος διαγορεύει. πάλιν οὖν διὰ τοῦ μεσαραίου αἱ φλέβες αὗται ἐδέξαντο, δύο γενόμεναι ἐκ πολλῶν ἐμβάλλουσιν εἰς τὸ ἧπαρ κατὰ τὰς λεγομένας αὐτοῦ πύλας. ἐν δὲ τῷ ἥπατι ἐξαιματουμένης τῆς τροφῆς, ὁμοῦ διακρίνεται ἕκαστον τῶν περιττωμάτων. καὶ ἡ μὲν ξανθὴ χολὴ ἐπὶ κύστιν τὴν ἐν τῷ ἥπατι φέρεται. ἡ δὲ μέλαινα ἐπὶ σπλῆνα. ἀπὸ δὲ ἥπατος ἐξαιματωθεῖσα ἡ τροφὴ εἰς τὴν δεξιὰν ἀναδίδοται τῆς καρδίας κοιλίαν. ἀπὸ δὲ τῆς καρδίας, διὰ μὲν τῶν σφαγιτίδων, ἐπὶ τὰ ἄνω τὸ αἷμα ἀναδίδοται. διὰ δὲ τῆς κοίλης φλεβὸς, ἐπὶ πάντα τοῦ σώματος τὰ μέρη. ἀπὸ γοῦν τῆς κοίλης φλεβὸς διακρινομένου τοῦ ἐῤῥώδους

nitentes et veluti ſubſtrato allevatae finiunt. Atque hoc pacto in ſingulis amfractibus ad hirudinum ſimilitudinem compoſitis, aperto ore jejuno inhiantes, omnem in eo alimoniam in ſuccum converſam exugunt. Simul autem inter exugendum protinus ipſum in ſanguinem mutant, qui ſuccus antea erat, dum in jejuno eſſet. Non enim aliunde vel pituitae vel ſanguinis vel alterius cujusdam vas eſſe natura indicat. Rurſus igitur duae factae ex multis venae, a meſaraeo acceptum, ad hepar per dictas ejus portas digerunt. In jecinore quum ſanguinis naturam nutrimentum induit, recrementa ſingula pariter ſecernuntur. Flava bilis ad veſicam ei inhaerentem deſertur: atra ad lienem. Jam vero ab hepate verſum in ſanguinem alimentum in dextrum cordis ventriculum diſtribuitur. A corde ſanguis per jugulares venas ad ſuperiores corporis partes derivat. Per cavam autem venam in univerſum corpus diffunditur. Ab hac rami duo, ſanguine jam a ſero diſcreto, ad renes perreptant, qui lumbis ſub clunium carnibus, per quas

ἀπὸ τοῦ αἵματος, ἀποσχίδες ἐπὶ νεφροὺς φέρουσιν, οἵ κεῖνται κατὰ τὴν ὀσφὺν ὑπὸ τὰς ψόας, δι' ὧν διηθεῖται τὸ οὖρον. ἐπὶ τὴν κύστιν δὲ παραγίνεται, διὰ τῶν λεγομένων οὐρητήρων. ἡ δὲ κύστις δέχεται μὲν κατὰ τοῦ σώματος αὐτῆς τὸ οὖρον. ἐκκρίνει δὲ διὰ τοῦ καυλοῦ εἰς τὰ ἐκτός. δίδυμοι δὲ τὴν μὲν σύστασιν ἀδενώδεις, δοχεῖα δέ εἰσιν καὶ ἐργαστήρια τοῦ γόνου, ὃς φέρεται ἐπ' αὐτοὺς διὰ τῶν κρεμαστήρων. καθήκουσι δὲ εἰς αὐτοὺς καὶ ἕτερα ἀγγεῖα τὰ τρέφοντα αὐτούς. περιέχεται δὲ ὑπὸ δύο χιτώνων, τοῦ τε ἐρυθροειδοῦς καὶ τοῦ δαρτοῦ λεγομένου. ἐπὶ δὲ τούτοις ἡ ὀσχή. ταῖς δὲ γυναιξὶν ἡ ὑστέρα ἔοικεν ὀσχῇ ἀνεστραμμένῃ. ἀνεστόμωνται εἰς τὸ ἔνδον αὐτῆς φλέβες, ὡς ὅτι πλεῖσται, δι' ὧν τὸ αἷμα ἀποκαθαίρεται, ὃ ἐν ταῖς συλλήψεσιν ἐπέχεται καὶ χωρεῖ εἰς τροφὴν καὶ διάπλασιν τοῦ ἐμβρύου· ἀπὸ γὰρ τῶν φλεβῶν τῶν πλεκουσῶν τὸ χορίον γενόμεναι δύο φλέβες καὶ ἀπὸ τῶν κατ' αὐτὸ ἀρτηριῶν δύο ἀρτηρίαι καὶ ἀπὸ τῶν νεύρων νεῦρον ἓν συνελθόντα ἀποτελεῖ τὸν οὐραχὸν, ὃς ἐμβάλλει εἰς τοῦ ἐμβρύου τὸν ὀμφαλὸν, ἐξ οὗ καὶ ἐκαύεται καὶ ἀποκρεμᾶται. ἀπὸ δὲ ὀμφαλοῦ αἱ μὲν φλέβες

urina deftillat, inhaerent. Ad veficam autem per ureteras proficiscitur. Vefica corpore fuo urinam recipit et per colem foras excernit; tefticuli vero fubftantia glandulofi funt, conceptacula et officinae feminis, quod per cremafteres ad eos fertur. In quos etiam alia vafa ipfos nutrientia defcendunt. Caeterum duabus tunicis conteguntur, quarum tenuiorem erythroïdem, valentiorem dartum appellant. Ab his eft, quod fcrotum dicitur. Foeminis autem vulva fcroti converfi fimilitudinem refert Venae in partem ejus interiorem quam plurimae aperiuntur, per quas fanguis expurgatur: qui in conceptibus retinetur, ceditque in alimentum foetui et formationem. Nam a venis, quae fecundas implicant, binae aliae prodeuntes venae, ab arteriis ibidem fitis binae arteriae et a nervis unus nervus mutuo in unum congreffu urachum appellatum abfolvunt, qui infantis umbilico inferitur, ex quo et enafcitur et fufpenfus eft. Ab umbilico autem venae ad je-

ἐπὶ ἥπατος πύλας τὸ αἷμα διδόασιν ἐπὶ τῶν ἐμβρύων. αἱ δὲ ἀρτηρίαι κατὰ τὴν κύστιν εἰς τὴν παχεῖαν ἀρτηρίαν ἐμβάλλουσι. τὸ δὲ νεῦρον τοῦτο εἰς τὴν ῥάχιν.

[375] Κεφ. ιβ'. [Περὶ ὀστεολογίας.] Τῶν δὲ ὀστῶν διττὴ ἡ σύνθεσις, ἡ μὲν πρὸς τὸ κινεῖσθαι καὶ καλεῖται ἄρθρον, ἡ δὲ πρὸς τὸ ἀκίνητον καὶ καλεῖται συνάρθρωσις. εἴδη δὲ ταύτης τρία, ῥαφὴ, σύμφυσις, γόμφωσις, κατὰ ῥαφὴν μὲν οὖν σύγκεινται τὰ ἐκ τῆς κεφαλῆς ὀστᾶ. ῥαφαὶ δὲ εὑρίσκονται ἐπὶ τῶν πλείστων πέντε. στεφανιαία ἡ διὰ τοῦ βρέγματος. ὀβολιαία ἡ διὰ τῆς κορυφῆς. λαμβδοειδὴς, ἡ διὰ ἰνίου κροτάφιαι δύο καθ' ἑκάτερον κρόταφον μία. ὀστᾶ δὲ κρανίου ἑπτά· ἰνίου ἕν· κορυφῆς δύο· κροτάφων δύο· μετώπου ἕν. πολυμόρφου ἕν· ἐκφύσεις δὲ ἔχει ὁ ἐγκέφαλος δύο, ἑκατέρωθεν τῆς παρεγκεφαλίδος, αἳ καλοῦνται κορῶναι. ἐναρμόζονται δὲ εἰς τὰς τοῦ πρώτου σπονδύλου κοιλότητας, ἐν ᾧ καθάπερ ἐπὶ κνώδακος τῆς τοῦ δευτέρου σπονδύλου ἀποφύσεως, ἡ κεφαλὴ εἴς τε τὰ πλάγια ἐπιστρέφεται, ἀνανεύει τε καὶ ἐπινεύει. μετὰ δὲ ταῦτα, αἱ ὀστοειδεῖς ἀπο-

cinoris portas fanguinem in foetibus transmittunt: arteriae vero juxta veficam, craffiori arteriae: nervus hic fpinae inferitur.

Cap. XII. [*De ofteologia.*] Offium duplex compofitio, una ad motum accommodata nomen articuli habet: altera ad ftabilitatem, fynarthrofis appellatur. Hujus autem tres funt fpecies, futura, fymphyfis et gomphofis. Suturis igitur capitis offa conftant. Inveniuntur autem futurae in plurimis quinque. Prima per finciput, coronalis. Altera per verticem fagittalis. Tertia per occipitium, lambdoidea littera. Duae temporales, in utroque temporum una. Offa calvariae feptem numerantur, occipitis unum, verticis duo, temporum item duo, frontis unum, multiformis unum. Cerebrum duos ab utraque cerebelli parte proceffus obtinet quae coronae vocantur, qui in primae vertebrae cavitates infinuantur, in qua velut centro, fecundae vertebrae caput in latera movetur, annuit, renuitque, deinde offei dicti proceffus duo, paululum in-

φύσεις καλούμεναι δύο μικρὸν διεστῶσαι, δι' ὧν τένοντες καὶ νεῦρα καταφέρονται· εἶτα ἄλλα δύο ἐπάνω τῶν ἀκουστικῶν πόρων, τὰ ζυγοειδῆ καλούμενα ὀστᾶ· ὑπὸ δὲ ταῦτα λιθοειδῆ ὀστᾶ δύο καὶ ταῦτα. ἔμπροσθεν δὲ αἱ βελονοειδεῖς ἐκφύσεις. ἐγένοντο δὲ εἰς διάστασιν τοῦ φαρυγγέτρου. καὶ λέγεται ὑοειδὲς ὀστοῦν, καθ' ὃ χόνδρῳ συνδεῖται αὐτῶν τὰ ἄκρα. ἐπάνω δὲ τούτων τὰ ἀνώνυμα, ὧν κατὰ τὸ ἔμπροσθεν μέρος κεῖται τὸ πολύμορφον. κατὰ δὲ σύμφυσιν τὰ τῆς ἄνω γνάθου ὀστᾶ σύγκειται. συμφύσεις δὲ ἔχει τὸ πρόσωπον ἐννέα, μίαν μὲν κατ' εὐρυ- (379) χωρίαν ἑκατέραν τῶν ὀφθαλμῶν τεταγμένην· δύο δὲ ἐκ πλαγίων τῆς ῥινός. καὶ ἄλλην μέσην τὴν ῥῖνα ἐπ' εὐθείας τέμνουσαν. δύο δὲ κατὰ μῆλα καὶ δύο κατὰ τῆς ὑπερώας πλαγίας. μίαν δὲ ἐπ' εὐθείας διαιροῦσαν καὶ τέμνουσαν τὴν ὑπερώαν. κοιναὶ δὲ προσώπου καὶ κεφαλῆς αἱ ἐπὶ τῶν ζυγωμάτων. ὀστᾶ δὲ προσώπου δώδεκα, ῥινὸς δύο. ὀφθαλμῶν δύο. μήλων δύο, ὑπερώας τέσσαρα. τὰ τῶν φατνίων δύο, τὰ τοῖς πτερυγίοις ὅμοια. ἡ δὲ κάτω γνάθος κατ' ἐνίους μὲν δύο ἐστὶν ὀστᾶ

vicem diffidentes, per quos tendines et nervi deorfum feruntur. Poft alia duo offa fuper foramina, per quae facultas audiendi eft, emergunt, jugalia appellata. Sub his rurfus alia duo petrofa. Priore capitis parte proceffus funt ftiliformes. Facti autem funt ad faucium divifionem. Ubi fummae eorum partes cartilagine committuntur, os hyoeideum appellatur. Quae vero fuper his funt, nomen defiderant. Quorum in priore parte fitum eft os multiforme. Porro fuperioris maxillae offa fymphyfi conftant. Facies item fymphyfes novem habet. Prima in lato utroque oculorum fpatio fitum obtinet: duae a latere narium utroque. alia medias nares recta interfecat. Malae quoque fingulas habent. Duae rurfus obliquae palatum fecant, unaque in rectum idem palatum dividit. Communes autem faciei et capiti funt in offibus jugalibus. Jam quidem faciei duodecim offa funt, narium duo, oculorum quoque totidem, malarum fingula, palati quatuor, dentium receptaculorum duo, alis fimilia. Maxilla inferior quo-

συμπεφυκότα κατὰ τὸ γένειον· κατ' ἐνίους δὲ ἕν. κατὰ γόμφωσιν δὲ σύγκεινται οἱ ὀδόντες, ἐγγεγόμφωνται γὰρ τοῖς φατνίοις. εἰσὶ δὲ τὸν ἀριθμὸν λβ'. ἔν τε τῇ ἄνω καὶ κάτω γνάθῳ. τομεῖς ὀκτώ. κυνόδοντες τέσσαρες, μυλῖται εἴκοσι. τῶν δὲ ἄλλων ὀστῶν αἱ μὲν κλεῖδες πρὸς μὲν τὸ ἀκρώμιον συμφυεῖς δέδενται, πρὸς δὲ τὸ στέρνον μίγμα ἄρθρου καὶ συμφύσεως δοκοῦσιν ποιεῖσθαι. ἐοίκασι δὲ τῷ σχήματι τῷ ῥωμαϊκῷ σίγμα S, καὶ αὐτῷ ἡπλωμένῳ. ἑξῆς δὲ πλευραί. δώδεκα γὰρ αἱ πᾶσαι καθ' ἑκάτερον πλευρόν. ἑπτὰ δὲ αὐτῶν πρός τε τοὺς τῆς ῥάχεως σπονδύλους καὶ πρὸς τὸ στέρνον συνάπτουσιν ἑκατέρωθεν. αἱ δὲ λοιπαὶ πέντε τῇ μὲν ῥάχει συμβάλλουσιν ἐκ τῶν ὄπισθεν, κατὰ δὲ τὰ ἔμπροσθεν εἰς ἀλλήλας ἀνανεύουσαι, χόνδρῳ συνδέονται. οἱ δὲ σπόνδυλοι εἰκοσιτέσσαρες μὲν οἱ πάντες. διαιροῦνται δὲ τραχήλου μὲν ἑπτά· νώτου δώδεκα· ὀσφύος δὲ πέντε. ἐπὶ πᾶσι δὲ τὸ ἱερὸν ὀστοῦν, δοκοῦν ἐκ σπονδύλων συγκεῖσθαι συμπεφυκότων ἀλλήλοις. τὸ δὲ στέρνον ὁμοίως καὶ αὐτὸ δοκεῖ ἐκ τῶν ἑπτὰ ὀστῶν συγκεῖσθαι, συμπεφυκότων ἀλλήλοις ἐν τῷ

rundam fententia duo in mento connata habet offa, nonnullorum unum. Caeterum dentes gomphofi junguntur, quippe alveolis infixi funt. Sunt autem numero triginta duo. Ex his quaterni primi in fuperiore atque inferiore maxilla, quia fecant, incifores nominantur: canini quatuor, maxillares feu molares viginti funt. Reliquorum offium claviculae ad fummum humerum coëuntes deligantur: ad pectus autem articuli et fymphyfeos mixtionem facere videntur et Romanae literae S, ejusque fimplicis figuram oftendunt. Dein coftae duodecim utroque latere habentur. Septem ex eis cum fpinae vertebris, cumque offe pectorali utrinque coëunt. Reliquae quinque a pofteriori parte fpinae inferuntur, parte anteriori in fefe invicem refupinatae, cartilagine colligantur. Vertebrae vero omnes quatuor et viginti funt. Septem in cervice, dorfi duodecim, quinque lumborum: poft omnes os facrum, quod ex vertebris invicem fymphyfi junctis conftare videtur. Quin et pectus fimiliter ex feptem offibus fymphyfi conjunctis

ξιφοειδεῖ σχήματι. βραχίων δὲ ἑκάτερος κατὰ ἄρθρον διήρμοσται τῷ τοῦ ὤμου. [376] ἐμβάλλει δὲ τῇ ἑαυτοῦ κεφαλῇ πλαγίως εἰς τὴν κοιλότητα τῆς ὠμοπλάτης. ἐπίκεινται δὲ αἱ ὠμοπλάται μυσὶν τοῖς ὑπεστρωμένοις ταῖς πλευραῖς ἐκ τῶν ὄπισθεν. πῆχυς δὲ καὶ κερκὶς παράκεινται μὲν ἀλλήλοις κατὰ σύμφυσιν, συμβάλλουσιν δὲ καὶ τοῦ βραχίονος τῇ ἑτέρᾳ κεφαλῇ κατ' ἄρθρον. τρισὶ μὲν γὰρ ἑαυτοῦ κονδύλοις εἰς τὴν σιγματοειδῆ τοῦ πήχεος ἀναγλυφὴν ἐναρμόζεται ὁ βραχίων. τῷ δὲ τετάρτῳ κονδύλῳ ὡς περὶ κνώδακα ἡ κερκὶς περιστρέφεται. καρποῦ δὲ τὰ ὀστᾶ τρία μὲν ὄντα πρὸς μὲν ἄλληλα συμφύσει δέδενται πρὸς δὲ πῆχυν καὶ κερκίδα κατ' ἄρθρον διήρμοσται. τὰ δὲ τοῦ μετακαρπίου πέντε ἐστίν· ἄρθρον δὲ καὶ αὐτὰ ποιεῖ πρὸς τὰ τοῦ καρποῦ, πρὸς ταῦτα γὰρ συμπέφυκε. τὰ δὲ τοῦ καρποῦ πρὸς μὲν αὐτὰ καὶ πρὸς τὰ τοῦ μετακαρπίου συμφύσει συνέχεται, πρὸς δὲ τὰς πρώτας τῶν δακτύλων σκυταλίδας κατ' ἄρθρον συμβάλλονται. δακτύλων δὲ σκυταλίδες μὲν καθ' ἕκαστον τρεῖς, κατ' ἄρθρον δὲ ἡ σύνθεσις αὐτῶν. μηροῦ δὲ

ensis figura structum esse apparet. At brachium utrumque cum humero conjungitur articulo. Porro suo ipsius capite oblique in scapularum sinum immittitur. Caeterum scapulae musculis qui posteriore parte costis substernuntur incumbunt Cubitus et radius symphysi quidem sese contingunt, articulo vero alteri brachii capiti committuntur. Tribus enim sui condylis brachium in cubiti sigmoeidem cavitatem inseritur. Quarto jam condylo radius veluti circa axem volvitur. Carpi ossa tria mutua symphysi deligata sunt: ad cubitum tamen et radium articulum apte faciunt. Metacarpii quinque ossa videre licet, articulum cum carpi ossibus, quibus connata sunt, explentia. Carpi ossa invicem et metacarpi ossibus symphysi junguntur continenturque. Caeterum cum primis digitorum intermediis articulo junguntur: digitorum vero internodia singulorum tria, quae articulo componuntur. Femoris os unum est, cujus caput leniter reflexum in coxae profundum sinum conjicitur Quam commissuram nervus, qui e

ἓν μὲν ὀστοῦν. συμβάλλει δὲ επικεκαμμένη μετρίως τῇ κεφαλῇ αὐτοῦ εἰς βαθεῖαν κοτύλην τοῦ ἰσχίου καὶ νεύρῳ ἀπήρτηται ἐκφυομένῳ ἐκ μέσης τῆς κοτύλης καὶ ἐμφυομένῳ εἰς μέσην τὴν κεφαλὴν τοῦ μηροῦ. τὰ δὲ ἰσχία δύο ὄντα ὀστᾶ, ἐκ μὲν τῶν ὄπισθεν κατὰ σύμφυσιν παράκεινται τῷ ἱερῷ ὀστῷ· ἐκ δὲ τῶν ἔμπροσθεν ἀλλήλοις, ἔνθα καὶ ἥβης ὀστᾶ καλεῖται. κνήμης δὲ ἑκατέρας, δύο μὲν τὰ ὀστᾶ, τότε τῆς κνήμης καὶ τὸ τῆς περόνης. οὐκ ἐξικνεῖται δὲ ἡ περόνη πρὸς τὸ κατὰ γόνυ ἄρθρον, ἀλλὰ μόνον τὸ τῆς κνήμης ἄκρον, τέσσαρας ἔχον ἐν αὐτῷ ἐπιπολαίους τύπους, εἰς οὓς ὑποδέχεται τοὺς τοῦ μηροῦ κονδύλους δύο ὄντας. ἐπίκειται δὲ αὐτοῖς ἡ ἐπιγονατὶς, ἐκ τῶν ἔμπροσθεν ὀστάριον στρογγύλον, ὑπόπλατυ οἷον ἀσπιδίσκιον συνέχον αὐτῶν τὴν συμβολὴν, διὰ τὸ ἐπιπολαίως συνηρθρῶσθαι. τῆς δὲ περόνης τὸ μὲν ἄνω ἄκρον συμπέφυκε κατὰ τοῦ ἀντικνημίου ὑπὸ τὴν ἐπίφυσιν, κατὰ δὲ τὰ σφυρὰ ἐπὶ πέρατα τοῦ ἀντικνημίου καὶ τῆς περόνης, πρὸς μὲν ἄλληλα συνδεῖται νευροχονδρώδει δεσμῷ. ἐπιβέβηκε δὲ τῷ ἀστραγάλῳ, ἐντὸς αὐτοῦ συνέχον τὰ ὀστᾶ. ὁ δὲ ἀστράγαλος κατὰ μῆκος τοῦ

medio ſinu prodit et in medium femoris caput inſeritur, continet. Coxae, quae duo ſunt oſſa a poſteriore parte, cum oſſe ſacro; priore inter ſe coaleſcentiam habent: ubi et pubis oſſa vel pectinis nominantur. Tibiae utriusque oſſa duo, nempe tibiae et fibulae: non pervenit autem fibula ad genu articulum, verum ſola tibiae ſummitas quatuor in ſe ſuperficiales ſinus obtinens, quibus duos femoris nodos excipit. His incumbit ab anteriore parte parvum os rotundum, ſublatum, ſcuti brevis inſtar, commiſſuram eorum continens, quod in ſummo coarctetur. Fibulae ſuperior extremitas anteriori tibiae parti ſub inſertione connectitur: juxta malleolos autem, qua deſinunt utraque tibiae oſſa, ligamento nerveo cartilaginoſoque invicem colligantur: caeterum intus talo incumbit intra ſe oſſa continens. Talus, juxta pedis longitudinem ſitus, ſibulae inſidet eique firmiter coaptatus eſt. Caeterum ti-

ποδὸς κείμενος τῇ μὲν περόνῃ ἐπιβέβηκε καὶ συνήρμοσται ἀκινήτως. τοῖς δὲ τῆς κνήμης ὀστοῖς καὶ τῷ σκαφοειδεῖ κατὰ τὰ ἐμπρόσθια αὐτοῦ μέρη συμβάλλει κατὰ ἄρθρον. τὸ δὲ σκαφοειδὲς καθὰ μὲν συμβάλλει τῷ ἀστραγάλῳ κεκοίλωται, ὡς σκαφοειδὲς δοκεῖν εἶναι. ἐκ δὲ τοῦ ἀντικειμένου κυρτὸν ὂν ἔχει τρίβους τρεῖς, αἷς δέχεται τὰ χαλκοειδῆ ὀστᾶ τρία ὄντα· τὸ δὲ κυβοειδὲς ἔξωθεν μὲν τὴν θέσιν ἔχει· συνήρθρωται δὲ πρὸς τὸ σκαφοειδὲς καὶ τὴν πτέρναν. ἔχει δὲ καὶ ἔκφυσιν ἐκ τῶν κάτω εἰς τὸ ἔμπροσθεν, ὑφ᾽ ἣν ὑπελήλυθε τοῦ ταρσοῦ τὸ ὀστοῦν, πρὸς τὸ ἀνέχειν αὐτό. εἶτα τὸ καλούμενον πεδίον ἐκ πέντε καὶ αὐτὸ συγκείμενον ὀστῶν· εἶτα ἐφεξῆς εἰσιν οἱ πέντε δάκτυλοι τοῦ ποδὸς, ἐκ τριῶν ἅπαντες φαλάγγων, ὁμοίως τοῖς κατὰ τὰς χεῖρας συγκείμενοι πλὴν τοῦ μεγάλου, μόνος γὰρ αὐτὸς ἐκ δύο ἐγένετο. συνάγουσι δὲ τὰς μὲν τούτων διαρθρώσεις ὑμενώδεις τινὲς σύνδεσμοι, τὰς δὲ κατὰ τὸν ἀστράγαλόν τε καὶ τὴν πτέρναν ἰσχυροί τε πάνυ καί τινες ἐξ αὐτῶν στρογγύλοι τε ἅμα καὶ νευροχονδρώδεις.

[377] Κεφ. ιγ΄. [Περὶ χυμῶν τε καὶ δυνάμεων καὶ

biae offibus, tum naviformi, in anteriore ipfius parte articulo committitur. Rurfus naviforme, ubi cum talo coit, excavatum eft, ut fcaphae fpeciem referre videatur. E regione gibbum calles tres habet, quibus offa chalcoeidea, quae tria funt, inferuntur: porro cuboides extrinfecus fitum eft: coarctatum eft autem naviformi offi et calci. Proceffum quoque ex inferiori ad priorem partem obtinet, quam plantae os retinendi ipfius gratia fubiit. Deinde os dictum metatarfus et ipfum quinque conftat offibus. Tum deinde quinque pedis digiti habentur, ex tribus omnes internodiis, fimiliter iis, qui in manu funt, compofitis, fi magnum excipias: is enim folus duobus conftat. Contrahunt autem horum juncturas membranofa quaedam ligamenta: talum et calcem valida admodum et quaedam ex iis rotunda, fimul et nervea cartilaginofaque.

Cap. XIII. [*De humoribus, facultatibus, morbis,*

νόσων καὶ διαφορῶν αὐτῶν καὶ αἰτιῶν καὶ θεραπειῶν.] Οἱ δὲ ἐν τῷ σώματι χυμοὶ ἐκ πρώτης γενέσεως τέσσαρες ὄντες συμμιγεῖς μέν εἰσιν ἀλλήλοις καὶ ἀνακεκραμένοι τῷ σώματι. πλεονάζει δὲ ἄλλος ἐν ἄλλῳ μᾶλλον τόπῳ, τὸ μὲν αἷμα ἐν καρδίᾳ, τὸ δὲ φλέγμα ἐν τῇ κεφαλῇ· ἡ ξανθὴ δὲ χολὴ ἐν ἥπατι· καὶ ἡ μέλαινα ἐν σπληνί. τοῦ δὲ ἐμφύτου πνεύματος διττὸν εἶδος. τὸ μὲν φυσικὸν, τὸ δὲ ψυχικόν. εἰσὶ δὲ οἳ καὶ τρίτον εἰσάγουσι, τὸ ἑκτικόν. ἑκτικὸν μὲν οὖν ἐστι πνεῦμα, τὸ συνέχον τοὺς λίθους. φυσικὸν δὲ τὸ τρέφον τὰ ζῶα καὶ τὰ φυτά. ψυχικὸν δὲ τὸ ἐπὶ τῶν ἐμψύχων αἰσθητικά τε ποιοῦν τὰ ζῶα καὶ κινούμενα πᾶσαν κίνησιν. ἵδρυται δὲ ἐν τοῖς ζώοις· ἐκ γὰρ τῶν τριῶν συνέστηκε τὰ ζῶα. τὸ μὲν οὖν ψυχικὸν ἐν τῇ κεφαλῇ κατῴκισται. τὸ δὲ φυσικὸν ἐν καρδίᾳ. τὸ δὲ ἑκτικὸν ἐν παντὶ τῷ σώματι. φυσικαὶ μὲν οὖν εἰσιν ἐνέργειαι, ἀπὸ πρώτης γενέσεως κύησις καὶ διάπλασις, ἐπὶ δὲ τῶν ἀποτεχθέντων ὄρεξις καὶ κατάποσις, ἡ ἐν τῷ στομάχῳ πέψις, ἀνάδοσις, ἐξαιμάτωσις, διάκρισις, θρέψις, αὔξησις. διακρίνεται δὲ ἐν τῷ σώματι σκύ-

eorum differentiis, causis ac curationibus.] Humores corporis ex prima generatione quatuor, commixti invicem et contemperati sunt corpori. Exuperat autem alius in alio magis loco, sanguis in corde, pituita in capite, flava bilis in jecinore, atra in liene. Caeterum duplex spiritus innati species, alius naturalis, alius animalis. Non desunt tamen qui et tertium hecticum introducant. Hecticus igitur est spiritus, qui lapides continet. Naturalis animantia et stirpes nutrit. Animalis sentiendi omnisque motus facultatem animanti exhibet: situs autem est in animantibus: nam his tribus animalium natura constat. Itaque animalis in capite sedem habet, naturalis in corde: hecticus in toto corpore versatur. Naturae actiones sunt, a prima generatione impraegnatio foetusque formatio: in editis appetitus, cibi deglutitio; in ventriculo concoctio, digestio, in sanguinem alteratio, segregatio, nutritio et actio. Excernuntur autem in corpore stercus, pituita, utraque

βαλον, φλέγμα, χολαὶ, οὖρον, ἱδρῶτες, μύξαι, σίαλον, γάλα. ψυχικαὶ δὲ δυνάμεις, αἴσθησίς τε καὶ προαίρεσις. αἰσθήσεις μὲν οὖν εἰσι πέντε, ἃς τὰ ζῶα παρέχει διὰ τῶν τοῦ σώματος ὀργάνων, ὅρασις, ἀκοὴ, γεῦσις, ὄσφρησις καὶ ἁφή. προαιρεῖται δὲ ἡ ψυχὴ, τὰ μὲν ἄνευ τοῦ σώματος λογιζομένη, ἢ ἐνθυμουμένη· μετὰ δὲ τοῦ σώματος προαιρεῖται, κινοῦσα αὐτὸ πρὸς ὑποδοχήν τινων, ἢ ἔκκρισιν, ἢ τὴν κατὰ τόπους κίνησιν· ἡ δὲ ἀναπνοὴ σύνθετός τις ἐνέργεια δοκεῖ εἶναι, πὴ μὲν κατὰ προαίρεσιν, πὴ δὲ ἀπροαιρέτως καὶ φυσικῶς γενομένη, ὡς ἐν τοῖς ὕπνοις. υγιαίνει τοίνυν ὁ ἄνθρωπος, τῶν μὲν πρώτων ἐξ ων συνέστηκε τῶν στοιχείων καὶ τῶν δευτέρων ἐξ ὧν διεπλάσθη τῶν τεσσάρων χυμῶν, ποσότητός τε συμμέτρως ἐχόντων πρὸς ἄλληλα καὶ ταῖς ποιότησιν εὐαρμόστως· τῶν δὲ στερεῶν σωμάτων, ἐξ ὧν σύγκειται, (380) μήτε διαιρουμένων, μήτε καταπυκνουμένων, μήτε ἐξισταμένων ἐκ τῆς αὐτῶν χώρας. τῶν δὲ πνευμάτων μήτε ἐπιτεινομένων ἄγαν, ὡς ἐπὶ τῶν φρενιτικῶν, μήτε ἐκλυομένων, ὡς ἐπὶ τῶν ληθαργικῶν, ἢ ἐπὶ τῶν ἐν καρδιακῇ

bilis, urina, ſudores, muci, ſaliva et lac. Animalis vero facultates, ſenſus et voluntas. Senſus quidem ſunt quinque, quibus animantia per corporis inſtrumenta funguntur, viſus, auditus, guſtus, odoratus et tactus. Eligit autem anima quaedam ſine corpore, ut quum ratiocinatur vel reminiſcitur. Cum corpore vero, ubi id ad quorundam receptionem vel excretionem vel ad loca movet. Reſpiratio compoſita quaedam actio eſſe videtur, partim ex arbitrio, partim ſponte et naturaliter, ut in ſomnis facta. Sanus igitur homo eſt, primis, unde conſtat, elementis et ſecundis, unde formatus eſt, quatuor humoribus, tum quantitate, tum qualitate mediocriter invicem contemperatis: ſolidis autem partibus, ex quibus compoſitus eſt, nec diviſis, nec condenſatis, nec e loco ſuo motis: ſpiritibus nec intenſis nimium, ut in phreniticis, nec diſſolutis, ut in lethargicis, vel in iis, qui cardiaco affectu tenentur. His enim hecticus ſpiritus reſolvi vide-

διαθέσει ὄντων· τούτοις γὰρ τὸ ἐκτικὸν πνεῦμα ἔοικεν ἐκλύεσθαι. ἐν ὑγείᾳ δὲ συντηρητέον τὸν ἄνθρωπον, τοῖς τε συνήθεσι γυμνασίοις χρώμενον καὶ τροφαῖς ταῖς κατὰ χώραν ἐν ἑκάστῃ ὥρᾳ τετηρημέναις, τὸ πλῆθος αὐτῶν μόνον φυλαττόμενον, ἐξ οὗ ἀπεψίαι γίνονται, ἀφ' ὧν αἱ νόσοι συνίστανται. προφυλακτέον δὲ τὰς νόσους μελλούσας γίνεσθαι ἢ ἔσεσθαι. εἰ μὲν ἐκ πλήθους, ἀποσιτίαν παραλαμβάνειν, ἢ κάθαρσιν, ἢ φλεβοτομίαν· εἰ δὲ ἀπὸ καμάτου καὶ ἐνδείας, ἀναπαῦσαι καὶ ὑποθρέψαι σύμφορον. αἱ δὲ νόσοι γίνονται πᾶσαι καθ' Ἱπποκράτην αἱ μὲν ἔξωθεν ἐκ τοῦ περιέχοντος, αἱ δὲ ἔσωθεν ἐκ τῶν διαιτημάτων, ἃ προσφερόμεθα, ὑφ' ὧν ἢ πλεονάζει τις τῶν τεσσάρων χυμῶν, ἢ ἐλλείπει, ἢ κατὰ ποιότητα μεταβάλλει. ὑπὸ δὲ τούτων καὶ τὰ ἔμφυτα πνεύματα ἃ μὲν ἐπιτείνεται ἄγαν, ἃ δὲ χαλᾶται εἰς ὑπερβολήν. τὰ δὲ στερεὰ σώματα καὶ ἔνδοθεν καὶ ἔξωθεν πολλὰς αἰτίας ἔχει τοῦ ὑπομένειν πλείονα πάθη. κατὰ δὲ Ἐρασίστρατον καὶ Ἀσκληπιάδην, ὡς ἐπίπαν μίαν αἰτίαν ἐπὶ πάσης νόσου, καθ' ὃν μὲν ἡ παρέμπτωσις

tur. Sanus autem homo conſervandus eſt conſuetis exercitiis et cibis patriis quolibet anni tempore obſervatis, copia eorum ſolum vitanda eſt, ex qua cruditates oriuntur, quae morbos pariunt. Praecavendi morbi ſunt, vel qui jam imminent, vel futuri ſunt. Si ex plenitudine proveniant, inedia vel purgatione vel venae inciſione curandi ſunt. Si ex labore et indigentia, quieti corpus dare et nutrire convenit. Verum univerſi morbi ex Hippocratis ſententia partim extrinſecus ex aëre nos ambiente, partim intrinſecus ex cibis et potu proficiſcuntur: a quibus humorum aliquis vel abundat, vel deficit, vel qualitatem commutat. Ab his etiam ſpiritus inſiti nunc intenduntur nimis, nunc plus aequo relaxantur. Solida vero corpora foris et intrinſecus multas cauſas habent plures affectus ſuſtinendi. Eraſiſtratus autem et Aſclepiades in univerſum unam omni morbo cauſam tribuunt: hic ſanguinis in arterias coincidentiam, ille corporeae

εἰς τὰς ἀρτηρίας τοῦ αἵματος· [378] καθ' ὃν δὲ ἡ ἔκτασις τῶν ὄγκων ἐν τοῖς ἀραιώμασιν. σημεῖα δὲ πλήθους νοσοποιοῦντος, κύρτωσις ἀγγείων καὶ ἔρευθος ἐπὶ τὸ πρόσωπον καὶ ὄγκος ὅλου τοῦ σώματος καὶ τῶν σφυγμῶν τὸ μέγεθος μετὰ εὐτονίας. ἐνδείας δὲ οὔσης σύμπτωσις τοῦ ὄγκου καὶ ἰσχνότης περὶ τὸ πρόσωπον καὶ μικροσφυξία μετ' ἀτονίας. τὸν μὲν οὖν πυρετὸν οἱ παλαιοὶ πάθος, αὐτὸν καθ' αὑτὸν ἡγοῦνται. Ἐρασίστρατος δὲ καὶ τῶν νεωτέρων τινὲς ἐπιγένημα. πυρετὸς δέ ἐστι τροπὴ ἐμφύτου θερμοῦ ἐπὶ τὸ καυσωδέστερον, διὰ τὸ ἔνδον ἀποστρέφεσθαι καὶ ἐμποδίζεσθαι διαπνεῖν. σημειούμεθα δὲ τοὺς πυρέττοντας ἐκ τῆς θερμῆς τῆς ἐπιτεταμένης καὶ ἀπροΐτου οὔσης καὶ τῶν σφυγμῶν ἐν ἀρχῇ μὲν εἰσβολῆς ἀμυδρᾶς καὶ ἀνωμάλου κινήσεως μετὰ πυκνότητος, ἐν ἀκμῇ δὲ σφοδροτάτης μετὰ ἐπάρσεως καὶ τάχους ὑπερβάλλοντος. κατὰ δὲ τοὺς νεωτέρους ἡ ἐκ βάθους ἀναφερομένη θερμασία πλείων τῆς κατὰ φύσιν, δακνώδης καὶ δριμεῖα καὶ ἐπίμονος, μετὰ τῆς τῶν σφυγμῶν πυκνότητός τε καὶ σκληρότητος οὖσα, τὸν πυρετὸν ἀφορίζει. εἴδη δὲ πυρετῶν κατὰ πάντας δύο, ὅ τε συν-

molis in raritate extenſionem. Plenitudinis morbum facientis notae ſunt vaſorum tumor, faciei rubor, totius corporis tumor et pulſuum magnitudo cum robore. Indigentiae ſigna, molis corporeae concidentia, gracilitas in facie et exiguus pulſus cum imbecillitate. Itaque febrim veteres ipſam per ſe affectum arbitrantur. Eraſiſtratus et recentiorum nonnulli ſymptoma. Febris igitur eſt nativi caloris in ardentiorem converſio, eo quod intro averſus perſpirare prohibeatur. Indicia febricitantium colligimus ex calore intenſo et intolerabili; tum in acceſſionis principio, ex languido, inaequali et crebro pulſuum motu: in ſtatu, ex vehementiſſimo motu elato et veloci admodum. Juniores calorem naturali magis ardentem, mordacem, acrem et conſtantem, cum pulſuum frequentia et duritie, ex alto venientem, ſebrem eſſe definiunt. Sunt autem duae ejus ſpecies ex omnium mente continua et intermittens. Continua eſt quae non ad integritatem prius quam morbus

δεχὴς καὶ διαλείπων. συνεχὴς μὲν οὖν ἐστιν ὁ εἰς ἀπυρεξίαν, πρὶν τελέως λυθῆναι τὸ νόσημα, μὴ παυόμενος. πάλιν δὲ τοῦ διαλείποντος εἴδη εἰσὶν ἓξ κατὰ τοὺς ἀρχαίους, ἀμφημερινὸς, τριταῖος, τεταρταῖος, πεμπταῖος, ἑβδομαῖος, ἐναταῖος. ἀμφημερινὸς μὲν οὖν ἐστιν ὁ καθ' ἑκάστην ἢ νύκτα, ἢ ἡμέραν ἐπισημαίνων, ἢ ἀνιέμενος. τριταῖος δὲ ὁ παρὰ μίαν. τεταρταῖος δὲ ὁ παρὰ δύο. πεμπταῖος δὲ ὁ παρὰ τρεῖς. ἑβδομαῖος ὁ παρὰ πέντε. ἐναταῖος ὁ παρὰ ἑπτά. ὁ ἡμιτριταῖος γὰρ ὅτε μὲν ἐν συνεχείᾳ ἐπιφαίνεται, ὅτε δὲ ἐν τοῖς διαλείπουσι τάττεται. τῶν δὲ ἄλλων νοσημάτων εἴδη δύο, εἴτε σὺν πυρετοῖς εἴη εἴτε ἄνευ πυρετοῦ. τὰ μὲν γάρ ἐστιν ὀξέα, τὰ δὲ χρόνια. ὀξέα μὲν οὖν ἐστι τάδε, φρενῖτις, καῦσος, συνάγχη, πλευρῖτις, περιπνευμονία, καρδιακὴ διάθεσις, ἴκτερος, χολέρα, εἰλεὸς, κωλικὴ διάθεσις, ἀποπληξία, τέτανος, ὀπισθότονος ἐμπροσθότονος. τὰ μὲν οὖν ὀξέα ὡς ἐπίπαν ὑπό τε αἵματος καὶ χολῆς ξανθῆς συνίσταται, πλεοναζόντων ἔν τισι μέρεσι τοῦ σώματος, ἐν οἷς νοσοποιοῦσιν ἐκτρεπομένων ἐπὶ τὸ κάκιον, τὰ δὲ χρόνια ὑπὸ φλέγματος καὶ με-

ex toto ſolutus ſit venit. Intermittentis rurſum ſex ſpecies invenimus apud veteres, quotidianam, tertianam, quartanam, quintanam, ſeptimanam et nonanam. Quotidiana eſt, quae ſingulis diebus aut noctibus acceſſionem vel deceſſionem facit. Tertiana unum diem praeſtat integrum, tertio redit. Quartana duos dies intermittit, deinde revertitur. Quintana tres: ſeptimana quinque. Nonana ſeptem. Nam ſemitertiana modo inter continuas, modo inter intermittentes ponitur. Jam vero reliquorum morborum duo genera ſunt, vel cum febribus, vel ſine febribus. Quidam enim acuti, quidam longi ſunt. Acuti quidem hi, phrenitis, febris ardens, angina, pleuritis, peripneumonia, cardiacus affectus, regius morbus, cholera, volvulus, colicus dolor, apoplexia, tetanus, opiſthotonus, emproſthotonus. Acuti igitur a ſanguine fere et flava bile, in nonnullis corporis partibus, quas ii male habent humores, ſuperfluis et in deterius verſis conſtituuntur. Longi a pituita et atra bile, ſimiliter vel copioſioribus quam

λαίνης χολῆς ὁμοίως, ἢ πληθυνόντων πολὺ παρὰ τὸ κατὰ φύσιν, ἢ μεταβαλλόντων ἐπὶ τὸ δριμύτατον. θεραπευτέον δὲ τοὺς ἐκ πλήθους νοσοῦντας, κατὰ μὲν δίαιταν ἀφαιροῦντά τε τὸν ἐκ πλήθους νοσοῦντα, ἢ δι' ἀσιτίας, ἢ διὰ καθάρσεως, ἢ διὰ φλεβοτομίας. προστιθέντα δὲ καὶ προσφέροντα τοῖς ἐξ ἐνδείας εἰς τὴν νόσον ἐμπεσοῦσιν, οἷς δὲ ἀπεψία καὶ δριμύτης ὑγρῶν αἰτία ἐστὶ, συμπέττειν δεῖ ταῖς ἐπιβροχαῖς καὶ τοῖς καταπλάσμασι, κατακεραννύναι δὲ τὰ δριμέα καὶ εὐχύλοις καὶ ὑγραινούσαις τροφαῖς χρῆσθαι. οἱ δὲ καιροὶ τῶν βοηθημάτων ἔν τε ὅλῳ τῷ νοσήματι καὶ ταῖς μερικαῖς ἐπισημασίαις εἰσὶ τέσσαρες, ἀρχὴ, ἀνάβασις, ἀκμὴ, παρακμή. ἐν ἀρχῇ μὲν ὅλου τοῦ νοσήματος ἀποσιτία ἁρμόζει μέχρι τῆς διὰ τρίτης. ἐφ' ὧν δὲ καὶ ἀρχὴ παντὸς μέχρι τῆς διὰ τρίτης. φλεβοτομίαν δὲ ἐν ἀρχῇ μὲν κρίνουσιν οἱ νεώτεροι, μέχρι τῆς διὰ τρίτης, οἱ δὲ παλαιοὶ καὶ μετὰ τὴν τρίτην παραλαμβάνουσιν, ἐὰν τὰ τῆς δυνάμεως ὑφεστήκῃ καὶ τὸ νόσημα ἀπαιτῇ. τροφῆς δὲ καιρὸς μετὰ τὴν διάτριτον κατὰ τοὺς νεωτέρους, κατὰ δὲ τοὺς παλαιοὺς οὐκ

naturae modus exigit, vel in acerrimam qualitatem immutatis. Qui jam ex copia laborant, victus ratione vel inedia vel purgatione vel venae inciſione curandi ſunt. Qui ex abſtinentia in morbum incidere, alimentis eos reſtituere convenit. Quibus incoctio et humorum acrimonia morbi cauſam fecerunt, iis fomentis et cataplasmatis concoctio paranda eſt. Acria contemperanda ſunt et cibis boni ſucci atque humectantibus uti oportet. Caeterum quatuor in toto morbo particularibusque acceſſionibus tempora auxiliis afferendis dicata ſunt, initium, incrementum, vigor et inclinatio. Principio totius morbi inedia triduana convenit, quibus et in totum abſtinere triduo conducit. Venae ſectionem in initio recentiores ad tertium usque diem ſtatuunt: veteres etiam poſt tertium diem praecipiunt, ſi vires ſuppetant et morbus poſtulet. Nutrimenti tempus a triduo juniores: antiqui non omnibus, ſed iis, qui copia laborant, tum junioribus tum ſenioribus inſtituunt. Pueros ſtatim morbo invadente nutriunt.

ἐπὶ πάντων, ἀλλ' ἐπὶ τῶν ἐκ πλήθους νοσούντων καὶ ἐπὶ νέων καὶ ἐπὶ πρεσβυτέρων. ἐπὶ δὲ παιδίων ἀπ' ἀρχῆς τρέφουσιν καὶ ἐφ' ὧν ἔθος τοιοῦτον, ἢ διὰ χώραν, ἢ διὰ τὸ περιέχον. πρὸ δὲ τῆς τροφῆς τῶν μετὰ τὴν πρώτην διάτριτον ἐπιβροχαῖς χρηστέον τῆς κεφαλῆς καὶ τῶν μέσων. [379] ταῖς δὲ ἑξῆς καταπλάσμασι καὶ κλύσμασι. τὰς δὲ οὖν ἐμβροχὰς ἀεὶ καὶ τὰς ἐπὶ τῶν μέσων θερμὰς παραληπτέον καὶ ἁπλᾶς ἑψοῦντας κύμινον ἢ ξυλάνηθον, τὰς δὲ ἐπὶ κεφαλὴν θερμὰς μὲν ἐπὶ ληθάργου καὶ πάσης καταφορᾶς, ἐμψυχούσας δὲ ἐπὶ φρενιτίδων καὶ ἐπὶ παντὸς πυρετοῦ ὀξέος· τῶν δὲ καταπλασμάτων τὰ μὲν διὰ μόνου μέλιτος καὶ ἐλαίου κατασκευάζεται καὶ καλεῖται μαλακτικὰ, τὰ δὲ δι' ὑδρελαίου, ἅπερ ὀνομάζουσιν ὠμὴν λύσιν, τὰ δὲ ἐμπασσόμενα τούτοις, οἷά ἐστι γῦρις καὶ λινόσπερμον καὶ τῆλις. οἱ δὲ κλυσμοὶ δι' ὑδρελαίου καὶ μέλιτος καὶ ἁλῶν καὶ νίτρου βραχέος. καιρὸς δὲ τούτων ὁ πρὸ τῆς τροφῆς ἐν ἀνέσει τῶν ἐπισημασιῶν καὶ παρακμῇ. ἐπὶ δὲ τῶν συνεχῶν ὁ ὄρθρος. φρενῖτις μὲν οὖν ἐστιν ἔκστασις διανοίας μετὰ παρακοπῆς σφοδρᾶς καὶ χειρῶν ἀλόγου περιφορᾶς καὶ κροκυ-

Praeterea illos, quibus hujusmodi confuetudo eft, vel loci vel aëris circumflui gratia. Ante cibum, poft triduum primum, perfufiones capitis et praecordiorum ex ufu funt; fequentibus diebus cataplasmata et clyfteres. Perfufiones igitur in praecordiis calidas femper affumere oportet et fimplices ex cumini vel xylanethi decocto: ad caput calefacientes quidem in lethargo et in omni gravi fopore: refrigerantes autem in phrenitide et quavis acuta febre conveniunt. Cataplasmata quaedam folo melle et oleo conficiuntur, vocanturque emollientia. Quaedam ex aqua, cui oleum fit adjectum, fiunt, quae crudam dilutionem nominant. Alia his infperguntur, veluti pollen, lini femen et foenumgraecum. Clyfteres hydrelaeo, melle, fale et nitro modico praeparantur. Tempus eorum ante cibum eft, dum acceffiones remittuntur et inclinant. In continuis morbis diluculum. Phrenitis eft mentis alienatio. Notae funt, infania vehemens, temeraria manuum gefticulatio,

δισμοῦ καὶ καρφολογίας καὶ πυρετοῦ ὀξέος. γίνεται δὲ ἐξ αἰτίας ὡς ἐπὶ πολὺ χολῆς. συνίσταται δὲ περὶ ἐγκέφαλον, ἢ μήνιγγας, ἢ ὥς τινες λέγουσι περὶ φρένας, ὃ διάφραγμα καλεῖται. θεραπεία δὲ ἁρμόδιος ἥδε. εἰ μὲν προγνοίη τις ἐν ἀρχῇ διὰ φλεβοτομίας καὶ σικύας, ἀφαίρεσις δὲ καὶ κλυσμὸς καὶ ἀποσιτία ἁρμόδιος. ἐνστάντος δὲ τοῦ πάθους ἐπιβροχαὶ καρωτικαί τε καὶ ὑπνωτικὰ ἐπιχρίσματα καὶ τροφαὶ ὑγραίνουσαι. ὁ δὲ καῦσος εἶδος μέν ἐστι πυρετοῦ, τέτακται δὲ ὑπὸ μὲν Ἱπποκράτους ἐν τοῖς ὀξέσιν, ὡς τεταρταῖος ἐν τοῖς χρονίοις, ὑπὸ δὲ τῶν νεωτέρων οὐκ ἔτι. συνίσταται δὲ ἐκ χολῆς, οὐκ ἄγαν ξηρᾶς περὶ τὰ φλέβια, τὰ κατὰ τὸ ἧπαρ. θεραπεύεται δὲ φλεβοτομίᾳ ἐν ἀρχῇ καὶ ψυχροῦ δόσει ἐν ἀκμῇ, ἢ πόμασιν ἐμψύχουσιν, ἢ ἐπιθέσεσιν, οἷόν ἐστι τὸ δι' ὑδρελαίου ζεστοῦ. κυνάγχη δὲ καὶ συνάγχη φλεγμοναί εἰσι περὶ τὸν τράχηλον, ἡ μὲν περὶ τὸ ἐντὸς αὐτοῦ ὀξέως πνίγουσα, ἡ κυνάγχη· ἡ δὲ συνάγχη εἰς τὰ ἐκτὸς μᾶλλον νεύουσα καὶ διὰ τοῦτο ἧττον πνίγουσα καὶ ἧττον κινδυνώδης ἐστί. γίνεται δὲ ἑκάτερον πάθος ἢ ὑπὸ

floccorum et feftucarum collectio et febris acuta. Caufam habet magna ex parte bilem. Conftituitur in cerebro vel ejus membranis vel in fepto transverfo, quod diaphragma nominatur. Curatio haec convenit. Initio fi praescius fueris, venae incifio, cucurbitulae conveniunt, fubtractio et clyfter et abftinentia conveniens: inftante autem morbo perfufiones foporiferae, inunctiones, quibus fomnus accerfitur et humectantes cibi conducunt. Caufus febris fpecies ab Hippocrate quidem inter acutos, ut quartana inter longos morbos refertur, a recentioribus non item. Oritur ex bile non nimis ficca, circa venas quae ad jecur funt. Curatur in principio fanguinis miffione: in ftatu frigidae tum aliorum, quae refrigerandi vim obtinent, potio confert, vel epithema cujusmodi ex ferventi hydrelaeo praeparatur. Angina eft circa cervicem inflammatio. Ejus fpeciem unam cynanchen appellant, quae in interiore ipfius parte orta fubito ftrangulat: alteram fynanchen: haec in exteriorem partem incumbit, eoque minus ftran-

(381) χολῆς, ἢ ὑπὸ φλέγματος ἁλμυροῦ. συνίσταται δὲ ὁτὲ μὲν σὺν πυρετῷ ὀξεῖ, ὁτὲ δὲ χωρὶς πυρετοῦ. θεραπεία δὲ ἡ μὲν γενναιοτάτη καὶ ὀξυτάτη εὐθὺς ἐν ἀρχῇ διὰ φλεβοτομίας, μετὰ δὲ ταῦτα διὰ τῶν ἀποφλεγματιζόντων φαρμάκων καὶ τῶν ἔξωθεν ἐπιτιθεμένων κηρωτῶν. Ἀσκληπιάδης δὲ ἐπὶ τῶν ἄκρως πνιγομένων καὶ λαρυγγοτομεῖ. πλευρῖτις δέ ἐστι φλεγμονὴ περὶ τὸ πλευρὸν ἐκ τῶν ἔνδον, μετὰ πυρετοῦ ὀξέος καὶ ἀλγημάτων σφοδρῶν καὶ βηχός. γίνεται δὲ ὑπὸ χολῆς μάλιστα. θεραπεία δὲ ἐν ἀρχῇ μὲν φλεβοτομία, εἶτα ἡ διὰ τῶν καταπλασμάτων καὶ ξηρῶν πυριῶν, οἷον κέγχρων καὶ ἁλῶν τρίτη ἡ διὰ τῶν ἀνακαθαιρόντων ἔνδοθεν φαρμάκων πλευριτικῶν ἐπιγραφομένων. φυλάττεσθαι δὲ ἐπὶ τούτων τὰς τῆς κοιλίας ῥύσεις. ἡ δὲ περιπνευμονία τοῖς μὲν δοκεῖ φλεγμονὴ βαρεῖα εἶναι περὶ πνεύμονα καὶ τῷ βάρει τοῦτο διαδείκνυται. τοῖς δὲ οὐ δοκεῖ ὁ πνεύμων δύνασθαι φλεγμαίνειν, τὰ πλησίον δὲ αὐτοῦ φασὶν ἐν τοιαύτῃ διαθέσει γινόμενα οὕτως ὀνομάζεσθαι αὐτὴν ποιεῖ. συνίσταται δὲ τὸ πάθος τοῦτο μετὰ πυρετοῦ ὀξέος καὶ ὑπὸ

gulat minusque periculofa eft. Uterque affectus vel a bile vel a pituita falfa nafcitur, idque nonnunquam cum febre acuta, nonnunquam fine febri. Remedium et generofiffimum et praefentiffimum eft fanguinis ftatim in principio miffio: deinde medicamenta pituitam per os educentia et cerata foris impofita. Afclepiades ultimum auxilium pofuit in iis qui maxime fuffocantur laryngem incidere. Pleuritis lateris ab interiore parte inflammatio eft. Huic febris acuta, dolor vehemens et tuffis accedit: a bile potiffimum generatur. Praefidio eft in initio adhibita venae incifio: deinde cataplasmata et ficca fomenta, nempe milii et falis: poftremo medicamenta intrinfecus purgantia, quae pleuritica nominantur. Cavenda vero in his funt ventris profluvia. Peripneumonia nonnullis auctoribus inflammatio gravis eft circa pulmonem, idque gravitate oftenditur. Quibusdam pulmo inflammationem pati non poffe videtur, fed vicina ejus loca, cum in difpofitione ejusmodi funt, ea ut ita nominetur faciunt. Habet au-

τῶν αὐτῶν αἰτίων ὧν ἡ πλευρῖτις· κατὰ δέ τινας ὑπὸ φλέγματος. θεραπεία δὲ τὰ πολλὰ ὁμοία τῇ πλευρίτιδι. ἡ δὲ καρδιακὴ διάθεσις οὐκ ἀπὸ τοῦ περὶ καρδίαν εἶναι τὸ πάθος οὕτως ὠνομάσθη, ἀλλ' ἐπεὶ καρδίαν οἱ παλαιοὶ τὸν στόμαχον ἐκάλουν. τούτου δὲ ἀναλυομένου ἐν πυρετῷ ὀξεῖ συμβαίνει τοὺς κάμνοντας διαφορεῖσθαι. γίνεται δὲ τὸ πάθος ὡς ἐπὶ τὸ πολὺ μὲν ἐκ τῶν ἀμέτρων ἀποσιτιῶν, ἢ ἐκ φλεβοτομίας ἀκαί- [380] ρου, ἤ τινος ἀφαιρέσεως ἀλόγου παραληφθείσης. διὸ τροφῆς δέονται τῆς εὐαναδότου καὶ ἀναθερμαινούσης, ὥσπερ δι' οἴνου καὶ χιόνος καὶ τῶν στερεῶν ὅσα τροφιμώτερα καὶ τὸν στόμαχον τονοῦν δυνάμενα. ἔστι δὲ ὅτε καὶ φλεγμαινόντων τῶν ἔνδον, μάλιστα δὲ τοῦ ἥπατος, τοῦτο γίνεται, ὅτε τοὐναντίον, ἀφαιρέσεως δεῖται καὶ καταπλάσεως τῆς ἐπὶ τῶν φλεγμαινόντων. ἴκτερος δέ ἐστιν ἀνάχυσις χολῆς εἰς τὴν ἐπιφάνειαν, ὁτὲ μὲν σὺν πυρετῷ ὀξεῖ, ὁτὲ δὲ καὶ ἄνευ πυρετοῦ, μετὰ ἐγκαύσεως τῶν ἔνδον καὶ κακοστομαχίας. δεῖται δὲ, εἰ μὲν τὰ μέσα φλεγμαίνει, καταπλασμάτων πρῶτον καὶ εἰ πλῆθος ὑποκέοιτο φλε-

tem hic morbus febrem acutam comitem. Eadem ipfius caufa, quae pleuritidem concitat, fecundum alios tamen pituita. Remedium fere huic cum fuperiore malo commune eft. Cordis affectus nominatur, non quod in corde affectus fit, fed quoniam ftomachum veteres cor appellabant, quo in febri acuta refoluto, aegrotos immodice diffolvi contingit. Accidit fere ex immodica abftinentia vel parum tempeftiva venarum fectione vel cum aliquid praeter rationem corpori adimitur. Quare alimento, quod facile diftribui queat et recalfacere, fuccurrendum eft: quemadmodum ex vino ac nive: cibo qui ex valentiore materia eft et ftomachum corroborare poteft. Eft cum vifceribus inflammatis, potiffimum jecinore, hic morbus eveniat: cum e contrario ablatione et cataplasmatis inflammationi dicatis opus eft. Regius morbus eft bilis in fummam cutem redundantia. Interim cum febri acuta oboritur, interim fine illa, cum interiorum aduftione et ftomachi vitio. Si praecordia inflammantur, cataplasmata

βοτομίας, εἰ δὲ μὴ, τῶν τὴν χολὴν κενούντων ἢ διὰ κοιλίας καὶ ἐντέρων, ἢ δι' οὔρων, ἢ διὰ ῥινῶν, ἢ δι' ἱδρώτων. ἡ δὲ χολέρα διττή ἐστι καθ' Ἱπποκράτην, ἡ μὲν ὑγρὰ, ἣν καὶ πολλοὶ ἴσασι μετ' ἐκκρίσεως σφοδρᾶς καὶ χολώδους καὶ κάτωθέν τε καὶ ἄνωθεν καὶ στροφῶν χαλεπῶν μετὰ τῶν ἐπιγινομένων σπασμῶν καὶ συνολκῶν κατὰ τὰς γαστροκνημίας μάλιστα· ἐπιμέλεια δὲ ἐπιβροχῶν μὲν θερμῶν κατὰ τῶν συνελκομένων· καὶ λουτροῦ μετὰ τὴν ἀποκάθαρσιν καὶ τροφῆς εὐδιοικήτου τε καὶ εὐανοδότου καὶ εὐστομάχου. τὸ δὲ ἕτερον εἶδος ξηρὰν χολέραν καλεῖ ὁ Ἱπποκράτης, ὑπὸ μὲν τοῦ αὐτῷ αἰτίου γινομένην καὶ περὶ τὰ αὐτὰ συνισταμένην, ἄνευ μέντοι ῥύσεως κοιλίας καὶ ἐμέτων. διὸ καὶ δεῖται προανέσεώς τε καὶ διὰ καταπλασμάτων καὶ οὐ προσφορᾶς, ἀλλὰ τοὐναντίον ἐνδείας. εἰλεὸς δὲ καὶ κωλικὴ διάθεσις φλεγμοναί εἰσιν ἐντέρων, ἡ μὲν τοῦ λεπτοῦ, ἡ δὲ τοῦ κώλου. διὸ καὶ ἀποκλείεται τά τε διαχωρήματα καὶ αἱ φῦσαι ἐνειλούμεναι τοῖς ἐντέροις, τῷ μὴ ἔχειν τὴν ἔξοδον,

primum defiderant: fi copia fubfit, venae fectionem: fin minus, medicamenta, quae bilem evacuant aut ventris ductione et inteftinorum, aut per urinas aut per fudores aut per nares. Cholera duplex eft fecundum Hippocratem: altera humida, in qua, uti omnes norunt, vehemens eft excretio, bilis fupra infraque erumpit, inteftina graviter torquentur. Accedunt convulfiones, faepe etiam crurum furae contrahuntur. Remedio contractionibus funt perfufiones calidae in iis, quae contrahuntur, balneum poft expurgationem, tum alimenta, quae ex facili difponuntur digeruntur que et ftomachum adjuvant. Alteram ficcam choleram vocat Hippocrates, ab eadem provenientem caufa ac circa eadem confiftentem, at citra ventris fluorem et vomitum. Ideoque remiffionem praecedentem et per cataplasmata requirit, nec cibi ingeftione, fed contra inedia opus eft. Volvulus et colicus dolor inteftinorum inflammationes funt, quorum alter tenuioris, alter plenioris. Quare dejectiones includuntur et flatus inteftinis involuti,

ἀλγήματα σφοδρὰ παρέχουσι καὶ στρόφους. ὀξύτερον δὲ καὶ τῇ διαθέσει καὶ τοῖς συμπτώμασιν ὁ εἰλεὸς καὶ κινδυνωδέστερος. ἔμετοί τε γίνονται τῶν εἰλεωδῶν, τοῖς ἐσχάτως ἔχουσιν ἑκάτερον τὸ πάθος. ἐν ἀρχῇ μὲν φλεβοτομίᾳ ὁ εἰλεὸς μάλιστα ἰᾶται, τὰ πολλὰ δὲ ἀσιτίαις καὶ καταπλάσμασι τοῖς ἀνιεῖσι καὶ λύουσι τὰς φλεγμονάς. ἐνεργέστερον δὲ βοηθεῖ τὰ ἔνδοθεν ἐνιέμενα κωλικὰ φάρμακα. τῶν τε γὰρ ἀλγημάτων ῥύεται καὶ ὕπνον ἐπάγει καὶ τὴν διαχώρησιν κινεῖ. ἀποπληξία δὲ γίνεται μὲν διὰ πλῆθος ὑγρῶν παχέων, ἐμφραττόντων τὰ ἀπὸ τῆς κεφαλῆς ἀγγεῖα, τὰ διαδιδόντα εἰς πᾶν τὸ σῶμα τὴν αἴσθησιν καὶ τὴν κίνησιν, διὸ καὶ ἀναίσθητοι καὶ ἄφωνοι καὶ ἀκίνητοι γίνονται ἀπόπληκτοι. λέγει δὲ Ἱπποκράτης περὶ τοῦδε τοῦ πάθους. ἀποπληξίην ἰσχυρὴν μὲν λύειν ἀδύνατον, ἀσθενέα δὲ οὐ ῥηΐδιον. φλεβοτομεῖν δὲ εὐθὺς τοὺς κεκρατημένους, ἐὰν καὶ τὰ τῆς ἡλικίας συνᾴδῃ καὶ ἡ δύναμις ὑπακούῃ. τέτανος δὲ καὶ ὀπισθότονος καὶ ἐμπροσθότονος περὶ τὰ νεῦρα πάθη. εἶδος δέ ἐστιν ἑκάτερον σπασμοῦ τῶν ἀπὸ τῆς κεφαλῆς νεύρων, δι᾽ ὧν τὴν

eo quod exitum non habent, dolores vehementes et tormina concitant. Volvulus autem difpofitione et accidentibus acutior, magisque periculofus eft. Alterutro autem morbo extreme laborantibus vomitus concitantur. Auxilium eft volvuli maxime fanguinis miffio per initium, plerumque abftinentia et cataplasmata mitigantia et inflammationem difcutientia. Efficacius juvant medicamenta, quae colica nominant, intro per fedem immiffa. Nam dolores auferunt, fomnum conciliant et alvum movent. Apoplexia ex humorum crafforum copia generatur, qui capitis vafa, unde corpori fentiendi movendique facultas advenit, obftruunt. Quamobrem apoplexia correpti fenfu, voce et motu privantur. Hippocrates de hoc vitio fcribit, *Apoplexiam*, inquiens, *validam folvere non licet*, *imbecillem haud facile*. Sanguis mittendus ftatim jam oppreffis, fi modo et aetas confentiat et vires fuftineant. Tetanus, opifthotonus et emprofthotonus, nervorum morbi exiftunt: verum utraque fpecies eft convulfionis nervorum, qui a

κίνησιν διαδίδωσιν εἰς τὸ σῶμα. γίνεται δὲ δι' ἔμφραξιν ὑγρῶν παχέων τῶν νεύρων, ὁτὲ μὲν εἰς τοὔπισθεν, ὥστε μὴ συννεύειν, καὶ καλεῖται ὀπισθότονος, ὁτὲ δὲ τῶν εἰς τὸ ἔμπροσθεν, ὥστε μὴ ἀνανεύειν, καὶ καλεῖται ἐμπροσθότονος, ὁτὲ δὲ ἐπ' εὐθείας, ὥστε μὴ συγκάμπτεσθαι, καὶ τέτανος προσωνόμασται. θεραπεύεται δὲ ὑπὸ φλεβοτομίας, εἰ πλῆθος ὑπόκειται, ὡς ὁ παρ' Ἱπποκράτει καταπεσὼν καὶ τὴν κεφαλὴν τραυματισθείς. ἴαται δὲ αὐτοὺς καὶ ψυχροῦ πολλοῦ κατάχυσις, θέρους ὥρᾳ μάλιστα, εἰ μὴ ἰσχνὸς, ἀλλ' εὔσαρκος εἴη ὁ πάσχων. θέρμης γὰρ ἐπανάκλησιν ποιεῖται. [381] ὡς δὲ οἱ πολλοὶ χρῶνται κηρώμασι τοῖς ἠρέμα θερμαίνουσι καὶ χαλῶσι καὶ ἀλείμμασι τοῖς ὁμοίοις καὶ ἐρίων ἠλαιωμένων ἐπιθέσει καὶ πυρίαις καὶ καταπλάσμασι θερμοῖς. χρόνια δὲ πάθη περὶ τὰ ἐντὸς συνίσταται τάδε. κεφαλαία, ἐπιληψία, ἴλιγγοι, σκοτώματα, μανία, μελαγχολία, λήθαργος, κόρυζα, βράγχος, κατάῤῥους, αἵματος ἀναγωγὴ, ἐμπύημα ἐν θώρακι, φθίσις, απόστημα ἐν μεσοπλευρίῳ, ἀπόστημα ἐν κατακλεῖσιν, ἠπατικὴ διάθεσις, τεινεσμὸς, δυσεν-

capite descendentes corpori motum distribuunt. Nam si viscosi humores eos obstruant, affectio talis oritur. Quae si scapulis caput annectat, quo minus possit annuere, opisthotonum: quum mentum pectori contrahit, ut renuere nequeas, emprosthotonum: quum rectam et immobilem cervicem tendit, tetanum appellant. Sanat venae sectio, si copia subest: ut videre licet apud Hippocratem in illo, qui prolapsus vulnus in caput acceperat. Medetur enim eis et frigidae copiosae infusio, si aestas sit, praesertim si non gracilis, sed quadratus existat aeger: nam caloris revocationem molitur. Multi sane ceratis modice recalfacientibus et relaxantibus utuntur, ad haec inunctionibus similibus, necnon lanis oleo imbutis, atque impositis et fomentis et cataplasmatis calidis. Longi morbi interioribus accidunt hi, cephalaea, morbus comitialis, vertigines, oculorum caligationes, insania, melancholia, lethargus, distillatio, raucitas, gravedo, sanguinis eruptio, suppuratio in thorace, tabes, abscessus in medio latere, abscessus in

τερία, ἕλμινθες αἱ πλατεῖαι, ἕλμινθες αἱ στρογγύλαι, ἀσκαρίδες, ἰσχιὰς, ἀρθρῖτις, ποδάγρα, ἐλεφαντίασις. δοκεῖ δὲ τῶν ἐκτὸς εἶναι. τῶν οὖν χρονίων κεφαλαία ἐστὶ κεφαλῆς ἄλγημα ἐνδιάθετον περιοδικῶς ἐνίοτε, τὰ πολλὰ κινούμενον, ὑπὸ φλέγματος γινόμενον, ὁτὲ δὲ εἰς ἓν μέρος τῆς κεφαλῆς τὸ ἄλγημά ἐστι καὶ καλεῖται ἑτεροκρανία ἴασις δὲ ἀμφοτέρων δι' ἀφαιρέσεως αἵματος, ἢ διὰ σικύας ἐπὶ τὸ ἰνίον καὶ ἀποφλεγματισμοῦ καὶ διὰ κοιλίας κάθαρσιν καὶ ἐπιθεμάτων, ὅσα ἀναγράφεται ἐν καταπλάσματος τρόπῳ, ἢ ἐν μαλάγμασιν, ἢ ἐπιχρίσμασιν, τὸ δὲ τελευταῖον σιναπισμῷ ἀναξηραίνεται τὸ αἴτιον. ἐπιληψία δὲ, ἣν καὶ ἱερὰν νόσον καλοῦσι, συνίσταται μὲν περὶ τὰς ἀρχὰς τῶν ἀπὸ κεφαλῆς νεύρων, δι' ὧν ἡ αἴσθησις καὶ ἡ κίνησις εἰς πᾶν τὸ σῶμα διαδίδοται. αἰτία δὲ τοῦ πάθους, ὡς ὁ Πλάτων καὶ Ἱπποκράτης φασὶ, φλέγμα καὶ χολὴ μέλαινα, διὸ καταπίπτουσιν οἱ τῷ πάθει ἐχόμενοι, ἐμφραττομένων αὐτοῖς τῶν ὁδῶν τῆς τε αἰσθήσεως καὶ τῆς κινήσεως, ἀφρῶσι δὲ διὰ τὸν κλόνον τῶν ὑγρῶν, ὃς γίνεται ἀπὸ τοῦ σπασμοῦ τῶν νεύρων, διὸ

claviculis, jecinoris affectus, tenesmus, dyſenteria, lumbrici lati, lumbrici rotundi, aſcarides: coxarum dolor, articularis morbus, podagra, elephantiaſis ad exteriores partes ſpectare videntur. Ex longis morbis cephalaea internus capitis dolor eſt, qui in circuitu interdum affligit a pituita naſcens: interim unam capitis partem infeſtat: tunc heterocraniam nominant. Auxilium utriusque eſt ſanguinis detractio, vel cucurbitulae occipitio impoſitae, eductio pituitae per os, per alvum purgatio et epithemata, quae inter cataplasmata vel malagmata vel illitus inſcribuntur, poſtremo cauſa ejus ſinapismo reſiccatur. Morbus comitialis, quem et ſacrum vocant, circa nervorum, qui a capite deſcendentes ſenſum motumque univerſo corpori diſtribuunt, originem conſiſtit. Cauſam ejus Plato et Hippocrates pituitam et bilem atram indicant. Homo concidit, qui hoc malo detinetur, quoniam ei ſentiendi movendique meatus obturantur, ſpuma iis os ob humorum commotionem, quae a nervorum convulſione provenit. Qua de

Ed. Chart. II. [381.] Ed. Baf. IV. (381. 382.)

ἔστιν ὅτε καὶ οὖρον ἐκκρίνουσιν ἀπροαιρέτως. ἴαται δὲ τὸ πάθος ἐπὶ μὲν τῶν πρὸ ἥβης παίδων, ἡ φύσις ἐκλάμψασα περὶ ἥβην καὶ κρίσιν τοῦ νοσήματος ἐργασαμένη, τῷ ἐμφύτῳ θερμῷ ἀναξηράνασα τὰ αἴτια. τοῖς δὲ μετὰ τὴν ἥβην δυσίατον, ἢ καὶ ἀνίατον τὸ πάθημα. τὰ δὲ σκοτώματα καὶ αἱ ἴλιγγες συγ- (382) γενῆ ἐστιν τῆς ἐπιληψίας καὶ ὑπὸ τῶν αὐτῶν αἰτίων γινόμενα καὶ περὶ τὰ αὐτὰ χωρία συνιστάμενα. ἐπιπολαία μέντοι ἡ κατασκευὴ αὐτῶν καὶ οὐκ ἐνδιάθετος, διὸ καὶ εὐιατοτέρα καθάρσεσι ταῖς ἀπὸ κοιλίας, μάλιστα τῇ ἱερᾷ, ἔπειτα ἀποφλεγματισμοῖς καὶ ἐμέτοις ἐν κύκλῳ παραλαμβανομένοις, τοῖς μὲν ἀπὸ δείπνου, τοῖς δὲ νήστεσιν. ἐπὶ πᾶσι δὲ κατορθοῦται ἐλλεβόρῳ. τῆς δὲ περὶ τὴν διάνοιαν ἐκστάσεως, δύο μὲν τὰ ἐξέχοντα εἴδη μανία τε καὶ μελαγχολία. πολλαὶ δὲ καὶ ἐν τούτοις αἱ διαφοραὶ, ἀκατωνόμαστοι οὖσαι. συνίσταται μὲν οὖν περὶ κεφαλὴν πᾶσαν ἔκστασις διανοίας. αἰτία δὲ τῆς μὲν μανίας ξανθὴ χολή. διὰ τοῦτο ταραχώδεις καὶ ἔκφοροι καὶ πρόχειροι ὑβρισταί τε οἱ τούτῳ ἐχόμενοι τῷ πάθει. τῆς δὲ μελαγχολίας

caufa interim urina fine voluntate prorumpit. Praefidium affert pueris impuberibus natura circa pubertatem efflorefcens et morbum humoribus nativo calore exiccatis terminat. Qui pubertatem exceſſerunt, aegre aut nunquam fanantur Caligines oculis offufae et vertigines cognata funt vitia morbo comitiali, ab eisdemque caufis prodeunt, atque easdem fedes occupant. Hoc tamen intercedit difcriminis, quod illae in fuperficie corporis, non intus accidant, ob quod facilius, quam hic, curantur alvi ductione, praefertim per hieram, adminiftrata, deinde apophlegmatismis et vomitibus per circuitum partim a coena, partim jejunis adhuc excitatis. Omnium maxime veratro fuccurritur. Mentis alienatio duplici fpecie infigni conftat: mania et melancholia. Complures vero et harum exiftunt differentiae, nominum adhuc indigae. Conftituitur itaque mentis alienatio circa totum caput. Caput infaniae flava bilis eft. Ob hoc qui tali vitio laborant, tumultuofi, praecipites, manu prompti contumeliofique fiunt. Melancholia

αἰτία μέλαινα χολὴ, ψυχρότερος χυμὸς καὶ ζοφώδης. διὸ ζοφοειδεῖς τέ εἰσι καὶ δύσθυμοι οἱ τοιοῦτοι. ὕποπτοι δὲ εἰς πάντα καὶ μισάνθρωποί τε καὶ ἐρημίαις χαίροντες, οἷος ὁ Βελλοροφόντης ἱστορεῖται.

Ἤ τοι ὁ καππεδίον τὸ Ἀλήϊον οἶος ἀλᾶτο,
Ὃν θυμὸν κατέδων, πάτον ἀνθρώπων ἀλεείνων.

Ἴασις δὲ διὰ καθάρσεως τῶν ἀπὸ κοιλίας καὶ μάλιστα ἡ δι' ἐμέτων. ἐπὶ πᾶσι δὲ ἐλλέβορος ἑκάτερος λύσις. ὁ δὲ λήθαργος ἐναντίον πάθος ἐστὶ τῇ φρενίτιδι. καταφορὰ γάρ ἐστι βαθεῖα καὶ δυσανάκλιτος. οἱ κάμνοντες ἐπιλανθανόμενοι πάντων ὅσα λέγουσι. ταῦτα δὲ ἐν πυρετῷ αὐτοῖς συνεδρεύει. τόπος μὲν οὖν τοῦ πάθους ἡ κεφαλή. περὶ γὰρ μήνιγγας αὐτῆς συνίσταται. αἴτιον δὲ τούτου φλέγμα, χυμὸς ψυχρὸς, καὶ τῇ ψύξει [382] καὶ τῇ ὑγρότητι εἰς ὕπνον αὐτοὺς κατάγον. θεραπεία δὲ ἁρμόδιος, ἡ ὑπεναντία τῇ φρενίτιδι, ἀνάτριψις τῶν ἄκρων, διά τινων δριμέων καὶ νυσσόντων, ὀσφραντῶν τε προσαγωγαὶ ἀνεγειρόντων. τροφαί τε ὁμοίως

nafcitur ex atra bile, humore frigido et tenebrofo. Unde melancholici tenebriones ac lucifugae triftesque apparent, de omnibus fufpiciofi, hominum confuetudinem oderunt, folitudinibus gaudent, quemadmodum Bellerophontes a Poëta defcribitur.

Qui mifer in campis errabat folus Aleis,
Ipfe fuum cor edens, hominum veftigia vitans.

Medetur per ventrem purgatio et maxime, quae per vomitum excitatur: adhuc his magis utrumque veratrum folvit. Lethargus morbus eft phrenitidi contrarius: eft enim profunda in fomnum delatio et inexcitabilis. Hoc vitio correpti omnium quae dicuntur oblivifcuntur, atque haec in febri ipfos comitantur. Locus igitur affectionis caput eft: nam in membranis cerebri conftituitur. Caufa ipfius pituita eft, humor frigidus, frigiditate ac humiditate fomnum inducens. Curatio conveniens ea eft, quae contraria ei quae phrenitidi. Frictio fuperiorum corporis partium per acria quaedam et pungentia et admotio rerum fuaveolen-

διαχέουσαι καὶ τέμνουσαι τὸ φλέγμα, ἐπιβροχαί τε τῆς κεφαλῆς διὰ τῶν ἀναξηραινόντων καὶ καταπλάσματά ἐστιν ὅπου κατὰ τῶν μέσων. πολλάκις γὰρ ταῦτα φλεγμαίνοντα πιέζει καὶ τὴν ἐν τῇ κεφαλῇ ἀρχὴν εἶναι νεύρων. κόρυζα δὲ καὶ βράγχος καὶ κατάῤῥους ἀπὸ κεφαλῆς μὲν ἄρχεται τὰ πάθη πληρουμένης, εἶτα κατασταζούσης, ὁτὲ μὲν εἰς ῥῖνας, καὶ καλεῖται κόρυζα, ὁτὲ δὲ εἰς βρόγχον, καὶ βράγχος ὀνομάζεται τὸ πάθος, ὁτὲ δὲ εἰς θώρακα, καὶ κατάῤῥους λέγεται. εὐίατον μὲν οὖν καὶ πρόσκαιρον ἡ κόρυζα· δεύτερον ὁ βράγχος. ὀλιγοσιτίαι γὰρ καὶ θερμαὶ τροφαὶ καὶ σιτώδεις ἐρύσαντο πολλάκις τῶν παθῶν. δυσίατον δὲ ὁ κατάῤῥους καὶ πολλάκις ἀνίατος. ἐκ γὰρ κατάῤῥου δριμέος καὶ ἁλμυροῦ διεσθιομένων τῶν σωμάτων αἵματος ἀναγωγὴ γίνεται. αἰτίαι δὲ αἵματος ἀναγωγῆς τρεῖς· ἢ γὰρ κατ' ἀνάβρωσιν τῶν ἀγγείων, παραῤῥέοντος τοῦ αἵματος εἰς τὴν τραχεῖαν ἀρτηρίαν, ἀνάγεται διὰ τοῦ στόματος, ἢ διὰ δύναμιν ῥήξεως γενομένης, ἢ δι' ἀσθένειαν καὶ ἀτονίαν τῶν ἀγγείων οὐ στεγόντων, ἀλλ' ἀνεστομωμένων διαπηδῶντος τοῦ αἵματος.

tium. Cibi fimiliter difcutientes fecantesque pituitam perfufiones capiti admoventur, quae exiccandi vim obtinent et cataplasma aliquando praecordiis. Crebro namque haec inflammatione vexata nervorum quoque in capite principium conftringunt gravantque. Gravedo, raucitas et catarrhus funt affectus qui fiunt ab humore qui ab oppleto cerebro decumbit; quum in nares, vocatur gravedo, quum in afperam arteriam, raucitas nominatur, quum in thoracem, catarrhus appellatur. Gravedini itaque facile et brevi fuccurritur, deinde raucitati modico fane et calido victu, qui frumentacei generis exiftat. Deftillatio in thoracem non ex facili curatur, imo faepe immedicabilis eft. Nam ab ea acri et falfa partibus exefis, fanguinis eductio fequitur: cujus tres caufae referuntur. Vel enim vafa erofionem paffa funt, ideoque fanguis in afperam arteriam defcendens per os rejicitur: vel rupta funt violenter: vel ob imbecillitatem non continent, fed adaperta oscula eum transmittunt. Differunt fanguinis excretio et

διαφέρει δὲ αἵματος ἔκκρισις καὶ αἵματος ἀναγωγή. ἡ μὲν γὰρ ἢ ἀπὸ πνεύμονος ἢ ἀπὸ τῆς τραχείας ἀρτηρίας γίνεται· ἡ δὲ ἀπὸ στομάχου καὶ τὸ αἷμα μελάντερον φαίνεται, τὸ δὲ ἀπὸ θώρακος ξανθότερον καὶ ἀφρίζον, ἔπειτα τῷ τὸ μὲν μετὰ βηχὸς ἀνάγεσθαι, τὸ δὲ ἄνευ βηχός. πολλάκις δὲ καὶ ἀπὸ κεφαλῆς διὰ τῶν τῆς ὑπερῴας τρημάτων εἰς τὸ στόμα καταφερόμενον τὸ αἷμα, ἀναγωγῆς φαντασίαν παρέχει οὐκ οὖσαν. τόποι δὲ ἐξ ὧν κυρίως τὸ αἷμα ἀνάγεται τρεῖς, πρῶτος μὲν τὸ φαρύγετρον, καὶ ἀκινδυνοτέρα καὶ εὐιατοτέρα ἐντεῦθεν ἡ τοῦ αἵματος ἀναγωγή, δεύτερος ἀπὸ τῆς τραχείας ἀρτηρίας, καὶ δυσίατος αὕτη ἡ διαφορὰ καὶ κινδυνώδης, τρίτος ἡ ἀπὸ τοῦ πνεύμονος πασῶν δυσιατοτέρα καὶ κινδυνωδεστέρα, ἐφ' ᾗ μάλιστα καὶ τὸ ἐμπύημα καὶ ἡ φθίσις, ὥς φησιν Ἱπποκράτης. ἐφ' αἵματος πτύσει πύου πτύσις· ἐπὶ πύου πτύσει φθίσις· ἐπὶ φθίσει θάνατος. δοκεῖ δέ τισι καὶ ἀπὸ πλευροῦ αἷμα ἀνάγεσθαι. ἀμφίβολος δὲ οὗτος ὁ τρόπος. ἴασις δὲ αἵματος ἀναγωγῆς ἐπισχεθῆναι τὸ αἷμα, ἢ διὰ φλεβοτομίας μετοχετεύσαντα καὶ

rejectio. Haec etenim vel a pulmone vel aſpera arteria provenit: illa a ſtomacho et ſanguis apparet nigrior. Qui ex thorace rejicitur, flavus magis et ſpumans: deinde hic cum tuſſe, alter ſine illa ſpuitur. Saepenumero etiam a capite per palati foramina in os defertur ſanguis, praebetque eductionis falſam imaginem. Loci, ex quibus proprie ſanguis educitur, tres ſunt. Primus fauces, unde minore cum periculo ſanguis rejicitur, faciliusque ſiſtitur. Secundus aſpera arteria, atque hic morbus curationem difficulter accipit, plenusque periculi eſt. Tertius pulmo, ubi minus omnibus praeſidii, plus periculi affectus habet. Comitatur enim maxime ſuppuratio et tabes, ut ait Hippocrates, cujus verba haec ſunt. *Sanguinis ſpuitionem puris ſpuitio, hujus ſpuitionem tabes, tabem mors ſequitur.* Nonnulli etiam ex latere ſanguinem educi arbitrantur. At hoc ambiguum eſt. Salus vitii hujus eſt, ſanguinem reprimere vel venae ſectione alio ducentem, idque potiſſimum in juvenibus, vel poſca ſiſtentem vel inedia copiam

μάλιστα ἐπὶ τῶν νέων, ἢ διὰ ὀξυκράτου στήσαντα, ἢ ἀποσιτίᾳ μειώσαντα τὸ πλῆθος, ἢ διά τινος τῶν ἁπλῶν φαρμάκων, οἷον ἀκακίας, ὑποκυστίδος, βαλαυστίου, ἀρνωγλώσσου χυλοῦ καὶ τῶν ὁμοίων. ἐμπυήματος δὲ ἴασις ἡ μὲν παλαιὰ διὰ καυστηρίων ἀναξηραινόντων τὸν θώρακα καὶ εἰς τὰ ἐκτὸς μεταῤῥευματίσαι, ἡ δὲ νεωτέρα συμπεπᾶναι τοῖς τε καταπλάσμασι καὶ τοῖς ἐκλεικτοῖς, ἔπειτα ἀνακαθᾶραι ταχέως τοῖς διὰ στόματος διδομένοις φαρμάκοις, πρὶν ἢ καθαιρεθῆναι τὸ σῶμα. ἐπιγράφεται δὲ τὰ φάρμακα ἰδίως, πρὸς ἐμπυικούς. τὰ δὲ ἐν μεσοπλευρίοις συνιστάμενα ἐμπυήματα τεμνόμενα ἰδίως πρὸς μοτὸν ἔχει τὴν ἔκκρισιν τοῦ ὑγροῦ· ἡ γὰρ ἀθρόα ἀναιρεῖ. γίγνεται δὲ ἐμπυήματα καὶ ὑπὸ τὸ διάφραγμα, ἃ λέγουσιν ἐν κατακαλύψει ἀποστήματα, οὐχ ὁμοίως κινδυνώδη, οὐδὲ δυσίατα, τὰ πολλὰ ἐντὸς ῥηγνύμενα ταύτῃ ἐκκρίνεται, ἢ διαιρουμένων τῶν ἐκτὸς σωμάτων. ἱστορεῖ δὲ Διοκλῆς καὶ τὰ ἐν θώρακι ἐμπυήματα, ἔστιν ὅτε συῤῥηγνύμενα εἰς τὴν ἐπὶ νεφροὺς καὶ κύστιν φέρουσαν ἀρτηρίαν, ταύτῃ

ejus imminuentem, vel fimplici quodam medicamento, ut acacia, hypociftide, balauftio, plantaginis fucco, atque id genus aliis. Suppurationis praefidium vetus funt ferramenta candentia, quae thoracem exiccent, fluoremque in exteriores partes dirigant. Recentiores confueverunt mitigare cataplasmatis et delingendis medicaminibus, deinde cito repurgare medicamentis per os affumptis prius, quam corpus exedatur. Infcribuntur autem proprie medicamenta ad purulentos. Quae fuppurationes medio latere conftituuntur, refectae proprie ad linamentum, humoris excretionem habent: quae fi univerfum fiat, hominem interimit. Accidunt vero fuppurationes quoque fub transverfo fepto, quae fe intus occultantes abfceffus nominantur, non ex aequo periculofi, nec curationi refiftentes, plerumque intus rupti hac excernuntur, vel partibus exterioribus divifis. Diocles memorat etiam thoracis fuppurationes erumpentes interim in arteriam, quae ad renes ac veficam tendit, fimul cum urinis excerni. Tabes proprie dicitur

ἀποκρίνεσθαι σὺν τοῖς οὔροις. [383] φθίσις μὲν κυρίως λέγεται ἡ ἐν πνεύμονι, ἢ εἰς τὸν θώρακα ἐπὶ τῶν ἐμπυημάτων σύντηξις τοῦ σώματος. δυσίατον δὲ τὸ πάθος, ἢ καὶ ἀνίατον. γαλακτοποσία τε ἐν αὐτῇ τῇ ἀκμῇ καὶ τόποι ξηρότεροι καὶ τῆς Αἰγύπτου τὰ ἄνω καὶ ἡ Λιβύα ἰῶνται μάλιστα τὸ πάθος. λέγεται δὲ καὶ ἰσχιαδική τις φθίσις ὑπὸ Ἱπποκράτους, ἡ ἐπὶ τοῖς περὶ τὸ ἱερὸν ὀστοῦν ἐμπυήμασι σύντηξις τοῦ σώματος. ὁμοίως δὲ καὶ ἡ νεφριτική. αἱ δὲ περὶ τὸ ἧπαρ καὶ σπλῆνα φλεγμοναὶ, εἰ μὲν εἰς ἐμπύημα μεταβάλλοιεν, συντήκουσι καὶ αὗται μετρίως τὸ σῶμα. εὐιατότερα δὲ ταῦτα τὰ ἐμπυήματα τῶν ἐν πνεύμονι καὶ ἀκινδυνότερα. εἰ δὲ μὴ μεταβάλλοιεν, ἀλλ' ἄπεπτοι μένοιεν αἱ φλεγμοναὶ καὶ σκιῤῥώδεις καχεξίας ἐπιφέρουσαι τῷ σώματι καὶ τελευτῶσαι ὕδρωπας ἐπιφέρουσι. μέχρι δὲ ἁπλαῖ φλεγμοναί εἰσιν, ἡ μὲν περὶ ἧπαρ πυρετοὺς ἐπιφέρει συνεχεῖς, ἡ δὲ περὶ σπλῆνα τεταρταίους ὡς ἐπὶ τὸ πολύ. αἰτία γὰρ τοῦ τύπου τούτου μέλαινα χολὴ, ἧς ἀγγεῖον ὁ σπλὴν, ὅθεν ἴαμα τεταρταίου, πρὸ μὲν τοῦ ῥίγους, πυ-

in pulmone vel in thorace, corporis ob ſuppurationes colliquatio: difficilis ejus ſalus eſt aut nulla. Lactis uſus potui datur, dum conſiſtit: loca ſicciora conveniunt. Superior Aegyptus et Libya maxime huic malo medentur. Hippocrates tabis cujusdam coxendicum meminit, iſchiadicam vocans, qua in ſuppurationibus circa os ſacrum accidentibus corpora colliqueſcunt. Similiter alterius renum nephriticae. Porro jecinoris et lienis inflammationes ſi in pus vertuntur et ipſae mediocriter corpus conſumunt. At hae ſuppurationes multo citius curantur, minusque periculoſae ſunt, quam quae pulmonem affligunt. Verum ſi minus in ſuppurationes mutantur inflammationes, ſed crudae et in ſcirrhi natura permanſerint, malum habitum corpori aſſerentes, tandem aquam inter cutem afferunt. Quatenus autem ſimplices extiterint, in jecinore, febres continuas afferunt: in liene, quartanas magna ex parte: nam hujus ſpeciei cauſa bilis atra eſt, quae in liene tanquam vaſe continetur. Unde quartanae auxilium eſt, ante

ριῶντα τὰ ἄκρα διὰ τὴν ψυχρότητα τοῦ χυμοῦ, ἐν δὲ τοῖς διαλείμμασιν ἡ δι' ἐμέτων ἀγωγή. ὑδρώπων δὲ τριττὸν εἶδος κατὰ τοὺς νεωτέρους, ὁ μὲν ἀσκίτης, ὁ δὲ τυμπανίτης, ὁ δὲ ὑποσαρκίδιος. κατὰ δὲ Ἱπποκράτην δύο φύσεις. ὁ γὰρ ἀσκίτης καὶ ὁ τυμπανίτης τῆς αὐτῆς ἰδέας ἐστί. ἐφ' ἑκατέρᾳ γὰρ παρέγχυσίς ἐστιν τῆς ἐξυδαρουμένης τροφῆς εἰς τὸν μεταξὺ τόπον τῶν τε ἐντέρων καὶ τοῦ περιτοναίου· ἀλλ' ἐπὶ μὲν τοῦ ἀσκίτου πλεῖον τὸ ὕδωρ, ἔλαττον τὸ πνεῦμα. ἐπὶ δὲ τοῦ τυμπανίτου πλεῖον τὸ πνεῦμα, ἔλαττον τὸ ὑγρόν. ὁ δὲ ὑποσαρκίδιος κατὰ πᾶν ἐστὶ τὸ σῶμα ἀνάλυσις τῶν στερεῶν σωμάτων εἰς ὕδατος φύσιν. τοῦτον καὶ Ἱπποκράτης ἀνίατόν φησιν. καλεῖται δὲ καὶ λευκοφλεγματίας. αἰτία δὲ παντὸς ὑδέρου, ὡς μὲν Ἐρασίστρατός φησιν, φλεγμονὴ ἥπατος, ἢ σπληνὸς (383) χρονισθεῖσα καὶ σκιῤῥωθεῖσα. ἐμποδίζουσα γὰρ τῆς τροφῆς τὴν ἐν τοῖς σπλάγχνοις τούτοις κατεργασίαν τε καὶ ἀνάδοσιν εἰς πᾶν τὸ σῶμα ἐξυδαρεῖ αὐτὴν, καταψυχθεῖσα δὲ παρεγχεῖται μεταξὺ ἐντέρων καὶ περιτοναίου. κατὰ δὲ Ἱπποκράτην καὶ αὐτὴ μὲν

rigorem fummas partes propter humoris frigiditatem fomentis tueri. In intermiffionibus eductio per vomitum. Hydropis tres funt fpecies ex fententia neotericorum, afcites, tympanites et anafarca. Hippocrates duas ftatuit, nam tympanites et afcites funt ejusdem fpeciei, quoniam in utraque nutrimentum in aquam redactum inter inteftina et peritonaeum transfunditur. Sed in hac aquae plus, quam fpiritus, in unum intus contrahitur: in illa copiofior fpiritus, minor humiditas eft: in reliqua folidae totius corporis partes in aquae naturam tranfeunt: hanc et Hippocrates medicabilem effe fcribit, vocatur autem et leucophlegmatia. Caufa vero cujusque hydropis eft, auctore Erafiftrato, inflammatio jecinoris vel lienis, temporis fpatio in fcirrhum indurata. Nam quum alimenti in his vifceribus confectionem atque in totum corpus digeftionem impediat, in aquae fubftantia ipfum commutat, quod ita refrigeratum inter inteftina et peritonaeum transmittitur. Hoc quoque malum Hippocrati falutis fpem nullam

ἀνίατος· εἰ δὲ καὶ ἄνευ φλεγμονῆς γινόμενον ὕδερον καὶ μάλιστα τὸν ὑποσαρκίδιον τοῦ ἐμφύτου θερμοῦ καταψυχομένου καὶ οὐκ ἔτι κρατοῦντος τὴν ἐν τοῖς ἀγγείοις τροφὴν, διὸ καταψυχόμενον τὸ αἷμα ἐξυδαροῦται καὶ παραῤῥεῖ διὰ τῶν φλεβῶν, ὡς ἐκ τῶν ἀσκῶν, τὸ ἔλαιον διαπηδήσει. μέχρι μὲν γὰρ ἐν ταῖς φλεψὶν αἷμά ἐστιν, ἀκριβῶς ὑπὸ τοῦ σώματος τῶν φλεβῶν συνέχεται. ὅταν δὲ ἡ ἐν αὐτῷ λιπαρότης πλεονάσῃ, ὡς ἐπὶ τῶν πιμελῶν, παρεγχεόμενον τοῦτο πιμελὴν ποιεῖ. ἢ ἐξυδαρούμενον τὸ αἷμα, ἢ μὴ στεγνόμενον διαῤῥεῖ, ἢ εἰς τὸν μεταξὺ τόπον τῶν ἐντέρων καὶ τοῦ περιτοναίου, ἢ κατὰ πᾶν τὸ σῶμα. ἴασις δὲ τῶν δύο ἑτέρων ὑδρώπων, ἢ διὰ μαλαγμάτων ἀναξηραινόντων, ἢ διὰ φαρμάκων διουρητικῶν, ἢ διὰ καθαρτικῶν ὑπηλάτων. νεφροὶ δὲ πεπονθότες ἀλγήματα μὲν σφοδρὰ ἐπιφέρουσιν, δυσδιάκριτος δὲ ἐπ᾽ αὐτῶν ὁ πεπονθὼς τόπος διὰ τὸ συμπεφυκέναι αὐτὸν τοῖς ἔξωθεν σώμασι καὶ ἐπικεῖσθαι τὸ κῶλον αὐτοῖς· διὸ ἐν πυήσει γινόμενοι φαντασίαν παρέχουσι φλεγμονῆς, ἤ τοι περὶ τὰ ἐκτὸς ἢ κωλικῆς διαθέσεως. πολλάκις δὲ

habet. Quod ſi vel absque inflammatione hydrops, praeſertim anaſarca eveniat, calore genuino refrigerato, nec alimentum in venis amplius edomante, ſanguis caloris inops aquae naturam induit et ex venis, ceu oleum ex utribus deſluit. Quousque enim ſanguis exactus in venis eſt, ab earum corpore continetur. Ubi vero in eo pingue exuperaverit, ut in obeſis, ſanguis effuſus adipem generat, aut in aquam verſus, aut dum non continetur, difſluit in locum qui medius eſt inter inteſtina et peritonaeum, aut per univerſum corpus effunditur. Tolluntur duo alii hydropes vel ex malagmatis exiccantibus, vel medicamentis urinas cientibus, vel hypelatis purgandi facultate praeditis. Renes affecti dolores magnos pariunt. Locus autem male habens non ex facili poteſt diſcerni, quod exterioribus partibus cohaereat et colon ipſis incumbat, quare dum in eis eſt abſceſſus, vel inflammationis partium externarum vel colici doloris ſpeciem praebent. Non raro eodem affecto inteſtino renes conſentientes dolent.

καὶ κώλῳ συμπάσχουσιν οἱ νεφροί. πάθη δὲ συνίστανται περὶ νεφροὺς ταῦτα, φλεγμονὴ, ἕλκωσις, λιθίασις, πάρεσις. [384] φλεγμονῆς μὲν οὔσης, οὐδὲν διασημαίνει δι᾽ οὔρων· ἀλλὰ μᾶλλον ἀλγήματα ἐπιφέρει, οὐκ ἀκριβῶς ἐπιφαίνοντα τὸν πρωτοπαθοῦντα τόπον δι᾽ ἃ ἔφαμεν. δυσπαραμύθητοι δὲ αἱ ὀδύναι, οὔτε καταπλάσμασιν εἴκουσαι, οὔτε τῇ διὰ σικύας ἀφαιρέσει ἐνδιδοῦσαι, μόνον δὲ εἴπερ τοῖς ἔνδοθεν διδομένοις τισὶ νεφριτικοῖς φαρμάκοις. εἰ δὲ ἕλκωσις εἴη, ὅτε μὲν πυώδη διὰ τῶν οὔρων ἀποκρίνεται, ὅτε δὲ αἱματώδη. λιθιάσεως δὲ οὔσης, ὁτὲ μὲν αἱματώδη ἀποκρίνεται, τραχυνομένων τῶν σωμάτων ὑπὸ τοῦ λίθου, ὁτὲ δὲ ψαμμία ὑφίστανται τῷ οὔρῳ, εἰ εὔθρυπτος εἴη ὁ λίθος, ἢ καὶ γενέσεως ἀρχὴν ἔχοι. ἐπὶ δὲ παρέσεως αἱματῶδες τὸ οὗρον ἀποδίδοται, ὡς ἂν οὐ διακρινόμενον. περὶ δὲ τὴν κύστιν ταῦτα συνίσταται τὰ πάθη, πάρεσις, πιτυρίασις, λιθίασις, ἕλκωσις, περὶ τὸν τράχηλον μάλιστα. ἐπισυμβαίνει δὲ τούτοις ἰσχουρία, στραγγουρία, δυσουρία, ἀπό τε τούτων καὶ ἐξ ἄλλων αἰτίων. φλεγμονὴν μὲν οὖν δηλοῖ τὰ περὶ τὸ ἐφή-

Affectus autem, qui in eis conſiſtunt, hi ſunt, inflammatio, exulceratio, calculi, imbecillitas. Quum inflammatio renes exercet, nihil per urinam innoteſcit, ſed dolores excitantur potius, non exacte locum primum dolentem oſtendentes, ob eam, quam dixi, rationem, verum intolerabiles: quippe qui nec cataplasmatis cedant, nec detractione per cucurbitulas facta remittantur: ſola medicamenta nephritica intus accepta praeſidio ſunt. Si exulceratio eos infeſtat, interdum purulenta per urinas excernuntur, interdum cruenta. Quum ineſt calculus, aliquando cruenta, partibus videlicet ab eo exaſperatis, ejiciuntur, aliquando arenulae in urina ſubſident, ſi friabilis ſit lapis vel etiam recens modo naſcatur. In imbecillitate ſanguinolenta urina redditur, quaſi nondum ſegregata. Veſicae affectus hi ſunt, imbecillitas, furfuratio, calculus, exulceratio, circa collum maxime. His accedit urinae ſuppreſſio ejusque difficultas et ſtillicidium. Ex his vero aliisque cauſis pro-

βαιον ἀλγήματα καὶ δυσχέρεια περὶ τὴν τοῦ οὔρου ἔκκρισιν. λύει δὲ φλεγμονὴν κύστεως κατάπλασμα καὶ ἐπιβροχαὶ καὶ ἔνδεια τροφῆς. εἰ δὲ ὑπερβάλλοι καὶ ἀφαίρεσις αἵματος διὰ φλεβοτομίας. ἕλκωσιν δὲ σημαίνει, ποτὲ μὲν αἱματώδη ἐκκρινόμενα, ποτὲ δὲ πυώδη, ἔστι δὲ ὅτε μυξώδη καὶ τὰ περὶ τὸ ἐφήβαιον ἀλγήματα. ἴασις δὲ διὰ τῶν ἐπιθεμάτων καὶ μάλιστα γλυκυχυμία καὶ εὔχυμος τροφὴ προσφερομένη. καὶ τὰ ἔνδοθεν διδόμενα πρὸς ἕλκωσιν κύστεως καὶ τὸ Βισσίνου φάρμακον. πάρεσιν δὲ κύστεως, δηλοῖ μὲν καὶ ἡ τῶν οὔρων ἀπροαίρετος ἔκκρισις. δυσίατον δὲ, ἢ καὶ ἀνίατον τὸ πάθος. λίθον δὲ ἐν κύστει ὄντα, σημειοῦνται μὲν ἀκριβέστατα οἱ δάκτυλοι καθιέμενοι εἰς τὸ ἀπευθυσμένον ἐπὶ τῆς ἕδρας, ὥς τε ἐπικάμπτεσθαι τὸν λιχανὸν δάκτυλον ἐπὶ τὸν μέσον τοῖς ἄκροις καὶ ἐπὶ τὸ ἔμπροσθεν ἐπὶ τὴν κύστιν, ἔνθα καὶ ἐντυγχάνουσι τῷ λίθῳ ἐμπλέοντι καὶ ἀναφέρουσιν αὐτὸν εἰς τὸν τράχηλον τῆς κύστεως. λίθων δὲ διαφοραὶ πλείονες· οἱ μὲν γὰρ αὐτῶν προσφυεῖς, οἱ δὲ ἀπόλυτοι, καὶ οἱ μὲν εὔθραυστοι, οἱ δὲ δύσθραυστοι. δυσίατοι μὲν οὖν

ficiscuntur. Inflammationis notae ſunt circa pubem dolores, urinae excernendae difficultas. Solvitur cataplasmatis, perſuſionibus et a cibo abſtinentia. Quod ſi excedat, ſanguinem quoque per venam mittere convenit. Exulcerationis indicia ſunt, ſanguinolenta excretio interdum, interdum purulenta, nonnunquam mucoſa et circa pubem dolores. Auxiliantur epithemata, maximeque dulcis bonique ſucci alimentum ad haec, quae intus adhibentur adverſus ulcerationem veſicae et Byſſini medicamentum. Imbecillitatem veſicae innuit et urina, cum citra mejentis voluntatem effluit. Difficilem morbus curationem, aut nullam recipit. Lapidem in veſica eſſe, digiti in rectum inteſtinum per ſedem immiſſi exquiſitiſſime deprehendunt, ſed ita, ut index ad medium in ſummo reflectatur, atque in priorem veſicae partem, ubi et lapidem innatantem contingunt, referuntque in veſicae cervicem. Calculorum differentiae plures ſunt, quidam enim illorum adnati ſunt, alii poſſunt auferri. Rurſus aliqui facile frangi poſſunt,

ὡς ἐπὶ τὸ πολὺ οἱ προσφυεῖς. τῶν δὲ ἄλλων τοὺς μὲν εὐθραύστους, τὰ φάρμακα δύνανται διαλύοντα ἐκκρίνειν. τοὺς δὲ στερεοὺς καὶ δυσλύτους οἱ χειρουργοὶ κομίζονται, διαιροῦντες τῆς κύστεως τὸ σαρκοειδὲς τοῦ τραχήλου. ἰσχουρία μὲν οὖν ἐστιν ἡ τελεία ἐποχὴ τῶν οὔρων. στραγγουρία δὲ, ἡ κατὰ στράγγα οὔρησις. καὶ δυσουρία τὸ αὐτὸ τοῦτο μόνον ποιοῦσα, δυσχέρειαν τοῦ ἀπουρεῖν. γίνεται δὲ ταῦτα διὰ πολλὰς αἰτίας, ὁτὲ μὲν διὰ τὸν λίθον ἐσφηνωμένον τῷ τραχήλῳ τῆς κύστεως καὶ τελέως ἐμφράττοντα τὸν πόρον ἢ ἔνδον τι καταλιπόντα ἢ ἐννηχόμενον τῇ κύστει. γίνεται δὲ ἰσχουρία διὰ φλεγμονὴν κύστεως ὑπερβάλλουσαν καὶ διὰ πλήρωσιν ἄμετρον, οὐ δυναμένης περισταλῆναι τῆς κύστεως καὶ διὰ δριμύτητα τῶν οὔρων τοῦ τραχήλου ἀκριβῶς συστελλομένου τῇ δήξει καὶ διὰ θρόμβον αἵματος ἀποκλείοντα τὴν δίοδον καὶ διὰ παχύτητα οὔρων προσισχομένων. πεπεμμένων οὖν τῶν ἐκκρινομένων ὄντων, τὴν τοιαύτην παχύτητα ἀποσπᾶσθαι χρὴ, τὸν δὲ θρόμβον διαλύειν τοῖς δυ-

nonnulli non poſſunt. Itaque magna ex parte adnati difficulter curantur. alii qui facile franguntur, alii qui difficile; itaque vix ſanabiles ſunt ut plurimum adnati. Ex aliis autem, qui facile franguntur, diſſolventibus medicamentis excerni poſſunt. Duros vero et vix ſolubiles chirurgi tollunt, carunculam dividentes veſicae cervicis. Iſchuria ſumma eſt urinarum retentio: ſtranguria urinae ſtillicidium: dyſuria urinae difficultas. Atque haec multis e cauſis proveniunt, aliquando calculo veſicae cervici impacto, ac meatum in totum obſtruente, vel ſi intus quippiam relictum ſit aut veſicae innatet. Urinae retentio propter veſicae inflammationem nimiam aut repletionem immodicam accidit, veſica ſcilicet ad excretionem imbecilla, aut cervice vehementer ex urinarum acrimonia per morſum contracta, aut ex grumis ſanguinis iter occludentibus, aut ex urinarum adhaerentium craſſitie. Coctis igitur iis quae excernuntur, ejusmodi craſſitiem trahere oportet, grumum vero medicamentis liquefaciendi vim haben-

ναμένοις τήκειν. τὴν δὲ πλήρωσιν κενοῦν τῷ Ἐρασιστρατείῳ καθετῆρι. ἔστι δὲ οὗτος προσεοικὼς τῷ ῥωμαϊκῷ σίγμα. σ, ἡ δὲ περὶ κοιλίαν καὶ ἔντερα ἀρχὴ, ὁ στόμαχός ἐστι καὶ κατὰ φύσιν ἐχόντων καὶ παρὰ φύσιν διατιθεμένων. στομάχου τοίνυν παθήματα φλεγμονὴ, ἕλκωσις, αἵματος ἀναγωγὴ, ἐμπνευμάτωσις, πλάδος, ἀνορεξία, ἀκράτεια τῶν προσφερομένων. φλεγμονὴν μὲν οὖν σημαίνει τὸ ἄλγημα ἐγκείμενον. [385] ἐπιμέλεια δὲ δι' ἐπιβροχῶν καὶ καταπλασμάτων καὶ τροφῶν σιτωδῶν καὶ εὐδιοικήτων. ἕλκωσιν δὲ ἐν στομάχῳ δηλοῖ ἰδίως σῆψις καὶ δῆξις καὶ δυσκαταποσία. ἴασις δὲ διά τε τῶν ἔξωθεν ἐπιτιθεμένων καὶ διὰ τροφῶν εὐχύλων, αἷμα δὲ ἀπὸ στομάχου ἀναγόμενον ἐπέχει διδόμενα, τὰ πρὸς αἵματος ἀναγωγὴν τὴν ἀπὸ θώρακος, τὰ προγεγραμμένα. ἐμπνευμάτωσιν δὲ διαλύουσι στομάχου αἱ ἐξόποροι καὶ ὅσα ἐρυγὴν κινεῖ. πλάδον δὲ ἀναξηραίνει, ξηροφαγία τε καὶ ἀψινθίου πόσις. ἀνορεξία δὲ ἡ μέν τις γίνεται διὰ φλέγμα παρακείμενον καὶ δεῖ ἀναξηραίνειν τὸ αἴτιον, ἢ διὰ χολὴν ἐπιπολάζουσαν καὶ δεῖ ἀνακαθαίρειν

tibus diſſolvere. Plenitudinem vacuare ferramento, quod Eraſiſtratus catheterem nominat Romanae literae S ſimili. Stomachus ventris et inteſtinorum principium eſt, ſive naturaliter, ſive praeter naturam afficiantur. Stomachi igitur vitia ſunt, inflammatio, exulceratio, ſanguinis eductio, inflatio, humiditas flaccida, cibi faſtidium, ingeſtorum ciborum incontinentia. Inflammationem ergo notat dolor incumbens. Succurritur perfuſionibus et cataplasmatis, alimentis frumentariis et quae facile poſſint digeri. Exulcerationem in ſtomacho notant proprie putredo, mordicatio, deglutiendi difficultas. Auxiliantur his extrinſecus impoſita, cibique probe ſucculenti. Sanguinis e ſtomacho eductio iisdem medicamentis ſiſtitur, quibus ex thorace: ejusdem rejectio, iis quae ſuperius adnotata ſunt. Inflationem diſſolvunt diſcutientia et quae ructus movent. Humiditatem ſiccorum eſus et abſinthii potio tollunt. Cibi faſtidium aut ex pituita adjacente oritur, ideoque exiccare illam ex uſu eſt: aut a bile ſupernatante, unde ſtomachus

Ed. Chart. II. [385.] Ed. Baſ. IV. (383.)

τὸν στόμαχον, ἢ ἀδυνατοῦντα τὴν φυσικὴν ἐνέργειαν ἀποδιδόναι τὴν ὀρεκτικὴν, ὡς καὶ ὀφθαλμοὺς ἀμβλυωπεῖν δι᾽ ἀτονίαν τοῦ ὁρατικοῦ πνεύματος. πρὸς δὲ τὴν τοιαύτην ἀνορεξίαν χρὴ τὰ προκλητικὰ καὶ ὑπομνηστικὰ τῆς ὀρέξεως προσφέρειν. ἀκρατὴς δὲ γίνεται ὁ στόμαχος τῶν προσφερομένων καὶ διὰ πλάδον, μάλιστα δὲ δι᾽ ἀτονίαν καὶ ἀσθένειαν, ὡς καὶ χεὶρ παρειμένη οὐκ ἴσχει ὧν ἂν ἐφάπτηται. χρὴ οὖν τονοῦν αὐτὸν καὶ ἰσχυροποιεῖν, τότε ὅλον τὸ σῶμα ἀνατρέφειν. περὶ δὲ κοιλίαν γίνεται μὲν πολλὰ τῶν περὶ τὸν στόμαχον πλὴν τῆς ἀνορεξίας. τὸ δὲ μὴ πέπτειν τὰ σιτία ἴδιον αὐτῆς καὶ τὰ πλεῖστα περὶ αὐτὴν γίνεται, ᾧ πάθος ἕπεται ἡ διάῤῥοια. τὰ μὲν οὖν ἄλλα ὁμοίως ἰατέον τοῖς περὶ τὸν στόμαχον. τὴν δὲ διάῤῥοιαν ἀκριβῶς ἐξεταστέον, δι᾽ ἣν αἰτίαν ἀπεπτηθείσης τῆς τροφῆς γίνεται. καὶ εἰ μὲν διὰ φλεγμονὴν, καταπλάττειν καὶ ἐπιβρέχειν, εἰ δὲ διὰ φλέγμα παρακείμενον ποιοῦν τὸν πλάδον, ἀναξηραίνειν τῇ διαίτῃ τὴν ὑγρότητα, εἰ δὲ παρὰ χολῆς πλῆθος, τὴν χολὴν καθαίρειν, εἰ δὲ δι᾽ ἀτονίαν, ὡς τοῖς ἀτονοῦσι τόνον

purgandus eſt: aut non potente naturali functione appetitum reddere. Nam oculi quoque propter ſpiritus viſorii imbecillitatem hallucinantur. Adverſum cibi faſtidium hujusmodi adhibenda ſunt, quae appetitum provocent ſuppeditentque. Stomachus autem non continet accepta propter humiditatem, maxime vero ob impotentiam ac imbecillitatem, ſicut dimiſſa manus non continet, quae attingit. Expedit igitur corroborare, fortioremque ipſum reddere, tum univerſum corpus reficere. Ventrem multa vitia ſtomacho communia infeſtant, praeterquam appetentiae pravitas. Sed concoctionis male obita functio ventriculo propria tribuitur, ut quae potiſſimum in eo adminiſtretur: quem affectum diarrhoea ſequitur. Reliqua igitur pari modo cum iis, quae ſtomachum cruciant, curabis. Fluxus exacte diſquirendus eſt, cur alimento incocto accidat: et ſi inflammatio eam pepererit, cataplasmatis et profuſionibus occurretur. Si pituita humiditatis illius flaccidae parens, victus ratione exiccanda eſt. Si bilis exuperet, eam

ἐμποιεῖν τῷ σώματι. εἰ δὲ παρ' αὐτὴν τὴν ποιότητα τῶν προσενεχθέντων δυσπέπτων ὄντων, ἢ εὐφθάρτων, ἤ τι ἐχόντων ἀλλό- (384) τριον, ἀποθεραπεύσαντα παραιτεῖσθαι τὰ τοιαῦτα. δυσεντερία δέ ἐστι πάθος περὶ τὰ ἔντερα· γίνεται δὲ ἐπὶ διαῤῥοίᾳ χρονιζόντων τῶν διεφθαρμένων καὶ διεσθιόντων καὶ ἑλκούντων τὰ ἔντερα. γίνεται δὲ καὶ ἄνευ διαῤῥοίας ἐξ ἀρχῆς, ὑπὸ χυμοῦ τινος δριμέος διαφαγόντος τὸ ἔντερον. ἔστι δὲ ὅτε καὶ ἐπὶ λύσει νοσήματος γίνεται ἡ δυσεντερία, ἣν ἀπαγορεύει ὁ Ἱπποκράτης ἰᾶσθαι, μὴ ἐκ τῆς ἐποχῆς ἕτερόν τι μεῖζον ἐπιγίνηται νόσημα. τὴν μὲν οὖν ἐκ διαῤῥοίας γενομένην ἰᾶται τοῖς στέλλουσι καὶ ἱστᾶσι τὸ ῥεῦμα, τὴν δὲ ἔκ τινος δήξεως χυμοῦ δριμέος ἰᾶται τοῖς καταγλυκαίνουσι καὶ κατακεράσαι δυναμένοις, ἐκκλύζων τε τὰ αὐτὰ τὰ ἡλκωμένα τοῖς ὁμοίοις. χρονίζοντος μέντοι τοῦ πάθους νομώδη καὶ σεσηκότα εἴωθεν διαχωρεῖν, ὅτε ἁρμόζουσιν οἱ ἐνιέμενοι τροχίσκοι, οἱ διὰ σανδαράχης καὶ τιτάνου καὶ ἀρσενικοῦ καὶ τῶν τοιούτων συντιθέμενοι. μὴ

purgare utile eſt. Si ex imbecillitate provenit, ut infirmis, robur corpori faciendum eſt. Si ab ipſa qualitate eorum, quae concoctu difficilia aſſumpta ſunt vel quae prompte corrumpuntur vel quid alienum habent, poſt curationem talia oportet interdicere. Dyſenteria inteſtinorum eſt affectus generatus in ventris profluvio, humoribus corruptis immorantibus, erodentibus et exulcerantibus inteſtina. Fit etiam ſine fluxu, primum ab humore acri inteſtina intus exedenti. Eſt cum in morbi deceſſione dyſenteria contingat, quam curari Hippocrates prohibet, ne ſuppreſſio alium quempiam morbum majorem acceſſat. Illam quae ex fluore nata eſt, reprimentibus et ſiſtentibus fluorem medicatur: aliam, cujus origo ex acris cujusdam humoris roſione eſt, dulcorantibus et quae mitigare poſſint, abluendo ipſa exulcerata, ſimilibus. Diuturno tamen morbo depaſta ulceris ramenta et putrida ſolent dejici, tum proſunt immiſſi paſtilli ex ſandaracha, calce, auripigmento, atque id genus aliis compoſiti. Ubi vero non

ὄντων δὲ νομωδῶν τῶν διαχωρουμένων, μὴ χρῆσθαι τούτοις, ἐπεὶ σπασμὸν ἐπιφέρουσιν. εἰ δὲ καὶ ἀνωτέρω ἡ τοιαύτη ἕλκωσις τῶν ἐντέρων εἴη, οὐδὲ οὕτως χρηστέον τοῖς τροχίσκοις. οὐ γὰρ φθάνουσιν ἐπὶ τὰ πεπονθότα ἐξικνεῖσθαι. τῶν γὰρ ὑγιεινῶν καθαπτόμενοι ὄλεθρον ἐργάζονται, ἀνωτερικοῖς δὲ φαρμάκοις χρῆσθαι, τοῖς πρὸς δυσεντερίαν ἀναγεγραμμένοις. λειεντερία δὲ γίνεται μὲν ἀπὸ τῆς δυσεντερίας, ὅταν πολλῆς ἑλκώσεως οὔσης ἐπὶ τὰ ἔντερα οὐλαὶ πολλαὶ ἐπιγένωνται, δι᾽ ἃς οὐ κρατεῖ τὰ ἔντερα τῆς τροφῆς, ὅθεν λειεντερία εἴρηται ἐκ τῆς περὶ τὰ ἔντερα λειότητος. διὸ καὶ ἀνίατος ἡ τοιαύτη λειεντερία. οὐλὰς γὰρ οὐκ ἔστιν ἰᾶν. χαλεπὴ δὲ καὶ δυσίατος ἡ δι᾽ ἀτονίαν ἐντέρου γινομένη. ἐγχειρεῖν δὲ τῇ θεραπείᾳ, τόνον ἐντιθέντα τῷ τε ὅλῳ τῷ σώματι καὶ τοῖς ἐντέροις. [386] γίνεται δὲ καὶ λειεντερία καὶ διὰ φλέγμα ἐπικλύσαν τὰ ἔντερα καὶ ὄλισθον ἐμποιοῦν αὐτοῖς. καὶ δεῖ ἀναξηραίνειν ἀποσιτίᾳ τε καὶ τροφῇ τῇ πρὸς φλέγμα ἀντιτασσομένῃ. τεινεσμὸς δὲ ἰδίως περὶ τὸ ἀπευθυσμένον γίνεται. φλεγμαῖνον γὰρ τοῦτο συνεχεῖς

fit ramentofa ulceris dejectio, non his utendum eft, quoniam convulfionem faciunt. Quod fi talis inteftinorum exulceratio in fuperiore quoque parte confiftat, neque fic paftillorum ufus eft: non enim ftatim ad affectos locos perveniunt: nam ubi fanos contingunt, perniciem eis faciunt: verum medicamentis utendum eft, quae fuperioribus locis conveniunt, quorumque titulus eft adverfus dyfenteriam inditus. Ex dyfenteria inteftinorum laevitas oritur, ubi ex magna ulceratione multae cicatrices inteftinis oboriuntur, propter quas cibum non retinent: unde ex inteftinorum laevitate vocata eft leienteria. Quamobrem talis eft infanabilis, cicatrices namque non fanefcunt. Si vero ex inteftini imbecillitate contigerit, tum quoque gravis eft, nec ex facili tollitur. Remedium autem erit, fi moliaris robur univerfo corpori ac inteftinis adjungere. Caeterum caufa etiam morbi pituita eft, inteftinis lubricitatem illuendo generans. Succurrit inedia reficcando et cibi pituitae contrarii. Tenesmus proprie morbus eft re-

ἐντάσεις καὶ προθυμίας πρὸς διαχώρησιν ἐμποιεῖ καὶ τοῦτό ἐστιν ὁ τεινεσμός. ἴασις δὲ διὰ πυριαμάτων κάτωθεν τῶν στυφόντων καὶ τροφὴ σιτώδης καὶ σταλτική. εἰ δὲ ἐπιμένει καὶ ἐνέματα διὰ πτισάνης χυλοῦ καὶ στέατος τραγείου χρηστέον. ἕλμινθες δὲ πάθος ἐντέρων. τρισσὸν δὲ εἶδος ἑλμίνθων· αἱ μὲν γὰρ στρογγύλαι σπιθαμιαῖαι τὸ μῆκος, ἢ καὶ μείζους, αἳ καὶ μέχρι στομάχου νέμονται. αἱ δὲ βραχεῖαι καὶ ἐμφερεῖς σκώληξι μακροτέροις, καλοῦνται δὲ ἀσκαρίδες, συνίστανται δὲ περὶ τὸ ἀπευθυσμένον. αἱ δὲ πλατεῖαι καὶ ἐπιμήκεις, ὥστε ὅλῳ τῷ ἐντέρῳ παρατείνονται. λέγονται δὲ καὶ κειρίαι ἐκ τοῦ ἐμφερεῖς εἶναι κειρίαις. ὁμοίως δὲ καὶ ταινίαι, εὐίατοι μὲν οὖν στρογγύλαι. πληθύνουσι γὰρ ἐπὶ παιδίων. αἱ δὲ ἀσκαρίδες πλεονάζουσιν ἐπὶ τῶν παρηβώντων, δυσίατοι δὲ καὶ δυσέκκριτοι, μόνον ὑπὸ τῶν δριμυφαγιῶν καὶ φαρμάκων τῶν διὰ πικρᾶς συντεθειμένων καὶ ἑλενίου, ὡς ἐπὶ τὸ πλεῖστον ἐμβαλλομένων. ἰσχίας δὲ καὶ ἀρθρῖτις καὶ ποδάγρα μεγέθει μόνον ἀλλήλων διαφέρουσι, ταῖς δὲ αἰτίαις

cti inteſtini. Hoc enim inflammatione laborans, crebrae inanesque egerendi cupiditates et impetus exercent. Proſunt ei ſomenta parti inferiori adhibita, ſtringentia, tum alimentum ex frumentacea materia et reprimens. Quod ſi perſeveret nihilque imminuatur, enematibus ex ptiſanae cremore et hircina adipe utendum eſt. Lumbricorum qui inteſtina excruciant triplex eſt ſpecies. Quidam enim teretes, palmi longitudine vel etiam majore, ad ſtomachum usque proſerpunt. Quidam breves et minusculis vermibus ſimiles, aſcarides appellantur, circa rectum vero inteſtinum generantur nonnulli lati et oblongi adeo ut in totum exporrigantur inteſtinum: quos faſcias vocant, quod ſimiles faſciis ſint. Teretes itaque ad remedia faciles, maxime autem in pueris: aſcarides in iis, qui ſub pubertatem ſunt, abundant: aegre praeſidiis cedunt et excernuntur, niſi cibis acrioribus et medicamentis ex hiera compoſi is et helenio maxima ex parte injectis. Iſchias, arthritis vitia et podagrae ſola inter ſe magnitudine differunt: caeterum

καὶ τοῖς τόποις τοῖς πρωτοπαθοῦσι τὰ αὐτά ἐστιν. ὑπό τε γὰρ φλέγματος ὡς ἐπὶ πολὺ γίνονται καὶ περὶ τὰ νεῦρα συνίστανται, τὰ συνέχοντα τὰ ἄρθρα καὶ τὴν κίνησιν αὐτοῖς παρέχοντα. ἀλλ᾽ ἡ μὲν ἰσχίας περὶ τὸ ἄρθρον τὸ κατὰ ἰσχίον γίνεται. διατείνεται δὲ πολλάκις μέχρι σφυρῶν. ἴασις δὲ διὰ φλεβοτομίας ἀπὸ σφυροῦ. καὶ διὰ σικύας ἀπὸ τοῦ ἰσχίου καὶ διὰ κλυσμῶν δριμέων καὶ δι᾽ ἃ δυσεντερίας τρόπον τινὰ ποιοῦσι καὶ τὰ ἔξωθεν καταπλάσματα ἄκοπα καὶ μαλάγματα. ποδάγρα δὲ περὶ μόνους τοὺς πόδας συνίσταται καὶ ἐπισημαίνει ἐν ἀκμῇ μὲν πυρετῶδες ἄλγημα, διὸ τῶν ἐμψυχόντων δεῖται, παρακμῇ δὲ ναρκῶδες καὶ μετὰ ψύξεως, ὅθεν τῶν θερμαινόντων δεῖται. ἀρθρῖτις δὲ ταὐτὸν πάθος τοῖς προειρημένοις περὶ πάντα τὰ ἄρθρα συνιστάμενον. φαρμάκων δὲ δεῖται θεραπευτικῶν τῶν ἀλεαινόντων κηρωμάτων καὶ τῆς καταλλήλου διαίτης. ἡ δὲ ἐλεφαντίασις τὸ πάθος ἔσχε τὸ ὄνομα ἀπὸ ὁμοιότητος τῆς πρὸς τὸν ἐλέφαντα. τὸ γὰρ δέρμα τῶν ἐν τῷ πάθει τούτῳ κατεσχημένων παχύτερόν τε καὶ σκληρότερόν ἐστιν, ἐμφέρειαν ἔχον πρὸς τὸ τῶν

caufis et locis, qui affectum primum fentiunt, iisdem conftant: a pituita namque plerumque fiunt: circa nervos confiftunt, quibus articuli conferuntur, motumque recipiunt. Ac ifchias in ipfius coxae articulo ortus ad talos usque non raro extenditur. Praefidio erit fanguis ex talo miffus, cucurbitulae coxis admotae, clyfteres acres, quique inteftinorum tormina quodammodo faciunt. Et foris cataplasmata acopa et malagmata adhibita profunt. Podagra folos pedes affligit. In ftatu quidem febrilis dolor intenditur, eoque refrigerantibus opus eft. In declinatione torpor cum frigore hominem occupat, ob quod calefacientia conducunt. At arthritis vera praedictis fimilis affectus eft, circa articulos omnes confiftens: medicamenta curatoria, mitigantia ceromata et victus rationem aptam defiderant. Elephantiafis affectus eft, qui ab elephanti fimilitudine nomen fortitus eft. Nam qui hoc vitio laborant, cutem craffam, duram, elephantorum modo afperatam habent. Originem mali excitat pituita craffa et atra

ἐλεφάντων δέρμα. αἴτιον δὲ τοῦ πάθους φλέγμα παχὺ καὶ χολὴ μέλαινα, ἢ βλεννώδης μάλιστα ἐνσπειρομένη. οἱ γὰρ χυμοὶ οὗτοι θηριῶδες αὐτὸ ἀποφαίνουσιν. διὸ καὶ μόνη θεραπεία ἀνύσιμος ἐπὶ τῶν ἐλεφαντιώντων, ἡ δι' ἐλλεβόρου λευκοῦ καὶ μέλανος. τινὲς δὲ τῶν παλαιοτέρων εἰς ἓξ διαιροῦσι τὸ πάθος αὐτὸ, εἰς ἐλεφαντίασιν, λεοντίασιν, ὀφίασιν, λέπραν καὶ ἀλωπεκίαν καὶ λώβην. ἐλεφαντίασιν μὲν οὖν λέγουσι τὴν ἐμφερῆ κατὰ τὸ δέρμα καὶ κατὰ τοὺς πόδας ἐλέφαντι· παχεῖς γὰρ καὶ οὗτοι τοὺς πόδας ἔχουσιν οἱ τῷ πάθει τούτῳ περιπεσόντες δηλονότι, ὥσπερ ἐκεῖνοι· λεοντιᾷν δέ φασι τοὺς ὀχθώδεις ἐπαναστάσεις ἔχοντας, ἢ καὶ οἰδηματώδεις καὶ πυῤῥοτέρους ὄντας δίκην λεόντων. ὀφίασιν δὲ τὴν ἐκδέρουσαν τοὺς ἁλόντας ὡς ὄφεις. ἀλωπεκίαν δὲ ἀπὸ μεταφορᾶς τῶν ζώων ἐκείνων· λώβην δὲ, τὴν τὰ ἄκρα χειρῶν τε καὶ ποδῶν διαφθείρουσαν καὶ τοὺς τῶν τοιούτων μελῶν ἐστερημένους, λελωβημένους. λέπραν δὲ τὴν τραχύνουσαν τὸ δέρμα καὶ οἷον ὁρᾶται ἐπὶ τῶν λεπρῶν, ποιουμένην. ὁ δὲ λειχὴν πάθος μὲν καὶ αὐτὸς δέρματος.

bilis vel mucofa, maxime diffeminata. Hi enim humores ferinum ipfum denunciant. Quare folum veratrum five nigrum, five album, praefens elephantiafis eft remedium. Quidam ex veterioribus affectum illum in fex *partes* dividunt, in elephantiafin, leontiafin, ophiafin, alopeciam et mutilationem. Elephantiafin igitur appellant affectum in cute et pedibus elephanti fimilem, hi enim craffos pedes habent qui fcilicet hoc morbo corripiuntur non fecus ac illi. Leontiafi vero laborare dicunt eos qui tumentes eruptiones habent aut oedematofas et qui leonum inftar fulvi funt. Ophiafin autem *vocant* affectum, quo correpti pelle ut ferpentes exuuntur. Alopeciam vero deducta metaphora ab illis animalibus. Mutilationem, quae fumma manuum et pedum labefacit, privatos quoque ejusmodi partibus, mutilatos *appellamus*. Lepram quae cutem exafperat, quemadmodum in leprofis fieri videmus. Impetigo vero et ipfa cutis affectus eft. Impetiginis duae fpecies

διττὸν δὲ εἶδος λειχῆνος, ὁ μὲν ἥμερος καὶ πρᾳότερος, ὁ δὲ ἄγριος καὶ χαλεπώτερος. ἀφίστανται δὲ ἐπὶ τούτων καὶ λεπίδες τοῦ δέρμα- [387] τος καὶ ὁ ὑπὸ τὰς λεπίδας τόπος ἐνερευθέστερος καὶ ἐγγὺς ἡλκωμένοι φαίνεται. γίνεται δὲ τὸ πάθος ὑπὸ φλέγματος ἁλμυροῦ καὶ χολῆς τῆς ξανθῆς· ἔνθεν ὡς ἐπὶ τῶν ἁλμῶν τῶν κεραμίων ἀφίστανται τοῦ δέρματος αἱ λεπίδες. ἴασις δὲ ἥ τε διὰ φαρμάκων φλεγμαγωγῶν καὶ τῶν ἔξωθεν ἐπιχρίστων. λέπρα δὲ πάθος μὲν καὶ αὐτὴ δέρματος ἐπὶ τὸ λευκότερον καὶ τραχύτερον τρεπόμενον. ἡ δὲ τραχύτης οἷον ψυδρακίων ἐπανεστώτων. ἡ δὲ ψώρα ἐστὶν ἑλκωδεστέρα. γίνεται δὲ ἑκάτερον ἰδίως ὑπὸ φλέγματος ἁλμυροῦ. ἴασις δὲ ἥδε διὰ φλεγμαγωγῶν φαρμάκων καὶ τῶν ἔξωθεν ἐπιχρισμάτων, ὅσα πρὸς λέπραν καὶ ψώραν ἀναγέγραπται. ὁ δὲ ἀλφὸς διττόν ἐστι πάθος, ὁ μὲν λευκὸς, ὁ δὲ μέλας. γίνεται δὲ ὁ μὲν μέλας ὑπὸ μελαίνης χολῆς· διὸ καὶ μελαγχολικὰ τὰ πολλὰ ῥύεται ὁ δὲ λευκὸς ὑπὸ φλέγματος γίνεται, οὐχ ἁλυκοῦ. ἡ δὲ λεύκη ὅμοιον μὲν τὸ πάθος ἀλφῷ λευκῷ, μᾶλλον δὲ ἐπισημαίνει γῆν λευκοτάτην.

ſunt, quae cutem moleſtant: una tolerabilis mitiorque eſt: altera effera, quae difficilius tollitur. Squamulae in his ex cute abſcedunt, ſub quibus locus rubicundior fereque exulceratus apparet. Gignitur affectus a pituita ſalſa et flava bile: unde, ceu in ſalſugine vaſis fictilibus, ex cute ſecedunt ſquamae. Succurritur medicamentis pituitam moventibus et quae extrinſecus corpori illinuntur. Lepra quoque cutis vitium eſt, ſed magis ſubalbidum asperiusque apparet. Ea vero asperitas eſt veluti pſydraciorum erumpentium. Pſora vero exulcerata magis eſt. Pituita ſalſa utrumque malum proprie producit. Medicamenta pituitam cientia, tum quae extrinſecus illinuntur, quibus ad lepram et ſcabiem titulus eſt, iisdem ſuccurrunt. Vitiligo duas habet ſpecies, albam et nigram. Haec ab atra bile generatur, ob quod magna ex parte medicamina melancholiae dicata conveniunt: alba a pituita non ſalſa. Leuce habet quiddam ſimile vitiligini albae, ſed magis colore terram albiſſimam refert: a lepra variat,

λέπρας δὲ διαφέρει τῷ λεῖον εἶναι καὶ μὴ τραχύνεσθαι τὸ δέρμα, ὡς ἐπὶ λέπρας. ῥύεται δὲ τούτων ἁπάντων τὰ φλεγμαγωγὰ φάρμακα καὶ τὰ ἔξωθεν σμήγματα.

Κεφ. ιδ΄. [Περὶ συνθέσεως ἀρίστης καθαρσίου.] Συντίθεται δὲ ἡ πρὸς τὰ ἐντὸς φαρμακεία ἀπό τε ἀποφρακτικῶν καὶ τμητικῶν καὶ λεπτυντικῶν καὶ προοδοποιητικῶν καὶ προτρεπτικῶν καὶ καθαρτικῶν καὶ κολαστικῶν τῆς τῶν φαρμάκων κακίας, εὐστομάχων τε καὶ ἐφεκτικῶν τῆς ἀλόγου φορᾶς. ἀποφρακτικὰ μὲν οὖν ὅσα τοὺς πόρους ἀραιοῖ καὶ τὰ σώματα εὔροα ποιεῖ· τμητικὰ δὲ ὅσα τέμνει τοὺς χυμοὺς καὶ πέπτει τοὺς μὲν παχύνοντα, τοὺς δὲ λεπτύνοντα. προοδοποιητικὰ δὲ ὅσα προάγει καὶ προπέμπει τὰ φάρμακα εἰς ἃ βουλόμεθα μόρια, ὡς ἐπὶ μὲν τῶν ἧπαρ καθαίρειν βουλομένων, σάνδαλα· τῶν δὲ σπλῆνα, σκολοπένδριον· νεφροὺς δὲ καὶ ἰσχία, κενταύριόν τε καὶ θλάσπι· τὰ ὄπισθεν τῆς κεφαλῆς, παιωνία καὶ στοιχάς· τὰ ἐμπρόσθιά τε καὶ σάμψυχον καὶ τὰ τοιαῦτα· στήθη καὶ πνεύμονα καὶ θώρακα καὶ καρδίαν καὶ μετάφρενα καὶ ἔντερα, γλυκύῤῥιζον

quod lenior huic cutis minusque aspera quam in illa ſit. Omnia hujusmodi curant medicamenta pituitae trahendae idonea, tum ſmegmata foris adhibita.

Cap. XIV. [*De optimae purgationis compoſitione.*] Componitur autem ad internos humores purgans medicamentum ex deobſtruentibus, incidentibus, attenuantibus, vias reſerantibus, impellentibus, purgantibus et edomantibus vitium medicamentis et ſtomacho utilibus et immoderatum profluvium compeſcentibus. Deobſtruentia itaque ſunt quaecunque laxant et corpora meabilia efficiunt. Incidentia vero, quae humores incidunt et alios quidem incraſſando, alios vero attenuando concoquunt. Vias autem reſerantia ſunt, quae deducunt ac praemittunt medicamenta in quas volumus partes, ut ad hepar quum purgare volumus, ſandala, ad lienem vero ſcolopendrium; ad renes vero et iſchia centaurium et thlaſpi; ad poſteriorem capitis partem paeonia et ſtoechas; ad anteriorem vero et ſampſuchus et ſimilia; ad ſternum et pulmonem et thora-

καὶ στύραξ καὶ σπέρμα τήλεως· ἀμύγδαλά τε καὶ κρόκος καὶ σπέρμα λινοζώστεως καὶ τοὺς ἁρμοὺς καὶ τὰ ἄρθρα, ἑκάτερον ἑρμοδάκτυλον καὶ ἄλλοις ἄλλα, ἅπερ ἐκ τῶν εἰρημένων δεῖ συντεκμαίρεσθαι. προτρεπτικὰ δὲ ὅσα κινεῖ καὶ προτρέπει τὰ φάρμακα, ὡς μὲν ἀγαρικὸν, ἶρις, ῥέον δὲ Ἰνδικὸν, στάχυς· ἐντεριώνην δὲ κολοκυνθίδος, τραγάκανθα· σκαμμωνίαν δὲ, ἀλόη, ἢ χυλὸς κράμβης, ἢ ῥόδων, ἢ σπέρματα. ὡσαύτως ἅλας ὀρυκτόν· τὸ ἐπίθυμον, ὥσπερ εὐφόρβιον, βδέλλιον καὶ τὸν ἐλλέβορον· ῥαφανῖδος σπέρμα καὶ τὴν ἀλυπαίαν· ὄξος ἢ χρυσοβάλανος καὶ τὰ μυροβάλανα· βρυωνία καὶ τὸ ἐλατήριον ἅλας. καὶ μὲν δὴ καὶ τῆς πιτυούσης τὴν ῥίζαν, ἑρμοδάκτυλον τὸ στογγύλον καὶ τοῖς ἄλλοις ὡσαύτως τὰ παραπλήσια, ἅπερ ἐν τῷ περὶ ἀρίστης συνθέσεως φαρμάκων κατὰ μέρος διήλθομεν καὶ δεῖ ἐκεῖθεν νομίζεσθαι τὰ ἐλλείποντα. καθαρτικὰ δὲ ὅσα καθαίρει κἀνταῦθα κἀν τῷ περὶ ἁπλῶν φαρμάκων ἡμῖν γέγραπται. κολασιικὰ δὲ τῆς κακίας ὅσα τοῖς δηλητηρίοις τῶν φαρμάκων

cem et cor et metaphrenum et inteſtina glycirrhiza, ſtyrax, ſemen ſoenugraeci, amygdala, crocus et ſemen mercurialis; ad commiſſuras et articulos uterque hermodactylus et ad alias partes alia, quae ex dictis conjicienda ſunt. Impellentia ſunt quaecunque medicamenta movent ac impellunt, ut agaricum, eris, rheum Indicum, ſtachys, interior pars colocynthidis, tragacantha, ſcamonium, aloë vel ſuccus braſſicae vel roſarum vel ſemina; ſimiliter ſal foſſile, epithymum, quemadmodum euphorbium, bdellium et helleborus, radiculae ſemen, turpetum, chryſobalanus et myrobalana, bryonia et elaterion ſal, quibus quidem annumeramus pytyuſae radicem, hermodactylum rotundum et aliis peraeque ſimilibus, quae in libris de optima compoſitione ſecundum partes declaravimus; ac quae deſunt inde ducenda ſunt. Purgantia vero ſunt quaecunque hic purgant et quae in opere de ſimplicibus medicamentis a nobis ſcripta ſunt. Edomantia autem malitiam ſunt quaecunque medicamentorum noxis adverſantur proprie, ut

ἀντικεῖσθαι ἰδίωμα, ὡς ἀγαρικοῦ μὲν ζίγγιβερ, σκαμμωνίας δὲ ὀποῦ, μαστίχη ἢ κόμμι Ἀραβικὸν, ἢ καφουρὰ, ἢ κυδωνίων μήλων χυλός· κολοκυνθίδος δὲ ἀμυγδάλων ἔλαιον· ἀλυπαίας δὲ νᾶπυ· ὥσπερ ἐλλεβόρου καστόριον, ἢ ὑδρόμελι· καὶ εὐφορβίου κιννάμωμον. ἀλόης δέ γε μαστίχη· ὥσπερ αὐτὴν προτρέπει τὸ σμύρνιον· καὶ τἄλλα ὅσα ἡμῖν ἐν τῷ [388] περὶ ἀρίστης συνθέσεως εἴρηται. εὐστόμαχα δὲ καὶ ἐφεκτικὰ τῆς ἀλόγου τῶν φαρμάκων φορᾶς, ὅσα τονοῖ καὶ συνέχει καὶ τὰς φυσικὰς διεγείρει ἐνεργείας. τὸ δὲ κατὰ μέρος ταῦτα ἐπεξεργάσασθαι περισσὸν νῦν ἡμῖν ἔδοξε.

Κεφ. ιε΄. [Περὶ διαιρέσεως τῆς διὰ φαρμάκων θεραπείας.] Ἡ δὲ φαρμακεία διττή ἐστιν, ἡ μὲν πρὸς τὰ ἐντὸς πάθη, ᾗ μάλιστα χρῆται ὁ διαιτητικός· ἡ δὲ πρὸς τὰ ἐκτὸς, ἧς οὐκ ἄνευ συντελεῖται τὰ κατὰ χειρουργίαν. τῆς μὲν οὖν πρὸς τὰ ἐντὸς φαρμακείας εἴδη ἐστὶ δεκαδύο. τὸ μὲν τῶν ἐν τῇ κεφαλῇ παθῶν· τὸ δὲ τῶν στοματικῶν· τὸ

agarici noxae Zingiber, fucci fcammoniae, mastiche vel gummi Arabicum vel caphura vel malorum cotoneorum fuccus, colocynthidis vero amygdalinum oleum; turpeti autem fynapium; ut hellebori caftorium vel mulfa et euphorbii cinnamomum. Aloës vero maftiche, quemadmodum ipfam promovet fmyrnium et caetera quae a nobis in opere de optima compofitione dictum eft. Euftomacha five quae ftomachum roborant, ephectica quae immoderatam medicamentorum vacuationem reprimunt, quae roborant ac continent et fufcitant naturales facultates. Sed in particulari, ut ea quae modum excedunt eximant, jam a nobis demonftratum eft.

Cap. XV. [*De curationis per medicamenta divifione.*] Pharmacia duplex eft. Prima interiores morbos curat, qua potiffimum victus ratione fanans utitur: altera exteriores, citraque illam manu nihil peragitur. Medicaminum ad interiora pertinentium fpecies duodecim exiftunt. Quaedam capitis affectibus dicata medicamina: quaedam

Ed. Chart. II. [388.] Ed. Baf. IV. (384. 385.)

δὲ τῶν πεπτικῶν· τὸ δὲ τῶν βηχικῶν· τὸ δὲ τῶν ἀνωδύνων τὸ δὲ τῶν ἀλεξιφαρμάκων· τὸ δὲ τῶν καθαιρόντων. καὶ τὰ μὲν ἡπατικὰ ἰδίως· τὰ δὲ σπληνικά· τὰ δὲ νεφριτικά· τὰ δὲ πρὸς τοὺς ἐν τῇ κύστει λίθους καὶ ἕλκη· τὰ δὲ πρὸς ὑστέραν· τὰ μὲν δὴ στοματικά ἐστι, τὰ δὲ πρὸς οὖλα αἱμασσόμενα, σηπόμενα, βεβρωμένα καὶ ὀδόντας καὶ ὅσα πρὸς ἄφθας καὶ ἐσχάρας, ὅσα τε πρὸς σταφυλὴν κεχαλασμένην. τῶν δὲ πεττικῶν τὰ μέν ἐστι πρὸς ἀτονίαν στομάχου, ἢ κοιλίας· τὰ δὲ πρὸς ἐμπνευμάτωσιν τούτων· τὰ δὲ πρὸς αἵματος ἀναγωγήν· τὰ δὲ πρὸς πλευριτικοὺς, ἢ περιπνευματικούς· τὰ δὲ πρὸς φθισικούς· τὰ δὲ πρὸς ἀσθματικοὺς, ἢ ὀρθοπνοϊκούς· τὰ δὲ πρὸς τραχύ- (385) τητά τε ἀρτηρίας καὶ φωνῆς ἐκκοπήν. τῶν δὲ ἀνωδύνων τὰ μὲν πρὸς νεφριτικοὺς, τὰ δὲ πρὸς κοιλίας ῥύσεις καὶ δυσεντερίας καὶ πρὸς κωλικοὺς καὶ εἰλεώδεις. κοινῶς δὲ πάντα πρὸς πᾶσαν ὀδύνην. τὰ δὲ ἀλεξιφάρμακα τὰ μὲν ἁπλᾶ, ἄλλα πρὸς ἄλλο δηλητήριον. ἡ δὲ θηριακὴ πρὸς πάντα καὶ προσλαμβανομένη καὶ ἐπιδιδομένη. τῶν δὲ καθαιρόντων τὰ μὲν ἄνωθεν κα-

oris vitiis accommoda dicuntur. Alia concoquunt: alia bechica. Alia anodyna, alia alexipharmaca ſunt: alia purgant. Nonnulla proprie hepatica, ſic ſplenica, nephritica. Sunt quae adverſus veſicae calculos et ulcera nomen habent, ſimiliter ad vulvam. Jam vero ſtomatica ſunt, quae ad gingivas cruentas, putridas, eroſas et dentes faciunt. Eodem referuntur, quae aphthas et cruſtas, tum quae uvam deſcendentem ſanant. Quae concoquunt, partim ad ſtomachi vel ventriculi imbecillitatem conducunt, partim ad horum inſlammationem, quaedam ad ſanguinis rejectionem e pectore. Quaedam ad pleuriticos vel peripneumonicos: alia ad tabidos, alia ad aſthmaticos vel qui orthopnoici vocantur. Aliqua ex his aſperitatem arteriae et vocis abſciſſionem auferunt. Porro anodyna nunc renum affectus ſedant, nunc ventris profluvia: alias dyſenterias, alias colicum dolorem, coli et ileum, id eſt communiter omnia quemvis dolorem mitigant extinguntque. Alexipharmaca ſimplicia, alia ad aliud venenum uſurpamus: theriace ad-

θαίρει, ὡς τὰ δι' ἐλλεβόρου καὶ ἐμετικὰ πάντα, τὰ δὲ κάτωθεν παραλαμβάνεται, ὡς τὰ διὰ σκαμμωνίας καὶ ἀλόης καὶ ἐλατηρίου καὶ κολοκυνθίδος καὶ εὐφορβίου καὶ κόκκου κνιδίου καὶ τῶν τοιούτων. τρίτα δὲ τούτοις τετάχθω καὶ τὰ πρὸς ἕλμινθας πλατείας, οἷά ἐστι τὸ διὰ κέρατος ἐλαφείου καὶ ἡδυόσμου καὶ πεπέρεως. ἔστι δὲ καὶ τέταρτον εἶδος τῶν κεφαλὴν μόνην καθαιρόντων διὰ στόματος καὶ ῥινῶν ἃ παραλαμβάνεται ἰδίως. ἐπί τε τῶν ἐν τῇ κεφαλῇ καὶ τοῖς ὀφθαλμοῖς παθῶν καὶ τὰ πλεῖστα ἐπὶ ἰκτέρων. ἁρμόζουσι δὲ αἱ μὲν διὰ τῶν ἄνω καθάρσεις πρὸς ἀνασκευὴν τῶν χρονίων. καιρὸς δὲ αὐτῶν τὰ διαλείμματα. αἱ δὲ κάτωθεν, πρὸς τὰ ὀξέα νοσήματα κατάλληλοι, πλευρίτιδας καὶ περιπνευμονίας. καιρὸς δὲ αὐτῶν πάντων ἡ ἄνεσις τῶν ἐπὶ μέρους παροξυσμῶν. τῆς δὲ πρὸς τὰ ἐκτὸς φαρμακείας εἴδη ἐστὶν ἕνδεκα. τὰ μὲν γὰρ αὐτῶν διαφορητικὰ, τὰ δὲ συμπεπτικὰ, τὰ δὲ ἔναιμα, τὰ δὲ πυοποιὰ, τὰ δὲ ἀνακαθαρτικὰ, τὰ δὲ ἀναπληρωτικὰ, τὰ δὲ κατασταλτικὰ, τὰ δὲ

verfus omnia et prius et poft fumitur. Inter purgantia quaedam per fuperiores corporis partes agunt, quemadmodum quae veratro conftant, vomitumque cientia omnia. Per inferiores, quae ex fcammonia, aloë, elaterio, colocynthide, euphorbio, cocco gnidio atque his fimilibus. Tertio ordine ab his ponantur quae lumbricos latos repellunt: cujusmodi medicamentum eft quod cervi cornu, menta et pipere praeparatur. Eft et quarta fpecies caput tantum per os atque nares purgantium, quae in capitis oculorumque affectibus proprie fumuntur. Ad haec quae in arquato crebro in ufu funt. Convenit autem per fuperiora purgatio morbis longis demoliendis. Tempus hujus eft, cum morbi intermittunt. Inferiori parte adhibita, acutis, ut pleuritidi et peripneumoniae. Tempus vero univerfae eft particularium acceffionum remiffio. Exteriorum remedia undecim fpecies continent, alia difcutiunt, alia concoquunt, alia cruentis ftatim imponuntur, alia pus movent, alia repurgant, alia implent, alia reprimunt, alia

Ed. Chart. II. [388. 389.] Ed. Baf. IV. (385.)

ἐπουλωτικὰ, τὰ δὲ ὀφθαλμικὰ, τὰ δὲ ἐν ὅλῳ τῷ σώματι, τὰ δὲ καυστικὰ ἐπὶ ἐρυσιπέλατα καὶ ἕρπητας καὶ ἄνθρακας· τὰ δέ εἰσιν ἀλείμματα ἄκοπά τε καὶ θερμαντικὰ πρὸς παραλύσεις ποιοῦντα καὶ ἀρθριτικοὺς καὶ ποδαγρικοὺς καὶ πᾶσαν νεύρων πῆξιν καὶ τετανικοὺς καὶ ὀπισθοτονικούς. τὰ δὲ σμηκτικὰ τῶν εἰς τὴν ἐπιφάνειαν ἐξανθούντων, λεύκης, ἀλφοῦ, λειχῆνος καὶ λέπρας. τὰ οὖν διαφορητικὰ καὶ συμπεπτικὰ ἐπὶ φυμάτων καὶ παντὸς ἀποστήματος τοιούτου ἁρμόζει. διαφορητικαὶ δέ εἰσιν αἱ διὰ [389] ἁλῶν πᾶσαι καὶ ὅσαι διὰ νίτρου, ὡς τὸ Κτησιφῶντος. συμπεπτικὰ δὲ τὰ διὰ ῥητίνης καὶ χαλβάνης καὶ ἀμμωνιακοῦ θυμιάματος· τῶν δὲ ἐναίμων φαρμάκων αἱ μὲν φαιαὶ ἐπὶ τῶν κατὰ τοῦ σώματος προσφάτων τραυμάτων ἁρμόζουσιν. αἱ δὲ ἰδίως χλωραὶ καὶ μέλαιναι, ὡς ἡ βάρβαρος, πρός τε τὰ ἐν τῇ κεφαλῇ καὶ πρὸς τὰ κυνόδηκτα. ἐπὶ δὲ ἑλκῶν τοῖς μὲν πυοποιοῖς ἐπὶ τῶν φλεγμαινόντων χρηστέον, ὡς τῇ τετραφαρμάκῳ. τοῖς δὲ ἀνακαθαίρουσιν ἐπὶ τῶν ῥυπαρῶν, ὡς τῇ χλωρᾷ ἀνειμένῃ. τοῖς δὲ ἀναπληροῦσιν ἐπὶ τῶν κοίλων. τοῖς

cicatricem inducunt, alia oculis, alia univerfo corpori adhibentur, alia adurunt, eryfipelatis, herpetibus carbunculis idonea. Alia funt, quae illinuntur, acopa et excalfacientia, quae ad nervorum refolutiones faciunt, articulorum morbos, podagras, tetanos, opifthotonos omnemque nervorum morbum. Alia piftulas fumma cute orientes leucen, alphum, impetiginem et lepram abftergunt. Quae digerunt et concoquunt, phymatis et cuilibet id genus abfceffui auxilio funt. Digerentia funt omnia, quae conftant fale et quaecunque etiam nitro, ut Ctefiphontis compofitio teftatur. Concoquentia, refina, galbano, ammoniaco thymiamate. Quae cruentis imponuntur pharmaca, fufci coloris, ad recentia corporis vulnera valent. Quae proprie viridia et nigra funt, ut barbarum, capitis mala et canum morfus fanant. In ulceribus partim pus educentibus in his, quae laborant inflammatione, utendum eft, ut tetrapharmaco: in fordidis vero repurgantibus, ut viridi diluto: in cavis replentibus: in carne fupercrefcenti

δὲ καταστέλλουσιν ὡς ἐπὶ τῶν ὑπερσαρκούντων, ὡς τοῖς διὰ μίσυος καὶ λεπίδος, ἃ καὶ ἐπὶ τῶν δυσεπισχέτων αἱμοῤῥαγιῶν ἁρμόζει. τοῖς δὲ καυστικοῖς ὁτὲ μὲν πρὸς τὸ διελεῖν καὶ ἀναπτύξαι σώματα χρώμεθα, ὡς ἐπὶ τῶν ἀποστημάτων τὴν περιοχὴν, ὁτὲ δὲ ἐπὶ τῶν κεχαλασμένων βλεφάρων ἀντὶ ἀναῤῥαφῆς, ἀφαιροῦντες τὸ σύμμετρον τῆς οὐλῆς, ἀνασπῶμεν τὸ κεχαλασμένον. ὁτὲ δὲ ἐπὶ κεφαλαίας δυσιάτου παραλαμβάνομεν, διὰ βαθείας ἐσχάρας μεταβάλλοντες εἰς τὰ ἐκτὸς ῥεύματα. ὕλη δὲ τῶν καυστικῶν κονία, ἄσβεστος ζῶσα καὶ ἀρσενικὸν καὶ σανδαράχη καὶ φέκλα καὶ τὰ τοιαῦτα. τῶν δὲ κεφαλικῶν τὰ μὲν πρὸς ἀχῶρας καὶ πίτυρα καὶ ἐκβράσματα ἁρμόζει, τὰ δὲ πρὸς κεφαλαλγίαν καὶ ἑτεροκρανίαν. τῶν δὲ ὠτικῶν τὰ μὲν πρὸς φλεγμονὴν ὤτων, τὰ δὲ πρὸς ἕλκωσιν· τὰ δὲ πρὸς πυοῤῥοοῦντα· τὰ δὲ πρὸς δυσηκοΐαν· τὰ δὲ πρὸς ὦτα τεθλασμένα. τῶν δὲ ὀφθαλμικῶν φαρμάκων εἴδη εἰσὶν ἑπτά. τὰ μὲν γὰρ πρὸς ἀρχομένας ὀφθαλμίας ἁρμόζει, ὡς τὰ διὰ γλαυκίου καὶ τὰ διὰ κρόκου καὶ τὰ κυκνάρια· τὰ δὲ πρὸς τὰς διαθέσεις, ὡς τὰ νάρδινα καὶ τὰ θεο-

reprimentibus, ut quae ex mify et fquama conficiuntur, in vehementi quoque fanguinis fluore fiftendo non parum efficacibus. Adurentibus interim in diducendis partibus ac aperiendis utimur, velut in abfceffuum comprehenfione, interim in palpebris quum fumma cutis relaxatur et procidit vice futurae pilis mediocriter ablatis, partem relaxatam retrahimus. Aliquando in cephalaea per altas cruftas humores in exteriorem educentes affumimus. Adurentium materia, lixivium, calx viva, auripigmentum, fandaracha, faecula, atque id genus alia. Ex cephalicis medicamentis, ad achoras, capitis furfures et eruptiones valent alia: ad capitis dolorem et heterocraniam alia. Aurium remedia partim earum inflammationem, partim exulcerationem, partim puris effluxum, partim difficilem auditum, partim contufionem juvant. Oculorum pharmaca feptem fpecies habent. Quaedam enim ad incipientes lippitudines, ut quae ex glaucio et ex croco et cycnaria infcribuntur. Quaedam ad eorum difpofitiones, ut nardina

δότια καλούμενα. τὰ δὲ πρὸς ῥεύματα, ὡς τὰ διὰ λιβάνου καὶ ἀκακίας καὶ ἐρείκης καρποῦ. τὰ δὲ πρὸς τραχώματα, ὡς τὰ διὰ τῶν μεταλλικῶν, οἷον κεκαυμένου χαλκοῦ καὶ χαλκίτεως καὶ λεπίδος χαλκοῦ. πέμπτον δέ ἐστι τὸ πρὸς ξηροφθαλμίας καὶ ψωροφθαλμίας εἶδος τῶν κολλυρίων καὶ ξηρῶν ὀξυδερκικῶν, ἃ τῆς αὐτῆς ὕλης ἐστὶ τοῖς προγεγραμμένοις. ἕκτον δὲ τῶν ὑγρῶν εἶδος, τῶν πρὸς ὑποχύσεις ἀναγεγραμμένων, ἃ διὰ χολῶν σκευάζονται καὶ μάλιστα δι' ὑαίνης. ἕβδομον δὲ τὸ τῶν καταπλασμάτων εἶδος, ἃ παραλαμβάνεται ἐπὶ τῶν ἄκρως φλεγμαινόντων ὀφθαλμῶν καὶ περιοδυνώντων. ἔστι δὲ τάδε διὰ μελιλώτων καὶ γλυκέος καὶ τήλεως καὶ τὰ τοιαύτης ὕλης. περιχρίομεν δὲ τὰ βλέφαρα ἐν ἀρχῇ μὲν τοῖς ἀποκρουστικοῖς, οἷά ἐστι τὰ διὰ γλαυκίου καὶ τοῖς διὰ κρόκου καὶ αὐτῷ μόνῳ γλαυκίῳ. ἐπὶ δὲ τῶν ἐνδιαθέτων τοῖς ἀναξηραίνουσι καὶ παραμυθουμένοις, οἷον ναρδίνοις καὶ θεοδοτίοις. ὅσα δὲ πρὸς εὐμορφίαν ἐπιχρίεται, ὡς τὰ διὰ σάνδυκος καὶ ἡδυχρόου, οὐκ ἰατρικῆς, ἀλλὰ καλλωπιστικῆς ἐστιν ἴδια.

et theodotia appellata. Quaedam ad fluorem, quae ex thure, acacia et ericae fructu componuntur. Quaedam ad fcabritiem, ut ex metallis confecta, nempe ufto aëre, chalcitide et aeris fquama. Quinta ad ficcam lippitudinem et fcabiofam collyriorum fpecies eft, tum ficcorum oxydercicon, ejusdem cum fuperioribus materiae. Sexta humidorum, quae ad fuffufiones infcribuntur, ex fellis generibus hyaenaeque potiffimum compofita. Septima cataplasmatum fpecies in oculis vehementer inflammatis et circundolentibus ufurpatur, ex meliloto, paffo, foenugraeco fimilibusque materiis confecta. Oblinimus palpebras initio repellentibus et cujusmodi funt quae ex glaucio et croco medicamina: etiam folo ipfo glaucio. Interius affectis exiccantia lenientiaque admovemus, ut nardina, theodotia. Quae vero ad colorem decoremque formae conciliandum illinuntur, qualia hedychroo et fandice conftituuntur, non medicinae, fed artis cultui ac elegantiae dicatae funt propria.

Κεφ. ιστ'. [*Περὶ τῶν ἐν ὀφθαλμοῖς συνισταμένων παθῶν.*] *Πάθη δὲ περὶ μὲν τὸν ὅλον ὀφθαλμὸν συνίσταται τάδε. τάραξις, ὀφθαλμία, ἐπιφορὰ, φλεγμονὴ, οἴδημα, ἐμφύσημα, σκίῤῥωσις, χήμωσις, ἄνθραξ, στραβισμὸς, σπασμὸς, παλμὸς, μυωπίασις, γάγγραινα, σηπεδὼν, ἕλκος, σῦριγξ, ξηροφθαλμία, ψωροφθαλμία, σκληροφθαλμία, πρόπτωσις, ἀτροφία. περὶ δὲ τοὺς ὑμένας τάδε. ῥῆξις, διάβρωσις, διάτασις, ἀναστόμωσις, παχύτης, πυκνότης, ῥύσωσις, ἔκτασις, ἀραιότης. περὶ δὲ τὰ ἐντὸς μὲν βλεφάρων τραχύτης, παχύτης, σύκωσις, τύλωσις, σκληρία, χαλάζωσις, πλαδαρότης, μύδησις, σάρκωσις, πωρίασις. περὶ δὲ τὰ ἐκτὸς τῶν βλεφάρων* [390] *ὑδατίδες, λιθίασις, φθειρίασις, μελικηρὶς, γάγγραινα, φύματα, κολοβώματα. περὶ δὲ τὴν στεφάνην κριθὴ καὶ ποσθία, τριχίασις, διστιχία, τριστιχία, φαλάγγωσις, πύρωσις, πτίλωσις, ψωρίασις, μαδαρότης, παράλυσις. κοινῶς δὲ πρὸς ὅλα τὰ βλέφαρα, παράλυσις, πρόπτωσις, ἐκτροπή. περὶ δὲ τοὺς κανθοὺς, ἐγκανθὶς ἀγκύλη, πτερύγιον, ῥοιὰς, πρόσφυσις. ἔξωθεν δὲ αἰγίλωψ, ἀγχίλωψ.*

Cap. XVI. [*De oculorum affectibus.*] Affectus, qui totum oculum exercent, hi funt, perturbatio, lippitudo, epiphora, inflammatio, oedema, inflatio, durities, chymofis, carbunculus, ftrabismus, convulfio, palpitatio, myopiafis, gangraena, putredo, ulcus, fiftula, xerophthalmia, pforophthalmia, fclerophthalmia, procidentia, atrophia. In membranis hi confiftunt, ruptura, exefio, diftentio, anaftomofis, craffities, denfitas, corrugatio, extenfio, raritas. Interiores palpebrarum partes infeftant afpritudo, craffities, fycofis, tylofis, durities, chalazofis, pladarotes, mydefis, farcofis, poriafis. Exteriores hydatides, lithiafis, phthiriafis, meliceris, gangraena, phymata, colobomata. In corona crithe, pofthia, trichiafis, diftichia, triftichia, phalangofis, pyrofis, ptilofis, pforiafis, madarotes, paralyfis. Communes toti palpebrae paralyfis, procidentia, inverfio. Angulis hi accidunt, encanthis, ancyle, pterygion, rhoeas, profphyfis. Extrinfecus aegilops, anchilops.

περὶ δὲ τὸ λευκὸν ψυδράκιον ἕλκος, ὑπόσφαγμα, ἀπόστασις, χήμωσις, κοίλωμα, πτερύγιον, φάκωσις, ἴκτερος, πῶρος. περὶ δὲ τὴν ἶριν ἄργεμον, νεφέλιον, ἀχλὺς, ἐπίκαυμα, ἕλκος, βοθρίον, φλυκτὶς, μυιοκέφαλον, σταφύλωμα, ὑπόπυον, ῥῆξις, οὐλὴ, λεύκωμα, κοίλωμα, πρόπτωμα, ὄνυξ, πύωσις, ἕλκωσις. περὶ δὲ τὴν κόρην ὑπόχυσις, γλαύκωσις, μυδρίασις, φθίσις, σύγχυσις, πλατυκορίασις, ἀμαύρωσις, ῥυτίδωσις, νυκτάλωψ, ἡμεράλωψ, μυωπίασις, διαπύησις. περὶ δὲ τοὺς πόρους ἀπόῤῥηξις, παρέμπτωσις, σύμπτωσις, ἕλκωσις, ἀνθράκωσις. τάραξις μὲν οὖν ἐστιν, ὅταν συγκινηθεὶς ὁ ὀφθαλμὸς ἐπιπολαίως καὶ μετρίως ἐπὶ τὸ ἐρυθρότερον καταστῇ τελέως. ὀφθαλμία δέ ἐστιν, ὅταν τὸ λευκὸν ἐνερευθὲς ᾖ καὶ τὰ βλέφαρα ἐπηρμένα μετὰ τοῦ τήν τε μύσιν τῶν βλεφάρων ἐπαλγῆ εἶναι καὶ τὴν τῶν χειρῶν ἐπαφὴν ἐπώδυνον. φλεγμονὴ δέ ἐστιν ἐπίτασις τοῦ (386) τε ἐρυθήματος καὶ τῆς ἐπάρσεως τῶν βλεφάρων, ὡς ἐπιπόνως ἀναβλέπειν. ἐπιφορὰ δὲ κοινὸν ὄνομα ἐπὶ παντὸς τοῦ σώματος καὶ φλεγμονῆς σφοδρᾶς ἐπιφερομένης καὶ ῥευμάτων

Album affligunt pſydracion ulcus, hypoſphagma, abſceſſus, chemoſis, coeloma, pterygion, phacoſis, icterus, tophus. Iridem oculi infeſtant, argemon, nephelion, achlys, epicauma, ulcus, bothrion, phlyctis, myocephalon, ſtaphyloma, hypopyon, ruptura, cicatrix, leucoma, coeloma, proptoma, unguis, pyoſis, exulceratio. In pupilla eſſe ſolent effuſio, glaucoſis, mydriaſis, phthiſis, ſynchyſis, platycoriaſis, amauroſis, rhytidoſis, nyctalops, hameralops, myopiaſis, diapyes. Meatus exercent aporrhexis, paremptoſis, ſymptoſis, helcoſis, anthracoſis. Perturbatio igitur eſt, quum oculus leviter ac mediocriter commotus tandem rubicundior evadit. Ophthalmia vero eſt quum album rubeſcit et palpebrae attolluntur, cum dolore connivent aegreque manus admotas ferunt. Inflammatione oculorum rubor intenditur, palpebrae magis elevantur, ut non niſi magno negotio queas ſuſpicere. Epiphora tum inflammationis magnae univerſo illatae corpori, tum largae fluxioni commune nomen eſt: proprie vero de ocu-

λάβρων ἐπιῤῥεόντων. ἰδίως δὲ ἐπὶ ὀφθαλμῶν λέγεται, ἐπειδὰν μετὰ φλεγμονῆς μεγίστης καὶ ῥεύματος πλῆθος ἐπιῤῥυῇ. οἴδημα δέ ἐστιν, ὅταν ἐπηρμένος καὶ ἀχρούστερος, ἢ καὶ δυσκίνητος ἐπιφαίνηται. ἐνίοτε δὲ καὶ τὸ λευκὸν ὑπὲρ τὸ μέλαν ἐπαίρεται. ἐμφύσημα δέ ἐστιν, ὅταν ἄφνω οἰδίσας ὁ ὀφθαλμὸς ἀχρούστερος καὶ φλεγματωδέστερος γένηται. γίνεται δὲ ὡς ἐπίπαν πρεσβύταις, μάλιστα θέρους. σκίῤῥωσις δὲ γίνεται κατ' ἐπίτασιν φλεγμονῆς χρονίου τῆς σαρκὸς αὐξανομένης καὶ ὑποπελιαζούσης. ῥευματίζεται δὲ ὁ ὀφθαλμὸς, ὅταν μὴ μόνον ἐρυθρὸς ᾖ, ἀλλὰ καὶ ὅταν πολὺ δάκρυον ἐκκρίνῃ. ξηροφθαλμία δέ ἐστιν, ὅταν οἱ κανθοὶ ἑλκώδεις καὶ τραχύτεροι καὶ κνησμώδεις εἰσὶ καὶ τὰ βλέφαρα ἐρυθριᾷ καὶ δάκρυον ἁλμυρὸν καὶ νιτρῶδες διαστάζει. σκληροφθαλμία δέ ἐστιν, ὅταν τὰ βλέφαρα σκληρότερα ᾖ καὶ αὐτὸς ὁ ὀφθαλμὸς δυσκίνητος καὶ ἐνερευθής. πρόπτωσις δέ ἐστιν, ὅταν ὁ ὀφθαλμὸς κινητὸς μετὰ φλεγμονῆς προπέσῃ. ἀτροφίαν δὲ λέγουσιν ὀφθαλμοῦ, ὅταν ἐξ ἀῤῥωστίας μακρᾶς, ἢ ἔκ τινος ἀδήλου αἰτίας, ὥσπερ ὀλίγον ἔξω-

lis effertur, ubi cum maxima inflammatione etiam humoris copia influxerit. Oedema nominant, quum elevatus apparet oculus et colorem amifit, vel etiam aegre movetur: interim album quoque fupra nigrum attollitur. Inflatio dicitur, cum fubito tumefcens oculus decolor fit, exuperante pituita: ut plerumque fenibus aeftate potiffimum folet accidere. Scirrofis ex inflammationis diuturnae vehementia oritur, carne increfcente et fublivida. Rheumatismo laborat oculus, cum non folum rubet, fed multas quoque lachrymas excernit. Xerophthalmia eft, cum anguli ulcera et afpritudinem pruritumque contraxerunt, palpebrae rubent et lacrima falfa et nitrofa profluit. Sclerophthalmia eft cum palpebrae duriores funt, oculi rubent et cum difficultate quadam moventur. Proptofis appellatur ubi cum inflammatione moti fede fua procidunt. Atrophiam nominant, cum ex longa imbecillitate, vel alia quadam latente caufa paululum quafi propulfus, deinde cavatus ad radicem cum dolore minor evadit, ob-

θούμενος, εἶτα κοιλαινόμενος κατὰ τὰς ῥίζας ἀλγῶν μικρότερος γίνηται καὶ ἀμυδρῶς, ἢ μηδ᾽ ὅλως βλέπῃ τραχέα δὲ τὰ βλέφαρα λέγεται, ὅταν ἐκστραφέντα ἐναιμότερα φαίνηται καὶ τραχύτερα καὶ σαρκωδέστερα καὶ κεγχραμίσιν ὅμοια. παχέα δὲ βλέφαρα τὰ ἐκστραφέντα τῶν κατὰ φύσιν καὶ σκληρότερα καὶ σαρκωδέστερα τῶν τραχέων φαινόμενα. σύκωσις δέ ἐστιν, ὅταν τὸ ἐντὸς τῶν βλεφάρων σαρκωθείη σαρκὶ παραπλήσιον μετὰ ὑπεροχῆς καὶ ὁ ὀφθαλμὸς ἅπας δυσκίνητος ᾖ. τύλωσις δέ ἐστιν, ὅταν τὰ ἐν τοῖς βλεφάροις τραχώματα διὰ παλαιότητα παχύτερα καὶ λευκότερα καὶ δυσαίσθητα ᾖ καὶ διὰ τοῦτο δυσαπότριπτα γένηται. σκληρίασις δέ ἐστιν ἔπαρμα μετ᾽ ἐρυθήματος ἐπὶ τὸ βλέφαρον καὶ ὀδύνης, δυσαπότριπτον καὶ χρονιώτερον φλεγμονῆς. χαλάζωσις δέ ἐστι περιφερῆ τινα ἔνδοθεν τοῦ βλεφάρου ἐπάρματα περιγεγραμμένα, ἐοικότα τῇ χαλάζῃ. πλαδαρότης δέ ἐστι μαλακὰ οἷον σώματα παλαιά γε καὶ ἄχρούστατα κατὰ τὰ ἐντὸς τῶν βλεφάρων οὔπω τὸ τραχὺ ἔχοντα, διὸ πλαδαρότης καλεῖται. [391] μύδησις δὲ κοινὸν ὄνομά ἐστι

ſcureque aut nihil omnino videt. Aſperae dicuntur palpebrae, cum everſae ſanguinolentiores apparent et magis aſperae carnoſaeque et ſici acinis ſimiles. Craſſae vocantur, ubi everſae duriores iis, quae naturaliter ſe habent, exiſtunt et ſcabris magis carnoſae. Sycoſis accidit, cum in palpebrarum parte interiore carni quid ſimile enatum fuerit, quod emineat et oculus totus aegre moveatur. Tyloſis eſt, cum in palpebris aſpritudines ex ſenectute craſſiores, albidiores et parum ſenſiles extiterint, eoque minus deteri poſſunt. Scleriaſis eſt tumor palpebrae cum rubore doloreque, difficulter aboletur: durat magis quam inflammatio. Chalazia vel chalazoſis orbicularia quaedam intra palpebras tubercula ſunt circumſcripta: nomen a ſimilitudine grandinis acceperunt. Pladarotes ſunt mollia veluti corpora vetuſta, decolora, palpebrarum parte interna nondum aſpredinem habentia, propterea pladarotes vocatur. Mydeſis commune nomen eſt partium, quae ex pu-

σώματος, ἐκ σήψεως ἀπολλυμένων. γίνεται δὲ τὸ αὐτὸ τοῦτο καὶ περὶ τὰ βλέφαρα καὶ ὀγκωδέστερα φαίνεται καὶ συνεχῶς ῥευματίζεται, πλείονος πιμελῆς περὶ αὐτὰ γινομένης. κριθὴ δὲ, ἢ καὶ ποσθία λέγεται, ὅταν τὸ ἐντὸς τῶν βλεφάρων πρὸς ταῖς στεφανιαίαις ὑπόπυον παράμηκες, ὅμοιον κριθῇ κατὰ τὸ σχῆμα γένηται. γίνεται δὲ καὶ ἄλλα μείζονα κατὰ μέσα βλέφαρα κριθὴ λεγόμενα. λιθίασις δέ ἐστιν, ὅταν ἐκστραφέντων τῶν βλεφάρων ὅμοια πώροις περὶ τὰ βλέφαρα ὑπάρχῃ λευκὰ καὶ παχέα καὶ οἷον λίθοις ἐμφερῆ νύσσοντα τὸν ὀφθαλμόν. φθειριᾷν δέ φαμεν τὰ βλέφαρα, ὅταν περὶ τὰ τετριχωμένα πλατέες πολλαὶ φθεῖρες σμικραὶ γίνωνται. διτριχιᾷν δὲ λέγεται ὁ ὀφθαλμὸς, ὅταν ὑπὸ τὰς κατὰ φύσιν τρίχας ἄλλαι ὑποφυεῖσαι νύσσωσι τὸν ὀφθαλμὸν καὶ ῥευματίζωσι. πτίλωσις δέ ἐστιν, ὅταν ἄλλαι μὲν ὑποφύουσιν, αὗται δὲ αἱ κατὰ φύσιν συμπεσοῦσαι καὶ κατακλασθεῖσαι νυγμοὺς παρέχουσι. φαλάγγωσις δέ ἐστιν, ὅταν διστιχία, ἢ τριστιχία τῶν ὑποφυομένων τριχῶν ᾖ ἐν τῷ ἄνω, ἢ ἐν τῷ κάτω βλεφάρῳ. παραλελύσθαι δὲ λέγεται ὁ ὀφθαλμὸς, ὅταν

trefactione corrumpuntur. Palpebrae quoque eadem laborant, ubi et tumentiores apparent et affidue diffluunt, adipem paulo copiofiorem fortitae. Crithe, quae et pofthia dicitur, quum parte interna palpebrarum in ambitu fuppuratum oblongum, figura hordeo fimile fit, unde appellatum eft. Generantur alia quoque majora in mediis palpebris eodem appellata nomine. Lithiafis, albida quaedam et craffa, callis lapillisque fimilia, quae oculum pungunt in palpebris retortis oftendit. Phthiriafim vocamus, quum palpebrarum pilos multi, lati exiguique pediculi infeftant. Ditrichiafi laborat oculus, quum pilis naturalibus alii fubnafcentes ipfum pungunt fluoremque concitant. Ptilofis eft, quum alii quidem fubnafcuntur, naturales autem collapfi fractique ftimulant ac pungunt. Phalangofis, quum pilorum fubnafcentium duplex triplexve acies vel in fuperiore vel in inferiore palpebra provenit. Refolutus oculus dicitur, ubi naturali motu deftitutus, neque furfum

αὐτὸν ἐπιλείπωσιν αἱ φυσικαὶ κινήσεις καὶ μὴ δύνηται ἀναβλέπειν, ἢ κάτω βλέπειν, ἀναίσθητος δὲ ᾖ. πολλάκις δὲ καὶ περὶ μέρη τινὰ τοῦ ὀφθαλμοῦ τοῦτο συμβαίνει. ἐκτετράφθαι δὲ λέγουσι τὰ βλέφαρα, ὅταν ἐπὶ πλέον ἐκτραπῇ ἑλκωθέντων ἐξοφθαλμιῶν. ἐγκανθίδα δὲ λέγουσιν, ὅταν ἐξ ἑλκώσεως ὑπερσαρκώσῃ ὁ κανθὸς πρὸς τὴν ῥῖνα. πάσχουσι δὲ τοῦτο μάλιστα οἱ θαλασσουργοί. πτερύγιον δὲ λέγουσιν, ὅταν ἐπὶ πλέον ἑλκωθέντος καὶ ὑπερσαρκώσαντος τοῦ λευκοῦ ὑμὴν λεπτὸς καὶ νευρώδης ἐπιδράμῃ τὸν ὀφθαλμὸν, ἀρξάμενος ἀπό τινος τῶν κανθῶν, ἕως τοῦ μέλανος καὶ τῆς κορυφῆς ἐφάψηται. ῥοιὰς δέ ἐστιν ἐπὶ ὀφθαλμῷ, ὅταν ἔκ τινος αἰτίας ἀδήλου ὁ κανθὸς παρέλθῃ, ἢ ἐκ χειρουργίας ἀρθῇ καὶ μηκέτι στέγειν τὸ δάκρυον οἷόν τε ᾖ, ἀλλὰ ῥευματίζεται. προσφύεται δὲ τὰ βλέφαρα ἢ τῷ λευκῷ ἢ τῷ μέλανι ἐξ ἑλκώσεως. καὶ ἐὰν μὲν τῷ μέλανι προσφυῇ, τελέως κωλύει τὴν ὅρασιν, ἐὰν δὲ τῷ λευκῷ, ἧττον· καλεῖται δὲ ἀγκύλωσις. αἰγίλωπα δὲ λέγουσιν, ἢ ἀγχίλωπα, ὅταν ἀπόστημά τι γένηται πρὸς τῷ κανθῷ τῷ παρὰ τῇ ῥινὶ πῦον περιέχον, ἢ

neque deorſum intendi poteſt, verum ſentiendi expers conſiſtit: frequenter hoc mali partibus etiam oculi accidit. Inverti autem dicuntur palpebrae, quum ex ulceratis oculis plus extra feruntur. Encanthis, ubi ex ulcere caro in angulis juxta nares ſupercreverit; nautae ac piſcatores hoc vitii peculiare habent. Unguis vero eſt in albo oculi praeter modum exulcerato, carneque oppleto membranula tenuis et nervoſa: quae orta ab angulorum aliquo ad nigrum et verticem ejus pervenit. Rhoeas, cum angulus ex latente quadam cauſa receſſerit, aut prava curatione ſublatus fuerit, ut lacrimas continere non amplius poſſit, ſed humorem dimittat. Cohaereſcunt palpebrae cum albo oculi vel nigro ex ulceratione. Et ſi nigro cohaereant, viſus omnino prohibetur: ſin albo, minus. Hoc malum angyloſim appellant. Aegilops vel anchilops abſceſſus quidam eſt ad angulum, qui naribus propior eſt, pus continens, quod erumpens aut os exedit aut ad angulum

λιπαῖνον τὸ ὀστέον συῤῥηγνύμενον, ἢ εἰς κανθὸν, ἢ εἰς ῥῖνα περιχεῖ τὸ ὑγρόν. ψυδράκιον δ' ἐστὶ κοινῶς λεγόμενον περὶ πᾶν τὸ σῶμα καὶ περὶ τὸ λευκὸν τοῦ ὀφθαλμοῦ γίνεται, οἷον ἐξάνθημα ἐξ ἄκρου ἐρευθές. ἕλκος δὲ γίνεται περὶ τὸ μέλαν, ἢ τὸ λευκὸν, ὅταν ἡ ἐπιδερμὶς διαιρεθῇ μηνοειδὴς, ἢ στρογγύλη τὸ σχῆμα, κοιλότερον, ὁμόχρουν ἢ ὑπόλευκον. ὑπόσφαγμα δὲ λέγουσιν, ὅταν ὑπὸ πληγῆς ῥαγέντων τῶν ἐν τῷ πρώτῳ χιτῶνι ἀγγείων μεταξὺ τῆς κτηδόνος τοῦ λευκοῦ καὶ τοῦ ἐντὸς χιτῶνος αἷμα ὑπέλθῃ, καὶ παραχρῆμα μὲν ἔναιμον ᾖ τὸ χρῶμα τοῦ ὀφθαλμοῦ, ὕστερον δὲ πελιδνόν. χήμωσις δέ ἐστιν, ὅταν ἐκ φλεγμονῆς σφοδροτέρας ἀμφότερα τὰ βλέφαρα ἐκτραπῇ καὶ μὴ ὅλον σκέπῃ τὸν ὀφθαλμόν. κυρίως δὲ χήμωσις λέγεται, ὅταν τὸ λευκὸν ἑκατέρωθεν τῆς ἴριδος φλεγμάνῃ, κατὰ δὲ τὴν ἶριν κοιλαινόμενον, ὅμοιον τοῖς σχήμασι τῇ καλουμένῃ χήμῃ. κοιλώματα δὲ λέγεται ἐπὶ ὀφθαλμοῦ ὅσα στρογγύλα καὶ κοῖλα ἕλκη πλατύτερα τῶν βοθρίων γίνεται ἐν αὐτῷ περὶ τὴν ἶριν. ἄργεμον δέ ἐστιν, ὅταν κατὰ τὸν τῆς ἴριδος κύκλον καὶ τὸ λευ-

vel usque ad nares diftillat. Pfydracion communi vocabulo circa corpus totum et circa album oculi fit. Eft autem velut puftula in fummo rubicundum. Ulcus oritur in albo vel nigro, quum cuticula divifa lunae figuram vel rotundam cavam, fimilis coloris vel fubalbidi acceperit. Hypofphagma vocant, quum vafis in prima tunica ruptis ab ictu fanguis intra albi fpatium et interiorem tunicam coierit, atque oculi color ftatim cruentus, poft lividus exiftat. Chemofis ex inflammatione vehementiore utrasque palpebras in exteriorem partem detorquet, ne totum oculum contegant. Proprie vero chemofis dicitur, quum album utraque iridis parte inflammatione afficitur, juxta irim autem cavum hiatularum fimilitudine apparet. Coelomata funt rotunda et cava ulcera, bothriis latiora, quae in oculis circa irim nafcuntur. Argemon, in iridis circulo vel in albo, interdum etiam nigro, ulcus rotundum et fubalbidum oritur. Nephelion fummae cutis ulcus paulo

κὸν, ἐνίοτε δὲ καὶ τὸ μέλαν, ἕλκος γίνηται στρογγύλον καὶ ὑπόλευκον. νεφέλιον δέ ἐστιν ἕλκος ἐπιπόλαιον καὶ μικρῷ μεῖζον ἀργέμου καὶ λευκόν. ἀχλὺς δέ ἐστι περὶ ὅλον τὸ μέλαν ἀπὸ ἑλκώσεως ἐπιπολαίου, οὐλὴ λεπτοτάτη ἀέρι ἀχλυώδει παραπλησία. ἐπίκαυμα δέ ἐστιν, ὅταν ἐξ ἐπιπολῆς ἡ ἐπιδερμὶς ἐπικαυθεῖσα ἑλκωθῇ, ἢ καὶ βραχὺ βαθυτέρα γένηται ἐξ ἐπιφορᾶς μεγάλης ἐγγινομένη. [392] βοθρίον δέ ἐστιν ἕλκος κοῖλον καθαρὸν, στενὸν, κεντήμασι στρογγύλοις ὅμοιον, βαθύτερον ἑλκυδρίου. φλύκταιναν δὲ λέγουσιν, ὅταν ἐξ ἑλκώσεως, ἢ καὶ ἄνευ ἑλκώσεως, ἐξ ἐπιπολῆς τοῦ κερατοειδοῦς χιτῶνος, ὑμὴν λεπτότατός τε καὶ μετέωρος ἀρθεὶς παραδέξηται μεταξὺ αὐτοῦ ὑγρασίαν, ἢ καὶ ὑπὸ τὴν κτηδόνα τοῦ χιτῶνος παχυτέρα ὑποδραμοῦσα ὑγρασία καὶ τὴν φλύκταιναν ἀποτελέσασα. μυοκέφαλον δέ ἐστιν, ὅταν ἐξ ἑλκώσεως διαβρωθέντος τοῦ πρώτου χιτῶνος κατὰ τὴν ἶριν προκύψῃ ὁ δεύτερος χιτὼν, ὡς οἷον μυίας κεφαλῇ ἐοικέναι. σταφύλωμα δὲ λέγεται, ὅταν ἡ (387) κόρη τοῦ ὀφθαλμοῦ μετεωρισθῇ μετὰ φλεγμονῆς καὶ πόνου καὶ γίνηται ὅμοιον ῥαγὶ σταφυλῆς, λευκὸν τῇ χροιᾷ. ὑπόπυον δέ ἐστιν, ὅταν

majus argemo et albidum. Achlys eſt circa totum nigrum a ſuperficiaria ulceratione cicatricula tenuiſſima, aëri caliginoſo aſſimilis. Epicauma, quum in ſuperficie cuticula aduſta ulcus contraxerit vel etiam paulo profundior fiat ex epiphora magna originem habens. Bothrion eſt ulcus cavum, purum, anguſtum, puncturis rotundis ſimile, ulcuſculo altius. Phlyctaenam vocant, ubi per exulcerationem vel etiam ſine hac exterior corneae tunicae membrana tenuiſſima et ſublimis elata intra ſe humorem collegerit, aut ſub tunicae ſpatio craſſior humor currens phlyctaenam pariat. Myocephalon morbus eſt, quum tunica priore juxta irim, exulcerationis vitio exeſa, ſecunda prociderit, ut ceu muris caput referre videatur. Staphyloma dicitur, quando oculi pupilla cum inflammatione et dolore attollitur et album colore et acino uvae ſimile redditur. Hypopyon univerſam irim pure occupat, vel ejus dimidium.

πῦον ὅλην τὴν ἶριν περιλάβῃ, ἢ τὸ ἥμισυ. ῥῆξις δέ ἐστιν ἕλκωσις ὑπὸ πληγῆς ἢ ἄλλης τινὸς αἰτίας κατὰ βάθος ἐπιφέρουσα ὡς ἐπὶ τὸ πολὺ, τὴν διαίρεσιν τῶν ὑμένων ὅλων, ὥστε ἐκχεῖν καὶ τὰ ὑγρὰ οἷς βλέπομεν. οὐλὴ δέ ἐστιν, ὅταν ἐπὶ τῷ μέλανι τοῦ ὀφθαλμοῦ ἐξ ἕλκους βαθέος ὄντος παχύτης ὑμένος ἐπιγένηται καὶ ἡ χροιὰ λευκοτέρα φαίνηται. συνίσταται δὲ καὶ ἐπὶ τοῦ λευκοῦ ὑμένος καλουμένου, ἀλλ' οὐ διαδείκνυται. λεύκωμα δὲ ταὐτὸν μὲν τῇ καλουμένῃ οὐλῇ ἐστι, διαφέρει δὲ τῷ ἐξ ἑλκώσεως μεγάλην οὐλὴν μείζονα καὶ παχυτέραν ἐπιγίνεσθαι ἐπὶ τῆς ἴρεως, ἣν καλοῦσι λεύκωμα. ἧλος δέ ἐστιν ἡ μετὰ λείας καὶ λευκῆς, οἷον οὐλὴ σαρκώδης, ὑπεροχὴ τοῦ μέλανος στερεά· πολλάκις δὲ καὶ ἐπὶ τῷ λευκῷ τῷ μέλανι συνάπτοντι ἐπανισταμένη. ὑποκεχύσθαι δὲ λέγουσί τινες, ὅταν συμβῇ παρέγχυσιν ὑγροῦ τινος γενέσθαι κατὰ τὴν κόρην καὶ πῆξιν πολλάκις, ὥστε κωλῦσαι τὸ ὁρᾷν, ἢ καὶ ἀμαυροῦσθαι ἐν τῷ φαίνειν. γλαύκωσις δέ ἐστι τοῦ κρυσταλλοειδοῦς ὑγροῦ εἰς λευκὴν καὶ ὑδατώδη χροιὰν μεταβολὴ, δι' ἣν τὸ βλέπειν κωλύεται. μυδρίασις δὲ λέγεται, ὅταν ἡ κόρη τῷ μὲν χρώματι μηδὲν

Rhexis eſt exulceratio ab ictu vel alia quadam cauſa in alto totas ſubinde membranas dividens, ut etiam humores, quibus videndi facultas adminiſtratur, effundat. Cicatrix appellatur, ubi nigro oculi ex alto ulcere membranae craſſities ſupervenit et color albior apparet; accidit quoque albae membranae dictae, ſed non perſpicitur. Albugo nihil a cicatrice differt, niſi quod ex ulcere major cicatrix ſimul et craſſior in iride naſcitur, quam albuginem nominant. Clavus eſt carnoſus nigri exceſſus ſolidus, cum levi albaque velut cicatrice, frequenter etiam in albo nigro cohaerenti conſurgens. Suffuſionem quidam interpretantur, quum humor quidam in pupillam deſtillaverit, concreveritque ſaepe adeo, ut viſum offendat vel in apparentibus hebetet. Glaucoſis eſt humoris cryſtallini in album atque aqueum colorem mutatio, cujus gratia viſus impeditur. Mydriaſis dicitur, quum pupilla quidem nihil

παραλλάττῃ, πλατυτέρα δὲ ᾖ πολλῷ τοῦ κατὰ φύσιν, ὥστε ἐγγίζειν τῷ κύκλῳ τῆς ἴρεως καὶ ἐμποδίζειν τὸ βλέπειν. φθίσις δὲ λέγεται στενουμένης τῆς κόρης, ὡς κεντήματι ἐοικέναι καὶ ἀμαυροτέρας καὶ ῥυσοτέρας γινομένης, ἢ ἐξ ἀσθενειῶν ἐπικινδύνων, ἢ κεφαλαλγιῶν ἐπιτεταμένων. σύγχυσις δέ ἐστιν, ὅταν τὰ ἐν τῷ ὀφθαλμῷ ὑγρὰ μὴ κατὰ χώραν μένῃ, τὴν ἰδίαν τάξιν σώζοντα, ἀλλὰ τεταραγμένα ᾖ. ἀμαύρωσις δέ ἐστιν, ὅταν παντελὴς παρεμποδισμὸς ᾖ τοῦ ὁρᾷν, χωρὶς φανερᾶς αἰτίας. νυκτάλωπας δὲ λέγουσιν, ὅταν ἡμέρας μὲν βλέπωσιν ἀμαυρότερον, δυομένου δὲ ἡλίου λαμπρότερον· νυκτὸς δὲ ἔτι μᾶλλον· ἢ ὑπεναντίως, ἡμέρας μὲν ὀλίγα, ἑσπέρας δὲ ἢ νυκτὸς οὐδ᾽ ὅλως. μύωπας δὲ λέγουσι τοὺς τὰ μὲν σύνεγγυς βλέποντας, τὰ δὲ πόῤῥωθεν μὴ ὁρῶντας. διαπύησις δέ ἐστι βραχυτέρου ὑγροῦ σύστασις περὶ αὐτὴν τὴν κόρην, δυσεξάτμιστος καὶ δυσδιαφόρητος, ὑποχύματος ξηροτέρα. ἀπόῤῥηξις δὲ γίνεται τοῦ πόρου περὶ ὀφθαλμὸν, ὅταν ὁ διατείνων ἀπὸ τοῦ ἐγκεφάλου καὶ μήνιγγος πόρος ἐπὶ τὸν ὀφθαλμὸν ἀποῤῥαγῇ, ὡς ἀβλεψίαν τελείαν γενέσθαι προηγησαμένης πληγῆς περὶ τὴν κε-

colore variat, dilatatur autem magis quam natura poſcat, ut iridis circulo fiat proxima et viſioni noceat. Phthiſis appellatur, dum pupilla arcte coit vel ſtimulo aſſimilis fit, tum rugoſior aut ex imbecillitate periculoſa, aut ex capitis dolore vehementi. Confuſio, dum humores oculorum ſuo loco non conſiſtunt, proprium ordinem ſervantes, ſed huc illucque feruntur. Hebetudo ſumma viſionis ſine cauſa evidenti offenſio. Nyctalopes vocantur qui die vident obtuſius, ſole occiduo acrius, nocte magis adhuc: vel contra die parum, veſperi aut nocte prorſus nihil. Myopes vicina vident, remota non item. Suppuratio humor exiguus in pupilla collectus, qui difficulter evaporat ac diſcutitur, ſuffuſione ſiccior. Abruptio eſt, quando meatus a cerebro et meninge in oculum deſcendens ex ictu capitis vel caſu ex alto diruptus eſt ita ut abſolutam caecitatem afferat. Coincidentia, ubi in meatum, qui a baſi cerebri

κεφαλὴν, ἢ ἀφ᾽ ὕψους πτώματος, ἀφ᾽ οὗ γίνεται ἡ τοῦ πόρου ἀπόῤῥηξις. παρέμπτωσις δέ ἐστιν, ὅταν εἰς τὸν πόρον, κατ᾽ ἀναστόμωσιν, ἢ ῥῆξιν ἀγγείου, τὸ ὑγρὸν παρεμπέσῃ καὶ ἐμφράξῃ τὸν πόρον ἀπ᾽ αὐτῆς τῆς βάσεως τοῦ ἐγκεφάλου, ὅθεν καὶ τῷ ὀφθαλμῷ ἡ τοῦ ὁρᾷν δύναμις, ὥστε μετ᾽ ἀλγημάτων καὶ τὸ ὁρᾷν ἐμποδίζεσθαι. σύμπτωσις δὲ γίνεται μὲν ὑπὸ τοῦ πόρου στενουμένου καὶ συμπίπτοντος δι᾽ ἀτροφίαν καὶ πάρεσιν. σπάνιον δὲ τοῦτο τὸ πάθος καὶ δυσίατον. ἀνθράκωσις δέ ἐστιν ἕλκος ἐσχαρῶδες μετὰ νομῆς καὶ ῥεύματος καὶ βουβῶνος ἐνίοτε καὶ πυρετῶν γινομένων περὶ τὸ ἄλλο πᾶν σῶμα, ἔστι δὲ ὅτε καὶ περὶ ὀφθαλμούς.

[393] Κεφ. ιζ΄. [Περὶ τῶν ἐκτὸς τῆς κεφαλῆς παθῶν.] Περὶ δὲ τὰ ἐκτὸς τῆς κεφαλῆς συνίστανται τάδε, ἃ οὐκ ἀναγέγραπται ἐν τοῖς χρονίοις, περὶ τῶν ἐν τῇ κεφαλῇ καταγμάτων τοῦ κρανίου. διαφοραὶ δὲ αὐτῶν εἰσι πέντε, ῥωγμὴ, ἐγγείσωμα, ἐκπίεσμα, ἀπήχημα, καμάρωσις, διάτασις ῥαφῶν, ὑδροκέφαλον, ἀχῶρες, πιτυρίασις, μελικηρὶς, ἀθέρωμα, κηρίον. περὶ δὲ τὸ τετριχωμένον τῆς κεφαλῆς καὶ τοῦ γενείου ἀλωπεκία, ὀφίασις, μαδαρότης, φαλάκρωσις.

veniens oculo videndi facultatem tribuit, humor adaperto vel rupto vafe incidit, obturatque eum: unde cum dolore vifus offenditur. Symptofis accidit, quum meatus ex atrophia vel refolutione fit arctior conciditque. Quod vitium ut rarum eft, fic remediis aegre cedit. Carbunculus cruftofum eft ulcus, depafcens cum fluore et bubone, aliquando etiam cum febribus, interdum in toto corpore, interdum in oculis factum.

Cap. XVII. [*De exterioribus capitis affectibus.*] Circa capitis exteriores partes confiftunt ii, qui inter longos afcripti non funt. Calvariae autem fracturarum differentiae quinque exiftunt, rhogme, engifoma, ecpiesma, apechema et camarofis, diftenfio futurarum, hydrocephalon, achores, pityriafis, meliceris, atheroma, favus. Porro eam partem, quae capillo tegitur et mentum occupant alopecia, ophiafis, calvities, madarofis. Pili omnes fluunt,

τρίχες δὲ πᾶσι ῥέουσι, λεπτύνονται, θραύονται, σχίζονται, αὐχμῶσι, χνοΐζονται, ὑπόξανθοι γίνονται, πολιοῦνται. τὰ δὲ περὶ ὀφθαλμοὺς κατ' ἰδίαν ἀναγέγραπται. τὰ δὲ περὶ τὰ ὦτα, περίθλασις, πτερυγώματα, κάταγμα χόνδρου, κυψελίδος πλεονασμὸς, ἢ ἔλλειψις, βαρυηκοΐα, κώφωσις, πύου ῥύσις, ῥεῦμα δυσῶδες. περὶ δὲ ῥῖνα τάδε συνίστανται, ὄζαινα, πολύπους, ἕλκος, κάταγμα, διαστροφὴ, ἔνθλασις, σίμωσις. περὶ δὲ στόμα σῆψις οὐλῶν, βρῶσις ὀδόντων, ὀδονταλγία, φατνωμάτων ἔκπτωσις, ἀπόστημα ἐπὶ γλώττης, ἐπουλὶς, παρουλὶς, ἄφθαι, ἐσχάρωσις, παρίσθμια, σταφυλὴ, σύκωμα. περὶ δὲ τὸ πρόσωπον ἔφηλις, ἴονθοι, φακός. κάταγμα ὀστέων. διάτασις τῶν συμφύσεων. ἐξαρθρήματα τῆς κάτω γένυος ἀπὸ τῆς ἄνω. περὶ δὲ τὸν τράχηλον συνάγχη, κυνάγχη, ἀγχόνη, ἔξωσις σπονδύλων, χοιράδες, στεατώματα. περὶ δὲ ὤμους τοῦ ἀκρωμίου κάταγμα, διάστασις. περὶ δὲ ἀγκῶνα μελικηρὶς, ἀθέρωμα, στεάτωμα, ὑγρὸν ὑδατῶδες. περὶ δὲ καρποὺς γαγγλία. περὶ δὲ δακτύλους χειρὸς καὶ ποδὸς χείμεθλα, παρωνυχία. τοπικὰ δὲ ὅπου ἂν

extenuantur, quaſſantur, ſcinduntur, ſqualleſcunt, in pulverem rediguntur, ſubflaveſcunt, caneſcunt. Oculorum morbi ſeparatim conſcripti ſunt. Aurium contuſio, pterygomata, fractura cartilaginis, ſordium vel exuperantia vel defectus, gravis auditus, ſurditas, puris fluor, fluxus graveolens. Nares excruciant ozaena, polypus, ulcus, fractura, perverſio, compreſſio, ſimitas. Os infeſtat gingivarum putredo, dentium eroſio, eorumque dolor et cum ſede ſua excidunt, abſceſſus in lingua, epulis, parulis, aphthae, cruſtae, tonſillae, uva, ficus. Faciem occupant ephelis, vari, lentigo, oſſium fractura, diſtentio commiſſurarum, luxationes maxillae inferioris a ſuperiore gena. Cervicem habent ſynanche, cynanche, ſtrangulatio, vertebrarum expulſio, ſtrumae, ſteatomata. Humeros male habet verticis ipſorum fractura, diſtentio. Juncturam cubiti occupant meliceris, atheroma, ſteatoma, humor aqueus. Carpum ganglia. Digitos manus et pedis chimethla, red-

τύχη τοῦ σώματος, φλεγμονὴ, οἴδημα, ἐμφύσημα, σκλήρωμα, ἀπόστημα, ἕλκος καθαρὸν, ἕλκος ῥυπαρὸν, κοῖλον ἕλκος, ὑπερσαρκοῦν, ἐσχαρῶδες, ἕλκος ξηρὸν, ῥευματιζόμενον, ὑπόνομον, τετυλωμένον, σεσυριγγωμένον, μύδησις, φῦμα, δοθιὴν, θέρμινθες, φύγεθλον, χάλαζα, φαγέδαινα, φλυκτίδες, ἄνθρακες, ἐπινυκτίδες, ἐρυσίπελας, ἕρπητες. περὶ δὲ τοὺς μαζοὺς ἰδίως καὶ περὶ τὰ αἰδοῖα γυναικὸς καὶ ἀνδρὸς καρκινώματα. συνίσταται δὲ καὶ ὅπου ἂν τύχῃ τοῦ σώματος καρκίνωμα κρυπτὸν, καρκίνωμα ἡλκωμένον, θηρίωμα. περὶ δὲ βουβῶνας βουβῶνες ἁπλοῖ, φύματα ἐκπυΐσκοντα. περὶ δὲ γόνατα γουναλγίαι, ῥευματισμοὶ, πῶροι. περὶ δὲ ἰγνὺν στεατώματα, ἀγκύλη. περὶ δὲ κνήμην κιρσοί. ἐν γαστροκνημίᾳ σκίῤῥωμα, χειρώνεια ἕλκη. περὶ δὲ ἄκρα ποδὸς μελανίαι, νεκρώσεις, ποδάγρα, σύριγγες. περὶ δὲ πτέρνας λεπίδες.

Κεφ. ιη'. [*Περὶ τῶν τοῦ δέρματος παθῶν.*] *Περὶ* δὲ τὸ δέρμα καὶ τόπους καθ' ὅλου τοῦ σώματος λέπρα, ψώρα, ἀλφὸς λευκὸς, ἀλφὸς μέλας, λεύκη, λειχὴν ἁπλοῦς,

uvia. Quamcunque corporis partem inflammatio, oedema, inflatio, durities, abfceffus, ulcus purum, ulcus fordidum, cavum, carne fupercrefcens, cruftofum, ficcum, fluens, fubpafcens, callofum, fiftulofum, mydefis, phyma, dothien, therminthes, phygethlon, chalaza, phagedaena, phlyctides, carbunculi, epinyctides, eryfipelas, herpetes. Mammillas peculiariter, tum naturaliter fexus utriusque vexant carcinomata. Quamlibet corporis partem impetunt carcinoma occultum, carcinoma ulceratum, therioma. Inguina bubones fimplices, phymata purulenta invadunt. Genu gonyalgiae, rheumatifmi, tophi. Poplites fteatomata, ankyle. Tibiam varices. Suram fcirrhoma, chironia ulcera. Summam pedis partem nigredines, necrofis, podagra, fiftulae. Calcem fquamae.

Cap. XVIII. [*De cutis affectibus.*] Cutem totiusque corporis partes exagitant lepra, pfora, alphus albus, alphus niger. leuce, impetigo fimplex, impetigo fera, dra-

λειχὴν ἄγριος, δρακοντίασις, ἀκροχορδόνες, θύμοι, μυρμηκίαι, ἧλοι, πῶροι. οἱ μὲν ἐκ ποδάγρας καὶ ἀρθρίτιδος, οἱ δὲ καὶ καθ' ἑαυτούς. περὶ δὲ ἕδραν αἱμοῤῥοΐδες τυφλαὶ, ῥαγάδες, πρόπτωσις, κονδυλώματα, πυλίδες. γίνεται δὲ καὶ μήτρας ὅλης πρόπτωσις εἰς τὰ ἐκτός. περὶ δὲ ὄσχεον ἐντεροκήλη, κιρσοκήλη, ἐπιπλοκήλη, σαρκοκήλη, πωροκήλη, στεατοκήλη. περὶ δὲ τὰ ἐν ὅλῳ τῷ σώματι ὀστᾶ, τερηδὼν, σφάκελος, κάταγμα ἄνευ τραύματος, ἢ σὺν τραύματι, ἐκβύρσωσις. [394] διαφοραὶ δὲ καταγμάτων πέντε, σχιδακηδὸν, καυληδὸν, ῥαφανηδὸν, καρυηδὸν, ἀλφιτηδόν. μελαίνεται δὲ ὀστᾶ ποτὲ μὲν ἐν κατάγμασιν, ποτὲ δὲ ἄνευ τούτων. περὶ δὲ τὰ ἄρθρα πάντα παραγωγαὶ, παρακινήματα, ἐξαρθρήματα, παραρθρήματα, σύνδεσις, πώρωσις, ῥευματισμοὶ, διάστασις συμφύσεων.

(388) Κεφ. ιθ'. [Περὶ χειρουργίας εἰδῶν.] Χειρουργία ἐστὶν ἄρσις ἐμμέθοδος τοῦ ἰδίως λεγομένου ἀλλοτρίου, διὰ τομῶν καὶ καταρτισμῶν μετὰ τῆς τῶν τραυμά-

contiafis, acrochordones, thymi, myrmeciae, clavi, calli. Quaedam horum ex podagra et articulari morbo, quaedam ex fefe oriuntur. Sedem afficiunt haemorrhoides caecae, fiffurae, procidentia, condylomata, pylides. Advenit etiam toti vulvae procidentia, cum in exteriora procidit. Scrotum habent enterocele, cirfocele, epiplocele, farcocele, porocele, fteatocele. Totius corporis offa patiuntur cariem, fphacelum, fracturam fine vulnere vel cum vulnere, ecbyrfofin. Fracturarum differentiae quinque funt. Prima fchidacedon facta, per rectitudinem: altera per transverfum, cauledon. Tertia raphani in morem, raphanedon. Quarta caryedon, in modum nucis. Poftremo alphitedon in fpeciem farinae. Nigrefcunt interdum offa in fracturis interdum fine his. Articulis omnibus accidunt paragoge, e fede propria motio, luxatio, intertrigo, colligatio, porofis, rheumatifmi, diftentio commiffurarum.

Cap. XIX. [*De chirurgiae fpeeiebus.*] Chirurgia eft alieni, ut proprie vocant, per incifiones concinnationesque cum via quadam et ratione ablatio: ad haec vul-

των καὶ ἑλκῶν θεραπείας, ἐπ' ἀνθρώπου σώματι παραλαμβανομένη. χειρουργίας δὲ καθολικαὶ μὲν ἐνέργειαι δύο, σύνθεσις καὶ διαίρεσις. ἔστι δὲ τούτων εἴδη πολλά. καὶ συνθέσεως μὲν εἴδη συνθετισμὸς τῶν κατεαγότων ὀστέων καὶ ἐπίδεσις καὶ ἀρθρέμβολον τῶν ἐξηρθρηκότων καὶ τάξις τῶν προπεπτωκότων ἐντέρων καὶ μήτρας καὶ ἀπευθυσμένου καὶ γαστροῤῥαφία καὶ ἐπαγωγὴ τῶν κολοβωμάτων, ὡς ἐπὶ ῥινῶν καὶ χειλῶν καὶ ὤτων. διαιρέσεως δὲ εἴδη ἁπλοτομία καὶ περιαίρεσις, ὑποσπαθισμὸς, περισκυθισμὸς, ἀγγειολογία, ἐκκοπὴ, καῦσις, ξύσις, ῥίνησις, ἔκπρισις. ἁπλοτομίᾳ οὖν χρώμεθα ἐπὶ τῶν ἀποστημάτων πάντων. χρὴ δὲ διαιρεῖν ἐπ' εὐθείας τοῦ κώλου καὶ μὴ ἐγκαρσίως. περιαιρέσει δὲ ἐπὶ τῶν ἐν μασχάλαις καὶ βουβῶσι καὶ γλουτοῖς καὶ ἕδρᾳ, μυρσινοειδῶς περιαιροῦντες. ὑποσπαθισμῷ δὲ κατὰ το μέτωπον ἐπὶ τῶν ῥευματιζομένων ὀφθαλμῶν, καὶ περισκυθισμῷ, ἐπὶ τῶν κατὰ τοῦ βρέγματος καὶ ἐπὶ πόσθης μελανθείσης. ἐκκοπῇ δὲ ἐπί τε τῶν κώλων μελαινομένων καὶ ἐπὶ τῶν ἐν τῇ κεφαλῇ καταγμάτων. ἐπὶ δὲ

nerum atque ulcerum curatio: quae in corpore humano adminiſtratur. Primariae ejus actiones duae ſunt, compoſitio et diviſio. Harum rurſus multae ſunt ſpecies. Compoſitionis quidem fractorum oſſium ſynthetiſmus et deligatio, arthrembolum luxatorum, inteſtinorum quae prociderunt taxis, ad haec vulvae et recti inteſtini. Gaſtrorraphia. Curtorum epagoge, ut in naribus, labris atque auribus. Diaereſeos ſpecies, ſimplex inciſio, periaereſis, hypoſpathiſmus, periſcythiſmus, angeiologia, eccope, adustio, raſio, limatio, ſectio per ſerram. Simplici ſectione in abſceſſibus univerſis utimur. Dividendum vero membrum eſt recta linea, non transverſa. Periaereſi locus eſt in alis, inguinibus, naribus et ano inſtar myrti adhibitae. Hypoſpathiſmo in fronte, cum oculi fluunt. Periſcythiſmo in ſincipite et colis pellicula, quam praeputium vocant, nigricante. Eccope in membris nigreſcentibus et capitis fracturis. In omnibus autem, quae ad oſſa pertinent, aliisque multis uſtio, raſio, limatio, ſerrae uſus utiles

πάντων περὶ τὰ ὀστᾶ ἥ τε καῦσις καὶ ξύσις καὶ ἡ ῥίνησις καὶ ἡ πρίσις εὔχρηστοι καὶ ἐπ᾽ ἄλλων πολλῶν. καύσει δὲ τῇ διὰ καυτήρων χρώμεθα, ἰδίως μὲν ἐπὶ τῶν νεμομένων ἤδη πάντων καὶ ἐπὶ τῶν ῥευματιζομένων ὀφθαλμῶν, ἰσχίων, ἢ καὶ τῶν ἐντός. καὶ γὰρ ἐπὶ φθισικῶν παραλαμβάνονται καυστῆρες καὶ ἐπὶ σπληνικῶν καὶ ἐπὶ τῶν εἰς μασχάλην μελετησάντων ἐκπίπτειν βραχιόνων καὶ ἐπὶ αἰγίλωπος καὶ ἐπὶ τῶν μελαινομένων, ἢ πριζομένων διὰ τὰ ἀναστομούμενα ἀγγεῖα καὶ ἐπὶ τῶν ἄλλως αἱμοῤῥαγούντων. περὶ μὲν οὖν κεφαλὴν ταῦτα συνίσταται των ὑπαγομένων χειρουργίαις. καταγμάτων δὲ περὶ κεφαλὴν εἴδη πέντε, ῥωγμὴ, ἐγγείσωμα, ἐκπίεσμα, ἀπόχημα, καμάρωσις κατὰ δέ τινας ἓξ καὶ τριχίασις, ἡ ἐπιπόλαιος δηλονότι τῶν ὀστῶν ἐγχάραξις. ὑδροκεφάλων δὲ εἴδη τέσσαρα. τὸ μὲν μεταξὺ ἐγκεφάλου καὶ μήνιγγος. τὸ δὲ μεταξὺ μήνιγγος καὶ ὀστοῦ. τὸ δὲ μεταξὺ ὀστοῦ καὶ περικρανίου. τὸ δὲ μεταξὺ ὀστοῦ καὶ δέρματος. συνίστανται δὲ περὶ τὸ δέρμα μελικηρὶς, ἀθέρωμα, καὶ ἔξωθεν ἀλωπεκίασις. τὰς μὲν οὖν ἀλωπεκίας ἀμύσσομεν,

ſunt. Uſtio candentia ferramenta requirit, proprie in iis jam malis omnibus, quae depaſcuntur et oculis rheumaticis, coxis vel etiam interioribus. Etenim in tabidis candentia ferramenta aſſumuntur et in lienoſis: tum in brachiis, quae in alam excidere conſueverunt: inſuper in aegilope, in nigricantibus vel iis quae reſecantur, propterea quod aperiantur vaſa: poſtremo in aliis ſanguinis profluxionibus. Haec itaque in capite conſiſtunt, quibus manus auxiliantur. Fracturarum autem capitis genera ſunt quinque: rhogme, engiſoma, ecpieſma, apochema et camaroſis. Nonnullorum ſententia additur et ſexta, trichiaſis, per ſumma oſſium inſculptio. Hydrocephalon quatuor ſpecies obtinet: unam cum intra cerebrum et meningem humor ſubſidet: alteram, cum inter meningem et oſſa: tertiam, cum intra os et pericranium: reliquam ubi os et cutem interiacet. Circa cutem oriuntur meliceris, atheroma et extrinſecus alopeciaſis. Itaque alopecias laniamus: meliceridas et atheromata myrti modo vel ſimpliciter ſum-

τὰς δὲ μελικηρίδας καὶ τὰ ἀθερώματα μυρσινοειδῶς, ἢ καὶ ἁπλῶς διαιροῦντες τὴν ἐπιφάνειαν, εἶτα ἀποδέροντες τοῖς δακτύλοις τοὺς χιτῶνας, σὺν τοῖς ἐνοῦσιν ὑγροῖς κομιζόμεθα. τὰ δὲ ὑδροκέφαλα τὰ μὲν ὑπὸ τὸ δέρμα καὶ τὸ περικράνιον δύο που ἢ τρισὶν εὐθείαις διαιρέσεσι κενοῦμεν. τὰ δὲ ὑπὸ τὰ ὀστᾶ ἐκκόπτοντες. τὰ δὲ μεταξὺ μήνιγγος καὶ ἐγκεφάλου ἀθεράπευτα. πᾶν δὲ εἶδος τῶν ἐν κεφαλῇ καταγμάτων τῇ ἐκκοπῇ ὑπάγεται διὰ ἐκκοπέων περιαιρουμένων τὸ κατεαγὸς τῶν ὀστῶν. οἱ μὲν οὖν παλαιοὶ χοινικίοις πρίοντες ταῖς διὰ τῆς περιστρεφομένης ἐξέκοπτον αὐτά· οἱ δὲ μετὰ ταῦτα κεφαλοτρυπάνοις, ἕδρας παρέχοντες τοῖς ἐκκοπεῦσιν. [395] οἱ δὲ νῦν μόνοις τοῖς ἐκκοπεῦσιν ἀρκοῦνται. τῶν δὲ περὶ ὀφθαλμοὺς παθῶν ταῦτα χειρουργίαις ὑπάγεται, τριχίασις, ὑδατίδες, ἐγκανθίδες, πτερύγια, σταφυλώματα, ὑποχύματα, ῥεύματα χρόνια καὶ ὑπερβάλλοντα, λιθίασις περὶ τὰ βλέφαρα, σύμφυσις εἰς αὐτὸ τῶν περὶ τοὺς ὀφθαλμοὺς αἰγίλωψ. τὰ μὲν οὖν κεχαλασμένα βλέφαρα ἀναῤῥάπτομεν καὶ καταῤῥάπτομεν ἀφαι-

mam cutem dividentes, deinde tunicas digitis avellentes, cum ipſis humoribus, qui inſunt, auferimus. Hydrocephalon ſub cute et pericranio duabus vel tribus rectis lineis incidentes evacuamus. Quod ſub oſſibus eſt, excidimus. Quod tandem intra meningem cerebrumque incidit, inſanabile eſt. Omnis fracturarum calvariae ſpecies excisione adminiſtratur, exciſoribus id, quod in oſſibus fractum eſt, auferentibus. Veteres igitur modiolis per circumverſionem ſecantes ipſa excidebant. Poſteri terebris uſi ſunt, aegros in ſedile, tum ſectores collocantes. Hac tempeſtate exciſoribus tantum ſedem exhibent. Ex oculorum vitiis haec manus praeſidium expetunt, trichiaſis, hydatides, encanthides, ungues, ſtaphylomata, ſuffuſiones, fluores diuturni et excedentes, palpebrarum calculi, coagmentatio oculos ambientium in idem, aegilops. Palpebras itaque relaxatas conſuimus, faſciolam ab ipſis auferentes, quantam commenſuratio juxta palpebrarum figuram poſtulat. In palpebris non relaxatis pilos per acum

ροῦντες αὐτῶν ταινίδιον τὸ σύμμετρον καὶ κατὰ τὸ σχῆμα τῶν βλεφάρων. ἐπὶ δὲ τῶν μὴ κεχαλασμένων ἀναβροχίζοντες τὰς τρίχας διὰ βελόνης. τὰς δὲ ὑδατίδας κομιζόμεθα κατ' ἰδίαν βάλλοντες. τὰς δὲ ἐγκανθίδας καὶ πτερύγια καὶ τὰ σταφυλώματα περιαιροῦμεν, τὰ μὲν σταφυλώματα λίνον διείραντες καὶ ἀποβροχίζοντες, τὰ δὲ πτερύγια καὶ τὰς ἐγκανθίδας ἢ λίνῳ ἀνατείναντες, ἢ ἀγκίστρῳ. τὰ δὲ ὑποχύματα κατάγομεν, παρακεντοῦντες περὶ τὴν ἶριν, ἐκ τοῦ πρὸς τῷ μικρῷ κανθῷ μέρους μέχρι κενεμβατήσει καὶ παρακεντήσει· εἶτα πλαγιάζοντες ἐπὶ τὴν ἶριν τῷ ἄκρῳ αὐτοῦ τὸ συνεστὸς κατὰ τὴν κόρην ὑγρὸν κατάγομεν ξύοντες καὶ σφίγγοντες, ὥστε μὴ ἀναβλέψαι. τὸ δὲ ῥεῦμα ἵστησιν ὑποσπαθισμός τε καὶ περισκυθισμὸς καὶ ἀγγειολογία. ὁ μὲν οὖν ὑποσπαθισμὸς γίνεται τριῶν διαιρέσεων ὑπὲρ μετώπου διδομένων· εἶτα τῆς σπαθομήλης διεκβαλλομένης διὰ τῶν μεταξὺ σωμάτων. ὁ δὲ περισκυθισμὸς τοιοῦτός ἐστι διαιρεῖται ἐπὶ ἐγκαρσίαις διαιρέσεσι τὸ μέτωπον, οἷον στεφανιαία. καθ' ἕτερον δὲ μέρος αὐτῆς, μικρὸν ἀνωτέρω τῶν κροτάφων ἀφαιρεῖταί τινα τρίγωνα, ἐοικότα τὸ σχῆμα τῷ Δ στοιχείῳ. ἡ δὲ ἀγγειολογία ἐπιτελεῖται τῶν κεκρυμμένων

illaqueamus. Hydatidas ſingulatim tollimus. Encanthides, ungues et ſtaphylomata praecidimus et auferimus. Staphylomata quidem filo transmiſſo ablaqueantes. Ungues et encanthidas vel lino vel hamulo attrahimus. Suffuſiones deducimus pungentes circa irim ex minori angulo, donec acus penetrarit et loco vacuo excipiatur: deinde per obliquum ad iridem perducentes ſumma ejus parte compactum circa pupillam humorem deducimus, deligantes et ſtringentes, ut non aſpiciat. Hypoſpathiſmus, periſcythiſmus et angeiologia fluorem ſiſtunt. Hypoſpathiſmus itaque tribus ſit ſupra frontem diviſionibus. Deinde lato ſpecillo per corpora quae interiacent transmiſſo. Periſcythiſmus eſt, quum transverſis lineis coronae modo frons ſecatur. Altera ipſius parte paulo ſuperius, quam tempora ſunt, quaedam triangula amputantur, litterae Δ ſimilia. Angeiologia perſicitur vaſis latentibus a tempore ad

ἀγγείων ἀπὸ κροτάφου ἐπὶ κρόταφον διαιρουμένων εἰς βάθος. τὴν δὲ τῶν βλεφάρων λιθίασιν ἰώμεθα διαιροῦντες τὸ βλέφαρον ἐπὶ πολὺ καὶ κομιζόμενοι τὸν λίθον ἀσκύλτως. τὰ δὲ συμπεφυκότα βλέφαρα ἀναπτύξαντες σμίλῃ διαστέλλομεν τιλτοῖς ξυροῖς τοὺς δὲ αἰγίλωπας περιαιροῦντες μέχρι ὀστοῦ καυτῆρσι διακαίομεν. εἰσὶ δὲ οἳ ἀντὶ καυστηρίου κεφαλοτρεπάνῳ τιτρῶσι τὸ ὀστοῦν, ὡς ἐπὶ τὴν ῥῖνα. τὰ δὲ ἐν ῥινὶ συνιστάμενα, πολύποδας μὲν περιαιροῦμεν στενῷ σμιλαρίῳ καὶ ξυστῆρι ὕστερον ἀποξύομεν τὰς ῥίζας. αἱ δὲ ὄζαιναι ὡς ἐπὶ τὸ πολὺ ἀθεράπευτοι· ἡ δὲ αὐτὴ ἐγχείρησις καὶ ἐπὶ τούτων. τῶν δὲ ἐν τῷ στόματι ἐπουλίδας μὲν καὶ παρουλίδας διαιροῦμεν, ὅταν πυοποιήσωμεν. τὰς δὲ κεχαλασμένας σταφυλὰς ἀμέτρως ἐκτέμνομεν μυδίῳ λαβόμενοι, τοὺς δὲ ὀδόντας ἐξαιροῦμεν περιχαράσσοντες. τοὺς δὲ ἐν παρισθμίοις ὑπεραίροντας τὸ κατὰ φύσιν ἀδένας περιαιροῦμεν τοῖς ἀντιοτόμοις. τὰ δὲ ἐν τῷ τραχήλῳ στεατώματα καὶ χοιράδας διαιροῦντες τὴν ἐπιφάνειαν καὶ ἀποδέροντες τοῖς δακτύλοις, λύοντες τὴν πλοκὴν τῶν ἀγγείων

tempus in profundum divifis. Palpebrarum calculis medemur magna ipfarum divifione, qua lapides integre auferimus. Concinnatas palpebras fcalpello aperientes fubjectis linamentis diducimus. Aegilopas ad os usque excidentes ferramentis candentibus adurimus. Sunt autem qui loco ferramentorum candentium terebra os forant usque ad nares. Polypum, qui in naribus nafcitur, angufto fpecillulo ab offe refolvimus et raforio cultello poftea radices abradimus. Ozaenae raro ad fanitatem perducuntur: curatio vero earum in iisdem verfatur. In ore epulidas et parulidas dividimus, ubi fuppuratio fe oftenderit. Uvas demiffas five collapfas nimium incidimus, volfella prehendentes. Dentes eximimus fcarificatione circa eos facta. Adenas excedentes naturam in tonfillis adverfis plagis amputamus. In cervice fteatomata et ftrumas, cute divifa et digitis avulfa, tum vaforum complexu diffoluto tollemus. Ganglia, quae in metacarpiis magna ex parte eveniunt et mulieribus lana victum quaeritantibus, plerumque

κομιζόμεθα. τὰ δὲ γαγγλία ἐν τοῖς μετακαρπίοις μὲν ὡς ἐπὶ τὸ πολὺ γίνεται καὶ γυναιξὶν ἐριουργοῖς τὰ πλεῖστα ἐκθλῶμεν, ἃ δὴ καὶ κηρώμασιν ἐκμαλασσόμενα καθίσταται. τὰ δὲ ἐν μασχάλαις φύματα καὶ χοιράδας μετὰ περιαιρέσεως τέμνομεν. ὁμοίως δὲ καὶ τὰς ἐν βουβῶσι. τὰ δὲ ἐν μεσοπλευρίῳ ἀποστήματα διαιροῦντες οὐκ ἀθρόως ποιούμεθα τοῦ πύου τὴν ἔκκρισιν, ἀλλὰ πρὸς μέτρον. εἰσὶ δὲ οἳ καὶ διακαίουσιν αὐτά. καρκινώματα γίνεται μὲν ἐν πολλοῖς μέρεσι τοῦ σώματος, μάλιστα δὲ περὶ τοὺς μασθούς. περιαιρεῖται δὲ ἔνθ' ἂν ᾖ καὶ καυστηρίοις διακαίεται οὐ σφόδρα πεπυρωμένοις. εἰσὶ δὲ οἳ ξυραφίοις πεπυρωμένοις ὁμοῦ τέμνουσι καὶ διακαίουσιν. ἐξόμφαλοι δὲ πάντες μὲν οἱ ἔχοντες ἐν ὑπεροχῇ τὸν ὀμφαλὸν λέγονται. διαφορὰς δὲ ἔχουσι τρεῖς. οἱ μὲν γὰρ αὐτῶν πνευματόμφαλοι, οἱ δὲ ἐντερόμφαλοι, οἱ δὲ ὑδρόμφαλοι. πᾶσαι δὲ αἱ διαφοραὶ ὑπάγονται χειρουργίαις, λίνου διπλοῦ διὰ βελόνης διεμβαλλομένου καὶ περισφιγγομένου τοῦ ὀμφαλοῦ. τοὺς [396] δὲ ὑδεριῶντας παρακεντοῦμεν μικρὸν ὑπὸ τὸν ὀμφαλὸν, ἐκ τῶν εὐωνύμων σιδηρᾷ μυρ-
(389) σίνῃ μέχρι κενεμβατήσῃ. τῶν δὲ λειποδέρμων διττὴ

extendimus, interim ceratis mollita curamus. In aliis phymata et ſtrumas praecidimus: ſimiliter in inguinibus. Abſceſſus in ſpatio intercoſtali dividentes non univerſim, ſed moderate paulatimque puris excretionem molimur. Sunt et qui medicamentis aridis ſcindant ſimul et adurant eos. Carcinomata in multis corporis partibus, maxime circa mammas oriuntur. Praecidimus ubicunque fuerint et ferramentis peruruntur non admodum ignitis. Non deſunt qui raſoriis ferramentis ignitis ſimul ſecantibus et adurentibus utuntur. Exomphali omnes quibus umbilicus exuberat, appellantur. Differentia triplici comprehenduntur, quidam enim pneumatomphali. Alii enteromphali. Reliqui hydromphali. Omnes differentiae manu ſanantur, lino duplici per acum immiſſo et umbilico circumſtricto. Hydropicos paululum ſub umbilico a ſiniſtris pungimus, ferro inſtar myrti facto, donec inania penetraverit. Appellarum duplex curatio, horum, qui intrinſecus excorian-

ἡ χειρουργία, τῶν μὲν ἔνδοθεν ὑποδερομένων, τῶν δὲ ἔξωθεν ἐπιπολῆς διαιρουμένων ἐν κύκλῳ, ἵνα ἔνδον ἡ πόσθη ἐπισπασθῇ. οἱ δὲ πεφιμωμένοι τὴν ἀκροποσθίαν χειρίζονται, ἐπαναγομένης τῆς ἀκροποσθίας ἐφ᾽ ὅσον δύναται. εἶτα τῶν προφαινομένων τύλων ἀπολυομένων φλεβοτόμῳ ἐξ ἐπιπολῆς. ὑποσπαδίαι δέ εἰσιν οἱ ἐκ γενετῆς ἔχοντες τὴν οὐρήθραν κάτωθεν, ὑπὸ τὸν λεγόμενον κύνα. θεραπευτέον δὲ τετρημένης τῆς βαλάνου ἄκρας καὶ σωληνιδίου ἐντιθεμένου. οἱ δὲ λεγόμενοι ἄτρητοι, εἴτε τρῆμα ἔχοιεν λεπτὸν εἴτε μηδ᾽ ὅλως, οὕτω συγχειρίζονται. τὸ ὀξὺ τοῦ φλεβοτόμου καθιέντες προσαναπτύσσομεν, εἶτα τὸν δάκτυλον ὑποβάλλοντες πανταχόθεν ἀπολύομεν. τοὺς δὲ λίθον ἔχοντας ἐν κύστει τέμνομεν σφηνώσαντες μὲν τὸν λίθον ἐν τῷ τῆς κύστεως τραχήλῳ, ἐπικόπῳ δὲ τῷ λίθῳ χρώμενοι διαιροῦμεν ἀθρόως τὰ ἐπικείμενα σώματα καὶ λιθολάβῳ τὸν λίθον κομιζόμεθα. τοὺς δὲ ῥυαδικοὺς, τοὺς ὁπωσοῦν γεγονότας, ἐὰν μέγας λίαν ὁ τύλος ᾖ, περιαιροῦντες ἀνασκευάζομεν. οἷς δὲ ἐποχὴ οὔρου διὰ τὸ πλῆθος ἐνοχλεῖ, περιτεινομένης τῆς κύστεως

tur, illorum, qui extrinſecus orbiculatim in ſumma cute dividuntur, ut praeputium intus attrahatur. Qui per anguſtias praeputii exerere glandem nequeunt, ſumma ejus pellicula quantum licet retracta, dein callis, qui in conſpectum prodeunt, ſcalpello per ſumma avulſis curantur. Hypoſpadei ſunt, qui ex generatione urinae iter inferius ſub dicto cane habent: curantur autem ſumma glande perforata et canaliculo immiſſo. Qui dicuntur atreti, ſive foramen habeant tenue, ſive nullum omnino, auxilium capiunt hoc pacto: acuto ſpecilli immiſſo adaperimus, deinde digitum ſubmittentes undique abſolvimus. Lapides in veſica habentes ſecamus, calculum in veſicae collum adigentes, qui rei incidendae ſupponitur, lapide utentes, ſemel ſuperjacentes particulas dividimus et inſtrumento lapidi excipiendo idoneo calculum auferimus. Quoquo modo factos rhyadicos, ſi magnus callus fuerit, praecidendo ipſum curamus. Quibus urina propter copiam non reddi-

καὶ συστέλλεσθαι μὴ δυναμένης, διὰ καθετῆρος κομιζόμεθα τὸ οὖρον. ἔοικε δὲ ὁ καθετὴρ τῷ ῥωμαϊκῷ σίγμα S. καθίεται δὲ εἰς τὸν καυλὸν διὰ τῆς οὐρήθρας μέχρι τῆς κύστεως, ἔχοντες ἐν αὐτῷ ῥάμμα ἐπ᾿ ἄκρου ἔχον ἐρίου βραχὺ προκύπτον προβρεχόμενον τῷ οὔρῳ, ἔπειτα ἑλκόμενον εἰς τὰ ἐκτός· συνέπεται δὲ αὐτῷ τὸ οὖρον, εἰς ἔκκρισιν οἷον ὁδηγοῦν τι αὐτῷ. τῶν δὲ περὶ ὄσχεον συνισταμένων ὄγκων εἴδη εἰσὶν ἑπτὰ, ὑδροκήλη, πωροκήλη, στεατοκήλη, σαρκοκήλη, ἐπιπλοκήλη, κιρσοκήλη, ἐντεροκήλη. εἰσὶ δὲ ἐφ᾿ ὧν καὶ ἐπιπλέκεται ταῦτα, οἷον ὑδρεντεροκήλη, σαρκοεπιπλοκήλη. ἐπὶ μὲν οὖν τῶν ὑδροκηλικῶν διελόντα δεῖ τὸ ὄσχεον καὶ κατὰ τὸ φλεβωδέστατον ἐντυχόντα τῷ χιτῶνι τῷ τὸ ὑγρὸν περιέχοντι κενῶσαι καὶ τὰ περισσὰ τοῦ χιτῶνος ἐπαφαιρεῖν. ἐφ᾿ ὧν δὲ ἄνευ τοῦ χιτῶνός ἐστιν, ἐκκρίναντες τὸ ὑγρὸν ἀρκούμεθα. τὰς δὲ στεατοκήλας καὶ πωροκήλας τέμνειν χρὴ, ὁμοίως ὑπερβάλλοντας τῇ ἀριστερᾷ χειρὶ τὸ ὄσχεον, ἔπειτα διαιρεῖν ἐξ ἐπιπολῆς ἕως ἐντύχωμεν τῷ στέατι, ἢ πώρῳ, ἢ ὅ τι ἂν ᾖ καὶ τοῦτο κομι-

tur, vesica distenta, ut remittere se nequeat, per cathetera urinam elicimus. Porro huic instrumento ad Romanae literae S figuram facto, quod in urinae iter usque ad vesicam demittitur, inditur filum, quod in summo habens lanae paululum procumbens, urina madefactum, deinde foras extrahitur, quod urina tanquam ducem viae sequitur. Tumorum qui scroto accidunt septem species sunt, hydrocele, porocele, steatocele, sarcocele, epiplocele, cirsocele, enterocele. A quibusdam hae complicatae adduntur, hydrenterocele, sarcoepiplocele. In his qui hydrocele laborant, scrotum diducendum est et ubi maxime venosum est, inventaque tunica, humorem ea comprehensum evacuare oportet et tunicae supervacanea auferre: in quibus sine tunica est, excernere humores sufficit. Steatocelas et porocelas similiter sinistra manu scrotum extendentes secare convenit, postea in superficie diducere, donec adipi vel callo vel alii cuicunque incidamus et hoc auferamus.

ζόμεθα. καὶ οἱ σαρκοκηλικοὶ δὲ ὁμοίως χειρίζονται. δεῖ μόνην τὴν πρὸς δὲ τὴν ὑποπίπτουσαν σάρκα λευκανθίζουσαν περιαιρεῖν, τὴν δὲ ἐρυθρὰν ἀποδέροντα καὶ ἀπαλλοτριοῦντα τότε ἀφαιρεῖν τὰ ἐγκαταλείμματα. ἐπὶ δὲ τῶν κιρσοκηλῶν ἀνατείνας ἀγκίστρῳ ἐξ ἐπιπολῆς διαιρῶν καὶ ἀναλαβὼν τὸν κιρσὸν καὶ ἀποδείρας ἀπολιπὼν ὡσεὶ μικροῦ δακτύλου τὸ πλάτος, τὸ δὲ λοιπὸν ἀνατείνων ἀπόκοπτε. φυλακτέον δὲ ἀκριβῶς ἐπὶ τῶν συμπεπλεγμένων κρεμαστήρων, ἢ διδύμων. τοὺς δὲ ἐντεροκηλικοὺς καὶ ἐπιπλοκηλικοὺς οὕτω τέμνομεν ἀναπιέσαντες τὸ ἔντερον, ἢ τὸν ἐπίπλουν ἀκριβῶς, εἶτα τὸν σπερματικὸν πόρον ἀφαιροῦμεν ὅσον δυνάμεθα. εἰ δὲ μὴ τὸ περιτόναιον ἐπισπασάμενοι καὶ ἐπιβροχήσαντες περιαιροῦμεν. τὰς δὲ αἱμοῤῥοΐδας λίνον λεπτὸν διπλοῦν, διὰ τῶν βάσεων αὐτῶν διείροντες ἀποσφίγγοντες, μετὰ δύο ὥρας ἀποτέμνομεν. τῶν δὲ συρίγγων αἱ μὲν εἰσιν ἀσύντρητοι, μόνον τὸ στόμα ἔχουσαι. αἱ δὲ συντετρημέναι, ἢ ἔνδον εἰς τὸν δακτύλιον, ἢ ἔξωθεν. ἐπὶ μὲν οὖν τῶν συντετρημένων εἰς τὸν δακτύλιον διαβάλλων τὴν μηλωτίδα, εἶτα τὸν δάκτυλον καθεὶς εἰς τὴν

Pari modo ſarcocelici tractantur. Oportet autem ſubjacentem carnem albicantem praecidere, rubram excoriare et detrahere, ac tunc reliquias adimere expedit. In cirſocelis extendes varicem hamulo in ſuperficie diviſum, exceptumque avelles, relicta ceu digiti parvi latitudine, reliquum extenſum abſeca. Cura vero non mediocris adhibenda eſt in illis complicatis cremaſteribus et teſticulis. Enterocelicos et epiplocelicos ita ſecamus, reprimentes inteſtinum vel omentum diligenter, mox ſeminarium meatum auferemus quam fieri poterit commode: ſin minus peritonaeum attrahentes et laqueo excipientes praecidimus. Haemorrhoides lino duplici per ipſarum baſes traducentes conſtringentesque poſt horas duas abſcindimus. Fiſtularum nonnullae perſoratae non ſunt, os tantum habentes. Quaedam perſoratae vel intus in anum vel extrinſecus. In perforatis in anum ſpecillum immittes, mox digitum in ſedem inſeres, inteſtinum attrahes mucrone ſpecilli,

ἕδραν, ἐπισπάσαι τὸ ἔντερον ἄκρῳ τῆς μηλωτίδος καὶ περιαίρει κάτωθεν ἀρχόμενος. ὁμοίως δὲ καὶ ἐπὶ τῶν ἐκτὸς τῆς ἕδρας. ἐπὶ δὲ τῶν μὴ συντετρημένων τῷ ὀξεῖ τῆς [397] μηλωτίδος διαπερᾷν ἅπαντα τὰ ὑγιῆ σώματα. εἰσὶ δὲ οἳ ἀντὶ τοῦ ἀνακείρειν, ἢ περιαιρεῖν τὰ μεταξὺ τῶν συντρήσεων λίνον βύσσινον συνεστραμμένον ἐν ἄκρῳ τῆς μηλωτίδος, ἔχοντα τὰ διῃρημένα τούτῳ ἀποσφίγγοντες τὰ μεταξὺ σώματα, ἑκάστης ἡμέρας περιτείναντες τὰ ῥάμματα, διακόπτουσι τὰ μεταξὺ καὶ ἐκτυλώσαντες τῇ Αἰγυπτίᾳ ἐπουλοῦσιν. ἀναγέγραπται δὲ καὶ παρ' Ἱπποκράτους πρώτου ὁ τρόπος οὗτος. τοὺς δὲ ἐν τοῖς σκέλεσι κιρσοὺς πρῶτον ἔξωθεν ἐπισημηνάμενοι δι' ὅλου ἐγχαράξεσιν, εἶτα κλίναντες, ἐξ ἐπιπολῆς λαβόμενοι τοῦ δέρματος, αὐτὸ πρῶτον διαιροῦμεν, εἶτα ἀγκίστρῳ ἐπισπώμενοι τὸν κιρσὸν διαδέομεν καὶ μετὰ πάσας τὰς διαιρέσεις τοῦτο ποιήσαντες, ἢ κιρσουλκῷ ἐξαιροῦμεν διακόπτοντες τὰ ἄκρα, ἢ διπυρήνῳ διαλαβόντες λίνῳ διὰ τῆς κοιλίας τοῦ κιρσοῦ κατ' ἀναστροφὴν ἐξέλκομεν. τά τε λεγόμενα δρακόντια ὅμοιά ἐστι τοῖς κιρσοῖς· μεγάλην δὲ ἀλγηδόνα ἐπιφέρει κινούμενα, μικρὸν προκύπτοντα.

idque amputabis, ab inferiore loco incipiens, fimiliter et in exterioribus ani. In non perforatis fpecilli acumine omnes fanas particulas penetrare convenit. Sunt qui loco recifionis praecifionisque partium foramina interjacentium lino byffino in fummitate fpecilli converfo divifa avellunt, intermedias partes quotidie circumtendentes fila amputant et callum mollientes medicamento Aegyptio cicatricem inducunt. Hic modus primum ab Hippocrate confcriptus eft. Varices in cruribus primum extrinfecus incifuris per totum infignitos, deinde inclinantes fumma cute prehenfa, ipfam primam dividimus et mox hamulo attractum varicem illigamus, quo poft omnes divifiones facto vel varicum extractorio inftrumento eximimus fumma difcindentes vel bicipiti fpecillo exceptum lino per ipfius ventriculum fecundum everfionem extrahimus. Dracontia varicibus fimilia funt, magnum vero dolorem, dum paululum prominentes moventur, concitant. Oportet autem divifis,

δεῖ οὖν διελόντα ὡς ἐπὶ τῶν κιρσῶν ἀποδέρειν καὶ οὕτως ἐξαιρεῖν. τοὺς δὲ ἥλους καὶ τύλους καὶ ἀκροχορδόνας καὶ θύμους καὶ μυρμηκίας ἐκτέμνοντες ἐπικαίομεν, ἢ τῷ ψωρικῷ ἐπιπάσσομεν. τὰ δὲ κολοβώματα, τὰ περὶ μυκτῆρας, ἢ ὦτα, ἢ χείλη οὕτως εἰς τὸ κατὰ φύσιν ἀποκαθίσταται, τὰ μὲν χείλη σμιλαρίῳ πανταχόθεν ἀναδέροντες αἱμάσσομεν, εἶτα προσάγοντες ῥάπτομεν πυκνότερον. πρὸς δὲ τὰς σιαγόνας ἐξ ἑκατέρου πέρατος τῶν χειλῶν, καθ' ἃ συμπέφυκεν ἀλλήλοις, ἔνδοθέν τε καὶ ἔξωθεν διαιροῦμεν καὶ τίλμασι διαστέλλομεν, πρὸς τὸ μὴ τὴν σάρκα φυεῖσαν, χάλασμα παρασχεῖν· τὰ δὲ ἐν τοῖς ὠσὶν ἢ μυκτῆρσιν κολοβώματα, ὅταν ὁ χόνδρος ᾖ διῃρημένος, ἐκχονδρίζειν δεῖ καὶ οὕτως διαῤῥάπτειν ἐρείῳ ῥάμματι.

Κεφ. κ'. [Περὶ καταγνυμένων κώλων καὶ ἐξαρθρουμένων μορίων.] Τὰ δὲ καταγνύμενα κῶλα ἐκ διατάσεως μὲν εὐθετίζεται, ἐξ ἐπιδέσεως δὲ πωροῦται. τὰ μὲν οὖν περὶ κεφαλὴν κατάγματα ποσαχῶς τε γίνεται καὶ ὅπως θεραπεύεται εἴρηται. κἂν ἐν προσώπῳ κάταγμα γένηται, ὡς τὰ ἐν τῇ κεφαλῇ θεραπεύειν, ἐκκόπτοντα τὸ πεπονθὸς ὀστοῦν.

ut varicibus, ſummam cutem detrahere ſicque praecidere. Clavos, callos, acrochordonas, thymos, myrmecias excindentes adurimus vel pſorico illinimus. Curta in naribus, auribus, oculis hoc modo ad naturalem habitum reſtituuntur: labra ſcalpello undique deradentes cruentamus, deinde adducentes denſius ſuimus: juxta maxillas autem ex utroque labrorum extremo, qua invicem coëunt, intus et extrinſecus dividimus diſtendimusque volſellis, ne caro inde relaxetur. Quae auribus vel naribus curta accidunt, quum fuerit cartilago diviſa, producere aliam convenit, ſicque conſuere lanae filo.

Cap. XX. [*De artubus confractis partibusque a ſuo articulo dimotis.*] Fracti artus ex diſtentione quidem in rectum reſtituuntur: ex deligatura callo obducuntur. Calvariae ergo fractiones quot modis accidant et quomodo curentur, diximus. Et ſi in faciem fractura contingat, ut in capite ſanare convenit, oſſe quod aſſe-

εἰδέναι δὲ χρὴ καὶ ὅσα τῶν καταγνυμένων ὀστῶν ἀθεράπευτα. ἐὰν μὲν οὖν ῥὶς κατεάγῃ, οὐκ ὀρθοῦται. καὶ οὖς δὲ κατάγνυσθαί φησιν Ἱπποκράτης, ὅτι καὶ ὁ χόνδρος ὀστοῦν μιμεῖται καὶ δυσαποκατάστατος εἶναι δοκεῖ εἰς τὸ ἀρχαῖον σχῆμα. ἀλλὰ κᾂν ἐξ ὑπερώας μεσίζῃ ἡ ῥὶς, ὥς φησι, σιμοῦται ἀθεράπευτος. ἐὰν δὲ κλεὶς κατεάγῃ, ἢ κατακλεὶς, ἤ τις πλευρὰ καὶ ταῦτα, ὡς ἐπὶ τὸ πολὺ δυσαποκατάστατα. ἐπιτιθέναι δὲ χρὴ ἐπὶ τῶν κατακλείδων μάλιστα καὶ ἐπιδεῖν ἀπὸ μασχάλης ἐπὶ μασχάλην. ἐὰν δέ τι τῶν μειζόνων κώλων κατεάγῃ, ἢ τῶν μικροτέρων μερῶν, οἷον δακτύλων σκυταλίδες, ἢ καρποῦ ὀστᾶ, ἢ μετακαρπίου, ἢ ταρσοῦ, πάντα μεγαλομερῶς μὲν κατάγνυται, καυληδὸν, ἢ ῥαφανηδὸν, ἢ σχιδακηδόν. ἐπὶ λεπτὸν δὲ καρυηδὸν ἢ ἀλφιτηδόν. πρότερον μὲν οὖν χρὴ ἐπιδέοντα πάντα καταγνύμενα καὶ διατείνοντα πάνυ ἰσχυρῶς καὶ βεβαίως διαστῆσαι καὶ πολὺ ἀποστῆσαι ἀλλήλων, ἵνα εὐθετισθῇ καὶ ἀποκατασταθῇ εἰς τὸ ἀρχαῖον σχῆμα. εὐθετίζειν δὲ χρὴ τὰ ὀστᾶ, οὐκ ἐπὶ εὐθὺ πάντα, ἀλλὰ πρὸς σχῆμα τοῦ ὁμοζύγου κώλου. [398] ἐὰν μὲν εὐθὺ

ctum eſt exciſo. Sciendum autem eſt quae oſſa fracta curationem non recipiant. Si igitur nares confractae ſunt, non recte poſſunt reſtitui. Aurem etiam frangi ſcribit Hippocrates, quoniam et cartilago imitatur os, aegerrimeque in priſtinam figuram reducitur. Verum ſi ex palato fracturam accipiant nares, ſimae, ut inquit, evadunt et inſanabiles. Porro ſi clavicula frangatur vel jugulum vel coſta aliqua, et haec frequenter reſarciri non poſſunt. Epithemata in jugulo adhibenda ſunt, ipſumque ab ala ad alam deligandum eſt. Caeterum ſi quod majorum membrorum fractum ſit vel minorum partium aliqua, ut digitorum nodi vel oſſa carpi vel metacarpii vel tarſi, omnia quidem in magna fruſta cauledon vel raphanedon et ſchidacedon franguntur: in minuta caryedon vel alphitedon. Omnia ergo fracta deligantes extendentesque admodum vehementer et valide diducere et multum invicem ſeparare oportet, ut juſtum ſitum priſtinamque figuram recipiant. Non autem in rectum omnia reſtitui de-

ᾖ, ἐπ' εὐθείας, ἐὰν δὲ καμπύλον ἢ ἄλλως πως σκαμβὸν, ὁμοίως. τρόπος δὲ παρασκευῆς ἐστιν ἐπιδέσεως εἰς πάντα, ἐπίδεσμον ποιεῖν ἐξ ὀθονίων παλαιῶν, (390) πρός τε τὸ πλάτος καὶ τὸ μέγεθος τοῦ κώλου. πλάτος μὲν ἐπὶ τῶν μεγίστων δακτύλων τεσσάρων ἢ πέντε, ἐπὶ δὲ τῶν ἰσχνοτέρων μὴ ἔλασσον δακτύλων τριῶν. ἐπιδέσεως δὲ νόμος τοιοῦτος. ἡ πρώτη ἐπίδεσις ἀπὸ τοῦ κατάγματος ἐπὶ τρεῖς ἐπιδέσεις ἄνω νέμεται ὡς ἐπὶ τὸ πλεῖστον. ἡ δὲ δευτέρα ἀπὸ τοῦ αὐτοῦ τόπου ἄρχεται, ἀλλασσομένων τῶν ἐπιδέσεων, κάτω μὲν νέμεται, ἐπὶ τὰ ἄνω δὲ ἀνάγεται, ὥστε εἶναι διπλῆν τῆς πρώτης. διάβροχον δὲ εἶναι ὑδρελαίῳ, ἢ οἰνελαίῳ ἢ γλυκελαίῳ μέχρι πρώτης διὰ τρίτης, ἔπειτα κηρωτῇ λελυμένῃ καὶ ὑγρᾷ, ὡς παχὺ ἔλαιον εἶναι. πιέζειν δὲ μηδὲ πάνυ ἄγαν, ἵνα μὴ νεκρωθῇ, ἀλλ' ὥστε προκεῖσθαι καὶ προσερηρεῖσθαι, μήτε κεχαλασμένως, ἵνα συνέχῃ καὶ ἀποκρούηται τὰ ἐπιῤῥέοντα, πρὸς τὸ μὴ φλεγμαίνειν. ἔπειτα σπλῆνας τριπτύχους ἢ τετραπτύχους ποιοῦντας ἐπιτιθέναι, πληροῦντας τοῦ κώλου τὸ πάχος, ὥστε μήτε ἐπιπίπτειν

bent, fed ad proximi cui cohaerent membri figuram. At fi os rectum fit, in rectum: fi obliquum vel alio quovis modo curvum, fimili modo. Modus autem deligationis ad omnia praeparandae hic eft. Fafcia eft linteis veteribus facienda, quae tum latitudine, tum magnitudine membro refpondeat. Latitudine quidem in maximis digitorum quatuor vel quinque. In tenuioribus non minus digitorum trium. Deligationis haec ratio. Prima fafcia ter nobis in fractura furfum verfus fertur, ut plurimum. Altera dimidio longior ab eodem loco incipit, evariantibus deligationibus deorfum quidem tribuitur, fed ad fuperiora reducitur: irrigari hydrelaeo vel oenelaeo vel glycelaeo adusque triduum expedit; poft cerato diluto et liquido, ut oleum craffum videatur. Verum fafcia ita paretur ut non nimium premat, ne membrum emoriatur, fed quoad adjacet apteque adhaereat: neque fit laxa, ut contineat et repellat influxus, ne oboriatur inflammatio. Poft fplenia triplicia quadrupliciaque adhibeantur, quae artus

ἀλλήλοις μήτε ἀφεστῶτας διαλείμματα ποιεῖν· ἐπὶ δὲ τούτοις ἐπιδεσμίδα τρίτην ἐπιβάλλοντας ἀπὸ τοῦ κατάγματος κάτω νέμεσθαι ἐπὶ τὰ ἄνω χωρεῖν καὶ ἐκεῖ τερματίζεσθαι. αἱ δὲ ἐπιλύσεις αἱ μὲν πρῶται διὰ τρίτης· αἱ δὲ μετὰ τὴν ἑβδόμην διὰ πλειόνων πρὸς τὰς ἐπειγούσας χρείας. ναρθηκίζουσαι δὲ, ἀπὸ νάρθηκος ἀληθινοῦ, ἐπὶ τῆς ἐσχάτης ἐπιδεσμίδος, ἐρίου προστιθεμένου, ἐκ διαστημάτων τασσομένων τῶν ναρθήκων· ὅταν ἀκριβῶς ἀφλέγμαντον ᾖ, τῶν μὲν κυρτῶν αὐτοῦ ἔξωθεν αἰρουμένων, τοῦ δὲ λείου ἐπιβάλλοντος ἔνδοθεν ἀμματίῳ, ἐπ' αὐτοῖς ἀμματιζομένων ἢ ταινιδίων ἢ ναυτικοῦ ῥάμματος. ἐπὶ δὲ τῶν μετὰ τραύματος καταγμάτων, ἀντὶ τούτων πάντων, σπλῆνας διπτύχους, ἢ τριπτύχους ποιοῦντας, ἕκαστον πληροῦντα τὸ πάχος ἐν κύκλῳ τοῦ κώλου, ὡς χωρίζεσθαι τὰ πέρατα αὐτοῦ, ἐπιπίπτοντα ἀλλήλοις, ἅπαν τε κῶλον τούτοις ἐπὶ δέον συγκείμενον ἔχοντες· πρώτως μὲν τοῖς σοῖς ἐπιβάλλουσι τῷ σώματι διαβρόχους εἶναι τῶν προειρημένων· ἐπὶ δὲ τούτοις προϋποκείμενα ἔχουσιν ἔρια καὶ ἀποδεσμίδας ἁπλῶς ἐπὶ τοῖς ἐρίοις

craffitiem impleant: quo nec fibi mutuo incidant, nec diffidentes intervallum relinquant. Ab his fafcia convenit triplex, quae a fractura deorfum veniens furfum feratur, ibique finiat. Solutiones membri primae tertio quoque die faciendae: poft feptimum vero diebus intermiffis pluribus, prout neceffitas exiget. Inde licebit ferulas circumponere; fed ita ut ad ultimam fafciam lana apponatur et ex intervallis ferulae collocentur, quum membrum ab inflammatione eft prorfus immune, curva ipfarum parte extrinfecus fublata, levi autem intus deligatione injecta; quibus fuperligabuntur vel chordulae vel nauticum filum. In fracturis cum vulnere pro his omnibus fplenia duplicia vel triplicia facientes per fingula craffitiem membri circulatim implebimus, ut termini ipfius invicem incumbentes feparentur, totumque membrum his contineatur. Primum fane ex praedictis impofita madida effe convenit: deinde lanas propofitas et fafcias poft lanas habere per fubjectam fedem canalis aperti. Maxime is modus deli-

κατὰ τῆς ὑποτιθεμένης ἕδρας τοῦ ἀνοίκτου σωλῆνος· μάλιστα δὲ οὗτος ὁ τρόπος τῆς ἐπιδέσεως ἁρμόδιος ἐπὶ τῶν ἀλφιτηδὸν καταγνυμένων, μετὰ τραυμάτων καὶ πολλῆς περιθλάσεως τῶν μυῶν, ἐφ' ὧν καὶ μοτὰ χρὴ προϋποτιθέναι διάβροχα τοῖς ἁρμόζουσι. μοτῶν δὲ εἴδη πέντε· στρεπτὸς, ξυστὸς, τιλτὸς, ἐλλυχνιωτὸς, πριαπισκωτός. ἐπὶ δὲ τῶν ἐξαρθρούντων δεῖ μὲν καὶ τῆς διατάσεως προηγουμένης· ἡ δὲ ἐμβολὴ καθ' ἕκαστον οἰκεία μετὰ τὴν διάτασιν παραλαμβάνεται. πάντα δὲ ἐπὶ τοῦ Ἱπποκρατείου βάθρου καταρτίζεται, ὁμοῦ τε διατεινόμενα καὶ συμβαλλόμενα. ἐξαρθροῖ δὲ κεφαλὴ μὲν, ἐνήρθρωται γὰρ τῷ πρώτῳ σπονδύλῳ τοῦ τραχήλου πρὸς τὸν δεύτερον. ἡ δὲ κάτω γνάθος ἐξίσταται μὲν τοῦ κατὰ μῆλα ζυγώματος, ἐμβάλλεται δὲ μόναις ταῖς χερσὶ παραγομένη ἔνθεν κἀκεῖθεν ἐπὶ τὰ συνερειδόμενα πρὸς τῇ ἄνω. τοῦ δὲ ὤμου εἰς μασχάλην μόνην ὀλισθάνοντος ἡ δι' ἄμβης ἐμβολὴ μετὰ διατάσεως. εἰσὶ δὲ καὶ ἄλλαι παλαιστρικαὶ λεγόμεναι. ἀγκῶνος δὲ ἐξαρθρημάτων διαφοραὶ τέσσαρες, ἡ μὲν ἔσω, ἡ δὲ ἔξω, ἡ δὲ εἰς τὰ ἔμπροσθεν,

gationis confert iis, quae alphitedon fracta ſunt cum vulneribus et multa contuſione muſculorum, in quibus etiam linamenta liquoribus competentibus madentia imponenda ſunt. Linamentorum ſunt quinque ſpecies, aliud flexile, aliud raſile, aliud vulſorium, aliud lucernarium, aliud priapiſcotum appellant. In luxatis vero diſtentione quidem antecedente opus eſt: repoſitio pro quolibet membro propria aſſumitur: omnia in Hippocratico ſubſellio reſtituuntur, ſimul et tenſa et commiſſa. Caput luxatur, nam prima cervicis vertebra coarctatur ad ſecundam. Maxilla inferior ex jugali, quod eſt ad malas, excidit; ſolis autem manibus in ſedem ſuam compellitur, hinc illincque ad ſuperiorem adducta. Humerus in alam tantum excidit, capitulo rotundo et leniter cavo, cum diſtenſione in ſedem reducitur. Sunt et aliae *inferiores*, quas palaeſtricas nominant. Quatuor ſunt exciſionum cubiti differentiae; una ad intra, altera ad extra, tertia ad anteriora, quarta ad poſteriora. Cubitus in omnes quatuor partes excidere

ἢ δὲ εἰς τὰ ὄπισθεν· τὰς μὲν εἰς τὰ ἐκτὸς ἢ εἰς τὰ ἐντὸς, μετὰ διατάσεως ἀντιπαράγοντες τὰ ἐξεστῶτα ὀστέα οὕτως καθιστῶμεν, τὰς δὲ εἰς τοὐπίσω, ἢ εἰς τὸ ἔμπροσθεν, ἄνευ διατάσεως· ἡ μὲν γὰρ ἐκ συγκάμ- [399] ψεως ἀθρόας, ἐντιθεμένου τινὸς τῇ συγκάμψει τοῦ ἀγκῶνος, καθίσταται· ἡ δὲ ἐκτάσεως σφοδροτέρας. καρποῦ δὲ καὶ μετακαρπίου καὶ δακτύλων ἐξαρθρήματα ἐκ βραχείας διατάσεως τῶν χειρῶν εὐθετίζεται. ῥάχεως δὲ πᾶσα διαστροφὴ, ἥ τε ὕβωσις καὶ εἴσωσις καὶ σκολίωσις, ἀδιόρθωτα. μηροῦ δὲ ἡ πρὸς τὰ ἰσχία κεφαλὴ ἢ ἔσωθεν εἰς τὸ περιτόναιον ἐμπίπτει, ἢ ἔξωθεν εἰς τὸ ἀντικείμενον, ὀπίσω τε εἰς γλουτὸν καὶ ἔμπροσθεν εἰς βουβῶνα. ἀνίατοι δὲ τέσσαρες διαφοραί. κατὰ δὲ τὸ γόνυ συνεχὴς μὲν ἡ εἰς τὸ ἔξω ἐξάρθρησις καὶ ῥᾳδία ἡ ἀποκατάστασις διὰ συγκάμψεως. ἔλαττον δὲ εἰς τὰ ἐντὸς καὶ γίνεται καὶ ἀποκαθίσταται. ἔτι δὲ σπανιώτερον ἡ εἰς τουπίσω. ἡ δὲ εἰς τοὔμπροσθεν οὐδὲ ὅλως γίνεται. οὐδέποτε γὰρ ἐξίσταται τὰ ὀστᾶ διὰ τὴν συνέχουσαν ἐπιγονατίδα, πλὴν εἰ μὴ καὶ αὕτη κατεάγῃ κατὰ δὲ τὰ σφυρὰ βραχεῖα μὲν παρεναλλαγὴ γινομένη δυσαποκατάστατος. πολλὴ

potest: si in exteriorem interioremve, cum distensione dimota ossa sic reponimus: si in priorem vel posteriorem, sine distensione restituimus: nam haec ex subita inflexione quodam imposito flexurae cubiti consistit: illa extensione vehementiori. Carpus et metacarpium, ad haec digiti luxati, modica distensione reponuntur. Quaevis spinae perversio, curvitas et inclinatio et distorsio instaurari non possunt. Femur ad coxas vel intro ad peritonaeum, ut extra ad oppositam partem prolabitur, retro ad clunes et ante in inguina, atque hae quatuor differentiae immedicabiles. Genu quoque crebro in exteriorem partem prolabitur et facile ex flexura restituitur: minus in interiora excidit, reditque multo rarius in posteriora, in anteriora nunquam: quippe ossa propter patellam, quae continet (nisi et ipsa fracta fuerit) nullo tempore elabuntur. Talus modice prolapsus aegre restituitur. Si magna sit luxatio et violenta, ne sustinet quidem instaurationem. Periculosa

δὲ καὶ βίαιος οὐδὲ ἀνέχεται τὴν διόρθωσιν. ἐπικίνδυνος γὰρ σφόδρα καὶ εἰ μετὰ τραύματος γένηται· δάκτυλοι δὲ ποδὸς ἐξαρθρήσαντες, ὡς τῶν χειρῶν ἀπευθύνονται. αἱ δὲ τῶν συμφύσεων αὐτῶν πᾶσαι διαστάσεις, ὡς ἐπὶ προσώπου καὶ πήχεως καὶ κερκίδος κνήμης τε καὶ περόνης, μετακαρπίου τε καὶ ταρσοῦ καὶ ἔτι εἰς τὸ ἀρχαῖον ἀποκαθίστανται. τὰ δὲ μελαινόμενα καὶ νεμόμενα, εἴτε ἐκ καταγμάτων εἴτε βιαίου σφίγξεως, ἐκπρίζομεν ὅλα τὰ κῶλα πολλάκις. ὁμοίως δὲ καὶ τὰ ὑπὸ τῶν ἰοβόλων ἤδη προκατειλημμένα. ἔπειτα καυτῆρσιν ἄγαν πεπυρωμένοις ἱστῶμεν τὴν νομήν. μετὰ δὲ τοὺς καυτῆρας πράσῳ τῷ χλωρῷ καταπλάσσομεν μεθ' ἁλῶν, εἶτα ὅταν καθαρθῶσιν αἱ ἐσχάραι, ὡς ἕλκη θεραπεύομεν. τὰ δὲ τῶν ἰοβόλων δήγματα οὐδὲ ταχὺ ἐπουλοῦσθαι βουλόμεθα, ἀλλ' ὡς ἐπὶ τὸ πλεῖστον ῥευματίζεσθαι τὰ ἕλκη σπουδάζομεν.

enim nimis et ſi cum vulnere accidit. In digitis nihil ultra fieri debet quam quod in iis, qui ſunt in manu, poſitum eſt. Omnes vero coagmentationum eorum ſeparationes, ut in facie, cubito et radio, tibia et ſura, metacarpio, tarſo, in veterem figuram reſtituuntur. Porro quae membra nigreſcunt vel depaſcuntur, ſive ex fracturis ſive violenta aſtrictione, tota ſaepe reſecamus. Similiter in iis facimus, quos venenatae ferae momorderunt, mox ferramentis prope candentibus paſtionem ſiſtimus, poſt ferramenta, porro viridi cum ſale illinimus. Deinde ubi cruſtae ablatae fuerint, tanquam ulcera curamus. Venenatorum morſus neque cito ad cicatricem ducimus, ſed frequentius ulcera diu ſtillare in iis curamus.

Printed in the United States
By Bookmasters